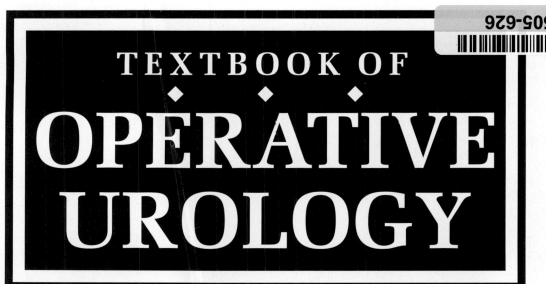

TEXTBOOK OF
◆ ◆ ◆
OPERATIVE
UROLOGY

Editor:

Fray F. Marshall, MD
Professor of Urology
James Buchanan Brady
Urological Institute
Director, Adult Urology
Johns Hopkins Medical Institutions
Baltimore, Maryland

Section Editors:

Louis R. Kavoussi, MD
Associate Professor of Urology
Chief, Department of Urology
Director, Division of Endourology
Johns Hopkins Bayview Medical Center
Baltimore, Maryland

Jack W. McAninch, MD
Professor and Vice Chairman
Department of Urology
University of California, San Francisco
Chief of Urology
San Francisco General Hospital
San Francisco, California

Craig A. Peters, MD
Assistant in Surgery (Urology)
Assistant Professor of Surgery
Children's Hospital
Harvard Medical School
Boston, Massachusetts

W.B. SAUNDERS COMPANY

A Division of Harcourt Brace & Company
Philadelphia   London   Toronto   Montreal   Sydney   Tokyo

W.B. SAUNDERS COMPANY
A Division of Harcourt Brace & Company

The Curtis Center
Independence Square West
Philadelphia, Pennsylvania 19106

Library of Congress Cataloging-in-Publication Data

Textbook of operative urology / editor, Fray F. Marshall; section editors, Louis R.
Kavoussi, Jack W. McAninch, Craig A. Peters.—1st ed.

  p. cm.

ISBN 0–7216–5510–6

1. Genitourinary Organs—Surgery.   [DNLM: 1. Urologic Diseases—Surgery.
2. Genital Diseases, Male—Surgery.   WJ 168 T3554 1996]

RD571.T495 1996
617.4′6—dc20

DNLM/DLC   95–17717

TEXTBOOK OF OPERATIVE UROLOGY   ISBN 0–7216–5510–6

Printed in the United States of America.

Last digit is the print number: 9   8   7   6   5   4   3   2   1

*To my wife, Lindsay,
and children, Wheatley and Brooks,
because a man is only as strong as his family
and I am fortunate to have a good one.*

Contributors

JOHN B. ADAMS II, M.D.
Assistant Professor of Surgery (Urology) and Chief of Endourology, Medical College of Georgia, Augusta, Georgia
Laparoscopic Surgery of the Ureter

MARK C. ADAMS, M.D.
Assistant Professor of Urology, Indiana University School of Medicine; Active Staff, James Whitcomb Riley Hospital for Children, Indianapolis, Indiana
Augmentation Cystoplasty

DAVID M. ALBALA, M.D.
Associate Professor of Urology, Loyola University Stritch School of Medicine, Maywood, Illinois; Staff Urologist, Hines Veterans Hospital, Hines, Illinois
Laparoscopic Adrenalectomy

TERRY D. ALLEN, M.D.
Professor of Urology, University of Texas Southwestern Medical Center; Chief of Pediatric Urology, Children's Medical Center of Dallas, Dallas, Texas
Ureterosigmoidostomy

ALEX F. ALTHAUSEN, M.D.
Associate Clinical Professor of Surgery (Urology), Harvard Medical School; Senior Urologist, Massachusetts General Hospital, Boston, Massachusetts
Colon Conduit

GERALD L. ANDRIOLE, M.D.
Associate Professor of Urologic Surgery, Washington University School of Medicine, St. Louis, Missouri
Penectomy and Inguinal Lymphadenectomy for Carcinoma of the Penis

KENNETH W. ANGERMEIER, M.D.
Attending Staff, Department of Urology, The Cleveland Clinic Foundation, Cleveland, Ohio
Penile Prosthesis Implantation

RODNEY A. APPELL, M.D.
Head, Section of Voiding Dysfunction and Female Urology, Department of Urology, The Cleveland Clinic Foundation, Cleveland, Ohio
Periurethral Injections in the Treatment of Intrinsic Sphincteric Dysfunction

WILLIAM J. ARONSON, M.D.
Assistant Clinical Professor, UCLA School of Medicine, Los Angeles, California; Chief of Urology, Sepulveda Veterans Administration Medical Center, Sepulveda, California
Ileal Ureter

ANTHONY ATALA, M.D.
Assistant Professor, Harvard Medical School; Assistant in Surgery, Children's Hospital, Boston, Massachusetts
Congenital Urethral Duplication

RICHARD K. BABAYAN, M.D.
Professor of Urology, Boston University School of Medicine; Active Staff, Boston University Medical Center Hospital, Boston, Massachusetts
Flexible Cystoscopy

DEMETRIUS H. BAGLEY, M.D.
Professor of Urology and Radiology, Jefferson Medical College, Thomas Jefferson University, Philadelphia, Pennsylvania
Ureteroscopy (Diagnostic)

DAVID M. BARRETT, M.D.
Professor and Chair, Mayo Foundation/Mayo Medical School, Rochester, Minnesota
Artificial Sphincter in the Treatment of Male Urinary Incontinence; Artificial Sphincter in the Treatment of Female Urinary Incontinence

JOHN M. BARRY, M.D.
Professor of Surgery and Chairman, Division of Urology and Renal Transplantation, Oregon Health Sciences University; Attending Surgeon, University Hospital, Portland, Oregon
Donor Nephrectomy

RICHARD BIHRLE, M.D.
Associate Professor, Indiana University School of
Medicine, Indianapolis, Indiana
Retroperitoneal Lymphadenectomy

MICHAEL L. BLUTE, M.D.
Associate Professor of Urology and Consultant in
Urology, Mayo Foundation/Mayo Medical School,
Rochester, Minnesota
Percutaneous Nephrolithotomy

STUART D. BOYD, M.D.
Professor of Urology, University of Southern
California School of Medicine; Chief of Urology,
USC University Hospital, Los Angeles, California
Kock Pouch Urinary Diversion

CHARLES B. BRENDLER, M.D.
Professor and Chief, Section of Urology,
University of Chicago Hospitals and Pritzker
School of Medicine, Chicago, Illinois
*Vesical Diverticulectomy; Partial and Simple
Cystectomy; Urethrectomy with Preservation of
Potency*

MICHAEL C. CARR, M.D., PH.D.
Assistant Professor of Urology, University of
Washington School of Medicine; Attending
Surgeon, Department of Pediatric Urology,
Children's Hospital and Medical Center, Seattle,
Washington
*Gastrocystoplasty and Bladder Replacement with
Stomach; Cloacal Exstrophy*

SERGE CARRIER, M.D.
Assistant Professor of Surgery (Urology),
University of Montreal; Staff Urologist, Notre-
Dame Hospital, Montreal, Quebec, Canada
Surgery for Priapism

H. BALLENTINE CARTER, M.D.
Associate Professor of Urology and Oncology,
Johns Hopkins University School of Medicine,
Baltimore, Maryland
Ureterolithotomy

WILLIAM J. CATALONA, M.D.
Professor and Chief, Division of Urologic Surgery,
Washington University School of Medicine and
Barnes Hospital, St. Louis, Missouri
*Nerve-Sparing Radical Retropubic Prostatectomy;
Penectomy and Inguinal Lymphadenectomy for
Carcinoma of the Penis*

ROLAND N. CHEN, M.D.
Chief Resident, Department of Urology, The
Cleveland Clinic Foundation, Cleveland, Ohio
Therapeutic Ureteroscopy

ASHOK CHOPRA, M.D.
Fellow, Department of Reconstructive Surgery,
Neurourology, and Urodynamics, UCLA School of
Medicine, Los Angeles, California
*Vaginal Surgery for Female Incontinence and Vaginal
Wall Prolapse*

RALPH V. CLAYMAN, M.D.
Professor of Urology and Radiology, Washington
University School of Medicine and Barnes
Hospital, St. Louis, Missouri
Laparoscopic Nephrectomy and Nephroureterectomy

JOHN W. COLBERG, M.D.
Instructor, Division of Urologic Surgery,
Washington University School of Medicine, St.
Louis, Missouri
*Penectomy and Inguinal Lymphadenectomy for
Carcinoma of the Penis*

WILLIAM H. COONER, M.D. (deceased)
Professor of Surgery (Urology), Emory University
School of Medicine, Atlanta, Georgia
Needle Biopsy of the Prostate

ANTHONY DeFRANZO, M.D.
Assistant Professor of Plastic Surgery, Bowman
Gray School of Medicine, Wake Forest University,
Winston-Salem, North Carolina
Vascular Surgery for the Treatment of Impotence

JEAN B. DeKERNION, M.D.
Professor of Surgery (Urology), UCLA School of
Medicine; Surgeon, Urological Oncologist, and
Chief, Division of Urology, UCLA Medical Center,
Los Angeles, California
Ileal Ureter

CHARLES J. DEVINE, JR., M.D.
Professor Emeritus of Urology, Eastern Virginia
Medical School, Norfolk, Virginia
Total Penile Construction/Reconstruction

DAVID A. DIAMOND, M.D.
Professor of Oncology and Pediatrics, University
of Massachusetts Medical Center, Worcester,
Massachusetts
Reconstruction of Male Epispadias

STEVEN G. DOCIMO, M.D.
Assistant Professor of Pediatric Urology, James
Buchanan Brady Urological Institute, and
Attending Pediatric Urologist, Johns Hopkins
Hospital, Baltimore, Maryland
*Endoscopic Surgery in Children; Laparoscopic
Surgery in Children; Circumcision*

JOHN P. DONOHUE, M.D.
Distinguished Professor Emeritus of Urology,
Indiana University School of Medicine,
Indianapolis, Indiana
Retroperitoneal Lymphadenectomy

JAMES F. DONOVAN, JR, M.D.
Associate Professor of Urology, University of Iowa School of Medicine; Active Staff, Veterans Administration Medical Center, Iowa City , Iowa
The Laparoscopic Varix Ligation

JOHN W. DUCKETT, JR., M.D.
Professor of Urology (Surgery), University of Pennsylvania School of Medicine; Director, Division of Pediatric Urology, Children's Hospital of Philadelphia, Philadelphia, Pennsylvania
Mitrofanoff Principle in Continent Reconstruction of the Lower Urinary Tract; Penile Hypospadias

ASIM F. DURRANI, M.D.
Fellow, Division of Urology (Endourology), Duke University Medical Center, Durham, North Carolina
Endoscopic Management of Ureteral Strictures and Fistulas

JACK S. ELDER, M.D.
Professor of Urology and Pediatrics, Case Western Reserve University School of Medicine; Director of Pediatric Urology, Rainbow Babies' and Children's Hospital, Cleveland, Ohio
Orchiopexy and Herniorrhaphy; Diagnostic Laparoscopy for the Impalpable Testis

DAVID H. EWALT, M.D.
Assistant Professor of Surgery (Urology), University of Texas Southwestern Medical School; Attending Pediatric Urologist, Children's Medical Center of Dallas and Texas Scottish Rite Hospital for Children, Dallas, Texas
Distal Hypospadias

MARGIT FISCH, M.D.
Assistant Professor of Urology, University of Mainz School of Medicine, Mainz, Germany
Rectal Neobladders and Mainz Pouch II

RICHARD S. FOSTER, M.D.
Associate Professor of Urology, Indiana University School of Medicine, Indianapolis, Indiana
Retroperitoneal Lymphadenectomy

ANDREW FREEDMAN, M.D.
Fellow, Department of Pediatric Urology, Children's Hospital of Michigan, Detroit, Michigan
Simple and Radical Orchiectomy

JOHN P. GEARHART, M.D.
Associate Professor of Pediatrics and Pediatric Oncology and Director of Pediatric Urology, James Buchanan Brady Urological Institute, Johns Hopkins Hospital, Baltimore, Maryland
Surgical Repair of Exstrophy/Epispadias; Ambiguous Genitalia

GLENN S. GERBER, M.D.
Assistant Professor of Surgery (Urology), University of Chicago Pritzker School of Medicine, Chicago, Illinois
Laparoscopic Retroperitoneal Lymphadenectomy for Carcinoma of the Testis

J. MATTHEW GLASCOCK, M.D.
Resident, University of Iowa School of Medicine, Iowa City, Iowa
Laparoscopic Pelvic Lymph Node Dissection

MARC GOLDSTEIN, M.D
Professor of Urology, Cornell University Medical College; Director, Center for Male Reproductive Medicine and Microsurgery, Department of Urology, The New York Hospital–Cornell Medical Center; Staff Scientist, Center for Biomedical Research, The Population Council, New York, New York
Microsurgical Vasovasostomy

ERIK T. GOLUBOFF, M.D.
Chief Resident, Department of Urology, College of Physicians and Surgeons of Columbia University and Columbia-Presbyterian Medical Center, New York, New York
Simple Nephrectomy

LEONARD G. GOMELLA, M.D.
The Bernard Godwin, Jr. Associate Professor of Prostate Cancer, Jefferson Medical College, Thomas Jefferson University, Philadelphia, Pennsylvania; Consulting Physician, Surgical Service, Wilmington VA Hospital, Wilmington, Delaware
Prostatectomy: New Technologies Including Laser, Microwave, Ultrasound Surgery, and Stents

EDMOND T. GONZALES, JR., M.D.
Professor of Urology, Baylor College of Medicine; Head, Department of Surgery and Department of Pediatric Urology, Texas Children's Hospital, Houston, Texas
Lower Tract Surgery for Ureterocele and Duplication Anomalies

MICHAEL GRASSO, M.D.
Associate Professor of Urology, New York University School of Medicine; Director, Minimally Invasive Urologic Surgery Center, New York University Medical Center, New York, New York
Intracorporeal Lithotripsy: Ultrasonic, Electrohydraulic, Laser, and Electromechanical

LAURENCE M. HAREWOOD, M.B.B.S.
Associate Professor of Surgery, University of Melbourne; Urologist, The Royal Melbourne Hospital, Melbourne, Victoria, Australia
Laparoscopic Surgery for Stress Incontinence

RICHARD E. HAUTMANN, M.D.

Professor and Chairman, Department of Urology, University of Ulm, Ulm, Germany
The Ileal Neobladder

SEAN P. HEDICAN, M.D.

Resident, Department of Urology, James Buchanan Brady Urological Institute, Johns Hopkins Hospital, Baltimore, Maryland
Laparoscopic Surgery of the Ureter

TERRY W. HENSLE, M.D.

Professor of Urology, College of Physicians and Surgeons of Columbia University; Director of Pediatric Urology, The Babies' and Children's Hospital of Columbia-Presbyterian Medical Center, New York, New York
The Correction of Ureteropelvic Junction Obstruction; Reconstruction of the Lower Ureter: Psoas Hitch, Boari Flap, and Transureteroureterostomy; Colovaginoplasty for Vaginal Reconstruction in Children and Adults

RUDOLF HOHENFELLNER, M.D.

Professor and Chairman, Department of Urology, University of Mainz School of Medicine, Mainz, Germany
Rectal Neobladders and Mainz Pouch II

M'LISS A. HUDSON, M.D.

Assistant Professor of Urological Surgery, Washington University School of Medicine, St. Louis, Missouri
Transurethral Resection of Bladder Tumors

CHARLES LEE JACKSON, M.D.

Chairman, Department of Urology, Cleveland Clinic—Florida, Fort Lauderdale, Florida
Surgery for Renal Cysts and Renal Abscesses

ALI CUNEYID ISERI, M.D.

Visiting Fellow, Department of Urologic Surgery, Univesity of Minnesota School of Medicine, Minneapolis, Minnesota; Associate Professor, Gata Haydarpasa, Istanbul, Turkey
Sigmoid Neobladder

JONATHAN P. JAROW, M.D.

Associate Professor of Urology, Bowman Gray School of Medicine, Wake Forest University, Winston-Salem, North Carolina
Vascular Surgery for the Treatment of Impotence; Varicocelectomy, Hydrocelectomy, Spermatocelectomy, and Testicular Biopsy

THOMAS W. JARRETT, M.D.

Assistant Professor of Urology, The George Washington University School of Medicine, Washington, D.C.
Endopyelotomy and Percutaneous Renal Surgery

ROBERT D. JEFFS, M.D.

Professor of Pediatric Urology, Johns Hopkins Medical Institutions, Baltimore, Maryland
Surgical Repair of Exstrophy/Epispadias

ALAN D. JENKINS, M.D.

Associate Professor of Urology, University of Virginia School of Medicine, Charlottesville, Virginia
Extracorporeal Shock Wave Lithotripsy

GERALD H. JORDAN, M.D.

Professor of Urology, Eastern Virginia Medical School; Active Staff, Sentara Norfolk General Hospital, Leigh Memorial Hospital, Bayside Hospital, Children's Hospital of King's Daughters, and DePaul Hospital, Norfolk, Virginia
Laparoscopic Surgery in Children; Surgery of Anterior Urethral Structures; Total Penile Construction/ Reconstruction

DAVID B. JOSEPH, M.D.

Associate Professor of Surgery and Pediatrics, The University of Alabama at Birmingham; Chief of Pediatric Urology, The Children's Hospital of Alabama, Birmingham, Alabama
Pediatric Nephrectomy

LOUIS R. KAVOUSSI, M.D.

Associate Professor of Urology, Chief, Department of Urology; Director, Division of Endourology, Johns Hopkins Bayview Medical Center, Baltimore, Maryland
Therapeutic Ureteroscopy

MICHAEL A. KEATING, M.D.

Associate Professor of Urology, Indiana University School of Medicine; Attending Pediatric Urologist, James Whitcomb Riley Hospital for Children, Indianapolis, Indiana
Noncontinent Urinary Diversion; Continent Urinary Diversion in Children

WILLIAM A. KENNEDY II, M.D.

Fellow, Department of Pediatric Urology, Children's Hospital of Philadelphia, Philadelphia, Pennsylvania
Reconstruction of the Lower Ureter: Psoas Hitch, Boari Flap, and Transureteroureterostomy

ANDREW J. KIRSCH, M.D.

Chief Resident, Department of Urology, College of Physicians and Surgeons of Columbia University, New York, New York
The Correction of Ureteropelvic Junction Obstruction

EDUARDO KLEER, M.D.

Urological Surgery Associates, P.C., Ypsilanti, Michigan
Artificial Sphincter in the Treatment of Male Urinary Incontinence; Artificial Sphincter in the Treatment of Female Urinary Incontinence

HARRY P. KOO, M.D.
Assistant Professor of Surgery (Pediatric Urology), University of Michigan School of Medicine and C. S. Mott Children's Hospital, Ann Arbor, Michigan
Penile Hypospadias

STEPHEN A. KRAMER, M.D.
Professor of Urology, Mayo Medical School; Head, Section of Pediatric Urology, Mayo Clinic/Mayo Foundation, Rochester, Minnesota
Surgical Management of Pediatric Neoplasms

ROBERT J. KRANE, M.D.
Professor and Chairman, Department of Urology, Boston University School of Medicine, Boston, Massachusetts
Surgical Treatment of Peyronie's Disease

KENNETH A. KROPP, M.D.
Professor and Chairman, Department of Urology, and Professor, Department of Pediatrics, Medical College of Ohio, Toledo, Ohio
Urethral Fistula and Diverticula

EUGENE D. KWON, M.D.
Research Fellow, Laboratory of Kidney and Electrolyte Metabolism, National Heart, Lung, and Blood Institute, National Institutes of Health, Bethesda, Maryland
The Laparoscopic Varix Ligation

MILTON M. LAKIN, M.D.
Head, Department of Urology (Medical Urology), The Cleveland Clinic Foundation, Cleveland, Ohio
Penile Prosthesis Implantation

GARY E. LEACH, M.D.
Associate Clinical Professor of Urology, UCLA School of Medicine; Chief, Department of Urology, Kaiser Permanente Medical Center, Los Angeles, California
Urethral Reconstruction for Urinary Incontinence

HERBERT LEPOR, M.D.
Professor and Chairman, Department of Urology, New York University Medical Center, New York, New York
Idiopathic Retroperitoneal Fibrosis: Ureterolysis

JOHN A. LIBERTINO, M.D.
Faculty, Harvard Medical School, Boston, Massachusetts; Chairman of Urology and Chief of Surgery, Lahey Clinic Medical Center, Burlington, Massachusetts
Celiac Axis for Renal Revascularization: Splenorenal and Hepatorenal Arterial Bypass Procedures

GARY LIESKOVSKY, M.D.
Professor of Urology, University of Southern California School of Medicine; Active Staff, Kenneth Norris, Jr. Cancer Center and Research Insitute, Los Angeles, California
Kock Pouch Urinary Diversion

CRAIG W. LILLEHEI, M.D.
Assistant Professor of Surgery, Harvard Medical School; Associate in Surgery, Children's Hospital, Boston, Massachusetts
Surgical Considerations in Pediatric Renal Transplantation

FRANKLIN C. LOWE, M.D., M.P.H.
Clinical Associate Professor of Urology, College of Physicians and Surgeons of Columbia University; Associate Director, Department of Urology, St. Luke's/Roosevelt Hospital, New York, New York
Gangrene of the Male Genitalia

TOM F. LUE, M.D.
Professor of Urology, University of California, San Francisco, School of Medicine, San Francisco, California
Surgery for Priapism

JAMES MANDELL, M.D.
Professor of Surgery and Pediatrics and Chief, Division of Urology, Albany Medical College, Albany, New York
Partial Nephrectomy and Ureteropyelostomy

FRAY F. MARSHALL, M.D.
Professor of Urology, James Buchanan Brady Urological Institute; Director, Adult Urology, Johns Hopkins Medical Institutions, Baltimore, Maryland
Endoscopic Treatment of Urethral Strictures and Urethral Obliterations; Minilaparotomy Staging Pelvic Lymphadenectomy (Minilap); Radical Nephrectomy: Flank Approaches; Radical Nephrectomy with Excision of Vena Caval Tumor Thrombus; Partial Nephrectomy; Radical Cystectomy (Anterior Exenteration) in the Female; Total Bladder Substitution: Ileocolic Neobladder

VICTOR F. MARSHALL, M.D.
Emeritus Professor of Urology, Cornell University Medical College, New York, New York, and University of Virginia School of Medicine, Charlottesville, Virginia
Stress Incontinence in the Female

JACK W. McANINCH, M.D.
Professor and Vice Chairman, Department of Urology, University of California, San Francisco; Chief of Urology, San Francisco General Hospital, San Francisco, California
Renal Trauma: Evaluation and Surgical Treatment; Surgical Repair of Ureteral Injuries; Rupture of the Bladder: Surgical Treatment; Membranous Urethral Stricture: Use of Pubectomy in Repair; Surgical Repair of Genital Injuries

JOHN F. McCARTHY, M.D.
Instructor in Surgery (Urology), Washington University School of Medicine; Attending Physician, Barnes Hospital, Barnes West Hospital, The Jewish Hospital of St. Louis, John Cochran Veteran's Administration Hospital, and St. Louis Children's Hospital, St. Louis, Missouri
Nerve-Sparing Radical Retropubic Prostatectomy

W. SCOTT McDOUGAL, M.D.
Professor of Surgery, Harvard Medical School; Chief, Department of Urology, Massachusetts General Hospital, Boston, Massachusetts
Ureterocalicostomy; Total Pelvic Exenteration in the Male

ELSPETH M. McDOUGALL, M.D.
Assistant Professor of Urologic Surgery, Washington University School of Medicine; Active Staff, Barnes Hospital and Affiliates, St. Louis, Missouri
Laparoscopic Renal Surgery

EDWARD J. McGUIRE, M.D.
Professor and Director, Division of Urology, The University of Texas—Houston Medical School, Houston, Texas
Pubovaginal Slings

WINSTON K. MEBUST, M.D.
Valk Professor and Chairman, Department of Urologic Surgery, Kansas University Medical Center, Kansas City, Missouri
Prostatectomy

AGOSTINO MENEGHINI, M.D.
Fellow, Department of Urology, Institute of Urology, University of Padua, Padua, Italy
Extended Psoas Hitch

MANI MENON, M.D.
Professor and Chairman, Division of Urology, University of Massachusetts Medical Center, Worcester, Massachusetts
The Lumbodorsal Approach to the Kidney; Nephrostomy and Renal Biopsy

MICHAEL E. MITCHELL, M.D.
Professor of Urology, University of Washington School of Medicine; Chief, Division of Pediatric Urology, Children's Hospital and Medical Center, Seattle, Washington
Gastrocystoplasty and Bladder Replacement with Stomach; Cloacal Exstrophy

DROGO K. MONTAGUE, M.D.
Professor of Surgery (Urology) and Head, Section of Prosthetic Surgery, Department of Urology, The Cleveland Clinic Foundation, Cleveland, Ohio
Penile Prosthesis Implantation

JAMES E. MONTIE, M.D.
Professor of Urology, University of Michigan School of Medicine; Clinical Director, Urologic Oncology Program, University of Michigan Comprehensive Cancer Center, Ann Arbor, Michigan
Surgery for Renal Cysts and Renal Abscesses; Technique of Radical Cystectomy in the Male

ROBERT G. MOORE, M.D.
Assistant Professor of Urology, Johns Hopkins University School of Medicine; Active Staff, Johns Hopkins Bayview Medical Center, Baltimore, Maryland
Endoscopic Treatment of Urethral Srictures and Urethral Obliterations

JACEK L. MOSTWIN, M.D., PH.D.
Assistant Professor of Urology, Johns Hopkins University School of Medicine; Staff Urologist, Johns Hopkins Hospital, Baltimore, Maryland
Surgery of the Kidney and Ureter in Pregnancy; Burch Colposuspension; Paravaginal Repair

STEPHEN Y. NAKADA, M.D.
Assistant Professor of Surgery (Urology) and Head, Section of Endourology and Stone Disease, University of Wisconsin Medical School and University of Wisconsin Hospital and Clinics, Madison, Wisconsin
Laparoscopic Nephrectomy and Nephroureterectomy

MICHAEL J. NASLUND, M.D.
Assistant Professor of Urology, University of Maryland School of Medicine; Director, The Maryland Prostate Center, Baltimore, Maryland
Vesical Fistulas; Vasectomy

H. NORMAN NOE, M.D.
Professor of Urology and Chief, Department of Pediatric Urology, University of Tennessee, Memphis, College of Medicine; Chief, Department of Urology, LeBonheur Children's Medical Center, Memphis, Tennessee
Posterior Urethral Valves

ANDREW C. NOVICK, M.D.
Chairman, Department of Urology, The Cleveland Clinic Foundation, Cleveland, Ohio
Radical Nephrectomy: Anterior Approach; Renal Arterial Grafts and Renal Bench Surgery

CARL A. OLSSON, M.D.
Professor and Chairman, Department of Urology, College of Physicians and Surgeons of Columbia University; Chief, Department of Urology, Columbia-Presbyterian Medical Center; Chief, Squier Urological Clinic, New York, New York
Simple Nephrectomy

FRANCESCO PAGANO, M.D.
Chief and Chairman, Institute of Urology, University of Padua, Padua, Italy
Extended Psoas Hitch

FARHAD PARIVAR, M.D.
Chief Resident, University of California, San Francisco, School of Medicine, San Francisco, California
Surgery for Priapism

ALAN PARTIN, M.D., Ph.D.
Instructor of Urology, Johns Hopkins University School of Medicine; Active Staff, Johns Hopkins Hospital, Baltimore, Maryland
Minilaparotomy Staging Pelvic Lymphadenectomy (Minilap)

DAVID F. PAULSON, M.D.
Professor of Surgery and Chief, Department of Urology, Duke University Medical Center, Durham, North Carolina
Radical Perineal Prostatectomy; Seminal Vesiculectomy

LUIS M. PÉREZ, M.D.
Assistant Professor, Division of Urology, Department of Surgery, The University of Alabama at Birmingham; Assistant Professor, Pediatric Urology, The Children's Hospital of Alabama, Birmingham, Alabama
Prune-Belly Syndrome

CRAIG A. PETERS, M.D.
Assistant in Surgery (Urology), Assistant Professor of Surgery, Children's Hospital, Harvard Medical School, Boston, Massachusetts
Ureteral Reimplantation: Including Megaureter Repair; Urinary Undiversion: Surgical Considerations and Strategies; Surgical Management of Testicular Torsion; Surgical Considerations in Pediatric Renal Transplantation; Surgical Management of Fetal Uropathies

GLENN M. PREMINGER, M.D.
Professor of Urologic Surgery and Director, Comprehensive Kidney Stone Center and Urology Laboratories, Duke University Medical Center, Durham, North Carolina
Endoscopic Management of Ureteral Strictures and Fistulas

JACOB RAJFER, M.D.
Professor of Surgery (Urology), UCLA School of Medicine, Los Angeles, California; Chief, Department of Urology, Harbor–UCLA Medical Center, Torrance, California
Simple and Radical Orchiectomy

SHLOMO RAZ, M.D.
Professor of Surgery (Urology), UCLA School of Medicine, Los Angeles, California
Vaginal Surgery for Female Incontinence and Vaginal Wall Prolapse

PRATAP K. REDDY, M.D.
Professor and Acting Chairman, Department of Urologic Surgery, University of Minnesota; Chief, Department of Urology, Veterans Affairs Medical Center, Minneapolis, Minnesota
Sigmoid Neobladder

JAMIL REHMAN, M.D.
Fellow, Department of Urology, Albert Einstein College of Medicine and Montefiore Medical Center, Bronx, New York
Surgery for Priapism

BRUCE A. REITZ, M.D.
Norman E. Shumway Professor and Chairman, Department of Cardiothoracic Surgery, Stanford University School of Medicine; Active Staff, Stanford Health Services, Stanford, California
Radical Nephrectomy with Excision of Vena Caval Tumor Thrombus

MARTIN I. RESNICK, M.D.
Professor and Chairman, Department of Urology, Case Western Reserve University School of Medicine, Cleveland, Ohio
Pyelonephrolithotomy

ALAN B. RETIK, M.D.
Professor of Surgery (Urology), Harvard Medical School; Chief, Division of Urology, Children's Hospital, Boston, Massachusetts
Ureteral Reimplantation: Including Megaureter Repair; Proximal Hypospadias

JEROME P. RICHIE, M.D.
Elliott C. Cutler Professor of Surgery, Harvard Medical School; Chairman, Harvard Program in Urology (Longwood); Chief of Urology, Brigham and Women's Hospital, Boston, Massachusetts
Nephroureterectomy for Carcinoma of Renal Pelvis and Ureter

RICHARD C. RINK, M.D.
Associate Professor, Department of Urology, Indiana University School of Medicine; Chief, Department of Pediatric Urology, James Whitcomb Riley Hospital for Children and Indiana University Medical Center, Indianapolis, Indiana
Augmentation Cystoplasty

TIMOTHY M. RODDY, M.D.
Clinical Faculty, University of Washington School of Medicine, Seattle, Washington; Active Staff, Stevens Memorial Hospital, Edmonds, Washington
Surgical Treatment of Peyronie's Disease

RANDALL G. ROWLAND, M.D., PH.D.

Professor of Urology, Indiana University School of
Medicine, Indianapolis, Indiana
Cutaneous Continent Ileocecal Reservoir

DANIEL B. RUKSTALIS, M.D.

Associate Professor and Chairman, Department of
Surgery (Urology), Medical College of
Pennsylvania, Philadelphia, Pennsylvania
*Laparoscopic Retroperitoneal Lymphadenectomy for
Carcinoma of the Testis*

ARTHUR I. SAGALOWSKY, M.D.

Professor of Surgery (Urology), University of Texas
Southwestern Medical School; Chief of Urologic
Oncology and Surgical Director Renal
Transplantation, Children's Medical Center of
Dallas, Dallas, Texas
Renal Transplantation and Autotransplantation

W. HOLT SANDERS, M.D.

Assistant Professor of Surgery (Urology), Emory
University School of Medicine, Atlanta, Georgia
Needle Biopsy of the Prostate

JAY I. SANDLOW, M.D.

Assistant Professor of Urology, University of Iowa
School of Medicine, Iowa City, Iowa
The Laparoscopic Varix Ligation

IHOR S. SAWCZUK, M.D.

Associate Professor of Urology, College of
Physicians and Surgeons of Columbia University;
Associate Attending in Urology, Columbia-
Presbyterian Medical Center, New York, New York
Simple Nephrectomy

PETER N. SCHLEGEL, M.D.

Assistant Professor of Urology, Cornell University
Medical College; Visiting Associate Physician,
Rockefeller University Hospital; Assistant
Attending Urologist, The New York Hospital; Staff
Scientist, The Population Council, Center for
Biomedical Research, New York, New York
*Preperitoneal Hernia Repair During Urological
Surgery; Vasoepididymostomy, Epididymal Sperm
Retrieval, and In Vitro Techniques for Male Factor
Infertility*

STEVEN M. SCHLOSSBERG, M.D.

Associate Professor of Urology and Anatomy,
Eastern Virginia Medical School, Norfolk, Virginia
Total Penile Construction/Reconstruction

RICHARD N. SCHLUSSEL, M.D.

Assistant Professor of Urology, Mt. Sinai Medical
Center School of Medicine, New York, New York;
Englewood Medical Center, Englewood, New
Jersey; Elmhurst Medical Center, Queens, New
York
*Urinary Undiversion: Surgical Considerations and
Strategies*

ERIC K. SEAMAN, M.D.

Chief Resident, Department of Urology, Columbia-
Presbyterian Medical Center, New York, New York
*Colovaginoplasty for Vaginal Reconstruction in
Children and Adults*

JOSEPH W. SEGURA, M.D.

Carl Rosen Professor of Urology and Consultant in
Urology, Mayo Foundation/Mayo Medical School,
Rochester, Minnesota
Percutaneous Nephrolithotomy

ELLEN SHAPIRO, M.D.

Professor of Urology, New York University School
of Medicine, New York, New York
Ileal Conduit Urinary Diversion

DONALD G. SKINNER, M.D.

Professor and Chairman, Department of Urology,
University of Southern California School of
Medicine; Chief of Surgery, Kenneth Norris, Jr.
Cancer Center and Research Institute, Los
Angeles, California
Kock Pouch Urinary Diversion

EILA SKINNER, M.D.

Assistant Professor of Urology, University of
Southern California School of Medicine; Active
Staff, Kenneth Norris, Jr. Cancer Center and
Research Institute, Los Angeles, California
Kock Pouch Urinary Diversion

ARTHUR D. SMITH, M.D.

Professor of Urology, Albert Einstein College of
Medicine, Bronx, New York; Chairman,
Department of Urology, Long Island Jewish
Medical Center, New Hyde Park, New York
Endopyelotomy and Percutaneous Renal Surgery

JOSEPH A. SMITH, JR., M.D.

Professor and Chairman, Department of Urology,
Vanderbilt University School of Medicine;
Surgeon-in-Chief, Vanderbilt University Hospital,
Nashville, Tennessee
Laser Treatment of Bladder Cancer

ROBERT B. SMITH, M.D.

Professor of Surgery (Urology), UCLA School of
Medicine; Surgeon and Urologic Oncologist,
UCLA Medical Center, Los Angeles, California
Ileal Ureter

HOWARD M. SNYDER III, M.D.

Professor of Urology (Surgery), University of
Pennsylvania School of Medicine; Associate
Director, Division of Pediatric Urology, Children's
Hospital of Philadelphia, Philadelphia,
Pennsylvania
*Mitrofanoff Principle in Continent Reconstruction of
the Lower Urinary Tract*

MITCHELL S. STEINER, M.D.

Associate Professor of Urology and Pharmacology, University of Tennessee School of Medicine; Active Staff, William F. Bowld Hospital, Memphis, Tennessee

Minilaparotomy Staging Pelvic Lymphadenectomy (Minilap)

LYNN STOTHERS, M.D., M.H.Sc.

Fellow, Department of Reconstructive Surgery, Neurourology, and Urodynamics, UCLA School of Medicine, Los Angeles, California

Vaginal Surgery for Female Incontinence and Vaginal Wall Prolapse

RAY E. STUTZMAN, M.D.

Associate Professor of Urology, Johns Hopkins University School of Medicine; Director of Outpatient Urology, James Buchanan Brady Urological Institute, Johns Hopkins Hospital, Baltimore, Maryland

Suprapubic Prostatectomy

BRETT A. TROCKMAN, M.D.

Clinical Instructor of Urology, Loyola University Medical Center, Maywood, Illinois

Urethral Reconstruction for Urinary Incontinence

S. VAIDYANATHAN, M.D.

Active Staff, Division of Urology, University of Massachusetts Medical Center, Worcester, Massachusetts

The Lumbodorsal Approach to the Kidney; Nephrostomy and Renal Biopsy

E. DARRACOTT VAUGHAN, JR., M.D.

James J. Colt Professor of Urology and Senior Associate Dean for Clinical Affairs, Cornell University Medical Center; Urologist-in-Chief, The New York Hospital, New York, New York

Adrenal Surgery

PATRICK C. WALSH, M.D.

David Hall McConnell Professor and Chairman, Department of Urology, Johns Hopkins University School of Medicine; Urologist-in-Chief, James

Buchanan Brady Urological Institute, Johns Hopkins Hospital, Baltimore, Maryland

Preperitoneal Hernia Repair During Urological Surgery; Urethrectomy with Preservation of Potency

ROBERT WAMMACK, M.D.

Faculty, Department of Urology, University of Mainz School of Medicine, Mainz, Germany

Rectal Neobladders and Mainz Pouch II

GEORGE D. WEBSTER, M.B.

Professor of Urologic Surgery, Duke University Medical Center, Durham, North Carolina

Reconstruction of the Membranous Urethral Stricture; Management of Voiding Dysfunction Following Incontinence Surgery

HOWARD N. WINFIELD, M.D.

Associate Professor of Urology, University of Iowa School of Medicine; Associate Professor of Urology, University of Iowa Hospitals and Clinics, Iowa City, Iowa

Laparoscopic Pelvic Lymph Node Dissection

J. CHRISTIAN WINTERS, M.D.

Clinical Assistant Professor, Louisiana State University Medical Center, New Orleans, Louisiana

Periurethral Injections in the Treatment of Intrinsic Sphincteric Dysfunction

BRAD A. WOLFSON, M.D.

Practicing Urologist, Palm Springs, California

Simple and Radical Orchiectomy

JOHN R. WOODARD, M.D.

Director of Pediatric Urology, Emory University School of Medicine; Chief of Pediatric Urology, Egleston Children's Hospital, Atlanta, Georgia

Prune-Belly Syndrome

GANG (KEVIN) ZHANG, M.D.

Assistant Professor, University of Minnesota School of Medicine; Staff Physician, Veterans Affairs Medical Center; Consultant, Park Nicollet Clinic, Minneapolis, Minnesota

Sigmoid Neobladder

Preface

In this information age, surgical innovation and technological change continue to accelerate. As I have stated previously, much of what I do now in urology did not exist when I was in my urology residency. This training, however, provided the framework for incorporation of these new surgical and technological advances into practice. Extracorporeal shock wave lithotripsy, percutaneous nephrolithotomy, microsurgical vasovasostomy, continent urinary diversion, cardiopulmonary bypass with renal tumors, endoscopic reconstruction of membranous urethral transections, and laparoscopy are all examples of these new procedures.

The *Textbook of Operative Urology* was designed to be the most comprehensive, informative book that could be devised on the operative management of the urological patient. The best experts in the field were selected to describe the indications for the operation, the preoperative evaluation and management, the operative technique, the postoperative management, and the complications for each procedure. It is hoped that this book will be a valuable resource to anyone interested in operative urology.

FRAY F. MARSHALL, M.D.

Acknowledgments

This book has been a major undertaking and has been greatly facilitated by the subeditors, Dr. Louis Kavoussi, who is the section editor on Endourology; Dr. Jack McAninch, the section editor on Urological Trauma; and Dr. Craig Peters, the section editor on Pediatric Urological Surgery. In addition, Mary Nori has been superb in helping organize this book and has received aid from Darlyn Tucker. Sandra Valkhoff of W.B. Saunders has also been excellent in her careful review and management of this text for W.B. Saunders. Richard Zorab of W.B. Saunders is to be thanked for his belief in this text.

The Editors and Publisher wish to acknowledge that many of the illustrations appearing in this new text originally appeared in *Operative Urology*, edited by Fray Marshall, M.D., and published by W.B. Saunders in 1991.

Contents

SECTION II ADULT UROLOGICAL SURGERY

SECTION IV SURGERY AFTER UROLOGICAL TRAUMA

SECTION V PEDIATRIC UROLOGICAL SURGERY

SECTION I

ENDOUROLOGY

Part I

Endoscopy and Extracorporeal
Shock Wave Lithotripsy

Part II

Adult Laparoscopy

Part III

Pediatric Endoscopy
and Laparoscopy

Part I

ENDOSCOPY AND EXTRACORPOREAL SHOCK WAVE LITHOTRIPSY

Chapter 1

Flexible Cystoscopy

Richard K. Babayan

HISTORICAL BACKGROUND

Cystoscopic inspection of the bladder was formerly a hospital-based procedure performed in specialized cystoscopy suites, often with the patient under general anesthesia. As cystoscopy has made the transition largely to an office-based procedure, both for diagnostic purposes and in selected therapeutic instances, flexible fiberoptic instruments have gradually replaced the rigid cystoscope as the endoscope of choice, especially among younger urologists. There are several reasons for this trend. Since the mid-1980s, there has been an increasing awareness on the part of urologists of the utility of flexible instruments in the urinary tract. As urologists became accustomed to flexible nephroscopes in viewing areas of the upper tracts difficult to gain access to with rigid scopes, it was a natural transition to use similar flexible instruments to view the bladder and urethra. During this period, purpose-built flexible cystoscopes have appeared offering distinct advantages over standard rigid cystoscopes in terms of procedure cost, simplicity, speed of performance, and patient comfort (Fig. 1–1). Since urologists have gained familiarity with the nuances of flexible fiberoptic cystoscopy and the versatility of the instrumentation, it is not surprising to understand the rapid acceptance of flexible cystoscopy as an office procedure.

The internal construction of the typical flexible cystoscope is significantly more complex than that of its rigid counterpart.[1] Three fiberoptic bundles, two for illumination and one for imaging, along with the irrigation/instrumentation channel, form the central core of the shaft of the flexible scope. Stainless steel cables run alongside these central elements from the handle to the distal deflection apparatus. The core elements are wrapped by intertwining helical steel bands that are in turn enveloped by a thin layer of wire meshlike material. An impermeable polymer skin forms the outer coating of the flexible cystoscope shaft and provides a waterproof skin that offers minimal friction to passage through the urethra (Fig. 1–2).

PREOPERATIVE PREPARATION

Although the initial cost of instrumentation is more expensive for flexible than for rigid cystoscopes, the daily care, preparation, and average procedure costs are significantly decreased with flexible cystoscopy, which also requires little in the way of set-up. The procedure is performed with the patient in the supine position lying on a standard office examining room table. A special cystoscopy table with drain pan, with the patient in the dorsal lithotomy position is unnecessary. Flexible cystoscopy requires less irrigating fluid than rigid cystoscopy (usually less than 250 ml). Like office-based endoscopy, flexible cystoscopy is also more versatile than rigid cystoscopy in that it can be performed at the bedside of a hospitalized

2

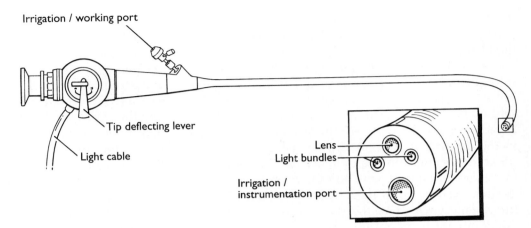

Figure 1–1. Basic design of a flexible cystoscope, illustrating features of the handle and tip of the shaft *(inset).*

patient as well as in situations that would preclude proper positioning for rigid cystoscopy (e.g., patients with frozen pelves or in traction).[2] Flexible cystoscopy allows access to the bladder via suprapubic cystotomy tracts and may be used to view urinary conduits and continent catheterizable urinary pouches, all with minimal discomfort to the patient. General anesthesia or intravenous sedation is seldom, if ever, required for the performance of flexible cystoscopy. Topical transurethral application of lidocaine jelly is usually sufficient local anesthesia in males, and females often require nothing more than simple lubricating jelly.

Indications for diagnostic flexible cystoscopy are virtually identical to those for rigid cystoscopy. Although the instrumentation channel and choice of accessories is more limited than with rigid cystoscopy, most therapeutic cystoscopic maneuvers, including retrograde catheterization of the ureteral orifices, placement and removal of ureteral stents, biopsy, and fulguration of the bladder can all be performed with flexible cystoscopes. A relative contraindication to flexible cystoscopy, however, is the presence of gross hematuria with clots. Flexible cystoscopes have a much smaller irrigation channel than do their rigid counterparts, and as such do not have sufficient irrigation flow to enable the bladder

to be adequately examined in the presence of gross hematuria or to irrigate out the clots.

Flexible cystoscopes may be either gas sterilized or soaked in disinfectant solutions before use. A separate valve or cap is usually present to switch back and forth. It is important to avoid soaking the flexible cystoscope with the vent open, or gas sterilizing when the vent is not engaged. Either condition will lead to serious damage to the scope. Emersion in disinfectant solutions for excessive lengths of time may lead to build-up of a film, which will impair the optics, and in extreme cases result in corrosion of the instrument.[3]

OPERATIVE TECHNIQUE

Flexible cystoscopy is performed with males in the supine position; females are generally placed in a frog-leg position to allow better access to the urethral meatus. No special cystoscopy table is required: a simple office examining room table suffices. An exception to this rule is when the cystoscopy is to be performed for ureteral catheterization immediately before a percutaneous nephrostolithotomy. In this instance, patients of either sex may be cystoscoped in the prone position to obviate the need for reposition-

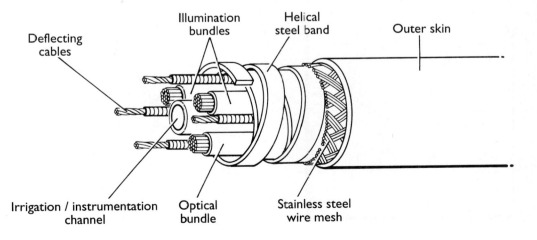

Figure 1–2. Internal construction of a flexible fiberoptic cystoscope.

ing on the operating/fluoroscopy table. Obviously, in male patients, prone cystoscopy is possible only with the flexible cystoscope.

The genitalia are prepared with povidone-iodine solution and draped with a fenestrated sheet. A Foley catheter insertion prep kit may be used in the office setting. Local anesthesia is introduced in the form of 2 percent lidocaine jelly, 10 ml of which is instilled in the urethral meatus. A Zipser clamp may be applied for several minutes to allow the lidocaine jelly to remain in contact with the urethral mucosa. The flexible cystoscope is then introduced into the urethra, being grasped in the dominant hand with the nondominant hand guiding the shaft up the urethra. If a nurse or assistant is available, they may assist by holding the phallus taut. If no assistant is available, the operator may use his fourth and fifth fingers to grasp the penis, while advancing the shaft of the scope with the thumb, index, and middle fingers (Fig. 1–3). With the irrigation running, the pendulous and bulbous urethra are well visualized. As the flexible cystoscope passes through the external sphincter, it is often useful to ask the patient to try to void, thus relaxing the external sphincter and bladder neck musculature. As a result of the small caliber of the irrigation channel, the flow through most flexible cystoscopes is less than ideal for distention and visualization of the prostatic urethra during initial passage of the cystoscope. It is therefore recommended that

the prostatic urethra be viewed at the end of the procedure when the flexible cystoscope is being withdrawn from the partially distended bladder.

Upon entering the bladder, the phallus is released and an orderly inspection of the bladder begins. To gain proper orientation, it is suggested that the inspection begin at the dome, which is readily identified by the presence of an air bubble (Fig. 1–4). The tip of the flexible cystoscope deflects in two directions, usually up and down, with a maximal deflection of 180 to 220 degrees in one direction and a lesser deflection in the opposite direction. It is necessary to rotate the shaft 90 degrees in order to flex the tip of the scope left or right, and it may be necessary to rotate the shaft 180 degrees to position the direction of maximal deflection in the proper orientation (Fig. 1–5). Thus, one hand moves the shaft of the flexible cystoscope in and out from the bladder neck to the posterior wall, and at the same time controls right and left angulation. With the other hand controlling tip deflection, the entire mucosal surface of the bladder may thus be visually inspected within minutes.

The flexible cystoscope has a unique ability that makes it even more distinct from the rigid cystoscope: it can retroflex and look back upon itself (Fig. 1–6). Not only can the flexible cystoscope be deflected 180 to 220 degrees by active deflection, but there is also a passive deflection mechanism that

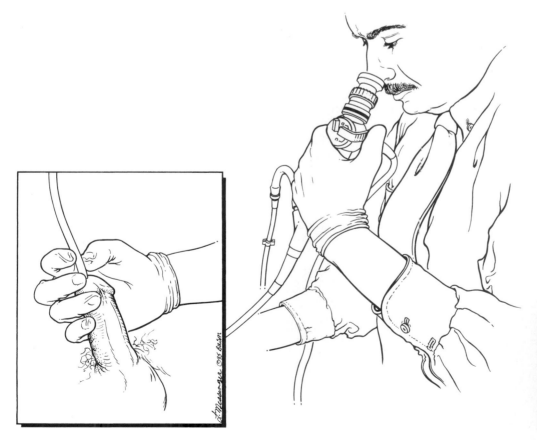

Figure 1–3. Customary positioning of the hands on the flexible cystoscope upon insertion into the male urethra. Note how the urethra is kept taut while the shaft of the cystoscope is introduced into the meatus *(inset)*. (Illustration drawn by L. Messinger. Copyright 1995, Boston University Medical Campus.)

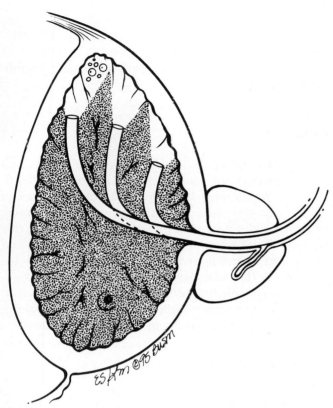

Figure 1–4. Inspection begins at the dome posteriorly with the flexible cystoscope brought back and forth toward the bladder neck. (Illustration drawn by ES/LM. Copyright 1995, Boston University Medical Campus.)

allows the more proximal shaft of the cystoscope to deflect off the back wall of the bladder, literally look back upon itself, and view the more proximal shaft as it comes through the bladder neck. This feature is especially useful in surveillance cystoscopy for bladder cancer when a recurrence is suspected near the bladder neck at the dome.

A number of flexible accessories that will pass through the instrumentation port of the flexible cystoscope are available. These accessories have profiles of 3 Fr. to 5 Fr. in circumference. Grasping and biopsy forceps, fulgurating electrodes, electrohydraulic lithotripsy probes, and laser fibers are among the most widely used accessories. It must be remembered that the turning radius of the tip deflection will be significantly reduced when an accessory is passed through the flexible cystoscope. In addition, it may not be possible to pass larger accessories through the instrumentation port when the tip of the cystoscope is fully deflected. Also, since the irrigation/instrumentation port is a single channel, there will be markedly reduced flow when an accessory is present within that channel, and this may significantly affect visualization, especially in the presence of gross hematuria.

Flexible cystoscopy is particularly useful for surveillance cystoscopies of patients with histories of

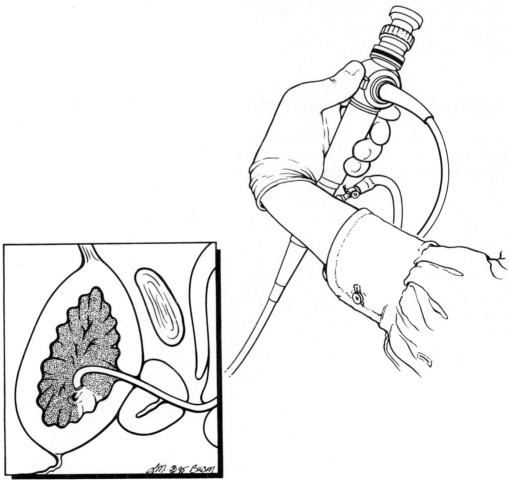

Figure 1–5. To achieve maximal deflection toward the floor of the bladder, the handle and shaft are rotated 180 degrees. (Illustration drawn by LM. Copyright 1995, Boston University Medical Campus.)

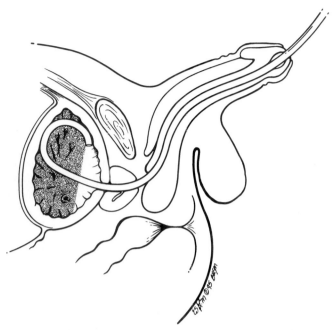

Figure 1–6. Retroflection of the flexible cystoscope against the posterior wall of the bladder allows the urologist to view the proximal shaft as it comes through the bladder neck. (Illustration drawn by ES/LM. Copyright 1995, Boston University Medical Campus.)

transitional cell carcinoma or carcinoma in situ. Bladder barbotage for cytology or flow cytometry may be performed using a large-bore syringe attached to the irrigation port of the flexible cystoscope. If an area suspicious for carcinoma in situ is visualized, the barbotage may be directed at that site to obtain exfoliated cells.

POSTOPERATIVE MANAGEMENT

After removal of the flexible cystoscope, there is little urethral or bladder discomfort for most patients. The transient dysuria often associated with rigid cystoscopy is seldom encountered after flexible cystoscopy. Most patients are able to resume normal activities within minutes of the procedure, and most of those who have undergone both rigid and flexible cystoscopy prefer the latter.

Summary

Flexible cystoscopy has challenged the domination of rigid cystoscopy since the mid-1980s. Flexible fiberoptic instruments have clearly become the ones of choice for office-based cystoscopy, especially among urologists who have completed their training in this period. The versatility of the instrumentation and its obvious patient acceptance make it a valuable addition to the urologist's endoscopic arsenal. As advances in fiberoptic technology continue, and with the prospect of future digital imaging on the horizon, the role of flexible cystoscopy is likely to expand.

Editorial Comment

Fray F. Marshall

Flexible cystoscopy has helped revolutionize office-based urology. Although we utilize flexible cystoscopy very frequently, it is not performed routinely in all patients. Patients with a high bladder neck, a median lobe, or a large prostate and young patients are more suited to flexible cystoscopy, which produces less discomfort.

REFERENCES

1. Babayan RK. Flexible fiberoptic endoscopy of the upper urinary tract. In de Vere White RW, Palmer JM, eds. New Techniques in Urology. Mt. Kisco, NY, Futura, 1987, p 29.
2. Rittenberg MH, Bagley DH. Flexible cystoscopy in the inaccessible but catheterizable urethra. J Endourol: 1:161, 1987.
3. Babayan RK. Flexible cystoscopy for office procedures. Contemp Urol 42, December 1990.

Chapter 2

Prostatectomy

Winston K. Mebust

INDICATIONS

The prevalence of benign prostatic hyperplasia (BPH) increases progressively with age. The prevalence of histologically identifiable BPH for 60-year-old men is greater than 50 percent and by age 85 is approximately 90 percent.

In 1968, Lytton et al[1] estimated that a man aged 40 had a 10 percent chance of requiring a prostatectomy during his lifetime. In 1985, Glynn et al[2] revised this estimate to 29 percent. Arrighi et al,[3] in reviewing the Baltimore Longitudinal Study of Aging (BLSA), felt that men over age 60 had a 39 percent chance of needing surgery in the next 20 years, that men 50 to 59 years of age had a 24 percent chance, and that in those aged 40 to 49 the likelihood of having prostatectomy within the next 20 years was 13 percent.

The usual indications for surgery are the symptoms of prostatism, which include symptoms of bladder outlet obstruction and bladder irritability. In the American Urological Association (AUA) Cooperative Study, symptoms of prostatism were the most common indication for prostatectomy, but over 70 percent of men had more than one indication, such as urinary retention and recurrent infections.[4] To determine the relationship among urological symptoms, prostate size, and subsequent prostatectomy, Arrighi et al[5] analyzed a symptom questionnaire and physical examination of 1057 men followed for up to 30 years in the BLSA Study. They noted that men with prostate enlargement and obstructive symptoms, especially those of diminished size and force of urinary stream and a sensation of incomplete emptying, were found to be five to eight times more likely to require prostatectomy over the next few years than those of the same age who did not. Epstein et al[6] found that nocturia and hesitancy predicted a surgical outcome more commonly in men ages 49 to 59, but beyond age 62 nocturia was the only predictive symptom.

To quantify symptoms so that they could be used in the decision process, whether to treat or not treat a man with BPH, Barry et al[7] developed a symptom severity questionnaire consisting of seven questions with a possible total of 35 points. This became known as the AUA-7 Symptom Index. It was to be self-administered by patients, who were classified as having mild symptoms with a score of 0 to 7, moderate symptoms with 8 to 19, and severe symptoms with 20 to 35.

In the Agency for Health Care Policy and Research (AHCPR) Guideline on BPH, it is recommended that a formal assessment of patient symptoms be made using the AUA Symptom Severity Index.[8] The questionnaire is not disease specific and does not differentiate patients with from those without BPH. It is a way of quantifying symptoms to help determine whether treatment is necessary. In addition to the severity of symptoms, the disease-specific quality of life must be considered. A global question on the disease-specific quality of life was incorporated with the AUA-7 Symptom Index and adopted by the World Health Organization as the International Prostate Symptom Score (I-PSS). Barry et al[9] have expanded this single quality-of-life question to a total of four questions referred to as the BPH Impact Index. Fowler[10] noted that 80 percent of patients who had severe symptoms had improvement in quality of life after treatment, but patients did vary as to how much a certain symptom bothered them. The AHCPR Guideline on BPH also requires that the patient be informed of the risks and benefits of each treatment modality.[8] Therefore, the indication to treat will be in patients with moderate to severe symptoms, and informed patients will participate in the decision to treat and with the choice of appropriate treatment.

In addition to symptoms being an indication for surgical intervention, the complications of an obstructing prostate, such as acute or chronic urinary retention, recurrent infection, hematuria, bladder stones, and postrenal azotemia, may make evident the need to treat.

PREOPERATIVE MANAGEMENT

In the general evaluation of the patient being considered for a transurethral prostatic resection (TURP), the Agency's guideline points out that there must be a detailed history that would help exclude patients with disease entities that could mimic the symptoms of prostatism, such as diabetes. Also, comorbidity factors had to be identified in the patient assessment. In the AUA study, 77 percent of the patients undergoing TURP had preexisting comorbidity factors.[4] A focused physical examination should be performed, including a digital rectal examination to help identify (1) patients with prostate carcinoma and (2) those with a very large prostate who might be candidates for an open procedure rather than TURP.

Laboratory tests commonly obtained are a complete blood count, blood chemistry profile, chest radiograph, electrocardiogram, urinalysis, and, if indicated, culture and sensitivity. Creatinine is specifically recommended in the guideline because of the increased morbidity and mortality associated with patients who are azotemic. It was noted in the AUA study that the incidence of complications was 25 percent in patients with a serum creatinine level greater than 1.5 mg/dl compared with 17 percent when the level was less than 1.5 mg/dl.[4]

The guidelines for diagnosis and treatment of BPH do not recommend a routine serum prostate-specific antigen (PSA) test.[8] Rather, it was left as an option because of (1) the guideline panel's concern over the significant overlap in PSA values between men with BPH and men with pathologically organ-confined prostate cancer, (2) a lack of consensus concerning the optimal evaluation of the minimally evaluated PSA, and (3) the lack of evidence showing that PSA testing reduces the morbidity or mortality rates in men with prostatic disease. The panel also recommended that imaging of the urinary upper tract not be done routinely but rather reserved for patients with a history of hematuria, urinary tract infection, renal insufficiency, stones, or previous genitourinary surgery. The BPH panel advised against the routine use of preoperative cystometrography, in the belief that it added little that could not be obtained from the patient's history. Determination of maximal urinary flow rate was left as an option because, if the patient had a peak flow rate over 15 ml/sec, the outcome was not as good as in those with a lesser flow rate. Furthermore, patients with significant symptoms of prostatism and a flow rate higher than 15 ml/sec might need pressure flow studies. Rollema and Mastrigt[11] and Schafer[12] have advocated pressure flow studies to differentiate between patients who are obstructed and those who are nonobstructed. They pointed out that as many as 20 percent of patients undergoing a TURP may not be obstructed, although many do have improvement in symptoms after surgery. Pressure flow studies are invasive and are not readily available to all urologists but are left as an option for them.

Postvoid residual urine has been used by many as an indication for surgical intervention. However, this test is extremely variable when performed repetitively in the same patient and it correlates poorly with signs and symptoms of prostatism. Furthermore, the amount of postvoid residual urine that would mandate intervention such as surgery, or that would cause the patient irreparable bladder damage if allowed to continue, has not been determined. Determination of postvoid urinary residuals has been left as an option that may be of use in following some patients who have elected not to undergo intervention.

Urinary tract infection is found in 8 to 24 percent of patients preoperatively and should be treated before surgery. The use of prophylactic antibiotics is somewhat controversial, but they were given to over 60 percent of patients in the AUA study.[4] The incidence of complications related to infection was significantly lower in this study than in previously reported studies. Other authors have also noted that prophylactic antibiotics used with transurethral prostatectomy significantly lower the incidence of complications.

Immediately before surgery it is recommended that the patient have a meal of clear liquids and a simple cleansing enema or Dulcolax suppository, because a difficult bowel movement in the immediate postoperative period could cause significant hematuria.

SURGICAL OPTIONS

Transurethral prostatectomy remains the gold standard with which other therapeutic modalities have been compared. Ninety percent of patients undergoing surgery for BPH have a transurethral prostatectomy. It is associated with low mortality (0.2 percent), but it does carry a significant morbidity of up to 18 percent. However, TURP gives the greatest degree of improvement in the patient's symptoms and in urinary flow rate in comparison with other forms of therapy.

The BPH Guideline Panel considered transurethral incision of the prostate (TUIP) a greatly underutilized procedure. Best used in glands under 30 gm, it is an easy technique to learn, has a shorter operating time than TURP, and involves less incidence of sexual dysfunction. Retrograde ejaculation occurs in 6 to 10 percent of cases and impotence in 0 to 4 percent. The disadvantage of TUIP is that it cannot be easily used in larger glands (over 30 gm) or in patients with a prominent median lobe and in whom there is no tissue obtained for histologic evaluation. However, Christensen and Miller and their respective colleagues[13, 14] have reported satisfactory durable long-term results, although the improvement in flow rate is less than that observed after TURP.

Larger prostate glands are traditionally treated by open prostatectomy. However, there have been reports of successful TURPs in patients having more than 80 gm of tissue resected. The symptomatic improvement is 94 to 98 percent after an open prostatectomy, and morbidity is 7 to 43 percent.

Balloon dilation initially provoked a wave of enthusiasm because it was a simple procedure done on an outpatient basis, and there appeared to be improvement in the patients' symptoms and maximum flow rate. However, Donatucci et al[15] pointed out that the durability of objective responses (e.g., flow rate) was not observed, with patients returning to pretreatment urinary flow rates within 1 year after surgery. Its use has therefore waned over the last few years.

A number of new surgical as well as medical options are becoming available. Surgical options include thermotherapy, microwave hyperthermia, high-frequency focus ultrasound, transurethral needle ablation of the prostate, and lasers. All of these are investigational and except for lasers are not readily available in the United States. The exact role of these new therapeutic tools in the armamentarium of the urologist will depend on outcome studies comparing them with the standard transurethral prostatectomy.

OPERATIVE TECHNIQUE

Stage 1

In stage 1 (Fig. 2–1), after the observational endoscopy and introduction of the resectoscope, the bladder and fossa are again inspected. The bladder is distended with approximately 100 ml of fluid to demarcate more readily among prostate, bladder neck, and bladder wall. Anteriorly, at 12 o'clock, an initial cut is made with the resectoscope loop and is continued deeper, until the seemingly circular fibers at the bladder neck are exposed as well as the fibers of the prostatic capsule. Depending on the size of the gland, a full loop length or less will be required.

The resection is then continued from 12 o'clock anteriorly to approximately 3 o'clock. Cuts are made from the prostatic urethra out toward the surgical capsule until the fibers of the capsule are identified. When the 3 o'clock position is reached, bleeding that has not been controlled to improve vision should be treated. Resection is similarly carried out from 12 to 9 o'clock; resection is now continued posteriorly from 3 to 9 o'clock.

The median lobe or, in some instances, the vesical

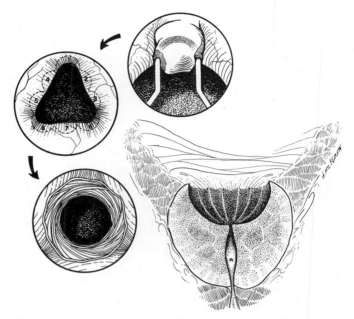

Figure 2–1. Stage 1 of a transurethral prostatectomy. Resection at the bladder neck, starting at 12 o'clock (cut no. 1 and continuing in a stepwise fashion. (From Mebust WK, Foret JD, Valk WL. Transurethral surgery. In Harrison JH, Gittes RF, Perlmutter AD, et al, eds. Campbell's Urology, 4th ed. Philadelphia, WB Saunders, 1979, p 2370.)

median bar is now resected. At this point, manipulation of the floor with the finger in the O'Connor shield will facilitate the resection. Care must be taken, however, not to undermine the trigone, which may result in extravesical extravasation. The ureteral orifices should have been identified and carefully preserved during the resection. The resection is carried down only to the circular fibers, and the floor tissue is removed only to the point that the neck now becomes pliable and falls away from the endoscope. If the bladder neck is still prominent after the resection, the neck is incised at 6 o'clock.

Stage 2

In stage 2 (Fig. 2–2) the scope is placed essentially on, or in front of, the verumontanum, depending on the length of the gland. The resectionist once again starts at the 12 o'clock position. Resection of the quadrant, covering 12 to 3 o'clock, is now accomplished down to the surgical capsule, controlling the bleeding points as necessary, but preserving final control when capsule fibers are fully exposed. Similarly, the 12 to 9 o'clock quadrant is resected; the 3 to 6 o'clock quadrant is resected, starting in the center of the prostatic urethral; and the adenoma is resected, proceeding laterally to the capsule.

In some instances, continuing the resection down along the plane between the capsule and the adenoma is advisable, but care must be taken not to inadvertently resect a large portion of adenoma, thus

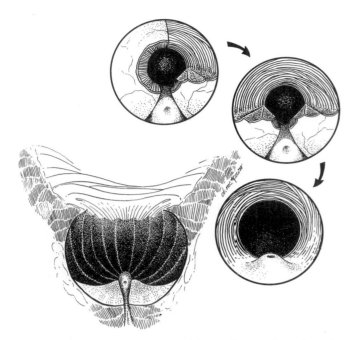

Figure 2–2. The second stage or midprostatic resection, where the adenoma is removed quadrant by quadrant. (From Mebust WK, Foret JD, Valk WL. Transurethral surgery. In Harrison JH, Gittes RF, Perlmutter AD, et al, eds. Campbell's Urology, 4th ed. Philadelphia, WB Saunders, 1979, p 2370.)

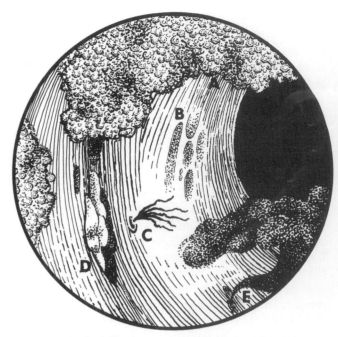

Figure 2–3. The resected prostatic fossa: A, glandular-appearing adenoma; B, striated capsule; C, arterial bleeders; D, capsular perforation with protruding fat; and E, venous bleeders. (From Mebust WK, Foret JD, Valk WL. Transurethral surgery. In Harrison JH, Gittes RF, Perlmutter AD, et al, eds. Campbell's Urology, 4th ed. Philadelphia, WB Saunders, 1979, p 2371.)

making its removal difficult at the end of the procedure. I have found that after removal of the bulk of the lateral lobe, it is usually more advisable to swing over to the other quadrant and continue it down, such as from the 9 to the 7 o'clock position.

The floor tissue can now be resected by using the finger in the rectum with the O'Connor shield. The adenomatous tissue is resected to such a point that the floor becomes pliable. Fibers identified on the roof and the lateral walls are no longer that readily apparent. One can usually feel the loop moving on the floor through the rectal shield. During this portion of the resection, one must be careful not to resect into the proximal neck portion, which might result in extravasation. If the resection is indeed carried too deeply into the prostatic capsule, venous sinuses will become apparent. Small fenestrations of fat globules may be noted (Fig. 2–3). These consist of minor extravasation and are usually of little clinical significance. If multiple areas are exposed, however, the surgical procedure may have to be terminated and catheter drainage instituted. In resection of glands heavier than 45 gm, a common error is to resect too deeply into the capsule, thus exposing the venous sinuses and causing fluid absorption, hyponatremia, and the so-called transurethral resection (TUR) syndrome. Extraprostatic extravasation can occur but is usually uncommon at this point. If the patient should complain suddenly of pain or demonstrate suprapu-

bic tenderness and shock, extravasation should be considered and confirmed by cystography.

Stage 3

Once hemostasis is satisfactory, the third stage may begin (Fig. 2–4). In contrast to an early original description of starting the primary incision at 12 o'clock anteriorly, I prefer to groove the verumontanum. The external sphincter is identifiable because it is immediately adjacent to the distal portion of the verumontanum. A fold or wrinkles can be seen between the relatively mobile prostate and the fixed external sphincter (Fig. 2–5). After identification of the external sphincter by the wrinkle mark and the presence of the verumontanum, the resectoscope is carefully placed at the 7 o'clock position. Resection is now begun from 7 to 12 o'clock. By means of a lateral-to-median sweep, in response to the concavity of the gland, the adenomatous tissue is carefully removed. Care must be taken not to advance the scope inward and, more important, not to retract the scope outward during this resection. The scope is locked into position by the resectionist. After emptying of the bladder, the surgeon immediately becomes reoriented by locating the external sphincter and verumontanum, and continues.

Bleeding should be well controlled during this

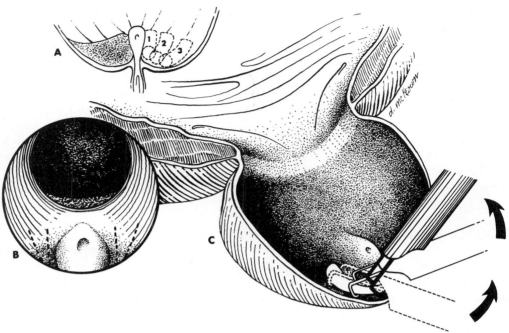

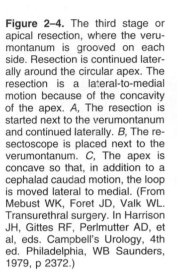

Figure 2–4. The third stage or apical resection, where the verumontanum is grooved on each side. Resection is continued laterally around the circular apex. The resection is a lateral-to-medial motion because of the concavity of the apex. *A,* The resection is started next to the verumontanum and continued laterally. *B,* The resectoscope is placed next to the verumontanum. *C,* The apex is concave so that, in addition to a cephalad caudad motion, the loop is moved lateral to medial. (From Mebust WK, Foret JD, Valk WL. Transurethral surgery. In Harrison JH, Gittes RF, Perlmutter AD, et al, eds. Campbell's Urology, 4th ed. Philadelphia, WB Saunders, 1979, p 2372.)

stage to avoid cutting the external sphincter. The verumontanum is now grooved on the other side at the 5 o'clock position, and the resection is carried to the 12 o'clock position. Upon completion of this stage, the scope is withdrawn into the bulbous urethra, so that the sphincter, verumontanum, and prostatic fossa can be observed. Not uncommonly, mucosal tags will drop in the upper two quadrants (Fig. 2–6). These may be resected but will probably be sloughed in the immediate postoperative period. However, the surgeon should be certain that these are indeed mucosal tags and not adenomatous ones. At this point, also, tissue may be seen to fall in from the upper quadrants, more proximal to the external sphincter. This usually indicates that the surgeon has not resected to the roof capsular fibers. Upon resection, this tissue, not uncommonly lateral lobe tissue that had not been noted previously, now falls into

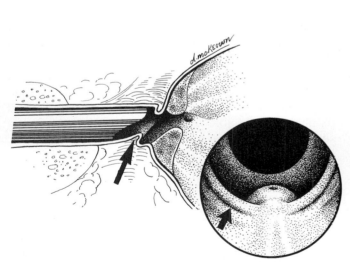

Figure 2–5. The external sphincter is identified as relatively immobile compared with the prostate and the more distal urethra. With advancement of the resectoscope, the urethral mucosa will appear to wrinkle just distal to the sphincter. The wrinkle sign identifies the junction of the relatively mobile prostate and fixed external sphincter, and is the urethral mucosa just distal to the verumontanum but cephalad to the external sphincter and perineal diaphragm. (From Mebust WK, Foret JD, Valk WL. Transurethral surgery. In Harrison JH, Gittes RF, Perlmutter AD, et al, eds. In Campbell's Urology, 4th ed. Philadelphia, WB Saunders, 1979, p 2372.)

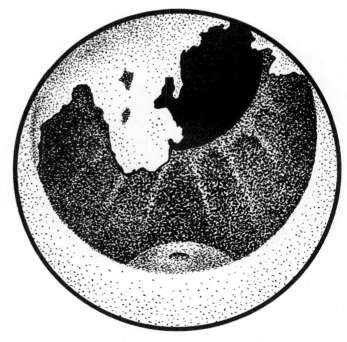

Figure 2–6. Mucosa tags may drop into view as the resectoscope is moved into the more distal urethra beyond the prostate apex. (From Mebust WK, Foret JD, Valk WL. Transurethral surgery. In Harrison JH, Gittes RF, Perlmutter AD, et al, eds. Campbell's Urology, 4th ed. Philadelphia, WB Saunders, 1979, p 2373.)

view and will also have to be resected. The fossa is inspected meticulously for arterial bleeding points and residual adenomatous tissue. The chips are carefully removed with the Ellik evacuator.

If the bladder neck needs to be incised, I prefer making the incision at 6 o'clock. With a Collings knife the incision is carried through the prostate to the verumontanum. The incision should be deep through the prostatic floor and into the capsule of the prostate. The surgeon should see the filmy fibers of the prostatic capsule while cutting through it, and occasionally the periprostatic fat.

POSTOPERATIVE MANAGEMENT

After surgery a 22 or 24 Fr., three-way Foley catheter is used, with saline for irrigation. The rate of inflow is enough to keep irrigation a light pink, or approximately 400 ml/hr. The catheter is attached to a closed drainage system that incorporates an irrigation system, e.g., the Travenol Cystopump, which may be necessary for clot evacuation in the postoperative period.

Patients resume a normal diet as soon as they have recovered from the anesthetic, and are ambulated as soon as possible. In addition to antibiotics, they are given a stool softener. The catheter is removed as soon as the urine is only slightly tinged with blood or light pink, usually on the second postoperative day. Patients are cautioned not to engage in strenuous activities for 1 month, to reduce the risk of delayed bleeding and clot retention.

OPERATIVE COMPLICATIONS

Intraoperative complications occur in 6.9 percent of patients, the most common being bleeding (2.5 percent), TUR syndrome (2 percent), cardiac arrhythmia (1.1 percent), and extravasation (0.9 percent).[4]

Bleeding

Bleeding is related to the size of the prostatic gland and the length of the operative time. The incidence of transfusion, for patients with over 45 gm of glandular tissue, is 10 percent, as compared with 1 percent for those with less than 45 gm. Operative time of more than 90 minutes is also associated with increased intraoperative bleeding. Arterial bleeding is controlled by cauterizing specific points as each stage of the operation is completed. Resection should leave a smooth prostatic fossa. Ragged irregular tissue may hide bleeding points.

Venous bleeding is usually associated with cutting

the prostatic surgical capsule too thin, exposing the venous sinuses. The surgeon cannot identify individual venous bleeding points because the pressure of the irrigating fluid is usually slightly higher than the venous pressure. However, as the surgeon empties the bladder, a dark, bloody discharge is noted through the resectoscope, indicating significant venous bleeding. This is best managed by placing the catheter on traction, with the balloon overinflated. Traction is usually applied for 10 minutes in the operating room. If the patient is in the recovery room and venous bleeding recurs, prolonged catheter traction may be necessary.

Transurethral Resection Syndrome

The TUR syndrome consists of dilutional hyponatremia. Therapy usually takes the form of a loop diuretic and intravenous fluid replacement with normal saline. In a severely hyponatremic patient who is symptomatic, the quickest and most effective therapy is the slow infusion of hypertonic (3 percent) saline. The amount given is calculated by knowing the patient's body weight and calculating the normal amount of extracellular fluid. The change in serum sodium can then be used to calculate the amount of excess extracellular fluid. The amount of sodium required to return the serum sodium to normal is then determined.[16]

Extravasation

Although many patients have small perforations of the surgical capsule, about 1 percent have clinically significant perforations. Usually, 90 percent of these can be managed by stopping the surgery and leaving the patient on catheter drainage. However, if the patient has severe abdominal pain, nausea, vomiting, a palpable suprapubic mass, or infected urine, simple suprapubic drainage may be necessary.

POSTOPERATIVE AND LONG-TERM COMPLICATIONS

The incidence of immediate postoperative complications is 18 percent. The most common complications are failure to void (6.7 percent), secondary to a hypotonic bladder; clot retention (3.5 percent), from venous bleeding; bleeding (3.3 percent); and urinary infection (2.3 percent).[4]

Long-term complications include urethral stricture (2.5 percent), vesical neck contracture (2.7 percent), stress incontinence (1.7 percent), and total incontinence (0.5 percent).

It is beyond the scope of this chapter to discuss the cause, prevention, and management of these complications. However, one long-term complication does deserve comment: sexual dysfunction, which has been reported to occur in 0 to 40 percent of patients postoperatively. Approximately 50 percent of patients experience retrograde ejaculation, which decreases fertility but should not impair erectile ability. It is extremely difficult to obtain objective data on the incidence of impotence after transurethral prostatectomy, since it depends on the presence or absence of an active sexual partner, and the patient's own perception of his sexual ability or disability.[17] In one study an objective evaluation of patients, pre- and postoperatively, did not correlate with their perception of ability or disability in all cases.[18] Nevertheless, erectile impotency of unclear etiology probably occurs in about 4 percent of cases.

Summary

Transurethral prostatectomy is a commonly performed operation in patients with clearly defined indications. It is associated with very low mortality and morbidity rates. The results appear to be excellent, at least in the short-term evaluations made. In the few studies completed, in which patients are evaluated over a period of several years after surgery, the majority continue to do well.[19] However, the operation remains one of the most difficult procedures for the surgeon to learn, even with the use of a video camera.

Editorial Comment

Fray F. Marshall

Many urologists develop their own adaptations to transurethral surgery. I have tended to use the No. 24 resectoscope sheath increasingly rather than a larger sheath in hope of avoiding stricture disease. The position of the resectoscope table is usually level during the resection. The resection is less likely to move into the area of the sphincter if the table is not tilted.

We have used sorbitol as an isotonic irrigating agent.

REFERENCES

1. Lytton B, Emery JM, Harvard BM. The incidence of benign prostatic obstruction. J Urol 99:639, 1968.
2. Glynn RJ, Campion EW, Bouchard GR, Gilbert SE. The development of benign prostatic hyperplasia among volunteers in the normative aging study. Am J Epidemiol 121:278, 1985.
3. Arrighi HM, Metter EJ, Guess HA, et al. Natural history of benign prostatic hyperplasia and risk of prostatectomy: The Baltimore Longitudinal Study of Aging. Urology 38(Suppl 1):4, 1991.
4. Mebust WK, Holtgrewe HL, Cockett ATK, et al. Transurethral prostatectomy: Immediate and postoperative complications. A cooperative study of 13 participating institutions evaluating 3,885 patients. J Urol 141:243, 1989.
5. Arrighi HM, Guess HA, Metter EJ, Fozard JL. Symptoms and signs of prostatism as risk factors for prostatectomy. Prostate 16:253, 1990.
6. Epstein RS, Lydick E, deLabry L, et al. Age-related differences in risk factors for prostatectomy for benign prostatic hyperplasia: The VA normative aging study. Urology 38(Suppl 1):9, 1991.
7. Barry MJ, Fowler FJ Jr, O'Leary MP, et al. The American Urological Association symptom index for benign prostatic hyperplasia. J Urol 148:1549, 1992.
8. Benign Prostatic Hyperplasia Guideline Panel. Benign prostatic hyperplasia diagnosis and treatment. Clinical Practice Guideline No. 8, Agency for Health Care Policy and Research Publication No. 94-0582, U.S. Department of Health and Human Services, Public Health Service, Rockville, MD, February 1994.
9. Barry MJ, Fowler FJ Jr, O'Leary MP, et al. Measuring disease-specific health status in men with benign prostatic hyperplasia. Med Care 33(Suppl):AS145, 1995.
10. Fowler FJ. Patient reports of symptoms and quality of life following prostate surgery. Eur Urol 20(Suppl 2):44, 1991.
11. Rollema HJ, Mastrigt RV. Improved indication and followup in transurethral resection of the prostate using the computer program CLIM: A prospective study. J Urol 148:111, 1992.
12. Schafer W. Urodynamics in benign prostatic hyperplasia (BPH). Arch Ital Urol Androl 65:599, 1993.
13. Christensen MM, Aagaard J, Madsen PO. Transurethral resection versus transurethral incision of the prostate: A prospective randomized study. Urol Clin North Am 17:621, 1990.
14. Miller J, Edyvane KA, Sinclair GR, et al. A comparison of bladder neck incision and transurethral prostatic resection. Aust N Z J Surg 62:116, 1992.
15. Donatucci CE, Berger N, Kreder KJ, et al. Randomized clinical trial comparing balloon dilatation to transurethral resection of prostate for benign prostatic hyperplasia. Urology 42:42, 1993.
16. Sacks SA. The transurethral (TUR) syndrome. AUA Update Series 4(40):2, 1985.
17. Hargreave TB, Stephenson TP. Potency and prostatectomy. Br J Urol 49:683, 1977.
18. So EP, Ho PC, Bodenstab W, et al. Erectile impotence associated with transurethral prostatectomy. Urology 19:259, 1982.
19. Brusekewitz RC, Larsen EH, Madsen PO, Dorflinger T. Three-year followup of urinary symptoms after transurethral resection of the prostate. J Urol 136:613, 1986.

Chapter 3

Transurethral Resection of Bladder Tumors

M'Liss A. Hudson

Bladder cancer is often discovered in patients presenting with gross, painless, intermittent hematuria[1] and has been found in up to 10 percent of patients with microscopic hematuria.[2] Irritative voiding symptoms—urgency, frequency, and dysuria—are frequently noted in those with carcinoma in situ of the bladder or invasive tumors.[3]

The initial evaluation of patients with hematuria and/or irritative voiding symptoms should include studies such as intravenous pyelography (IVP), urinary cytology, and office cystoscopy, which usually establish the diagnosis of bladder cancer. These studies are important in the preoperative evaluation of the patient with bladder cancer. The results of these initial studies will direct the use of additional studies in patients in whom invasive or upper tract disease is suspected.

PREOPERATIVE EVALUATION

Intravenous Pyelography

An IVP is recommended for patients with signs and symptoms suggesting bladder cancer. It is not a sensitive means of detecting bladder cancer but is useful for assessing the upper urinary tracts for lesions causing hematuria, including urothelial tumors. The likelihood of finding an upper tract tumor if a filling defect is noted in the bladder is about 10 percent[4] (Fig. 3–1). Bladder tumors may be detected as filling defects on the cystogram phase of the IVP; however, only 60 percent of bladder tumors are usually found with this study[5] (Fig. 3–2). Obtaining an early bladder filling film, a distended bladder filling film, and a postvoid film facilitates the diagnosis of bladder tumors. Other findings that are helpful in evaluating bladder cancer include ureteral obstruc-

tion with hydronephrosis or a nonvisualizing kidney. These findings are associated with invasive disease in 90 percent of cases[6] (Fig. 3–3).

Urinary Cytology

Cytological examination of the urine is highly accurate (95 percent) in the diagnosis of high-grade transitional cell carcinoma and carcinoma in situ.[7] It is less helpful (10 to 50 percent accurate) in diagnosing low-grade tumors. Quantitative fluorescent image analysis (QFIA) quantitatively measures the DNA content of the individual cell. QFIA has proved more sensitive (76 percent) than conventional cytology for the detection of low-grade bladder cancer.[8] Cytological examination can be helpful when mucosal abnormalities without overt tumors are seen cystoscopically. Urinary cytological tests are useful in detecting residual tumor[9] and may predict tumor recurrence after transurethral resection.[10]

Flow cytometry, which measures the DNA content of cell lines, can be a useful adjunct in detecting abnormal cell populations. Aneuploid cell lines are usually seen with high-grade tumors, including carcinoma in situ, while diploid cell lines are usually seen with low-grade tumors. DNA ploidy has been correlated with the risk of tumor recurrence, progression, and cancer-specific survival.[11, 12]

Diagnostic Cystoscopy

The initial cystoscopy is usually performed in the office. The purpose of this evaluation is to determine whether a bladder tumor is present, and if so to evaluate its physical characteristics. Bladder mapping of the tumor and any associated lesions is help-

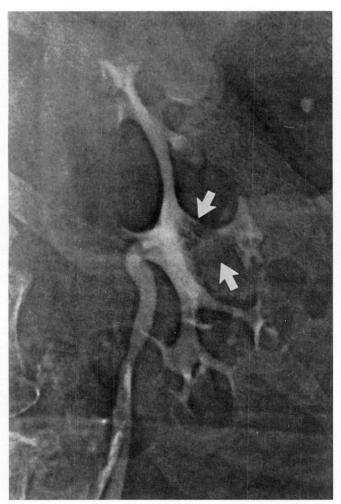

Figure 3–1. Intravenous pyelogram showing a filling defect in the left renal pelvis *(arrows),* which proved to be transitional cell carcinoma of the upper tract.

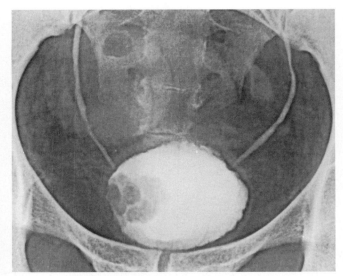

Figure 3–2. Cystogram phase of an intravenous pyelogram demonstrating a filling defect that proved to be a bladder tumor.

turia is present. Rigid cystoscopy may therefore improve visualization of the bladder when there is gross hematuria.

With either cystoscope, it is imperative that a careful, systematic approach be used to inspect the entire bladder mucosa. Ureteral orifices should be observed for bloody or clear efflux and for structural abnormal-

ful both for planning current treatment and for review if future tumors develop (Fig. 3–4). The location of the tumor(s); size; solid versus papillary architecture; proximity to ureteral orifices; and associated red, granular, velvety, inflamed, ulcerated, or other lesions can be recorded.

The visual appearance of the tumor often provides prognostic information. Large, solid, or nodular tumors are more likely to be high grade and invasive than papillary tumors on a fibrous stalk. The presence of dysplastic lesions or carcinoma in situ, a size greater than 3 to 5 cm, and tumor multiplicity have all been associated with increased risk of both tumor recurrence and progression.[6]

Office cystoscopy can be performed with either a flexible or rigid cystoscope; the former is more common today. Its advantages over the rigid cystoscope include less patient discomfort and improved visualization of the anterior bladder neck and trigone (Fig. 3–5) in those with prostatic enlargement. The rigid cystoscope allows for irrigation and potentially clot evacuation with a Toomey syringe when gross hema-

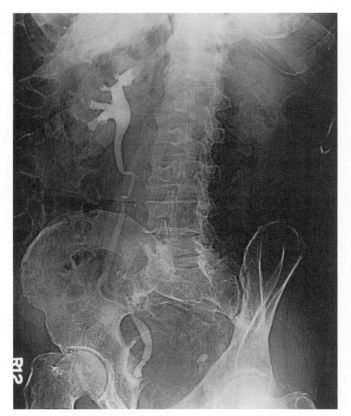

Figure 3–3. Large filling defect in the bladder causing obstruction and resulting hydroureteronephrosis of the right ureter, which was found to be a muscle-invasive bladder tumor.

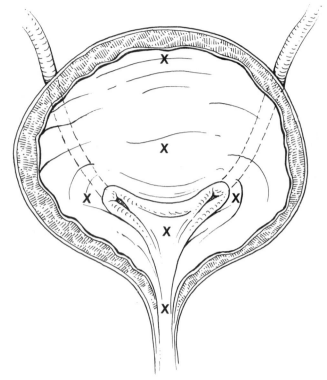

Figure 3–4. Bladder map for recording location, size, and characteristics of bladder tumor(s). The Xs represent the sites recommended for selected site mucosal biopsies.

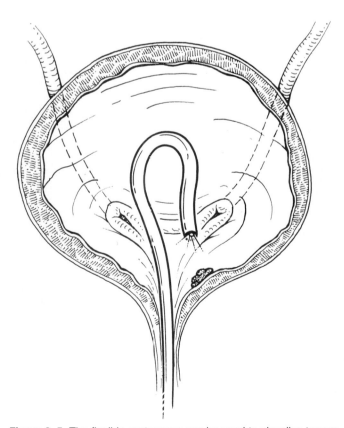

Figure 3–5. The flexible cystoscope can be used to visualize tumors on the anterior bladder neck.

ities. Bloody efflux is suggestive of upper tract pathology. If adequate visualization is not achieved in the office setting, repeated formal cystoscopy in the endoscopy suite or operating room under an anesthetic is recommended so as not to miss a tumor.

Computed Tomography

When the characteristics of the tumor found on the initial screening studies suggest invasive cancer, computed tomography (CT) before transurethral resection allows more accurate clinical staging. Focal bladder wall thickening suggests muscle-invasive cancer (Fig. 3–6). Its presence after transurethral resection is less accurate for predicting the depth of tumor invasion, as postoperative edema may cause similar changes. CT criteria for detection of extravesical bladder tumor extension include loss of the perivesical fat plane. For detection of extravesical extension, CT has a diagnostic accuracy of about 80 percent.[13, 14]

For detection of lymph node metastases, CT scanning relies primarily on size criteria (greater than 1 cm) to deem nodes suspicious for metastatic disease. CT misses approximately one third of nodes harboring micrometastases.[15]

Magnetic Resonance Imaging

The introduction of magnetic resonance imaging (MRI) brought the hope that the depth of bladder wall tumor penetration and the presence of extravesical extension could be determined more accurately. As with CT, the accuracy of staging is improved when postsurgical changes are not present. Gross involvement of the bladder wall is identified as disruption of a portion of the low-intensity signal line representing the bladder wall on T2-weighted images (Fig. 3–7). Perivesical fat invasion appears as an area of diminished signal intensity within the adjacent high-intensity fat. Although early studies[13, 16, 17] suggested improved staging with MRI compared with CT, not all studies have confirmed these results.[18] The overall accuracy of MRI staging of bladder cancer is about 85 percent.

Bimanual Examination

The bimanual examination should be performed with the patient under anesthesia before tumor resection. In male patients, the examiner places an index finger in the rectum and the opposite hand in the suprapubic region. In females, two fingers are placed in the vagina and the opposite hand in the suprapu-

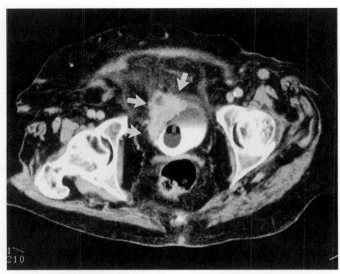

Figure 3–6. Computed tomography demonstrating marked thickening of the bladder wall from a large bladder tumor *(arrows)* found to extend into the perivesical adipose tissues.

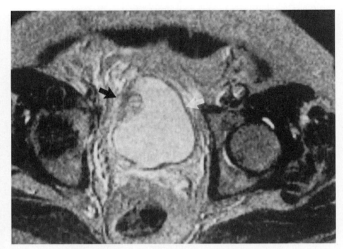

Figure 3–7. T2-weighted magnetic resonance image demonstrating the low-intensity line *(white arrow)* of the bladder wall and its focal disruption *(black arrow)* from a bladder tumor.

bic region. The presence of a mass should be noted, along with induration or fixation to adjacent structures. If the mass is fixed or indurated, muscle-invasive disease is more likely. However, in patients who have undergone previous radiation therapy or have pelvic inflammatory disease, fixation is an unreliable means to differentiate benign from malignant disease.[19]

Retrograde Pyelography

If the upper tracts are not fully imaged on the IVP, or if a contrast allergy precludes intravenous administration of contrast material, retrograde pyelography is indicated. Although the likelihood of inducing an allergic reaction to contrast is reduced with retrograde pyelography, pretreatment with diphenylhydramine hydrochloride and steroids and the use of nonionic contrast are also appropriate. Nonionic contrast is suitable when urine is to be collected for cytological examination or when brush biopsies are performed, to reduce the likelihood of contrast artifact.

Retrograde pyelography is best performed with a bulb-tipped ureteral catheter through a rigid cystoscope. Care must be taken to clear air from the catheter before injection of the ureter, as air bubbles will appear as filling defects within the collecting system. Use of the bulb-tipped catheter allows distention of the entire ureter and renal collecting system. The normal collecting system usually holds 5 to 7 ml of contrast. Contrast should be diluted 1:3 with saline, because full-strength contrast may be dense enough to obscure small, partial filling defects. The injection is best monitored under fluoroscopic guidance to pre-

vent overdistention of the collecting system resulting in pyelolymphatic or pyelovenous backflow.

Alternatively, when the filling defect is in the renal pelvis and the ureter is known to be normal, a 5 Fr. ureteral catheter can be passed under fluoroscopic guidance to the renal pelvis. Before the injection of contrast, urine and renal pelvis washings (barbotage) can be obtained for cytological examination. Use of nonionic contrast for the retrograde injection will confirm the presence of the filling defect and delineate the area for a brush biopsy, as discussed below (Fig. 3–8).

It is debatable whether retrograde pyelography is best performed before tumor resection or after the bladder has been cleared of all visible tumor. My preference has been to assess the upper urinary tract as fully as possible before any treatment of existing tumor if technically feasible. Occasionally a large tumor obscures a ureteral orifice that becomes visible after resection of the tumor. I subsequently evaluate the upper tract in this circumstance. Retrograde pyelography is about 75 percent accurate in establishing the diagnosis of an upper tract tumor.[20]

Antegrade pyelography is to be avoided in patients with bladder cancer whenever possible, as complete ureteral obstruction is more likely to be associated with high-grade, invasive tumors and the risk of tumor spread is increased. In exceptional circumstances when the cause of the obstruction cannot be defined on any other study or the patient has incipient renal failure, antegrade pyelography and nephrostomy tube placement is necessary.

Brush Biopsy

With this technique, a fine brush mounted on a guidewire is introduced through a ureteral catheter.

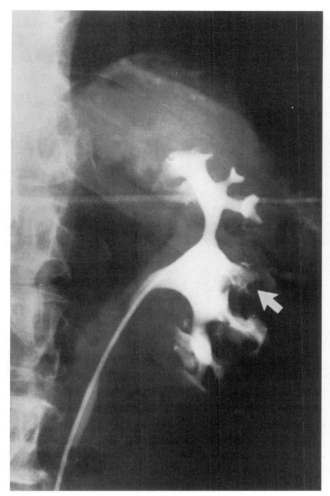

Figure 3–8. Retrograde injection through a 5 Fr. ureteral catheter using nonionic contrast to demonstrate the filling defect in the left renal pelvis.

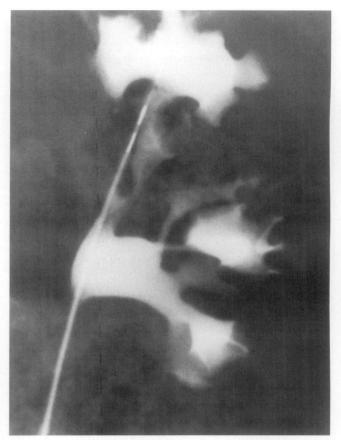

Figure 3–9. Brush biopsy being performed on an irregular lesion in the upper pole infundibulum.

Fluoroscopy is used to monitor sampling of the lesion with the brush (Fig. 3–9). The sample is withdrawn through the catheter and sent for cytological examination. Brush biopsies carry a possible risk of seeding other areas of the urinary tract, but complications are rare. They are about 80 to 90 percent accurate in diagnosing upper tract tumors.[21]

Ureteroscopy

Ureteroscopy has been used increasingly to establish the diagnosis of upper tract lesions or to assess unilateral hematuria after conventional diagnostic techniques have failed. The major concerns with the use of ureteroscopy are the risk of ureteral perforation with extravasation of tumor cells or denudation of the ureteral mucosa with tumor implantation. The reported accuracy of diagnosis of renal pelvis tumors is 86 percent and of ureteral tumors 90 percent, with an overall complication rate of 7 percent.[21]

Selected-Site Mucosal Biopsies

Many urologists advocate routine selected-site mucosal biopsies from the areas adjacent to the tumor(s), as well as from the dome, posterior wall, right and left lateral walls above the ureteral orifices, trigone, and prostatic urethra in men. Use of cold cup biopsy forceps rather than a resection loop is recommended to preserve cellular architecture and avoid cautery artifact. However, biopsy of the prostatic urethra is more readily obtained with the resection loop so that the biopsies include the deep ducts and stroma. Endoscopically, normal-appearing urothelium may show changes ranging from dysplasia (13.5 percent) to frank carcinoma in situ (4.5 percent). Red, velvety lesions or granular, mossy patches may contain dysplasia or carcinoma in situ in 15 to 40 percent of cases.[22] In one study the likelihood of tumor recurrence within 5 years was 67 percent if associated dysplasia or carcinoma in situ was found on biopsies compared with 32 percent if the mucosal biopsies were normal.[23] A number of studies have shown that abnormal random biopsies indicate an increased incidence of recurrence and a higher chance of progression.

Not all authors agree that routine biopsies are advisable, and some suggest that they may be hazardous because they may foster tumor implantation at sites of urothelial disruption.[24] Their prognostic value has also been questioned when normal-appearing mucosa is present.[25] My personal practice is to perform selected-site mucosal biopsies in all quadrants of the bladder and prostatic urethra, as well as in any other abnormal areas within the bladder.

TUMOR RESECTION

Before the planned resection, a preoperative evaluation should document the sterility of the patient's urine. The patient should undergo routine laboratory testing, including a complete blood count, electrolytes, clotting parameters, and a clot sample to be sent to the blood bank. Any electrolyte or clotting abnormalities should be corrected preoperatively. Severe anemia may require preoperative transfusion.

The patient is placed in the lithotomy position, care being taken that the lower extremities are padded and there is no pressure on the popliteal fossa. Many surgeons administer prophylactic broad-spectrum antibiotics. General anesthesia with muscle-paralyzing agents is preferred to avoid obturator spasms.

Three types of electrical current are used in transurethral resection: cutting, coagulation, and blended. The keenest current for cutting is the undamped current generated by a tube oscillator circuit. Coagulation is accomplished with a highly damped spark-gap current generated from a spark-gap oscillator circuit. A blended current combines the two currents. The usual application of a blended current is to reduce bleeding when resecting vascular tissue by adding the coagulating effect of a spark-gap current to a tube cutting current. Too high an increase in the coagulating current impairs the cutting efficiency of the unit.[26] The current density varies with the surface area of the loop. Loops are made in five sizes: 10, 12, 15, 18, and 20. The numbers refer to the diameter of the loop (thousandths of an inch). Finer-caliber loops project a more concentrated current and cut more easily; larger-caliber loops produce better hemostasis but do not cut as readily. Incrustation of the loop with tissue interferes with transmission of the current and impedes both cutting and coagulation. The zone of tissue destruction with a cutting current is negligible, and thus the use of a more powerful cutting current adds little danger to the procedure. A rapid cutting stroke, in addition to reducing operating time, prevents charred tissue from adhering to the loop. The higher the moisture content of the tissue, the easier the resection is to perform.[26]

Coagulation currents are more destructive. The longer the time of application, the wider is the zone of tissue destruction. Excess tissue destruction leads to prolonged sloughing of tissue, secondary bleeding, and delayed healing.[26]

The requirements of an irrigating fluid are that it be sterile and nontoxic, have a low coefficient of electrical conductivity, and be delivered at room temperature. Some surgeons prefer to use sterile water as the irrigating medium for resection of bladder tumors. Water causes hemolysis, which may allow a clearer field of vision in the bladder during a resection. The irrigating medium will be intravascularly absorbed during the resection. When water is used as the irrigating fluid, hemolyzed blood can be found in the patient's blood serum. Although small amounts of hemolyzed blood are usually not harmful, massive hemolysis from absorption of large quantities of water can cause death. Isotonic solutions such as glycine, sorbitol, or mannitol reduce the risk of hemolysis. When blood comes into contact with these solutions, however, a pink solution that obscures vision may be produced. Excessive absorption of these solutions is not without risk, however, as other electrolyte abnormalities may be produced.[26]

Resectoscope sheaths are commonly made of Bakelite, a material that insulates the working element from the urethra. Sheaths come in sizes of 24, 26, and 28 Fr. The larger sheath allows use of a larger resecting loop, which in turn allows resection of larger tumor fragments and may lead to a shorter operating time. Calibration of the urethra with a sound should determine the appropriate size sheath to be used. The sheath should slide easily within the urethra; if not, urethral complications are likely.[26]

The distal end of the sheath is beveled to allow for excursion of the loop. Sheaths are made with either a short or a long bevel. The short bevel is more maneuverable and provides better access to the tissue being resected. The long bevel affords better protection of the loop, because it keeps more tissue away from the loop, but can be dangerous in that it may inadvertently gouge the tissue, leading to perforation or bleeding.

The working element of the resectoscope consists of the Foroblique lens and a cutting loop mounted on either a rachet-type or spring-loaded instrument. The rachet-type instrument requires the use of both hands to operate. It responds to the lightest touch and is the most precise for cutting. The spring-loaded devices are operated by a thumb control and are manipulated with one hand, allowing use of the other hand for pressure in the suprapubic region as needed to facilitate tumor resection. The spring-loaded units are also more compact.

The surgeon should be comfortably seated on a rolling stool. After calibration of the urethra with a sound, the resectoscope sheath is passed with the obturator in place following the natural course of the urethra. No resistance should be encountered. If the urethral meatus is small, a meatotomy should be performed. It is preferable to have the bladder partially full when the resectoscope sheath is passed. The working element is then introduced. The resectoscope should be held lightly but securely with both hands (Fig. 3–10). Some surgeons advocate intravenous administration of methylene blue or indigo carmine at the start of the resection to aid in identification of the ureteral orifices.

A good method for resecting a bladder tumor is to resect the superficial, exophytic portion first in an orderly fashion, starting at one end of the tumor and proceeding to the other.[27] The principle of using the resectoscope is to cut tissue in long segments the length and depth of the loop. In excising fragments the section is not of uniform thickness and is shallower at the end of the cut. The loop is fully extended and engaged over the projecting tissue, and the cut is made straight back to the beak of the sheath. The bladder should be sufficiently distended so that the tissue is not folded on itself. Overdistention of the bladder thins out the bladder wall and can lead to perforation (Fig. 3–11). The cutting motion with the resectoscope should follow the contour of the bladder wall. Initially, the tumor should be resected to the level of the bladder mucosa (Fig. 3–12). It is not prudent to resect a large tumor on a stalk by simply cutting it at the base. Tumors that are too large to fit through the resectoscope but are free-floating in the bladder are more difficult to cut into pieces. These tumors should be resected in appropriately sized fragments down to the base of the tumor. The superficial tissue should be sent for pathological analysis as a separate specimen. Tumor fragments can be evacuated from the bladder using either an Ellik evacuator

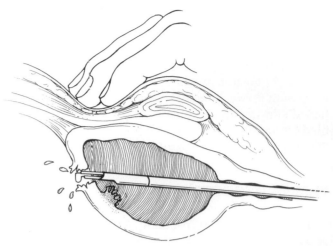

Figure 3–11. Perforation of the bladder with the resectoscope occurs when the bladder is overdistended and/or when the loop is extended and used in a manner that does not follow the bladder contour.

or a Toomey syringe. The deep part of the tumor, along with some underlying muscle, is next resected and sent as a second specimen. Superficial papillary tumors can be easily resected from the bladder surface along with the superficial muscularis propria (Fig. 3–13). Muscle-invasive tumors are more difficult to resect entirely, particularly if the tumor invades

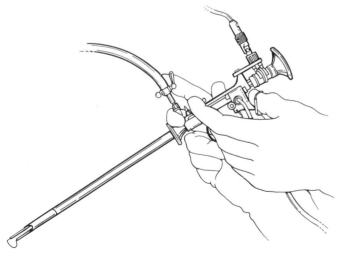

Figure 3–10. Proper positioning of the hands when using a spring-loaded resectoscope.

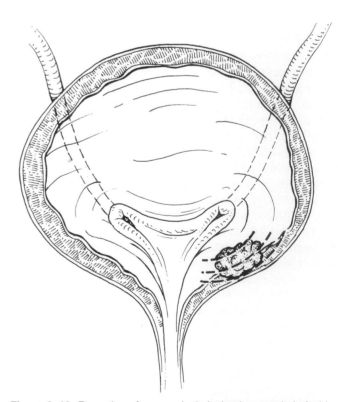

Figure 3–12. Resection of an exophytic lesion in an orderly fashion from one end to the other. The base of the lesion is then resected into the muscularis propria and sent as a separate specimen. The resection should be performed in a manner following the contour of the bladder wall.

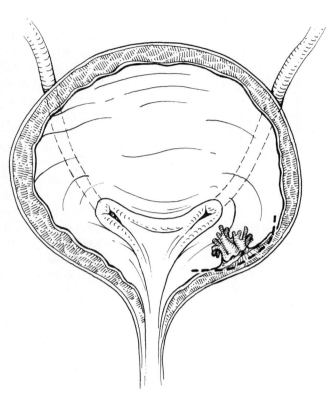

Figure 3–13. Resection of a superficial papillary tumor and underlying superficial muscle.

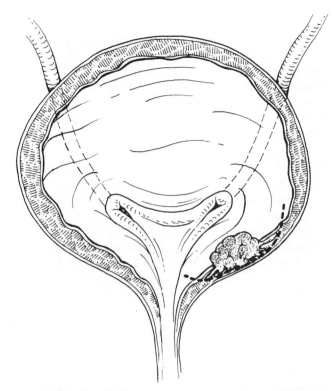

Figure 3–14. Resection of a muscle-invasive tumor is often less complete because of tentacular tumor extension and the concern that bladder perforation will occur.

the muscularis propria with tentacular extensions (Fig. 3–14). The base of the tumor bed, along with an adjacent 1-cm rim of tissue around the tumor site, should be fulgurated. A roller ball electrode can replace the cutting loop and is useful for this purpose. These maneuvers accomplish complete removal of the tumor and provide accurate, detailed diagnostic information about its grade and stage.

Hemostasis should be well maintained throughout the resection to prevent excessive blood loss and maintain a clearly visible operative field. Sometimes, large vessels feeding the base of a tumor can be seen in the adjacent mucosa. These are fulgurated before the tumor resection is begun. Resection and hemostasis should be achieved in one segment of tissue before proceeding to the next area of resection. When multiple tumors are present, complete resection of one tumor with hemostasis of the tumor bed should be achieved before attempting to resect another. It is prudent to resect tumors in less accessible areas of the bladder such as the anterior bladder and dome first, as these will be more difficult to find if bleeding partially obscures one's vision. Air introduced into the bladder or gas formation during the resection also make resection in the dome of the bladder more difficult as the surgery proceeds. Resection in the dome of the bladder is facilitated by external pressure in the suprapubic region and minimal filling of the

bladder (Fig. 3–15). Placing the patient in a prone position has been described[28] but requires a perineal urethrotomy in males. Bleeding is stopped by placing the loop directly on the bleeding point and activating the coagulating current for a brief period. Excessive coagulation leads to necrotic tissue and should be avoided.

Sometimes a bleeding vessel is obscured by intervening tissue that must be resected before the bleeding vessel can be located and fulgurated. Like-

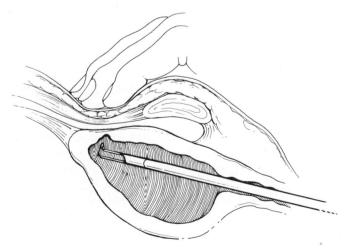

Figure 3–15. The resectoscope is inverted and suprapubic pressure applied to facilitate resection on the dome or anterior bladder wall.

wise, blood clots may have to be scraped away with the loop to accurately pinpoint the site of bleeding. Arterial bleeding may be so vigorous that it completely obscures a "head-on" view. This type of bleeding vessel may be located by a sideways approach along the wall of the bladder. The loop can then be extended to compress the spurting vessel, and the coagulating current can be activated to stop the bleeding. Occasionally, bleeding whose source is difficult to locate is coming from the prostatic urethra. Although resection has not taken place in this area, manipulation of the sheath can injure mucosal vessels here.

Attempts to achieve complete resection may be ill advised in patients with extensive, broad-based, sessile tumors that are obviously invasive or metastatic and therefore certain to require additional therapy. In these cases, sufficient tumor should be resected to establish the tumor grade and presence of muscle invasion. The adequacy of the specimen can be confirmed by frozen section at the time of surgery. Vigorous attempts at tumor resection that risk bladder perforation, excessive blood loss, or excessive absorption of irrigating fluid resulting in electrolyte abnormalities should be avoided. However, large, superficial tumors may occasionally require repeated transurethral resections to render the patient tumor free.

Tumors encroaching on a ureteral orifice should generally be resected without regard to the orifice. However, it is important not to fulgurate the orifice after resecting the tumor. Some authors have advocated leaving a ureteral stent in place for a few days after resection to prevent obstruction of the ureteral orifice. Others feel that ureteral stents may allow reflux of tumor cells into the upper urinary tracts where implantation may occur in areas of mucosal disruption. A higher incidence of upper tract tumors has been noted in patients with vesicoureteral reflux.[29] Attempts to resect around a ureteral stent may preserve the orifice but prevent adequate tumor resection. I prefer not to leave a ureteral stent in place when resecting tumors encroaching on an orifice.

Resection of tumors on the lateral bladder walls can stimulate the ipsilateral obturator nerve, resulting in violent contractions of the adductor muscles of the leg. A sudden movement of the patient during the resection may cause the resectoscope to perforate the bladder and even injure the iliac vessels. Resection of lateral wall tumors should be performed with the patient under a general anesthetic with concomitant administration of muscle-paralyzing agents. Lowering the current on the diathermy unit and resecting with the bladder only partially filled reduce the risk of obturator nerve stimulation. Transvesical or direct injection of the obturator canal with lidocaine has also been described.[30]

At the conclusion of the resection, a systematic inspection of the bladder should be made. Previously controlled vessels may have restarted bleeding, particularly if the patient's blood pressure has risen. All tissue fragments and blood clots should be evacuated. Efflux from the sheath should be essentially clear. The ureteral orifices should be inspected for injury.

Most surgeons place a Foley catheter to gravity drainage at the conclusion of the procedure. If small, superficial tumors have been resected, catheter drainage may not be necessary. Catheter drainage serves several purposes, including monitoring the amount of postoperative hematuria and urinary output, lessening the likelihood of perforation if the bladder wall was significantly thinned from the resection, and reducing the chance of clot retention, as the bladder is not required to contract to empty. Bladder contraction may activate bleeding. Continuous bladder irrigation is occasionally used but generally should be avoided after bladder tumor resection. Unlike bleeding from the prostatic fossa due to oozing from a venous sinus, bleeding from the bed of a resected bladder tumor is not controlled by compression from the catheter and irrigation.

Several technological advances have improved the standard resectoscope for the resection of bladder tumors.[27] A continuous-flow resectoscope allows the resectionist to maintain bladder filling at a constant level and avoid overdistention. Video units eliminate the need for the surgeon to place an eye to the lens and lessen the risk of exposure to bodily fluids. They may also facilitate viewing difficult areas of the bladder such as the anterior bladder neck.

Tumors in a Diverticulum

Tumors arising in a bladder diverticulum, by definition, have no muscular layer between the tumor and bladder serosa. Since the bladder wall is thinned and unsupported, attempted transurethral resection might perforate the bladder. Accordingly, tumors arising in a diverticulum should be treated with partial or total cystectomy.

Recurrent Tumors

Complete tumor resection may not be necessary in all situations. In patients in whom a low-grade, superficial tumor with a similar cystoscopic appearance has been previously diagnosed, the recurrent tumor may be treated with simple fulguration. Laser ablation has also been used in this clinical setting. The disadvantage of this approach is that it does not provide histological documentation of tumor grade and stage. Intravesical treatment, including bacille Calmette-Guérin immunotherapy and intravesical chemotherapy with agents such as mitomycin C and thiotepa, has been successfully used to eradicate residual tumor after incomplete resection.

POSTOPERATIVE CARE

Postoperatively, the patient's catheter is removed when the hematuria has resolved, usually the morning after surgery. Catheter drainage is maintained for longer periods, often 3 to 7 days, when the tumor resection extends to the limit of the bladder wall, or when a perforation has occurred. Antibiotics are not required, but many physicians give oral antibiotics prophylactically for 3 to 5 days. Pain medications such as phenazopyridine hydrochloride and antispasmodics are helpful for dysuria and bladder spasms, respectively.

COMPLICATIONS

Bladder Perforation

Bladder perforation is usually caused by resection with the cutting loop through the wall of the bladder. Occasionally it is done purposely in resecting a muscle-invasive tumor that has extended into the perivesical fat (the so-called radical procedure). Such vigorous resections are not standard therapy. Perforation may rarely occur from overdistention of the bladder with irrigating fluid, or from the beak of the resectoscope. Rarely the tip of the Foley catheter is pushed through the thinned bladder wall at the conclusion of surgery.

Signs and symptoms of bladder perforation include lack of free and ample return of the irrigating fluid; abdominal pain if the patient is under spinal anesthesia; and a distended, tense, or rigid abdomen. The patient appears pale, sweaty, and tachycardic. A precipitous rise in blood pressure followed by a sharp decrease and signs of cardiovascular collapse ensue. When perforation leads to extravasation and intravascular absorption, hemolysis, water intoxication, hyponatremic shock, and cardiorespiratory difficulties arise.

Perforations may occur either extra- or intraperitoneally. When a bladder perforation is suspected, a cystogram should be obtained, including a postirrigation film. Small extraperitoneal perforations rarely cause difficulty and can be managed with catheter drainage and broad-spectrum antibiotic coverage. Intra- or large extraperitoneal bladder perforations should be explored and formally repaired. Late com-

plications include renal failure and pelvic abscess or peritonitis.

Hematuria and Clot Retention

The time to control bleeding is at the time of the operation. It is improper to conclude the transurethral resection when gross hematuria is persistent. If hemostasis is obtained and drainage from the catheter remains free, the chances of serious bleeding are small.

When the patient complains of suprapubic pressure or an urge to void, or when drainage from the catheter is not observed, the first maneuver is to irrigate the catheter with 50 to 100 ml of sterile saline in a catheter-tipped syringe. If the catheter does not irrigate freely, the position of the catheter should be checked by deflating the balloon, inserting the catheter to the meatus, reinflating the balloon and again attempting to irrigate the catheter. Small clots may be removed by repeated irrigation of the catheter. Such irrigation should continue until clear urine is obtained.

When numerous large, thick clots are encountered, there is nothing to be gained by prolonged attempts to evacuate the bladder through a catheter. It is more effective to return the patient to the cystoscopy suite and, under an anesthetic, evacuate the clots through a resectoscope sheath. The bladder is again carefully inspected and any bleeding points are fulgurated. Simple evacuation of the bladder may allow the bladder wall to contract, which will terminate bleeding. All old clots should be removed, as these may subsequently obstruct the catheter. Bleeding points may also be found under areas of organized clot.

Bleeding patients should also have coagulation parameters checked and necessary blood products replaced. Epsilon-aminocaproic acid (Amicar), which helps stabilize fibrin clot, may be useful when administered intravenously or orally. Amicar is usually administered in a 5-gm loading dose, followed by 1 gm each hour until bleeding is controlled, usually about 8 hours. Maintenance doses of 1 gm every 4 to 6 hours are then instituted. The total dose in 24 hours should not usually exceed 24 gm, although overdoses have not been described. If bleeding continues, Amicar may cause the formation of large, rubbery clots that are difficult to evacuate. Irrigation solutions such as alum (0.25 to 0.5 percent) or silver nitrate (0.25 to 1 percent) may rarely be indicated to control bleeding. Laser coagulation has also been applied for this purpose.

Obstruction of a Ureteral Orifice

Obstruction of a ureteral orifice can occur when the coagulation current is used in the area around the orifice. Use of the cutting current across the orifice causes gaping of the orifice and possible reflux but does not usually result in stricture formation. Ureteral obstruction may go undetected because the resultant hydronephrosis is slow and painless in its development. This complication should be suspected in a patient complaining of flank pain. It would be prudent to obtain an IVP about 4 to 6 weeks postoperatively even in an asymptomatic patient when the ureteral orifice has been resected, to document prompt drainage from the kidney. Obstruction of a ureteral orifice is best treated early with balloon dilation and possible incision. If these endoscopic measures are not successful, ureteral reimplantation will be required.

Absorption of Excess Irrigation Fluid/Hemolysis

Several problems result from the entry of irrigation fluid into the circulation: (1) volume overload, (2) fluid and electrolyte imbalances, and (3) intravascular hemolysis leading to acute renal failure.

Volume overload leads to cardiopulmonary difficulties, in particular pulmonary edema, necessitating treatment with diuretics, supplemental oxygen, and fluid restriction.

Several forms of electrolyte disturbances may be seen with absorption of excess irrigation fluid. Severe hyponatremia can lead to cerebral edema and death. Lesser degrees of hyponatremia can be treated with fluid restriction and diuretics. Severe hyponatremia, with a serum sodium level of less than 120 mEq/L, often requires salt replacement. The appropriate treatment for hyponatremic shock is replacement of sodium chloride with an intravenous 3 percent solution: 250 to 500 ml of 3 percent sodium chloride is usually sufficient.

Intravascular hemolysis often results in acute renal failure, heralded by characteristically sudden oliguria (less than 400 ml of urine in 24 hours). Oliguria may persist for a few days or weeks, with progressive uremia, hyperkalemia, and increased total body water. Symptoms include nausea, vomiting, weakness, low-grade fever, hypertension, abdominal distention, and mental status changes. Appropriate treatment consists of fluid restriction, administration of furosemide to convert oliguric to nonoliguric renal failure, monitoring of electrolytes, and dialysis, if necessary. As renal function improves, a postobstructive type of diuresis may ensue.

Urethral Strictures

Urethral strictures may develop at any point in the urethra but are most common at the narrowest points:

the external meatus, fossa navicularis, and bulbomembranous junction. Trauma and infection are predisposing factors. Use of too large an instrument or forceful placement of the instrument can lead to stricture formation. Prolonged catheter drainage has also been implicated. Strictures occur more commonly in patients undergoing repeated tumor resections.

Treatment of urethral strictures may include urethral dilations, internal urethrotomy, and (rarely) formal urethroplasty.

Editorial Comment

Fray F. Marshall

Transurethral resection of bladder tumors is covered in excellent detail. It is rare that open exploration is required for perforations. It is clearly preferable to avoid an open exploration, especially if partial or total cystectomy might be considered. Urologists need to be careful about the use of Amicar unless there is documented fibrinolysin activity. Otherwise, the clots that are formed can be very tenacious and difficult to irrigate.

REFERENCES

1. Varkarakis MJ, Gaeta J, Moore RH, et al. Superficial bladder tumor: Aspects of clinical progression. Urology 4:414, 1974.
2. Payne P. Sex, age, history, tumour type, and survival. In Wallace DM, ed. Tumors of the Bladder. Edinburgh, Churchill Livingstone, 1959, p 285.
3. Wallace DM, Harris DL. Delay in treating bladder tumours. Lancet 1:332, 1965.
4. Mahadevia PS, Alexander JE, Rojas-Corona R, et al. Pseudosarcomatous stromal reaction in primary and metastatic urothelial carcinoma: A source of diagnostic difficulty. Am J Surg Pathol 13:782, 1989.
5. Czerniak B, Deitch D, Simmons H, et al. Ha-ras gene codon 12 mutation and DNA ploidy in urinary bladder carcinoma. Br J Cancer 62:762, 1990.
6. Badalament RA, Ortolano V, Burgers JK. Recurrent or aggressive bladder cancer: Indications for adjuvant intravesical therapy. Urol Clin North Am 19:485, 1993.
7. Zein TA, Milad MF. Urine cytology in bladder tumors. Int Surg 76:52, 1991.
8. Parry WL, Hemstreet GP III. Cancer detection by quantitative fluorescence image analysis. J Urol 139:270, 1988.
9. Harving N, Wolf H, Melsen F. Positive urinary cytology after tumor resection: An indicator for concomitant carcinoma in situ. J Urol 140:495, 1988.
10. Schwalb DM, Herr HW, Fair WR. The management of clinically unconfirmed positive urine cytology. J Urol 150:1751, 1994.
11. Gustafson H, Tribukait B, Esposti PL. DNA profile and tumour progression in patients with superficial bladder tumours. Urol Res 10:13, 1982.
12. Blomjous ECM, Schipper NW, Baak JPA, et al. The value of morphometry and DNA flow cytometry in addition to classic prognosticators in superficial urinary bladder carcinoma. Am J Clin Pathol 91:243, 1989.
13. Buy JN, Moss AA, Guinet C, et al. MR staging of bladder carcinoma: Correlation with pathologic findings. Radiology 169:695, 1988.
14. Husband JES, Olliff JFC, Williams MP, et al. Bladder cancer: Staging with CT and MR imaging. Radiology 173:435, 1989.
15. Bryan PJ, Butler HE, Lipuma JP, et al. CT and MR imaging in staging bladder neoplasms. J Comput Assist Tomogr 11:96, 1987.

16. Fisher MR, Hricak H, Tanagho EA. Urinary bladder MR imaging. Part II: Neoplasm. Radiology 157:471, 1985.
17. Rholl KS, Lee JKT, Heiken JP, et al. Primary bladder carcinoma: Evaluation with MR imaging. Radiology 163:117, 1987.
18. Wood DP Jr, Lorig R, Pontes JE, Montie JE. The role of magnetic resonance imaging in the staging of bladder carcinoma. J Urol 140:741, 1988.
19. Proppe KH, Scully RE, Rosai J. Postoperative spindle cell nodules of genitourinary tract resembling sarcomas: A report of eight cases. Am J Surg Pathol 8:101, 1984.
20. Murphy DM, Zincke H, Furlow WL. Management of high grade transitional cell carcinoma of the upper urinary tract. J Urol 125:25, 1981.
21. Blute ML, Segura JW, Patterson DE, et al. Impact of endourology on diagnosis and management of upper urinary tract urothelial cancer. J Urol 141:1298, 1989.
22. Skinner DG, Lieskovsky G. Management of invasive and high-grade bladder cancer. In Skinner DG, Lieskovsky G, eds. Diagnosis and Management of Genitourinary Cancer. Philadelphia, WB Saunders, 1988, p 295.
23. Weldon TE, Soloway MS. Susceptibility of urothelium to neoplastic cellular implantation. Urology 5:824, 1975.
24. Whitmore WF Jr, Batata MA, Hilaris BS, et al. A comparative study of two preoperative radiation regimens with cystectomy for bladder cancer. Cancer 40:1077, 1977.
25. Blackard CE, Byar DP. Results of a clinical trial of surgery and radiation in stages II and III carcinoma of the bladder. J Urol 108:875, 1972.
26. Weyrauch HM. Transurethral prostatectomy. In Weyrauch HM, ed. Surgery of the Prostate. Philadelphia, WB Saunders, 1959, p 303.
27. Soloway MS, Patel J. Surgical techniques for endoscopic resection of bladder cancer. Urol Clin North Am 19:467, 1992.
28. Nachtsheim DA, So EPH, Greene LF. Transurethral resection of lesions in the dome of the bladder. Urology 18:84, 1981.
29. Amar AD, Das S. Upper urinary tract transitional cell carcinoma in patients with bladder carcinoma and associated vesicoureteral reflux. J Urol 133:468, 1985.
30. Augspurger RR, Donohue RE. Prevention of obturator nerve stimulation during transurethral surgery. J Urol 123:170, 1980.

Chapter 4

Laser Treatment of Bladder Cancer

Joseph A. Smith, Jr.

Since they were first introduced into clinical practice almost 15 years ago, lasers have been used for ablation of transitional cell carcinoma of the bladder. Justification for the use of lasers as an alternative to standard methods of electrocautery resection has been based on theoretical therapeutic advantages as well as an observed decrease in treatment-related morbidity. The development of new laser wavelengths and instrumentation has facilitated and expanded the use of lasers in a number of areas of urological surgery, including treatment of bladder cancer.

TISSUE EFFECTS

The tissue effects of surgical lasers depend on transformation of light energy into heat. Laser light is monochromatic (i.e., composed of a single wavelength) and travels in a unidirectional manner. The light can be deflected for projection onto tissue surfaces. The laser beam is coherent, although most surgical laser fibers are designed to provide a certain angle of divergence.

The active medium determines the wavelength of a particular laser. Atoms in the active medium are stimulated from the ground state to an excited state, usually by an electrically powered flashlamp. When the atoms spontaneously return to the ground state, a photon is emitted. The photons are deflected from a totally reflecting mirror at one end of the laser cavity and exit as a parallel beam through a partially reflecting mirror at the other end. The beam may pass directly from the laser or be transmitted by a flexible quartz fiber. The absorption characteristics of a particular wavelength influence the tissue effects.

Energy Density

In addition to wavelength, other parameters can be used to predict and, to some extent, control the tissue effects and depth of penetration of a particular laser. Stated simply, energy density is the amount of energy delivered to a given area of tissue. It is determined by the formula:

$$\text{power (watts)} \times \text{duration (seconds)}/\text{area}^2 \text{ (cm}^2)$$

The power output of a particular laser is controlled from the instrument panel. Duration can be modified by controlling the time length of a particular pulse or by varying the speed with which the beam is moved across the tissue surface.

An influential component of the formula for energy density is the size of the treatment area. Surgical laser fibers with a wide angle of divergence produce a lower energy density by treating a larger surface area for a given power and time. In addition, distance between the fiber tip and the tissue surface influences the surface area being treated. Contact fibers, by limiting the treatment surface area, increase energy density.

Coagulation

When tissues are heated to less than 60°C for only a few seconds, tissue warming without irreversible damage is observed. Between 60° and 100°C, protein denaturation occurs with tissue coagulation. Although the tissue injury with coagulation is irreversible and destructive, immediate tissue removal does not occur. The thermally injured tissue either sloughs or resorbs secondarily. Hemostasis is usually excellent as the coagulation process extends to blood vessels within the volume of treated tissue. Poorly absorbed wavelengths, such as neodymium:yttrium-aluminum-garnet (Nd:YAG), cause primarily tissue coagulation. Also, coagulation is increased by lowering the energy density. In general, low-power, long-duration laser exposure increases the amount of coagulation and the depth of tissue injury compared with higher power used for a short duration.

Vaporization

When high tissue temperatures (generally exceeding 100°C) are achieved, immediate tissue vaporization ensues. Some surface carbonization may be observed and a smoke plume generated. Some degree of coagulation accompanies carbonization, so hemostasis is usually good, although less than that observed with pure coagulation techniques. Under water, vaporization is more difficult to achieve than in an air environment. This is particularly pertinent in the bladder as the irrigating fluid causes surface cooling. Excessive charring of the tissue surface results in scatter of the beam and limits further penetration of the energy into the tissue. Vaporization is increased by using highly absorbed wavelengths, by using a high laser power output, or by decreasing the treated surface area (as with contact tips).

CHOICE OF LASER

Laser instruments differ primarily in the wavelength of the emitted light.[1] Wavelength is a function of the active medium, which may be a solid, liquid, or gas. In addition, crystals may be interposed to change the wavelength of the emitted light.

Neodymium:YAG Laser

Since its introduction into clinical practice in 1979, the Nd:YAG has been and remains the most frequently used laser in urological surgery. The active medium consists of neodymium ions contained within an yttrium-doped aluminum-garnet lattice. It emits light with a wavelength of 1060 nm. Light at this wavelength is poorly absorbed by water and body pigments. Because of this poor absorption, the light penetrates deeply into the tissue before the thermal energy is extinguished.

When a noncontact, free-beam mode is used, Nd:YAG laser energy penetrates bladder tissue 3 to 5 mm, depending on the power and, in particular, duration of exposure. In a fluid environment, the poor absorption of the laser energy results in thermal coagulation of the tissue. However, the tissue maintains its structural and architectural integrity. A certain percentage of the energy is transmitted as both forward and backward scatter. Thus, the thermal effects may extend to adjacent organs beyond the bladder wall without actual perforation of the bladder itself.

After Nd:YAG laser treatment of the bladder, hemostasis is usually total. The coagulated tissue takes on a white, fluffy appearance. The tissue sloughs secondarily, although complete healing may take up to 2 months.

Carbon Dioxide Laser

The 10,600 nm wavelength of a carbon dioxide (CO_2) laser is strongly absorbed by water. Thus, the energy is rapidly extinguished, creating high temperatures in the surface tissue. Vaporization is observed along with carbonization. The depth of penetration is limited.

The relatively long wavelength of the CO_2 laser creates problems for transmission via flexible fibers. Attempts have been made to develop cystoscopes using a series of reflecting mirrors, but so far a practical CO_2 laser cystoscope has not been developed.

Argon Laser

An argon laser has a spectral emission with a wavelength between 488 and 514 nm. Light at this wavelength is poorly absorbed by water but strongly absorbed by body pigments such as melanin and hemoglobin. Consequently, the depth of penetration is intermediate between that of an Nd:YAG and a CO_2 laser. Argon lasers have been used to treat superficial transitional cell carcinoma of the bladder. However, commercially available surgical argon lasers have a relatively limited power output and generally can be used only for small tumors less than 1 cm in size.

KTP Laser

A KTP 532 laser uses a crystal to double the frequency of an Nd:YAG laser, thereby producing a wavelength of 532 nm. This provides an intermediate level of vaporization and coagulation. The energy can be transmitted by means of a small, flexible fiber. Tissue effects are similar to those achieved with an argon laser, although greater power can be produced than with most surgical argon lasers.

KTP lasers have been used to treat superficial bladder cancer. Some authors consider that the KTP provides an increased safety margin compared with an Nd:YAG laser because of limited penetration depth. However, treatment is also slower than with an Nd:YAG laser and there may be less effective overall treatment for large tumors.

Holmium:YAG

The holmium:YAG laser emits light in the mid-infrared region of the electromagnetic spectrum (2100 nm). This laser is absorbed by water and thus has more vaporizing and cutting effects than an Nd:YAG laser. Because more vaporization occurs, the hemostatic abilities are less than those of an Nd:YAG laser. The energy is readily transmitted by a flexible fiber.

Argon Dye Laser

Dye lasers can be used to produce light at a specific wavelength that provides excitation of photosensitized tissue. These principles are used for photodynamic therapy.

DELIVERY SYSTEMS

With the exception of the CO_2 laser, all the laser wavelengths that have been used to treat bladder cancer are transmitted via small, flexible fibers.[2] The fibers can be inserted through either rigid or flexible cystoscopes. Most can be produced in a size small enough to also be introduced satisfactorily through ureteroscopes. Since energy density is influenced significantly by the area of treatment, the angle of emergence of the laser light from the fiber tip, as well as the distance between the tip and the tissue surface, affects the depth of penetration.

Noncontact Fibers

Most reported laser treatments of bladder cancer have used noncontact (free-beam) laser fibers. The standard Nd:YAG laser fiber used to treat bladder cancer is an end-fire device with an angle of divergence of 5 to 15 degrees. The multiple fibers currently being investigated for treatment of benign prostatic hyperplasia usually use a side-firing fiber. In addition, the angle of emergence most often is much greater and may be up to 90 degrees. These same fibers may be used for treatment of bladder cancer, but in general a smaller angle of divergence is preferable for specific application of energy to a papillary bladder tumor.

Contact Vaporization

Increasing the energy density of an Nd:YAG laser also increases the vaporizing effects of this wavelength. This can be accomplished most readily by placing the fiber tip in direct contact with the tissue. Free-beam fibers can be used for this purpose. In addition, specialized tips have been developed for contact laser vaporization; the depth of penetration is less than with a free-beam method. Vaporization is increased and hemostasis decreased. The technique is most applicable to small papillary tumors, and the contact probe can be used in a manner similar to that used with a Bugbee electrode.

PATIENT SELECTION

Although some investigators still believe that tumor recurrence rate is decreased after laser treatment compared with electrocautery resection,[3] laser therapy for superficial bladder cancer is performed more often because of the observed decrease in morbidity and duration of hospitalization. Patients with superficial bladder cancer undergoing laser treatment usually have a history of recurrent low-grade papillary transitional cell carcinoma that has been biopsied previously. When papillary tumors are seen on a routine surveillance cystoscopy, laser treatment can be an effective, low-morbidity method for eradication of these recurrent lesions.

Laser vaporization or coagulation results in tumor destruction, which does not allow retrieval of tissue for adequate histological examination. Preoperative cold cup biopsies can partially address this issue, allowing pathological examination to determine tumor grade and provide some staging information. In general, though, sessile-appearing tumors in which invasion cannot be excluded reasonably by visual inspection should be treated by electrocautery resection, with biopsies of the underlying muscle tissue of the bladder wall. Some investigators also consider that first-time tumors should be treated by electrocautery resection rather than laser treatment so that adequate histological material is available.[4]

Tumor size is another consideration. Lesions larger than 1 to 2 cm are difficult to treat with laser alone and may require a debulking electrocautery resection before a laser treatment of the tumor base. This may, however, obviate many of the practical advantages of laser if electrocautery resection is required anyway.

Tumor location is a relatively minor issue. Virtually all parts of the bladder are accessible for laser treatment. Extra caution is appropriate for tumors on the bladder dome where loops of small bowel may be adjacent. Treatment of tumors overlying the ureteral orifice appears to be associated with a very low risk of stricture and obstruction of the ureter.

TREATMENT TECHNIQUE

A number of different treatment techniques have been described for laser destruction of bladder tumors. There are also differences relating to the laser wavelength. Finally, the amount and manner of energy delivery depend on the preoperative assessment of tumor stage.

Superficial Tumors

Laser treatment of superficial transitional cell carcinoma of the bladder (stages Ta to T1) is usually performed on an outpatient or ambulatory surgery basis. When treatment is performed without anesthesia, the patient is able to perceive the laser energy and often describes it as a burning type of discomfort. However, treatment seems to be tolerated far better than electrocautery resection. The exact reason for this is uncertain. However, laser energy probably results in rapid heating and destruction of nerve fibers in a well-defined volume of tissue. Electrocautery resection is associated with more irregular propagation of the energy along nerve and muscle bundles. The decision to perform laser therapy with general or regional anesthesia is based primarily on the surgeon's experience, the personality of the patient, and the size, number, and location of the tumors.

When a rigid cystoscope is used, the patient is placed in a standard lithotomy position. Most cystoscope instrument companies have a laser insert that adapts to the standard cystoscope with either a 19 Fr. or 21 Fr. sheath. The laser insert allows stabilization of the fiber tip and a watertight entry port. The laser fiber is inserted through the channel and the tip of the laser fiber is positioned just beyond the end of the visualizing telescope. With a noncontact Nd:YAG end-fire probe, the fiber is positioned 3 to 5 mm from the tumor surface. Either sterile water, normal saline, or amino acid solutions can be used for irrigation. A continuous flow system is not required: the irrigant can generally be turned off since bleeding is usually nonexistent.

When an end-fire probe with a 5- to 15-degree angle of divergence is used, the tip is positioned 3 to 5 mm from the surface of the tumor. With an Nd:YAG laser, 35 to 40 watts of energy is usually sufficient. The duration of the treatment is generally controlled by the speed with which the fiber tip is moved across the tumor surface. The laser can be operated in a continuous mode whereby energy is emitted whenever the foot pedal is depressed. An aiming beam, either from a flashlamp or from a helium neon laser, marks the point of impact, since the Nd:YAG laser beam is invisible to the human eye.

Laser treatment is best performed as a dynamic process rather than a series of adjacent static impulses. The beam is slowly moved across the surface of the tumor in a "painting" fashion. The tumor undergoes a white discoloration indicative of adequate thermal necrosis (Fig. 4–1). Care should be taken to avoid excessive laser energy application in any given area. Usually 2 to 3 seconds of duration are required in a given area for complete thermal coagulation to be evident. Techniques have been described wherein a ring of coagulated tissue is created around the tumor base to seal blood and lymphatic vessels. Practically, this is unnecessary, as bleeding does not occur even if the energy is applied initially to the center of the exophytic portion of the tumor.

It is not necessary to treat the tumor base initially, but it is important to make certain that all aspects of the lesion have been thermally coagulated. After the papillary frondular tissue is coagulated, it can usually be dislodged with the tip of the fiber or the cystoscope to expose deeper portions and the tumor base. It is best to treat the tumor with the bladder in as collapsed a state as possible to avoid excessive thinning of the bladder wall. If an air bubble overlies the tumor, this can either be evacuated or the patient can be tilted in one way or another to remove the tumor from the air bubble. If this proves to be difficult, treatment can be performed through the air bubble itself, but there is usually some surface carbonization and smoke production. The temperature of the irrigating fluid does not seem to be a major factor in determining tissue or treatment effect.

Subsurface boiling may be observed during treatment, producing a popcorn-like effect. These microexplosions, although sometimes dramatic, carry no particular significance. If the fiber tip inadvertently touches the bladder wall, there is usually some superficial carbonization and a cratering effect. The foot pedal is simply released and the fiber withdrawn from the tissue surface. If there is any tissue adherent to the fiber tip, it should be wiped away with a moist sponge before proceeding with therapy.

The depth of penetration cannot be monitored satisfactorily intraoperatively but is generally predicted preoperatively on the basis of the known characteristics of the wavelength, the power and duration of the laser output, and the spot size. Under most circumstances, 3 to 5 mm of penetration can be anticipated.

If a small amount of bleeding occurs, especially after a cold cup biopsy, hemostasis is usually accomplished in the course of treatment. However, even a relatively small amount of blood undergoes rapid carbonization and can both obscure and prevent effective energy delivery to the tumor surface.

Superficial tumors in bladder diverticula can be treated satisfactorily with a laser. Even though, by definition, there is no muscular backing to a diverticulum, actual free perforation of the diverticulum and bladder wall is uncommon. Usually, there is some

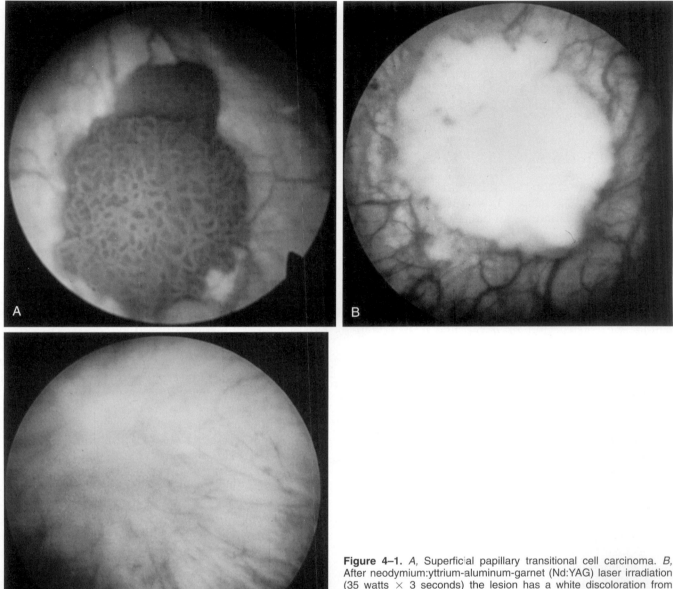

Figure 4–1. *A,* Superficial papillary transitional cell carcinoma. *B,* After neodymium:yttrium-aluminum-garnet (Nd:YAG) laser irradiation (35 watts × 3 seconds) the lesion has a white discoloration from thermal coagulation. *C,* Three months later a pale white scar is seen with no evidence of residual tumor.

shriveling of the mucosa of the diverticulum as the coagulation process occurs. The iliac blood vessels and obturator nerve are often adjacent to diverticula, but if appropriate energy densities are used, direct injury is unlikely. The obturator nerve is not stimulated by laser energy. Obturator spasm and a leg jerk, as may be observed with electrocautery, do not occur.

Treatment of tumors directly overlying the ureteral orifices is performed in the same manner as if the tumor were located elsewhere in the bladder. Stents should be removed from the ureteral orifice before treatment is performed, as the laser energy may melt the stent itself. Metal guidewires can be used alternatively. After an extensive treatment overlying the ureteral orifice, postoperative management with a stent may be advisable because of temporary edema. However, the long-term risk of ureteral stenosis appears to be low.

A postoperative Foley catheter is usually not necessary because of the lack of bleeding. The thermally coagulated tissue either sloughs as imperceptible particles or is resorbed. If the treatment is thought to have been adequate and proceeded satisfactorily, follow-up cystoscopy can be performed according to the routine for a particular patient, depending on tumor grade, stage, and history.

Intravesical drugs can be used after laser treatment, and the indications for their use should be the same as after electrocautery resection. However, since raw surfaces of the bladder wall are not exposed after laser treatment, intravesical drugs such as bacille Calmette-Guérin (BCG) or chemotherapy can be introduced more rapidly after treatment, with an apparently decreased risk of systemic absorption.[5]

Invasive Tumors

The ability of an Nd:YAG laser to produce transmural coagulation without perforation has allowed laser treatment of some invasive bladder cancers, although even in a controlled setting the depth of penetration is variable.[6] However, application of energy to both the inner and outer bladder wall through both a cystoscope and a laparoscope allows overlapping zones of thermal necrosis and complete transmural coagulation.[7] The location of most invasive bladder tumors on the trigone makes laparoscopic visualization and energy application somewhat difficult.

Patients being considered for laser treatment of invasive bladder cancer should first undergo a standard transurethral electrocautery resection. This accomplishes two purposes: first, it allows accurate histological examination for tumor staging, and second, it debulks the surface of the tumor. Logically, if laser is considered a method for extending the margin of resection, the electrocautery resection should extend deeply into the bladder muscle.

Under most circumstances, it is best to delay laser treatment for at least 3 to 5 days after an electrocautery resection to allow any bleeding to cease and overlying clot to lyse. Active bleeding or blood clot interferes with the delivery of energy. General or regional anesthesia is usually required, since relatively large amounts of laser energy are needed. The irregular appearance of the resection crater does not permit visual determination of treatment adequacy. Therefore, there should be systematic application of laser energy to the entire resection crater as well as an adequate surrounding margin.

Since the goal of treatment is transmural necrosis, energy output of up to 45 or 50 watts may be appropriate. When an end-fire probe with a 5- to 15-degree angle of divergence is used, the energy is maintained in a given area for 2 to 3 seconds. If a laparoscope has been inserted, small bowel can be displaced from the treatment area. After adequate energy has been applied through the cystoscope, the Nd:YAG laser fiber can be inserted through the laparoscope and energy applied to the intraperitoneal surface of the bladder in the same region if visualization is adequate.

The most appropriate candidates for laser treatment of invasive bladder cancer are patients with minimally invasive lesions.[8, 9] Lasers have been used to treat bulky, invasive bladder cancers. However, the surface effect obtained in this circumstance usually offers no demonstrable benefit compared with electrocautery debulking and cauterization of the tumor surface.

A catheter is not required postoperatively but may be used, depending on the amount of bladder surface area requiring treatment. Follow-up cystoscopy is performed after 1 month to assess the healing and detect any obvious residual tumor. Re-epithelialization of the bladder surface overlying residual cancer is feasible, but usually there is no residual tumor when complete re-epithelialization occurs within 2 to 3 months of treatment.

COMPLICATIONS OF LASER TREATMENT

Laser treatment of bladder cancer is used most often because of the observed decrease in patient morbidity and treatment-related complications. Usually, there is minimal discomfort after treatment. A distinct advantage is the almost complete lack of bleeding with coagulative procedures. Bleeding that may be present from a preoperative biopsy is usually coagulated adequately during the course of energy application. The coagulation that occurs from the laser energy itself causes virtually no bleeding as either an immediate or a delayed phenomenon.

The most feared complication of laser treatment of bladder cancer is perforation of an adjacent viscus. The small bowel or colon may lie in direct approximation with the peritoneal surface of the bladder. Thus, the risk of bowel perforation is greatest with laser therapy on the posterior bladder wall or dome.

Most patients with bowel perforation present with signs and symptoms within 8 to 24 hours of treatment, but symptomatic presentation has been delayed for as long as 2 weeks. Abdominal pain, physical findings consistent with an acute abdomen, and free intraperitoneal air are all associated with bowel perforation from laser therapy. It is important to recognize that bowel perforation may occur in the absence of any evident bladder perforation. A cystographic picture may be normal. The thicker muscle wall of the bladder makes it less prone to perforation, and forward scatter of the energy places the bowel at risk.

Immediate laparotomy is indicated if small bowel or colon perforation is suspected. The site of laser energy is identified. The zone of tissue injury may be far greater than is visibly evident, so resection of the affected site is generally indicated.

Although bladder perforation can occur, its incidence has been low. Hofstetter and colleagues treated over 500 tumors and reported only two incidences of small bowel perforation, in at least one of which excessive energy levels were used inadvertently.[3] Smith and associates have had no cases of small bowel perforation in over 150 laser treatments of superficial bladder tumors.[4]

RESULTS

Initially, laser treatment of superficial bladder cancer was promoted as a means to decrease the recurrence rate.[10, 11] Since anecdotal clinical observation and some experimental data[12] support the contention that some recurrences of superficial bladder cancer are due to implantation of viable tumor cells dislodged at the time of resection, the thermal, noncontact coagulation achieved with the laser has the potential to favorably affect the recurrence rate from implantation.

Both prospective and retrospective clinical series have generally failed to support any strong evidence of a favorable effect of laser treatment on the recurrence rate of bladder cancer.[13, 14] In most retrospective series, the patient population under study is one of the most influential factors in determining recurrence rate. This complicates comparisons of laser-treated patients with historical series of those undergoing electrocautery resection. Prospective studies have shown no apparent salutary effect of laser treatment on the overall recurrence of superficial bladder cancer.

On the other hand, there is good evidence attesting to the effectiveness of laser therapy in eradicating existing and visible superficial bladder tumors. Multiple series have shown a local recurrence rate of around 5 to 10 percent, a figure that compares favorably with electrocautery resection. In a randomized prospective study, Beisland and Seland found a local recurrence rate of 43 percent for stage T1 transitional cell carcinoma treated with electrocautery resection alone, compared with only 7 percent for Nd:YAG laser treatment.[13]

There are no studies comparing various laser fibers, wavelengths, or contact versus noncontact treatment of superficial bladder tumors. There has been only a single published report on holmium:YAG treatment of bladder tumors.[14] If adequate vaporization or coagulation of the lesion occurs, good results can be anticipated in terms of local eradication of visible tumors with any of the laser wavelengths. Overall, though, the Nd:YAG laser has proved the most versatile and allows treatment of larger tumors.

PHOTODYNAMIC THERAPY

The treatment results discussed above rely on the pure thermal effects of lasers in producing either vaporization or coagulation of tissue. Photodynamic therapy involves photoactivation of sensitized cells.

There are a number of potential photosensitizing agents. The one studied initially and most extensively is hematoporphyrin derivative (HPD). The mechanism of the photocytotoxic action of HPD is uncertain but may occur at both a cellular and vascular level. Excitation of HPD-sensitized cells produces a singlet oxygen, which is toxic to cellular components.

After intravenous administration, HPD concentrates in dysplastic or frankly malignant cells.[15] However, HPD photosensitization has been associated with severe bladder contracture in a small percentage of patients and with skin photosensitivity. The drug is poorly absorbed when administered intravesically.

Newer photosensitizing agents have the potential for a decrease in both systemic and local complications. In addition, it may be possible to instill them locally. Further studies of photodynamic therapy are ongoing but investigational.

Summary and Recommendations

Laser therapy is firmly established as an effective treatment for superficial bladder cancer. The ability to eradicate existing, visible tumors is comparable with or, perhaps, superior to results obtained with electrocautery resection. Overall, however, there is no demonstrable favorable effect on tumor recurrence. Therefore, the indications for adjuvant intravesical treatment with either BCG or cytotoxic drugs after laser therapy are unchanged in comparison with standard treatment recommendations.

Laser treatment of superficial bladder cancer has been associated with an observed decrease in treatment-related morbidity. Bleeding is almost nonexistent and catheter drainage of the bladder is not required. Treatment can be performed more readily on an ambulatory basis. A complication unique to laser therapy, perforation of an adjacent viscus, is unusual if appropriate treatment parameters are used. A number of laser wavelengths and fibers have been used successfully to treat superficial bladder cancer. None has proved inherently superior to another, although an Nd:YAG laser used in a noncontact manner produces the optimal coagulation. There is no evidence that other laser treatment techniques offer an increased margin of safety.

The primary limitations of laser treatment of superficial bladder cancer are the lack of tissue available for histological examination and the difficulty in treating with laser alone tumors that exceed 2 cm in size. Laser treatment of invasive bladder cancer is limited by difficulties and inaccuracies with clinical staging of invasive transitional cell carcinoma and by the inability to predict and control the depth of penetration. Combined cystoscopic and laparoscopic application of energy may have a favorable effect on results, as reliable transmural coagulation can be achieved.[7] The location of most invasive tumors on the bladder trigone makes laparoscopic visualization and accessibility for laser treatment difficult and somewhat limits such a combined approach.

Editorial Comment

Fray F. Marshall

The advantages of the laser are presented here by Dr. Smith. The expense of laser equipment, the lack of pathological material, and the competition from standard transurethral resection have slowed the widespread acceptance of the laser for the treatment of bladder cancer.

REFERENCES

1. Stein BS. Laser tissue interaction. In Smith JA Jr, ed. Lasers in Urologic Surgery. St. Louis, Mosby-Year Book, 1993, p 10.
2. Milam DF. Surgical laser fibers. In Smith JA Jr, ed. Lasers in Urologic Surgery. St. Louis, Mosby-Year Book, 1993, p 26.
3. Hofstetter A, Frank K, Keiditsch E. Laser treatment of the bladder: Experimental and clinical results. In Smith JA Jr, ed. Lasers in Urologic Surgery. St. Louis, Mosby-Year Book, 1985, p 63.
4. Smith JA Jr. Endoscopic applications of laser energy. Urol Clin North Am 13:405, 1986.
5. Cho YH, Chi SH, Hernandez AD, et al. Adriamycin absorption after Nd:YAG laser coagulation compared to electrosurgical resection of the bladder wall. J Urol 147:1139, 1992.
6. Smith JA, Landau S. Neodymium:YAG laser specifications for safe intravesical use. J Urol 141:1238, 1989.
7. Scaletscky R, Milam DF, Smith JA. Combined laparoscopic and cystoscopic Nd:YAG laser photocoagulation of the porcine bladder wall. San Antonio, TX, Abstracts of the American Urological Association, 1993.
8. Smith JA Jr. Treatment of invasive bladder cancer with a neodymium:YAG laser. J Urol 135:55, 1986.
9. Beisland HO, Sander S. Neodymium:YAG laser irradiation of stage T2 muscle-invasive bladder cancer: Long-term results. Br J Urol 65:24, 1990.
10. Hofstetter A. Treatment of urological tumors by neodymium: YAG laser. Eur Urol 12 (Suppl):21, 1986.
11. Malloy TR, Wein AJ, Shanberg A. Superficial transitional cell carcinoma of the bladder treated with neodymium:YAG laser: A study of the recurrence rate within the first year [abstract]. J Urol 131:251A, 1984.
12. Soloway MS, Masters S. Urothelial susceptibility to tumor cell implantation. Cancer 46:1158, 1980.
13. Beisland HO, Seland O. A prospective randomized study on neodymium:YAG laser irradiation versus TUR in the treatment of urinary bladder cancer. Scand J Urol Nephrol 20:209, 1986.
14. Smith JA Jr. Current concepts in laser treatment of bladder cancer. Prog Clin Biol Res 303:463, 1989.
15. Benson RC Jr. Treatment of diffuse transitional cell carcinoma in situ by whole bladder hematoporphyrin derivative photodynamic therapy. J Urol 134:675, 1985.

Chapter 5

Ureteroscopy (Diagnostic)

Demetrius H. Bagley

Early attempts at ureteroscopy were limited to diagnosis by observation alone because the flexible endoscopes available did not have a channel for working instruments. Rigid ureteroscopes with adequate channels were limited to the distal ureter. After a working channel was incorporated into flexible ureteroscopes and small working instruments became available, the potential for interventional ureteroscopic procedures, both diagnostic and therapeutic, became a reality.

The diagnostic applications of ureteroscopy have evolved along with the endoscopes and working instruments. The major diagnostic indications include filling defects in the upper urinary tract, ureteral obstruction and narrowing, unilateral gross hematuria, and "the elusive calculus." Variations of ureteroscopic techniques may be applied to each of these indications to optimize the yield from the diagnostic effort.

FILLING DEFECTS

The most common, and potentially the most important, ureteroscopic diagnostic indication is the upper tract filling defect. Typically, the patient has been studied for hematuria or some unrelated finding and has been found to have a filling defect on excretory urography. Since it is usually impossible to diagnose a filling defect definitively by excretory urography alone, other radiographic studies are employed. A diagnosis of a lucent calculus can be confirmed by either ultrasound examination, which may demonstrate a hyperechoic lesion with acoustic shadowing typical of a calculus, or a computed tomographic (CT) scan, which can demonstrate the high density of the calculus. Noncalculus filling defects, however, cannot be fully defined radiographically. Endoscopy can usually provide a firm diagnosis. Visualization alone can often distinguish between calculi and neoplasms. Simple visualization can also give some suggestive differential diagnosis of soft tissue filling defects. For instance, low-grade transitional cell carcinoma in the upper tract has the same typical papillary appearance as those seen in the bladder. Inverted papillomas may have a smooth surface, and ureteritis cystica has a more typical smooth, yellowish cystic appearance. The distinction can be confirmed by biopsy (Figs. 5–1 to 5–3).

Several techniques are now available for biopsy with the larger- or smaller-diameter rigid ureteroscopes or the small-diameter flexible endoscopes. Successful diagnosis by biopsy depends on several factors. An attempt should be made to obtain the largest piece of tissue possible and the most cellular and largest volume of fluid if tissue sampling is not feasible. The optimal yield from the samples available depends on close cooperation between urologist and pathologist.

In a series examining the yield from various ureteroscopic biopsy techniques of upper tract neoplasms, Abdel-Razzak et al[1] found that the techniques employed were related to the diagnostic yield. After inspection of the lesion in the collecting system, a sampling device should be passed to remove a fragment of the lesion. For papillary transitional cell carcinoma, a flat wire basket proved to be the most effective instrument to remove a large, potentially diagnostic sample. Other devices, including cup forceps and graspers, were also effective. Brushes tended to move the tissue when placed under vision but were not very efficient in obtaining a sample. Washing with saline was not effective in all patients but did give a diagnosis in some in whom the other sampling techniques did not provide a diagnostic yield. More sessile lesions may be better sampled with cup forceps and/or a brush. Our present sampling scheme includes multiple biopsy and irrigation samples (Table 5–1).

After the optimal sample has been provided to the pathology laboratory, cytology slides are prepared, and when there are any tiny fragments of tissue grossly visible, a cell block is also prepared. In a

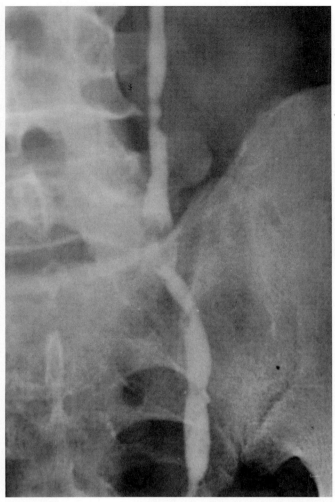

Figure 5–1. A filling defect in the middle ureter shown on retrograde pyelography was found to be a low-grade transitional cell carcinoma on ureteroscopic biopsy.

study of biopsy techniques, the cell block often provided the diagnosis.[2, 3] Since the tissue architecture and histological pattern can be seen in the hematoxylin and eosin preparations from the cell block, the transitional cell tumors can be graded.

Low et al[4] reported that techniques that remove tissue can be used most effectively to sample upper tract tumors. They compared several different sampling techniques, including brush biopsy, fine needle aspiration, and forceps biopsy. The last was the most accurate technique, giving a diagnostic accuracy of 100 percent, although it gave adequate tissue in only 56 percent of the patients sampled.

In general, to provide a diagnosis, the most successful technique of ureteroscopic biopsy is to obtain the largest piece of tissue possible or the most cellular fluid sample. These can then be processed by the cytopathology laboratory most efficiently to avoid loss of any sample. The basket or grasper should not be closed fully because of the risk of shearing the sample from the grasping device. For the same rea-

son, the device with the sample should not be withdrawn through the working channel of the ureteroscope. If it is removed in this way, any tissue extending from the cup or from the basket will be lost as the device enters the working channel. The sample of tissue should be removed along with the ureteroscope and sampling device. The entire unit can be removed from the patient to retrieve the sample. The ureteroscope can then be replaced into the ureter to sample the area again, to irrigate and aspirate at the level of the lesion, or to treat the lesion.

When the ureteroscopic procedure is initiated for evaluation of a filling defect, a safety guidewire should be left in the ureter. After removal of the ureteroscope and the tissue sample, the ureteroscope can be replaced. A rigid ureteroscope can be passed under direct vision and the guidewire used as a landmark into the ureteral orifice. If a flexible ureteroscope is being used, a second wire or a working wire can be introduced by using a double-lumen catheter placed over the safety wire or with a dilator sheath used for the same purpose. The flexible ureteroscope can then be placed over this working wire.

URETERAL NARROWING AND OBSTRUCTION

Ureteral narrowing is another indication for endoscopic evaluation. Ureteral obstruction can be consid-

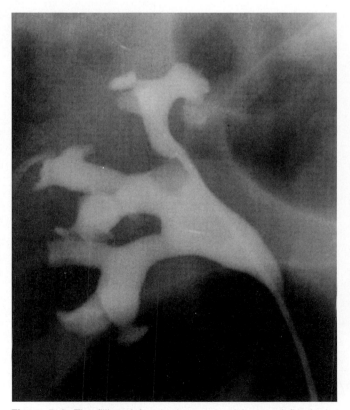

Figure 5–2. The filling defect in the renal pelvis was defined as a low-grade transitional cell carcinoma and treated ureteroscopically.

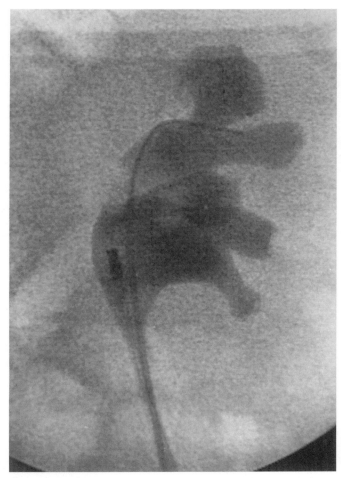

Figure 5–3. A flexible ureteroscope is seen in the fluoroscopic image showing a filling defect in the upper infundibulum.

ered a special instance of ureteral narrowing, one so severe that the small lumen remaining is inadequate for passage of urine.

Direct visual inspection of an area of ureteral narrowing is an important step for diagnosis. The quality and color of the mucosa can be inspected and the ureteral lumen gauged. It is often evident from direct endoscopic inspection whether there is intrinsic narrowing in the structure of the ureter or whether there is some external compression. Intrinsic narrowing limits the size of the lumen, and the narrow site can be seen, just as urethroscopy can reveal a stricture in the urethra. The extent of the narrowing may be evident if it is short, but with a long narrowing the full extent may not be appreciated visually. In comparison, extrinsic compression may show distortion or displacement of the ureter, and the adequacy of the true lumen may be evident. The extent and diameter of the narrowing may be appreciated more fully by simultaneously injecting contrast material through the working channel of the ureteroscope during direct inspection. Simultaneous fluoroscopy or a radiogram can outline the full stricture, while endoscopic visualization and visual inspection give some apprecia-

tion of the mucosa itself. Edema, papillary neoplasm, erythema, and pallor can be seen. Occasionally, a calculus may be noted, surrounded by edema or obscured by a narrowing of the ureter. Even in these cases, the calculus may be evident within the lumen beyond a narrow segment.

Direct endoscopy of a narrow segment or ureteral obstruction also offers a chance for interventional procedures. The site in question can be sampled. Since the tissue involved in narrowing of the ureter is often more solid than seen with filling defects, other sampling techniques are more successful. For instance, a brush can remove tissue from the surface, and this device also has the advantage of a size that can be placed into the lumen of a very narrow segment. A cup forceps can take a sample from a firmer lesion within the narrowed ureter. In the rare circumstance when a papillary tumor obstructs the ureter, the sampling techniques with a basket or grasper are more effective.

Endoscopy also provides the opportunity for various options in treatment. The first step may be endoscopic placement of a guidewire through the narrowed segment or through an obstruction. Often, under direct vision, the guidewire can be directed effectively to enter and pass a segment otherwise inaccessible to retrograde manipulation. Once control has been gained with a guidewire, the full range of possibilities for treatment are available. A catheter or stent can be passed for urinary drainage. A narrow segment can be dilated to allow passage of an endoscope proximally in an attempt at therapy. This segment can also be incised if desired. It can be biopsied or resected, and a calculus retrieved or fragmented. In this way, the initial visual diagnosis can direct immediate therapy.

GROSS UNILATERAL HEMATURIA

Ureteroscopy has also proved extremely valuable in evaluation of patients with gross unilateral hematuria, also known as benign essential hematuria.[4, 5]

TABLE 5–1. Ureteroscopic Biopsy: Sample Collection

1. Bladder urine
2. Ureteral urine
3. Aspirate at lesion
4. Irrigate and aspirate at lesion
5. Biopsy with one or more:
   a. basket
   b. forceps
   c. grasper
   d. other
6. Aspirate
7. All to cytopathology

These patients have gross hematuria but have no pathological lesion detected by standard radiological and cytological studies. They have usually undergone contrast studies with excretory urography and/or retrograde pyelography. The renal parenchyma has been studied with ultrasound or CT scan. Patients have often undergone renal arteriography also. Studies of patients with gross hematuria have included clotting parameters and urinary cytology. By definition, the patients have undergone cystoscopy to define the ureteral source of the bleeding. Those with microscopic hematuria alone or without any evidence lateralizing the gross hematuria may not benefit from ureteroscopic study.

Operative Technique

Cystoscopy is first performed to look at the bladder again and to lateralize the hematuria if it persists. A cone-tip retrograde ureteropyelogram is then performed to define the collecting system. Particular care should be taken to avoid overfilling of the intrarenal collecting system, with resultant pyelolymphatic and venous backflow and bleeding. Overfilling also causes ecchymosis in the mucosa of the renal collecting system, which can be confused with other sources of bleeding.

Ureteroscopy is next performed to visualize the entire collecting system from the distal ureter to the entire intrarenal system. The distal ureter should be inspected with a small-diameter rigid ureteroscope, which can be passed into the ureteral lumen without dilation. It can be advanced as far as possible within the ureter, with a guidewire placed as the endoscope is removed. Care should be taken to place the wire only into the middle to proximal ureter, and to avoid placing it into the intrarenal collecting system where it may traumatize the mucosa.

The flexible ureteroscope is then advanced over the guidewire. It should be used to inspect the middle and proximal ureter and any portion not seen with the rigid ureteroscope. The ureteroscope is then advanced into the renal pelvis and intrarenal collecting system. The pelvis should be inspected as thoroughly as possible, and the instrument then advanced into the infundibula and calices in a systematic fashion. The upper infundibula are first inspected, followed by each subsequently lower infundibulum. The most inferior calices should be reserved until last, since secondary deflection of the ureteroscope may be needed to bring it to that level. The endoscope impinging on the upper portion of the renal pelvis may cause ecchymosis, which can be confused with other lesions that may have been the source of hematuria.

The ureteroscope is followed fluoroscopically as irrigation is maintained with saline containing radiographic contrast. In this way the collecting system is outlined for fluoroscopic localization. Care should be taken to avoid mixing irrigants within the visual field; if these solutions of different density are mixed, the light is refracted to disturb the visual field. If the collecting system is overfilled and does not drain well along the ureter outside the ureteroscope, the fluid can be aspirated through the working channel of the ureteroscope. Aspirate from the collecting system as well as bladder urine should be submitted for cytological study.

There has been a remarkable similarity in the yield found in series using total ureteroscopy to study patients with gross unilateral hematuria.[4, 5] The most common finding in each series has been a small hemangioma or some other small vascular lesion. These are most commonly associated with the renal papillae and have been located throughout the kidney. Therefore, it is clear that the intrarenal collecting system must be inspected with an actively deflectable, flexible ureteroscope. Rarely, patients have been found to have a papillary transitional cell carcinoma or a calculus as a source of the hematuria (Table 5–2).

Overall, a lesion responsible for the hematuria could be detected in approximately two thirds of patients. In approximately one third, no source was found. The hematuria frequently cleared in these patients after the endoscopic procedure. Among those in whom there was a discrete causative lesion, endoscopic treatment was successful. The most common lesion, a hemangioma, was treated by fulguration or laser ablation with excellent long-term success.

THE ELUSIVE CALCULUS

The clinical setting termed "the elusive calculus" is uncommon but certainly not rare. In this situation, the patient experiences pain consistent with, and even strongly suggestive of, a calculus. Often, there is microscopic hematuria, but radiological studies, particularly excretory urography, do not demonstrate

TABLE 5–2. Chronic Unilateral Hematuria: Endoscopic Diagnosis

	Bagley	Kumon
Discrete Lesions	16	9
Hemangioma	11	4
Minute venous rupture	2	4
Papillary tumor	1	1
Varices	1	0
Calculus	1	0
Nonspecific Lesions	7	1
Submucosal erythema	5	1
Abnormal papillary tip	1	0
Dilated collecting duct	1	0
No Lesion Seen	5	2

a stone. These patients are often studied exhaustively with other radiological tests that may have demonstrated a stone in some patients and other causes of the pain in others. There remains a group of patients with symptoms without objective evidence of disease except for hematuria. In these, the final definitive study may be endoscopy of the urinary tract.

Evaluation in these patients includes cystoscopy, retrograde ureteropyelography, and ureteroscopy. Cystoscopy may detect a small calculus that has recently passed into the bladder. Retrograde ureteropyelography may outline a calculus not appreciated on excretory urography. Complete ureteroscopy should be performed in these patients. The distal ureter is inspected with a small rigid endoscope without previous instrumentation, if possible. The entire lumen of the ureter must be inspected: it is not sufficient just to pass the ureteroscope proximally within the ureter without inspecting the entire lumen, since small calculi can be passed. After ureteroscopy of the distal ureter, a guidewire is left in place to permit introduction of a flexible ureteroscope to inspect the middle and proximal ureter and even the intrarenal collecting system. Any freely moving calculus, no matter how insignificant it appears, should be removed, both to eliminate it as the possible source of symptoms and to prevent its future growth. In atraumatic ureteroscopy, the need for a stent or catheter postoperatively can be determined by the presence of any bleeding or ureteral dilation for the procedure, either of which would be an indication for internal drainage.

Accuracy of Fragmentation

Shortly after shock wave lithotripsy of ureteral or renal calculi, there are often fragments remaining in the ureter. In an otherwise normal ureter, a decision for intervention or treatment may be based on the usual indications regarding stone progression, obstruction, or pain. However, in patients with an indwelling stent, it can be very difficult to estimate the discrepancy between the size of the stone and the ureter. Frequently the fragments of stone pass after removal of the stent, but often they become obstructive. It is impossible to make a decision to remove the stent in these cases of nonprogressing ureteral stone fragments without the patients' input. Many prefer to give the fragments a chance to pass after simply removing the stent, while many others do not want to risk having pain with obstruction from the fragments. It is this latter group who can benefit from ureteroscopy at the time of stent removal. The ureteral stone fragments can then be retrieved or, if necessary, fragmented further. The lumen should be cleared of any fragments larger than about 1 to 2

mm. The kidney should also be inspected to remove fragments that may be too large to pass. Endoscopy in these patients with ureteral fragments after shock wave lithotripsy of calculi can clear the fragments and ensure a course without ureteral obstruction. It should be considered and offered to patients with fragments who fail to progress alongside an indwelling stent. Endoscopy is particularly valuable if the fragments are of a size similar to or slightly greater than the stent itself.

Adequacy of Chemolysis

A similar clinical setting is seen in the patient with a stone that has been treated by chemolysis. These are usually patients with uric acid stones who have been treated by oral alkalinization. Radiolucent stones can usually be seen on ultrasound examination. If they have passed into the proximal ureter or broken into several pieces, they may not be appropriately visualized by sonography alone. A CT scan with thin cuts offers greater accuracy but still may not be conclusive.

Ureteral endoscopy can provide a definitive observation of the presence or size of stone fragments, whether they are radiolucent or poorly opaque, and regardless of their location. Many of these patients have an indwelling stent that has been previously placed either for relief of obstruction or to prevent obstruction as the stone decreases in size. When the stone is no longer detected by sonography, it is appropriate to remove the stent. If the patient wants to be absolutely certain that the stone has cleared or if it has disappeared in a time that seems clinically inappropriate, there may be concern for a possible larger fragment lurking in the middle to proximal ureter. Endoscopy is then appropriate.

Ureteroscopic inspection of the ureter can be performed at the same time as removal of the stent. The ureter and intrarenal collecting system can be inspected as noted above, both for unilateral hematuria and for the elusive calculus. Again, all residual fragments larger than 1 to 2 mm are removed or fragmented further. This should be performed as atraumatically as possible in the dilated ureter to avoid the need for postoperative stenting. In this way, the patient can be relieved of the stent and assured of a stone-free collecting system.

The Submucosal Calculus

There is another small group of patients who show radiographic evidence of a calculus and may have obstruction, but in whom endoscopy has demonstrated no stone within the ureter. They have usually undergone some previous lithotripsy for a ureteral stone, but they fail to clear fragments or may have relief of symptoms followed by recurrent obstruction. Endoscopy may indeed demonstrate a portion of the calculus within the lumen or obstruction with intact mucosa. Placement of an indwelling ureteral stent for a few weeks may result in resolution of the mucosal edema at the level of the calculus or erosion of the stone through to the lumen, so that subsequent ureteral endoscopy can recognize the calculus.

For the truly submucosal calculus, the ureteral lumen remains free of stone even on repeat endoscopy. It may be possible to determine the location of the calculus with different radiographic views, such as lateral or oblique, with simultaneous endoscopy. More often, this is unfruitful. Endoluminal ultrasonography has located these stones extremely accurately and permitted their grouping into categories.[6] The three groups are those that frequently cause strictures; those that can be observed; and others that have a single or only a few very superficial (less than 3 mm) calculi within the substance of the ureteral wall, and should be treated by endoscopic removal of the fragments. Stones deeper than 4 mm can be left in place without obstruction or reaction. Multiple fragments embedded within the wall of the ureter are a major problem and have been associated with long-term stricturing in some patients.

Endoluminal Ultrasound

Endoluminal ultrasound in the ureter has been performed with ultrasound transducers mounted in catheters of 3.5, 4.8, or 6.2 Fr. size. The transducers rotate 360 degrees at 30 revolutions per second. They have an ultrasonic frequency of 12.5 or 20 MHz and a cross-sectional view with a penetration of 1.5 to 2 cm. The larger probe can be passed cystoscopically or percutaneously into the ureter and renal collecting system using either a round-tip probe or over a guidewire model. The smaller probes can be passed through endoscopes with an appropriate channel. By combining endoscopic visualization with the ultrasonic view, it is possible to see both within the lumen and deep to the surface.[8] Thus, with endoluminal ultrasound, another dimension is added to endoscopic diagnostic imaging.

Summary

In summary, rigid and flexible ureteroscopy has been extremely successful in extending endoscopic diagnostic techniques into the upper collecting system. Techniques combined with the use of cytopathological evaluation can often provide a diagnosis of lesions requiring biopsy. The combination of endoluminal ultrasound with ureteral endoscopy offers another dimension that has proved particularly useful in patients with submucosal calculi.

Editorial Comment
Louis Kavoussi

This chapter demonstrates the various ways in which ureteroscopy has markedly broadened the urologist's ability to diagnose pathological conditions of the upper urinary tract. Although this procedure is useful, significant injury can occur if caution is not exercised. A safety wire is crucial, all manipulations should be performed under direct vision, and excessive force should be avoided when passing instruments. Most important, all surgeons must realize their limitations and the shortcomings of available equipment.

REFERENCES

1. Abdel-Razzak OM, Ehya H, Cubler-Goodman A, Bagley DH. Ureteroscopic biopsy in the upper urinary tract. Urology 44:451, 1994.
2. Chaubal A, McCue PA, Bagley DH, Bibbo M. Multimodal cytologic evaluation of upper urinary tract urothelial lesions. J Surg Pathol 1:31, 1995.
3. Bian Y, Ehya H, Bagley DH. Cytologic diagnosis of upper urinary tract neoplasms by ureteroscopic sampling. Acta Cytol 1995 (in press).
4. Low RK, Moran ME, Anderson KR. Ureteroscopic cytologic diagnosis of upper tract lesions. J Endourol 7:311, 1993.
5. Bagley DH, Allen J. Flexible ureteropyeloscopy in the diagnosis of benign essential hematuria. J Urol 143:549, 1990.
6. Kumon H, Tsugawa M, Matsumura Y, Ohmon H. Endoscopic diagnosis and treatment of chronic unilateral hematuria of uncertain etiology. J Urol 143:554, 1990.
7. Grasso M, Goldberg BB, Liu JB, Bagley DH. Submucosal calculi: Endoscopic and endoluminal ultrasonographic diagnosis and treatment options. J Urol 153:1384, 1995.
8. Bagley DH, Liu JB, Goldberg BB. The use of endoluminal ultrasound of the ureter. Semin Urol 10:194, 1992.

Chapter 6

Therapeutic Ureteroscopy

Roland N. Chen and Louis R. Kavoussi

Advances in fiberoptic technology have allowed for the development of small rigid and flexible endoscopes that can be passed transurethrally into the upper urinary tract. Adequate-sized working channels have made these instruments useful for both the diagnosis and treatment of upper urinary tract pathology. Neoplasms, ureteral and renal calculi, arteriovenous malformations, caliceal diverticula, and strictures have all been successfully approached ureteroscopically. This chapter discusses ureteroscopic techniques for the management of these lesions, ureteroscopic management of upper tract foreign bodies such as displaced ureteral stents, and standard retrograde ureteroscopy and percutaneous antegrade techniques.

PATIENT PREPARATION

All patients must be free of infection and able to tolerate general or regional anesthesia. Because bleeding can affect visualization, coagulopathies should be corrected. For rigid ureteroscopy, patients must be able to tolerate a modified dorsal lithotomy position. The ipsilateral lower extremity is straightened and lowered and the contralateral lower extremity is raised and abducted at the hip. This allows the eyepiece of the ureteroscope adequate room to swing under the contralateral leg during endoscopy. Flexible ureteroscopy, however, can be performed with the patient supine. Occasionally, simultaneous percutaneous antegrade and retrograde ureteroscopic access is necessary, in which case patients can be positioned prone, using a table on which the legs can be split (Fig. 6–1).

Endoscopy of the urinary tract is a clean, not sterile procedure, and thus patients should receive a broad-spectrum antibiotic 1 hour before surgery. Normal saline irrigation is used for routine ureteroscopic procedures to reduce the risk of electrolyte abnormalities in the event of ureteral perforation. Normal saline can also be used during electrohydraulic lithotripsy (EHL). Glycine or water is needed only when electrocautery is being used.

Radiographs pertaining to the pathologic condition should be available in the operating room, which should be equipped with fluoroscopy equipment capable of taking hard copies. The surgeon should have direct control over the operation of the fluoroscopy unit and positioning of the operating table. Retrograde ureteropyelography may be useful in select cases in which preoperative studies fail to demonstrate pathology adequately. This study also provides a "road map" of the ureter, allowing one to anticipate areas of ureteral narrowing or tortuosity that may impede passage of the ureteroscope.

All equipment, including endoscopes, cameras, and light sources, should be checked before initiation of the procedure. In addition, the surgeon should be certain that all accessory equipment such as ureteral catheters, guidewires, stents, dilators, graspers, and stone baskets is readily available.

On occasion, patients have a nephrostomy tube in place before ureteroscopy. For ureteroscopic management of stones, the nephrostomy tube should be clamped to prevent proximal stone migration. For management of fixed lesions such as upper tract tumors and arteriovenous malformations, the nephrostomy tube should be left open to drainage, providing for continuous irrigation to facilitate visualization.

INSTRUMENT SELECTION AND URETERAL ACCESS

The choice of endoscope is based on the location of the lesion and the goals of the surgeon. For example, flexible deflectable ureteroscopes provide the greatest access to the entire collecting system; however, only a limited number of accessories will pass through their relatively small working channels. Rigid ureteroscopes cannot reach all portions of the upper

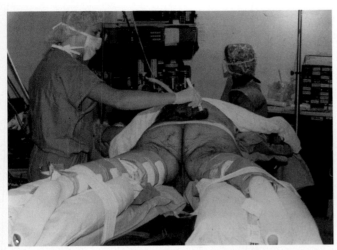

Figure 6–1. Prone position for simultaneous percutaneous and retrograde ureteral access. Note the split position of the legs to allow room for the surgeon.

itate use of the flexible ureteroscope when treating pathology above the iliac vessels. The ureteral access sheath should first be passed over the working wire (Fig. 6–3). The flexible ureteroscope can then be advanced through the sheath under direct vision. It is important not to pass the sheath over the iliac vessels, as this may result in stricture formation.

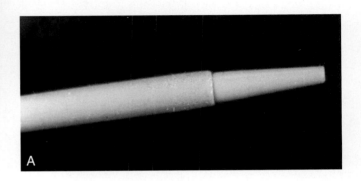

A

urinary tract. On the other hand, rigid endoscopes provide superior optics, possess larger working and irrigation channels, and allow for intraureteral resection and cold knife incision. Remember that more than one endoscope may be required to accomplish a given task. In general, if the pathology is in the distal ureter, a rigid ureteroscope should be used. For lesions above the iliac vessels, the flexible deflectable ureteronephroscope is preferred.

Once the patient is adequately anesthetized, cystoscopy is performed and a floppy-tip guidewire coiled in the renal pelvis. When a miniureteroscope (less than 7.2 Fr. distal tip) is used, no further manipulation of the ureteral orifice may be necessary. The endoscope can be advanced alongside the guidewire, which is secured to the glans or the labia minora with a 2-0 silk suture. When passage of a larger endoscope is required, one must dilate the ureteral orifice to obtain access. An 8/10 Fr. Amplatz coaxial dilation set, containing two tapered dilators that are 8 and 10 Fr., is needed to pass a second "working wire" (Fig. 6–2A). The 8 Fr. dilator is first passed over the floppy-tip wire into the orifice. The 10 Fr. dilator is then passed over the 8 Fr. dilator, and the latter is removed. This allows passage of a second Super Stiff wire through the lumen of the 10 Fr. dilator (Fig. 6–2B). The 10 Fr. dilator is removed and the initial safety wire secured to the glans or the labia minora with a 2-0 silk suture. A balloon dilator can then be passed over the super-stiff wire to dilate the ureteral orifice. A 5-mm balloon is usually sufficient to allow ureteral access.

For approaching pathology above the iliac vessels, a flexible ureteroscope is recommended. The flexible endoscope can be difficult to pass directly into the ureteral orifice, and it may be cumbersome to perform maneuvers that require repeated passage of the endoscope. Placement of a ureteral access sheath can facil-

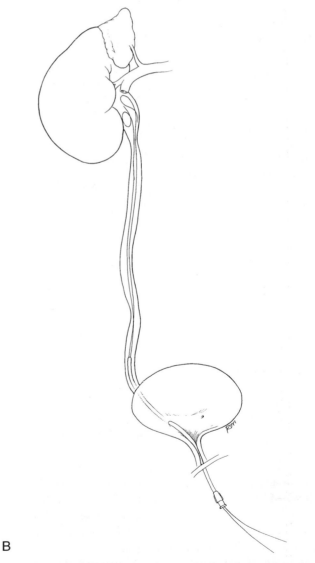

B

Figure 6–2. *A,* Tapered 8/10 Fr. Amplatz dilator. *B,* Diagram demonstrating that two wires can be passed once the 8 Fr. dilator is removed.

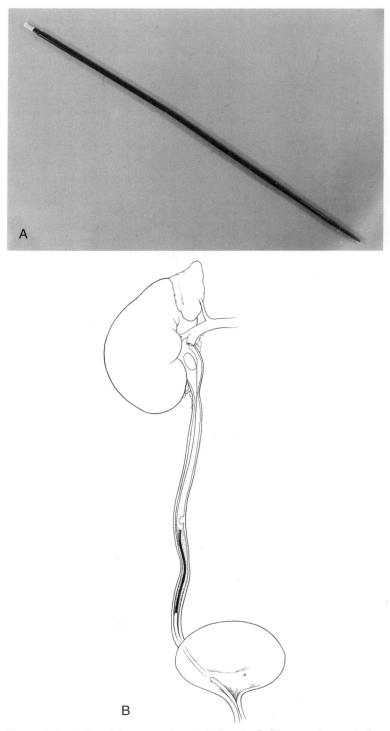

Figure 6–3. *A,* Tip of the ureteral access sheath. *B,* Diagram demonstrating passage of the flexible ureteroscope through the access sheath.

Fluoroscopy is helpful in negotiating tortuous regions of the ureter. If difficulty in passing the endoscope is encountered, contrast material should be injected into the irrigation channel and fluoroscopy utilized to assess the area of obstruction. Any narrow segments of the ureter may be dilated with a 5-mm balloon dilator. Pressurized irrigation separates the ureteral lumen, providing adequate visualization.

URINARY CALCULI

Ureteroscopy remains a useful adjunct for management of urinary calculi, particularly distal ureteral stones. Impacted stones and Steinstrasse may require endoscopic management. Stones in patients in whom extracorporeal shock wave lithotripsy (ESWL) is contraindicated or has failed may require endoscopic removal. Ureteroscopic management is also indicated when upper tract calculi are associated with distal anatomical obstruction. In such a setting, the obstructing lesion can be simultaneously approached.

Once the ureteroscope has been advanced under both direct vision and fluoroscopy to the level of the stone, the calculus can be directly extracted or managed by intracorporeal shock wave lithotripsy (ISWL). A number of stone baskets and graspers are available for the manipulation of upper urinary tract calculi, including single and double round wire spiral baskets and flat wire baskets that range in size from 1.7 to 4.5 Fr. Basket selection is based on the size of the working channel, the size of the stone, and personal preference. To engage smaller stones, a basket with more wires may be necessary. Many urologists prefer flat wire baskets for stone manipulation because they can open to a greater degree in the ureter for stone manipulation.

Once the stone is in view, a basket is advanced over the guidewire beyond the stone and opened. The basket is slowly withdrawn toward the ureteroscope while being gently twisted or manipulated back and forth under direct vision until the stone is engaged; this may require several passes of the basket. Once captured, the stone is pulled against the tip of the ureteroscope. The stone, basket, and ureteroscope are then slowly withdrawn together as a unit under both direct vision and fluoroscopy. If resistance is met while the stone is being extracted, it is critical to stop withdrawing the instrument in order to avoid ureteral injury or avulsion. If binding between the stone and ureteral mucosa occurs, one of the methods of ISWL should be performed to break the stone into smaller fragments before extraction. Most baskets are designed so that the handle can be detached, allowing the ureteroscope to be removed while leaving the stone and basket in situ (Fig. 6–4). The ureteroscope can then be passed alongside the basket and the stone fragmented. Alternatively, when using a ureteroscope with two separate working channels, a laser or EHL probe can be passed through the second channel. A side-arm adapter is used for continuous irrigation.

Because of the possibility of basket entrapment in the ureter, some surgeons prefer to use graspers; both three- and four-pronged versions are available. Four-pronged graspers provide a better purchase on the stone. Graspers in which the sheath retracts are preferable to prevent stone migration.

The goal of any form of ISWL is to fragment a large stone into pieces that may be removed or passed spontaneously. Energy is applied to the stone under direct vision by means of a variety of rigid, flexible, or wire transducers. Lithotripsy may be performed in situ or the stone may be secured at the end of the instrument in a basket. It may also be helpful to pass a basket above a stone before ISWL to prevent

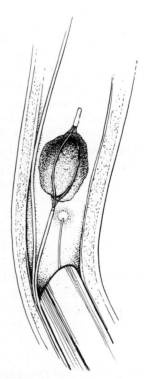

Figure 6–4. When a stone is too large to be removed via a basket or is trapped, the handle may be removed and the ureteroscope withdrawn and passed alongside the basket. Intracorporeal shock wave lithotripsy can then be used to fragment the stone.

proximal stone migration and to catch fragments. After lithotripsy, larger residual fragments should be extracted, whereas small fragments may be left to pass spontaneously. An impacted ureteral calculus that is only partially fragmented but dislodged from its position and irrigated back up into the renal pelvis can be treated with ESWL. If a nephrostomy tube is in place, proximal stones or fragments may be flushed distally. Detailed application of the available methods of ISWL is provided in Chapter 10.

ANTEGRADE URETEROSCOPY

An antegrade ureteroscopic approach may be useful in select cases. A flexible instrument is needed to obtain antegrade access to the ureter. This technique is helpful in approaching proximal ureteral calculi associated with a large renal stone burden, and when retrograde ureteroscopy is anatomically unfeasible, as in patients with urinary diversions or previous ureteral reimplantation. An antegrade approach may also be considered for impacted proximal ureteral calculi. The collecting system above the stone is often dilated, facilitating access.

Puncture of an upper or middle calix provides the best angle to gain access to the proximal ureter. Once access has been established, two guidewires are advanced down the ureter beyond the calculus. One serves as the working wire and the second as the safety wire. Once the ureteral calculus is identified, standard stone removal techniques are employed (Fig. 6–5). As with retrograde stone basketing, the endoscope, basket, and stone are removed as a unit under direct vision and fluoroscopy. After treatment of any renal calculi present, a flexible nephroscope or ureteroscope is advanced to the distal ureter to make certain that no fragments remain.

Patients with urinary diversions present a special challenge for ureteroscopy. One should be prepared to utilize both an antegrade and a retrograde approach. The patient should be positioned so that the surgeon has access to the affected side and stoma.

In patients with continent diversions, it may be necessary to place a percutaneous tract into the reservoir. This is accomplished by filling the pouch with saline through a catheter. An 18-gauge splenic needle is passed percutaneously into the reservoir and a 0.035 Fr. Bentson guidewire is coiled in the pouch. A 1-cm skin incision is made down into the fascia, a 30 Fr. balloon dilating catheter is passed over the wire and inflated, and an access sheath previously backloaded over the balloon is then slipped into the pouch.

A flexible cystoscope is usually needed to locate the ureteral orifices. A floppy-tip wire is passed into the upper tract and an 8/10 Fr. Amplatz dilator sys-

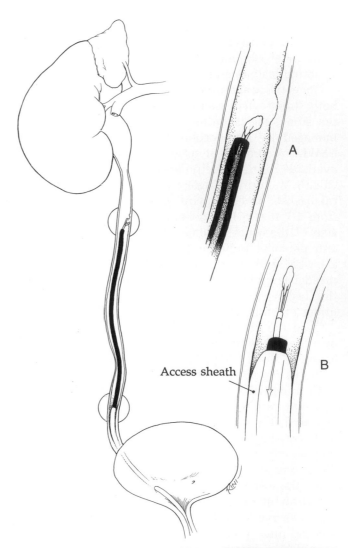

Figure 6–6. Steps used to take a biopsy. *A,* Once grasped, tissue may be pulled through the ureteroscope. *B,* Alternatively the entire ureteroscope may be removed. This will allow for larger biopsy specimens.

tem is used to place a second Super Stiff wire. A flexible ureteroscope can then be passed over the wire.

If percutaneous access has been achieved initially, an antegrade guidewire can be advanced into the conduit or pouch and grasped through a flexible cystoscope. The ureterointestinal anastomosis may be balloon dilated, providing access to the ureter for a flexible instrument or a retrograde stone basket. The stone may then be fragmented or extracted via an antegrade and/or a retrograde approach.

UPPER TRACT TUMORS

The indications for endoscopic management of upper tract transitional cell carcinoma remain controversial. Although nephroureterectomy remains the "gold standard" of therapy for these tumors, patients

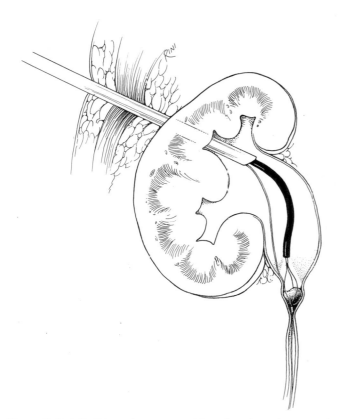

Figure 6–5. A flexible endoscope used to gain antegrade access to a ureteral stone.

with small, low-grade, noninvasive tumors, particularly when present in a solitary kidney, are reasonable candidates for endoscopic biopsy and fulguration or resection. Ureteroscopic management, compared with percutaneous management, is performed in a closed system, thus minimizing the theoretical risk of tumor spillage. The techniques for ureteroscopic management of upper tract tumors are similar to the cystoscopic management of bladder tumors, but there are some important differences. The wall of the ureter is very thin, so attempts at performing deep biopsies or resection should be avoided. In addition, because the ureter is a tubular structure, the instruments will be parallel, not perpendicular, to the wall of the ureter.

A retrograde ureteropyelogram is performed to delineate the pathologic condition. When treating tumors with a flexible ureteroscope, a ureteral access sheath should be used to facilitate tissue retrieval during repeated passage of the endoscope, which is necessary with currently available instrumentation. Upper tract tumors should be biopsied during the first pass of the ureteroscope (Fig. 6–6). The ureteroscope is advanced until the lesion is identified. A biopsy is performed with a 3 or 5 Fr. cup forceps under direct vision. The forceps are opened and ad-

vanced into the lesion until the tumor surface is deformed. The jaws are closed, and the ureteroscope and forceps are withdrawn as a unit, freeing the tumor from the ureteral wall. If a rigid ureteroscope is used, the ureteroscope lens should be removed before forceps withdrawal to provide additional room for the specimen. Otherwise, the specimen must be withdrawn through the working channel of the instrument, and portions of the specimen lying beyond the jaws of the forceps may be lost within the channel. The specimen should be immediately placed in a fixative. Ideally, five or six specimens should be obtained.

Alternatively, small lesions on a stalk may be amenable to basket extraction (Fig. 6–7A). The basket is opened and advanced adjacent to the lesion and manipulated until the tumor is entrapped within the wires. The basket is closed and the tumor is freed from the ureteral wall by avulsing the stalk. The instrument, basket, and tumor are removed together as a unit.

Fulguration of the tumor base is performed after biopsy using glycine irrigation (Fig. 6–7B). The biopsy forceps are replaced with a Bugbee electrode, and the remaining tumor and tumor base are fulgurated under direct vision.

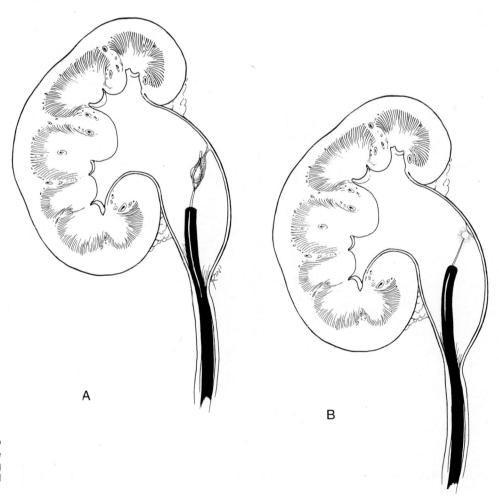

A

B

Figure 6–7. *A,* A basket may be used to remove tumors on a stalk. Care must be taken not to crush the specimen during removal. *B,* A Bugbee electrode is used to fulgurate the base.

As an alternative to biopsy and fulguration of an upper tract tumor, ureteroscopic resection may be performed with a rigid instrument (Fig. 6–8). Again, one must bear in mind that the ureteral wall is very thin, and deep bites beyond the ureteral mucosa should be avoided. The rigid ureteroscope is advanced to the level of the tumor, and the resectoscope loop is extended just beyond the tumor base. With glycine irrigation and the cutting current, the intra-luminal tumor can be resected parallel to the ureteral wall down to the level of the ureteral mucosa. The tumor base is then fulgurated with the resectoscope loop or a Bugbee electrode.

FULGURATION OF ARTERIOVENOUS MALFORMATIONS AND HEMANGIOMAS

Diagnostic ureteroscopy for essential hematuria occasionally reveals an arteriovenous malformation or hemangioma as the cause of the hematuria. These superficial mucosal lesions are usually on the tips of the renal papillae. Once access to the bleeding site is obtained via a flexible ureteroscope, the lesion can be fulgurated with a 1.9 Fr. Bugbee electrode under direct vision using coagulation current. Irrigation should be changed to glycine or water for the procedure.

FOREIGN BODY EXTRACTION

Proximal migration of ureteral stents and broken equipment such as portions of stone baskets, EHL probes, or laser fibers may require ureteroscopic management. To remove these foreign bodies, the ureteroscope is advanced until the distal end of the foreign body is visualized. A 3 Fr. biopsy or grasping forceps is manipulated until the foreign body is within the grasp of the forceps. The forceps, foreign body, and ureteroscope are removed together. Alternatively, a 3 or 5 Fr. ureteroscopic basket can be opened and advanced around the foreign body (Fig. 6–9). The basket

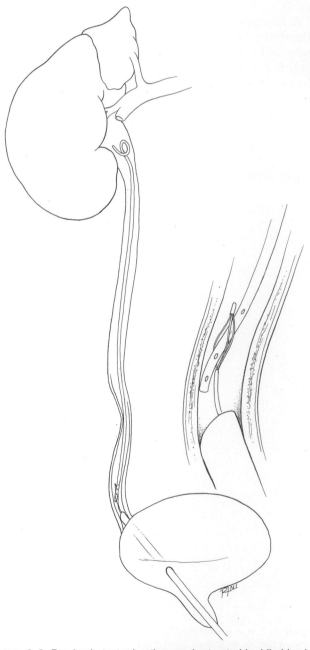

Figure 6–9. Proximal stent migration can be treated by blind basket or ureteroscopic-guided removal. A basket or grasper can be manipulated under direct vision to remove the stent.

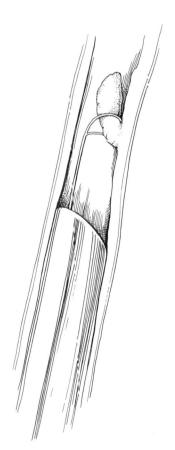

Figure 6–8. Ureteral tumors may be removed with a ureteroscopic resectoscope.

is closed, and the ureteroscope, basket, and foreign body are removed en bloc.

CALICEAL DIVERTICULA AND INFUNDIBULAR STENOSES

Although percutaneous management of caliceal diverticula and infundibular stenoses is preferable, ureteroscopic management of these lesions is feasible in select patients. A flexible ureteroscope is usually necessary to reach the intrarenal collecting system. The neck of the diverticulum or stenotic infundibulum must first be identified ureteroscopically and cannulated with a Terumo or floppy-tip guidewire (Fig. 6–10). The tip of the wire should be coiled within the diverticulum or the dilated calix. The ureteroscope is removed, and a low-profile 4-mm balloon dilator is advanced under fluoroscopic guidance until it lies across the stenotic segment. The balloon is inflated and deflated two or three times, each inflation cycle lasting 5 to 10 minutes. Alternatively, the neck may be incised using a 2 Fr. electrocautery probe or a neodymium:yttrium-aluminum-garnet or KTP laser probe. Multiple shallow radial incisions are recommended to avoid significant hemorrhage. Once access is obtained, the diverticulum or calix is inspected under direct vision. If a calculus is identified above the obstructed segment, it can be managed using the techniques described above. In the case of

a caliceal diverticulum, an attempt should be made to fulgurate the mucosal lining with a 1.9 Fr. electrode. At the conclusion of the procedure, a large (12 Fr.) double-pigtail indwelling ureteral stent is placed with the proximal end in the affected diverticulum or calix.

POSTOPERATIVE MANAGEMENT

At the end of any ureteroscopic procedure, a retrograde ureteropyelogram should be performed to determine the extent of any extravasation. If no significant ureteral injuries are noted and the ureteral orifices were not dilated, no stent may be necessary. Alternatively, a whistle-tip catheter may be placed over the safety wire and secured to the Foley catheter. The ureteral catheter can be removed the morning after surgery. If extravasation is noted on the retrograde ureteropyelogram or if the ureteral orifices are dilated, a double-pigtail stent should be placed over the safety wire and left indwelling for 1 week. For large perforations, longer drainage is advisable. Patients should be maintained on perioperative broad-spectrum parenteral or oral antibiotics for two doses. A longer course of treatment may be individualized. Foley drainage is maintained overnight. The diet is advanced on the first postoperative day as tolerated. An intravenous urogram should be obtained 6 weeks after the procedure to demonstrate resolution of the pathology and adequate ureteral healing.

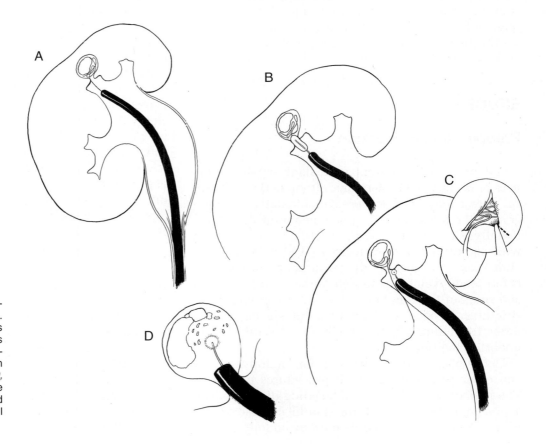

Figure 6–10. Ureteroscopic access to the caliceal diverticulum. *A,* Under direct vision a wire is passed. *B,* A low-profile balloon is used to dilate the orifice. *C,* Radial incisions are made to open the neck of the diverticulum. *D,* Once access is obtained, the stone can be fragmented and evacuated. The diverticulum wall is ablated by gentle fulguration.

Chapter 7

Endopyelotomy and Percutaneous Renal Surgery

Thomas W. Jarrett and Arthur D. Smith

Endopyelotomy has become a time-tested alternative to open pyeloplasty in the treatment of ureteropelvic junction (UPJ) obstruction with success rates of 75 to 89 percent[1-3] and lower morbidity.[4] Early skepticism concerned the durability of results, but an 8-year follow-up has shown few late failures. The procedure is based on a concept described by Davis in 1943 and Oppenheimer et al in 1955 whereby an incision through a diseased segment of ureter is followed by segmental regeneration of mucosa and smooth muscle over a stent provided that there is continuity in the region and adequate blood supply (Fig. 7–1). The chief advantages of endopyelotomy are the avoidance of open surgery and nondisruption of the ureteral blood supply.

ENDOPYELOTOMY

Preoperative Evaluation

Patients usually present with flank or abdominal pain or urinary tract infections, although the anatomical defect may be discovered incidentally on sonographic or other studies. Documentation of a functionally significant UPJ obstruction is established with an intravenous pyelogram (IVP) or a radionuclide scan. A retrograde pyelogram is performed just before endopyelotomy to determine stricture length and rule out concomitant calculus, tumor, and distal strictures. In equivocal cases a Whitaker test is performed to eliminate the possibility of a dilated but unobstructed renal pelvis.

The preoperative evaluation for endopyelotomy and other percutaneous renal procedures is similar. The patient is screened for a bleeding diathesis, and a preoperative urine culture should confirm sterile urine. Relative contraindications to endopyelotomy are renal function less than 15 percent of the total, upper ureteral and long strictures (greater than 2 cm), and small patient size (due to stent limitations). A high-inserting ureter and aberrant vessels are not contraindications.

Operative Technique

Step 1: Cystoscopy/Stent Insertion

Antibiotics are administered and, with the patient under general anesthesia in the lithotomy position, cystoscopy with retrograde pyelography is performed. An open-ended 6 Fr. ureteral catheter is advanced into the renal pelvis if possible under fluoroscopic control (Fig. 7–2). If passage into the renal pelvis is not possible, the UPJ can usually be negotiated with the aid of a cobra catheter and glidewire. It is worthwhile spending extra time maneuvering the catheter into the renal pelvis because the catheter will eventually be used to place a guidewire from the nephrostomy site to the urethral meatus. If passage into the kidney is not possible, the catheter is left in the ureter just abutting the renal pelvis. A Foley catheter is then placed and the ureteral catheter is secured to it with a silk suture.

Step 2: Renal Puncture

The patient is moved to the prone position and supportive bolsters are placed at the head, thorax, knees, ankles, and feet (Fig. 7–3). The C-arm fluoroscopy unit is brought into place from the contralateral side (Fig. 7–4) and contrast material is injected through the ureteral catheter to outline the caliceal anatomy. A posterior upper or middle pole calix is chosen (Fig. 7–5), and accurate and safe percutaneous

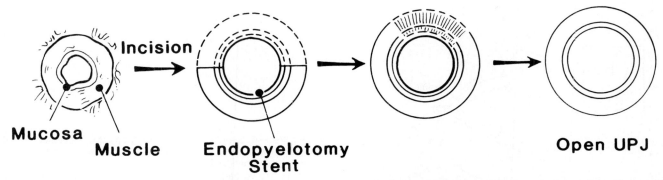

Figure 7–1. Incision through the diseased segment results in regeneration of both mucosa and muscular layers over a stent. The resultant ureteropelvic junction (UPJ) is nonobstructing and of larger diameter.

puncture is made employing fluoroscopically controlled needle manipulation with keen anatomical appreciation of the kidney and surrounding organs. The C-arm is rotated to 115 degrees and the tip of an 18-gauge diamond-tipped needle is superimposed over the chosen calix; this location should be just lateral to the paraspinal musculature and below the twelfth rib to minimize the risk of damage to adjacent organs (Fig. 7–6). The needle is advanced in the 115-degree plane directly into the desired location. This route of entry (approximating the Brödel line) provides the most direct and safest access to the posterior collecting system. Needle passage through the renal parenchyma minimizes injury to the hilar vessels and seals the nephrostomy tract from urine leakage.

Adequate depth of needle penetration cannot be assessed with a one-plane fluoroscopic view. Therefore, once the trocar needle appears properly posi-

tioned in the 115-degree view, the C-arm is rotated back to the 90-degree position (see Fig. 7–4). Using the second plane, the depth of penetration can be assessed and final positioning performed. Any difficulties in positioning can be managed by repeating the process of two-plane fluoroscopic visualization.

After adequate needle placement, the stylet is removed, and aspiration of urine and contrast from the collecting system confirms proper positioning. A

Figure 7–2. An open-ended 6 Fr. ureteral stent is advanced cystoscopically into the renal pelvis. Contrast material can be injected through the catheter to define caliceal anatomy and aid in renal puncture.

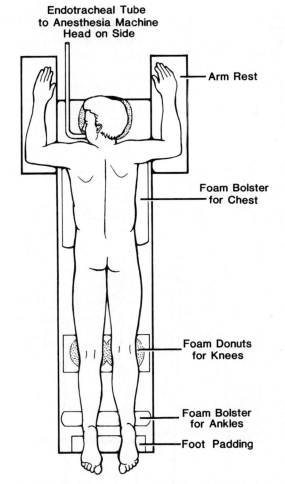

Figure 7–3. Proper prone positioning for all percutaneous procedures with foam supports at pressure points.

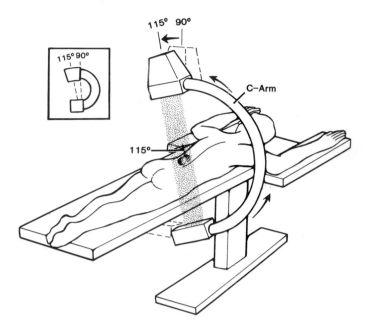

Figure 7–4. Standard C-arm fluoroscopy unit positioned from the contralateral side. The initial puncture is performed at a 115-degree inclination directly over the chosen calix; the unit is then rotated to 90 degrees to give two-plane visualization and assess the depth of needle penetration.

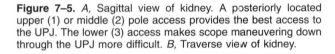

Figure 7–5. *A,* Sagittal view of kidney. A posteriorly located upper (1) or middle (2) pole access provides the best access to the UPJ. The lower (3) access makes scope maneuvering down through the UPJ more difficult. *B,* Traverse view of kidney.

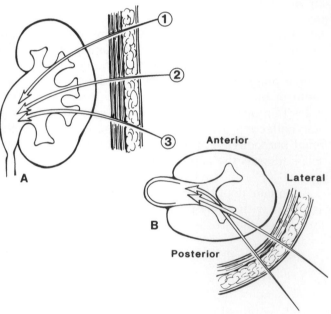

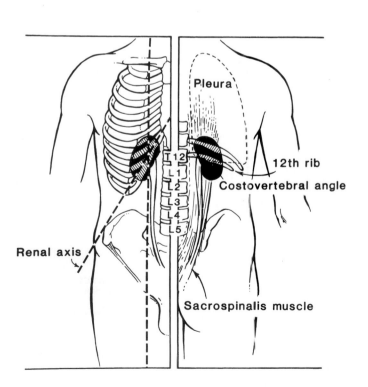

Figure 7–6. Normal position of the kidneys in a patient lying prone. Puncture is lateral to the paraspinal musculature and should be below the twelfth rib to avoid injury to the pleura.

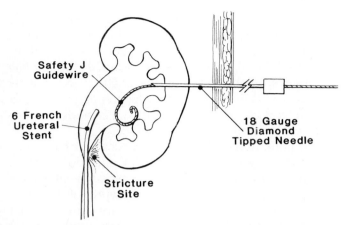

Figure 7–7. The stylet is removed from the 18-gauge trocar and a safety J-tipped guidewire is coiled in the renal pelvis.

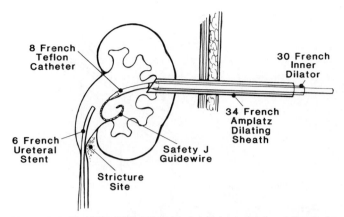

Figure 7–8. The 8 Fr. Teflon-coated sheath is passed over the J wire and the tract is sequentially dilated to the 30 Fr. inner dilator. The 34 Fr. sheath is then positioned in the renal pelvis, and the inner dilator and Teflon sheath are removed. A second (safety) guidewire can be placed through a 10 Fr. sheath, if desired, just before dilation.

0.038 safety J-tipped guidewire is advanced through the trocar and coiled in the collecting system (Fig. 7–7). Passage down the ureter is rarely possible owing to the nondependent, eccentrically located UPJ.

Step 3: Nephrostomy Tract Dilation

The initial puncture site is widened with a 1.5-cm skin incision and the tract is dilated. Dilation can be performed with fascial, metal coaxial, or balloon dilators. Our experience suggests that the disposable fascial dilators are the best: the Amplatz fascial dilator system has inner dilators of 6 to 30 Fr. and Teflon-coated outer sheaths of 28 to 34 Fr., which are left in place for nephroscopy.

Tract dilation is performed in a straight path over the guidewire with fluoroscopic assistance. Great care is essential, as misdirection may result in loss of access, kinking of the wire, or perforation of the renal capsule. Dilation begins with a stiff 10 Fr. dilator that when removed allows passage of a long 8 Fr. Teflon catheter; this catheter serves as a low-friction inner sheath that facilitates dilation by providing rigidity and protecting the guidewire from kinking. If desired, a second (safety) guidewire can be passed through a 10 Fr. sheath into the renal pelvis at this time. The larger dilators (12 to 30 Fr.) are then passed over the Teflon catheter using a twisting motion. The tract is sequentially dilated up to the 30 Fr. inner dilator, and the corresponding 34 Fr. sheath is positioned in the renal pelvis. The inner dilator is then removed, providing direct endoscopic access to the renal pelvis (Fig. 7–8).

Step 4: Endopyelotomy

Control of the renal pelvis with a guidewire is essential before incision of the stricture. This can be accomplished in three ways. First, if a ureteral catheter was successfully passed into the renal pelvis dur-

ing cystoscopy, the catheter can be grasped using the nephroscope and brought out of the nephrostomy tract (Fig. 7–9). A 0.038 torque guidewire is passed antegrade through the catheter until it emerges at the catheter's distal end (the urethral meatus). The catheter is then removed from below, leaving the guidewire in place with access from both proximal and distal ends. Second, if the catheter could not be manipulated into the renal pelvis cystoscopically, we suggest retrograde passage of a guidewire through the catheter to the point of obstruction. Nephroscopy is performed and a peanut grasper is used to bluntly dissect the UPJ, under fluoroscopic control, until the guidewire is visible. The tip of the guidewire is grasped and brought out of the nephrostomy tract. Third, as a last resort, a flexible ureteroscope is passed through a "peel-away" sheath to the point of obstruction. The light should be visible with the endopyelotome, and a cold knife incision to the light

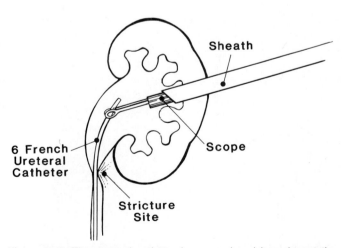

Figure 7–9. The ureteral catheter is grasped and brought out the nephrostomy tract. A 0.038-inch torque guidewire is passed through the ureteral catheter and out of the distal urinary tract; this establishes retrograde and antegrade control of the UPJ.

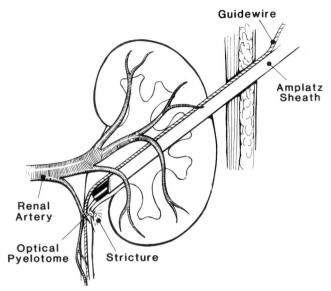

Figure 7–10. Using the endopyelotome with the hook blade, a posterolateral incision is made through the diseased UPJ. This incision avoids the renal and upper ureteral blood supply.

is performed. If the light is not visible, methylene blue is injected and the ureter is incised toward the dye. These last maneuvers run a significant risk of ureteral disruption and should be performed only as a final resort in experienced hands.

Once control of the UPJ is secured, the diseased segment is enlarged to 14 or 16 Fr. using the Amplatz fascial dilators under fluoroscopic guidance. If any renal calculi are present, they should be removed at this time. A hook-shaped cold knife (Storz) endopyelotome is used to create a posterolaterally located incision. The posterolateral approach avoids the hilar vessels and ureteral blood supply that emanates anteromedially from the basilar segment of the renal artery (Fig. 7–10). The incision is made through the diseased segment to bridge the healthy ureter at its proximal and distal ends and deep enough to reveal periureteral fat. After incision the UPJ should be wide open with a funnel-like appearance.

The hook knife allows the obstructing tissue to be lifted and inspected (especially for pulsations) before the incision. The area can be reassessed after each sweep for adequate length and depth of incision. After the initial incision, the tissue may intussuscept and distort the anatomy; further incisions should not be performed until the problem is resolved. In these cases the ureteral guidewire can be manipulated so as to straighten out any kinks. The "hot knife" is no longer used because of the high incidence of restenosis secondary to thermal injury.

Step 5: Ureteral Stenting

After endopyelotomy the area is intubated with an endopyelotomy stent. We now use a polyurethane stent that tapers from 14 Fr. in the kidney and proximal ureter to 8.2 Fr. in the distal ureter and bladder for adults, and from 10 to 5 Fr. for children. The stent is advanced over the torque guidewire until the proximal drainage holes are within the renal pelvis, with the distal portion of the guidewire extending outside the bladder. A portion of the distal endopyelotomy stent usually extends beyond the bladder and into the urethra (Fig. 7–11A). To solve this problem,

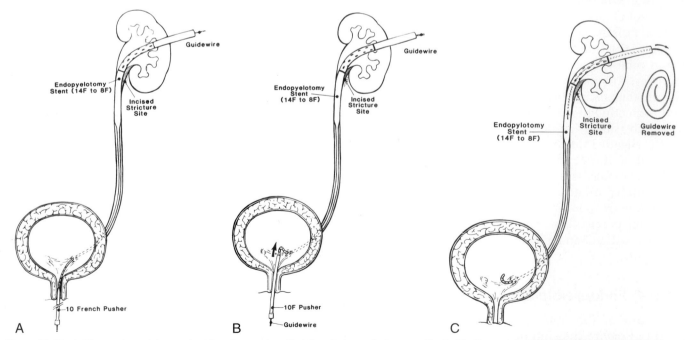

Figure 7–11. *A,* The endopyelotomy stent is advanced so that the drainage holes are situated in the renal pelvis. Usually the distal portion of the stent extends into the urethra; a 10 Fr. dilator can be fashioned into a pusher and used to push the distal stent back into the bladder *(B).* The distal stent will then coil in the bladder *(C)* when the guidewire is removed.

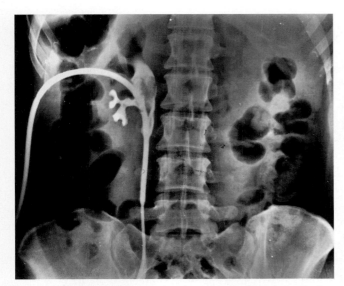

Figure 7–12. Postoperative nephrostogram showing proper stent position and no extravasation.

the nephrostomy tube and the Foley are placed to gravity drainage.

Postoperative Management

A hematocrit is drawn in the recovery room and a chest radiograph obtained if a supracostal access was used. A nephrostogram is obtained 48 hours postoperatively to ensure proper stent placement and urinary drainage, assess extravasation, and ensure complete removal of all calculus if present preoperatively (Fig. 7–12). The stent is clamped overnight, and if this is tolerated without leakage, the patient is discharged the next morning with the stent capped under a sterile dressing, with instructions on how to open the nephrostomy in the event of stent failure. Antibiotics are continued throughout the hospitalization.

The patient returns in 4 to 6 weeks for a nephrostogram and stent removal and then returns 3 months later. At this time, symptoms are reassessed and an IVP is obtained and compared with the preoperative study to identify improved drainage and definition of the renal contour (Fig. 7–13). If there is no improvement, a diuretic renal scan is obtained to permit a more precise assessment of renal function and urinary drainage.

a pusher can be fashioned by cutting off the distal end of the 10 Fr. dilator from the Amplatz set. The pusher is used in a retrograde fashion to place the distal stent into the bladder (Fig. 7–11B). The guidewire is then removed and the distal portion of the stent should curl in the bladder (Fig. 7–11C). The stent is then secured at the nephrostomy site with a silk suture. A Foley urethral catheter is inserted, and

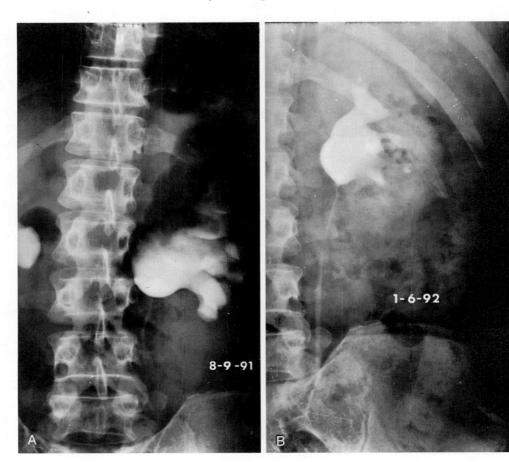

Figure 7–13. A, Preoperative and B, postoperative intravenous pyelogram (IVP) showing a good result.

Postoperative Complications

The immediate complications of endopyelotomy are essentially those of all nephroscopic procedures and are primarily related to the percutaneous access. Venous bleeding is the most common immediate complication and can usually be managed by temporarily clamping the nephrostomy tube. This allows the bleeding to tamponade; the nephrostomy is unclamped the following morning and will drain urine when all clot in the tube has lysed. Persistent bleeding despite this maneuver is usually arterial. In these cases the hematocrit should be followed closely and selective arterial embolization performed if bleeding persists.

Late complications are more common and usually related to stent movement. Stents frequently migrate and require repositioning with fluoroscopic assistance at a later date. Other more serious complications, including strictures of the ureterovesical junction, were seen before the advent of the latest 14/8.2 Fr. tapered endopyelotomy stents, but have not been a problem recently.

The most common long-term complication of endopyelotomy has been failure to achieve adequate patency of the UPJ. In our latest series, we report a 15 percent failure rate.[2] Failures should be treated by open pyeloplasty, which is not associated with greater morbidity than pyeloplasty de novo[4]; repeat endopyelotomy is usually unsuccessful and not recommended. Failures are most frequently due to angulation of the UPJ that prevents adequate drainage and not to a small strictured lumen.

PERCUTANEOUS APPROACH TO CALICEAL DIVERTICULUM

Preoperative Evaluation

A caliceal diverticulum is a nonsecretory, urothelium-lined cystic cavity within the renal parenchyma that usually communicates with the renal pelvis or a calix through a narrow channel. It is usually seen as an incidental finding on IVP. If it is suspected, delayed films may be necessary to allow retrograde filling of the diverticulum with contrast from the adjacent collecting system (Fig. 7–14). In some cases retrograde pyelography, computed tomography (CT), and renal sonography can help differentiate these diverticula from renal cysts, abscesses, hydronephrosis, or neoplasms.

No treatment is needed for asymptomatic patients, but intervention is required for pain, recurrent urinary tract infection, symptomatic calculi, gross hematuria, or progressive renal damage. When intervention is necessary, the percutaneous approach is the procedure of choice, as it has the highest success rates with the least morbidity to the patient.[6] The only exception is with anteriorly located diverticula, which are difficult to reach percutaneously and may be best approached laparoscopically.

Operative Technique

Step 1: Cystoscopy and Nephrostomy Tract

A ureteral catheter is placed, the patient is moved to the prone position, and direct needle puncture to the caliceal diverticulum is performed (Fig. 7–15A); contrast medium may be injected through the ureteral catheter to aid in localization. A safety J-tipped guidewire is coiled within the diverticulum (Fig. 7–15B) and the tract is dilated to accommodate a 34 Fr. sheath, using the Amplatz fascial dilating system. A subcostal approach is preferred because of the lower complication rate.

Step 2: Stone Extraction

The 26 Fr. nephroscope is passed into the diverticulum and the stone is extracted. If the calculi are too large to pass through the sheath, lithotripsy is required before removal (Fig. 7–16). The ultrasonic lithotripsy is preferable, but other forms such as electrohydraulic and laser lithotripsy are acceptable.

Step 3: Fulguration of Diverticular Wall

The diverticular wall and neck should be well visualized at this time; blue dye infused through the ureteral catheter can help localize the narrow neck. Once this is done, a guidewire is negotiated through the neck and into the main collecting system (preferably down the ureter) with the aid of fluoroscopy. If a communication through the neck cannot be established, one should proceed directly to fulguration. The caliceal lining is completely fulgurated using low current through the nephroscope or a resectoscope (Fig. 7–17).

Step 4: Dilation of Diverticular Neck

The diverticular neck is dilated over the guidewire to size 30 Fr. using the Amplatz system (Fig. 7–18). If access to the ureter has not been previously established with an antegrade guidewire, continuity with the normal collecting system is established by blunt dissection. The ureteral catheter is identified, grasped with the nephroscope, and exchanged for a guidewire.

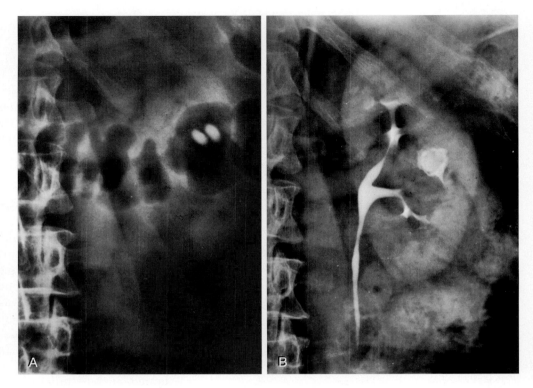

Figure 7–14. *A,* Scout and *B,* delayed film from an IVP showing a caliceal diverticulum of the middle calix with two symptomatic calculi. (From Jarrett TW, Smith AD. Percutaneous treatment of calyceal diverticuli. In Smith AD, ed. Controversies in Endourology. Philadelphia, WB Saunders, 1995, p 153.)

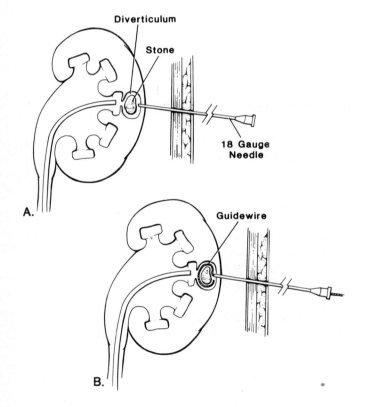

Figure 7–15. *A,* A ureteral catheter is placed and a direct puncture into a caliceal diverticulum is performed under fluoroscopic guidance. *B,* A 0.038-inch J-tipped guidewire is then coiled in the diverticular cavity. (From Jarrett TW, Smith AD. Percutaneous treatment of calyceal diverticuli. In Smith AD, ed. Controversies in Endourology. Philadelphia, WB Saunders, 1995, p 154.)

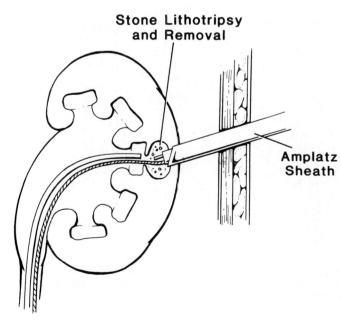

Figure 7–16. Stone lithotripsy and removal using the ultrasonic lithotripsy device. (From Jarrett TW, Smith AD. Percutaneous treatment of calyceal diverticuli. In Smith AD, ed. Controversies in Endourology. Philadelphia, WB Saunders, 1995, p 155.)

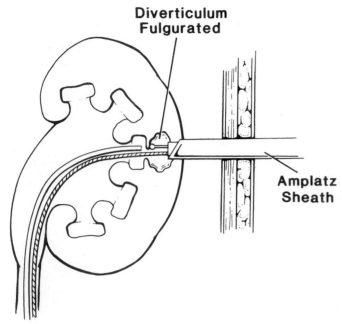

Figure 7–17. Fulguration of the diverticular cavity. (From Jarrett TW, Smith AD. Percutaneous treatment of calyceal diverticuli. In Smith AD, ed. Controversies in Endourology. Philadelphia, WB Saunders, 1995, p 155.)

At the conclusion of the procedure, a 24 Fr. nephrostomy re-entry tube is passed through the diverticulum with its dilated neck and down the ureter. A nephrostogram should confirm proper positioning.

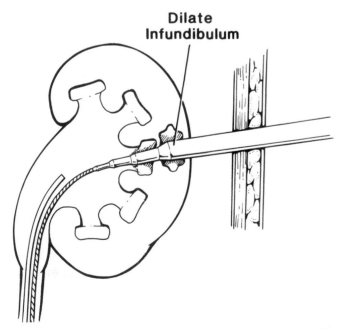

Figure 7–18. The neck of the diverticulum is identified and dilated to size 30 Fr. over a guidewire. (From Jarrett TW, Smith AD. Percutaneous treatment of calyceal diverticuli. In Smith AD, ed. Controversies in Endourology. Philadelphia, WB Saunders, 1995, p 156.)

Certain modifications may be necessary for anteriorly located diverticula. Direct puncture in these cases is usually possible, but because of the acute angle of the nephrostomy tract and calix, endoscopic vision is limited and safe access to the diverticular neck is not possible. In these patients the diverticular lining is fulgurated but the neck cannot be dilated. For these reasons, the laparoscopic approach may be more useful.

Postoperative Management

Immediate care is similar to that for all percutaneous procedures and is outlined above. A nephrostogram is performed 48 hours postoperatively and the nephrostomy tube is removed if there is no evidence of retained stones, extravasation, or obstruction. The patient is discharged when flank drainage has ceased and returns 3 months postoperatively for follow-up. At this time evaluation is made for persistence of symptoms, and an IVP and urine culture are obtained. If the studies show obliteration of the diverticular cavity, no further follow-up is necessary. If the cavity persists, the patient returns in 6 months for repeat IVP and retrograde pyelography to further evaluate the anatomy.

Postoperative Complications

Postoperative bleeding should be treated as with any percutaneous procedure; early bleeding should be controlled by clamping the nephrostomy tube; delayed arterial bleeding may necessitate arterial embolization. Persistent extravasation may require ureteral catheter placement to facilitate nephrostomy tract closure. Failure to obliterate the cavity should be treated with a repeat percutaneous approach only if there is persistence of symptoms.

PERCUTANEOUS MANAGEMENT OF TRANSITIONAL CELL CARCINOMA

Transitional cell carcinoma (TCC) involves the upper urinary tract in 5 to 10 percent of cases.[7] The tendency of upper tract TCC toward multifocality and recurrence has led to nephroureterectomy with a cuff of bladder as the "gold standard" treatment. In some patients the morbidity of radical surgery and the loss of renal function may increase the risk due to chronic renal failure and hemodialysis and lower the quality of life to unacceptable levels. In these cases, organ-sparing therapy may be considered as an alternative to radical surgery.

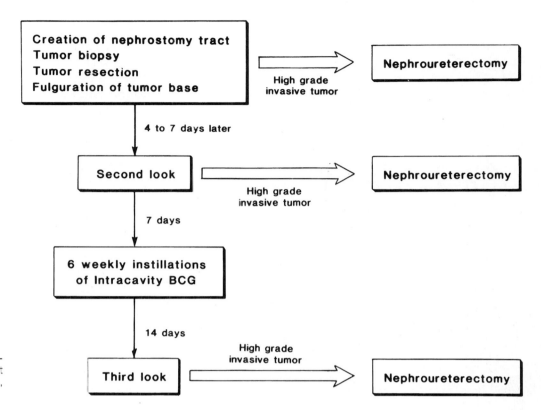

Figure 7–19. Protocol for percutaneous treatment of upper-tract transitional cell carcinoma. BCG, bacille Calmette-Guérin.

Preoperative Evaluation

Diagnosis is based on characteristic radiological findings as well as cytological study of the urine. The tumors are usually seen as a filling defect on an IVP or retrograde ureteropyelogram. In some cases a CT scan, ultrasonography, selective cytology, or ureteroscopy may be needed to establish the diagnosis. Patients initially selected for endourological management had one or more of the following indications: solitary kidney, chronic renal insufficiency, bilateral disease, or increased risk of morbidity or mortality from a major open surgical procedure. Recently, selected informed patients with two normal kidneys and without major comorbidities who wish to avoid radical surgery have been included as candidates for percutaneous management. All patients are impressed with the necessity of vigilant follow-up. As with any percutaneous procedure, preoperative evaluation should confirm sterile urine and rule out any bleeding diathesis.

Operative Technique

Our approach to treating TCC of the upper urinary tract is represented in Figure 7–19.[7] Although there were minor variations, all cases incorporated the principles of complete resection followed by second-look nephroscopy with repeat resection and fulguration of the tumor base, and finally a third-look nephroscopy to confirm the absence of tumor. Technically unresectable, high-grade, or invasive disease prompted immediate nephroureterectomy with a cuff of bladder if the patient was medically fit.

Step 1: Cystoscopy and Nephrostomy Tract

A ureteral catheter is placed, the patient is moved to the prone position, and needle puncture to the desired calix is performed as outlined in the previous section. The percutaneous approach to upper tract TCC is similar to that for renal calculi (Fig. 7–20). Tumors in the upper ureter or renal pelvis must be approached via an upper or middle pole access so that the endoscope can be maneuvered into the pelvis and through the UPJ as needed. If the tumor is in a peripheral calix, direct puncture is performed. The tract is dilated with Amplatz fascial dilators and the 34 Fr. sheath is left in place. Nephroscopy is performed with the 26 Fr. endoscope and the ureteral catheter is grasped, brought out of the nephrostomy tract, and exchanged for a torque safety guidewire. Any suspicion of upper ureteral involvement warrants flexible antegrade ureteroscopy at this time.

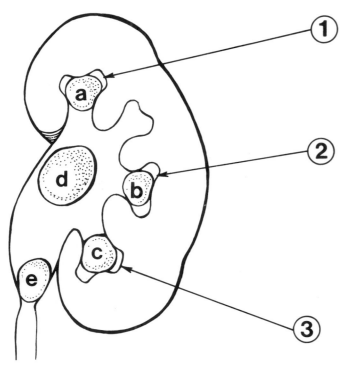

Figure 7–20. Points a, b, and c represent single tumors in peripheral calices; these are best approached by direct puncture to the diseased calix. Points d and e are tumors in the renal pelvis and upper ureter; an upper (1) or middle (2) pole approach is necessary for the surgeon to gain access to these tumors safely.

Step 2: Tumor Resection

After the collecting system is inspected and the location of the TCC noted, cup biopsy forceps or a cutting loop of a resectoscope are used to resect the tumor burden (Fig. 7–21). A Bugbee electrode through the nephroscope or a resectoscope is then used to coagulate bleeding and fulgurate the base. A pyeloscope is preferable to a standard resectoscope, which has a long beak and is more difficult to maneuver in the limited space of the renal pelvis. A 24 Fr. nephrostomy tube is placed and the correct position confirmed with an intraoperative nephrostogram.

Step 3: Second Look

Nephroscopy with resection of residual disease and random biopsies is performed 4 to 7 days later. Old and new tumor sites are fulgurated with electrocautery or the neodymium:YAG laser.

Step 4: Intracavitary Bacille Calmette-Guérin

In an effort to further reduce recurrences, since 1988 we have given six weekly instillations of intracavitary bacille Calmette-Guérin (BCG); therapy is begun 1 to 2 weeks after the second look if hematuria has resolved.

The patient is admitted and intravenous antibiotics are administered. Infusion of 0.9 percent normal saline with a pressure monitoring system (set to limit the maximum allowable pressure to 25 cm H_2O) is then begun at a rate of 10 ml/hr and gradually increased to 50 ml/hr. Next, 50 ml containing 1×10^8 colony forming units of BCG is infused over 1 hour.

Patients are instructed to void the bladder 1 hour after completion of the infusion, at which time the

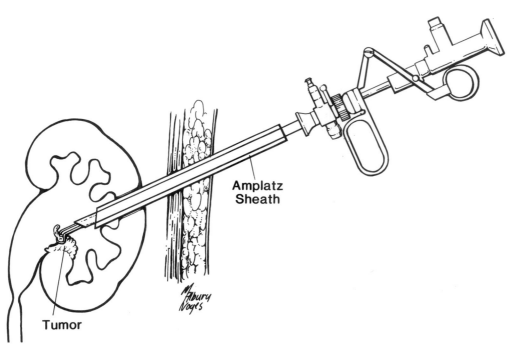

Figure 7–21. Percutaneous resection of tumor in the renal pelvis with a pyeloscope.

nephrostomy tube is clamped. They are closely monitored for any adverse effects; if there are none, they are discharged the next day. A chest radiograph and SMA-18 are obtained every other week to rule out systemic effects.

Step 5: Third Look

Nephroscopy with random biopsies is performed 1 to 7 days after the final BCG therapy. The nephrostomy tube is removed several days later.

Follow-up

Vigilant follow-up is imperative. Patients are evaluated every 3 months for the first year, every 6 months for the next 4 years, and then yearly. Follow-up visits consist of history taking and physical examination, urine cytology, and either IVP or retrograde ureteropyelography (more or less aggressive follow-up may be chosen, depending on the grade and stage of tumor). Other tests such as ureteroscopy are performed when clinically indicated. Patients unwilling or unable to conform to rigorous follow-up should not be considered for this form of treatment.

PERCUTANEOUS APPROACH TO SIMPLE RENAL CYSTS

Preoperative Evaluation

The presence of a simple renal cyst should be confirmed with ultrasonography or CT and the patient should be symptomatic; most cysts are incidental findings and require no further treatment. Ideal candidates for percutaneous surgical therapy are patients with large, peripheral, posteriorly located cysts. Anteriorly located cysts can be treated with laparoscopic excision.

Operative Technique

There are two approaches to renal cysts, both of which begin with direct puncture into the cyst cavity (intraoperative sonography may be helpful in cyst localization). Aspiration of clear fluid and injection of a contrast medium should confirm the proper position within the cyst wall. The tract is dilated with Amplatz dilators and a sheath positioned in the cyst cavity. There are two options at this time. First, with blunt dissection, internal drainage can be established by providing continuity with the renal collecting system. In this case, an endopyelotomy stent is left passing through the cyst and down the ureter for several weeks to ensure proper drainage. Second, a resectoscope is used to either resect or fulgurate the cyst wall (Fig. 7–22). In this case, a drain is left in the obliterated cyst cavity and removed when drainage has ceased.

In our experience, we have not performed this procedure in conjunction with other percutaneous procedures (e.g., percutaneous stone extraction) owing to excessive postoperative bleeding. In these cases, the cyst cavity fills with blood and does not tamponade, causing prolonged bleeding.

INFUNDIBULAR STENOSIS

The approach to infundibular stenosis is similar to that for a caliceal diverticulum in that direct punc-

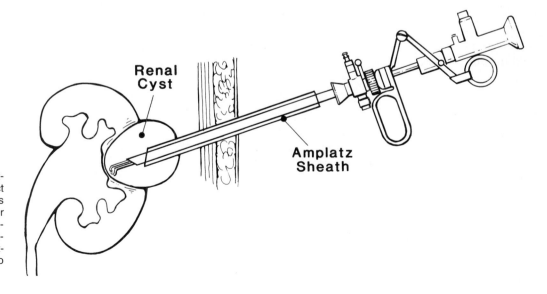

Figure 7–22. Percutaneous obliteration of a renal cyst. Direct puncture into the cyst cavity is performed, and the wall is either fulgurated or resected with a resectoscope. Alternatively, communication with the renal collecting system can be established to provide internal drainage.

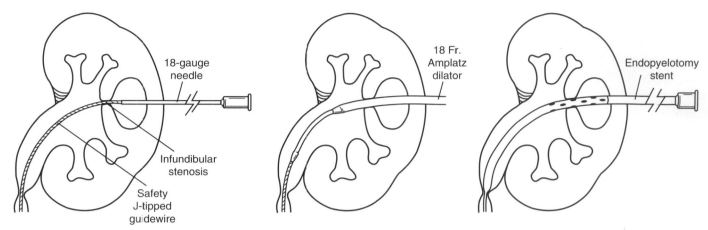

Figure 7–23. Percutaneous treatment of infundibular stenosis. A ureteral catheter is placed and direct puncture to the dilated calix is performed; a guidewire is then passed through the stenotic infundibulum and down the ureter. The infundibulum is dilated to size 16 to 18 Fr. with the Amplatz dilating system, and an endopyelotomy stent is passed through the infundibulum and down the ureter.

ture to the dilated calix is performed (Fig. 7–23) and a nephrostomy tract established. A guidewire is passed through the narrowed infundibulum and the stenotic segment is dilated to size 16 to 18 Fr. with the Amplatz dilating system. A 14/8 Fr. endopyelotomy stent is placed across the stenotic segment with the drainage holes positioned in the dilated infundibulum. The stent is subsequently removed after several weeks.

An IVP should be obtained after 3 months to document patency of the infundibulum.

Summary

The percutaneous nephrostomy tract has allowed access to the kidney in much the same way as the urethra to the bladder. Endourologic manipulations within the kidney have decreased the morbidity of most surgical procedures in the kidney. As a result, open stone surgery, nephrostomy, and pyelostomies have become outmoded surgical procedures. We hope that the procedures outlined in this chapter will similarly lead to greater general acceptance and benefit to all our patients.

Editorial Comment
Fray F. Marshall

The versatility of percutaneous renal surgery is well demonstrated in this chapter. Not only can endopyelotomy be performed, but endoscopy can be used to treat TCCs and caliceal diverticula. Cutting to the light is probably not advisable if a guidewire cannot be passed. There have been reports of tumor seeding of the tract, particularly with high-grade TCCs.

REFERENCES

1. Cassis AN, Brannen GE, Bush WH, et al. Endopyelotomy: Review of results and complications. J Urol 146:1492, 1991.
2. Motola JA, Badlani GH, Smith AD. Results of 221 consecutive endopyelotomies: An 8 year follow-up. J Urol 149:453, 1993.
3. Wickham JEA, Kellet MJ. Percutaneous pyelolysis. Eur J Urol 9:122, 1983.
4. Karlin GS, Badlani GH, Smith AD. Endopyelotomy versus open pyeloplasty: Comparison in 88 patients. J Urol 140:476, 1988.
5. Motola JA, Fried R, Badlani GH, et al. Failed endopyelotomy: Implications for future surgery. J Urol 150:821, 1993.
6. Bellman GC, Silverstein JI, Blickensderfer S, Smith AD. Technique and follow-up of percutaneous management of calyceal diverticula. Urology 42:21, 1993.
7. McCarron JP, Mills C, Vaughan ED. Tumors of the renal pelvis and ureter: Current concepts and management. Semin Urol 1:75, 1983.
8. Sweetser PM, Jarrett TW, Weiss GH, Smith AD. Percutaneous approach. In Smith AD, ed. Controversies in Endourology. Philadelphia, WB Saunders, 1995, p 193.

Chapter 8

Percutaneous Nephrolithotomy

Michael L. Blute and Joseph W. Segura

The first percutaneous nephrostomy tract made for the specific purpose of removing a stone was established by Fernström and Johannson in 1976.[1] In the late 1970s, Smith and co-workers[2] in the United States and Alken and colleagues[3] in Germany began to remove stones in occasional patients. By the early 1980s, percutaneous nephrolithotomy (PL) was a standard procedure in the urological armamentarium.[4-8] It remains an important procedure in the management of surgical stone disease despite the pervasive role of extracorporeal shock wave lithotripsy (ESWL).

INDICATIONS

Who is a Candidate?

Because of the ubiquity of ESWL, the usual choice involves whether a given clinical situation can be managed by ESWL. The problem was addressed in 1988 at the National Institutes of Health (NIH) Consensus Conference on the Management of Stone Disease.[9] In general, patients with noncystine stones 2.0 cm or smaller in unobstructed collecting systems whose anatomy permits focusing on the stones are candidates for ESWL. We analyzed the kind of patient who underwent PL during the first year the shock wave machine was at the Mayo Clinic (Table 8–1).[10] Almost half the patients underwent PL because of a large volume stone, an indication that has become more common. Percutaneous nephrolithotomy is also used as a rescue procedure when other modalities fail to achieve stone removal.

Generally, PL is preferred in the following situations:

1. In the presence of obstruction, so that spontaneous passage of fragments is not likely.
2. For large stones, alone or combined with ESWL.
3. When the certainty of stone removal is important.

4. For cystine stones.
5. For patients whose body habitus precludes ESWL.
6. For other modality failures.
7. In children until the issue of long-term safety is settled.
8. In certain other miscellaneous situations.

Contraindications

Uncontrolled bleeding diathesis is the only absolute contraindication to PL. Some patients have anatomical abnormalities so that percutaneous access is not possible. Also, PL should not be performed in the presence of infection. It is also important to assess accurately the likelihood that a given problem can be solved with percutaneous surgery. Some stones are so large or the renal anatomy is so complicated that the stones cannot be removed by any reasonable number or combination of PL and ESWL procedures.

OPERATIVE TECHNIQUE

PL may be divided into two parts: access and stone removal. Where in the hospital these procedures are performed and by whom are products of the local situation and are not particularly germane to the final results. The methods outlined subsequently have worked well at the Mayo Clinic in 2600 patients, however.

The patient is admitted in the morning and is started on prophylactic intravenous (IV) antibiotics. Cephalosporin is usually chosen unless the stone is known to be an infected stone, in which case selection is predicated upon culture and sensitivity results. The radiologist performs percutaneous access in the radiology department using IV sedation and local anesthesia. These provide sufficient pain control except for the occasional patient with an obstructing ureteral stone in whom significant pain is often present as the guidewire passes by the stone.

TABLE 8–1. Indications for Percutaneous Techniques in 143 Patients

	No. (%)
Obstruction	23 (16)
Ureteral, 4	
Ureteropelvic junction, 14	
Infundibular, 5	
Stone Volume	66 (46)
Large pelvic stone volume, 17	
Staghorn, 18	
Combined ESWL and percutaneous, 31	
Body Habitus	10 (7)
Pt. too large, 7	
Pt. too small, 1	
Scoliosis, 2	
Other Modality Failures	21 (15)
Ureteroscopic failures, ureteral stones, 4	
ESWL failures	
Stone did not break, 3	
Retained significant fragments, 12	
Hemorrhage after ESWL, 1	
Hypotension in bath, 1	
Miscellaneous	23 (16)
Cystine, 11	
Cardiac pacemaker, 4	
Calcified renal artery aneurysm, 1	
Indwelling nephrostomy tube, 3	
Pt. requested percutaneous removal, 4	

From LeRoy AJ, Segura JW, Williams HJ Jr, Patterson DE. Percutaneous renal calculus removed in an extracorporeal shock wave lithotripsy practice. J Urol 138:704, 1987.

The technique of establishing the percutaneous access tract has been described by LeRoy and colleagues.[11] In a typical case, access is under the twelfth rib and through the lower pole calix, but the exact access point may not be important unless the target stone is in a particular calix or a special approach is preferred for some anatomical reason. Supracostal approaches may be employed if necessary, although we have tried to avoid them because of the risk of pleural injury. Honey[12] described a supracostal upper pole technique wherein a thoracoscopy is purposely performed in order to place a transpleural upper pole approach under direct vision using a flexible instrument to make sure that the lung is uninjured. We have not performed this, but there are certainly occasional cases when this would be appropriate.

We prefer the Cope Introducer system. In brief, with the patient in the prone position, a 22-gauge needle is passed through the posterior axillary line into the appropriate calix. After access is assured, the guidewire is wiggled down the ureter, an angiographic catheter is passed over the wire, and the patient is brought to the endourology room, where the remainder of the procedure is performed utilizing general anesthesia.

A urinary catheter is left indwelling. After induction of anesthesia, the patient is turned to the prone position and prepared and draped, using standard surgical sterile technique. It is impossible in these procedures to maintain strict sterile technique, and experience has shown that "starting out sterile and finishing up clean" generates no untoward result.

A guidewire is placed down the angiographic catheter and the catheter is discarded. The tract is dilated to a 24 Fr. diameter, employing flexible fascial dilators. Concentric steel dilators or the Amplatz system are preferred if dense scar tissue surrounds the kidney or if the tract is unstable because it traverses long stretches of retroperitoneal fat. At some point during the procedure, a second safety guidewire is placed down the ureter to maintain access in case the original wire is inadvertently damaged or removed. When a 24 Fr. diameter is reached, the Wolf nephroscope is introduced into the collecting system, with the nephroscope's sheath providing the insulation between the tract and the retroperitoneum. All procedures are carried out through this instrument (Fig. 8–1).

Storz nephroscopes are size 28 Fr., as are the newer Wolf instruments. Many urologists prefer to use these instruments through an Amplatz sheath. This technique works as well as using the nephroscope sheath to tamponade the flank, but there is less hydrostatic distention and somewhat more bleeding when the Amplatz sheath is used, albeit less risk of extravasation.

Methods of Power Lithotripsy

The simplest way to take out a stone is simply to grab it with a basket or forceps and directly extract it. This maneuver has the virtues of speed and efficiency, but many stones are too large for this method. When the stone is too large for extraction through the 24 Fr. sheath, we prefer some form of power lithotripsy to break the stone up into more manageable

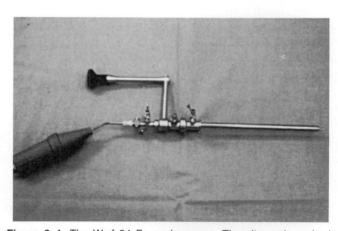

Figure 8–1. The Wolf 24 Fr. nephroscope. The ultrasonic probe is seen placed through the working channel. Any instrument that is about the same size as the probe, such as a forceps or basket, can also be used through the working channel.

fragments. Our personal preference is the ultrasonic probe because it rapidly removes pieces of stone as they are created and is, at least theoretically, effective for all stones (Fig. 8–2). The systems marketed by different manufacturers all vary slightly, but none of these dissimilarities are important in regard to their ability to break up and remove stone. Pressure must be exerted on the stone by the probe, or nothing is likely to happen. Too much pressure, however, may inadvertently result in a pelvic perforation if the probe slips off the stone or pokes through the stone.

Some stones are so large and hard that ultrasound cannot be expected to destroy them in a reasonable length of time. These stones are usually made of calcium oxalate monohydrate and are best managed with electrohydraulic lithotripsy. The probe is positioned adjacent to a crack or some other irregular point on the stone, and fired. Broken-off fragments can be extracted or further reduced with the ultrasonic probe.

The Swiss Lithoclast is a new device that uses compressed air and causes a probe to strike the stone rapidly and sharply. This is a very effective rapid method of stone destruction, but the pieces, once broken off, must be manually removed. A current modification of this device, called the Lithovac, can aspirate the fragmented pieces. At this writing, the Swiss Lithoclast is not approved for use in the United States.

The pulsed dye laser in the past has been limited in power, but new modifications raising the upper

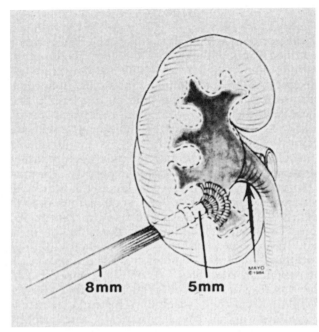

Figure 8–3. The nephroscope approach through the lower pole of the kidney. The first maneuver is to remove enough stone so that space is left for an indwelling nephrostomy tube if the procedure has to be aborted.

limit of power available to 125 millijoules has considerably broadened the spectrum of stones that may be broken up by the coumarin dye laser. The laser has no advantage over ultrasound or electrohydraulic lithotripsy for breaking up the average stone or the typical large stone in the renal pelvis, but when used through a flexible instrument it can have great utility in going after stones that cannot be seen directly with the rigid instrument.

Stone Removal

Exactly what is done next depends entirely on the characteristics of the stone. Below, we discuss the use of PL in several common situations.

Large Stones

The major advantage of PL in the treatment of large stones is rapid removal of easily accessible stony material. The ultrasonic probe should be selected for the most efficient removal, inasmuch as the probe removes the particles as they are created. Because most large stones fill the collecting systems in which they lie, the first maneuver for the surgeon is to remove enough stones so that if the procedure must be aborted, sufficient room is available for a nephrostomy tube (Fig. 8–3).

Every effort should be made to remove as much stone as possible (Fig. 8–4). First, it may be possible

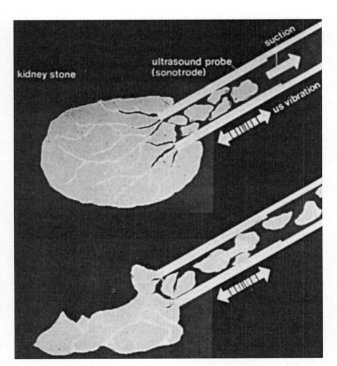

Figure 8–2. The ultrasonic probe batters the stone into small pieces. Suction is used to remove fragments, and aspiration moves them up the lumen so that the pieces are removed as they are created.

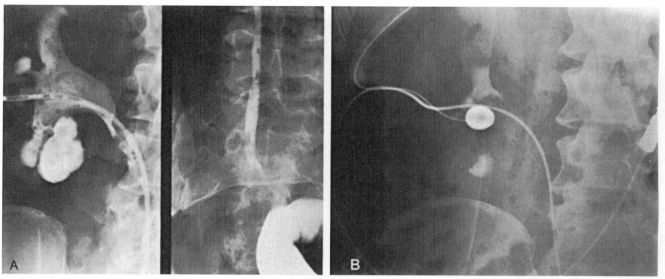

Figure 8–4. *A,* Infected staghorn in a paraplegic patient with an ileal conduit. Note the dilated lower pole calices. The broken fragments after extracorporeal shock wave lithotripsy (ESWL) are unlikely to pass. *B,* Considerable stone was removed after the first percutaneous nephrolithotomy (PL). Alternatives at this point were to repeat the PL or to perform ESWL, followed by percutaneous removal of fragments. In this case, we chose ESWL and percutaneous removal of the fragments.

to remove all the stone in one procedure. Second, if another procedure is necessary, either PL or ESWL, the amount of residual material that requires treatment will be smaller. Patients with staghorns, or stones with pieces difficult to reach, are good candidates for ESWL combined with PL. Once all possible material has been removed via PL, ESWL removes the stone located in places difficult or dangerous to reach. We learned that we could not depend upon broken-up stone to pass spontaneously.[13] It is essential that a last procedure be performed to ensure that all residual material is removed. This last procedure may be a second percutaneous maneuver utilizing the ultrasonic probe or the flexible instrument to examine all the collecting system, or it may be a simple irrigation of the collecting system through the nephrostomy tube. This last procedure cannot be omitted if a stone-free status is to be expected.

Use of PL followed by ESWL and then another percutaneous procedure has been called a sandwich technique or combined treatment. The literature examined by the American Urological Association Lithotripsy Committee revealed an overall stone-free rate of 82 percent, which is approximately the same rate achievable by open surgery. The committee determined that this in fact was the procedure of choice.

Prophylactic irrigation of the collecting system with hemiacidrin (Renacidin) has been advocated in the past but has not been our practice, mainly because of the extra in-hospital days required. While such irrigations may improve the stone-free rate, it should be possible to obtain the same stone-free rates by direct inspection of the collecting system.

Small Stones

Today, PL for a stone smaller than 2.0 cm is not a common practice. PL is usually performed when ESWL is contraindicated for some reason or is unavailable. Often, stones coexist with an obstructive uropathy that precludes ESWL, which can be managed percutaneously at the same time as removal of the stones (Fig. 8–5). These are, in fact, very straightforward cases with short operating times. When we used PL for a wide variety of cases, the shortest case consumed 6 minutes "skin to skin." If the stone is small enough, it is usually grasped and extracted. Larger stones are broken up with the ultrasonic probe and the pieces extracted.

Cystine Stones

Most patients with cystine stones have had multiple procedures, and most benefit greatly from a less invasive procedure. Cystine stones respond poorly to ESWL. Occasionally, small stones fracture into small pieces after ESWL, but this is not a consistent response. Our practice has been not to use ESWL in the treatment of cystine stones.

Most cystine stones that have failed medical therapy are large and obstructive and require surgery. Because they are large, considerable time may be needed to break them up, and repeat sessions are common. The ultrasonic probe is particularly useful because the pieces are removed as they are created, a process that seems to go faster after the shell of the stone is broken through.

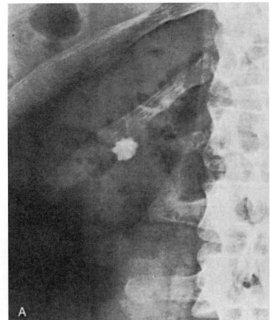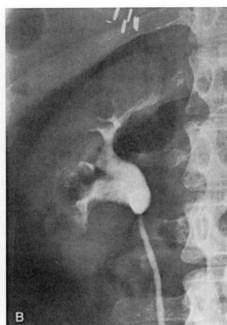

Figure 8–5. *A,* A jackstone-type calculus made of calcium oxalate monohydrate is evident. This type of calculus usually forms in an obstructive medium. *B,* Note the partial ureteropelvic junction (UPJ) obstruction. This patient should undergo percutaneous stone removal and endopyelotomy.

Many observers have noted that some cystine stones respond better to PL than others. Work by Bhatta and associates[14] suggests two varieties of cystine stone, a rough and a smooth, that vary in hardness. This possibility may explain the variability in response to PL. We find it useful to employ electrohydraulic lithotripsy to break off pieces of the stone, which are then further reduced with ultrasound.

Follow-up of these patients has demonstrated that medical therapy cannot be relied on to dissolve residual fragments. If the patient is to be rendered stone free, this task must be accomplished at the time of the original percutaneous procedure.[15]

Obese Patients

All too frequently, patients are of such configurations that maneuvering them into the focal point of the machine is not possible. Most such patients are obese, but scoliosis or some other abnormality may make such maneuvering impossible. These individuals may be good candidates for PL, because as long as access to the kidney can be achieved, removal of the stone is likely.

Ideally, the nephroscope traverses the distance to the stone. When this maneuver is possible, the stone is removed in the usual manner. Usually, however, the instrument is just barely long enough to reach the collecting system, resulting in limited therapeutic options. Two "tricks" will optimize the situation. In the first, an incision is made in the skin about 2.0 to

3.9 cm long. It is then possible to push the haft of the instrument an additional 1.0 to 2.0 cm into the flank, and this distance may be enough to accomplish the task. A second trick is simply to mature the tract for a few days with an indwelling 24 Fr. nephrostomy tube, after which access with flexible instruments is less difficult and the task can be accomplished.

Children

It is clear that ESWL in children is safe, at least in the short term. However, the long-term safety of ESWL in children has not been demonstrated, and so we have preferred to use PL in most children with stones.

Smaller instruments have been developed for these situations, but the difference in Fr. sizes is not great. We have been more confident using instruments with which we are most comfortable. Scrupulous care must be taken to avoid extravasation because of the risk of fluid overload in small young patients. Otherwise the techniques are the same.

POSTOPERATIVE MANAGEMENT AND COMPLICATIONS

Direct inspection and radiographical control will establish that the collecting system is free of stone. A nephrostomy tube should remain indwelling, and a removable stent is left down the ureter. This combination ensures tamponade of the tract to minimize the risk of postprocedure bleeding and permits reaccess to the collecting system, if necessary. Our practice is to obtain a radiograph and nephrostogram at 48 hours. If all is well, the stent is removed and the nephrostomy tube clamped in the morning. If the patient tolerates this, the nephrostomy tube is removed that evening, the patient leaves the hospital the next day, and the average individual returns to normal activity in about 1 week.

When PL was performed for a broader spectrum of patients, the significant complication rate was only 3 percent. This figure is higher in the group now forming the bulk of the patient load.[10]

Summary

PL is effective in the treatment of a wide variety of kidney and ureteral stones. The indications for PL are today restricted to particular situations in which appropriate management is impossible without it. PL remains safe and practical and is an integral part of an armamentarium that ensures safe, expeditious, and economical stone removal.

Editorial Comment
Fray F. Marshall

PL remains an important technique in the management of upper urinary tract calculi. Large stones, cystine stones, and anatomical obstructions are common indications for the use of this technique. With a large stone, we have not hesitated to use a large sheath, up to 26 to 28 Fr., because it facilitates removal of large fragments. We have also increasingly employed the electrohydraulic lithotrite with larger stones because this probe and the larger sheath allow more rapid extraction of abundant calculous material. Fortunately, the back-up of ESWL is always available when percutaneous procedures leave fragments behind. Hemiacidrin (Renacidin) irrigation or chemolysis of infected calculi remains another adjunct in management. Chemolysis can also be employed with cystine calculi.

REFERENCES

1. Fernström I, Johannson B. Percutaneous pyelolithotomy. A new extraction technique. Scand J Urol Nephrol 10:257, 1976.
2. Smith AD, Reinke DB, Miller RP, Lange PH. Percutaneous nephrostomy in the management of ureteral and renal calculi. Radiology 133:49, 1979.
3. Alken P, Hutschrenreiter G, Günther R, Marberger M. Percutaneous stone manipulation. J Urol 125:463, 1981.
4. Segura JW, Patterson DE, LeRoy AJ, et al. Percutaneous lithotripsy. J Urol 130:1051, 1983.
5. Segura JW, Patterson DE, LeRoy AJ, et al. Percutaneous removal of kidney stones: Review of 1000 cases. J Urol 134:1077, 1985.
6. Brannen GE, Bush WH, Correa RJ, et al. Kidney stone removal: Percutaneous versus surgical lithotomy. J Urol 133:6, 1985.
7. Reddy PK, Hulbert JC, Lange PH, et al. Percutaneous removal of renal and ureteral calculi: Experience with 400 cases. J Urol 134:662, 1985.
8. White EC, Smith AD. Percutaneous stone extraction from 200 patients. J Urol 132:437, 1984.
9. NIH Consensus Conference. J Urol 141:804, 1989.
10. LeRoy AJ, Segura JW, Williams HJ Jr, Patterson DE. Percutaneous renal calculus removal in an extracorporeal shock wave lithotripsy practice. J Urol 138:703, 1987.
11. LeRoy AJ, May GR, Bender CE, et al. Percutaneous nephrostomy for stone removal. Radiology 151:607, 1984.
12. Honey J. Personal communication.
13. Segura JW, Patterson DE, LeRoy AJ. Combined percutaneous ultrasonic lithotripsy and extracorporeal shock wave lithotripsy for struvite staghorn calculi. World J Urol 5:245, 1987.
14. Bhatta KM, Prien EL Jr, Dretler SP. Cystine calculi—rough and smooth: A new clinical distinction. J Urol 142:937, 1989.
15. Knoll LD, Segura JW, Patterson DE, et al. Long-term follow-up in patients with cystine urinary calculi treated by percutaneous ultrasonic lithotripsy. J Urol 140:246, 1988.

Chapter 9

Endoscopic Management of Ureteral Strictures and Fistulas

Asim F. Durrani and Glenn M. Preminger

Recent advances in endourological techniques have revolutionized the management of stones, soft tissue lesions, and obstructive processes within the ureter. However, the expanded role of endoscopic manipulation of the urinary tract has significantly increased the number of iatrogenic injuries to the ureter, with a resultant overall increase in the incidence of strictures and fistulas of the ureter.

Nonetheless, most ureteric lesions, whether naturally occurring or iatrogenic in origin, can be successfully managed by endoscopic means. Improved fiberoptic endoscope design combined with enhanced endoscopic instrumentation can now successfully treat most ureteric lesions via a minimally invasive endoscopic approach.[1] It is the goal of this chapter to review endoscopic techniques for the management of strictures and fistulas within the ureter.

ETIOLOGY OF URETERAL STRICTURES

Ureteral strictures may be classified as having an intra- or extraluminal cause. Strictures caused by intraluminal pathology are amenable to endoscopic surgery, but the latter is not appropriate for extraluminal pathology. A brief synopsis of some intraluminal causes of ureteral stricture formation follows.

Intraluminal Ureteral Strictures

POSTINSTRUMENTATION. Iatrogenic ureteral injury after endoscopic manipulation is currently the most common cause of ureteral stricture formation.[2-4] Anatomically the proximal ureter and renal pelvis are the least well supported portions of the ureter and thus are more prone to injury and perforation. Another key factor in the cause of endoscopic injury to the ureter is the size and flexibility of the endoscope used during ureteroscopy.[5] Significant mucosal injury with urinary extravasation after ureteral perforation may cause ureteral wall fibrosis that could induce stricture formation.[6]

The risk of ureteric injury is increased by poor endoscopic technique, if care is not taken to dilate the ureter when such a need exists, or if endoscopy is continued with poor visualization.

STONES. Ureteral stones, if present for a prolonged period, may result in injury to the mucosal lining of the ureter, and in due course fibrosis, even after stone removal, may cause stricture formation.

INFECTIONS. Fungal infections can induce ureteral strictures, especially infection with *Coccidioides immitis*. Ascending or opportunistic fungal infections in patients on long-term antibiotics, or in immunosuppressed or immunocompromised patients, may cause fungal ball formation in the ureter, the most common causative agent being *Candida* or *Aspergillus*. *Schistosoma haematobium* infestation in some parts of the world results in ureteral stricture formation; however, results from endoscopic management of such strictures are unsatisfactory.[7, 8] Ureteral stricturing may also result from genitourinary tuberculosis. Most tuberculous strictures occur in ureteropelvic or vesicoureteral junctions and rarely respond well to endoscopic techniques.

PREOPERATIVE EVALUATION

Appropriate preoperative evaluation is imperative not only to assess the severity of the problem, but also to select the appropriate treatment. Moreover, it is important both to determine the extent and location of a particular ureteral stricture or fistula and to fully assess the functional capabilities of the affected system.[9] Therefore, appropriate renal function studies may also be necessary in selected cases.

An intravenous pyelogram (IVP) remains an appropriate first-line study to assess obstruction or leakage from the ureter.[10] However, in certain circumstances the extent of a ureteral stricture or fistula cannot be fully assessed after injection of intravenous contrast material. Alternative contrast studies should therefore be employed, including either retrograde or antegrade ureterograms.

Occasionally it may be difficult to assess the severity or length of a ureteral stricture, depending on the extent of the lesion. In these selected cases, a combination antegrade-retrograde study can help define the exact length of the obstruction. In select cases in which a combined antegrade and retrograde ureterogram cannot define a tight ureteral stricture, passage of a small-caliber, low-pressure ureteral dilating balloon can more exactly define the extent of obstruction.

Functional assessment of an obstructed renal unit can be performed with a furosemide (Lasix) washout renal scan. In cases in which the scan may be equivocal, a Whitaker test can fully assess the degree of function of an obstructed renal unit. If significant renal impairment is suspected, the obstruction can be treated temporarily by placement of an internal ureteral stent or a percutaneous nephrostomy tube. After decompression of the kidney, a differential renal scan should be performed to lateralize renal function.

TREATMENT OPTIONS
FOR URETERAL STRICTURES

Endourological options for the management of ureteral strictures include balloon dilation alone or endoureterotomy with or without balloon dilation. Ureteral incision can be performed with a hot or cold knife, electrocautery, or various forms of laser energy. Additionally, a recently introduced "hot wire" device has also been used to incise ureteral strictures. After ureteral incision and/or dilation, the ureter is stented for approximately 4 to 6 weeks. Animal and clinical studies are currently under way to better determine the appropriate size of ureteral stent as well as the ideal length of time the stent should remain in place.

General Considerations

Proper selection of appropriate patients for endourological management is important. Reported results of endourological management of short ureteral strictures are encouraging, with success rates ranging from 65 to 85 percent patency at 6 months.[11] However, long ischemic strictures have responded poorly to endourological management and often require open surgical repair (ureteroureterostomy, transureteroureterostomy, or ileal-ureter replacement).[12] Moreover, ischemic strictures secondary to radiation therapy have also fared poorly with an endourological approach.

As noted previously, appropriate functional assessment studies should be performed before initiating endourological management. It is often helpful to decompress an obstructed collecting system by placement of either an internal ureteral stent or a percutaneous nephrostomy tube. Once the functional status of the affected side has been determined, appropriate endourological management may be initiated.

Before beginning balloon dilation or incision of the ureteral stricture, it is helpful to again perform a gentle retrograde ureterogram or an antegrade ureterogram (if a percutaneous nephrostomy tube is in place) to further document the location and extent of the ureteral stricture. However, gentle injection of contrast is often insufficient to accurately delineate the extent of the ureteral stricture. It is often better to place a low-pressure ureteral dilating balloon across the presumed area of obstruction and identify a definitive waist by gentle inflation of the balloon. Depending on the length of the stricture, various management options are available.

Balloon Dilation

Balloon dilation alone of a ureteral stricture is without question the most straightforward of all the endourological approaches. However, the results of ureteral dilation alone have been uniformly marginal.[9, 13, 14] A standard high-pressure ureteral dilating balloon (usually 6 mm—18 Fr. in the dilated state) is the preferred device for ureteral dilation. As stated, with gentle inflation of the balloon one should document a short waist of the ureter delineating the ureteral stricture. However, with full inflation the balloon should fully expand and the waist should disappear (Figs. 9–1 and 9–2). It is recommended that the balloon remain inflated for approximately 5 minutes. After deflation and removal of the balloon, a repeat ureterogram should be performed to document patency as well as the integrity of the dilated ureteral segment. A 7/14 Fr. endopyelotomy stent or standard 7 or 8 Fr. internal ureteral stent is then placed over the safety guidewire.

Endoscopic Incision

Various methods of endoscopic incision of ureteral strictures have been described. A "cold" Collings

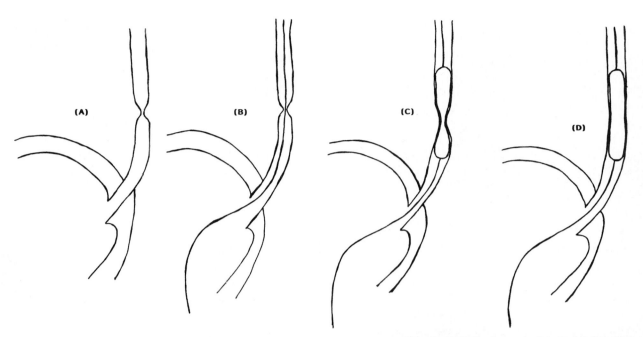

Figure 9–1. *A,* Short, smooth stricture in the distal ureter. *B,* After retrograde ureterography, a guidewire is manipulated past the stricture. *C,* A standard high-pressure balloon is passed over the guidewire and gently inflated. Note the waist at the site of the stricture. *D,* Full inflation of the balloon with disappearance of the waist.

knife can be used with a rigid ureteroscope.[15, 16] However, most ureteroresectoscopes are still quite large, measuring approximately 10 to 12 Fr. in diameter. If one wants to use a smaller-caliber, semirigid ureteroscope or flexible ureterorenoscope, flexible fibers must be utilized to incise the ureter. Electrocautery probes measuring 2.5 to 3.0 Fr. in diameter as well as 300- to 600-micron laser fibers can be used with semirigid and flexible ureterorenoscopes.[17] Studies have suggested that incision of the ureter with small (less than 3 Fr.) electrocautery probes, along with incision with neodymium:yttrium-aluminum-garnet laser fibers, produces the least amount of postoperative reaction to surrounding ureteral tissue.[18]

It is important to remember the position of the ureteral blood supply before initiating an incision of the ureteral stricture.[19] For strictures in the distal third of the ureter, the blood supply is primarily from the lateral position, and therefore the incision should be directed anteromedially (Fig. 9–3). For the middle and proximal ureter, a posterolateral or straight lateral incision is preferred to avoid damage to ureteral vasculature. When performing ureteral incision, it is important to obtain a through-and-through incision of the ureteral mucosa for approximately 1 cm above and below the stricture site. One should see fat through the incised ureter, denoting a full-thickness incision. As with all endourological procedures, a safety guidewire should be in place at all times to allow access to the renal collecting system should problems arise.[1]

Incision of ureteral strictures may be performed through either a retrograde or an antegrade approach, depending on the location of the stricture and whether or not a percutaneous nephrostomy tube has been placed to decompress an obstructed collecting system. An antegrade approach with a semirigid or flexible ureteroscope often provides better access to proximal and middle ureteral strictures than does a retrograde approach. Before beginning the incision, it is again helpful to accurately delineate the length of the ureteral obstruction. One useful technique is to pass a low-pressure ureteral dilating balloon across the strictured area. Gentle inflation will again demonstrate a waist denoting the ureteral stricture. This area may be marked on the fluoroscopy screen with a grease pencil. Marking the length of the stricture helps identify the site and length of incision once the ureteral dilating balloon has been removed.

After successful incision of the ureter, a ureteral dilating balloon should again be placed over the safety guidewire and gently inflated. If the incision has been appropriately incised, it should be possible to inflate the balloon to its full profile at low pressures (less than 1 atmosphere) with no evidence of a residual waist. Moreover, a retrograde ureterogram should also demonstrate extravasation, denoting a full-thickness incision through the ureteral wall. After confirmation of adequate incision, a 7/14 Fr. endopyelotomy stent or standard 7 or 8 Fr. internal ureteral stent is placed over the safety guidewire and positioned within the collecting system.

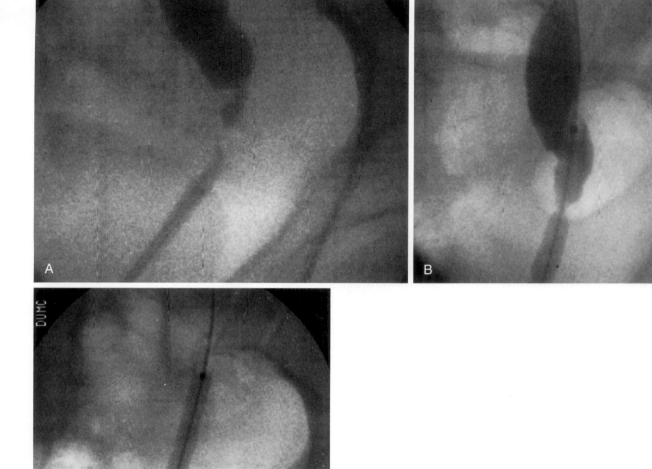

Figure 9–2. *A*, Retrograde ureterogram showing the ureteric stricture. *B*, With gentle inflation of the balloon, the waist identifies the exact extent of the ureteral stricture. *C*, Maximal inflation of the balloon will dilate the stricture and produce disappearance of the waist.

Cutting Balloon Catheter (Acucise)

Early results of endoureterotomy have been superior to those of balloon dilation alone for the treatment of ureteral strictures or ureteropelvic junction (UPJ) obstruction. However, initial techniques of endoureterotomy or endopyelotomy performed via an antegrade or a retrograde approach require the use of rigid or flexible nephroscopes or ureteroscopes and are often technically demanding.

A recently developed procedure for the treatment of ureteral strictures and UPJ obstruction utilizes an innovative ureteral cutting balloon catheter (Acucise).[20] This device may be used under fluoroscopic guidance alone, which significantly simplifies the procedure, with a concomitant reduction in operating time.

Device

The Acucise cutting balloon catheter is a 7 Fr. device incorporating both a monopolar electrocautery cutting wire and a low-pressure balloon that can be used for incising obstructions along the course of the ureter.[21] The balloon is used to define the area of stenosis and to carry the cutting wire into the area to be incised. The electrically active surface on the cutting wire is 3 cm in length. The device has radiopaque markers on the catheter body that assist in locating the position of the balloon in the cutting

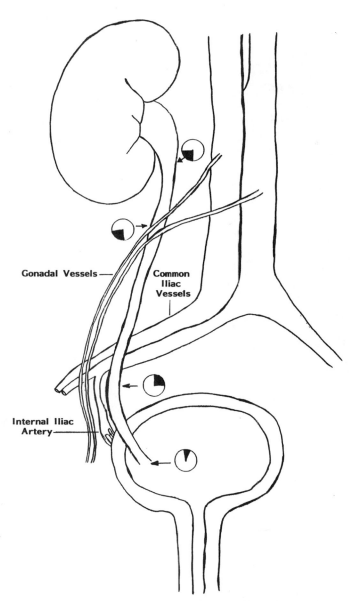

Figure 9–3. Recommended sites of ureteral incision. (Modified from Eshghi M. Endoscopic incisions of the urinary tract. Part II. Endoureterotomy. AUA Update Series, Vol 8, Lesson 38, 1989.)

Gonadal Vessels

Common Iliac Vessels

Internal Iliac Artery

wire. The position of the cutting wire, in relation to the inside guidewire, will facilitate alignment of the device in proper position before incision of the stenotic area. The profile of the balloon is 24 Fr. inflated and 13 Fr. deflated. The balloon is designed to accept a maximum of 2 ml of fluid. These Acucise cutting balloon catheters are intended for use with fluoroscopy and designed to interface with current marketed electrosurgical units.

Technique

The degree of obstruction should first be documented as being functional as well as anatomical by obtaining a furosemide washout renal scan and possibly a Whitaker test.

The Acucise cutting balloon catheter should be used only with fluoroscopy, not with static radiography. It is most easily positioned in a patient who has had an indwelling 6 or 7 Fr., standard internal ureteral stent placed for approximately 1 week before the planned endoureterotomy. Previous placement of an internal ureteral stent soft-dilates the ureter and allows easy passage of the cutting balloon catheter, as well as subsequent placement of a 7/14 Fr. endopyelotomy stent. Both the cutting wire and guidewire (located inside the catheter body) are radiopaque. Cystoscopically, the previously placed internal ureteral stent is withdrawn to the urinary meatus, and a 0.038-inch super-stiff guidewire can be passed through the internal ureteral stent and coiled within the renal collecting system, after which the stent is removed. The Acucise cutting balloon is then placed over the super-stiff guidewire. It is helpful to position the cutting wire in its correct rotational orientation before insertion. This maneuver will minimize the need for rotation of the device once it has been placed across the ureteral stricture.

Before removal of the ureteral stent and placement of the cutting balloon catheter, we have found it useful to perform a gentle retrograde ureterogram to again define the strictured area. Using fluoroscopy, the cutting balloon catheter is positioned over the super-stiff guidewire so that the stricture is within the two radiopaque markers. Only in the distal ureter is the cutting wire activated in a medial position (Fig. 9–4). In other sites along the ureter, the cutting wire should be positioned laterally. The proper position of the catheter is documented with the fluoroscope. C-arm fluoroscopy is useful to allow rotational views of the position of the cutting balloon within the ureter.

It is important not to use a safety guidewire during this procedure, as the electrical current could be transferred to the safety wire with potential damage along the course of the ureter. If one is unsure of the correct position of the balloon across the stricture, the balloon may be inflated with dilute contrast media. A waist should be demonstrated by inflation of the balloon with 2 ml of dilute contrast. The balloon is then deflated.

The cutting wire is activated at 75 to 100 watts (pure cut); simultaneously, dilute contrast is again instilled into the dilating balloon. As the balloon inflates, the stricture is incised. The waist of the stricture should be released and the balloon should now go to full inflation. The cutting wire should be activated for 5 seconds during the initial cut. If a waist is still present after instillation of 2 ml of contrast, the cutting wire may be reactivated for an additional 3 to 5 seconds. If a longer incision is required,

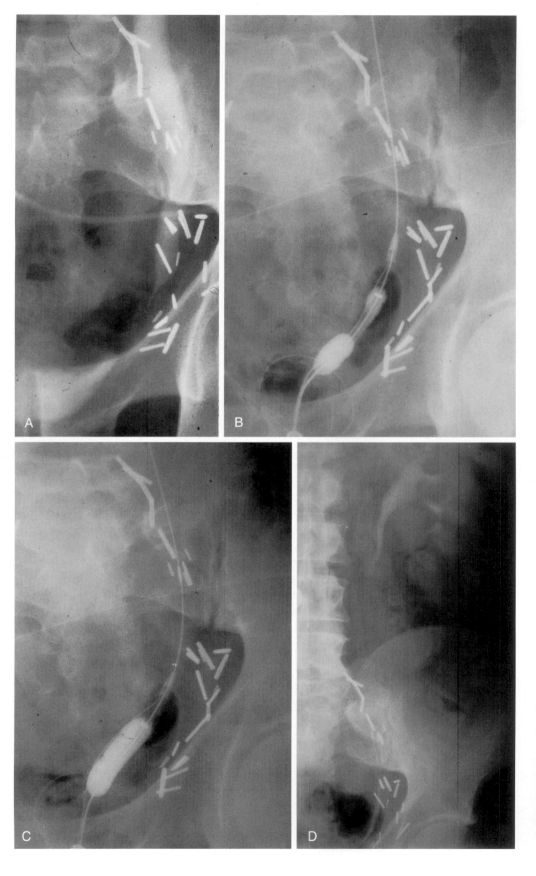

Figure 9–4. *A,* Intravenous pyelogram (IVP) demonstrating a tight distal ureteral stricture. *B,* Acucise cutting balloon catheter in place, positioned across the stricture. The balloon waist demarcates the extent of the stricture. Note that the cutting wire is positioned in a medial position in the distal ureter. *C,* After incising the stricture with the Acucise device, the balloon is fully inflated. *D,* Postoperative IVP demonstrates excellent flow of contrast through the distal ureter with resolution of hydronephrosis.

the balloon may be deflated and repositioned, and the cutting procedure repeated.

After the cutting is complete, a retrograde uretero-gram may be performed through the catheter to con-firm extravasation at the incision site. After the ade-quacy of the incision has been assured, the balloon is repositioned across the incised area and fully in-flated, and the tamponade is maintained for 10 min-utes. If significant bleeding occurs that cannot be controlled by the 24 Fr. balloon, a 30 Fr. (10-mm) balloon may be passed over the guidewire and posi-tioned to achieve tamponade. If bleeding is not con-trolled with the 30 Fr. tamponade balloon, underlying vessels may have been injured, necessitating angiog-raphy or open surgical exploration.

After the cutting balloon catheter is deflated and removed, a 7/14 Fr. endopyelotomy stent is placed over the super-stiff guidewire with its 14 Fr. end placed across the incised area. We have routinely left the endopyelotomy stent in place for 6 weeks postoperatively. However, studies are under way to further define the optimal length of time for postoper-ative stenting, as well as the ideal size of the postop-erative stent (standard 7 Fr. ureteral stent vs. 7/14 Fr. endopyelotomy stent). The endopyelotomy stent can be removed in the office with standard cystoscopic equipment or with a flexible cystoscope in male pa-tients. Patients return in 4 to 6 weeks after stent removal for a repeat IVP and/or differential renal scan with furosemide washout to confirm the efficacy of the endoureterotomy.

Results

Our experience with the Acucise cutting balloon catheter is limited to 18 patients who have been fol-lowed for an average of 21.2 months (16 patients for over 1 year).[22] The overall success rate, defined as resolution of obstruction radiographically and/or dis-appearance of symptoms, is 73 percent, with four overt failures (Fig. 9–4). In retrospect, three of these four patients were not ideal candidates for this proce-dure, in that they had either long (larger than 2 cm), ischemic ureteral strictures (in two patients) or a complex UPJ obstruction (crossing vessel found at open surgery) (in one patient). Treatment failures oc-curred within 3 months of the original procedure in 75 percent of patients.

All but one of the procedures were completed in 45 minutes or less, and 13 of the 15 patients were treated as outpatients. There were two significant complications. Both involved excessive bleeding, sec-ondary to an iliac vessel injury in one patient and probable incision of the lower pole of the kidney in a second patient. Both patients were managed angiog-raphically without long-term sequelae.

Endoluminal Stents

Endoluminal stents have been used for tight, irreg-ular, and/or long ureteric strictures, with encouraging results.[23] However, long-term follow-up is not avail-able in these patients at the present time. Placement of the endoluminal stent is a straightforward proce-dure. After the guidewire is manipulated past the stricture, ureteroscopy is performed and the endo-luminal stent placed across the stricture (Fig. 9–5). Once in place, the endoluminal stent is opened, keep-ing the ureter patent owing to its structural configu-ration. Preliminary studies in Europe suggest that the endoluminal stents become epithelialized, thereby re-ducing the chance of stone formation.

Combined Retrograde-Antegrade Technique

For extremely tight strictures in which retrograde or antegrade passage of a ureteral catheter is not pos-sible, one may attempt a combined antegrade and retrograde technique to approach the stricture from both directions. These patients usually have a percu-taneous nephrostomy tube placed to decompress the collecting system. Once functional assessment has determined that the collecting system is worth salvag-ing, the stricture may be approached from above through the percutaneous nephrostomy tract with a rigid or semirigid ureteroscope, and from below with a flexible ureteroscope. Of course, fluoroscopy is es-sential in these cases to ensure proper alignment of the retrograde- and antegrade-directed endoscopes. In most cases, injection of methylene blue, from either

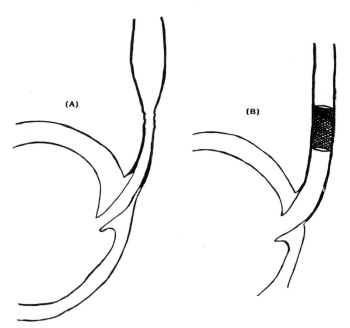

Figure 9–5. *A,* Tight irregular stricture. *B,* Endoluminal stent in place with patent ureter.

above or below, permits identification of the strictured ureteral lumen. However, when there is complete obstruction of the ureteral segment, one may "cut to the light" of either the retrograde or antegrade endoscope if it is determined that the strictured segment is short (0.5 mm or less) (Fig. 9–6). If the obliterated segment is larger than 1 cm, such a combined endoscopic technique is strongly discouraged in view of the extreme technical difficulties involved as well as the potential for poor postoperative results.

Stenting

After successful incision and/or balloon dilation of the ureteral stricture, an internal ureteral stent is placed. Currently a 7/14 Fr. endopyelotomy stent is preferred for postoperative stenting, with the 14 Fr. segment of the stent placed across the site of ureteral incision.[24] The stent is left in place for approximately 6 to 8 weeks to allow proper healing of the incised ureter.[25] However, more recent studies have suggested that placement of a standard 7 or 8 Fr. internal ureteral stent may provide results equivalent to those with the 7/14 Fr. endopyelotomy stent. Animal studies also suggest that the duration of stenting need not be 6 to 8 weeks but can be reduced to 1 or 2 weeks. Further animal and clinical studies are currently under way to further define the optimal size and duration of postoperative stenting after ureteral incision.

Postoperative Care

Most endoscopic procedures to manage ureteral strictures can be performed as day surgery or with 23-hour observation. A Foley catheter is usually left in place for 1 or 2 days to prevent extravasation of urine through the incised ureter. Moreover, if a percutaneous nephrostomy tube has been previously placed, this should also remain open for 1 or 2 days. Before removal of the percutaneous nephrostomy tube, a gentle antegrade nephrostogram should be performed to demonstrate that no extravasation is present.

The patient is placed on prophylactic antibiotic therapy for 5 to 7 days and then on suppressive antibiotics until the internal ureteral stent is removed. The previously placed internal ureteral stent is then removed in the office after an appropriate length of stenting (currently 6 to 8 weeks). The patient is instructed to expect a small amount of discomfort from ureteral edema once the internal ureteral stent is removed. Approximately 4 to 6 weeks after stent removal, the patient returns for follow-up IVP and/or differential renal scan with furosemide

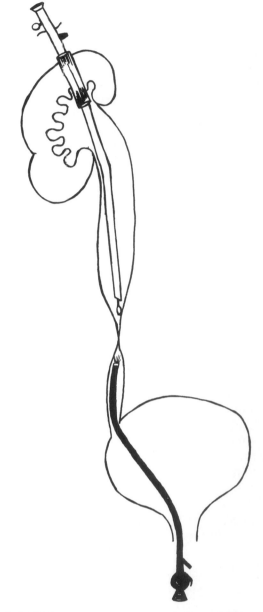

Figure 9–6. Rigid ureteroscope passed through an upper pole percutaneous nephrostomy tract and a flexible ureteroscope passed retrograde up the ureter. The light from the rigid ureteroscope is turned off and the stricture is incised by "cutting to the light."

washout to confirm the patency of the incised ureteral segment.

MANAGEMENT OF COMPLEX STRICTURES

Endourological management of postradiation and other ischemic strictures has yielded uniformly poor results. However, very little additional scarring is caused by endoscopical intervention, and if this is unsuccessful the open surgical repair does not appear to be significantly more difficult. Therefore, in some patients with complex ureteral strictures, an attempt at endourological management may be warranted. Recently, endoluminal stenting of such complex strictures has been performed with encouraging results.

Ureteroenteric strictures have also demonstrated a poor response to endoscopic management. Again, however, an antegrade percutaneous approach to the ureteroenteric stricture may be successful in a few patients and may therefore be an appropriate first choice in selected individuals.

MANAGEMENT OF URETERAL PERFORATION

Perhaps the most common complication of ureteroscopy is perforation of the ureter. Small ureteral perforations are often noted with passage of the smaller semirigid ureteroscopes as well as with the use of endoscopic baskets or intracorporeal lithotripsy probes. Assuming that a safety guidewire has been used during the ureteroscopic procedure, placement of a standard internal ureteral stent is the only treatment necessary to manage small ureteral perforations in most cases.[26]

However, if the ureteral perforation is quite large, if there is a significant tear of the ureter, or if one loses access to the renal collecting system, more aggressive procedures should be performed. Placement of a percutaneous nephrostomy tube decompresses the collecting system and usually prevents extravasation of urine through the perforation if an internal ureteral stent cannot be placed. If a stent or percutaneous nephrostomy tube cannot be positioned within the collecting system, open surgical repair of the ureteral perforation or tear is indicated.

MANAGEMENT OF URETERAL LIGATION

The ureter may be inadvertently ligated during pelvic surgery. It is important to again refer to the anatomical relations of the ureter within the pelvis (see Fig. 9–3). At the pelvic brim the ureter lies close to the vascular pedicle of the ovary. More distally its course is crossed by the uterine artery, and the ureter then resumes an intimate course to the cervix. Not only is the ureter at increased risk of ligation and division during the course of gynecological operations, but it can be ligated during endoscopic bladder neck surgery.

Ligation of the ureter may present as loin discomfort or pain, or as anuria if the patient has a solitary kidney. Initially, the patient may remain asymptomatic, or may present with urinary leakage from the wound or increased drainage from the drain site. Laboratory analysis of the fluid for determination of electrolytes, urea, and creatinine may help assess the nature of the increased drainage. Ultrasound may demonstrate hydronephrosis and complete obstruction, and leakage of contrast from the distal ureter at the site of injury may be seen by IVP.

Placement of a percutaneous nephrostomy tube will stabilize most of the immediate problems. If the injury is diagnosed within the first 24 to 48 hours, excision of the ligature is indicated, often necessitating open surgery. Endoscopic incision of the ligature has been described.[27] Alternatively, laparoscopic incision of the ligature may be performed. After incision of the ligature, an internal ureteral stent is placed within the ureter and should remain in place for 6 weeks. Even with prompt endoscopic management of a ligated ureter, the risk of stricture formation is high, and careful follow-up is warranted.

URETERAL FISTULAS

A ureteral fistula is a pathological communication between the ureter and another viscus, cavity, or skin. It may result as a complication of stone surgery, ureterointestinal anastomosis leak, or ureteral obstruction secondary to stricture disease or a neoplastic process.[28]

A urinary leak occurring from a fistulous tract after stone surgery will normally seal, given enough time. However, if there is no resolution of leakage within 10 to 14 days, further investigation should be made.[29] Earlier evaluation may be warranted if the patient has significant colic, since there may be a residual stone or stone fragment in the distal ureter, and the fistula will not dry up unless distal obstruction is corrected.

Evaluation should begin with plain films followed by contrast studies, including antegrade pyelography if a nephrostomy tube is already in place. Urinary fistulas may occur within the first week after creation of a ureterointestinal anastomosis. However, the incidence of such fistulas has been markedly reduced with the routine use of Silastic stents with the anastomotic procedures. Patient evaluation includes laboratory confirmation of urine collected from the drainage site, as well as contrast studies: IVP, antegrade nephrostogram, or retrograde ureterogram. If contrast studies show no definitive cause of obstruction (e.g., stone, tumor), the blockage may be due to mucosal edema, and internal stenting of the ureter will result in better drainage and healing of the fistula.

In open surgical cases when there is inadvertent damage to the ureter resulting in a ureteral fistula, internal stenting is beneficial if there is a partial tear in the wall of ureter. Another alternative is to place a percutaneous nephrostomy tube on the affected side to divert the urine and allow the fistula to heal.

In patients with ureterointestinal fistulas secondary to a ureterointestinal anastomotic leak, previously placed stents should be removed until the fistula heals. If the anastomosis was not performed with stents, percutaneous nephrostomy tubes should be placed bilaterally to allow time for both the anastomosis and the fistula to heal. Before removal of the nephrostomy tube, an antegrade nephrostogram and/or a fistulagram should be performed to make sure the leak has completely sealed.

URINOMAS

A retroperitoneal collection of urine or urinoma is most commonly secondary to urinary tract trauma or ureteral obstruction caused by the passage of a small ureteric calculus, which results in back pressure and forniceal rupture. Urinomas may also result from complications from endourological procedures (ureteroscopy, percutaneous stone removal).[4, 11] Retroperitoneal urine collections may be asymptomatic if they are small, as usually seen in cases of a forniceal tear after ureteral colic. No specific treatment is necessary if there is no longer any obstructing calculus and the urinoma is small and asymptomatic. However, if the urine collection is of significant size or causing discomfort, a more aggressive approach is indicated.

Urinomas may be detected by various imaging procedures, a computed tomographic scan being the most sensitive in delineating the extent of the urine collection.

Management of large, symptomatic urinomas is accomplished by removal of the fluid collection and relief of any existing obstruction. Urine drainage may often be successfully accomplished percutaneously. When drainage from the urinoma catheter has diminished, contrast media should be injected through the percutaneous tube to assess the size of the remaining cavity and determine whether continued drainage is indicated.

Editorial Comment
Fray F. Marshall

Endoscopic management of ureteral strictures and fistulas has become increasingly common. Typically, we have left a large-size 12 to 14 Fr. ureteral stent for at least 4 weeks after manipulation of a ureteral stricture.[1] If this endoscopic attempt fails, an open procedure is usually indicated. If a ureteral fistula is treated endoscopically, it is important to consider proximal urinary drainage with a nephrostomy tube and also placement of a stent. There is a high likelihood of ureteral stricture or obliteration at the site of injury when only a proximal nephrostomy tube is in place. New technological advances such as the Acucise balloon with a cutting wire on a balloon will facilitate management of many ureteral strictures without open surgery.

1. Chang R, Marshall FM, Mitchell S. Percutaneous management of benign ureteral strictures and fistulas. J Urol 137:1126, 1987.

REFERENCES

1. Preminger GM, Roehrborn CG. Special applications of flexible deflectable ureterorenoscopy. Semin Urol 7:16, 1989.
2. Biester R, Gillenwater JY. Complications following ureteroscopy. J Urol 136:380, 1986.
3. Altebarmakian VK, Caldamone AA, Davis RS, et al. Stricture of ureter caused by stone basket manipulation. Urology 19:13, 1982.
4. Lytton B, Weiss RM, Green DF. Complications of ureteral endoscopy. J Urol 137:649, 1987.
5. Silverstein JI, Libby C, Smith AD. Management of ureteroscopic ureteral injuries. Urol Clin North Am 15:515, 1988.
6. Whelan JP, Locke R, Newman RC, et al. Ureteral stricture secondary to endourologic procedures: A case leading to autotransplantation and review of treatment options. J Endourol 1:189, 1987.
7. Sabha M, Nilsson T, Bahar RH, et al. Endoscopic balloon dilation of bilharzial ureteric strictures. J Endourol 2:23, 1988.
8. Wishahi MM. The role of dilatation in bilharzial ureters. Br J Urol 59:405, 1987.
9. Ghoneim MO, Nabeeh A, El-Kappany H. Endourologic treatment of ureteral strictures. J Endourol 2:263, 1988.
10. Juul N, Brons J, Torp-Pedersen S, et al. Ultrasound versus intravenous urography in the initial evaluation of patients with suspected obstructing urinary calculi. Scand J Urol Nephrol (Suppl) 137:45, 1991.
11. Meretyk S, Albala DM, Clayman RV, et al. Endoureterotomy for treatment of ureteral strictures. J Urol 147:1502, 1992.
12. McQuitty DA, Boone TB, Preminger GM. Lower pole calycostomy for the management of iatrogenic ureteropelvic junction obstruction. J Urol 153:142, 1995.
13. Kramolowsky EV, Tucker RD, Nelson CM. Management of benign ureteral structures: Open surgical repair or endoscopic dilation? J Urol 141:285, 1989.
14. Kerbl K, Doblhofer F, Pauer W. Endoscopic balloon dilatation of postoperative strictured ureterosigmoidostomy. J Endourol 4:385, 1990.
15. Schneider AW, Conrad S, Busch R, et al. The cold-knife technique for endourological management of stenoses in the upper urinary tract. J Urol 146:961, 1991.
16. Selikowitz SM. New coaxial ureteral stricture knife. Urol Clin North Am 17:83, 1990.
17. Clayman RV, Denstedt JD. New technique: Ureterorenoscope urothelial endoureteroplasty: Case report. J Endourol 3:425, 1989.
18. Figenshau RS, Clayman RV, Wick MR, et al. Acute histologic changes associated with endoureterotomy in the normal pig ureter. J Endourol 5:357, 1991.
19. Schwalb DM, Eshghi M, Franco I, et al. Expanding the role of the ureteroscope. J Urol 143:485, 1990.
20. Chandhoke PS, Clayman RV, Stone AM, et al. Endopyelotomy and endoureterotomy with the Acucise ureteral cutting balloon device: Preliminary experience. J Endourol 7:45, 1993.
21. Aronson WJ, Barbaric Z, Fain J, et al. Cautery-wire/balloon catheter for fluoroscopically guided incision of ureteral strictures: A phase I study in pigs. J Endourol 5:337, 1991.
22. Gross M, Preminger GM. Incision of ureteral strictures with a cutting balloon catheter. J Urol 147:471A, 1992.
23. Cussenot O, Bassi S, Desgrandchamps F, et al. Outcomes of non–self-expandable metal prostheses in strictured human ureter. J Endourol 7:205, 1993.
24. Siegel JF, Smith AD. The ideal ureteral stent for antegrade and retrograde endopyelotomy: What would it be like? (review). J Endourol 7:151, 1993.
25. Babayan RK. Stents and catheters in percutaneous renal surgery. J Endourol 7:163, 1993.
26. Kramolowsky EV. Ureteral perforation during ureterorenoscopy: Treatment and management. J Urol 138:36, 1987.
27. Gigabhoy S, Kiely D. Ureteric obstruction by ligature treated by endoscopic diathermy. Br J Urol 67:662, 1991.
28. Cormio L, Battaglia M, Traficante A, et al. Endourological treatment of ureteric injuries. Br J Urol 72:165, 1993.
29. Mitty HA, Train JS, Dan SJ. Antegrade ureteral stenting in the management of fistulas, strictures, and calculi. Radiology 149:433, 1983.

Chapter 10

Intracorporeal Lithotripsy: Ultrasonic, Electrohydraulic, Laser, and Electromechanical

Michael Grasso

INDICATIONS FOR ENDOSCOPIC LITHOTRIPSY AND PREOPERATIVE PATIENT EVALUATION

Endoscopic lithotripsy is an accepted first-line therapy for upper urinary tract calculi. Extracorporeal shock wave lithotripsy (ESWL) is also a commonly employed, minimally invasive treatment. The correct modality and when to choose it continue to be debated. In an endeavor to obtain the most efficient overall treatment, guidelines have been developed with an accent on endoscopic technique.[1–3] Clinical presentations where endoscopic therapy is superior to ESWL include patients with large stone burdens (larger than 2.5 cm) and those with lower pole (dependent) renal calculi. Patients presenting with upper urinary tract calculi and obstruction secondary to either ureteropelvic junction (UPJ) stenosis or ureteral stricture are also best served when the underlying disorder is addressed (endo)surgically.[4]

Ureteral calculi are often successfully treated with ESWL. Endoscopic therapy, however, can be more efficient in that stones are fragmented and fragments extracted expeditiously rather than having their passage awaited. Impacted calculi and stones associated with a chronic urinary tract infection are best treated by endoscopic clearance and prompt drainage of the upper tract. Stone composition can also direct treatment. Patients with a history of calcium oxalate monohydrate, brushite, or cystine calculi have a lower success rate with extracorporeal therapy.[4, 5] In this setting, endoscopic access, fragmentation, and extraction of the stone fragments is a cost-effective alternative to serial ESWL treatments.

In a 1994 review of 110 ESWL failures, four groups emerged.[4] In the first group, calculi failed to fragment even after multiple sessions. These patients frequently had very dense, hard stone where the most common composition was calcium oxalate monohydrate. The second group consisted of patients with very large stone burdens who had postoperative upper urinary tract obstruction from many intercalating stone fragments log-jammed throughout the ureter (Steinstrassen, Fig. 10–1). Following the above guidelines, many of these patients should have undergone a relatively simple percutaneous procedure, but unfortunately they were left with rather complex stone burdens requiring vigorous endoscopic lithotripsy. The third group consisted of patients who had stones within poorly draining segments of the upper urinary tract, and as such they often experienced good fragmentation but virtually no clearance. These are patients with UPJ stenosis or ureteral strictures as well as those with caliceal diverticular stones. The final group consisted of patients whose stones were not adequately localized during extracorporeal therapy; these included both those with radiolucent stones and morbidly obese patients in whom localization for ESWL was substandard.

Endoscopic therapy can be a first-line treatment for any urinary calculi but is particularly useful in those who have failed previous shock wave lithotripsy. The lessons learned from the ESWL failures above should be applied in daily practice so that a treatment plan can be developed for each patient. Preoperative evaluation requires excellent imaging of the collecting system with either an intravenous pyelogram or a retrograde contrast study. Computed tomography and

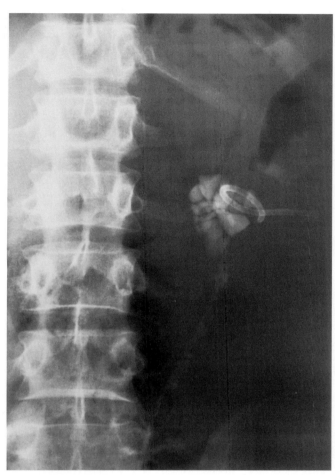

Figure 10–1. A 34-year-old patient with a large calcium oxalate monohydrate renal pelvic calculus underwent three extracorporeal shock wave lithotripsy sessions and was left with multiple ureteral and renal fragments (Steinstrassen) that did not clear over the course of 18 months. Multiple ureteral stents were exchanged during this period and then a nephrostomy tube was placed to improve drainage. Simultaneous antegrade and retrograde endoscopic lithotripsy was employed to clear the stone burden.

renal ultrasound can also be of benefit in special instances. All patients should undergo a urinalysis and a urine culture study. One must not assume that hematuria is de facto a product of the calculus, and a standard work-up to rule out urothelial malignancies must also be performed. In large patients or those with a body habitus that may inhibit extracorporeal therapy, it is often wise to perform an ESWL simulation to determine whether the calculus can be positioned in the second focal point of the ellipsoid.

Patients with lower pole caliceal calculi and those with distal third ureteral calculi represent two additional groups who may benefit from primary endoscopic therapy. Those with significant lower pole urinary calculi (larger than 1 cm) and a rather dependent caliceal system are frequently left with residual fragments after ESWL that fail to clear and may be symptomatic.[2] Patients with a lower pole caliceal calculus drained by a long narrow lower pole infundibulum

are less likely to clear stone fragments than those with a primary renal pelvic calculus.

Ureteroscopic treatment of an obstructing distal third ureteral calculus can be one of the most rewarding therapies for the endoscopist, as opposed to extracorporeal shock wave monotherapy where the results can be mixed and obstruction may persist as patient and physician await clearance of fragments. An 89 percent success rate in treating distal third ureteral calculi using the Dornier HM3 extracorporeal shock wave lithotriptor has been reported.[6] Unfortunately, only 40 percent of all stones within this series could be localized, and thus the author correctly acknowledged the merits of endoscopic therapy in this setting. ESWL failures have also been reported in greater frequency with the less powerful second- and third-generation lithotriptors.[4] Compared with ureteroscopic techniques in which very frequently the entire ureteral stone burden is cleared at one sitting, there is no question that endoscopic treatment can be more efficient.[7, 8]

Patients with a history of chronic urinary tract infection, and in particular those with known infectious calculi (struvite or magnesium ammonium phosphate), are more apt to suffer from perioperative urosepsis and must be carefully treated. Often these patients are elderly and diabetic, and even though their calculus may fragment well with ESWL, they run a significant risk of urosepsis. Good drainage of the upper urinary tract is essential. Serial urine cultures and sensitivities must be obtained and appropriate parenteral antibiotics prescribed perioperatively. Even when great care is taken, infectious urine and pyuria may persist after extracorporeal therapy. Postoperative fungal overgrowth of either *Candida* species or *Torulopsis glabrata* has been associated with urinary calculi and can represent the most morbid of postoperative complications.[9] For these reasons, it is thought that expeditious endoscopic therapy combined with superb drainage (either percutaneously or in retrograde fashion) and topical antibiotic or antifungal agents will lead to a better long-term outcome in these selected complex patients.

ENDOSCOPES AND ACCESS

Percutaneous nephrostolithotomy is a commonly employed technique for treating large renal calculi. In particular, large branched calculi, as well as infectious stones associated with upper urinary tract obstruction, can be treated efficiently with a percutaneous puncture into the collecting system and then a combination of rigid and flexible endoscopy. Pinpoint percutaneous access into a specific calix is frequently required, especially in patients with caliceal diverticular calculi.[3] The techniques for percutaneous access and nephroscopy are described in Chapter 7. It should be noted, however, that the combination of retrograde endoscopy with standard percutaneous techniques can lead to an efficient clearance of a large ureteral stone burden.[10] Steinstrassen treated in this fashion can be cleared expeditiously.

Ureteroscopic treatment of upper urinary tract calculi begins with standard cystoscopic techniques. The bladder urothelium is visualized with either a rigid or flexible cystoscope. Bladder pathology must be ruled out first, and the appropriate ureteral orifice carefully inspected. A cone-tipped retrograde ureteropyelogram may be performed if necessary. Care must be taken not to distort the ureteral orifice and thus complicate the ureteroscopic part of the procedure. Under fluoroscopic guidance, standard guidewires of various compositions can be passed up the ureter for access (Fig. 10–2). Teflon-coated, stainless steel guidewires with 3- to 8-cm floppy tips are commonly used. If the guidewires are unable to traverse an obstruction, a small-diameter, open-ended catheter is placed over the guidewire just to the level of obstruction, and the wire is then removed. Hydrophilic guidewires (Glidewire, Microvasive, Inc., Boston, MA) placed through the stabilizing catheter can often be passed beyond the obstruction. Angled and J-tipped guidewires combined with a directional torque vice are also helpful. Once the guidewire has been passed into the more proximal collecting system, the open-ended catheter should be advanced over the guidewire and radiopaque contrast instilled to verify the position of the catheter. In rare cases the guidewire may be forced submucosally or extraureterally, and this should be recognized promptly.

In patients with a tortuous collecting system, a standard guidewire should be manipulated into the renal pelvis and then, with an open-ended catheter, exchanged for a stiffer guidewire (Amplatz Super Stiff and Lunderquist guidewires, Cook Urologic, Spencer, IN). This will straighten the ureter and aid in endoscopic manipulation. Once a safety guidewire has been placed, a 10.5 Fr. double-lumen catheter (Stone Displacement Catheter, Microvasive, Inc., Boston, MA) can be used to place a second "working" guidewire (Fig. 10–2). This catheter gently dilates the intramural ureter and can be used to inject contrast material to opacify the collecting system. Standard graduated Nottingham dilators are used frequently to dilate the intramural ureter and thus allow endoscopic access. Balloon dilators are less often used, and in fact have decreased in outer diameter with endoscope downsizing.[11]

Rigid ureteroscopes are employed in both male and female patients. Owing to the configuration of the male pelvis with the ureter draping over the iliac vessels, it is often hazardous to pass a rigid ureteroscope into the more proximal ureter in men. Rigid endoscopes have evolved from rod lens to fiberoptic imaging. This change has allowed miniaturization

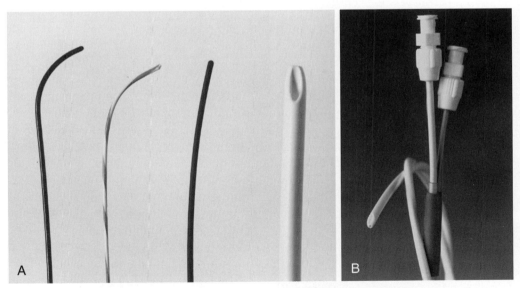

Figure 10–2. *A,* Various guidewires and catheters are employed to gain retrograde access to the upper urinary tract. The hydrophylic-coated, Glidewire is often employed to bypass impacted calculi and ureteral strictures *(far left)*. The angled tipped Zebra/Nitinol guidewire rarely kinks and is able to traverse many ureteral obstructions *(second from left)*. This nickel titanium guidewire has a thick Teflon coating that facilitates passage of the small-diameter flexible ureteroscope. Standard Teflon-coated, stainless steel guidewires are commonly used as safety guidewires *(second from right)*. The dual-lumen catheter (Microvasive stone displacement catheter) is a necessity during therapeutic flexible ureteroscopy. This catheter allows a working guidewire to be placed expeditiously and also enables the endoscopist to perform a retrograde pyelogram once a safety guidewire has been placed. *B,* Lateral view of a stone displacement catheter.

and added as much as 30 degrees of lateral flexibility to these once truly rigid endoscopes (Fig. 10–3). By preventing binding of endoscopic tools, endoscopes with two dedicated working channels have a theoretical advantage over those with one larger working channel. Semirigid endoscopes have been downsized to 6.9 Fr. with both a 3.4 and 2.2 Fr. working channel. By adapting a side-arm irrigating port (Urolock Adapter, Microvasive, Inc., Boston, MA), the endoscopist can first entrap a calculus within a basket and then fragment it with a variety of endoscopic lithotriptors while maintaining adequate irrigation (Fig. 10–3B).

Semirigid, fiberoptic ureteroscopes can often be passed in a retrograde fashion without intramural ureteral dilation. In patients in whom a guidewire cannot be passed beyond an impacted stone in the distal ureter, direct retrograde visualization can be employed. The next maneuver consists of endoscopic disimpaction with passage of a guidewire into the more proximal ureter. Proximal access with a safety guidewire is the essential next step before stone fragmentation. Once a guidewire is passed successfully into the more proximal ureter, the endoscope should be backed off and the guidewire secured to the drapes as a safety access. The rigid ureteroscope is then passed beside the safety guidewire and endoscopic lithotripsy is performed. If a safety guidewire cannot be passed with either fluoroscopically directed retrograde manipulation or direct endoscopic inspection, percutaneous decompression of the collecting system is the next step in the treatment algorithm. Endosurgical manipulation of the upper urinary tract without prompt postoperative drainage can lead to devastating urosepsis and pyonephrosis even with parenteral antibiotic therapy.

Actively deflectable, flexible ureteroscopy is reserved for proximal calculi. The flexible instrument can regularly be passed into each calix. Miniaturization has led to use of endoscopes of very small diameter while a standard-diameter working channel is maintained. The 7.5 Fr. actively deflectable, flexible ureteroscope is an excellent example of endoscope miniaturization with maintenance of a functional 3.6 Fr. working channel (Karl Storz Endoscopy).[11] It is important to note that the dimensions of the working channel do change with both active and passive endoscope deflection.[12] This limits the size of the endoscopic tools or lithotrites passed through the working channel. Note also that endoscopic instruments and lithotrites do inhibit the flexibility of the endoscope (Fig. 10–4). These variables must be addressed when

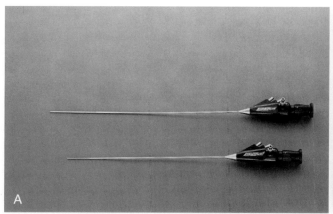

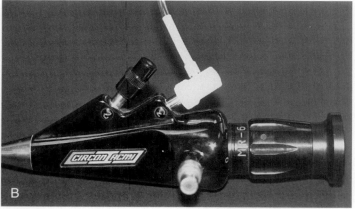

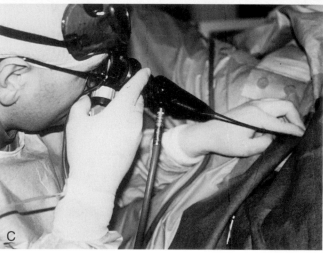

Figure 10–3. A, A 6.9 Fr semirigid flexible ureteroscope (MR-6, Circon ACMI, Stamford, CT). The progression from rod lens to fiberoptic imaging has led to endoscope miniaturization. B, Two working channels allow simultaneous passage of a grasper or basket and an endoscopic lithotrite without having the instruments bind on each other. Irrigating solution is also passed with the aid of a side-arm adapter (Urolok, Microvasive, Inc., Watertown, MA). C, Fiberoptic imaging has allowed these once "rigid" instruments to be deflected up to 30 degrees without damage to the patient or the endoscope.

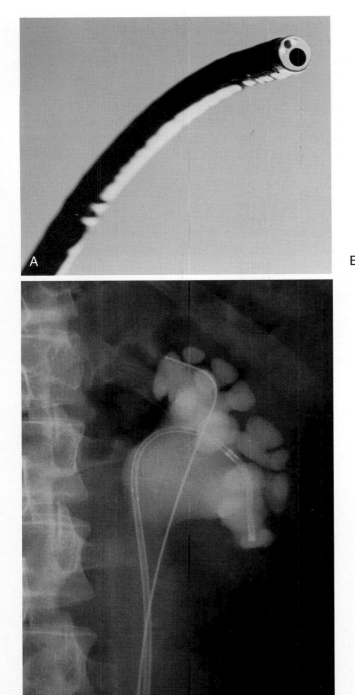

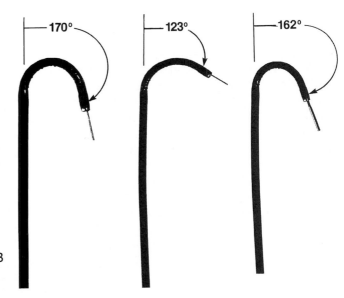

Figure 10–4. A 7.5 Fr. actively deflectable, flexible ureteroscope (Karl Storz Endoscopy). *A* and *B,* The small-diameter flexible ureteroscope has a single 3.6 Fr. working channel. By maintaining the working channel as close to center as possible, the channel's shape changes less during both active and passive deflection and facilitates easier passage of endoscopic instruments and lithotrites. Miniaturization of endoscopic tools and lithotripsy probes also aids passage through the working channel. *B,* A 1.6 Fr. electrohydraulic lithotripsy probe does not inhibit the actively deflecting portion of the endoscope *(left),* as compared with the somewhat stiff 320-μm laser fiber *(center).* The 3 Fr. electrohydraulic lithotripsy probe does inhibit the actively deflecting portion of the endoscope, but to a lesser degree than that noted with the quartz laser fiber. *C,* Secondary deflection refers to a proximal weakness in the durometer of the flexible ureteroscope, which allows the instrument to be banked off an upper pole infundibulum and placed into a dependent lower pole caliceal system. By first employing maximal active deflection and then advancing the endoscope, the secondary deflecting portion will allow the instrument to passively reflect off an upper pole infundibulum. By means of two-way deflection, the tip of the ureteroscope can then be directed laterally as necessary.

choosing the appropriate instrumentation for a specific clinical presentation. Where the stiff quartz fiber of the pulsed dye laser may inhibit endoscopic access to a peripheral lower pole caliceal calculus, use of small-diameter (1.6 and 1.9 Fr.) electrohydraulic lithotripsy probes often results in successful treatment. Access to the lower pole caliceal system is also dependent on secondary deflection (Fig. 10–4C). This refers to the inherent weakness in the durometer of the flexible ureteroscope, which allows the endoscop-

ist to bank the endoscope off the upper pole infundibulum and advance it into the lower pole caliceal system. Secondary deflection is required to reach the lower pole caliceal system in most patients.[11]

The flexible ureteroscope is always passed in a monorail fashion over a working guidewire. A safety guidewire is always placed initially, and then with a double-lumen catheter a second working guidewire is passed. A nonkinking, Teflon-coated, nickel titanium guidewire (Zebra/Nitinol guidewire, Microvasive

Inc., Boston, MA) has been found to be superior to standard stainless steel guidewires for passing a flexible ureteroscope.[11] Nitinol guidewires rarely kink and allow easier passage of the endoscope through the bladder and intramural ureter. The small-diameter flexible ureteroscope has a centrally located working channel and infrequently requires intramural ureteral dilation for placement when passed over a Nitinol guidewire. The working channel of the flexible instrument is then employed for both irrigation and passage of a lithotripsy probe or other endoscopic tool (e.g., graspers, baskets, biopsy forceps).

Inadequate upper urinary tract irrigation is an all too common source of frustration. Sterile saline irrigant is used for most upper urinary tract endoscopies. Gravity-fed irrigation lines are often inadequate owing to the significant resistance noted through the relatively long working channels of the commonly used ureteroscopes. For this reason, various irrigating devices have been developed. Some are mechanically driven pumps, while others are based on a hand-held piston syringe. The most cost-effective means of obtaining "power" irrigation is to use standard 60-ml syringes, a three-way stopcock, and extension tubing (Fig. 10–5). This combination allows for constant irrigation under the hand-held control of the assistant. With the endoscopist manipulating the endoscope under direct vision and with the aid of a beam-splitting camera head, the assistant is able to irrigate sufficiently to maintain adequate visualization for the entire team. With a small-diameter ureteroscope the renal pelvis will fill with irrigant promptly. Most of the irrigant will then pass around the endoscope into the bladder, which must be drained periodically. Small amounts of irrigant may be absorbed in either

the lymphatic or venous system. If sterile saline is used and the patient is treated preoperatively with antimicrobial agents, the overall risk of postoperative urosepsis is low.

Endoscopic tools include baskets, graspers, and biopsy devices (Fig. 10–6). Downsizing of endoscopic tools has increased the amount of irrigant passed simultaneously through a working channel, thus allowing better visualization. Baskets are frequently used through rigid endoscopes where a second working channel is available to place an endoscopic lithotrite if the entrapped calculus cannot be extracted. It is of utmost importance that once a calculus is entrapped in a basket, it be extracted under direct vision. This precaution should prevent ureteral avulsion. Inability to extract a calculus should lead to endoscopic fragmentation, resulting in an extractable core.

Flat-wire spherical baskets (Segura Baskets) are used in dilated collecting systems, while helical round-wire baskets are employed in narrow ureters or with impacted calculi. All baskets should be opened

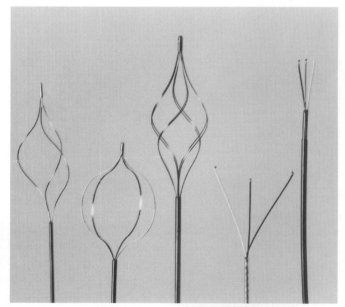

Figure 10–6. Commonly employed ureteroscopic tools. *Left*, The 1.9 Fr. Bagley helical basket can be passed easily through even relatively small working channels. *Second from left*, The 2.4 Fr. Segura flat wire basket is employed in dilated collecting systems to entrap a calculus. *Center*, The 3.0 Fr. double-wired Gemini helical basket is employed in narrow collecting systems and also to entrap impacted calculi. When open, this basket will dilate the ureter ever so slightly. The added space gained allows the basket to be easily rotated around the calculus, entrapping it. *Second from right*, A standard 2.4 Fr. three-pronged grasper is composed of three barbed wires and a single sheath. Stone fragments are engaged by first manipulating the wires around the fragment and then gently advancing the grasper as it is being closed. *Far right*, The nonretracting 2.4 Fr. three-prong grasper is composed of three barbed wires and two sheaths. With this device the grasper is not advanced during closing. Even though easier to manipulate onto a stone fragment, the smaller wires noted in this device are less apt to obtain an adequate purchase on a stone fragment than the standard variety.

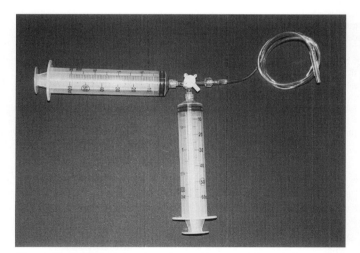

Figure 10–5. Saline irrigant can be easily passed through the working channel of the ureteroscope by employing two 60-ml syringes, a three-way stopcock, and extension tubing ("power" irrigation). Using a beam-splitting camera, the assistant can tailor the amount of irrigant administered, depending on the clarity of the field of view noted on the monitor.

beside a calculus if possible; opening one beyond a calculus may lead to ureteral perforation. Once the basket is opened beside a calculus, rotation of the endoscope and the basket simultaneously will expedite entrapment. Three pronged graspers consist of barbed-tip wires within a sheath. Those that are non-retracting are based on a double-sheath system in which the internal sheath extends out to close. The more standard three-pronged grasper has a single sheath and must be advanced while closing in order to engage a calculus. The nonretracting variety has smaller-diameter wires and thus is less likely to obtain an adequate purchase on a stone fragment for extraction. Graspers and baskets with Teflon coating can be passed more easily through the working channels of standard ureteroscopes than those with stiffer, more fragile polyamide coatings.

Endoscopic tools often used through the flexible ureteroscope include three-pronged graspers and very small 1.9 Fr. round-wire (Bagley Helical Basket) and 2.4 Fr. flat-wire baskets. Once a basket passed through a flexible endoscope has engaged a calculus, it is extremely difficult to simultaneously pass an endoscopic lithotrite through the same working channel. If the calculus is too large to extract, the next maneuver is to back the flexible ureteroscope off the basket and replace it beside the basket's sheath so as to employ an endoscopic lithotriptor. The importance of a safety guidewire in this setting cannot be overstated! Rather than entrapping a relatively large calculus in a basket passed through a flexible ureteroscope, it is safer to first direct the stone from the proximal ureter or renal pelvis to an upper or middle pole calix where it can be totally fragmented more efficiently. A three-pronged grasper can then be employed to extract the larger stone fragments (3 mm or more) that are thought to be too large to pass spontaneously.[13]

Correct patient positioning is essential for successful upper tract endoscopy. Patients are most commonly placed in a standard dorsal lithotomy position on a radiolucent operating table. Real-time fluoroscopy is an essential part of the procedure. Safety guidewires are always placed with at least fluoroscopic guidance; the endoscope's position can also be verified with fluoroscopy. This is important when inspecting the entire caliceal system with a flexible ureteroscope. Small amounts of radiopaque contrast can be added to the irrigant to faintly opacify the collecting system and help direct the flexible endoscope into the appropriate portion of the caliceal system. Purely diagnostic ureteroscopy can be performed under topical anesthetic, whereas therapeutic maneuvers, including endoscopic lithotripsy, often require a deeper anesthetic.

Complex stone burdens require varied patient positioning, depending on whether retrograde, antegrade, or a combination of endoscopic techniques is to be employed.[10] The flank-roll position entails placing the patient first in the lithotomy position and then rolling the shoulder on the side being treated up at approximately 45 degrees (Fig. 10–7A). The hip is also raised on the same side but to a lesser extent. This will expose an existing nephrostomy so that simultaneous antegrade and retrograde procedures can be performed. This position is used only when it is planned to pass flexible endoscopes in an antegrade fashion. If rigid endoscopes are required through a percutaneous tract, the prone split-leg position is employed (Fig. 10–7B). For this, the patient is first placed prone, chest rolls are used to aid in ventilation, and the lower extremities are padded and separated to allow access to the genitalia. In this position, flexible endoscopes are used in a retrograde fashion while both rigid and flexible endoscopes can be used for percutaneous nephroscopy (Fig. 10–7C). Both the flank-roll and prone split-leg positions are essential in treating complex upper urinary tract stone burdens, including large ureteral and renal stones and Steinstrassen.

ENDOSCOPIC LITHOTRIPTORS: THERMAL VERSUS NONTHERMAL

Endoscopic lithotrites continue to evolve, as do the ureteroscopes used to obtain retrograde upper urinary tract access. Mechanical lithalopaxy has all but disappeared and has been replaced by a variety of devices employed to fragment and sometimes evacuate a stone burden. The particular lithotrite employed must be adaptable to the endoscopes available in the operating suite. Endoscopic lithotripsy probes are either thermal or nonthermal based. Ultrasonic and electrohydraulic devices are hot to touch while in use and thus pose a theoretical risk of thermal damage to the ureter. The experimental holmium laser now in clinical trials actually vaporizes stones and has been suggested as a possible lithotrite for very hard calculi that do not respond well to other tools.[14] With all thermal-based lithotripsy probes, the risk of tissue coagulation is markedly diminished by adequate cooling irrigation. Other endoscopic lithotrites, including the coumarin-based pulsed dye laser and the mechanical (ballistic) lithotriptor, have no thermal effect on the urothelium. The merits of each specific lithotrite, as well as the risks of each technology, are addressed specifically below.

Ultrasonic Lithotripsy

Ultrasonic lithotripsy is based on an ultrasonic generator that vibrates stainless steel probes and, when

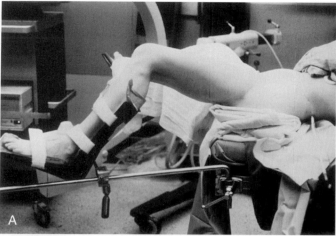
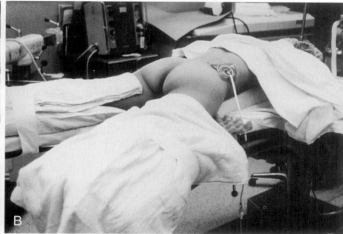
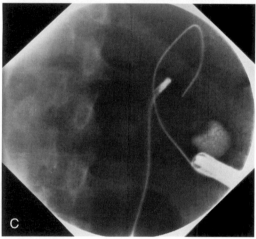

Figure 10–7. Simultaneous antegrade and retrograde endoscopy is often required when treating upper urinary tract stone burdens. *A*, The flank-roll position allows access to an existing nephrostomy site (for flexible antegrade endoscopy) during retrograde ureteroscopic treatment. *B*, The prone split-leg position allows the surgeon to perform flexible, retrograde endoscopy simultaneously with standard percutaneous techniques. *C*, Simultaneous rigid percutaneous nephrostolithotomy and flexible ureteroscopic lithotripsy allow a complex stone burden to be treated expeditiously. In this case the prone split-leg position allows a rigid nephroscope to clear a portion of a large stone burden, while the flexible endoscope addresses caliceal fragments.

endoscopically placed on a calculus, leads to fragmentation.[15] Ultrasonic lithotripsy has been employed for many years with both rigid nephroscopes and rigid ureteroscopes to clear large stone burdens. Hollow core probes not only fragment calculi but also have the added benefit of evacuating the small fragments produced. Using saline irrigant and suctions directed through the probe's central channel, a rather large stone burden can be efficiently cleared from the collecting system. The rotating burr-tipped design can fragment the hardest calculi (Karl Storz Endoscopy). The rotating tip is very powerful, and great care must be taken to avoid placing it directly on tissue while in operation. Also, with repeated use the burr tips have been noted to disengage from the end of the probe.[16]

The solid-wire ultrasound system is one of the most powerful ureteroscopic lithotrites available.[17] In general, ureteroscopic applications of ultrasonic lithotripsy are less commonly used, especially with the increasing popularity of the semirigid ureteroscope. Power delivery markedly decreases with modest angulation of the probes. This is particularly important when using the small semirigid and flexible ureteroscope, where significant angulation of the instrument

commonly occurs. With angulation of up to 15 degrees, the power available at the tip of the probe can drop off significantly.

Electrohydraulic Lithotripsy and the Electromechanical Impactor

Raney, working with Northgate Inc., was one of the first to describe a sparking electrode on the tip of a standard catheter that, when fired, created a cavitation bubble and thus led to an early form of shock wave lithotripsy.[18] The same principle is the basis for many extracorporeal shock wave lithotriptors. These probes are obviously not thermal free and are based on electrical current in a fluid medium causing a microexplosion. The initial experience with these probes supported their use in a dilute (1:6) saline solution to accentuate the shock wave effect. This has been refuted by subsequent researchers.[19] It has also been found that, with downsizing, the efficiency of endoscopic lithotripsy increases and the risk of thermocoagulation is diminished.[20] Commonly used ureteroscopic probes today range in size from 1.6 to 3.0 Fr. (Fig. 10–8).

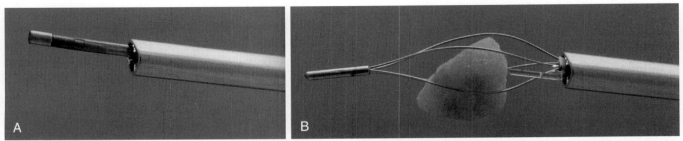

Figure 10–8. *A,* The MR-6 semirigid ureteroscope with a 3 Fr. electrohydraulic lithotripsy probe placed through the 3.4 Fr. working channel. *B,* A calcium oxalate dihydrate calculus entrapped within a 3 Fr. helical basket. The 320-μm quartz laser fiber is passed through the second working channel onto the calculus for fragmentation.

When a calculus is accessed endoscopically, the electrohydraulic probe should be placed just off the stone to maximize the benefits of the cavitation bubble and shock waves produced (Fig. 10–9). Care must be taken to keep the probe as far as possible from the safety guidewire to prevent arcing and thermal injury. Since the energy is delivered spherically from the tip of the probe, there is occasion to note ureteral ecchymosis and even small microperforations. To help prevent this, excellent visualization of the calculus and the tip of the probe is required throughout the endoscopic procedure. Fragments have been inadvertently pushed into the ureteral wall or extraureterally because of overzealous endoscopic technique. These fragments can be associated with ureteral obstruction and subsequent ureteral stricture.[21]

To minimize the side effects from electrohydraulic lithotripsy, the electromechanical impactor was developed by Drs. Bhatta and Dretler at Massachusetts General Hospital.[22] This device adds a shield over the sparking tip of the probe and directs the energy produced onto a spring-held bullet that moves along the long axis of the catheter, thus converting electrical energy to mechanical energy for fragmentation.

The major problem with this device is its overall size. This team has been unable to downsize the device so that it can pass through the available working channels of the small endoscopes commonly used.

Pulsed Dye Laser

The coumarin-based pulsed dye laser is a thermal free endoscopic lithotrite that allows light energy of 504 nm to be passed in a pulsatile fashion through optical quartz fibers. Both 320- and 550-μm fibers are employed with the larger fibers having higher available energy (up to 200 mJ). Standard energy for fragmentation of ureteral calculi ranges from 80 to 140 mJ, depending on stone composition. Harder calculi, especially calcium oxalate monohydrate stones, require the maximal energy for fragmentation.[13] The optical quartz fibers are somewhat rigid and do inhibit the flexibility of actively deflectable, flexible endoscopes to some degree (see Fig. 10–4*B*). The 320-μm laser fiber can frequently be passed throughout the collecting system to fragment calculi.[11] The larger 550-μm laser fiber does inhibit the actively de-

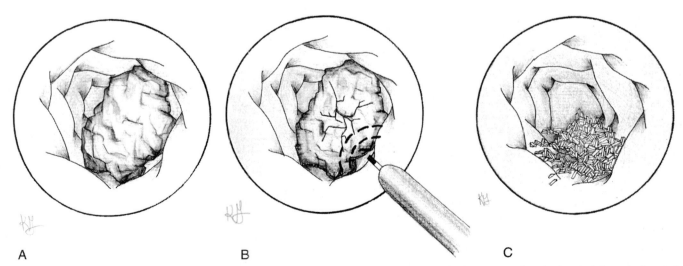

Figure 10–9. An impacted calcium oxalate dihydrate ureteral calculus. *A,* A semirigid endoscope is passed to the level of the calculus under direct vision, and then a small-diameter electrohydraulic lithotripsy probe is employed. *B,* The probe is placed just off the calculus to maximize the efficiency of this lithotrite. *C,* The small, sandlike fragments that remain are often left to pass spontaneously.

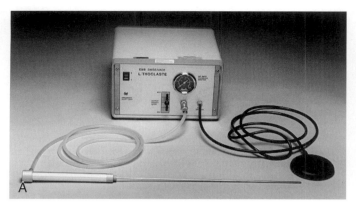

LITHOCLAST HAND PIECE

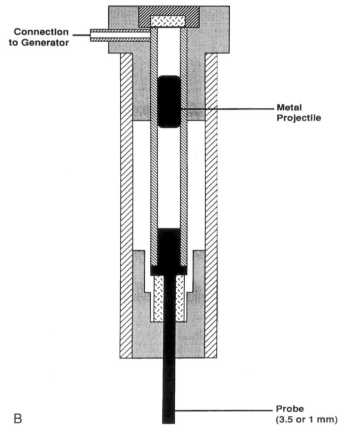

Connection to Generator

Metal Projectile

B

Probe (3.5 or 1 mm)

Figure 10–10. The ballistic, or jackhammer, mechanical lithotriptor (Lithoclast, Luzanne, Switzerland) is a pneumatically driven mechanical lithotrite. *A*, Compressed air drives a metallic projectile against a stainless steel probe, transforming kinetic energy into mechanical energy for fragmentation. *B*, The stainless steel probes are commonly placed through the working channels of both rigid and semirigid endoscopes. (Courtesy of John Denstedt, M.D.)

flectable portion of flexible endoscopes, and so this combination is never used. By altering the frequency of pulsations (in hertz), various fragmentation techniques can be employed. For stones that are mobile in dilated collecting systems, the frequency of pulsations should be lowered to prevent migration of the calculus. Impacted stones can be readily disimpacted

by increasing the frequency of pulsation. Large stones within the caliceal system can be pulverized efficiently with moderate to high frequency (6 to 8 Hz). When using high frequency it is important to clearly visualize the probe tip and calculus. It is an unfortunate endoscopist who moves too close to the calculus during fragmentation and unwillingly allows a portion of the fragmented stone to flip back and crack the endoscope's distal objective lens. There is little risk to the patient with this maneuver, but obviously this would be a terminal event for the endoscope!

Another laser lithotriptor currently under trial is the holmium-based pulsed dye laser (Coherent, Inc., Palo Alto, CA).[14] This is a truly thermal-based laser pulsed to combine both vaporization of the calculus and the fragmenting effect of pulsed light energy. Reviewing the early experience with lithotriptors, there is no question that it is an efficient lithotrite able to vaporize the hardest stones, including cystine, with short pulses of 400 to 1200 mJ of energy. In contrast, the coumarin-based pulsed dye laser has no effect on cystine stone where the light energy is transmitted through the crystalline matrix of the calculus rather than fragmenting it. The major concern with the holmium laser is similar to that raised with the ultrasonic or electrohydraulic lithotriptor: does the thermal effect lead to higher ureteral stricture rates?

Mechanical Stone Impactors and Ballistic Lithotrites

The ballistic or jackhammer mechanical lithotriptor (Lithoclast, Lausanne, Switzerland) is based on a pneumatically driven piston or bullet (Fig. 10–10).[23, 24] The piston strikes an endoscopically placed stainless steel probe and transmits kinetic energy onto a calculus, leading to fragmentation. Probes as small as 2 Fr. are available and have been successfully used through semirigid fiberoptic endoscopes. One concern is whether lateral probe vibration could fragment the fiberoptic pixels of commonly used semirigid endoscopes. Preliminary reports have not commented on this potential problem.

Purely mechanical lithotriptors can fragment the hardest urinary calculi. With rather dense stones, including calcium oxalate monohydrate and cystine, the calculus must first be entrapped within a basket before fragmentation to prevent retrograde migration. This endoscopic lithotriptor must also be employed carefully to prevent both migration of calculi and ureteral perforation.

The Lithoclast's stainless steel probes cannot be employed through an actively deflectable, flexible ureteroscope. Experimental work on a pneumatic impactor that can be delivered through a flexible endoscope is based on a different mechanical generator and nickel titanium probes (Browne Pneumatic Impactor, Minneapolis, MN).[25] Nitinol probes are flexible and minimally inhibit the deflectability of the endoscope. Animal studies have noted efficient stone fragmentation with the endoscope deflected up to 90 degrees. Retrograde migration of hard calculi before fragmentation is also noted with this device. This is prevented by first positioning the calculus within the caliceal system or engaging the stone within a grasper or hollow-core basket before fragmentation.

TECHNIQUES IN EFFICIENT ENDOSCOPIC LITHOTRIPSY AND POSTOPERATIVE MANAGEMENT

Calculi of various compositions fragment differently, depending on the endoscopic lithotrite employed. Very dense calculi, especially black calcium oxalate monohydrate, test the limits of most endoscopic lithotriptors. Other stones that are difficult to fragment include certain types of calcium phosphate (brushite) and cystine. Choosing the correct endoscopic equipment preoperatively decreases intraoperative time and increases the efficiency of each procedure. The density of the calculus on preoperative radiography loosely correlates with the difficulty of endoscopic lithotripsy. Stones of greater density than the bony spine are often difficult to fragment, but this is not an absolute rule. The composition of a calculus can also be estimated endoscopically, and thus the tools required for treatment can be employed expeditiously.[26] In 86 percent of cases hard stones can be differentiated from their softer counterparts by using a few simple endoscopic rules. Dark-colored and pure black mamillated calculi with internal laminations are by definition composed primarily of calcium oxalate monohydrate and are often very difficult to fragment. Bright yellow granular calculi are composed of either calcium oxalate dihydrate or uric acid and are easier to fragment. Mixed calcium oxalate and calcium phosphate calculi have variable endoscopic appearances and fragility.

An estimate of calculus composition can often be made endoscopically and a treatment plan developed accordingly.[13] When treating black mamillated calcium oxalate monohydrate calculi with the pulsed dye laser, the quartz probe should be placed off center for efficient fragmentation. High energies up to 140 mJ are required for fragmentation. By placing the laser fiber in a crack or groove, extractable fragments will be sheared from the stone's central core and expose internal lamination (Fig. 10–11). Calcium oxalate dihydrate calculi can be fragmented with lower energies with the laser fiber placed more centrally. The fragments produced in both settings are quite different. Calcium oxalate monohydrate fragments are often sharp and irregular, and if larger than 3 mm should be extracted. In comparison, the more fragile dihydrate calculi, when fragmented, often form small, sandlike dust that passes spontaneously (see Fig. 10–9). Calcium oxalate monohydrate fragments may embed and subsequently be overgrown by mucosa during vigorous endoscopic lithotripsy.[21] Submucosal fragments can be associated with persistent ureteral obstruction and hence a need for extraction at the time of initial endoscopic lithotripsy.

Ureteroscopic procedures are frequently performed in an outpatient setting.[27] Postoperative upper urinary tract drainage is essential for this to be success-

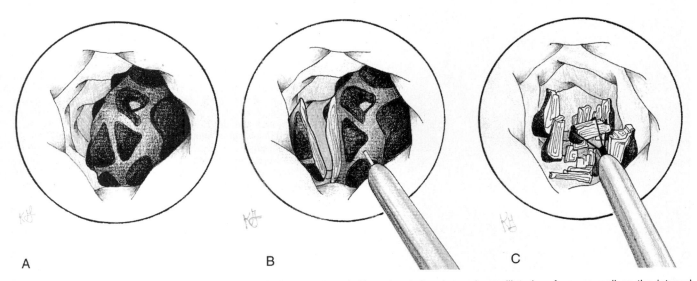

A   B   C

Figure 10–11. An impacted calcium oxalate monohydrate calculus. *A*, Note the dark color and mamillated surface, as well as the internal laminations. *B*, The quartz fiber of the laser lithotriptor is placed eccentrically in a crack or groove to shear fragments off the central core. *C*, To expedite clearance of the stone burden, the triangular fragments produced are often extracted with a basket or three-pronged grasper.

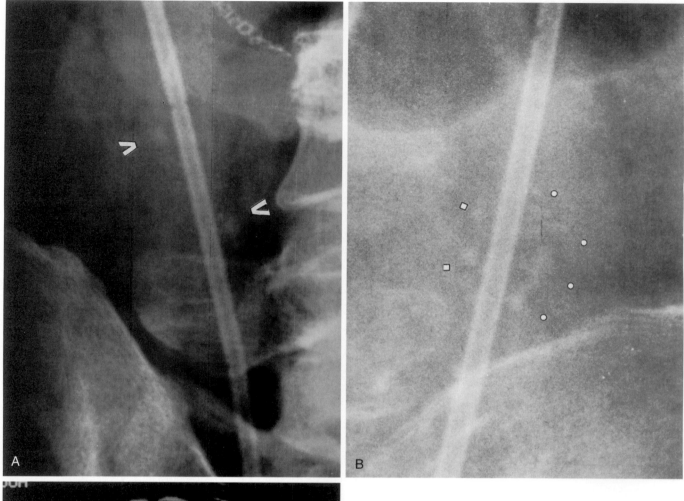

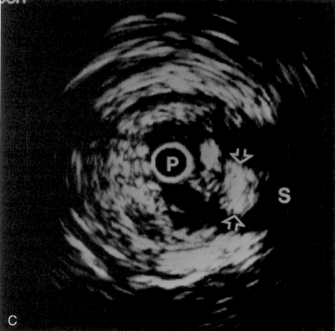

Figure 10–12. A submucosal stone fragment is most commonly calcium oxalate monohydrate in composition and may be the product of extracorporeal shock wave or endoscopy lithotripsy. *A,* A 35-year-old liver transplant recipient with persistent proximal ureteral obstruction 3 months after endoscopic lithotripsy. A plain radiograph is remarkable for two calcific bodies *(arrowheads)* adjacent to a ureteral catheter. No intraluminal stone fragments were noted on repeat upper urinary tract endoscopy. The position of stone fragments within the wall of the ureter was defined with intraluminal ultrasound examination. *B,* An elderly woman underwent extracorporeal lithotripsy monotherapy for an impacted ureteral calculus. A plain radiograph defined multiple calcific densities, as outlined, in the area of previous treatment. Ureteroscopy was initially nondiagnostic. Intraluminal ultrasound defined multiple small stone fragments within ureteral scarring. This was verified with ureteral biopsy. *C,* Sonographic image obtained with the 6.2 Fr., 12.5-mH intraluminal ultrasound probe (Microvasive, Inc., Watertown, MA). Probes passed in the upper urinary tract in either a retrograde or an antegrade fashion can image up to 1.5 cm laterally. The image presented is of a submucosal stone fragment that was associated with ureteral obstruction. This and other fragments were removed endoscopically, with subsequent resolution of hydronephrosis.

ful. Placement of an indwelling double-pigtail catheter allows for ureteral healing and for edema to subside. Depending on the nature of the endoscopic procedure, the catheters can be left in place for as little as 24 to 48 hours and as long as 6 weeks or more to facilitate ureteral healing and allow residual stone fragments to clear. Patients with complex stone burdens or infectious calculi often require careful hospital-based, postoperative monitoring and parenteral antibiotics. As an example, after treatment of an impacted distal third stone with an endoscopic lithotriptor, a ureteral catheter is frequently left in place for 7 to 10 days and then removed in the outpatient clinic. Patients are then followed up with serial plain radiographs to define any residual stone burden. Renal sonography should also be performed 4 to 6 weeks after removing the ureteral stent to rule out silent, progressive hydronephrosis from either a residual stone fragment or a ureteral stricture. Symptomatic patients require more invasive imaging (e.g., intravenous pyelography, retrograde ureteropyelography), which may lead to repeat endoscopy if there is a high index of suspicion for a residual fragment. Finally, careful attention to postoperative urinalysis is essential to rule out infection. Patients with a history of infectious calculi should have serial urine cultures and sensitivities obtained over at least the first 6 months postoperatively, and oral antibiotics prescribed accordingly.

COMPLICATIONS OF URETEROSCOPY

The evolution of endoscopic technique has decreased the overall complication rate of ureteroscopic lithotripsy. Downsizing of endoscopes and miniaturization of thermal-free lithotrites have also decreased intra- and postoperative problems. A relatively common complication is that of ureteral perforation from either a guidewire, a lithotripsy probe, or vigorous endoscopy. Small perforations are treated with an indwelling ureteral catheter drain and often heal spontaneously over the course of 4 to 6 weeks. Larger perforations and those associated with stone fragments may result in ureteral stricture and must be followed carefully with serial imaging.

Stone fragments associated with ureteral perforation may actually migrate into the periureteral tissue. If the stone fragments are outside the ureter they are frequently of no clinical significance, but if they are trapped within the ureteral wall they can be associated with obstruction and may lead to foreign body giant cell reaction and stricture.[21, 28] Persistent obstruction after endoscopic lithotripsy may be secondary to mucosal edema or a residual intraluminal fragment, but the possibility of a submucosal fragment or stricture must be part of the differential diagnosis.

Large-diameter (8 Fr. or more) ureteral stents may facilitate ureteral dilation and in fact can expose hidden stone fragments. If on a plain radiograph small, speckled calcifications or a larger radiopaque body are noted in the area of the ureter, and if these calcifications are not defined on direct endoscopic inspection, the diagnosis of a submucosal stone fragment should be entertained (Fig. 10–12A). Ureteral stone fragments can be diagnosed with intraluminal ultrasound and, when localized within the wall of the ureter, may be associated with postoperative obstruction (Fig. 10–12B).[21]

A 4 percent rate of major complications secondary to ureteroscopy was defined in 1988.[29] With endoscope miniaturization and thermal-free lithotrites, the complication rate has decreased and may approach 1 percent.

REFERENCES

1. Segura JW, Preminger GM, Assimos DG, et al. Nephrolithiasis Clinical Guidelines Panel summary report on the management of staghorn calculi. J Urol 151:1648, 1994.
2. Lingeman JE, Siegel YI, Steele B, et al. Management of lower pole nephrolithiasis: A critical analysis. J Urol 151:663, 1994.
3. Lam HS, Lingeman JE, Mosbaugh PG, et al. Evolution of the technique of combination therapy for staghorn calculi: A decreasing role for extracorporeal shock wave lithotripsy. J Urol 148:1058, 1992.
4. Loisides P, Beaghler M, Grasso M. Endoscopic Management of ESWL Failures. Presented at the Fourth World Congress of Endoscopic Surgery, Kyoto, Japan, June 1994.
5. Grasso M, Nord RG, Bagley DH. Shock wave lithotripsy failures treated with endoscopic laser lithotripsy. J Endourol 6:335, 1992.
6. Chaussy CG, Fuchs GJ. Extracorporeal shock wave lithotripsy of distal ureteral calculi: Is it worthwhile? J Endourol 1:1, 1987.
7. Seeger AR, Rittenberg MH, Bagley DH. Ureteropyeloscopic removal of ureteral calculi. J Urol 139:1180, 1988.
8. Blute ML, Segure JW, Patterson DE. Ureteroscopy. J Urol 139:510, 1988.
9. Wise GJ, Silver DA. Fungal infections of the genitourinary system. J Urol 149:1377, 1993.
10. Grasso M, Nord R, Bagley DH. Prone split leg and flank roll positioning: Simultaneous antegrade and retrograde access to the upper urinary tract. J Endourol 7:307, 1993.
11. Grasso M, Bagley DH. A 7.5/8.2 French actively deflectable, flexible ureteroscope: A new device for both diagnostic and therapeutic upper urinary tract endoscopy. Urology 43:435, 1994.
12. Bagley DH. Intrarenal access with the flexible ureteropyeloscope: Effects of active and passive tip deflection. J Endourol 7:221, 1993.
13. Grasso M, Shalaby M, el Akkad M, et al. Techniques in endoscopic lithotripsy using pulsed dye laser. J Endourol 37:138, 1991.
14. Webb DR, Kockelburgh R, Johnson WF. The Verapulse holmium surgical laser in clinical urology: A pilot study. Minimally Invasive Therapy 2:23, 1993.
15. Goodfriend R. Disintegration of ureteral calculi by ultrasound. Urology 1:260, 1973.
16. Dalton JR, Brutscher SP. Two cases of ureteroscopy and attempted stone disintegration complicated by disruption of the burr tip of the ultrasonic probe. J Urol 135:778, 1986.
17. Chaussy C, Fuchs G, Kahn R, et al. Transurethral ultrasonic ureterolithotripsy using a solid-wire probe. Urology 24:531, 1987.

18. Raney AM. Electrohydraulic lithotripsy: Experimental study and case reports with the stone disintegrator. J Urol 113:345, 1975.

19. Miller RA, Wickham JEA. Percutaneous nephrolithotomy: Advances in equipment and endoscopic techniques. Urology 23 (Suppl 5):2, 1984.

20. Denstedt JD, Clayman RV. Electrohydraulic lithotripsy of renal and ureteral calculi. J Urol 143:13, 1990.

21. Grasso M, Goldberg BB, Liu JB, et al. Submucosal calculi: Endoscopic and endoluminal ultrasonographic diagnosis and treatment options. J Urol 153:1384, 1995.

22. Bhatta KM, Rosen DI, Flotte TJ, et al. Effects of shielded and unshielded laser and electrohydraulic lithotripsy on rabbit bladder. J Urol 143:857, 1990.

23. Hofbauer J, Hobarth K, Marberger M. Lithoclast: New and inexpensive mode of intracorporeal lithotripsy. J Endourol 6:429, 1992.

24. Denstedt JD, Eberwein PM, Singh RR. The Swiss Lithoclast: A new device for intracorporeal lithotripsy. J Urol 148:1088, 1992.

25. Grasso M, Loisides P, Bagley DH, et al. Treatment of urinary calculi in a porcine canine model using the Browne Pneumatic Impactor. Urology 44:937, 1994.

26. Grasso M, Bagley DH. An endoscopic estimate of calculus composition directing laser lithotripsy techniques. J Endourol 6:1185, 1992.

27. Wills TE, Burns JR. Ureteroscopy: An outpatient procedure? J Urol 151:1175, 1994.

28. Dretler SP, Young RH. Stone granuloma: A cause of ureteral stricture. J Urol 150:1800, 1993.

29. Sosa RE, Bagley DH, Huffman JL. Complications of ureteropyeloscopy. In Huffman JL, Bagley DH, Lyon ES, eds. Ureteroscopy. Philadelphia, WB Saunders, 1988, p 157.

Chapter 11

Extracorporeal Shock Wave Lithotripsy

Alan D. Jenkins

INDICATIONS

Extracorporeal shock wave lithotripsy (ESWL) was first used clinically in 1980 and revolutionized the treatment of urolithiasis within a decade.[1] The use of ESWL was initially limited to calculi in the kidney and upper ureter, but lower ureteral and even bladder stones have been treated successfully. Open surgical removal of upper urinary tract calculi is rarely needed.

The goal of ESWL is to pulverize a calculus with shock waves generated outside the body. The resultant small particles pass spontaneously. A patient with a single renal pelvic calculus less than 2 cm in diameter is the ideal candidate for simple ESWL. Patients with larger stones and multiple stones can be treated, but complications are more likely. Isolated caliceal stones can be treated with ESWL, but the likelihood of complete particle passage is reduced for lower pole caliceal stones or stones in a caliceal diverticulum. This has led some investigators to advocate primary percutaneous removal for these calculi. A randomized study of ESWL versus percutaneous removal for the treatment of lower pole caliceal stones is under way, but patient acquisition has been difficult because patients are unwilling to undergo percutaneous removal of these small stones.

Staghorn calculi and large volume stones are usually approached with a combination of percutaneous lithotripsy and ESWL,[2] although staged ESWL with an indwelling double-pigtail catheter is used in some centers. The American Urological Association (AUA) Nephrolithiasis Guideline Panel reviewed the literature in 1994 and published recommendations regarding the management of staghorn calculi.[3] They advised that, for most standard patients, neither shock wave lithotripsy monotherapy nor open surgery should be first-line treatment, but rather a combination of percutaneous stone removal and shock wave lithotripsy.

The preferred method for treating stones in the upper ureter, above the iliac crest is ESWL.[4] Although ureteroscopy is the preferred method for removal of lower ureteral stones in the United States, ESWL is commonly used by urologists in Western Europe and is gaining wider acceptance in North America. In most situations, patient preference now determines whether lower ureteral calculi are treated with ESWL or ureteroscopy.

Radiolucent uric acid calculi that do not respond to a trial period of oral dissolution can be fragmented with ESWL.[5] Such stones can easily be treated with ESWL machines that employ ultrasound for stone localization, but a radiographic contrast agent must be administered intravenously or through a retrograde catheter if such stones are treated with a machine that uses fluoroscopic visualization. Uric acid calculi do not have to be finely pulverized. Even partial fragmentation results in a greatly increased surface-to-volume ratio that increases the efficacy of oral chemolytic agents. Shock wave fragmentation of uric acid calculi is especially valuable if a uric acid calculus has become coated with a layer of calcium phosphate during vigorous urinary alkalinization. Shock wave fragmentation will expose the central core of uric acid to the alkaline urinary milieu. The calcium phosphate shell is finely fragmented and should pass before the particles have an opportunity to grow.

Cystine calculi are resistant to shock wave fragmentation.[6] Renal calculi with diameters greater than 1 cm are probably best managed with percutaneous lithotripsy. Cystine stones that are impacted in the ureter are extremely resistant to ESWL: ureteroscopic lithotripsy or ureterolithotomy are better options.

The application of ESWL to bladder calculi has been described,[7] but transurethral lithotripsy or suprapubic cystolithotomy seem to be more efficient. Nevertheless, some patients may prefer this approach, and this option should not be summarily dismissed.

PREOPERATIVE MANAGEMENT

Patients who are potential candidates for ESWL should be evaluated with an excretory urogram or renal ultrasound. This evaluation is usually accomplished during the work-up of renal colic or hematuria. The purpose of the study is to evaluate the anatomy of the collecting system and to judge the capacity of the collecting system to pass all the crushed stone material. The likelihood of passing all the sand from a small renal pelvis is much greater than from a grossly dilated lower pole calix. A distal ureteral stricture would hinder passage of larger fragments. A stone proximal to this stricture would require finer pulverization or percutaneous removal.

The optimal treatment of stones in a caliceal diverticulum is controversial. The chance of rendering such patients stone free with ESWL alone is less than 50 percent. Nevertheless, the likelihood of rendering them symptom free (of pain, hematuria, or infection) is approximately 70 percent.[8] This needs to be discussed with patients. If they prefer to be rendered stone free, the best approach is primary percutaneous removal. If, however, they are not dismayed by the prospect of a few residual particles, primary ESWL is reasonable. If this option is chosen, however, the residual particles may regrow to form a new stone.[9] As long as patients understand the potential risks associated with ESWL, it seems reasonable to at least offer this as an initial treatment for a stone in an isolated caliceal diverticulum, especially in a patient whose symptoms are pain or hematuria.

The only absolute contraindications to ESWL are pregnancy and an uncorrectable bleeding disorder. A cardiac pacemaker or renal artery calcification is a relative contraindication. Such patients have been treated safely, but there must be a clear benefit of ESWL.[10]

The need for a general or regional anesthetic should be considered when evaluating patients for ESWL. Although a formal general or regional anesthetic is required with most treatments on an original Dornier HM-3 lithotriptor, lithotripsy on newer machines can be performed with only intravenous sedation or no anesthesia (piezoelectric lithotriptors). The availability of multiple lithotriptors has added another layer of complexity to the preoperative decision-making process. The optimal treatment of ureteral calculi provides an example. The standard management of ureteral calculi had been pre-ESWL placement of a ureteral catheter in an attempt to manipulate the stone back to the kidney. The availability of newer lithotriptors that require little, if any, anesthesia has made pretreatment cystoscopy unappealing. Patients and physicians must compare the appeal of in situ ESWL with the higher fragmentation rate achievable with ureteral catheterization and treatment on an original Dornier HM-3.

The limited availability of ESWL machines in some areas of the United States and the advent of mobile lithotripsy units that serve some hospitals only once or twice a month can delay the care of a patient. Patients with renal colic can be managed with a temporary indwelling double-pigtail catheter. Although these patients may have troublesome irritative bladder symptoms and intermittent flank discomfort from vesicoureteral reflux, the delay has no adverse effect on the ultimate success of ESWL.

Patients with asymptomatic ureteral calculi and mild obstructions have traditionally been observed for several weeks, or even months, in anticipation of spontaneous passage. Early investigators of ESWL found that ureteral stones that had been impacted for more than 6 weeks were more resistant to ESWL.[11] Consequently, patients with ureteral stones should be followed for no longer than 6 weeks. The popularity of in situ ESWL has probably led to the more rapid treatment of ureteral calculi. From the patient's point of view, in situ lithotripsy is preferable to an endoscopic procedure.

Some patients with upper urinary tract calculi may have concurrent urinary tract infections. Overt urosepsis should be managed aggressively and the patient should be stabilized before ESWL. It is paramount that any obstruction be relieved with a ureteral catheter or a percutaneous nephrostomy. Patients with branched calculi and presumed struvite stone formation should have pretreatment urine cultures taken, and the antimicrobial sensitivities of any isolated organisms should be determined. Because it is virtually impossible to sterilize the urine of such patients, long-term antibiotic treatment is not needed before ESWL. No adverse effects are seen if an appropriate antimicrobial agent is administered before the patient arrives in the lithotripsy suite. Some urologists administer prophylactic antibiotics to patients who have pretreatment cystoscopy and stone manipulation, even if the urine is sterile. This step may prevent urosepsis if bacteria are introduced during endoscopy and the patient develops an obstructing Steinstrasse ("stone street"; see Postoperative Management).

EQUIPMENT

Although the Dornier HM-3 lithotriptor was the machine that established ESWL as an accepted procedure, it is no longer manufactured. Older HM-3 machines are being replaced by second- and third-generation machines that require no anesthesia or only intravenous sedation. Nevertheless, some urologists still consider the HM-3 to be the best lithotriptor. This machine generates shock waves with an underwater spark discharge. The electrode tips are placed at one focus of a rotational ellipsoidal reflector, and the spherical shock waves converge at the second geometric focus of the ellipsoid. A patient is placed so that the stone is at the second focus, and multiple shock waves reduce the stone to particles 2 to 3 mm in diameter.

Since the introduction of the original Dornier lithotriptor in 1984, at least a dozen companies have developed extracorporeal shock wave lithotriptors. In spite of the number of devices, the machines can be classified on the basis of their method of shock wave generation and stone localization.[12]

Three basic means exist for the generation of shock waves. Most Dornier lithotriptors employ an underwater spark discharge and a rotational ellipsoidal reflector. Examples of other lithotriptors that utilize this technology are the Direx Nova and Tripter Compact, Dornier MFL-5000, EDAP Technomed Sonolith 4000, ESWL Products Delta 1000, Medas Lithoring Medstone STS, and Northgate SD-3.

A second means of generating shock waves is used in the Siemens Lithostar.[13] An electromagnetic coil generates planar shock waves at the base of a cylindrical shock head. The planar shock waves are focused with an acoustic lens and transmitted to the patient through a water-filled bellows. An electromagnetic shock wave generator is also used in the Siemens Lithostar Plus, Stortz Modulith SL-20, and Dornier Compact lithotriptors.

The third method of generating shock waves is with piezoelectric crystals.[14] The Wolf Piezolith 2500 and the EDAP LTO2 lithotriptor utilize an array of piezoelectric crystals mounted on a spherical plate. The application of an electric current to the crystals changes their shape. This shape change generates a shock wave that has a spherical configuration. The shock waves converge on the geometric center of the spheroidal plate. The OEC Medical Systems Therasonics LTS lithotriptor also employs piezoelectric shock wave generation technology, but a large piezoelectric crystal is attached to a spherical plate instead of mounting multiple small piezoelectric crystals on a plate. Piezoelectric lithotriptors have not gained popularity in the United States in spite of their ability to provide completely anesthesia-free lithotripsy.

The two basic methods of stone localization are radiographical and ultrasonic. The Dornier HM-3 and HM-4 lithotriptors and the Siemens Lithostar epitomized the use of a fixed biplanar x-ray system for stone localization. Radiographical localization is also used for the Dornier MFL-5000 and Medstone STS lithotriptors, but a single fluoroscopic system is rotated to provide two different views. All the newer lithotriptors, including the Direx machines, Tech-

nomed Sonolith 4000, Medstone STS, Stortz Modulith SL-20, and three piezoelectric lithotriptors, provide both radiographical and ultrasonic localization systems. Radiographical localization of stones is a less difficult skill to acquire, but ultrasonic localization of renal calculi can be just as successful as radiographical localization. Ultrasonic localization of stones in the juxtavesicular ureter can also be accomplished if the filled bladder is used as an ultrasonic window. Ultrasonic localization of stones in the ureter (other than in the juxtavesicular ureter or ureteropelvic junction) is extremely difficult, if not impossible. Ultrasonically visible ureteral catheters have been developed but are rarely used, because in situ lithotripsy of ureteral calculi is preferable to pretreatment passage of ureteral catheters.

One characteristic of all the newer lithotriptors is the need for less anesthesia. This effect is accomplished by decreasing the pressures generated at the focal area and by increasing the skin area through which the shock waves enter a patient. Little, if any, anesthesia is needed with the piezoelectric lithotriptors and is probably related to the large skin entrance area that is associated with shock waves generated with these machines. Although no anesthesia is needed, the patients can still feel the shock waves. This experience is not uncomfortable for most patients.

The makers of electrohydraulic lithotriptors have responded to this advantage by providing upgrades to their machines. These usually consist of ellipsoidal reflectors that are larger and result in skin entrance areas that are larger. One of the disadvantages of this approach is the reduction in size of the focal volume. Piezoelectric lithotriptors require that the stone be very precisely placed in the focal zone. The HM-3 lithotriptor is more tolerant, because its focal area is much larger. An analogy would be that the piezoelectric lithotriptors work like an ice pick to fragment stones, whereas the original electrohydraulic lithotriptors work like a hammer with a rather large face to fragment stones. In spite of the advantages of a large focal area (as with the Dornier HM-3), all newer lithotriptors can be used with intravenous sedation.

OPERATIVE TECHNIQUE

The shock waves produced by the original Dornier HM-3 lithotriptor are painful. Most patients require general or regional anesthesia. Some can be managed with local anesthesia or intravenous sedation, especially if the spark discharge voltage and resultant shock wave pressure are kept low.[15] The anesthetized patient is placed on a special chair or gantry, secured, and lowered into the water bath. A pair of orthogonal fluoroscopic systems is mounted so that their beams intersect at the second focus of the ellipsoidal reflector. The x-ray tubes are mounted beneath the tub, and the image intensifiers are suspended in two large canisters above the patient. The biplanar fluoroscopic system is used to accurately place the stone at the second focus and to monitor fragmentation during shock wave delivery.

The patient and chair are hydraulically moved until the stone is at the second focus, and shock wave delivery is initiated. Cardiac arrhythmias may occur with random discharge of the electrode. Electrode ignition is therefore triggered by the R wave of the patient's electrocardiogram. Shocks are given in groups of 100 or 200, interrupted by fluoroscopic verification that the crumbling stone material is still within the focal volume. A typical treatment consists of 1000 or 2000 shocks and lasts 30 to 45 minutes. Dornier recommends that a kidney be given a maximum of 2000 shocks during any 24-hour period. Although some urologists administer 3000 shock waves to a kidney during a single treatment,[16] most lithotripsy centers limit the single renal dose to 2400 shock waves.

A related problem is the safety of simultaneous bilateral ESWL treatments.[17] This approach was commonplace several years ago, but many urologists are now reluctant to perform simultaneous bilateral treatments. A major concern with this approach is the potential for bilateral ureteral obstruction. This concern is clinically unimportant unless the stone burden in each kidney is greater than 1.5 to 2 cm. There is some experimental evidence that bilateral ESWL treatments may be harmful to long-term renal function, but this is not accepted universally.[18] Bilateral ESWL treatment may be reasonable in a patient who has a 1-cm renal pelvic stone in one kidney and a 6-mm caliceal stone in the contralateral kidney. Bilateral treatment can probably be performed safely if the patient and urologist understand that there is the potential for bilateral ureteral obstruction and a higher incidence of the other complications associated with lithotripsy (because two kidneys are being treated in one patient).

The early application of ESWL to the treatment of ureteral stones led most urologists to pass a ureteral catheter in an attempt to manipulate the stone back into the kidney. If this was unsuccessful, the catheter was passed adjacent to a stone to provide an artificial "expansion space." Most urologists thought that a calculus would fragment more readily in a natural expansion space such as the renal pelvis or in an artificial expansion space provided by an adjacent ureteral catheter.

This approach was abandoned with the advent of second- and third-generation lithotriptors that can be used with intravenous sedation. Other studies have demonstrated effective fragmentation and stone clearance after in situ ESWL.[19]

In spite of the popularity of in situ ESWL, there are still advantages to pretreatment ureteral catheterization. A ureteral catheter can aid in the localization of a faint ureteral stone that is adjacent to the spine. The widespread availability of mobile lithotriptor units has also seen the use of double-pigtail catheters as a means of rendering patients pain and obstruction free while waiting for the arrival of the lithotriptor.

One of the most troublesome aspects of ESWL lies in determining the adequacy of fragmentation. One of the best indications of adequate pulverization is dispersion of the sand. This can occur only if the stone is in a cavity, such as the renal pelvis, that is larger than the stone. Caliceal stones or impacted ureteral stones may be adequately fragmented after 1500 shock waves, but the radiographical appearance may be unchanged. In such situations, it is best to stop after 2000 shock waves and follow the patient for 2 to 3 weeks. This time will allow edema to subside and the smallest particles to pass. The patient can be retreated if larger fragments are visible radiographically.

As a general rule, a calcium oxalate stone less than 2 cm in diameter should be sufficiently pulverized with 2000 shock waves at 18 to 22 kv (Dornier HM-3 lithotriptor). Calcium oxalate monohydrate calculi seem to be more resistant to fragmentation than calcium oxalate dihydrate stones.[20] Relatively pure calcium phosphate stones seem to be very resistant to the effects of shock waves, as do cystine stones. Up to 2000 shock waves may be needed to sufficiently fragment 1-cm cystine stones, although cystine stones that are relatively new may be easily pulverized. As a rule, struvite stones are easily fragmented with ESWL, but older struvite calculi can be very resistant to the effects of shock waves. An equivalent-sized stone usually requires more shock waves to achieve satisfactory fragmentation if a newer lithotriptor is used. It is not uncommon to use up to 5000 shock waves to fragment a 1-cm calcium oxalate stone with a Siemens Lithostar or a Dornier MFL-5000 lithotriptor.

TREATMENT OPTIONS

Ureteral Stones

Although the Dornier HM-3 lithotriptor was initially approved for the treatment of stones in the kidney or upper ureter, several investigators have successfully managed stones in the lower ureter. Stones in the upper ureter, that portion of the ureter above the superior border of the iliac crest, can be treated with the patient in the usual supine position. For practical purposes, the lower portion of the ureter can be divided into two portions. One is the presacral ureter, which passes over the sacroiliac (SI) joint (Fig. 11–1). The juxtavesicular ureter is that portion of the ureter between the lower margin of the SI joint and the bladder. Stones in the juxtavesicular ureter can be treated on the Dornier HM-3 lithotriptor with the patient in the sitting position (Fig. 11–2). The surrounding bony structures can make localization of these stones difficult. A retrograde ureteral catheter and a contrast-filled Foley balloon aid localization. Some investigators have reported ultimate stone-free rates as high as 98 percent with in situ ESWL of these lower ureteral stones.[21]

Initial attempts at treating stones in the presacral ureter were disappointing. Patients were treated in the standard supine position. Although some stones fragmented, most stones did not respond to the shock waves. The likely reason was that the shock waves had to traverse the thick sacral and iliac bones. Another problem with treating stones in the presacral ureter is that the stones often cannot be placed precisely in the focal area. The Dornier HM-3 lithotriptor was designed with a fixed focal distance of 13 cm between the top of the ellipsoidal reflector and the geometric focus. The distance between a presacral stone and a patient's back is often greater than 13 cm. The problems with accurate focusing and with shock wave absorption by bone can be overcome if a patient is treated in the prone position (Fig. 11–3). This maneuver requires a simple modification of the original gantry on the HM-3 lithotriptor.[22] Since the original description of this technique, several physicians have

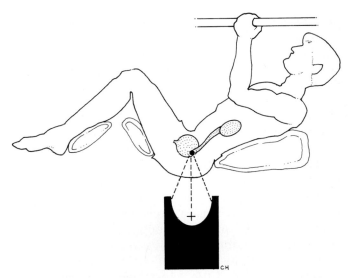

Figure 11–2. Sitting position used for juxtavesicular ureteral stones.

simply placed patients in a prone position on the newer mechanized gantries that are installed on most HM-3 lithotriptors. If patients with presacral stones are treated in the prone position, stone-free rates in excess of 90 percent can be achieved.

The limited focal distance of the HM-3 lithotriptor can also hinder the treatment of stones in ectopic pelvic kidneys or horseshoe kidneys. These kidneys tend to have a more anterior anatomical position. Patients with such kidneys can also be treated in the prone position.

Another way to treat stones in anteriorly placed kidneys is to use the "blast path."[23] This was described by Birdwell Finlayson and is based on an analysis of the various pressure vectors involved in the transmission of the shock waves. The blast path is the axis that extends from the base of the ellipsoid

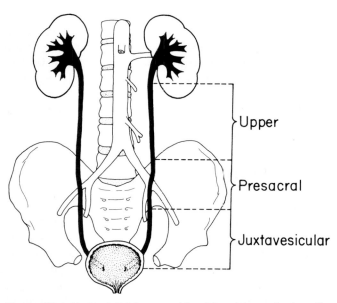

Figure 11–1. Ureteral divisions used for determining patient position during extracorporeal shock wave lithotripsy (ESWL).

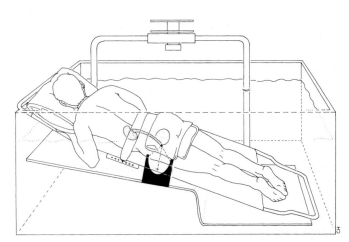

Figure 11–3. Prone position selected for presacral ureteral stones and stones in horseshoe or pelvic kidneys. (From Jenkins AD, Gillenwater JY. Extracorporeal shock wave lithotripsy in the prone position: Treatment of stones in the distal ureter or anomalous kidney. J Urol 139:913, 1989.)

and through the focal point. It is the major axis of the ellipsoidal reflector. Therapeutic stone fragmentation can be achieved if a stone is placed in the blast path, even if the stone is not exactly at the focal point. This therapeutic effect can be achieved up to 3 or 4 cm away from the geometric focal point, but more shock waves must be administered to achieve equivalent fragmentation.

Some theoretical reasons are given as to why management of stones on the blast path distal to the geometric focus may be more efficacious. Compressive forces are present in shock waves proximal to the focus, whereas tensile forces are present in shock waves that have passed through the focus. Kidney stones are much more sensitive to tensile forces than they are to compressive forces. Although this concept is very attractive, little experimental evidence has been provided that this technique works better than placing stones at the geometric focus.

Large Calculi

The early application of ESWL alone to large stones was fraught with problems. Patients with mean stone diameters greater than 2.5 cm were more likely to develop obstructions from stone fragments in the ureters. Percutaneous nephrostomies were placed after ESWL treatment in 29 percent of patients who had mean stone diameters greater than 2.5 cm. Only 1.8 percent of patients with stones smaller than 2.5 cm required a post-ESWL percutaneous nephrostomy.[24] These problems have led most urologists to favor a combination of percutaneous nephrostolithotomy and ESWL for large-volume renal calculi.

The approach to a large renal stone depends on several factors, one of which is stone composition. Large calcium oxalate stones (greater than 2 to 3 cm in mean diameter) are probably best treated with percutaneous nephrostolithotomy. Large uric acid stones can be managed with a combination of ESWL and oral chemolysis if an indwelling double-pigtail catheter is placed before ESWL. The fragmentation leads to a great increase in the surface-to-volume ratio of the stone. Adjuvant oral chemolysis with urinary alkalinization, fluids, and allopurinol will lead to a rapid dissolution of the stone material. Although cystine stones can be treated similarly, the chemolysis of these stones is not as rapid as that of uric acid stones. Percutaneous nephrostolithotomy is probably the best approach for large cystine stones.

Struvite calculi tend to fragment easily. The large volume of stone material, however, often leads to ureteral obstruction and the potential for urinary sepsis. Although obstruction from stone fragments can be managed, it seems to be more efficient to avoid this problem. The incidence of obstruction is related to the stone volume and the anatomy of the intrarenal collecting system. Some patients with normal upper tracts and small infundibuli and calices can undergo ESWL alone. The pretreatment placement of a double-pigtail catheter in this situation may prevent the development of an obstructive Steinstrasse and the need for post-ESWL auxiliary procedures.[25] ESWL monotherapy is advantageous for a partial staghorn calculus in the upper pole of a kidney with a nondilated collecting system. The upper pole location of these stones leads to rapid egress of the fragments. Although these stones can also be treated with percutaneous removal, their location may require placement of a nephrostomy tract very near, or even through, the pleural space. Partial staghorn calculi in a lower pole collecting system can also be treated with ESWL monotherapy, but the likelihood of rendering a patient stone free is lower than with an upper pole stone. Percutaneous removal of a lower pole partial staghorn calculus may be the best approach even if the stone burden is not great. A patient with a grossly dilated upper collecting system that is packed with stone material is best treated with initial percutaneous ultrasonic debulking followed by ESWL of any retained caliceal fragments. Another reasonable approach to these patients would be a formal surgical procedure, such as an anatrophic nephrolithotomy.

The AUA Nephrolithiasis Clinical Guidelines Panel has reviewed the management of struvite staghorn calculi.[3] They found that the expected stone-free rate for ESWL monotherapy was only 50 percent, while that for either percutaneous removal or combined ESWL and percutaneous removal was between 73 and 81 percent. They recommended that most patients with struvite staghorn calculi be treated with a combination of percutaneous stone removal and shock wave lithotripsy. ESWL monotherapy could be used for small-volume struvite staghorn stones in collecting systems that have a normal or near-normal anatomy. Open surgery would be appropriate in unusual situations in which an unreasonable number of percutaneous lithotripsy and/or ESWL procedures would be needed to remove the stone material.

POSTOPERATIVE MANAGEMENT AND COMPLICATIONS

A patient having undergone ESWL with a Dornier HM-3 lithotriptor often has a 2- to 3-cm diameter bruise on the back at the entrance site of the shock waves. Some bruising may also be evident on the anterior abdominal skin. Virtually all patients have gross hematuria for up to 24 hours after the procedure, even those who have been treated with second- or third-generation lithotriptors. Patients with stones in the renal pelvis often begin to pass sand the evening after treatment, which may be associated with irritative lower tract symptoms as the particles pass through the ureterovesical junction.

Patients should have postoperative radiographs to document the adequacy of stone fragmentation, and follow-up radiographs 1 month after ESWL. For all but the most simple stones, it is best to perform an excretory urogram or ultrasound to make sure that silent obstruction has not developed. A few reports have been made of nonfunctioning kidneys several months after ESWL.[26] Silent obstructions developed in these situations and, because the patients had no pain, they did not seek medical attention. It is important to emphasize to patients that they must come for medical follow-up, even when they feel fine.

Some patients may develop a column of sand in the ureter referred to as a Steinstrasse, which is the German word for "stone street." Surprisingly, many of these patients do not have renal colic. This lack of colic may be due to the presence of numerous particles that allow some urine to percolate through the ureter. Patients with a relatively asymptomatic Steinstrasse can be observed for 2 to 4 weeks. If the sand does not pass within this period or if the patient has an acutely symptomatic Steinstrasse, two techniques can potentially solve the problem. Patients can undergo cystoscopy and a ureteral catheter can be placed in the orifice. The application of pulsed-water irrigation with a syringe or even a Water-Pik device will flush many of the stone particles loose (Fig. 11–4).[27]

It is usually not safe to attempt to pass a ureteral catheter or even a guidewire, because the resistance to passage through this sand may be greater than resistance to passage of the guidewire through the ureteral wall. A patient may be obstructed because a large leading fragment is present. This fragment can be removed ureteroscopically. It is usually best not to attempt to remove all the material ureteroscopically. Vigorous efforts to remove all the sand may damage the ureteral mucosa and lead to a stricture. Some urologists have had very good success with pulsed dye laser lithotripsy of the particles.

A safer approach to the resolution of Steinstrassen is to place a percutaneous nephrostomy. Patients often begin to pass material after the nephrostomy. This effect may be related to more efficient ureteral peristalsis and coaptation of the ureteral walls after the hydroureteronephrosis has resolved. Antegrade pulsed water irrigation can also be used to loosen the fragments.[24]

Although the problem of Steinstrassen can be solved, it is usually best to prevent it by placement of double-pigtail catheters. These catheters seem to be most useful in patients with moderately large stone burdens (greater than 1.5 to 2 cm mean stone diameters). The low probability of developing obstructive Steinstrassen with stones smaller than 1.5 to 2 cm

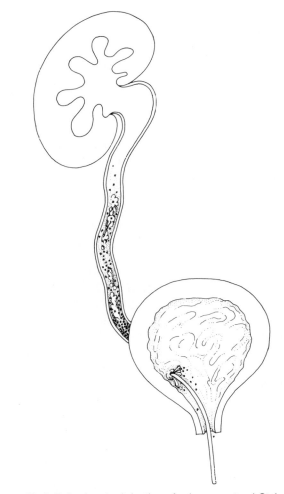

Figure 11–4. Pulsed water irrigation of a lower ureteral Steinstrasse ("stone street").

does not seem to merit the prophylactic placement of a double-pigtail catheter. The irritative lower tract symptoms associated with the catheters can be very aggravating. Removal of the double-pigtail catheters after treatment can be expedited if a monofilament suture is attached to the end of the catheter and permitted to exit from the urethra. Patients can remove the catheters themselves 3 to 4 days after treatment.

Many patients have nausea and vomiting after ESWL. These symptoms may be related to a small amount of retroperitoneal bleeding that occurs with ESWL. Approximately 0.3 percent of patients undergoing renal ESWL develop a clinically significant perinephric or subcapsular hematoma.[28] These patients may complain of severe flank pain after they have recovered from the anesthetic. Although the initial assumption is that this pain is due to renal colic from obstruction by stone fragments, one must always be suspicious of the development of a significant hematoma, which can be simply evaluated sonographically. Most patients who have symptomatic hematomas will not require blood transfusion or renal exploration. Nevertheless, reports have been made of the need for post-ESWL arterial embolization, nephrectomy, and late surgical drainage of a hematoma that did not spontaneously resolve.

Summary

ESWL has revolutionized the treatment of urolithiasis. Well over 90 percent of urinary tract calculi can be managed with ESWL. These include stones in the kidney and throughout the entire ureter.

ESWL machines and the application of this technology to clinical situations continue to evolve. Initial enthusiasm for ESWL monotherapy of staghorn calculi has waned, while that for in situ treatment of lower ureteral calculi has increased. The extensive efforts of the AUA Nephrolithiasis Clinical Guidelines Panel have led to the clarification of the role of ESWL and percutaneous nephrolithotomy in the treatment of staghorn calculi. Their future endeavors may lead to clarification of the proper role of in situ ESWL and ureteroscopy in the treatment of all ureteral calculi.

Editorial Comment
Louis R. Kavoussi

As pointed out in this chapter, most stones requiring surgical treatment are amenable to ESWL. However, each clinical presentation is different and treatment must be individualized. Not all stones should first be approached with lithotripsy, as this form of therapy has definite limitations and is expensive. The AUA Nephrolithiasis Clinical Guidelines Panel has clearly expressed that most patients with larger stones (e.g., staghorn calculi) be approached percutaneously or with sandwich therapy. Most ureteral stones being treated no longer require stenting. The relative roles of ureteroscopy and lithotripsy in the treatment of distal ureteral stones is still being debated as the benefits and costs are evaluated.

REFERENCES

1. Drach GW, Dretler SP, Fair WR, et al. Report of the United States cooperative study of ESWL. J Urol 135:1127, 1986.
2. Kahnoski RJ, Lingeman JE, Coury TA, et al. Combined percutaneous and extracorporeal shock wave lithotripsy for staghorn calculi: An alternative to anatrophic nephrolithotomy. J Urol 135:679, 1986.
3. Segura JW, Preminger GM, Assimos DG, et al. Nephrolithiasis Clinical Guidelines Panel summary report on the management of staghorn calculi. J Urol 151:1648, 1994.
4. Riehle RA, Naslund EB. Treatment of calculi in the upper ureter with extracorporeal shock wave lithotripsy. Surg Gynecol Obstet 164:1, 1987.
5. Royce PL, Fuchs GJ, Lupu AN, et al. The treatment of uric acid calculi with extracorporeal shock wave lithotripsy. Br J Urol 60:6, 1987.
6. Singh A, Marshall FF, Chang R. Cystine calculi: Clinical management and in vitro observations. Urology 31:207, 1988.
7. Ghatia V, Biyani CS. Extracorporeal shock wave lithotripsy for vesical lithiasis: Initial experience. Br J Urol 71:695, 1993.
8. Psihramis KE, Dretler SP. Extracorporeal shock wave lithotripsy of caliceal diverticula calculi. J Urol 138:707, 1987.
9. Fine JK, Pak CYC, Preminger GM. Effect of medical management and residual fragments on recurrent stone formation following shock wave lithotripsy. J Urol 153:27, 1995.
10. Goldsmith MF. ESWL now possible for patients with pacemakers (News). JAMA 258:1284, 1987.
11. Lupu AN, Fuchs GJ, Chaussy CG. Treatment of ureteral calculi by extracorporeal shock wave lithotripsy. UCLA experience. Urology 32:217, 1988.
12. Jenkins AD. A review of current ESWL technology. Urol Ann 4:265, 1990.
13. Wilbert DM, Reichenberger H, Noske E, et al. New generation shock wave lithotripsy. J Urol 138:563, 1987.
14. Marberger M, Turk C, Steinkogler I. Painless piezoelectric extracorporeal lithotripsy. J Urol 139:695, 1988.
15. Newman DM, Lingeman JE, Steele RE, et al. ESWL treatment using IV analgesia alone with an "unmodified Dornier HM-3" lithotriptor. J Urol 141:271A, 1989.
16. Spirnak JP, DeBaz BP, Green HY. Complex struvite calculi treated by primary extracorporeal shock wave lithotripsy and chemolysis with hemiacidrin irrigation. J Urol 140:1356, 1988.
17. Cohen ES, Schmidt JD, San Diego Kidney Stone Treatment Center. Simultaneous treatment of bilateral upper tract calculi with extracorporeal shock wave lithotripsy. J Endourol 3:37, 1989.
18. Thomas R, Roberts J, Sloane B, et al. Effect of extracorporeal shock wave lithotripsy on renal function. J Endourol 2:141, 1988.
19. Albala DM, Clayman RV, Meretyk S. Extracorporeal shock wave lithotripsy for proximal ureteral calculi: To stint or not to stint? J Endourol 5:277, 1991.
20. Dretler SP. Stone fragility—a new therapeutic distinction. J Urol 139:1124, 1988.
21. Jenkins AD. Dornier extracorporeal shock wave lithotripsy for ureteral stones. Urol Clin North Am 15:377, 1988.
22. Jenkins AD, Gillenwater JY. Extracorporeal shock wave lithotripsy in the prone position: Treatment of stones in the distal ureter or anomalous kidney. J Urol 139:911, 1988.
23. Whelan JP, Finlayson B, Welch J, et al. The blast path: Theoretical basis, experimental data, and clinical application. J Urol 140:401, 1988.
24. Tegtmeyer CJ, Kellum CD, Jenkins AD, et al. Extracorporeal shock wave lithotripsy: Interventional radiologic solutions to associated problems. Radiology 161:587, 1986.
25. Libby JM, Meacham RB, Griffith DP. The role of silicone ureteral stents in extracorporeal shock wave lithotripsy of large renal calculi. J Urol 139:15, 1988.
26. Hardy MR, McLeod DG. Silent renal obstruction with severe functional loss after extracorporeal shock wave lithotripsy: A report of 2 cases. J Urol 137:91, 1987.
27. Rubenstein MA, Norris DM. Variation on Water-Pik technique for treatment of steinstrasse after ESWL. Urology 32:429, 1988.
28. Knapp PM, Kulb TB, Lingeman JE, et al. Extracorporeal shock wave lithotripsy–induced perirenal hematomas. J Urol 139:700, 1988.

Chapter 12

Endoscopic Treatment of Urethral Strictures and Urethral Obliterations

Robert G. Moore and Fray F. Marshall

Urethral stricture disease is the most common urethral pathological condition requiring surgical intervention. A urethral stricture is defined as scar tissue causing contraction of the urethra that results in decreased urethral caliber.[1] Common etiological factors are trauma and inflammation. This chapter addresses the endoscopic treatment of urethral stricture disease.

PREOPERATIVE EVALUATION

Obstructive voiding symptoms with a history of predisposing factors (trauma, urethritis, catheterization, or instrumentation) are a common form of presentation for urethral stricture disease. This is usually confirmed by failure to pass a urethral catheter.

Bloody urethral discharge associated with pelvic trauma is a classic presentation for posterior urethral injury; others include perineal hematoma and/or difficult urethral catheterization in conjunction with pelvic trauma. A retrograde urethrogram is obtained for any of the above findings. A cystotomy is indicated for urinary drainage until posterior urethral continuity can be re-established in the pelvic trauma patient. Urethral realignment is deferred unless there is an associated injury of the rectum or bladder neck.

Before treatment of strictures, proper delineation is required of the length and location of the urethral stricture and the depth of the fibrosis of the corpus spongiosum. Urethroscopy, real-time ultrasound, and antegrade and retrograde urethrography are commonly used to assess these parameters.

A sterile urine culture should be obtained before any urethral manipulation. Antibiotic prophylaxis is given to prevent infection, which can lead to fibrosis and recurrent scarring.

The extent and anatomical location of the stricture can be delineated with a retrograde urethrogram. Standard intravenous contrast material is used as a precaution against extravasation, which can cause severe scarring and fibrosis.[2] Cystography is often needed to assess the length of an obliterated urethral segment, bladder neck competence, and bladder position after posterior urethral disruption.[3] During this study the patient must attempt to void to properly delineate the proximal prostatic urethra. Often the prostatic urethra does not fill but is still normal to the membranous urethra. Posterior urethral strictures less than 3 cm in diameter can be treated with endoscopic reconstruction. Normal prostate location on digital rectal examination correlates with an obliterated posterior segment of less than 3 cm.

The extent of fibrosis in the corpus spongiosum can be evaluated by physical examination, urethroscopy, and sonography. Urethroscopic findings of elasticity in the stricture generally indicate minimal fibrosis. Induration of the urethra overlying the stricture is the physical finding associated with fibrosis.

More recently, the depth of the urethral scarring has been evaluated by real-time ultrasound.[4–6] A 5- or 7.5-MHz linear-array probe is used to perform the examination. Sterile saline or 2 percent lidocaine jelly is injected in a retrograde fashion to delineate the urethra. Ultrasonic contrast gel is applied to the dorsum of the penis, scrotum, and perineum to examine the penile, bulbar, and posterior urethra, respectively. The urethra is scanned in both transverse and longitudinal images. Both stricture length and caliber are measured. The caliber (degree of stricture in the cross-sectional plane) is estimated by comparison of the strictured segment with the normal urethral segment. Densely fibrotic strictures demonstrate a hyperechoic area secondary to increased ultrasound reflection of the fibrotic tissues. Using this technique, treatment can be devised based on the degree of fibrosis.[7] As a rule, most strictures of mild or moderate fibrosis respond to endoscopic intervention.

ENDOSCOPIC DILATION OF URETHRAL STRICTURE

Urethral dilation is the earliest method used to treat urethral strictures[8] and has the advantage of being relatively easy to accomplish. Despite the immediate effectiveness of this technique, stricture recurrence is high, requiring frequent dilations.[9]

Technique

With the advent of the flexible cystoscope, urethral dilation can be performed with the patient in a supine position under endoscopic control. Two percent lidocaine jelly is used to anesthetize the urethra. The stricture opening is visualized and a 0.038-inch guidewire passed into the bladder under endoscopic control. Coaxial dilation is then utilized, using a graduated Amplatz renal dilator set or Nottingham ureteral dilation set.[10] Sequentially, dilators of increasing size are passed over the coaxial system until the desired caliber of dilation is accomplished. Care must be taken not to bend or kink the guidewire when passing dilators. If needed, a Councill catheter is passed over the guidewire into the bladder after successful dilation.

An alternative method for dilating the urethra is the use of a balloon dilator under endoscopic and fluoroscopic control. The advantages of balloon dilation are that it applies a stationary radial force and avoids the shearing force of traditional urethral sounds. Balloon dilation is excellent treatment for membranous urethral stricture to avoid injury to the external urinary sphincter (Fig. 12–1). It has also been helpful in dilating dense strictures in the entire urethra.

Stricture length is determined with a retrograde urethrogram under fluoroscopic guidance. The appropriate length of balloon is chosen (range, 5 to 10 cm). The diameter of urethral dilation balloons varies from 24 to 40 Fr. Most balloons currently used are available for other urological procedures (ureteral dilating balloons, nephrostomy tract dilating balloons). A smaller-diameter balloon is chosen for dense strictures, with increases in diameter with each sequential dilation.

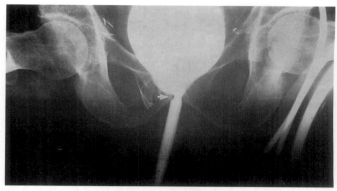

Figure 12–1. Balloon dilation of a membranous urethral stricture (arrow).

After a guidewire is passed through the stricture, the balloon dilator is passed over the guidewire and centered over the stricture. Radiopaque markers at either end of the balloon aid in placement. The balloon is typically inflated with contrast solution for 3 minutes at 5 atmospheres. The pressure can be monitored with a pressure gauge syringe, but this may not be essential. Occasionally, dense urethral strictures may require pressures as high as 50 to 75 pounds per square inch.[11] If a persistent waist is noted during dilation, repeat balloon dilation is performed until the waist is no longer visible. A Councill catheter can be passed over the guidewire into the bladder, but some investigators believe that catheterization is unnecessary.[12]

Postoperative Care

Endoscopic urethral dilation is performed as an office procedure. Patients should receive antibiotic prophylactics for 48 hours. If a Foley catheter is left in place, they may remove it at home after 48 hours. Patients can be placed on a self-catheterization program to prevent the high rate of recurrence. A coudé-tipped balloon catheter has been used for successful patient self-dilation.[13] Intermittent self-catheterization as a form of dilation works well especially in a patient who does not want any additional manipulations by physicians. Follow-up with a uroflow or retrograde urethrogram should take place to re-evaluate the need for subsequent urethral dilation.

Complications

The most frequent side effect is stricture recurrence, although some investigators have reported no such recurrence over a 4-year follow-up with balloon dilation.[14, 15] Bloody urethral discharge is occasionally encountered and can be treated by placing a urethral Foley catheter for 48 hours. Urethral false passage is a rare complication with endoscopic placement of dilators.

DIRECT VISUAL URETHROTOMY

Direct visual urethrotomy has been commonly used for endoscopic treatment of urethral strictures since the mid-1980s.[16, 17] This procedure is useful when there is only superficial spongiofibrosis.

Technique

The choice of anesthesia is dictated by the length and depth of stricture. The procedure is performed with the patient in the lithotomy position. By means of a urethrotome with a zero-degree lens, the stricture opening is visualized and a 5 Fr. ureteral catheter passed through it into the bladder. Saline irrigation is utilized to prevent inflammation from the extensive amount of extravasation of irrigation fluid.[2] Either a cold hook or knife blade can be used. We prefer a single 12 o'clock incision extending through the scar tissue, performed by extending the blade and moving the entire scope in an up-and-out direction (Fig. 12–2). This step is repeated until the complete length and depth of scar tissue is cut.[16, 17]

Fulguration of bleeding is rarely needed. A 0.035-inch guidewire is passed through the 5 Fr. ureteral catheter and a Councill catheter is placed into the bladder.

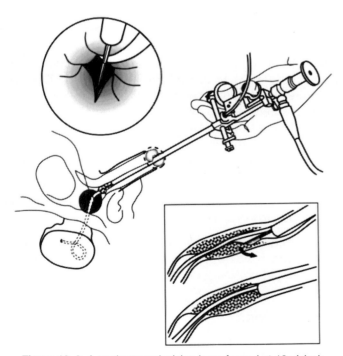

Figure 12–2. A urethrotomy incision is performed at 12 o'clock.

Postoperative Care

The length of catheterization depends on the extent and depth of the stricture. The catheter should remain in place until the urethrotomy incision has re-epithelialized. For superficial strictures the catheter can be removed within 48 hours; with long and dense strictures it should remain in place for 3 to 6 weeks.[2]

Complications

The incidence of complications after visual urethrotomy ranges from 3 to 25 percent.[18, 19] They include hemorrhage, sepsis, incontinence, priapism, chordee, penile pain, paresthesias of the glans penis, and impotence. The rate of recurrent stricture disease after direct visual urethrotomy is 29 to 50 percent.[16, 19, 20]

ENDOSCOPIC RECONSTRUCTION FOR URETHRAL OBLITERATION

The most challenging type of urethral stricture is complete urethral obliteration of the posterior urethra. Endoscopic reconstruction of urethral continuity for traumatic urethral obliteration has been performed since 1978.[21]

The maximal length of the stricture should not exceed 3 cm when endoscopic reconstruction is attempted.[3, 22] The timing of reconstruction is controversial. Some authors indicate that realignment should not be attempted until 3 to 6 months after the injury,[23] but endoscopic reconstruction has been performed after the patient stabilizes (1 to 3 weeks) in a limited number of cases.[24, 25] The proposed advantage to earlier establishment of urethral continuity is the avoidance of dense scar formation.

Three different forms of endoscopic reconstruction in posterior urethral obliterations are discussed here: (1) antegrade sound-assisted repair, (2) delayed bidirectional endoscopic reconstruction, and (3) early endoscopic reconstruction. The first two techniques are utilized when scar consolidation is present (more than 2 months after the injury). The third technique is used in the early postinjury period (1 to 3 weeks).

Antegrade Sound-Assisted Repair

Technique

The antegrade sound-assisted approach uses a cold knife optical urethrotome to incise the obliterated scar in a retrograde fashion.[26, 27] If the obliterating scar tissue is thin, the "cut to the light" approach is an option. The suprapubic tract is dilated with a nephrostomy tract dilating balloon, and a 30 Fr.

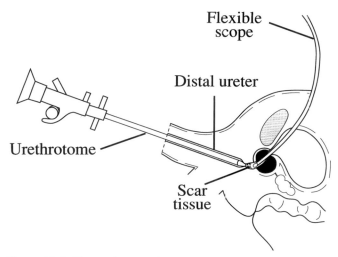

Figure 12–3. The urethrotomy incision is advanced toward the light of the flexible cystoscope. Blind cuts are discouraged. This is applicable only for short and thin obliterated urethral segments.

sheath is advanced over the balloon into the bladder. A flexible cystoscope is positioned into the proximal urethra, and the urethrotome incision is advanced toward the light until the endoscope is visualized (Fig. 12–3).

Unfortunately, a thicker scar is usually present, and the approach of advancing a Goodwin sound from the suprapubic tract is then applicable. The bulging of the tissue can be seen and used as a target for urethrotome incision (Fig. 12–4). After continuity has been established, a guidewire is passed through the Goodwin sound and the obstructing scar tissue can be incised, dilated, or resected. A 20 Fr. Councill

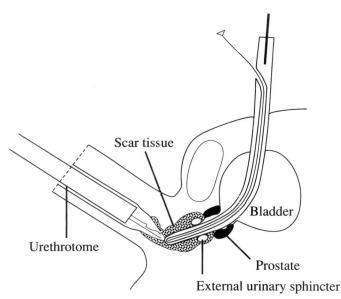

Figure 12–4. When the "cut to the light" procedure does not work, a Goodwin sound is placed at the proximal obliterated segment via the suprapubic tract, and the urethrotomy incision is directed toward the bulging tissue. If the sound is not easily appreciated, we recommend fluoroscopic alignment.

catheter is passed over the guidewire and positioned in the bladder. Unfortunately, this procedure has limited use because neither a "bulging sound" nor light in the proximal urethra may be seen.

Postoperative Care

The urethral Foley catheter is removed after 1 to 3 weeks. Suprapubic urinary drainage is maintained for another 2 weeks to confirm voiding.

Complications

The incidence of incontinence is 10 percent[26, 27] and in most cases is stress incontinence. Recurrent strictures have been noted in most patients requiring one or two additional urethrotomies. The incidence of impotence in this group was 13 percent.[26, 27]

Delayed Bidirectional Endoscopic Reconstruction

Technique

Bidirectional endoscopic reconstruction is accomplished with the aid of real-time imaging (fluoroscopy) and is generally preferred to "cut to the light" procedures. The patient is placed in the lithotomy position. After a suprapubic sheath is placed, a flexible endoscope is passed into the apex of the prostatic urethra. A 25 Fr. nephroscope is passed in a retrograde fashion up to the obliterated membranous urethral segment. Under fluoroscopic guidance a straight, narrow trocar (e.g., the Cook catheter needle set Rtan-5.OV-19-38) is passed into the prostatic ureteral apex (Fig. 12–5). After the trocar needle is visualized from the suprapubic endoscope, a 0.038-inch Rosen guidewire is passed and brought out the suprapubic tract. The scar tissue is dilated with Van Andel catheters (Fig. 12–6). The residual scar tissue is resected with a pediatric resectoscope.[28] A 22 to 24 Fr. Councill catheter is placed into the bladder (Fig. 12–7). Alternatively, the scar tissue can be resected with a pediatric resectoscope at a later date.

Postoperative Care

The urethral Foley catheter is removed 4 to 5 weeks postoperatively. Suprapubic drainage is continued until the patient can void.

Complications

Patients should be followed closely for recurrent strictures. Urethrotomy is usually required at least

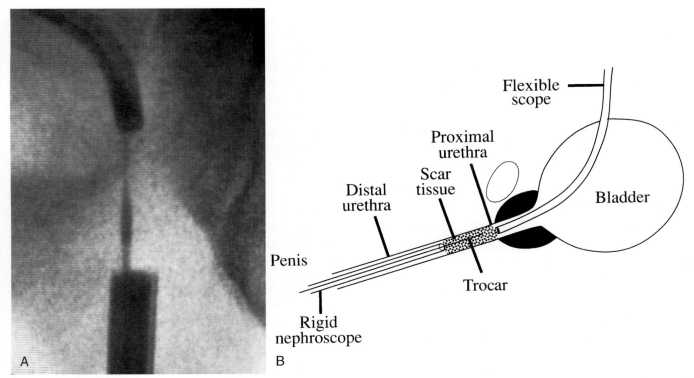

Figure 12–5. *A,* The proximal and distal obliterated urethral segments are fluoroscopically aligned. *B,* A straight, narrow trocar is passed through the nephroscope and into the obliterated scar. This technique provides controlled endoscopic reconstruction for urethral obliterations (<3 cm).

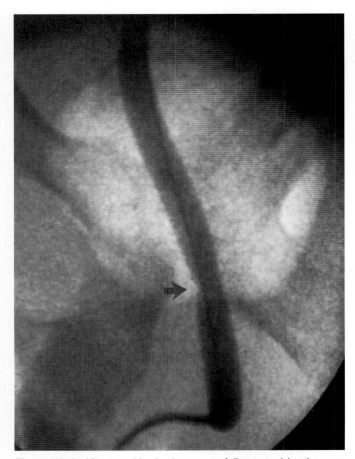

Figure 12–6. After a guidewire is successfully passed by the scar tissue, the obliterated urethral segment *(arrow)* is dilated.

once for recurrent stricture disease. The incidence of incontinence and impotence is 10 to 15 percent and 13 percent, respectively.[3, 22, 28–31] As long as the bladder neck is not injured, the incidence of incontinence is very low in our experience.

Early Endoscopic Reconstruction

Technique

Early endoscopic reconstruction of urethral obliteration is performed with general or regional anesthe-

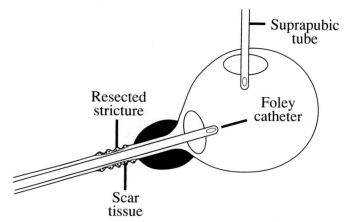

Figure 12–7. A Councill catheter is placed over the guidewire after dilation of the obliterated segment.

sia.[26, 27] A suprapubic sheath is placed as described earlier. A flexible cystoscope is passed into the prostatic urethra via a suprapubic sheath, and a rigid cystoscope is advanced in retrograde fashion toward the disrupted urethra under fluoroscopic guidance. Both scopes are aligned at their respective avulsed urethral ends. A 0.038-inch guidewire is then passed through the flexible cystoscope into the rigid cystoscope. A 20 Fr. Councill catheter is passed over the guidewire and across the defect.

Postoperative Care

A voiding cystourethrogram and cystoscopy are performed after 6 weeks to ensure patency before catheter removal. The patient is then started and maintained on a self-catheterization regimen for 12 to 18 weeks.

Complication

A stricture recurred in one of nine patients requiring visual urethrotomy.[24, 25]

EXPERIMENTAL AND NEW UNPROVEN METHODS

New techniques for the treatment of urethral stricture have been developed to decrease the morbidity of open urethral reconstruction. They include endoscopic urethroplasty and urethral stents. Both techniques have been reported to achieve short-term success in the treatment of urethral stricture disease, but long-term follow-up is lacking.

Endoscopic Urethroplasty

Endoscopic urethroplasty is a technique in which a skin graft is placed over the fresh bed of a urethrotomy incision.[32] The graft placement allows for rapid epithelialization, thus reducing the formation of scar tissue. It is not clear how often these grafts actually "take," and this procedure may represent no more than a urethrotomy. The procedure may be indicated when moderate to severe spongiofibrosis of the urethral stricture is present in a patient not desiring open urethroplasty.

Technique

Endoscopic urethroplasty is performed with the patient in the lithotomy position under regional or general anesthesia. A standard 12 o'clock cold knife urethrotomy incision is made through the scar down to periurethral fat. With dense urethral strictures, the entire scar may need to be resected. A full-thickness hairless skin graft from the thigh, forearm, or prepuce is harvested with a dermatome. Graft thickness should be about 0.45 mm. Graft length should be 2 cm longer than the length of the stricture to ensure correct placement over the entire stricture bed, since absolute accuracy of localization is frequently unattainable. The graft width should fit the circumference of a 20 to 22 Fr. Silastic Foley catheter (approximately 20 mm). The distance from the bladder neck to the proximal end of the stricture is measured to assess the location for graft fixation on the catheter.[32, 33] The graft is affixed to the estimated stricture point on the catheter and sutured in place with 4-0 chromic sutures (Fig. 12–8). The Foley catheter is positioned in the bladder. A compression dressing is applied to the penile shaft to help bring the graft into contact with the urethrotomy bed.

Alternatively, the graft can be secured to a purpose-built balloon that will carry the graft to the stricture site.[34, 35] Naude[35] described an alternative technique for graft fixation in which two 19-gauge spinal needles are passed from the perineum to the urethra. One needle is placed at the proximal end of the incised area, and the other distal to the urethrotomy site. Needle placement is confirmed endoscopically. Sutures are then passed through the needles, which are grasped and withdrawn from the urethra. These sutures are secured to the appropriate end of the graft. The graft carrier (Silastic Foley or balloon) is then drawn over the urethrotomy incision, using the proximal suture for traction. Cystoscopy is used to confirm correct placement when the balloon carrier is used. Both sutures are tied to a bolster placed on the perineal skin.

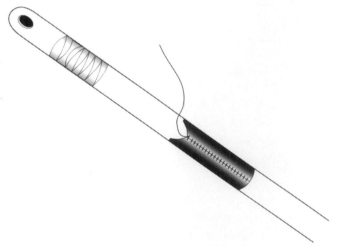

Figure 12–8. A full-thickness skin graft is affixed to a 20 Fr. Silastic Foley catheter.

The bladder is drained via a suprapubic catheter. If a balloon graft carrier is used, it is inflated enough to ensure moderate tension of the graft on the urethral wall.[35]

Postoperative Care

After the procedure the patient is placed on strict bed rest for 4 days when the balloon carrier is utilized, and 6 days when the Silastic Foley is used. The balloon carrier is removed under endoscopic control after 1 week.[35] If a Silastic Foley is used for the carrier device, it is removed 10 days postoperatively.[33] Suprapubic urinary drainage is maintained for 6 weeks. A voiding cystourethrogram is performed before removal of the suprapubic catheter.

Complications

Recurrent stricture was reported in 7 percent of patients undergoing endoscopic urethroplasty.[35] All case failures involved severe traumatic strictures.[32, 33, 35] In general, if these extensive endoscopic maneuvers are required, it may be more appropriate to perform open surgery, excise the scar, and reconstruct the urethra.

Urethral Stents

Cardiovascular physicians were the first group to use self-expanding stents to prevent restenosis of endoluminal obstruction after balloon angioplasty.[36] Both permanent and temporary stents have been applied for the treatment of outlet obstruction secondary to benign prostatic hypertrophy and recurrent urethral strictures.[37] Urethral stents are currently being evaluated by the Federal Food and Drug Administration for approval in the treatment of urethral stricture disease. This procedure should be considered for patients who have failed other forms of endoscopic therapy and do not wish to undergo an open urethroplasty.

Technique

Urethral stent placement can be performed with local, regional, or general anesthesia.[38, 39] Under endoscopic control a guidewire is placed through the stricture lumen into the bladder. The stricture is opened up to 30 Fr. by cold knife urethrotomy or urethral dilators.[40] The guidewire is then removed. The stent is preloaded in a compressed form on an applicator. With a zero-degree lens the stent is positioned across the stricture and released overlapping the distal and proximal portions of the stricture. One should realize that stent shortening occurs after disengagement: ap-

propriate compensation for this phenomenon must be made during stent placement. For a distal bulbar urethral stricture, stents should be positioned at least 0.5 cm from the external urinary sphincter to avoid urinary incontinence. They can be repositioned if correct endoscopic placement is not initially obtained. Proper positioning should always be confirmed by endoscopy before final release.

Postoperative Care

Patients should be followed up for stricture formation at the proximal and distal portions of the stent, encrustation of stent, and formation of occluding hypertrophic urothelium.

Complications

Most investigators report a greater than 90 percent success rate.[37-40] Failures are secondary to growth of fibroplastic tissue through the stent in the treatment of traumatic posterior urethral strictures. Early transient side effects include perineal discomfort and postvoid dribbling. These symptoms may or may not resolve after a few weeks. Additional side effects include stent encrustation, hematuria, and stress incontinence.[37] Significant longer-term complications of encrustation, recurrent stricture, and difficult removal make current urethral stent utilization more suspect as a long-term solution to urethral stricture disease.

Summary

Endoscopic treatment of urethral stricture disease can often be a challenging task. With careful patient selection, operative success and decreased morbidity can be accomplished with minimally invasive techniques.

REFERENCES

1. Yelderman JJ, Weaver RG. The behavior and treatment of urethral strictures. J Urol 97:1040, 1967.
2. Devine CJ Jr, Jordan GH, Schlossberg SM. Surgery of the penis and urethra. In Walsh PC, Vaughn D, Stamey J, Retik AB, eds. Campbell's Urology, 6th ed. Philadelphia, WB Saunders, 1992, p 2957.
3. Marshall FF. Endoscopic reconstruction of traumatic urethral transections. Urol Clin North Am 16:313, 1989.
4. Gluck CD, Bundy AL, Fine C, et al. Sonographic urethrogram: Comparison to roentgenographic techniques in 22 patients. J Urol 140:1404, 1988.
5. McAninch JW, Laing FC, Jeffrey RB Jr. Sonourethrography in evaluation of urethral strictures: A preliminary report. J Urol 139:294, 1988.
6. Merkle W, Wagner W. Sonographic evaluation of the distal male urethra—a new diagnostic procedure for urethral stricture: Results of a retrospective study. J Urol 140:1409, 1988.

7. Klosterman PW, Laing FC, McAninch JW. Sonourethrography in the evaluation of urethral stricture disease. Urol Clin North Am 16:791, 1989.
8. Attwater HL. The history of urethral stricture. Br J Urol 15:39, 1943.
9. Devereux MH, Burfield GD. Prolonged follow-up of urethral strictures treated by intermittent dilatation. Br J Urol 42:321, 1970.
10. Beaghler M, Grasso M, Loisides P. Inability to pass a urethral catheter: The bedside role of the flexible cystoscope. Urology 44:268, 1994.
11. Giesy JD, Finn JS, Hermann GD, et al. Coaxial balloon dilation and calibration of urethral strictures. Am J Surg 147:611, 1984.
12. Mohammed SH, Wirima J. Balloon catheter dilatation of urethral strictures. AJR 150:327, 1988.
13. Fishman JJ. Experience with a hydraulic balloon urethral dilator for office and self dilatation (abstract). J Urol 147:287A, 1992.
14. Daughtry JD, Rodan BA, Bean WJ. Balloon dilatation of urethral strictures. Urology 31:231, 1988.
15. Daughtry JD, Rodan BA, Bean WJ. Retrograde balloon dilatation of urethra. Urology 33:257, 1989.
16. Sacknoff EJ, Kerr WS Jr. Direct vision cold knife urethrotomy. J Urol 123:492, 1980.
17. Waterhouse K, Selli C. Technique of optical internal urethrotomy. Urology 11:407, 1978.
18. Asklin B, Petterson S. Visual internal urethrotomy with postoperative cystotomy or urethral catheter. Scand J Urol Nephrol 17:5, 1983.
19. Chilton CP, Shah PJR, Fowler CG, et al. The impact of optical urethrotomy on the management of urethral strictures. Br J Urol 55:705, 1983.
20. Aagaard J, Andersen J, Jaszcak P. Direct vision internal urethrotomy. A prospective study of 81 primary strictures treated with a single urethrotomy. Br J Urol 59:328, 1987.
21. Sachse H. Die Sichturethrotomie mit scharfean Schnilt. In Dikatim-Tecknick Ergebnisse. Urologe A 17:177, 1978.
22. Marshall FF, Chang R, Gearhart JP. Endoscopic reconstruction of traumatic membranous urethral transection. J Urol 138:306, 1987.
23. Leonard M, Emtage J, Perez R, Morales A. Endoscopic management of urethral strictures: "Cut to the light" procedure. Urology 35:117, 1990.
24. Cohen JR, Berg G, Carl GH, Diamond DD. Primary endoscopic realignment following posterior urethral disruption. J Urol 146:1548, 1991.
25. Towler JM, Eisen SM. A new technique for the management of urethral injuries. Br J Urol 60:162, 1987.
26. Lieberman SF, Barry JM. Retreat from transpubic urethroplasty for obliterated membranous urethra. J Urol 128:379, 1982.
27. Yashuda K, Yamanishi T, Isaka S, et al. Endoscopic re-establishment of membranous urethral disruption. J Urol 145:977, 1991.
28. Marshall FF. Endoscopic reconstructions of traumatic urethral transections. Urol Clin North Am 16:313, 1989.
29. Quint HJ, Stanisic TH. Above and below delayed endoscopic treatment of traumatic urethral disruptions. J Urol 149:484, 1993.
30. Chiou RK, Gonzales R, Ortlip S, Fraley EE. Endoscopic treatment of posterior urethral obliteration: Long-term follow-up and comparison with transpubic urethroplasty. J Urol 140:508, 1988.
31. Gupta NP, Gill IS. Core-through optical internal urethrotomy in management of impassable traumatic posterior urethral strictures. J Urol 136:1018, 1986.
32. Naude JH. Endoscopic urethroplasty. J Endourol 2:395, 1988.
33. Rosin RD, Edwards L. Endourethral urethroplasty. Br J Urol 51:584, 1979.
34. Gaur DD. Endourethral urethroplasty—use of a new catheter. J Urol 130:905, 1983.
35. Naude JH. Current concepts in the management of ureteral strictures. Surg Annu 23:69, 1991.
36. Dotter CT. Transluminally-placed coilspring endarterial tube grafts: Long-term patency in canine popliteal artery. Invest Radiol 4:329, 1969.
37. Parra RO, Boullier J, Cummings J. Endoluminal urethral stents: A review. J Endourol 7:117, 1993.
38. Parra RO. Experience with titanium urethral stents in men with urethral strictures and bladder outlet obstruction (abstract). J Endourol 5:S143, 1991.
39. Milroy EJG, Chapple C, Eldin A, Wallsten H. A new treatment for urethral strictures: A permanently implanted urethral stent. J Urol 141:1120, 1989.
40. Ashken MH, Coulange C, Milroy EJG, Sarramon JP. European experience with the urethral wall stent for urethral strictures. Eur Urol 19:181, 1991.

Part II

ADULT LAPAROSCOPY

Chapter 13

Laparoscopic Nephrectomy and Nephroureterectomy

Stephen Y. Nakada and Ralph V. Clayman

Laparoscopic nephrectomy was first performed at Washington University in 1990.[1] With a newly developed impermeable entrapment sack and a high-speed electrical tissue morcellator, a 190-gm tumor-bearing kidney (i.e, oncocytoma) was successully removed from an 85-year-old patient. Since then, this procedure has been performed both transperitoneally and retroperitoneally by laparoscopic urologists throughout the world.[2-8] Although it is primarily performed for benign renal disease, there have been subsequent reports of laparoscopic radical nephrectomy for renal cell carcinoma stages T1 through T3B.[6, 7, 9]

The advent of an effective laparoscopic gastrointestinal anastomotic (GIA) stapling device has enabled the urologist to couple laparoscopic nephrectomy with a total ureterectomy. The first laparoscopic nephroureterectomy was performed at Barnes Hospital, St. Louis, MO, in 1991 for a grade II transitional cell carcinoma (TCC) of the right collecting system. Since then, laparoscopic nephroureterectomy has been successfully accomplished at several other institutions.[2, 9, 10] However, given the relative rarity of conditions necessitating this type of surgery and the increased complexity of the procedure compared with a simple nephrectomy, its widespread use has been slow to develop.

LAPAROSCOPIC NEPHRECTOMY

Indications

The primary indication for laparoscopic nephrectomy is benign renal disease, including chronic obstruction, infection and flank pain associated with a poorly functioning renal moiety, renovascular hypertension, and the rare case of a symptomatic multicystic dysplastic kidney. However, an exception is xanthogranulomatous pyelonephritis, which is best treated by an open technique. With regard to nephrectomy for renal cell cancer, the usual indication is a clinical stage T1 renal cell carcinoma, but small T2 (i.e., <6 inches) and T3B tumors have also been removed laparoscopically.

Preoperative Patient Evaluation and Preparation

Routine preoperative laboratory studies include serum electrolytes, whole blood cell count, urinalysis, and urine culture. In patients with a renal malignancy, a metastatic evaluation is performed, including chest radiograph, computed tomography (CT) of the abdomen, and sometimes a bone scan. The last is mainly reserved for patients with symptomatic bone pain or an elevated level of serum calcium or serum alkaline phosphatase. The adequacy of contralateral renal function is assessed by serum creatinine levels and the renal appearance on CT. If there is any doubt about the ability of the contralateral kidney to function satisfactorily, a renal scan should be obtained.

Mechanical and antibiotic bowel preparation are carried out on an outpatient basis. This includes a clear liquid diet for 2 days; GoLYTELY, 4 to 6 L the day before surgery; neomycin, 2 gm, and metronidazole, 2 gm, orally at 7 and 11 PM the night before surgery; and prochlorperazine maleate (Compazine), 10 mg orally to limit nausea.[11] The patient is type- and cross-matched for 2 units of blood; autologous or donor-directed blood may be supplied, depending on the patient's wishes. With experience the bowel preparation can be reduced to a clear liquid diet and a Dulcolax suppository on the day before the planned surgery; also, a type and screen can be substituted for the type- and cross-match of 2 units. Informed consent is obtained for laparoscopy and simple or radical nephrectomy or nephroureterectomy. The patient is advised that there is a 10 percent possibility of an open laparotomy. A parenteral broad-spectrum antibiotic (e.g., cefazolin) is given on call to the operating room.

For the surgeon less experienced in laparoscopic nephrectomy, an arteriogram may be performed just before the procedure to identify the location and distribution of the renal vessels. At this time, the renal artery may be embolized to enable the surgeon to initially ligate the renal vein and thus simplify the hilar dissection.

Operative Technique: Laparoscopic Transperitoneal Simple Nephrectomy

Preliminary Procedure

Under intravenous sedation, the patient is placed in the dorsal lithotomy position and a 0.035-inch Bentson guidewire is passed up the ureter, over which a 7 Fr. 11.5-mm occlusion balloon catheter is positioned in the renal pelvis. The guidewire is removed and a retrograde pyeloureterogram performed with dilute contrast material. The balloon is inflated to 1 ml (34.5 Fr.), and a 0.035-inch Amplatz Super Stiff guidewire is passed through the catheter and affixed to its distal end with a side-arm adapter. A urethral catheter is inserted alongside the ureteral catheter, and both tubes are passed through a sterile plastic camera wrap and connected to closed sterile drainage. The patient is then transported to the main operating room.

Alternatively, stent placement can be performed in the main operating room via flexible cystoscopy, with the patient under general anesthesia in a lateral decubitus position. In this way, stent placement and pneumoperitoneum are performed in one step. Proper position of the ureteral catheter can be evaluated fluoroscopically.

Patient Positioning, Pneumoperitoneum, and Primary Port Placement

After induction with general anesthesia, the intubated patient is positioned supine on a beanbag mattress, with the iliac crest overlying the kidney rest and the break in the table. Pneumatic compression stockings are applied to both legs. In male patients a gauze wrap can be applied to the scrotum and penis separately to preclude a pneumoscrotum or pneumopenis during the procedure. A nasogastric tube is placed, and a pulse oximeter positioned on one hand to monitor blood flow. Both arms are placed on arm boards and the abdomen is insufflated via a closed or open umbilical approach. If a closed approach is used, the intra-abdominal pressure is allowed to rise to 25 mm Hg, after which a 12-mm port is inserted at the umbilicus. A 10.5-mm reducer, if not intrinsic with the sheath, is secured to the port; the 10-mm, 30-degree laparoscope is introduced and the abdominal cavity inspected to identify any visceral injury. Intra-abdominal pressure is reduced to 15 mm Hg.

The patient is turned into a lateral decubitus position, the contralateral arm is placed on an arm board, and an axillary roll is placed to protect the brachial plexus of the contralateral arm. The ipsilateral arm is then brought across the body and secured to an ether screen or a suspended arm board. A pillow is placed between the knees and thighs; the lower leg is flexed at the knees to 30 degrees while the upper leg is kept straight. Care is taken so that the surgeon has access to both the urethral and ureteral catheters; both catheters are prepared and draped into the surgical field.

The table is flexed and the beanbag deflated to secure the patient in a 70- to 90-degree lateral decubitus position. The patient is secured with chest and leg straps; soft rolls may be used to further support the patient, placed under the contralateral hip and upper thigh. The skin is prepared from the xiphoid process to the perineum and from the contralateral rectus muscle to the posterior axillary line. The urethral and ureteral catheters are included in the preparation; the camera wrap is carefully removed from the catheters, thereby keeping them sterile. A pulse oximeter is placed on one of the contralateral fingers.

For a transabdominal nephrectomy, the surgeon and camera holder are all aligned along the patient's front side (i.e., alongside the abdomen). The first assistant and scrub nurse stand facing the patient's back (Fig. 13–1). The primary monitor is positioned across the table in direct view of the surgeon and above the shoulder of the assistant. For the first assistant, a second monitor may be placed on the opposite side of the table just above the shoulder of the surgeon.

All laparoscopic instrumentation is placed on the nurse's table. The insufflator tubing and camera lines come off the assistant's side of the patient, while the irrigator/aspirator and electrosurgical lines come off the surgeon's side of the table (Fig. 13–1).

An alternative to this method is to place the patient initially in the lateral decubitus position and proceed to obtain a closed or open pneumoperitoneum by making an incision just lateral to the rectus sheath on a level with the umbilicus or subcostally in the midclavicular line. If this is done, it is helpful to make a 12-mm skin incision and then bluntly dissect

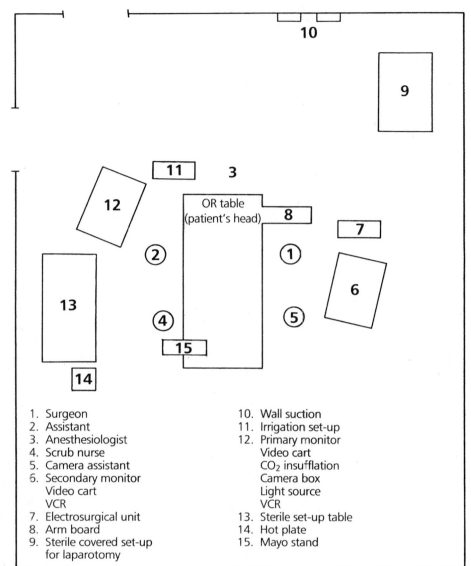

Figure 13–1. Operating room set-up for right laparoscopic transperitioneal simple and radical nephrectomy. Alternatively the scrub nurse unit (4, 13–15) can be placed on the surgeon's side of the table. In this case, the secondary monitor (6) and electrosurgical unit (7) move upward until they lie above the surgeon (1). (From Clayman RV, McDougall EM. Laparoscopic renal surgery. In Clayman RV, McDougall EM, eds. Laparoscopic Urology. St. Louis, MO, Quality Medical Publishing, 1993, pp 272–308.)

1. Surgeon
2. Assistant
3. Anesthesiologist
4. Scrub nurse
5. Camera assistant
6. Secondary monitor
   Video cart
   VCR
7. Electrosurgical unit
8. Arm board
9. Sterile covered set-up
   for laparotomy

10. Wall suction
11. Irrigation set-up
12. Primary monitor
    Video cart
    CO₂ insufflation
    Camera box
    Light source
    VCR
13. Sterile set-up table
14. Hot plate
15. Mayo stand

the subcutaneous fat. The abdominal wall fascia of the external oblique muscle can be grasped and elevated between two Kocher forceps. A 3- to 4-mm incision is made in the fascia and the Veress needle is introduced; its safe entry into the peritoneal cavity is facilitated by this maneuver. The usual guidelines for determining entry of the Veress needle into the peritoneal cavity also apply to lateral insufflation. This technique avoids the need to reposition the patient and provides a more lateral port for passage of the laparoscope, thereby facilitating delivery of the laparoscope to the area of the renal fossa.[6, 12, 13]

Secondary Port Placement

Five ports are used for laparoscopic nephrectomy. The incision for each is longitudinal with the exception of the initial umbilical port, which is U-shaped to conform to the natural skin contours of the umbilicus. The use of a no. 12 blade facilitates creation of a precise incision.

Under endoscopic guidance a 12-mm upper midclavicular line (UMCL) port is inserted just below the costal margin. The laparoscope is passed through this port, and the umbilical port site is inspected to rule out omental or visceral injury during initial port placement. A 5-mm lower midclavicular line (LMCL) port is placed 3 to 4 cm below the level of the umbilicus (Fig. 13–2A). After the line of Toldt is reflected, under endoscopic guidance, a 12-mm port is placed at the twelfth rib along the upper anterior axillary line (UAAL) and a 5-mm port at the level of the umbilicus along the lower anterior axillary line (LAAL) (Fig. 13–2B). Each port is sewn into place with a 0 Prolene suture to preclude inadvertent removal of the port from the abdomen.

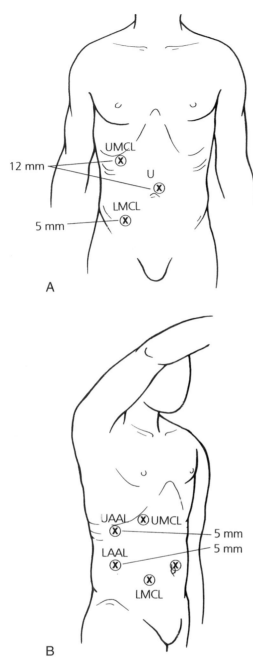

A

B

Figure 13–2. *A,* Initial port placement (supine). *B,* Axillary ports (12 mm and 5 mm) placed after reflection of the line of Toldt (lateral decubitus). If lateral insufflation is done, the U port is moved until it lies just lateral to the rectus muscle. U, umbilical; UMCL, upper midclavicular line; LMCL, lower midclavicular line; UAAL, upper anterior axillary line; LAAL, lower anterior axillary line. (From Clayman RV, McDougall EM. Laparoscopic renal surgery. In Clayman RV, McDougall EM, eds. Laparoscopic Urology. St. Louis, MO, Quality Medical Publishing, 1993, pp 272–308.)

Procedural Steps

A laparoscopic transperitoneal simple nephrectomy involves nine steps:

1. Incision of the line of Toldt
2. Securing the ureter
3. Dissecting the upper and lower pole of the kidney
4. Securing the hilar vessels
5. Incising the ureter
6. Intra-abdominal passage of the entrapment sack
7. Organ entrapment
8. Morcellation
9. Exiting the abdomen

Step 1: Incision of the Line of Toldt

The surgeon passes a 5-mm electrosurgical scissors through the 12-mm UMCL port and a 5-mm atraumatic forceps through the LMCL port. The white line of Toldt (i.e., lateral colonic peritoneal reflection) is identified and incised. After mobilization of the line of Toldt, the two AAL ports are placed. Next, the assistant can grasp and pull tissue laterally while the surgeon grasps and pulls tissue medially; the tissue in between the two forceps is pulled taut, thereby facilitating its incision (Fig. 13–3). The inferior extent of the incision in the peritoneum is the common iliac artery. The cephalad extent lies 5 to 10 cm above the hepatic or splenic flexure. During a right or left nephrectomy, the cephalad extension of the peritoneal incision, the right triangular and right anterior coronary ligaments or lienorenal and phrenicocolic ligaments, respectively, allows these organs to roll medially.

The surgeon and the assistant carefully advance their respective forceps cephalad along the cut edges of the peritoneum, placing the tissue under tension throughout the development of the retroperitoneal

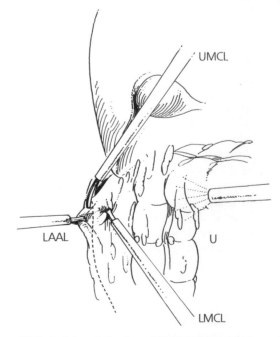

Figure 13–3. Incision of the line of Toldt (lateral colonic peritoneal reflection). (From Clayman RV, McDougall EM. Laparoscopic renal surgery. In Clayman RV, McDougall EM, eds. Laparoscopic Urology. St. Louis, MO, Quality Medical Publishing, 1993, pp 272–308.)

space. The surgical assistant uses the LAAL or UAAL port to improve lateral traction on the peritoneal reflection caudad and cephalad, respectively. The surgeon at this time may use the 5-mm forceps in the LMCL port to retract the transverse colon inferiorly. In performing a right nephrectomy, the surgeon now "T's" off of the lateral peritoneal reflection just beneath the liver and above the transverse colon. The peritoneal incision is continued medially, and a Kocher maneuver is performed to reflect the duodenum and thereby expose the anterior surface of the inferior vena cava. In a left nephrectomy the lienorenal and phrenicocolic ligaments must be electrosurgically coagulated and incised; if these structures appear to be substantial, 9-mm clips are placed before cutting them. This frees the spleen from the lateral side wall and allows it and the tail of the pancreas to roll medially away from the left kidney. The incision in the peritoneal reflection is continued medially, until the colon can be displaced medially, thus uncovering the kidney and the area of the renal hilum.

Step 2: Securing the Ureter

The scrub nurse slowly moves the occlusion balloon catheter and Amplatz Super Stiff guidewire back and forth; the ureter should now be seen moving in the retroperitoneum. The surgeon can also stroke the retroperitoneum horizontally with the 5-mm atraumatic forceps through the LMCL port to help identify the ureter. The forceps should be placed lateral to the

side wall of the aorta or inferior vena cava (IVC) and moved laterally across the retroperitoneum. The forceps will usually "bump" across the ureter, which has been made rigid owing to the placement of the occlusion balloon catheter. The ureter invariably lies more medial than expected, often tucked between the medial border of the psoas muscle and the lateral border of the IVC or aorta. If problems in identifying the ureter in the upper retroperitoneum persist, the surgeon should seek out the lower ureter where it crosses the common iliac vessels.

The assistant uses a 5-mm atraumatic grasper via the LAAL port to hold tissue laterally while the surgeon holds tissue medially through the LMCL port. Using the 5-mm electrosurgical scissors through the UMCL port, the periureteral tissue is divided and the ureter freed (Fig. 13–4A). A 1- to 2-cm window is created around the ureter, and a 4-inch umbilical tape is passed through the LAAL port and wrapped twice around the ureter; the two ends of the tape are secured with a 9-mm clip (Fig. 13–4B). The ends of the tape are secured with a 5-mm locking/grasping forceps via one of the AAL ports. The ureter can then be retracted laterally and rapidly dissected away from its retroperitoneal attachments. Alternatively, a 14-gauge Angiocath can be used to introduce a 30-inch strand of 0 suture material, which can be wrapped around the ureter. The end of the suture is retrieved by passing a loop of 0 nylon suture through the Angiocath and using it as a snare. A 5-mm grasper is passed through the loop, and the end of the suture is grasped and pulled through the loop; then as the loop

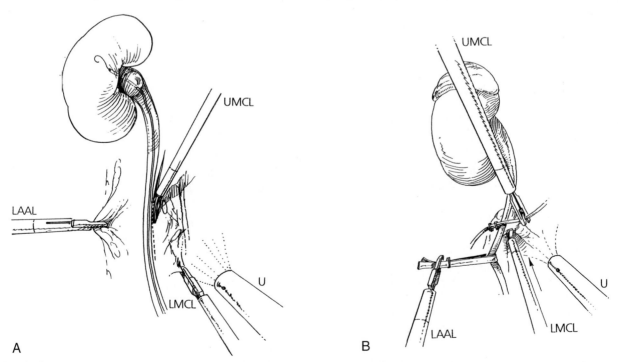

Figure 13–4. A, The ureter is freed by division of periureteric tissue. B, With an umbilical tape around the ureter, the gonadal vein is clipped. (From Clayman RV, McDougall EM. Laparoscopic renal surgery. In Clayman RV, McDougall EM, eds. Laparoscopic Urology. St. Louis, MO, Quality Medical Publishing, 1993, pp 272–308.)

is pulled through the Angiocath, the end of the suture is retrieved. The Angiocath is removed and tension on the ureter maintained by placing a small clamp on the two suspending sutures where they exit the skin. The same maneuver can be accomplished more simply by using a port closure needle device. Now the ureter can be suspended without having to use a standard 5-mm forceps through one of the five ports.

The gonadal vein is identified either crossing the right ureter anteriorly or lying medially alongside the upper left ureter. The right gonadal vein is dissected, creating a 360-degree window around the vein; via the UMCL port, the vein is clipped with four 9-mm clips and divided between the second and third clip (Fig. 13–4*B*). The left gonadal vein is left intact and followed cephalad to the renal hilum and renal vein. Once its juncture with the renal vein is dissected, the gonadal vein can be secured with four clips and incised between the second and third clips. This should be done at least 2 cm from the renal vein to avoid any problems with later placement of the vascular GIA stapler.

Rassweiler and Copcoat and their colleagues both describe early ligation of the ureter.[6, 8] This is done to further facilitate the renal hilar dissection. As such, the occlusion balloon catheter could be deflated at this point and, along with the Amplatz Super Stiff guidewire, withdrawn. The ureter is secured close to the ureteropelvic junction (UPJ) with four 9-mm clips and divided between the second and third clip. The cut end of the ureter is secured either with a 5-mm forceps or with a suture as described. Upward (i.e., lateral) traction on the ureter helps to expose the UPJ and renal hilum.

Step 3: Dissecting the Upper and Lower Pole of the Kidney

Once the ureter is freed up to the UPJ, Gerota's fascia is incised. The renal capsule overlying the lower pole of the kidney is identified, and the lower pole and lateral aspect of the kidney are dissected. As dissection is continued cephalad and medially, the adrenal gland is dissected away from the upper pole of the kidney. The upper pole is freed medially until its entire surface is exposed (Fig. 13–5).

In a right nephrectomy, dissection of the upper pole can be very difficult because of the encroaching edge of the liver. In this case, the surgeon should be certain that a sufficiently cephalad incision in the peritoneal reflection has been made; this allows the liver to rotate medially and also facilitates its cephalad retraction. The patient should be placed in a head-down position. The second assistant can use a 10-mm retractor through the UMCL port; the retractor should lie inside the upper cut edge of the peritoneal

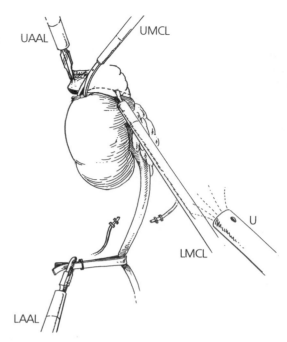

Figure 13–5. Freeing the upper pole of the kidney from the adrenal gland. (From Clayman RV, McDougall EM. Laparoscopic renal surgery. In Clayman RV, McDougall EM, eds. Laparoscopic Urology. St. Louis, MO, Quality Medical Publishing, 1993, pp 272–308.)

reflection. Thus, as the retractor is pushed cephalad to lift the liver, it is pushing directly on the underside of the incised peritoneum, thereby limiting any trauma to the liver from the retractor. Next, the surgeon can use the LMCL port to displace the upper pole of the kidney caudad. In a left nephrectomy, the spleen is retracted in a similar manner, so that any pressure on the spleen is indirectly applied through the peritoneum. Again, the cephalad extent of the peritoneotomy should extend superior to the spleen in order that it can be safely moved medially.

Step 4: Securing the Hilar Vessels

The renal hilum is placed on stretch by the assistant via lateral and upward traction on the ureter through the LAAL port, and lateral traction along the medial surface of the upper pole of the kidney via an atraumatic forceps passed through the UAAL port (Fig. 13–6). The surgeon operates with the electrosurgical scissors and the atraumatic forceps through the UMCL and LMCL ports, respectively. The dolphin-type and spoon forceps are useful for hilar dissection; the former are more pointed, which allows for finer, albeit potentially more traumatic, dissection of the perivascular tissues. In addition to the electrosurgical scissors, a right-angled hook electrode can be very helpful. With the tip end of the hook instrument, fine vessels and lymphatics surrounding the hilum can be lifted away from the hilar vessels and electrocoagu-

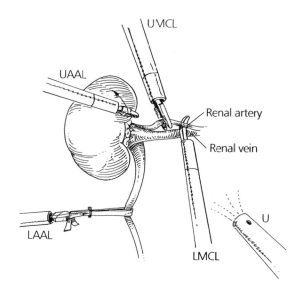

Figure 13–6. With the renal hilum on stretch via the axillary ports, the renal hilum is dissected free. Note that the renal artery is being clipped with a 10-mm multiload clip applier. (From Clayman RV, McDougall EM. Laparoscopic renal surgery. In Clayman RV, McDougall EM, eds. Laparoscopic Urology. St. Louis, MO, Quality Medical Publishing, 1993, pp 272–308.)

lated. The elbow of the hook electrode can then be used to bluntly dissect the underlying relatively avascular hilar fat.

Recently, Pearle and colleagues have been using a pneumodissector set at 4 atmospheres (atm) of pressure to bluntly dissect renal hilar tissues.[14] The pneumodissector is fired in brief bursts directly on the hilar tissue, thereby rapidly separating the hilar fat and exposing the main renal vessels. Any remaining perivascular tissue is then electrocoagulated via the hook electrode.[14]

The renal hilum is identified by moving cephalad along the medial aspect of the UPJ. The renal vein is seen first; dissection begins anteriorly, then continues inferiorly, superiorly, and posteriorly. Once the vein is dissected free and a 360-degree window created, the renal artery is identified and similarly dissected. A 10-mm right-angled dissector passed via the UMCL port facilitates creation of a 360-degree window around each renal vessel. For this task, the right-angled instrument is preferable to a curved dissector.

Typically, there is a single renal artery and vein on the right. However, on the left side the adrenal, ascending lumbar, and gonadal venous branches must be dissected and controlled separately. Again, four 9-mm clips are placed on each vein and the vein is incised between the second and third clips.

Once the renal vein and renal artery have been clearly dissected, the 10-mm multiload automatic feed clip applier is passed through the UMCL port. Five 9-mm titanium clips are applied to the renal artery and the artery is transected, leaving three clips on the stump side (Fig. 13–7).

In most cases the renal vein is too wide to be

secured with 9-mm or even 11-mm clips. In this situation the GIA vascular stapler is most useful; it simultaneously places six 3-cm long rows of staples and incises the renal vein between the third and fourth rows. Alternatively, the renal vein can be secured with free ties of 0 silk using extracorporeal knotting techniques.

Lastly, in some cases the GIA stapler has been used to secure the entire renal hilum en masse. Laboratory studies by Kerbl and associates have shown that this maneuver can result in a renal arteriovenous malformation.[16] Overall, it is safest to cleanly dissect both the renal artery and renal vein and to secure and divide them separately. These principles are the same as applied in the approach to the renal hilum during open surgery.

Step 5: Incising the Ureter

At this time the kidney's remaining retroperitoneal attachments are incised, leaving the ureter as the kidney's sole tether to the retroperitoneum. Next, the ureteral balloon catheter is deflated and removed along with the Super Stiff guidewire. The assistant now holds the ureter on tension via both AAL ports. Via the UMCL port, the 9-mm clip applier is passed, and four 9-mm clips are applied to the ureter 5 cm below the UPJ. The ureter is divided between the pairs of clips; the umbilical tape or suture used to retract the ureter is cut and removed via the UMCL port (Fig. 13–8). After ureteral division, a 5-mm traumatic locking/grasping forceps is passed through the UAAL port and secured to the proximal ureter. The ureter and attached kidney are then moved cephalad

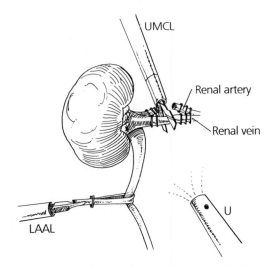

Figure 13–7. The renal artery has been transected, leaving three clips on the stump side; the renal vein has been secured similarly and is being transected. When the kidney is of normal size, a vascular GIA stapler is used to secure the renal vein. (From Clayman RV, McDougall EM. Laparoscopic renal surgery. In Clayman RV, McDougall EM, eds. Laparoscopic Urology. St. Louis, MO, Quality Medical Publishing, 1993, pp 272–308.)

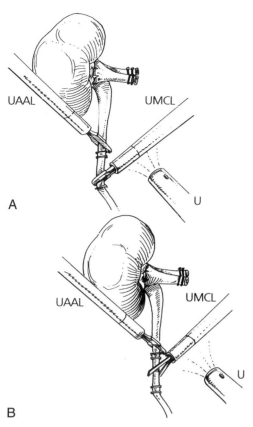

Figure 13–8. *A,* The ureter is clipped with four 9-mm clips, and divided between the two pairs of clips *(B).* (From Clayman RV, McDougall EM. Laparoscopic renal surgery. In Clayman RV, McDougall EM, eds. Laparoscopic Urology. St. Louis, MO, Quality Medical Publishing, 1993, pp 272–308.)

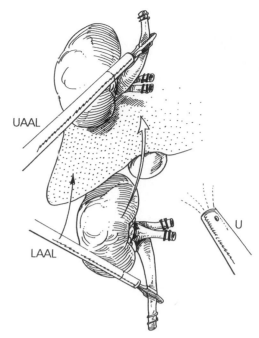

Figure 13–9. Using the traumatic locking/grasping forceps through the UAAL port, the ureter and attached kidney are moved to the ipsilateral upper quadrant, in this case onto the surface of the liver. (From Clayman RV, McDougall EM. Laparoscopic renal surgery. In Clayman RV, McDougall EM, eds. Laparoscopic Urology. St. Louis, MO, Quality Medical Publishing, 1993, pp 272–308.)

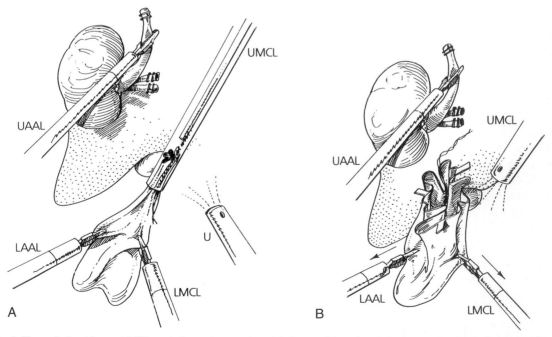

Figure 13–10. *A,* Through the 12-mm UMCL port, the entrapment sack is inserted into the abdomen. *B,* The entrapment sack is pulled deeper into the peritoneal cavity with two atraumatic 5-mm grasping forceps. (From Clayman RV, McDougall EM. Laparoscopic renal surgery. In Clayman RV, McDougall EM, eds. Laparoscopic Urology. St. Louis, MO, Quality Medical Publishing, 1993, pp 272–308.)

into the ipsilateral upper quadrant until the kidney rests on the surface of the liver or the spleen (Fig. 13–9). The 5-mm traumatic locking/grasping forceps is not released from the ureter.

Step 6: Intra-abdominal Passage of the Entrapment Sack

A variety of entrapment sacks are available. All except one, the LapSac (Cook Urology Inc., Spencer, IN), are made of a thin plastic, so that while they are easy to open, any manipulation of tissue within the sack results in the sack being torn. These thin-walled sacks are best used if the plan is to remove the benign kidney intact. In this case, however, the port site must be incised until it is large enough to allow the kidney and sack to be removed without any tension on the latter. However, if the plan is to morcellate the kidney, a 5- by 8-inch LapSac is introduced via the 12-mm UMCL port. The sack is rolled clockwise onto the forked introducer so that both tines remain outside the sack. It is also important to initially fold the drawstring down along the body of the sack, so that as the sack is wrapped around the tines, the drawstring is entrapped in the body of the sack. If this is not done, the drawstring may become enmeshed in the port's flap valve, greatly complicating introduction and subsequent opening of the sack. Via the 12-mm UMCL port, the loaded sack introducer is pushed into the abdomen up to its hub (Fig. 13–10A). This is done under continuous endoscopic monitoring. Us-

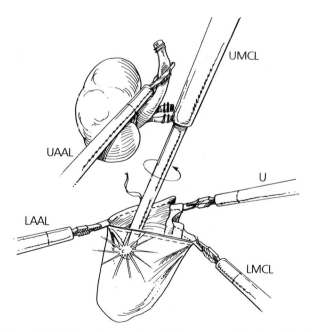

Figure 13–11. The entrapment sack is now opened using the shaft of the laparoscope through the UMCL port. (From Clayman RV, McDougall EM. Laparoscopic renal surgery. In Clayman RV, McDougall EM, eds. Laparoscopic Urology. St. Louis, MO, Quality Medical Publishing, 1993, pp 272–308.)

ing atraumatic 5-mm grasping forceps passed via the LAAL and LMCL ports, the bottom of the sack is pulled deeper into the peritoneal cavity (Fig. 13–10B). While the bottom of the sack is held with a 5-mm atraumatic forceps, the entrapment sack introducer is twisted counterclockwise and slowly removed. The blue drawstring should now be visible at the intra-abdominal end of the 12-mm UMCL port; the sack should lie entirely within the abdomen. The two atraumatic graspers can be used to gently pull the sack deeper into the abdomen and to unfurl the sack until it lies flat.

The 30-degree lens laparoscope is moved to the UMCL port. The entrapment sack is opened by passing three 5-mm traumatic locking/grasping forceps via the LAAL, umbilical, and LMCL ports and grasping the three equidistant tabs that lie along the mouth of the sack. The laparoscope is now pushed into the sack and then used to further open the sack by progressively widening circular motions of the shaft of the laparoscope (Fig. 13–11). To triangulate open the mouth of the sack, each grasper is pulled in a different direction: umbilical, slightly medial and cephalad; LAAL, lateral and slightly caudad; and LMCL, medial. This creates a slight bevel to the mouth of the sack so that the lower leading edge of the sack protrudes slightly forward of the upper edge.

Step 7: Organ Entrapment

The 5-mm locking/grasping forceps that still holds the ureter is now used to maneuver the proximal ureter and kidney into the sack (Fig. 13–12). With the sack opened as described, the assistant delivers the ureter high into the sack just beneath the upper edge tab held through the LAAL port. The kidney should now rest on the apron created by pulling the lower edge of the sack, via the umbilical port forceps, cephalad (Fig. 13–13). As the assistant is pushing the kidney deeper into the sack, the surgeon slowly lifts the umbilical port grasper laterally, closing the sack over the lower pole of the kidney.

Once the kidney is within the entrapment sack, the drawstrings are grasped with 5-mm locking/grasping forceps via the umbilical port. The assistant releases the ureter, withdraws the locking/grasping forceps from the sack, and then grasps the drawstring from the umbilical port grasper. The drawstring is pulled into but not through the sheath of the 12-mm UAAL port, thus closing the sack (Fig. 13–14). At this time the intra-abdominal pressure is lowered to 5 mm Hg and a careful search made for any bleeding site.

Step 8: Morcellation

The drawstring is now pulled through the 12-mm UAAL port, drawing the neck of the sack into the

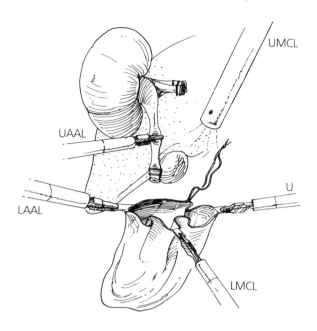

Figure 13–12. Using the 5-mm locking/grasping forceps on the ureter, the ureter and attached kidney are maneuvered into the open sack. (From Clayman RV, McDougall EM. Laparoscopic renal surgery. In Clayman RV, McDougall EM, eds. Laparoscopic Urology. St. Louis, MO, Quality Medical Publishing, 1993, pp 272–308.)

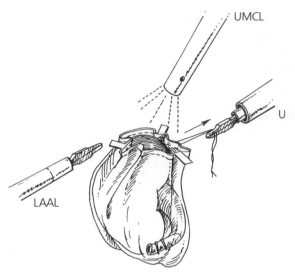

Figure 13–14. The sack is closed by pulling the drawstring. Once the neck of the sack is tightened, the drawstring is transferred from the U to the UAAL grasper and delivered onto the abdominal wall through that port. (From Clayman RV, McDougall EM. Laparoscopic renal surgery. In Clayman RV, McDougall EM, eds. Laparoscopic Urology. St. Louis, MO, Quality Medical Publishing, 1993, pp 272–308.)

barrel of the sheath (Fig. 13–15). The drawstring is released, and the forceps and the UAAL sheath are removed from the patient so that just the drawstring of the sack remains protruding through the 12-mm UAAL incision. Under endoscopic monitoring, the drawstring is pulled up until the entire neck of the sack rests on the abdomen (Fig. 13–16A).

Morcellation can be done either manually or with a high-speed electrical tissue morcellator. In the former

case a Kelly clamp and a ring forceps work extremely well. Either instrument is introduced into the sack and the kidney is fragmented. Pieces of renal tissue are then pulled from the sack. This is always done under continuous endoscopic control through the laparoscope to monitor for any perforation of the sack.

Alternatively, if the electrical tissue morcellator is available, it is plugged into a wall socket and its handle is connected to wall suction; the aspiration

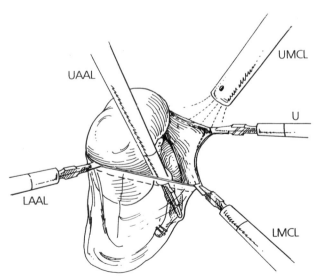

Figure 13–13. The ureter and attached kidney, resting on the lower edge of the sack, are being pushed into the sack by the assistant while the surgeon lifts the sack with the umbilical port forceps. (From Clayman RV, McDougall EM. Laparoscopic renal surgery. In Clayman RV, McDougall EM, eds. Laparoscopic Urology. St. Louis, MO, Quality Medical Publishing, 1993, pp 272–308.)

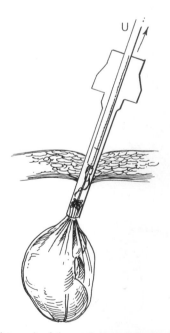

Figure 13–15. The neck of the sack is now drawn into the umbilical sheath by pulling the drawstring into the 12-mm UAAL port. (From Clayman RV, McDougall EM. Laparoscopic renal surgery. In Clayman RV, McDougall EM, eds. Laparoscopic Urology. St. Louis, MO, Quality Medical Publishing, 1993, pp 272–308.)

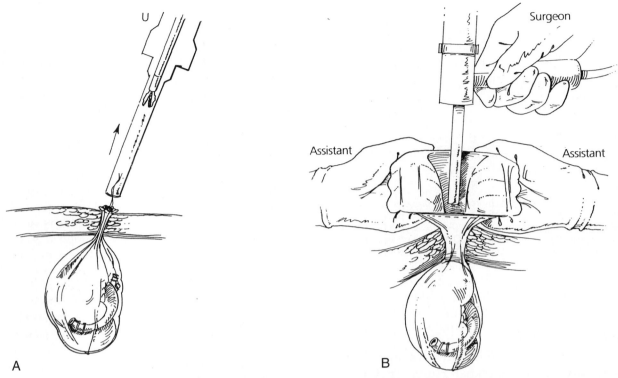

A   B

Figure 13–16. *A,* The drawstring is pulled upward until the entire neck of the sack rests on the abdomen. *B,* The neck of the sack is pulled upward by the assistant as the surgeon inserts the tip of the morcellator into the sack. (From Clayman RV, McDougall EM. Laparoscopic renal surgery. In Clayman RV, McDougall EM, eds. Laparoscopic Urology. St. Louis, MO, Quality Medical Publishing, 1993, pp 272–308.)

valve on the handle is turned off. The 10-mm metal barrel is placed into the sack by the surgeon until it touches the kidney; meanwhile the neck of the sack is pulled strongly upward by the assistant (Fig. 13–16*B*). The aspiration valve is turned to the "on" position and the morcellator is then activated by the foot controller. The 10-mm barrel is moved back and forth through the renal tissue, and the tissue is bluntly cored into the barrel of the morcellator, where it is cut by the recessed rotating blade. The renal fragments are aspirated into the morcellator's handle (Fig. 13–17).

Although the tip of the morcellator is blunt, it should not remain in contact with the sack for more than a second, otherwise the frictional heat may damage the sack. Short, controlled, to-and-fro motions are required to morcellate the tissue effectively. Systematic, clockwise movement of the morcellator all along the inside of the sack results in efficient and complete tissue morcellation. Throughout the morcellation process the assistant and surgeon provide upward traction on the sack to prevent any folds in the sack from being aspirated and cut by the morcellator (Fig. 13–18). In this regard, either a sudden drop in the pressure of the intra-abdominal pneumoperitoneum or loss of visibility indicates sack perforation. If this is suspected, morcellation must be stopped immediately to avoid serious injury to the bowel or other neighboring viscera.

Every 3 to 5 minutes morcellation is stopped, the handle of the morcellator is opened, and tissue is removed. This ensures that effective aspiration force is provided through the barrel of the morcellator. If

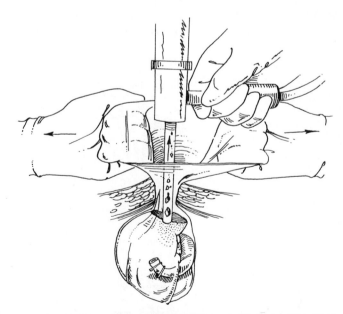

Figure 13–17. By moving the barrel of the morcellator back and forth through the renal tissue, the tissue is cored and cut and the renal fragments are aspirated into the handle of the morcellator. (From Clayman RV, McDougall EM. Laparoscopic renal surgery. In Clayman RV, McDougall EM, eds. Laparoscopic Urology. St. Louis, MO, Quality Medical Publishing, 1993, pp 272–308.)

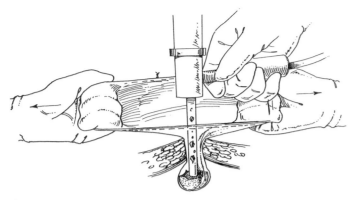

Figure 13–18. Throughout the morcellation process, the assistant and surgeon provide upward traction on the sack to prevent any folds in the sack from being aspirated or cut. (From Clayman RV, McDougall EM. Laparoscopic renal surgery. In Clayman RV, McDougall EM, eds. Laparoscopic Urology. St. Louis, MO, Quality Medical Publishing, 1993, pp 272–308.)

certain portions of the kidney are too fibrotic or too calcified to fragment, a blunt-tipped Kelly forceps or ring forceps can be used to grasp, crush, and remove the tissue.

Once the kidney is reduced to a 12-mm size, the sack and any remaining renal remnants are withdrawn (Fig. 13–19). A finger is placed over the UAAL incision to maintain the pneumoperitoneum.

Step 9: Exiting the Abdomen

The intra-abdominal pressure is again lowered to 5 mm Hg and the renal hilum is inspected a second time for bleeding. A 5-mm laparoscope is placed in the 5-mm LAAL port while the 12-mm ports (UMCL and umbilical) are removed under vision. Each 12-mm site is closed with a 0 absorbable figure-of-eight

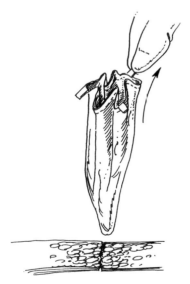

Figure 13–19. The sack is removed once the renal remnants are reduced to less than 12 mm in size. (From Clayman RV, McDougall EM. Laparoscopic renal surgery. In Clayman RV, McDougall EM, eds. Laparoscopic Urology. St. Louis, MO, Quality Medical Publishing, 1993, pp 272–308.)

suture placed under vision, using a Sinn retractor and Kocher clamp to facilitate exposure. The subcuticular tissues of the 12-mm ports are closed with 3-0 absorbable suture. The LMCL and UAAL trocars are removed under endoscopic vision and the LAAL port is removed last, with care to inspect the path of the port with the laparoscope. All skin sites are closed with adhesive strips.

Alternatively, a suture-carrying Veress-type needle, Maciol needle, Carter-Thomason device, or 14-gauge Angiocath technique can be used to close the fascia. Among the devices, the nondisposable Carter-Thomason apparatus has worked best in our hands. The suture placement is precise and there is no need to work with any forceps via another port. Also, if desired, a figure-of-eight fascial suture can be placed. The 10- or 12-mm guide tube is used to replace the port. The suture-carrying needle grasper is used to deliver a 0 absorbable suture through the upper hole on the guide tube. This suture is released in the abdomen, and the needle grasper is passed through the lower hole on the guide tube; the suture is grasped and pulled out of the abdomen. The guide tube is slid off the two ends of the suture, which are then tied securely.

A 14-gauge Angiocath technique for closure is helpful if none of the above-mentioned commercial devices are available. Under endoscopic monitoring, the 14-gauge sheathed needle is passed alongside the 12-mm port through the subcutaneous tissues and fascia. Upon entering the gas-filled abdomen, the needle is removed. A 0 Vicryl suture is passed through the 14-gauge sheath, and the sheath is removed and replaced over the introducer needle. The needle/sheath assembly is passed into the abdomen on the opposite side of the 12-mm port. The introducer needle is again removed. A 30-inch-long 0 Prolene suture is folded in half; the looped end is passed through the 14-gauge sheath. As more of the Prolene is fed through the sheath, the loop expands inside the peritoneal cavity. A 5-mm grasper is passed through one of the 5-mm ports and guided through the loop. The loose end of the 0 Vicryl suture is held with the 5-mm grasper and pulled through the loop of 0 Prolene. The loop is then pulled upward through the sheath, trapping the strand of Vicryl in the Prolene loop and pulling it through the sheath. The sheath is removed, as is the 12-mm port. The two ends of the Vicryl suture are tied to each other, thereby securely closing the abdominal wall fascia. Both 12-mm ports are closed in this manner.

Operative Technique: Laparoscopic Transperitoneal Radical Nephrectomy

In laparoscopic radical nephrectomy, most of the procedure is identical to what has already been described for laparoscopic simple nephrectomy. Indeed, there are only three differences: (1) Gerota's fascia is kept intact, (2) an adrenalectomy is performed if there is an upper pole tumor, and (3) the entrapped specimen is removed intact.

Right Adrenalectomy

The duodenum should previously have been completely mobilized off the anterior surface of the IVC. The peritoneotomy is extended cephalad by incising the triangular and posterior coronary ligament of the liver. The liver is retracted anteriorly, thereby uncovering the retrohepatic portion of the IVC. The adrenal vein is identified, dissected, and secured with only three 9-mm clips; it is incised so that two clips remain on the caval stump of the adrenal vein. In rare cases the short length of the adrenal vein may preclude placement of even three clips. In this event, two clips are applied and the adrenal side of the vein (i.e., the specimen side) is cut, grasped, and electrocoagulated, leaving two clips on the IVC stump of the adrenal vein. Once the adrenal vein is secured, any other minute attachments between the adrenal gland and the retroperitoneum can be electrocoagulated with a hook electrode. This electrode can be passed beneath the strands of tissue between the adrenal gland and IVC. It can then be gently lifted laterally and activated, thereby electrocoagulating each strand of tissue well away from the IVC. The lateral and inferior surfaces of the right adrenal gland are left undisturbed.

Left Adrenalectomy

On the left side, it is helpful to identify and secure the left adrenal vein. Four 9-mm clips are placed across the left adrenal vein, which is then cut between the two pairs of clips. The adrenal vein is then traced cephalad to the left adrenal gland, the medial surface of which can be mobilized, with a hook electrode, away from the aorta. Once this is done, the cephalad attachments of the adrenal can be dissected and electrocoagulated. The lateral and inferior surfaces of the left adrenal gland are left undisturbed.

Intact Removal

Once the specimen has been placed in an entrapment sack, the pneumoperitoneum is reduced to 5 mm Hg and a careful inspection is made for hemorrhage. If the LapSac has been used, the drawstring is grasped via the 5-mm LAAL port and pulled all the way into the port. Next the 5-mm port is removed and the drawstring is secured on the abdominal wall with a standard Kelly clamp. Via the 5-mm port incision, another Kelly clamp is placed into the abdomen. The clamp is turned so that it is concave toward the abdominal wall, and then opened. While monitoring the clamp laparoscopically, the surgeon extends the 5-mm port site transversely and anteriorly until it is 5 cm in length. This is done superficially with a skin knife, after which the deeper layers are incised with electrocautery. Next, Army-Navy right-angled retractors are placed superiorly and inferiorly along the wound. By pulling on the drawstring, the neck and upper body of the sack are manipulated into the wound. Then, by alternately pulling a retractor and the sack in opposite directions, the entire specimen and sack can be slowly molded and extruded through the 5-cm incision. The LapSac is strong enough to withstand tremendous force, thereby allowing the surgeon to deliver the specimen through a relatively small incision. However, if a thinner plastic sack is used, the wound needs to be enlarged to 7 or 8 cm so that the specimen can be delivered without exerting any force on the sack that might tear it.

Postoperative Management

If a scrotal or penile wrap was placed, it is removed now. The nasogastric tube is removed in the operating room and clear liquids are begun the evening of the procedure. The urethral catheter is removed on the first postoperative morning and at this time the patient is ambulated. Within the first 24 hours the patient is advanced to a regular diet. Pain control is achieved by parenteral morphine or a patient-controlled analgesic device. Oral analgesics should suffice by the second postoperative day. Parental antibiotics are continued for 24 hours postoperatively and the patient is usually discharged on the fourth postoperative day. The only prescription is for a non-narcotic analgesic.

Results

Laparoscopic Nephrectomy for Benign Disease

Laparoscopic simple nephrectomy for benign disease has spread to multiple medical centers. However, there are only seven reported series to date. Among these patients, the hallmark of the laparoscopic approach has been a brief hospital stay (3 or 4 days) and a short convalescence (1 to 2 weeks) (Table 13–1).[2–7, 17] In addition, the use of analgesics is markedly curtailed in the laparoscopic group. Kerbl and associates noted a fivefold decrease in the use of postoperative pain medications compared with similar patients undergoing an open nephrectomy (25 mg vs. 123 mg).[17] However, laparoscopic nephrectomy remains a time-intensive procedure requiring 3 to 6

TABLE 13–1. Laparoscopic Transperitoneal Simple Nephrectomy for Benign Disease

Author/Date	No. of Pts	OR Time (hrs)	EBL (ml)	Ureteral Catheter	Embolization +/−	Hospital Stay (days)	Convalescence (days)	Complications (%): Minor/Major
Copcoat 1992	21	4.5				4.8	12	
Dauleh 1994	12	3.8	70	−	−	<3	14	
Eraky 1994	60	3.5		+	−	3.2		31.6/6.6
Katoh 1993	26	4.4	459	+	+/−†	10	17	11.5/—0
Nicol 1994	5	3		−	−	2	7	20/0
Rassweiler 1993	9	3.8		+/−	−	6		22.2/11.1
Tse 1993	12	4.9		+	−	4.3		16.6/8.3
Wash. Univ 1994*	23	5.7		+	6	3.1	2.1	13/4

*Kerbl 1994.
†Some patients were embolized but number unknown.
EBL, estimated blood loss.

hours to complete. Complications have occurred in 22 percent of patients, including major problems such as pulmonary embolus (in one patient) and transient congestive heart failure; other less significant problems have included transient nerve palsies and epididymitis.[18] In addition, several authors have performed laparoscopic nephrectomy for benign disease successfully in children as young as 8 months of age.[19-21] Overall, this approach for benign disease has become widely accepted in all age groups and is being applied in an increasing number of patients.

Laparoscopic Nephrectomy for Malignant Disease

Laparoscopic radical nephrectomy for renal cell carcinoma has been reported by other groups (Table 13–2).[6, 7, 9, 12, 22] Experience with this approach is still limited, with only three groups reporting three or more patients and only one report of more than ten patients. Most of the tumors have been stage T1, but T2 and T3B tumors have also been removed laparoscopically. Operating room time has been 5 to 7 hours, hospital stay has been 3 to 8 days, and convalescence has required an average of 23 days. In the Washington University series, at 14 months' follow-up, there have been no reports of retroperitoneal recurrence or the development of metastatic disease. Complications have included prolonged ileus, paresthesias, and transient congestive heart failure. For upper pole tumors, ipsilateral adrenalectomy has been performed, but for lower pole tumors the adrenal gland has been left in situ. Work by Robey and Schellhammer, Gill and colleagues, and Sagalowsky and associates supports this approach for managing small lower pole tumors of the kidney.[23-25] At present, regional lymphadenectomy has not been performed with laparoscopic radical nephrectomy; its role in the

TABLE 13–2. Laparoscopic Radical Nephrectomy

	Copcoat 1992	Rassweiler 1993	Tse 1993	Kavoussi 1993	Ono 1993	Wash. Univ 1994*
No. of patients	3	3	4	8	2	11
OR time (hrs)	5.4	4.6	5	7.5	7	7
EBL (ml)				295	625	220
Urethral catheter				+	+	+
Embolization				−	−	1
Specimen wt. (gm)				347	405	399
Adrenalectomy		Yes		3	Yes	9
Grade				1–2	1–2	1–3
Stage		T2		T1	T1–T2	T1, T2, T3B
Oral intake			1	1		1
Hospital stay (days)	3	8	4.3	5.2	10	5.4
Return to normal activity (days)				21	16	23
Follow-up (mos)				15		14
Recurrence				0		0
Metastases				0		0
Death				0		0

*Unpublished data.

management of radiographically low-stage renal tumors remains controversial.

LAPAROSCOPIC RETROPERITONEAL NEPHRECTOMY FOR BENIGN RENAL DISEASE

Indications

The purely retroperitoneal approach to nephrectomy is primarily indicated in patients in whom the kidney is estimated to weigh 100 gm or less and in whom there has been no previous surgery in the retroperitoneum and no history of a perirenal or renal abscess. Ideal candidates for this approach include patients requiring nephrectomy for renal artery stenosis and associated hypertension, those with a hypoplastic kidney associated with pyelonephritis and chronic reflux, and those with a symptomatic multicystic dysplastic kidney. In addition, the retroperitoneal approach is excellent for renal cyst decortication, renal biopsy, and the rare case of a laparoscopic pyelolithotomy or ureteral lithotomy.

Preoperative Patient Evaluation and Preparation

Patient preparation for a retroperitoneal approach is less arduous than for a transperitoneal approach. Routine preoperative laboratory studies are obtained: cell blood count, serum electrolytes, and urine culture; the urine must be sterile before the procedure. In these patients, a mechanical and antibiotic bowel preparation is not necessary. A type- and cross-match for 2 units of blood is usually obtained.

Operative Technique

Preliminary Procedure

Immediately before retroperitoneal laparoscopic nephrectomy, a ureteral catheter is placed as described for transperitoneal laparoscopic nephrectomy.

Patient Positioning and Preparation

After endotracheal intubation and the initiation of general anesthesia, the patient is placed in a straight lateral decubitus position. The patient's back is placed as close to the edge of the table as possible. The contralateral (down-side) flank is well padded; in particular, an Action roll is placed beneath the

contralateral hip and upper thigh. It is essential that patient positioning be checked by surgeon and anesthesiologist to make certain that all pressure points are properly padded. The table is then flexed to approximately 30 degrees and the kidney rest is raised, maximally opening the space between the costal margin and the iliac crest. The patient is firmly secured to the table with appropriate straps or 2-inch adhesive tape. Each place where tape or a strap touches the body should be further cushioned by placing foam padding beneath the tape or strap. Pneumatic compression stockings are wrapped onto the patient's legs. The abdomen, flank, and genitalia are prepared and draped. The patient is draped particularly wide so that if it becomes necessary to convert to a pneumoperitoneum, this can be done without changing the patient's position. The previously placed ureteral and urethral catheters are likewise draped into the field.

The surgeon stands facing the patient's back. The main monitor as well as the insufflator and light source are placed on a cart opposite the surgeon. The assistant stands on the side facing the patient's abdomen. The camera person and scrub nurse stand on the same side as the surgeon, facing the patient's back.

Mandressi and associates have described an alternative, entirely prone approach to the retroperitoneum. The patient is positioned in a prone, jackknife position on the table; the abdomen is allowed to fall forward by placing two chest rolls laterally to support the ribs and the anterosuperior iliac spines. In this position the kidney falls forward and lies suspended from the renal hilum; however, if conversion to a transperitoneal approach becomes necessary, the patient needs to be rolled into a lateral decubitus or supine position and must be prepared and draped again. Likewise, emergency conversion to an open procedure would be more complicated with this approach.[26]

The instrumentation for performing a retroperitoneal laparoscopic nephrectomy is identical to that used during a transperitoneal nephrectomy. The only additional piece of equipment routinely used is a balloon dilator to develop space in the retroperitoneum. This can be most easily and inexpensively prepared by using either the middle finger of a No. 8 latex glove or a medical grade condom (we prefer the former). Either one is affixed with two silk sutures to the tip of a 16 Fr. red rubber Robinson catheter. The balloon-catheter assembly is then either inserted directly into the retroperitoneum if an open approach is used, or backloaded through a 30 Fr. Amplatz sheath if a closed Veress needle approach is used. Alternatively, commercially available retroperitoneal dissecting balloons can be purchased (Origin, Menlo Park, CA or GSI, Portola Valley, CA).

Procedural Steps

A retroperitoneal laparoscopic nephrectomy involves eight steps:

1. Obtaining the pneumoretroperitoneum
2. Port placement
3. Dissection of the ureter
4. Dissection of the upper and lower poles of the kidney
5. Securing the renal hilum
6. Occluding and dividing the ureter
7. Organ entrapment and morcellation
8. Exiting the retroperitoneum

Step 1: Obtaining the Pneumoretroperitoneum: Closed Technique

With this technique, a small incision is made at Petit's triangle (the inferior lumbar triangle) just above the iliac crest. A Kelly clamp is placed into the small incision, and the underlying fat is spread until the lumbodorsal fascia is palpated with the tip of the clamp. The fascia is grasped with a towel clip, after which the Veress needle is inserted. Usually there is only one area of resistance before the tip of the Veress needle springs into the fat of the retroperitoneum.

The same signs apply for entering the retroperitoneum as for entering the peritoneal cavity. A 10-ml syringe with 5 ml of saline is used to aspirate, irrigate, and then aspirate through the Veress needle to see if there has been any injury to the bowel or to a vascular structure. The saline should flow easily into the retroperitoneum and should not return during the second aspiration. After this, the syringe is removed from the Veress needle. As the patient inhales, any remaining saline in the hub of the needle should fall into the retroperitoneum.

The carbon dioxide (CO_2) line is then connected to the Veress needle. During inflow of the first 500 ml of CO_2 at 1 L/min, the retroperitoneal pressure should be less than 10 mm Hg. Next, the pressure limit is raised to 25 mm Hg. Typically, after 2 to 3 L of CO_2 is insufflated into the retroperitoneum, the 25 mm Hg pressure limit is reached.

A 12-mm trocar is passed at Petit's triangle. The side-arm stopcock is left open; as the trocar enters the gas-filled retroperitoneum, the surgeon can hear the rush of CO_2 from the side arm. The CO_2 line is connected to the side arm. The 10-mm, 30-degree lens laparoscope is inserted to confirm entry into the retroperitoneal space. All that should be seen is fatty tissue.

The 30 Fr. Amplatz sheath, which has been backloaded with the 16 Fr. retroperitoneal dissecting balloon, is passed into the 12-mm port. The back end of

the Amplatz sheath is held with a Kelly clamp so that it cannot be pushed too far into the 12-mm port. The 16 Fr. balloon-bearing catheter is advanced through the Amplatz sheath into the upper retroperitoneum. With a 60-ml catheter tip syringe, the balloon is repeatedly injected with saline until a volume of 1000 ml has been instilled. After this, the irrigator aspirator is used to decompress the balloon. The balloon and catheter are then pulled back into the Amplatz sheath, and the sheath and dissecting balloon are withdrawn from the 12-mm port.

If the balloon ruptures during the filling phase, there will be a sudden loss of resistance to instillation of saline. There will also be leakage of saline from the sheath. When the balloon ruptures, it is mandatory to perform careful laparoscopic examination of the retroperitoneum to identify and remove any pieces of latex.

Step 1: Obtaining the Pneumoretroperitoneum: Open Technique

The open technique for obtaining a pneumoretroperitoneum provides the neophyte laparoscopist with a little more security as it is a safer and surer method of gaining access to the retroperitoneum. A 2-inch incision is made posterior to the tip of the twelfth rib, overlying the superior lumbar triangle. The lumbodorsal fascia is identified and sharply incised. Two 0 silk sutures are placed on either side of the fascial incision. After this, the underlying muscle is spread until the retroperitoneum is entered. The surgeon should be able to readily palpate the pararenal fat lying outside Gerota's fascia.

The index finger of the surgeon is used to develop a space in the retroperitoneum. The 16 Fr. dissecting balloon catheter is then passed directly into the incision and inflated with 1000 ml of saline, as previously described. Next, the balloon's contents are aspirated; the balloon catheter is then removed. At this point, a 12-mm Hasson-type blunt trocar is introduced into the retroperitoneum and secured with the previously placed silk fascial sutures. In addition, a pursestring suture is placed into the lumbodorsal fascia to further secure the blunt trocar.

CO_2 insufflation is begun; the pressure limit is set at 25 mm Hg. The 10-mm, 30-degree lens laparoscope is inserted through the 12-mm port and the retroperitoneum is inspected. Usually, after balloon dilation, Gerota's fascia can be identified. In addition, if the assistant grasps the ureteral catheter at the urethral meatus, it now becomes possible to move the catheter back and forth. This maneuver usually clearly reveals the ureter. Sometimes, on the right side, the infrarenal portion of the IVC may be seen lying just medial to the ureter. It appears as a vertically running, somewhat flattened column of dull blue tissue.

Step 2: Port Placement

Two more trocars are placed, producing the following port arrangement: a 12-mm subcostal port in the inferior lumbar triangle just above the iliac crest, a 12-mm subcostal port in the superior lumbar triangle just posterior to the tip of the twelfth rib, and a 5-mm subcostal port two fingerbreadths posterior to the superior lumbar triangle. Proper entry of the initial 12-mm port is confirmed by inspection of the retroperitoneal entry site with the laparoscope passed through the second 12-mm port.

With the lens laparoscope in the lower 12-mm port, an electrosurgical scissors and an atraumatic 5-mm grasping forceps are introduced into the two subcostal ports. The peritoneum is dissected anteriorly as far as possible. A fourth port (5 mm) is placed subcostally, 2 or 3 fingerbreadths anterior to the tip of the twelfth rib. When all four trocars are properly placed, there should be three ports in horizontal alignment with the tip of the twelfth rib and one port directly inferior to the upper 12-mm port, thereby creating a T configuration.

Step 3: Dissection of the Ureter

The ureter is identified in the retroperitoneum. It is most easily seen along the lower medial border of the psoas margin; it is helpful for the assistant to again move the ureteral catheter where it exits the urethral meatus. The ureter is carefully dissected from the surrounding tissue and encircled with a Babcock clamp, a 4-inch length of umbilical tape, or a suture as described for a laparoscopic transperitoneal nephrectomy. If a suture is used to entrap the ureter using the 14-gauge needle/sheath method, the surgeon will still have all three remaining ports available for the passage of dissecting instruments.

The ureter is followed cephalad. On the right side the gonadal vein can be preserved, since it passes anterior to the ureter. On the left side the gonadal vein is taken between four clips; it then serves as a guide to the renal vein.

Step 4: Dissection of the Upper and Lower Poles of the Kidney

By following the ureter cephalad, Gerota's fascia should become apparent; it is sharply incised over the lower, lateral edge of the kidney. The perirenal fat is cleared away from the medial and posterior surfaces of the lower pole. Next the lateral surface of the kidney is cleared of fatty tissue. The dissection is continued over the upper posterior pole of the kidney and then medially until the medial surface of the upper pole of the kidney is likewise apparent. At all times the dissection closely follows the renal capsule.

Step 5: Securing the Renal Hilum

By exerting upward traction on the ureter as well as using the anterior 5-mm port to exert anterior traction on the upper pole, the kidney can be displaced laterally and anteriorly. This places the renal hilum on mild stretch. The surgeon, working through the upper 12-mm port and the posterior 5-mm port, can follow the ureter upward to the renal hilum.

On the *right* side the renal artery is encountered first (Fig. 13–20); the artery is carefully dissected with the electrosurgical scissors, hook electrode, and right-angled forceps. A 1- to 2-cm long, 360-degree window is developed around the renal artery. The artery is secured with five 9-mm titanium clips. At times, it is necessary to move the laparoscope to the 12-mm upper port and pass the clip applier via the lower 12-mm port in order to properly orient the clip applier to the renal artery. The renal artery is cut between the third and fourth clips so that three clips remain on the aortic stump of the renal artery.

After this, further anterior dissection provides a view of the broad right renal vein. The renal vein appears to lie further anterior than one might expect, and thus dissection anterior to the artery should proceed in a methodical, careful fashion. Once the renal vein is carefully dissected (i.e., creating a 2-cm long, 360-degree window around the vein), a vascular GIA stapler is introduced through the upper 12-mm port.

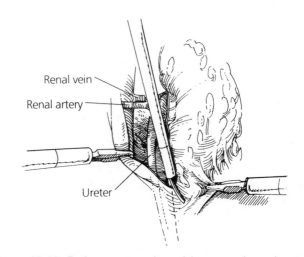

Figure 13–20. During a retroperitoneal laparoscopic nephrectomy, the right renal artery is encountered before the right renal vein. (From Clayman RV. Retroperitoneoscopy. In Clayman RV, McDougall EM, eds. Laparoscopic Urology. St. Louis, MO, Quality Medical Publishing, 1993, pp 321–370.)

The renal vein is then secured with the GIA vascular tissue stapler. The entire vein must lie within the jaws of the stapler, well proximal to the "cut" line, before the jaws of the stapler are closed. After the stapler is closed, the handle lock is released and the handles are tightly squeezed together, simultaneously occluding and incising the vein. The surgeon's grip on the handles is relaxed and the jaws of the stapler are opened. The vein should now be neatly cut; there should be no blood oozing from either cut end of the vein. If there is any oozing, a preformed loop laparoscopic suture is passed and secured over the bleeding stump of the renal vein.

If placement of the stapler around the vein is too difficult, the laparoscope should be moved to the upper 12-mm port and the stapler brought into the field via the lower 12-mm port. If problems continue, the surgeon should consider exchanging the 5-mm posterior port for a 12-mm port and passing the stapler through this "new" 12-mm port. If the space is still too tight and the stapler does not perfectly traverse the renal vein, with the "cut" line visible to the surgeon, the vein will have to be tied using intracorporeal suturing and extracorporeal knotting techniques.

On the *left* side the first vascular structure to be encountered is usually the ascending lumbar vein; because of the retroperitoneal approach and the lateral decubitus position of the patient, this vein will appear to be coming toward the surgeon. It is secured with four 9-mm titanium clips and incised between the second and third clips. *This should be done well away from the main renal vein, so that when the tissue stapler is applied to the renal vein, its path will not cross any clips.* Once the ascending lumbar vein is divided, the next vascular structure usually seen is the renal artery. The artery is dissected until a complete 1- to 2-cm long, 360-degree window has been created. The artery is occluded with five 9-mm titanium clips and then cut so that three clips remain on the aortic stump side.

The left gonadal vein should now appear as it courses into the surgical field just inferior to the renal vein. The gonadal vein is occluded with four 9-mm clips and divided. *Again, this should be done well away from the main renal vein, so that when the tissue stapler is applied, its path will not cross any clips.* Either the cephalad stump of the gonadal vein or the stump of the ascending lumbar vein can be traced to the inferior border of the renal vein. During dissection of the posterior surface of the renal vein, the adrenal vein is seen as it enters the upper edge of the renal vein. The adrenal vein is secured with four clips and cut so that two clips remain on either side. *Again, this should be done well away from the main renal vein, so that when the tissue stapler is applied, its path will not cross any clips.* Now the

renal vein is secured with the vascular GIA stapler as previously described. After this, the rest of the medial edge of the kidney can be freed. The anterior surface of the kidney is then rapidly dissected from the few remaining retroperitoneal attachments.

Step 6: Occluding and Dividing the Ureter

The kidney should now be attached only by its ureter. The retrograde ureteral occlusion balloon catheter is deflated, and the catheter and guidewire are removed. A locking/grasping forceps is passed through the anterior 5-mm port and used to grab the proximal ureter. The ureter is secured with four 9-mm titanium clips and divided between the second and third clips. The previously placed circumureteral umbilical tape or suture is cut and removed from the retroperitoneum. The kidney and proximal ureter are now suspended by the 5-mm locking/grasping forceps passed through the anterior port.

Step 7: Organ Entrapment and Morcellation

The pressure in the abdomen is now lowered to 5 mm Hg and a careful exploration made for any bleeding. If a closed approach was made to the retroperitoneum, an entrapment sack is passed into the superior lumbar 12-mm port. The technique of passing the sack is the same as described for a transperitoneal nephrectomy.

As soon as the sack has been passed into the upper 12-mm port, the 10-mm, 30-degree lens laparoscope is moved from the lower 12-mm port to the upper 12-mm port. As the laparoscope is advanced into the upper 12-mm port, it pushes the sack deeper into the retroperitoneum. Working with two 5-mm atraumatic grasping forceps via the inferior lumbar port and the posterior 5-mm port, the sack is pulled more caudal; the neck of the sack should then become clearly visible. Next, with two traumatic 5-mm graspers, two opposite tabs are grasped on the sack and pulled in different directions, thus opening the mouth of the sack.

Usually, since the kidney is small (less than 100 gm), the sack can be opened sufficiently with just two, rather than three, grasping forceps. The kidney, suspended by the anterior 5-mm port traumatic locking grasper, is then delivered into the open sack. By pushing the ureter as far down into the sack as possible, the kidney is dragged deep within the sack. Next the locking/grasping forceps is released from the ureter and slid out of the sack. After this, the laparoscope is returned to the lower 12-mm port. The drawstring is now grasped with a traumatic grasping forceps passed through the superior 12-mm port. The drawstring on the sack is delivered through the 12-mm port. Morcellation of the kidney can then proceed as previously described for laparoscopic nephrectomy for benign renal disease.

Alternatively, if an open access to the retroperitoneum was used, the entrapped kidney can be removed through the 2-inch (5-cm) incision that was initially made during placement of the upper 12-mm port; thus, the kidney is delivered intact. Indeed, the kidney is often small enough to be pulled directly through this wound without the need to entrap it in a sack.

Step 8: Exiting the Retroperitoneum

A 5-mm, 0-degree lens laparoscope is introduced into the posterior 5-mm port. With the intraretroperitoneal pressure lowered to 5 mm Hg, the two 12-mm ports are removed under endoscopic control. The fascia of the two 12-mm port sites is closed as previously described for transperitoneal laparoscopic nephrectomy. The 5-mm ports are also removed under direct endoscopic control, as previously described. The two 12-mm port skin sites are closed with a 4-0 absorbable subcuticular suture. All the skin sites are then closed with adhesive strips.

Postoperative Care

The postoperative care of a patient undergoing a retroperitoneal laparoscopic nephrectomy is identical to that rendered patients after a transperitoneal laparoscopic nephrectomy. The only difference is that with the retroperitoneal approach, shoulder pain is distinctly rare; likewise, the period of ileus and abdominal discomfort seems to be shorter.

Results

Retroperitoneal laparoscopic nephrectomy has been reported by three other groups (Table 13–3).[26–28]

At Washington University, 15 retroperitoneal nephrectomies were compared with 23 transperitoneal nephrectomies for benign disease. The patients who underwent retroperitoneal laparoscopic nephrectomy had small kidneys (103 gm); overall operating room time was decreased by 30 minutes, as was the time to oral intake (0.5 days) and the need for parenteral analgesics (19 mg morphine sulfate). The retroperitoneal nephrectomy group had a similar length of hospital stay (3.2 days) and convalescence (2.1 weeks).[18]

LAPAROSCOPIC NEPHROURETERECTOMY

Indications

Laparoscopic nephroureterectomy with excision of a bladder cuff is indicated in organ-confined upper tract TCC. Certain benign conditions, including renal tuberculosis with associated nonfunction, pyoureteronephrosis, and symptomatic nonfunctioning hydroureteronephrotic kidneys, may also be treated with laparoscopic nephrectomy and excision of the ureter down to the ureterovesical junction (UVJ).

Preoperative Evaluation and Preparation

Preoperative studies include complete blood cell count, serum creatinine, serum electrolytes, and a urine culture; the urine must be sterile before the operation. Metastatic evaluation for upper tract TCC usually includes liver function tests, bone scan, chest radiograph, and abdominal/pelvic CT scan.[29] An intravenous pyelogram should be taken to clearly visualize the contralateral kidney and rule out bilateral upper tract TCC. If visualization is inadequate, a retrograde ureterogram should be performed. All patients should also have undergone cystoscopy to rule out associated bladder cancer. Lastly, the presence of an upper tract filling defect, a positive cytologic study, and a normal cystoscopic picture are sufficient evidence of upper tract TCC to proceed to ablative surgery, but if the cytology is negative for malignant cells, ureteroscopy and biopsy of the lesion should

TABLE 13–3. Laparoscopic Retroperitoneal Simple Nephrectomy for Benign Disease

Author/Date	No. of Pts	OR Time (hrs)	EBL (ml)	Ureteral Catheter	Embolization +/−	Hospital Stay (days)	Normal Activity (days)	Complications (%): Minor/Major
Gaur 1993	1	2	100	−	−			0
Mandressi 1993	5	4.5	100	+	−	4		0
Rassweiler 1994	5	2.4	Minimal	−	−	7.8		20/0
Wash. Univ 1994*	15	5.3	200	+	−	3.2	2.1	11/11

*Unpublished data.

be performed to confirm the diagnosis of upper tract TCC.

The adequacy of contralateral renal function is verified before laparoscopic nephroureterectomy, usually by the excretory urogram or abdominal CT scan. If there is any doubt concerning the ability of the contralateral kidney to serve satisfactorily as a solitary unit, a renal scan with differential function should be obtained. If this scan reveals impaired function, nephron-sparing surgery can be considered: partial nephrectomy or local excision via an open, percutaneous, or ureteroscopic approach.

Preoperatively the patient should complete an outpatient antibiotic and mechanical bowel preparation. Two hours before the operation, intravenous antibiotics are given. The patient is type- and cross-matched for 2 units of blood or is given the option to donate autologous blood. Informed consent is obtained, with emphasis on the unique complications of laparoscopy, the possibility of converting to an open procedure, and the increased operative time attendant upon the laparoscopic approach.

Operative Technique

Preliminary Procedures

In the cystoscopy suite under intravenous sedation, the patient is placed in the dorsal lithotomy position, and with the flexible cystoscope a 0.035-inch Bentson guidewire is advanced up the ureter. A 7 Fr. 5-mm ureteral dilating balloon catheter is passed into the distal ureteral orifice, and the balloon is inflated to its full 15 Fr. size or until 1 atm of pressure is reached; no attempt is made to forcefully dilate the ureter, which would result in the ureter being torn. This is done under fluoroscopic control. The balloon is filled with dilute contrast material (a 50:50 mix of Conray 50 with saline). A 24 Fr. resectoscope, with an electrosurgical Orandi or Collings knife set at 50 watts pure cut, is passed alongside the shaft of the ureteral balloon. The ureteral orifice and tunnel are then unroofed by cutting from the outside inward toward the balloon at 12 o'clock along the ureteral orifice and tunnel. The incision is extended from the ureteral orifice to, but not through, the UVJ. This point usually lies just distal to the waist noted on fluoroscopy in the dilating balloon; the waist usually corresponds to the intramural ureter.

The ureteral balloon is deflated and advanced up the ureter until only the 7 Fr. shaft of the catheter rests alongside the incised ureteral tunnel and orifice. Now a roller electrode is attached to the 24 Fr. resectoscope; using coagulating current, the entire interior of the opened ureteral tunnel is electrocoagulated. Next, the deflated ureteral balloon catheter is removed and a 7 Fr. 11.5-mm occlusion balloon catheter

is advanced over the Bentson guidewire to the renal pelvis. The Bentson guidewire is removed and 3 to 5 ml of dilute contrast is gently instilled through the occlusion balloon catheter to outline the renal pelvis. Under fluoroscopic control the occlusion balloon is inflated with 1 ml of 1:4 diluted contrast; the catheter is then pulled caudally until it is snug at the level of the UPJ.

At this point the surgeon may elect to drain the renal pelvis; the amount of fluid drained is measured. At our institution, an equal volume of thiotepa (60 mg in 30 ml sterile water) is then instilled via the ureteral catheter. Next an Amplatz Super Stiff guidewire is passed up the ureter; a side-arm adaptor is attached to its distal end. A 16 Fr. urethral catheter is inserted and connected to sterile drainage; the ureteral and urethral catheters are coiled and placed in a sterile bowel bag.

Alternatively, Rassweiler and associates have described resection of the ureteral orifice and distal ureteral tunnel.[28] In this case the resection may be carried through the wall of the bladder, thereby detaching the ureter from the bladder. No ureteral catheter is placed. With this approach, removal of the ureter is greatly facilitated, as pulling on the proximal ureter detaches (Semple's pluck) the distal ureter, thus precluding dissection of the UVJ or laparoscopic closure of the bladder.[28] This eliminates the need for placing a sixth port (see below). However, hypothetical concerns have been raised about possible intraperitoneal as well as retroperitoneal seeding from tumor cells in the urine that extravasate from the cut end of the ureter.

Patient Positioning and Preparation for Operation

The patient is brought to the operating room and positioned supine on the table, with arms placed outstretched on an arm board.

To obtain a pneumoperitoneum, a Veress needle or open cannula approach is used at the umbilicus. Alternatively, if the patient is obese, a Veress needle pneumoperitoneum is obtained transumbilically, but the first 12-mm trocar is placed lateral to the rectus muscle several centimeters above the umbilicus. Otherwise, when the patient is turned to a lateral decubitus position, the drift of the pannus will displace the port medially and make it difficult for the camera operator to angulate and deliver the laparoscope to the surgical site. Alternatively, especially for the obese patient, lateral insufflation via a closed approach may be necessary, as previously described for nephrectomy.

Usually four trocars are inserted with the patient in the supine position. The patient is then placed in 70-degree lateral orientation and the table is flexed. Soft pads are placed beneath the contralateral hip and thigh. The ipsilateral arm is fixed to an ether screen or placed on pillows lying over the extended contralateral arm. An axillary roll is placed, beneath the contralateral arm, which lies in an outstretched position on an arm board. The contralateral leg is flexed and a pillow is placed between the knees. The ipsilateral leg is kept straight. Soft pads are placed beneath both ankles. When placed on the pillows, the ipsilateral leg should be level with the iliac crest, otherwise a "stretch" sciatic nerve injury can occur, especially in an obese patient. Safety straps are positioned to prevent the patient from rolling forward; a soft pad is again placed between the strap and where it would otherwise touch the patient. The position of the operating room equipment and personnel is the same as for a laparascopic nephrectomy.

Port Placement

While the patient is supine, four ports are placed: a 12-mm umbilical (or pararectus above the umbilicus), 12-mm midline suprapubic (SP) (halfway between the umbilicus and symphysis pubis), 12-mm UMCL, and 5-mm LMCL. The umbilical or pararectus port is for the camera, the two MCL ports are for the surgeon's use, and the SP port is for passage of a tissue GIA stapler for securing a cuff of bladder at the end of the procedure. Each port is passed 1 to 2 cm deep to the peritoneum and sutured to the skin with a No. 2 Prolene suture; thus, the port can be advanced but not inadvertently removed from the abdomen. As soon as a second 12-mm port is placed, the laparoscope is introduced through this port so that the entry of the initial "blind" trocar can be examined to rule out any inadvertent injury to the bowel or omentum.

Procedural Steps

A laparoscopic transperitoneal nephroureterectomy involves eight steps:

1. Distal ureteral dissection
2. Securing a cuff of bladder
3. Incision of the line of Toldt
4. Proximal ureteral dissection
5. Nephrectomy
6. Entrapment of the specimen
7. Specimen delivery
8. Exiting the abdomen

Step 1: Distal Ureteral Dissection

With the patient supine, the table is rotated until the ipsilateral side is tilted 30 degrees upward. The medial umbilical ligament (MUL) is located and a peritoneotomy is made medial to the MUL. The sur-

geon works with the electrosurgical scissors through the LMCL port while providing medial retraction via the SP port. As the retroperitoneal space is bluntly dissected posteriorly, the vas deferens in the male is found. This structure should be dissected free and divided using electrocautery. The round ligament must be similarly treated in the female, in order to rotate the ovary off the ureter.

The distal ureter is bordered by the bladder medially, the MUL laterally, and the vas deferens/round ligament anteriorly (Fig. 13–21). The ureteral catheter may be moved back and forth to help identify the ureter. A 360-degree window is created around the MUL, and through the SP port four 10-mm clips are applied to the MUL, two above and two below the level of the ureter. The MUL is divided between the pairs of clips. Next a 360-degree window is created around the distal ureter (Fig. 13–22).

A Babcock clamp is passed around the ureter via the SP port to allow retraction during dissection of the distal ureter and UVJ. Alternatively, a 4-cm umbilical tape or a suture may be used for ureteral retraction as described for laparoscopic nephrectomy. The patient is now repositioned in a full lateral decubitus position, as described earlier. The line of Toldt is dissected further cephalad. Two additional ports are then placed, both into the retroperitoneum: a 12-mm upper anterior axillary line port (UAAL) off the tip of the twelfth rib and a 5-mm lower anterior axillary line port (LAAL) just above the iliac crest.

Step 2: Securing a Cuff of Bladder

Through the 5-mm LAAL port the assistant retracts the distal ureter laterally as the surgeon passes the

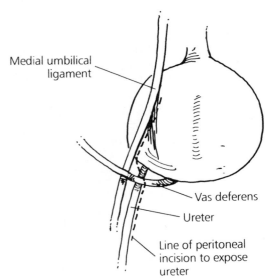

Figure 13–21. The distal ureter is bordered by the bladder medially, the medial umbilical ligament (MUL) laterally, and the vas deferens medially. (From Clayman RV. Retroperitoneoscopy. In Clayman RV, McDougall EM, eds. Laparoscopic Urology. St. Louis, MO, Quality Medical Publishing, 1993, pp 321–370.)

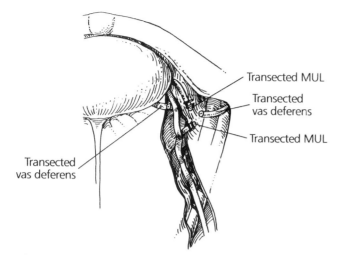

Figure 13–22. After transection of the medial umbilical ligament (MUL) and the vas deferens, the ureter is freed in a 360-degree window. (From Clayman RV. Retroperitoneoscopy. In Clayman RV, McDougall EM, eds. Laparoscopic Urology. St. Louis, MO, Quality Medical Publishing, 1993, pp 321–370.)

electrosurgery scissors through the LMCL port and forceps through the SP port. Now the bladder cuff may be dissected by following the ureter distally until it enters the detrusor muscle. The UVJ is cleared of perivesical fat over a 3- to 5-cm area (Fig. 13–23).

At this point the occlusion balloon is deflated and the ureteral catheter and Super Stiff guidewire are removed; the flexible cystoscope is inserted into the bladder by the second assistant while the nurse operates the laparoscope. The first assistant grasps the distal ureter through the LMCL port with traumatic locking/grasping forceps proximal to the UVJ, and

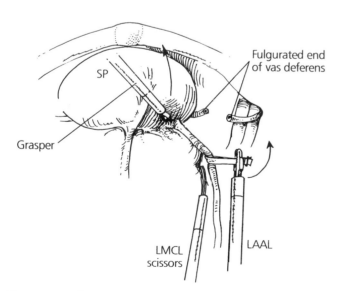

Figure 13–23. The ureterovesical junction (UVJ) is cleared of perivesical fat with the aid of traction on the ureter from the LAAL port. (From Clayman RV. Retroperitoneoscopy. In Clayman RV, McDougall EM, eds. Laparoscopic Urology. St. Louis, MO, Quality Medical Publishing, 1993, pp 321–370.)

cephalad and medial traction is applied to the ureter. Next, atraumatic forceps are passed through the 5-mm LAAL port by the first assistant; the bladder is retracted below the UVJ caudally and medially. The 12-mm laparoscopic tissue GIA stapler is passed via the SP port; the surgeon releases the stapler's control lever, opens the jaws of the stapler, and places them across the cuff of bladder just distal to the UVJ (Fig. 13–24A). The jaws are closed while the second assistant examines the bladder with the flexible cystoscope to verify that the ureter and cuff of urothelium are included and that the contralateral ureteral orifice remains undisturbed.

The surgeon now rotates the stapler 180 degrees to ensure that all tissue lies within the "cut" mark of the stapler (Fig. 13–24B). The safety lever is released and the handles of the GIA stapler are squeezed together. The GIA places six 3-cm rows of staples and cuts the tissue between the third and fourth rows. The locking lever is released. The bladder cuff should now be completely free of the bladder. The bladder is distended via the cystoscope; a note is made of any intravesically exposed staples. Laparoscopically the staple line is inspected for any leakage (Fig. 13–24C). If all looks well, the cystoscope is removed and the urethral catheter replaced.

An alternative method of transurethral ureteral detachment has been described by Rassweiler (see above). If this approach is used, a 9-mm clip is placed across the ureter as soon as it is identified to stop any urine from leaking into the abdomen and retroperitoneum. Also, with this approach the SP port is eliminated: the distal ureter can be delivered simply by pulling on the proximal ureter, since the tunnel has been resected and the distal ureter has actually been cystoscopically detached from the bladder wall at the outset of the procedure.

Step 3: Incision of the Line of Toldt

With the patient still in the lateral decubitus position, the table is tilted head down. The line of Toldt is identified and incised along the lateral gutter just as described for a laparoscopic nephrectomy. The caudal limb of the peritoneotomy joins the previous peritoneotomy at the level of the MUL.

Step 4: Proximal Ureteral Dissection

The assistant retracts the detached ureter by means of a Babcock clamp or umbilical tape through the UAAL port, or via the previously placed retracting suture. Countertraction on the retroperitoneal tissues is provided with an atraumatic grasping forceps through the LAAL port. The surgeon uses electrosur-

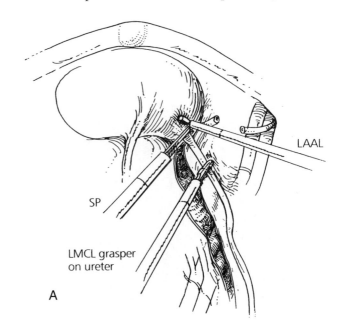

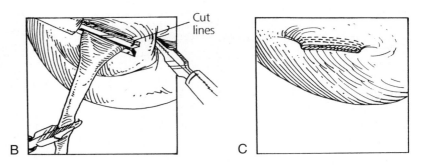

Figure 13–24. *A,* Via the SP port, the 12-mm laparoscopic tissue GIA stapler is positioned across the UVJ. *B,* Close-up view of the GIA stapler in position across the entire UVJ. *C,* Laparoscopically the staple line is examined for any leak while cystoscopy is performed to make note of any intravesical staples and to examine the contralateral ureteral orifice for injury. SP, suprapubic port. (From Clayman RV. Retroperitoneoscopy. In Clayman RV, McDougall EM, eds. Laparoscopic Urology. St. Louis, MO, Quality Medical Publishing, 1993, pp 321–370.)

gery scissors through the LMCL port and provides additional traction on the retroperitoneum through the SP port. The ureter is dissected free in the cephalad direction and the superior vesical artery is identified. This vessel is clipped (four 9-mm clips) and then cut so that two clips remain on both sides of the artery.

Care must be taken while attempting to dissect the ureter off the iliac vessels. If the ureter is adherent to the iliac vessels, the ureteral dissection should be started just above the iliac vessels. The surgeon operates with the electrosurgical scissors and a grasping forceps through the 12-mm LMCL and UMCL ports, respectively; the ureter is dissected proximally. Now the ureter can be retracted both caudal and cephalad to the iliac vessels, thereby facilitating a safer dissection along the underside of the iliac portion of the ureter. Once the ureter is freed from the iliac vessels, the remainder of the ureteral dissection is identical to that described for a laparoscopic nephrectomy.

Step 5: Nephrectomy

This part of the procedure is also identical to that described for laparoscopic radical nephrectomy.

However, unless the TCC resides in an upper pole calix or there is obvious invasion into the renal parenchyma, Gerota's fascia may be incised at the upper pole, thus sparing the adrenal gland.[30] Otherwise, the adrenal gland is included with the specimen. The technique is as described in the adrenalectomy portion of the section on laparoscopic radical nephrectomy (see above).

Step 6: Entrapment of the Specimen

The entrapment procedure is identical to a laparoscopic nephrectomy. However, if the tumor is in the ureter, the cuff of bladder is affixed to the inner lip of the sack with a 9-mm clip (Fig. 13–25).

Step 7: Specimen Delivery: Morcellation Versus Intact Removal

At this point in the procedure, the abdominal pressure is lowered to 5 mm Hg and a careful check made for hemostasis. Now, with the patient still in a lateral decubitus position, the drawstring is delivered onto

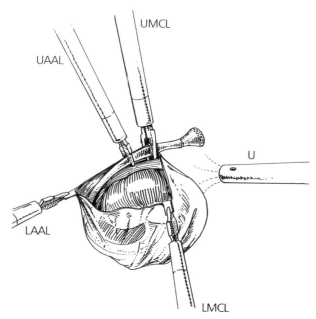

Figure 13–25. The cuff of bladder is clipped to the neck of the entrapment sack if there is tumor in the ureter. (From Clayman RV. Retroperitoneoscopy. In Clayman RV, McDougall EM, eds. Laparoscopic Urology. St. Louis, MO, Quality Medical Publishing, 1993, pp 321–370.)

the abdominal wall via the 5-mm LAAL port for TCC of the renal pelvis or calices (TCCP) or via the 12-mm UAAL port for TCC of the ureter (TCCU).

For TCCP, intact specimen delivery is indicated as described for laparoscopic radical nephrectomy (Fig. 13–26).

For TCCU, the clipped edge of the bladder cuff is freed from the exposed neck of the entrapment sack. The cuff of bladder and ureter are put on stretch and the proximal ureter is doubly clipped above the abdominal skin. The ureter is divided between the two clips and delivered separately, intact without spillage. The ureter can then be opened to ensure that the entire tumor has been removed with an adequate 1-cm margin. The remaining non–tumor-bearing kidney may now be morcellated as in laparoscopic nephrectomy for benign disease.

Step 8: Exiting the Abdomen

The abdomen is exited and the incisions are closed as previously described for laparoscopic nephrectomy.

Postoperative Management

Postoperative management is almost identical to that following a laparoscopic nephrectomy except that the urethral catheter is not removed on the first postoperative day. On the second or third postopera-

tive day a cystogram is obtained. If there is no extravasation, the urethral catheter is removed. If there is extravasation, the patient is discharged with an indwelling catheter; the cystogram is repeated 1 week later, and if there is no leakage, the catheter is removed. Follow-up for patients with TCCP or TCCU undergoing laparoscopic nephroureterectomy is identical to the regimen for patients undergoing standard open nephroureterectomy.

Results

Laparoscopic nephroureterectomy has been reported by four groups.[2, 9, 10, 31] The terminal ureter has been addressed by both adjunctive cystoscopic ureteral incision and resection. The juxtaureteral

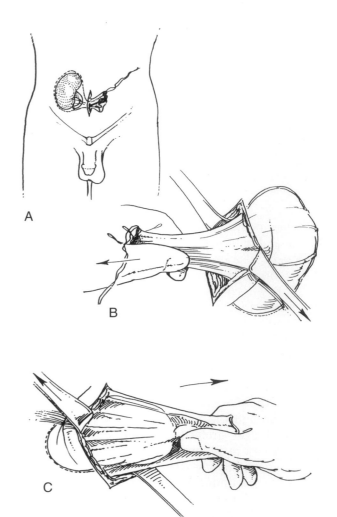

Figure 13–26. *A,* The entrapment sack is brought out through a 5-cm incision created by extension of the 12-mm SP port site. *B,* An Army-Navy right-angled retractor is positioned on either side of the incision. *C,* The entrapment sack and specimen are removed from the abdomen by alternately pulling a retractor and the sack in opposite directions. (From Clayman RV. Retroperitoneoscopy. In Clayman RV, McDougall EM, eds. Laparoscopic Urology. St. Louis, MO, Quality Medical Publishing, 1993, pp 321–370.)

TABLE 13–4. Laparoscopic Radical Nephroureterectomy for Transitional Cell Carcinoma

	Copcoat 1992	Chiu 1992	Dauleh 1994	Wash. Univ. 1994
No. of patients	1	1	2	10
OR time (hrs)	6	9	–	8.3
EBL (ml)	–	–	–	231
Ureteral tunnel*	1	2	1	2
Bladder closure†	1	3	2	2
Specimen wt. (gm)	–	–	–	408
Grade	–	3	–	2, 3
Stage	–	T3	–	Ta, T1, T2, T3
First oral intake (days)	–	4	–	1
Extravasation	–	–	–	0
Ambulation date (days)	–	1	–	–
Hospital stay (days)	–	5	–	5
Full recovery (wks)	–	–	–	42
Normal activity (days)	–	7	–	17
Follow-up (mos)	–	–	–	3–23
Recurrence	–	–	–	0
Bladder staples seen	–	–	–	1
Ureteral remnant	–	–	–	1
Metastases	–	–	–	1
Death	–	–	–	2
Complications				
Major	–	–	–	1
Minor	–	–	–	1

*1, resection; 2, incision.
†1, no closure; 2, staples; 3, sutures.

bladder tissue has been treated in various fashions: sutured bladder closure, stapled bladder closure, and no bladder closure (Table 13–4). Among the various reports, the average operative time was 8 hours and the average blood loss 231 ml. In our group of ten patients the average amount of parenteral morphine used by each patient was 22 mg and the average hospital stay 5 days. The patients returned to normal activity within 17 days, and full recovery occurred at 6 weeks. The number of patients treated remains small and the follow-up period is still brief. Nonetheless, with a follow-up of 6 to 40 months, superficial bladder tumors have developed in only two patients; no patients have developed distant metastatic disease. However, one patient with deeply invasive TCC, despite negative surgical margins, has developed a local retroperitoneal recurrence 1 year after surgery.

Postoperative Complications

Complications of laparoscopic nephroureterectomy and their management are basically similar to complications after laparoscopic nephrectomy. However, there are a few potential problems unique to the procedure. These include the risk of stone formation, leakage from the stapled bladder closure, and injury to the contralateral ureteral orifice. However, to date none of these complications have been reported among patients undergoing laparoscopic nephroureterectomy. Indeed, neither staples nor stones have

been found in the bladders of these patients despite surveillance cystoscopy for up to 3 years. In one patient a single staple is visible at the end of a 1-cm distal ureteral stump, yet after 3 years there is no evidence of stone formation. Also, through the performance of simultaneous cystoscopy and laparoscopic examination of the bladder during and after the bladder closure, extravasation as well as injury to the contralateral ureteral orifice should be precluded.

Summary

Laparoscopic nephrectomy and laparoscopic nephroureterectomy are safe and feasible procedures in the hands of the experienced laparoscopist. At this time, almost all nephrectomies for benign disease can be accomplished laparoscopically with less patient ileus, shorter hospitalization, less patient discomfort, and more rapid convalescence. Similarly, nephrectomy and nephroureterectomy for malignant disease can also be performed laparoscopically. However, although the short-term quality of life benefits to the patient are significant, longer follow-up is needed to determine whether this approach is as efficacious as its open surgical counterpart.

Editorial Comment
Fray F. Marshall

These authors are among the pioneers and have approached this surgery with imagination and originality. Laparoscopic nephrectomy and nephroureterectomy are more complicated than many of the simpler laparoscopic operations and demand more experience and expertise.

REFERENCES

1. Clayman RV, Kavoussi LR, Soper NJ, et al. Laparoscopic nephrectomy: Initial case report. J Urol 146:278, 1991.
2. Dauleh MI, Townell NH. Laparoscopic nephroureterectomy for malignancy: Arguments for morcellation or retrieval of intact specimens. Min Inv Ther 3:51, 1994.
3. Eraky I, El-Kappany H, Shamaa M, Ghoneim MA. Laparoscopic nephrectomy: An established routine procedure. J Endourol 8:275, 1994.
4. Katoh N, Kinukawa T, Hirabayashi S, et al. Review of laparoscopic nephrectomy in 26 patients. Jpn J Endourol ESWL 6:129, 1993.
5. Nicol DL, Winkle DC, Nathanson LK, Smithers B. Laparoscopic nephrectomy for benign disease. Br J Urol 73:237, 1994.
6. Rassweiler JJ, Henkel TO, Potempa DM, et al. The technique of transperitoneal laparoscopic nephrectomy, adrenalectomy and nephroureterectomy. Eur Urol 23:425, 1993.
7. Tse ETW, Knaus RP. Laparoscopic nephrectomy: The learning curve experience. Can J Surg 37:153, 1994.
8. Copcoat MJ, Joyce AD, Popert R, et al. Laparoscopic nephrectomy—the King's experience. Min Inv Ther 1S:67, 1992.
9. Copcoat MJ. Laparoscopy in urology: Perspectives and practice. Br J Urol 69:561, 1992.
10. Chiu AW, Chen MT, Huang WJS, et al. Case report: Laparoscopic nephroureterectomy and endoscopic excision of bladder cuff. Min Inv Ther 1:299, 1992.
11. See WA. Selection and preparation of the patient for laparoscopic surgery. In Clayman RV, McDougall EM, eds. Laparoscopic Urology. St. Louis, Quality Medical Publishers, 1993, p 7.
12. Kavoussi LR, Kerbl K, Capelouto CC, et al. Laparoscopic nephrectomy for renal neoplasms. Urology 42:603, 1993.
13. Figenshau RS, Clayman RV, Kerbl K, et al. Laparoscopic nephroureterectomy in the child: Initial case report. J Urol 151:740, 1994.
14. Pearle MS, Nakada SY, McDougall EM, et al. Laparoscopic pneumodissection: Initial clinical experience. Urology 45:882, 1995.
15. Gardner SM, Clayman RV, McDougall EM, et al. Laparoscopic

16. Kerbl K, Chandhoke PS, Clayman RV, et al. Ligation of the renal pedicle during laparoscopic nephrectomy: Comparison of staples, clips, and sutures. J Laparoendosc Surg 3:7, 1993.
17. Kerbl K, Clayman RV, McDougall EM, et al. Transperitoneal nephrectomy for benign disease of the kidney: A comparison of laparoscopic and open surgical techniques. Urology 43:607, 1994.
18. McDougall EM, Clayman RV. Advances in laparoscopic urology. Part 1: History and development of procedures. Urology 43:420, 1994.
19. Jordan G, Winslow B. Laparoscopic upper pole partial nephrectomy with ureterectomy. J Urol 150:940, 1993.
20. Koyle M, Woo H, Kavoussi L. Laparoscopic nephrectomy in the first year of life. J Pediatr Surg 28:693, 1993.
21. Ehrlich RM, Gershman A, Fuchs G. Laparoscopic renal surgery in children. J Urol 151:735, 1994.
22. Ono Y, Sahashi M, Yamada S, Ohshima S. Laparoscopic nephrectomy without morcellation for renal cell carcinoma: Report of initial 2 cases. J Urol 150:1222, 1993.
23. Robey EL, Schellhammer PF. The adrenal gland and renal cell carcinoma: Is ipsilateral adrenalectomy a necessary component of radical nephrectomy? J Urol 135:453, 1986.
24. Gill IS, McClennan BL, Kerbl K, et al. Adrenal involvement from renal cell carcinoma: Predictive value of computerized tomography. J Urol 152:1082, 1994.
25. Sagalowsky AI, Kadesky KT, Ewalt DM, Kennedy TJ. Factors influencing adrenal metastases in renal cell carcinoma. J Urol 140:352A, 1993.
26. Mandressi A, Buizza C, Antonelli D, et al. Retro-extraperitoneal laparoscopic approach to excise retroperitoneal organs: Kidney and adrenal gland. Min Inv Ther 2:213, 1993.
27. Gaur DD, Agarwal DK, Purohit KC. Retroperitoneal laparoscopic nephrectomy: Initial case report. J Urol 149:103, 1993.
28. Rassweiler JJ, Henkel TO, Stoch C, et al. Retroperitoneal laparoscopic nephrectomy and other procedures in the upper retroperitoneum using a balloon dissection technique. Eur Urol 25:229, 1994.
29. Catalona WJ. Urothelial tumors of the urinary tract. In Walsh PC, Retik AB, Stamey TA, Vaughan ED Jr, eds. Campbell's Urology, 6th ed. Philadelphia, WB Saunders, 1992, p 1144.
30. Richie JP. Nephroureterectomy for carcinoma of renal pelvis and ureter. In Marshall FF, ed. Operative Urology. Philadelphia, WB Saunders, 1991, p 41.
31. McDougall EM, Clayman RV, Elashrey O. Laparoscopic nephroureterectomy for upper tract transitional cell cancer. The Washington University experience. J Urol (in press).

pneumodissection. A unique means of tissue dissection. J Urol (in press).

Chapter 14

Laparoscopic Renal Surgery

Elspeth M. McDougall

Laparoscopic renal surgery paralleled the development of a surgical entrapment sack and a high-speed, 10-mm tissue morcellator to create a procedure in which the entire kidney was removed by a laparoscopic approach. Since the initial laparoscopic nephrectomy in 1990, this technology has been applied to other laparoscopic therapeutic surgical procedures on the kidney. The clinical work with laparoscopic renal surgery has subsequently been extended to include laparoscopic partial nephrectomy, wedge resection of small renal tumors, the treatment of perihilar and (rarely) peripheral renal cysts, and nephropexy for symptomatic renal ptosis. In this chapter, laparoscopic partial nephrectomy, wedge resection of the kidney, renal cyst decortication, and nephropexy are discussed.

PREOPERATIVE EVALUATION AND PREPARATION

Routine preoperative laboratory studies are obtained, including electrolyte values, blood cell counts, urinalysis, and a urine culture. In patients with renal cancer a metastatic evaluation is obtained: chest radiograph, bone scan, and computed tomographic (CT) scan of the abdomen. It must be shown that the renal vein and inferior vena cava (IVC) are free of any tumor thrombus. In patients undergoing partial nephrectomy, a renal angiogram is helpful in planning the proposed line of transection of the kidney. This examination will also define any lower or upper pole vessels that may be ligated to more accurately determine the line of incision for the partial nephrectomy. In patients with a renal cyst, a CT scan of the kidney also helps to accurately pinpoint the location of the cyst on the kidney. In the patient with an intraparenchymal renal cyst, the immediate preoperative placement of an 8 Fr. percutaneous tube into the cyst cavity may be considered. This allows easier identification of the cyst during the procedure,

as the cyst can easily be drained or filled with a solution stained with indigo carmine. This is also helpful in the patient with a perihilar cyst, since the cyst can be distinguished from the true collecting system. In addition, cyst fluid can be obtained for chemical and histologic analysis to preclude the unroofing of a malignant cyst.

On an outpatient basis, there is a full mechanical and antibiotic bowel preparation. The orders for the bowel preparation include a clear liquid diet 2 days before the procedure. The day before surgery patients should drink 4 to 6 L of chilled GoLYTELY (1 to 6 PM) until rectal effluent is clear; at 7 and 11 PM they receive neomycin, 2 gm orally, and metronidazole, 2 gm orally. Patients should be NPO status after midnight, with intravenous fluids and prochlorperazine maleate (Compazine), 10 mg orally at 2 PM the day before surgery to stop nausea. Patients are routinely type- and cross-matched for 2 units of blood if they are undergoing a partial nephrectomy or wedge resection of the kidney. Since this is an elective procedure, patients are offered the opportunity to provide 2 units of autologous blood. A type and screen is sufficient for patients in whom a renal cyst decortication or nephropexy is planned. On call to the operating room, patients are given a dose of a parenteral antibiotic (cephalosporin or an ampicillin/gentamicin combination).

OPERATIVE TECHNIQUE

In patients undergoing laparoscopic partial nephrectomy or renal cyst decortication, an external ureteral stent is placed. They are taken to the cystoscopy suite and placed in a dorsal lithotomy position. Flexible cystoscopy is performed and a 0.035-inch Bentson guidewire is advanced into the upper collecting system of the affected ureter. A 7 Fr. 11.5-mm occlusion balloon catheter is passed over the guidewire until the tip is positioned in the area of the renal pelvis. The guidewire is removed and a retrograde pyelogram is performed by injecting 5 to 10 ml of dilute contrast material (50:50 mix of saline and Conray 60). The balloon is inflated with saline by a one-way stopcock under fluoroscopic control and can be seen as a negative image in the contrast-filled renal pelvis. After insufflation of the balloon a 0.035-inch Amplatz Super Stiff guidewire is passed into the catheter. A side-arm adaptor is placed over the guidewire and fixed to the butt end of the occlusion balloon catheter. The side-arm adaptor is then screwed tightly down onto the Amplatz guidewire, securing it in place. A Foley urethral catheter is placed alongside the shaft of the occlusion balloon catheter to allow drainage of the bladder throughout the procedure. Both catheters are secured to drainage and placed in a sterile plastic bag, and the patient is transported to the main operating room. It is advisable to perform catheter placement under fluoroscopic control so that no inadvertent upper tract trauma occurs that could result in clot obstruction of the ureter or ureteral stent postoperatively.

All patients undergoing laparoscopic renal surgery are placed under general anesthesia with cuffed endotracheal control of the airway and nasogastric decompression of the stomach.

Laparoscopic renal surgery can be performed via a transperitoneal or retroperitoneal approach. The transperitoneal approach is better for patients with a large lesion, to facilitate access and use of the organ entrapment sack. However, the retroperitoneal approach is ideally suited to the patient undergoing wedge resection for a small renal lesion, decortication of a posterior renal cyst, or nephropexy. The retroperitoneal technique provides a more direct access to the retroperitoneum and involves less patient discomfort in the postoperative period.[1]

Transperitoneal Approach

For a transperitoneal approach to laparoscopic renal surgery, the patient is initially positioned supine and undergoes a full abdominal skin preparation. A pneumoperitoneum is created using a Veress needle through a small skin incision at the supraumbilical crease. A 12-mm port is then placed at the umbilicus or at the lateral border of the rectus abdominis muscle on the ipsilateral side at the level of the umbilicus. The laparoscope is inserted through this port and satisfactory positioning within the peritoneal cavity confirmed; the port is then secured to the skin with a No. 2 Prolene suture. The port is covered with a sterile towel and the patient is repositioned in the lateral decubitus position. After adequate padding has been placed under the axilla and the bony promi-

nence of the hip, the sterile draping is removed from the primary port. A second abdominal skin preparation is performed to include the entire abdomen from the xiphoid process to the symphysis pubis and from the ipsilateral paraspinal region posteriorly to the midclavicular line (MCL) on the contralateral side anteriorly. This preparation includes the primary port. The sterile plastic cover is removed from the urethral and ureteral catheters. These are prepared and separately draped, thereby ensuring ready access to the ureteral catheter throughout the procedure.

With the patient in the lateral decubitus position, the laparoscope is placed through the 12-mm port. Two additional ports are placed at the MCL if the primary port is in the umbilicus, or in the anterior axillary line (AAL) if the primary port has been placed lateral to the rectus abdominis muscles. These include a 12-mm port just below the costal margin and a 5-mm port 3 to 4 cm below the level of the umbilicus. With these two secondary ports, a grasping forceps and electrosurgical scissors are inserted and used to incise the line of Toldt. The incision is continued inferiorly until the common iliac artery is seen pulsating, and continued cephalad along the hepatic or splenic flexure. Blunt and sharp dissection is then performed to mobilize the bowel medially and expose the retroperitoneum. On the right side the duodenum is reflected medially to reveal the anterior surface of the IVC. On the left side, care must be used in dissection of the colon from the retroperitoneum in the area of the spleen. The splenorenal ligament must be incised to completely mobilize the splenic flexure medially. After exposure of the retroperitoneal space, additional ports may be placed in the posterior axillary line (PAL), if this is necessary for completion of the planned surgical procedure.

Retroperitoneal Approach

The patient is placed in a lateral decubitus position with the ipsilateral flank exposed. Skin preparation should include the abdomen from the xiphoid process to the symphysis pubis and from the ipsilateral paraspinal region posteriorly to the umbilicus anteriorly. The sterile plastic cover is removed from the urethral and ureteral catheters, which are prepared and separately draped, ensuring ready access to the ureteral catheter throughout the procedure. The Veress needle is inserted through the infero- or supero-posterior lumbar triangle in the PAL either just above the iliac crest or just below the tip of the twelfth rib. After development of the carbon dioxide (CO_2) pneumoretroperitoneum, a 12-mm port is inserted at this site. The dilating balloon catheter is created using a 16 Fr. red rubber catheter and the middle finger of a sterile size 8 latex surgeon's glove. The middle finger of the glove is placed over the tip of the catheter and secured in place with two 0 silk ligatures positioned so that the openings at the catheter tip are within the glove tip (Fig. 14–1). This balloon catheter is backloaded through a 28 or 30 Fr. Amplatz sheath until the balloon is retracted to just inside the sheath. The assembled unit is inserted through the 12-mm trocar until the tip of the sheath lies just at the port opening. The balloon catheter is advanced through the sheath, approximately 3 to 4 cm into the perirenal fat (i.e., outside Gerota's fascia). The balloon is then filled with 1 L of normal saline. After distention of the balloon the fluid is aspirated and the balloon catheter withdrawn into the Amplatz sheath, following which the balloon and sheath are removed from the 12-mm port. The port is then connected to the CO_2 insufflator at a set pressure of 12 to 15 mm Hg. The 10-mm 30-degree laparoscope is inserted and the retroperitoneal space examined. An additional two or three laparoscopic ports are inserted under endoscopic monitoring. A 12-mm trocar is placed just at the lateral border of the sacrospinal muscle, midway between the iliac crest and the costal margin. If the primary port is placed in the inferoposterior lumbar triangle, a 12- or 5-mm port is placed just below the twelfth rib in the PAL. If the primary port is placed at the tip of the twelfth rib, a 12- or 5-mm port is placed in the PAL just above the superior iliac crest at the area of the inferoposterior lumbar triangle. If a fourth port is required for suturing or retraction, a 5-mm port may be placed in the AAL midway between the twelfth rib and the superior iliac crest.

After balloon dilation of the retroperitoneal space, initial laparoscopic examination shows the psoas muscle and genitofemoral nerve clearly exposed. Usually, Gerota's fascia can also be appreciated. The ureter may at times also be seen; usually, minimal dissection in the area of the ureter is needed to expose this structure, medial to the psoas muscle.

LAPAROSCOPIC PARTIAL NEPHRECTOMY

The transperitoneal approach is usually preferred for the laparoscopic partial nephrectomy. This provides the larger space of the peritoneal cavity to facilitate insertion of the organ entrapment sack for removal of the surgical specimen.

After complete medial mobilization of the bowel, the ureter is identified in the retroperitoneal space by gently moving the retrograde ureteral catheter and indwelling guidewire back and forth within the ureter. The undulating ureter can usually be spotted lying immediately lateral to the IVC or aorta. The ureter does not need to be completely dissected or secured with a piece of umbilical tape. Instead, the ureter is dissected along its anterior surface until the lower pole of the kidney, within Gerota's fascia, is clearly identified. Gerota's fascia is incised and the perirenal fat tissue is dissected to expose the kidney. The anterior surface of the kidney is then exposed by further dissection of the perirenal fat. Dissection is continued over the lower or upper pole, depending on the segment of kidney to be resected. This area should be as completely dissected and mobilized as possible. Maintaining some of the retroperitoneal attachments of the kidney on the posterior aspect away from the area to be transected helps to stabilize the kidney during the dissection and excision of the diseased portion. If preoperative embolization has been performed in the polar vessels, the line of demarcation for transection of the kidney may be well defined. However, dissection will more likely require exposure of the renal hilum and the renal artery and vein to identify the appropriate line of transection. The renal vessels may be dissected to create a 360-degree window around each vessel, with a vessel loop placed around the structures for hemostatic purposes during the surgical procedure. However, this technique is not usually necessary, as the electrocautery and argon beam coagulator provide satisfactory hemostasis during resection of the renal tissue. The

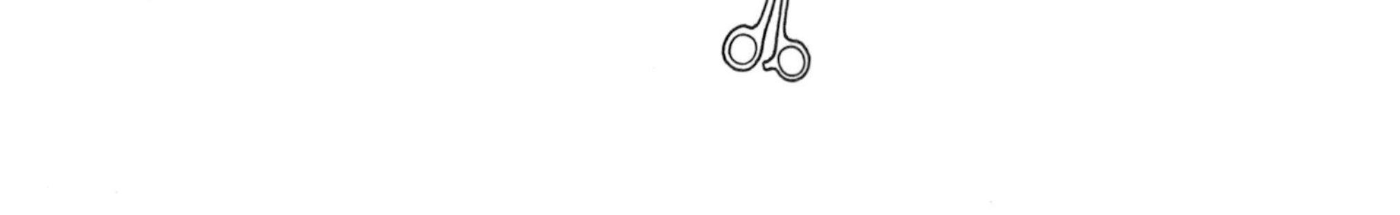

Figure 14–1. The dilating balloon catheter for retroperitoneoscopy is created by tying the middle finger of a size 8 latex surgeon's glove onto the tip of a 16 Fr. red rubber catheter. The balloon is inflated by injecting normal saline up to a maximum of 1000 ml. (From McDougall EM, Clayman RV, Vancaillie TG. Laparoscopic bladder neck suspension. In Rassweiler J, Janetschak G, Griffith DP, eds. Laparoscopic Surgery in Urology. Stuttgart, Germany, George Thieme Verlag (in press).)

laparoscopic 7-MHz ultrasound probe may be inserted through the 12-mm port and used to examine the kidney under laparoscopic control. If the partial nephrectomy is being performed for hydrocalix or a hypoechoic lesion, the ultrasound probe will assist in mapping the line of excision on the renal surface.

Once the area of kidney to be resected has been identified, the line of incision is marked circumferentially around the kidney, using the electrosurgical scissors to fulgurate this line. The assistant uses an aspirating, irrigating instrument to retract the tissue as it is resected and also to provide suctioning during the procedure. The surgeon alternates between the electrosurgical scissors and the 5- or 10-mm argon beam coagulator for transection and fulguration of the resected renal surface (Fig. 14–2). The electrosurgical scissors are used to incise the renal tissue, after which the argon beam coagulator is used to paint the transected surface to establish hemostasis. This procedure of alternating between the electrocautery scissors and the argon beam coagulator is continued until the intended resection of the renal parenchyma has been completed. The surgical specimen is secured in locking/grasping forceps and positioned away from the surgical site. The transected surface of the kidney is then examined, and the argon beam coagulator is used to fulgurate the transected surface

completely. When hemostasis is satisfactory, indigo carmine–stained normal saline can be injected through the ureteral catheter after removal of the Amplatz Super Stiff guidewire. During the injection of the saline, the transected surface is laparoscopically observed for any evidence of extravasation. If the integrity of the collecting system is not completely intact, the areas of extravasation are closed laparoscopically using an intracorporeal suturing technique. A 3-0 Vicryl (polyglactin 910) suture on an SH needle is passed through a needle introducer in the 12-mm port. With a locking/grasping forceps and a needle holder, the suture is then passed through the renal parenchyma in a figure-of-eight fashion to incorporate the open collecting system. An intracorporeal knot is created, snugging the suture down to close the collecting system. Three additional throws are placed on the knot to secure the closure. The needle holder is then introduced through the needle introducer in the 12-mm port. The suture is grasped just behind the needle and the suture is transected one quarter inch from the knot. The needle holder is then drawn into the needle introducer, drawing the needle with it until it is completely inside the needle introducer. The introducer, needle holder, and suture are all removed as one unit from the 12-mm port, and the needle and suture are retrieved. Indigo carmine–

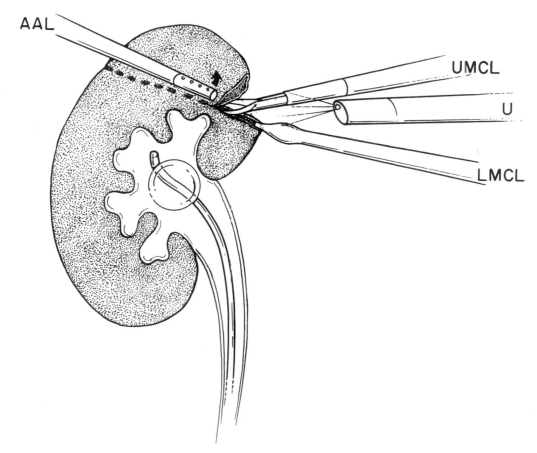

Figure 14–2. During a partial nephrectomy the assistant helps to retract the tissue and suction smoke generated during the electrosurgical excision by placing a suction/irrigator tip through the anterior axillary line (AAL) port. The surgeon works through the upper midclavicular line (UMCL) port and the lower midclavicular line (LMCL) port to transect and fulgurate the tissue along the demarcated cut line on the renal surface. U, umbilical.

stained saline is reinjected through the ureteral catheter. If there is any evidence of continued fluid leakage from the collecting system, the suturing procedure is repeated until closure of the collecting system has been achieved.

Animal studies have shown that the renal parenchymal vessels and collecting system can be satisfactorily occluded with just the argon beam coagulator.[2] If, after coagulation with the argon beam coagulator, there is no evidence of extravasation on injection of indigo carmine–stained normal saline through the ureteral catheter, suturing of the renal parenchyma is not necessary.

The resected surface of the kidney may be covered with perirenal fat or omentum to serve as a wick for any subsequent fluid that may develop at the surgical site and drain into the retroperitoneum (Fig. 14–3). A 10-mm hernia clip applier is passed through the 12-mm MCL port. The mobilized perirenal fat is placed over the surface of the resected kidney and fixed to the cut renal edge with the hernia clips. Alternatively, an intracorporeal suturing technique may be used to tack the fat onto the cut renal surface.

The pneumoperitoneum is reduced to 5 mm Hg or less pressure; a thorough check for hemostasis is performed. A 5-mm endoscope is placed through the 5-mm lower midclavicular line (LMCL) port. The two 12-mm ports are removed under laparoscopic visualization, and the fascia of each of these ports is closed in a figure-of-eight fashion using absorbable suture on a TT-3 needle. The 5-mm port is withdrawn under endoscopic control. The 5-mm laparoscope is pulled into the 5-mm port sheath until the tip of the endoscope is protruding just beyond the end of the sheath. The port and endoscope are then removed as one unit, allowing a clear view of the incision to ensure satisfactory hemostasis. The skin incisions of the 12-mm ports are closed with a subcuticular 4-0 absorbable suture. Adhesive skin strips are applied to all the port sites.

It is imperative that optimal drainage of the upper collecting system be established to ensure satisfactory healing and closure of the upper collecting system. The patient is therefore transferred to the cystoscopy suite. Under fluoroscopic visualization a guidewire is positioned through the balloon catheter. The balloon is deflated and the catheter removed, leaving the guidewire in position. A 7.1 pigtail external stent may be inserted into the upper collecting system and placed to drainage. On the second postoperative day a retrograde injection of contrast may be performed to confirm complete closure of the upper collecting system before removal of the stent. If extravasation occurs, the external stent may be exchanged for an

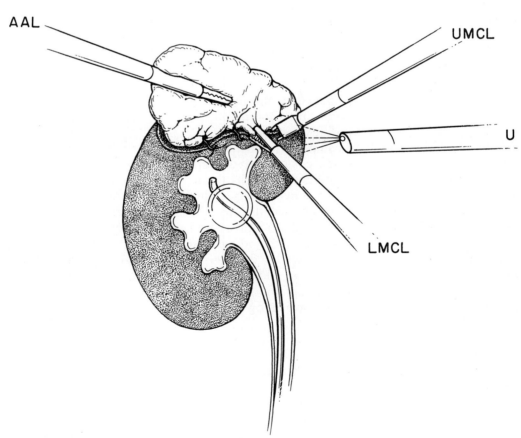

Figure 14–3. Perirenal fat may be placed over the resected surface of the kidney and fixed in place with a hernia clip applier.

indwelling ureteral stent and Foley catheter, which are maintained for 1 week, after which a repeat imaging study of the upper collecting system is performed. Alternatively, an indwelling ureteral stent and Foley catheter may be placed at the completion of the laparoscopic procedure. An 8/10 Fr. ureteral dilating catheter system is inserted over the guidewire until the 10 Fr. catheter is positioned in the distal third of the ureter. The 8 Fr. catheter is removed, leaving the guidewire and 10 Fr. in position in the collecting system. A double-pigtail ureteral stent is then placed over the guidewire and advanced, using a metal-tipped pusher, through the 10 Fr. catheter into the upper collecting system. The proximal coil of the stent is positioned within the renal pelvis, and the guidewire is partially withdrawn until satisfactory coiling of the stent within the renal pelvis is observed. The metal-tipped pusher is then positioned against the distal end of the stent. This position is fluoroscopically placed at the midpoint of the symphysis pubis. The 10 Fr. catheter is then removed, leaving the guidewire and stent in position in the upper collecting system. Maintaining the position of the pusher at the midpoint of the symphysis pubis fluoroscopically, the guidewire is removed. As the floppy tip of the guidewire approaches the distal end of the stent, this can be gently advanced into the bladder as the remaining wire is removed, allowing the distal tip of the stent to coil satisfactorily within the bladder. A Foley catheter is placed into the bladder and left to gravity drainage.

Postoperative Management

The nasogastric tube is removed in the operating room. The patient is started on clear liquids on the evening of the procedure and advanced to a regular diet by the end of the first postoperative day. Patient ambulation is started on the first postoperative morning. The Foley catheter is maintained to gravity drainage for 48 hours postoperatively. A cystogram is then taken. There will be reflux of contrast through the ureteral stent. If there is no evidence of extravasation from the operative site, the Foley catheter may be removed. If extravasation persists, the catheter is maintained to gravity drainage for an additional 5 to 7 days before repeating the cystogram. The Foley catheter is not removed until extravasation from the operative site has ceased.

Parenteral antibiotics are usually continued until the Foley catheter has been removed. Pain management is achieved initially with parenteral morphine sulfate. By the second postoperative day the discomfort can usually be completely controlled by oral analgesics. The patient is usually discharged, without any activity restrictions, on the third or fourth post-operative day. The ureteral stent may be removed with the flexible cystoscope 4 to 6 weeks after the surgical procedure.

Postoperative Complications

The main postoperative complication associated with laparoscopic partial nephrectomy is related to leakage of urine from the operative site. It is therefore important to provide upper tract drainage with an indwelling ureteral stent during the immediate post-operative period. However, clot obstruction of the stent may result in upper tract dilation and development of urinoma. If the patient develops fevers or flank pain, a CT scan will best delineate the presence and extent of a perirenal urinoma. Percutaneous drainage of the urinoma should be instituted. The ureteral stent may be replaced for patency, or nephrostomy tube drainage of the kidney may be required for more efficient decompression of the upper collecting system.

Bleeding from the operative site should be a rare complication if attention is directed to decreasing the pneumoperitoneum and examining this area before exiting the abdomen. However, if the patient's hematocrit is falling or if there is clinical evidence of hypovolemia (i.e., hypotension and tachycardia), a renal angiogram may delineate the site of bleeding and also facilitate selective embolization of the vessel. However, in an unstable patient, urgent open exploration may be required to achieve satisfactory hemostasis.

LAPAROSCOPIC WEDGE RESECTION OF THE KIDNEY

Recent advances in radiologic procedures to image the kidney have resulted in an increase in the incidental discovery of asymptomatic, low-stage, small renal cell carcinomas. The data from various studies support the efficacy of nephron-sparing surgery for selected patients with localized low-stage renal cell carcinoma.[3] However, it is now feasible to handle these small, low-stage renal masses, particularly those in a peripheral position, by a laparoscopic approach and to excise the lesion using wedge resection.

Laparoscopic wedge resection of a small renal mass may be ideally suited to a retroperitoneal approach.[4] There is no need to place a ureteral catheter before the planned procedure. The patient is placed in a lateral decubitus position with the flank exposed. Veress needle insufflation of the retroperitoneum is performed at the inferoposterior lumbar triangle. The first 12-mm port is inserted, and balloon dilation of the retroperitoneal space is performed through this port. Three additional ports are placed under direct endoscopic control: a 12-mm port at the lateral edge of the sacrospinal muscle, midway between the costal margin and iliac crest; a 5-mm port along the AAL just below the costal margin; and a 10-mm port just below the tip of the twelfth rib in the superoposterior lumbar triangle. The surgeon operates through the 12-mm port at the lateral edge of the sacrospinal muscle and the 10-mm port below the tip of the twelfth rib. The laparoscope is maintained through the inferoposterior lumbar triangle. The assistant operates through the 5-mm port at the AAL just below the costal margin. The surgeon uses atraumatic grasping forceps and electrosurgical scissors to incise Gerota's fascia overlying the kidney. The perirenal fat is carefully removed, exposing the posterior surface of the kidney from the upper to the lower pole. In doing so, a peripheral lesion will be well visualized in its position as confirmed by CT scan. If the lesion is within the deeper parenchymal tissues, a laparoscopic ultrasound probe (7 MHz) may be inserted through the 12-mm port at the lateral edge of the sacrospinal muscle. This will help delineate the area of the tumor and the surgeon can mark this on the renal capsule, using the electrocautery scissors. The line of the wedge resection is clearly delineated by a fulgurated line on the renal capsule. The assistant places an aspirating irrigating tip instrument through the 5-mm port in the AAL. This is used to help retract the renal tissue as it is incised and provide aspiration of smoke that may accumulate during electrocautery. Using the electrosurgical scissors through the superoposterior lumbar triangle port, the surgeon incises the renal parenchyma along the demarcated line of incision. A grasping forceps through the 12-mm port lateral to the sacrospinal muscle allows retraction and delineation of the line of transection. The electrosurgical scissors are alternated with the 10- or 5-mm argon beam coagulator to provide hemostasis of the transected renal surface as the wedge resection is being performed. The excised specimen is removed using the 10-mm spoon-shaped grasping forceps through the 10-mm port. The electrosurgical scissors are then replaced through this same port and used to resect the base of the incision site. The argon beam coagulator is again used for hemostasis after this excision. The specimen is sent for a frozen section to ensure that there is no evidence of tumor in the resected margin. The excision site is then systematically fulgurated with the argon beam coagulator. A plug of Avitene may be placed on the surgical site as an extra hemostatic precaution.[4]

The pneumoperitoneum is reduced to 5 mm Hg or less and a thorough check made for hemostasis. A 5-mm endoscope is placed through the upper AAL port. The larger than 5-mm ports are then sequentially removed under direct laparoscopic visualization. As each port is removed, the fascia is closed under direct visualization. The laparoscope is drawn backward into the end of the 5-mm port sheath. The port and laparoscope are removed as a unit under direct visualization to examine the incision site for satisfactory hemostasis. The larger than 5-mm port sites are closed in a subcuticular fashion with a 4-0 absorbable suture. Skin adhesive strips are applied to all port sites.

The nasogastric tube is removed in the operating room, and the urethral catheter is removed the morning after the procedure. Clear fluids are begun on the evening of the procedure. The patient's diet is advanced to regular by the end of the first postoperative day. Ambulation of the patient begins on the first postoperative morning.

Parenteral antibiotics are continued for the first 24 hours. Pain management is achieved with parenteral morphine sulfate or, as is more commonly required, an oral analgesic. The patient is usually discharged without any activity restrictions on the second or third postoperative day.

Postoperative Complications

If the patient's hemoglobin and hematocrit decrease during the postoperative period, or if clinical evidence of hypovolemia is observed (hypotension or tachycardia), bleeding from the operative site should be suspected. A CT scan will delineate any evidence of perirenal hematoma, which most often will be contained in the retroperitoneal space. Conservative management of the patient with clinical observation and repeat CT is usually sufficient. However, if continued bleeding is suspected, a renal angiogram will delineate the source of bleeding and also provide the opportunity for selective embolization.

In performing a wedge resection of deep parenchymal lesions, there is an increased risk of transection of the upper collecting system and subsequent urinary extravasation. In these patients, intraoperative ureteral catheterization and injection of indigo carmine–stained saline should be performed to rule out this type of injury. Argon beam fulguration of the tissues, combined with a postoperative indwelling ureteral stent, should allow complete closure of the collecting system postoperatively. However, if a large retroperitoneal urinoma develops, percutaneous drainage may be required. Optimal decompression of the upper collecting system with percutaneous nephrostomy and/or indwelling ureteral stenting may also be necessary.

RENAL CYST DECORTICATION

Laparoscopic decortication of renal cysts may be indicated in cysts that have been unresponsive to percutaneous drainage and sclerosis but remain symptomatic.[5] It is important for cyst puncture and sampling of the cyst fluid to be performed before any planned operative procedure. The fluid is sent for cytologic study and chemistry (protein, lactate dehydrogenase, culture) analysis to establish the benign nature of the cyst. For cysts in the posterior or polar region of the kidney, the retroperitoneal approach may be ideally suited for optimal access. However, for intraparenchymal or perihilar cysts, a transperitoneal approach may be more appropriate. The transperitoneal approach to renal cyst decortication will be discussed here. Pneumoperitoneum is developed as described, with the Veress needle at the umbilical site. A 10-mm primary umbilical port is placed and the patient placed in the lateral decubitus position. A 10-mm MCL subcostal port is positioned and a 5-mm MCL port is inserted 3 cm below the umbilicus. A 5-mm AAL subcostal port may also be used. The surgeon operates the two MCL ports while the surgical assistant operates through the AAL port. The laparoscope is positioned through the 10-mm umbilical port.

Before the laparoscopic procedure the patient undergoes cystoscopic insertion of an ipsilateral ureteral occlusion balloon catheter. This allows instillation of indigo carmine–stained normal saline into the upper collecting system after resection of the cyst, to confirm an intact renal collecting system.

The line of Toldt is identified, and the assistant, via the 5-mm AAL port, grabs and holds the peritoneum laterally while the surgeon, working through the two MCL ports, grasps the peritoneum medially. The line of Toldt is then incised with the endosurgical scissors, the incision being extended along the line of Toldt caudally to the level of the iliac vessels and cephalad to the level of the hepatic or splenic flexure. The bowel is mobilized medially off Gerota's fascia. The retrograde ureteral catheter is manipulated within the ureter, and the undulating ureter can be identified within the retroperitoneum lying lateral to the IVC or aorta. The ureter is dissected along its anterior surface until the lower pole of the kidney is identified within Gerota's fascia. There is no need to create a complete dissection of the ureter or to secure the ureter with a piece of umbilical tape.

The area of the renal cyst is identified and Gerota's fascia is opened overlying the cyst. Careful dissection of the perirenal fat is performed from the renal capsule to expose the outer cyst wall. Typical cysts have a blue dome appearance. This should be completely freed of any perirenal fat so that the adjacent normal renal parenchyma is identified circumferentially around the cyst. If a percutaneous cystotomy tube has been placed preoperatively into the cyst, indigo carmine–stained normal saline may be instilled through the nephrostomy catheter to facilitate recognition and dissection of the cyst.

After completely exposing the cyst, it may be helpful to decompress the interior of the cyst in order to perform the resection of the cyst wall. If a percutaneous tube is not present, an endoscopic needle is passed via the 10-mm upper midclavicular line (UCML) port to drain the cyst. If this has not already been done, the fluid should be sent for cytologic and chemistry analysis.

The surgeon uses a 5-mm grasping forceps via the LMCL port and a 5-mm electrosurgical scissors

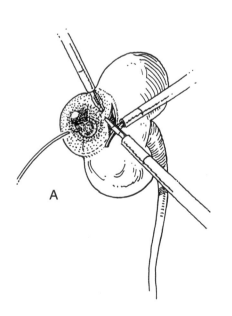

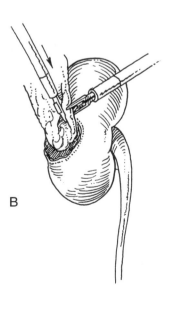

Figure 14–4. *A,* The cyst wall is circumferentially excised adjacent to the renal parenchyma. *B,* Perirenal fat is mobilized and placed into the base of the cyst. (From Clayman RV, McDougall EM. Laparoscopic renal surgery. In Clayman RV, McDougall EM, eds. Laparoscopic Urology. St. Louis, MO, Quality Medical Publishing, 1993, p 304.)

through the upper 10-mm port. The assistant, with a 5-mm atraumatic grasping forceps through the AAL port, grasps the collapsed outer wall of the cyst and retracts this laterally. The surgeon grasps the collapsed cyst wall and holds it taut. The cyst wall is then circumferentially incised immediately adjacent to the renal parenchyma (Fig. 14–4A). The edges of the cyst are electrocoagulated circumferentially. The excised outer cyst wall is secured with 10-mm grasping forceps through the 10-mm MCL port and removed as a surgical specimen for histologic evaluation.

The interior surface of the cyst is carefully inspected for any abnormalities. A biopsy is taken of any suspicious areas along the inner cyst wall. The biopsy site may be electrocoagulated. The 5- or 10-mm argon beam coagulator may be inserted through the UMCL port and used to fulgurate the interior of the cyst. The advantage of the argon beam coagulator is that this produces a superficial coagulation of the surface tissues, usually to a depth of 1 to 2 mm (140 watts, 4 L/min flow of argon).

If a perihilar cyst has been dissected and exposed, the cyst is carefully opened using just the scissors without any electrosurgical current. The outer wall is excised and sent as a specimen. The interior of the cyst is inspected and any suspicious areas may be sent for biopsy. However, because of the proximity of the cyst to the renal pelvis and vessels, biopsies should be utilized judiciously to avoid entering these structures. Electrofulguration should not be used on the interior of a perihilar cyst. Intraoperative ultrasound may be helpful to discriminate a perihilar cyst from the renal collecting system.

Perirenal fat is then mobilized and placed into the base of the cyst to serve as a wick so that any subsequent fluid that may develop from the interior surface of the cyst can drain out into the retroperitoneum (Fig. 14–4B). A 10-mm hernia stapling device may be passed through the 10-mm MCL port to secure the fat to the cut edge of the cyst wall.

Indigo carmine–stained normal saline should be injected through the ureteral catheter to ensure that there is no extravasation from the base of the cyst after fulguration of the cyst interior. If extravasation is noted, this should be closed using an intracorporeal suturing technique with a 3-0 or 4-0 Vicryl suture on an SH needle.

The pneumoperitoneum is reduced to 5 mm Hg or less and the surgical site examined for satisfactory hemostasis. A 5-mm endoscope is placed through the 5-mm LMCL port. The two 10-mm ports are removed under laparoscopic visualization, and the fascia is closed with a figure-of-eight 0 absorbable suture on a TT-3 needle. The 5-mm AAL port is withdrawn under laparoscopic control. The 5-mm laparoscope is drawn back into the 5-mm port sheath, allowing the tip of the endoscope to protrude beyond the end of the sheath. The sheath and the laparoscope are then removed as a unit, providing clear visualization of the incision site as the port is withdrawn. The skin incisions of the 10-mm ports are closed in a subcuticular fashion with a 4-0 absorbable suture. Adhesive skin strips are applied to all port sites.

If there is any doubt over the integrity of the collecting system after decortication and fulguration of the cyst base, optimal drainage of the upper collecting system should be provided. The patient is returned to the cystoscopy suite, where a 0.035-inch Bentson guidewire is passed through the occlusion balloon catheter into the upper collecting system. The balloon catheter is removed and an 8/10 Fr. ureteral dilating set inserted. The 8 Fr. catheter is removed, leaving the 10 Fr. catheter in position in the distal ureter with the guidewire in the upper collecting system. A double-pigtail ureteral stent is then placed over the guidewire and advanced through the 10 Fr. catheter to position the proximal coil of the stent within the renal pelvis. The metal-tipped pusher is placed behind the stent to maintain the position in the upper collecting system, and the 10 Fr. catheter is removed from the ureter. The guidewire is then removed from the stent under fluoroscopic visualization, maintaining the metal-tipped pusher at the midpoint region of the symphysis pubis. As the guidewire is removed and the floppy end positioned in the distal stent, the pusher can advance the distal stent into the bladder, allowing it to coil satisfactorily within the bladder. A Foley catheter is placed and left to gravity drainage.

Postoperative Management

After the laparoscopic procedure, the nasogastric tube is removed in the operating room. Clear liquids are begun on the evening of the procedure, and patients are usually advanced to a regular diet by the morning of the first postoperative day. They are ambulated on the first postoperative morning. The urethral catheter may be removed the morning after the procedure unless there is concern over urinary extravasation from the upper collecting system. If this is the case a cystogram should be performed before the planned removal of the Foley catheter to confirm that there is no evidence of contrast extravasation. A Foley catheter should be maintained until the upper collecting system is completely closed. Parenteral antibiotics are continued for the first 24 hours. Pain management is achieved with parenteral morphine sulfate or, more commonly, only oral analgesics. The patient is usually discharged, without any activity restrictions, on the second or third postoperative day.

Postoperative Complications

The main postoperative complication is related to unsuspected urinary leakage from the upper collecting system. For this reason, it is advisable to leave a double-pigtail ureteral stent in position in all patients for 2 to 4 weeks after cyst decortication. However, if the patient presents with fever or flank pain, this complication should be suspected. A CT scan usually delineates the location and extent of the perirenal urinoma. Percutaneous drainage of the urinoma will be necessary. A cystogram will confirm reflux through the ureteral stent and identify the area of extravasation. If the stent is occluded, this may require replacement by a patent ureteral stent and/or insertion of a percutaneous nephrostomy tube for decompression of the upper collecting system.

LAPAROSCOPIC NEPHROPEXY

Nephroptosis is characterized by a downward displacement of the kidney by more than two vertebral bodies (greater than 5 cm) when the patient moves from a supine to an erect position. This rare condition is most commonly found in thin young adult women and can be the cause of significant flank pain and a palpable abdominal mass. Supine and erect intravenous pyelography or supine and erect furosemide renography is most helpful to document functionally significant nephroptosis. The kidney becomes hydronephrotic when it descends to its pelvic position. On renographic studies, the T1/2 may show an obstructive pattern, and there may be diminished blood flow to the kidney when the patient is erect. The pain associated with obstruction should be relieved in these patients by placement of a ureteral stent.

The retroperitoneal approach is again ideal for the laparoscopic nephropexy. After the patient is placed in the lateral decubitus position and the retroperitoneum reached for CO_2 insufflation with the Veress needle, balloon dilation of the retroperitoneal space is performed. A 10- or 12-mm port is placed at the inferior posterior lumbar triangle site. A 5-mm port is placed just at the lateral border of the sacrospinal muscle, midway between the iliac crest and costal margin. An additional 12-mm port is placed on the AAL midway between the iliac crest and costal margin. The surgeon works through the 5-mm posterior port and the 12-mm AAL port. The laparoscope is positioned through the posterior lumbar triangle port. The surgeon uses an atraumatic grasping forceps through the posterior port and electrosurgical scissors through the anterior port. After balloon dilation of the retroperitoneal space, Gerota's fascia is usually easily identified. This is incised posteriorly and the perirenal fat is dissected from the kidney, exposing it

along the posterior aspect from the upper to the lower pole. The kidney is then dissected anteriorly and posteriorly to completely free it within the retroperitoneum. It is important to free the kidney completely in order to mobilize it and allow elevation to the most superior aspect of the retroperitoneum, and to secure it in this position. Once the kidney has been completely mobilized, it is best to place the patient in a head-down position to allow the kidney to fall cephalad as far as possible. A 6-inch length of 0 Vicryl suture on an SH needle is used to perform the nephropexy. A polydioxanone suture clip (Lapra-Ty, Ethicon Endosurgery Inc., Cincinnati) is placed on the distal end of the suture length, leaving a quarter-inch tail. The needle and suture is then passed via a needle introducer through the 12-mm anterior port. A locking/grasping forceps is used through the posterior port. The suture is then passed through the fascia of the psoas or quadratus lumborum muscle as far cephalad within the retroperitoneum as possible. The suture is pulled through until the Lapra-Ty clip is snugged up against the fascia. The suture is then passed through the renal capsule at the posterior border of the upper pole of the kidney. The suture is tightened down, drawing the upper pole of the kidney up against the suture site on the muscle fascia. The needle and suture are then passed for a second time through the fascia of the psoas muscle and snugged down tightly. The suture is held by the grasping forceps through the posterior port. A Lapra-Ty suture clip positioned in the clip applier is inserted through the 12-mm anterior port, placed onto the suture as it exits the psoas muscle, and secured. Alternatively, an intracorporeal knot may be tied to secure the kidney in position. The clip applier is removed and a needle holder passed via a needle introducer through the 12-mm anterior port. The suture is grasped just behind the needle, and the grasping forceps is released from the suture. A scissors is placed through the posterior port and used to transect the suture approximately one quarter inch from the Lapra-Ty clip. The needle holder is then drawn into the needle introducer, drawing the needle inside the introducer, and then the introducer, needle holder, and suture are removed as one unit through the 12-mm port. The suture and needle are retrieved. This technique is repeated at the posterior aspect of the midpolar kidney region to secure it to the fascia of the psoas, and similarly at the posterior aspect of the lower pole of the kidney. After the four to six sutures have been placed, the retroperitoneal pressure is reduced to 5 mm Hg or less and a thorough examination of the surgical site performed to confirm adequate hemostasis. A 5-mm endoscope is placed through the posterior 5-mm port. The 12-mm anterior port is removed under laparoscopic visualization. The remaining 12-mm port is similarly removed under endoscopic visualization. The 5-mm scope is pulled back into the 5-mm port sheath until the tip of the endoscope is protruding just beyond the end of the sheath. The sheath and the laparoscope are then removed as a unit, providing clear visualization of the incision site to ensure satisfactory hemostasis. The skin incisions of the 12-mm ports are closed in a subcuticular fashion with a 4-0 absorbable suture. Adhesive skin strips are applied to all the skin incisions.

Postoperative Management

After the laparoscopic procedure, the nasogastric tube is removed in the operating room. The urethral catheter is removed the morning after the procedure. Patients are started on clear fluids and advanced to a regular diet on the evening of the procedure or on the first postoperative day. They are ready to ambulate on the first postoperative morning. There is usually minimal requirement for postoperative analgesia. This is usually completely satisfied by oral analgesics, although occasionally a dose of parenteral morphine sulfate may be required. Patients are usually discharged on the first or second postoperative day.

Postoperative Complications

The most common postoperative complication after laparoscopic nephropexy is related to the positioning of the patient during the procedure. As these patients are invariably very thin, great care must be taken to pad and protect bony prominences in the region of the hips, elbows, and axilla. Prolonged unprotected pressure in these regions may result in tissue bruising or nerve palsies. These complications usually resolve with conservative management and physiotherapy over several weeks to months but are best avoided if possible. Retroperitoneal bleeding may occur postoperatively from the sutures placed in the psoas muscle or the renal parenchyma. This is usually self-limited and the retroperitoneal hematoma will resolve spontaneously. Only patients with clinical manifestations of hypovolemia, tachycardia, or syncope will require transfusions or angiography and selective embolization.

Summary

Since the first laparoscopic nephrectomy in 1990 at Washington University School of Medicine the application of laparoscopy has been used for numerous other surgical procedures on the kidney. Laparoscopic renal surgery necessitates a highly skilled surgical team. However, the advantages of the reduced postoperative discomfort, the short hospital stay, and the rapid return to regular activities make this an attractive surgical alternative for the patient. Urologists must provide this surgical option for patients requiring therapeutic renal surgery, or patients will seek laparoscopists from other surgical disciplines who can perform these procedures.

REFERENCES

1. Clayman RV, McDougall EM, Kerbl K, et al. Laparoscopic nephrectomy: Transperitoneal vs. retroperitoneal (abstract 459). J Urol 151:342A, 1994.
2. McDougall EM, Clayman RV, Chandhoke PS, et al. Laparoscopic partial nephrectomy in the pig model. J Urol 149:1633, 1993.
3. Licht MR, Novick AC. Nephron sparing surgery for renal cell carcinoma. J Urol 149:1, 1993.
4. McDougall EM, Clayman RV, Anderson K. Laparoscopic wedge resection of a renal tumor: Initial experience. J Laparoendosc Surg 3:577, 1993.
5. Morgan C, Radar D. Laparoscopic unroofing of a renal cyst. J Urol 148:1835, 1992.

Chapter 15

Laparoscopic Surgery of the Ureter

Sean P. Hedican and John B. Adams II

Laparoscopic surgical procedures were traditionally employed in the diagnosis and management of gynecological disease. The development of a laparoscopic method for cholecystectomy in general surgery demonstrated that reduced incision size had a definite impact on postoperative analgesic requirements, length of hospital stay, and duration of convalescence.[1] The application of laparoscopic methods in urology began with diagnostic pelvic lymph node dissections in prostate cancer patients and has progressed rapidly.[2] Improvements in instrumentation and the introduction of methods for intracorporeal knot tying further expanded the realm of the laparoscopic surgeon to include ureteral reconstruction. Laparoscopic management of ureteral malignancies, ureteropelvic junction (UPJ) obstruction, impacted ureteral calculi, and retroperitoneal fibrosis is now an acceptable treatment option. The preoperative evaluation, surgical technique, and preliminary results of laparoscopic pyeloplasty, ureterolysis, ureterectomy, and ureterolithotomy are presented in this chapter.

A detailed understanding of ureteral anatomy is essential for a laparoscopic approach. For surgical purposes, a ureter is divided into an abdominal and a pelvic portion. The abdominal ureter runs from the kidney to the iliac vessels. It originates from the UPJ and courses along the top of the psoas muscle, crossing the genitofemoral nerve at the level of the fourth lumbar vertebrae. The gonadal vessels pass anterior to the ureter as it extends toward the pelvic brim to cross the external iliac vessels on the right and the common iliac on the left. The pelvic ureter runs from the iliac vessels to the bladder (Fig. 15–1). Once it has entered the pelvis, the ureter courses posterior and medial to the medial umbilical ligament (MUL) and enters the detrusor muscle just posterior to the superior vesical artery. Other important structures adjacent to the distal ureter include the vas deferens in males and the round ligament, uterine artery, and broad ligament in females. These structures may need to be divided to gain access to the distal ureter (see Fig. 15–12).

PREOPERATIVE EVALUATION

Preoperative evaluation includes identification of patients who are unsuitable for a laparoscopic approach. Relative contraindications to laparoscopy include large abdominal aortic aneurysms, previous retroperitoneal surgery, extensive previous abdominal surgery, bleeding abnormalities, and intrauterine pregnancy. Preoperative laboratory testing should include a complete blood cell count, a standard electrolyte panel, prothrombin time, partial thromboplastin time, and a urine sample for microscopical evaluation and culture. A type and screen is obtained, and patients should avoid the use of aspirin and aspirin-like compounds before surgery. If a patient has taken these compounds within 5 days of the operation, a template bleeding time is documented. Informed consent is obtained and the patient is made NPO status after midnight. A single intravenous dose of a third-generation cephalosporin or a combination of ampicillin and gentamicin is administered on arrival to the operating room. Radiographical studies should be visible on the operative viewbox.

LAPAROSCOPIC PYELOPLASTY

The "gold standard" for repair of UPJ obstruction remains open pyeloplasty. Success rates in excess of 90 percent have been reported in most series.[3, 4] The significant morbidity associated with a large flank

144

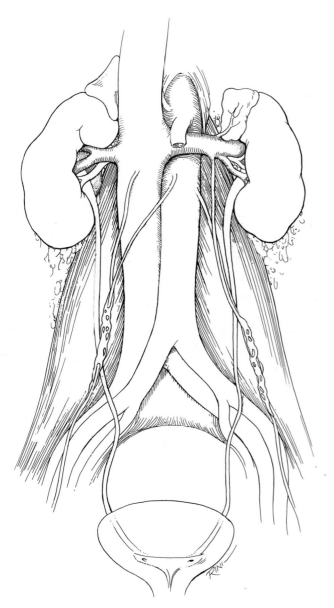

Figure 15–1. Normal course of the abdominal and pelvic ureter.

incision has, however, led to the development of several minimally invasive retrograde and antegrade approaches to UPJ repair. A percutaneous antegrade endopyelotomy was described by Wickham and Kellet in 1983, and a retrograde technique, initially devised to treat failed open pyeloplasties, was later introduced as an alternative primary repair.[5, 6] Success rates of 70 to 80 percent have been reported for these endoscopic techniques.[7, 8] The development of a fluoroscopically placed ureteral cutting balloon (Acucise) provided another alternative to open pyeloplasty.[9]

Laparoscopic pyeloplasty was first reported by Schuessler and colleagues in 1993 as a means of reconstructing the UPJ under direct vision without the associated postoperative pain, prominent skin incision, or prolonged convalescence of an open procedure.[10] The ideal candidates for this technique were those likely to fail a primary endoscopic approach. These included patients with a large redundant renal pelvis, a high ureteral insertion, or a lower pole crossing vessel.

Preoperative Evaluation

Evaluation of patients with UPJ obstruction should include an intravenous pyelogram (IVP), a diuretic renal scan, and a retrograde pyelogram. An IVP outlines the anatomy of the upper collecting system on the affected side and gives an indication of the degree of obstruction. It also provides information about the anatomy of the contralateral collecting system. A nuclear renal scan quantifies the degree of obstruction (clearance half-time) and documents relative percentage function of the two kidneys. Calculations of function in a highly obstructed system before stenting or nephrostomy tube placement will need to be repeated after the kidney is drained. A retrograde pyelogram performed either before or at the time of laparoscopic intervention is essential to evaluate the distal ureter and delineate the length of obstruction.

Technique

After general anesthetic administration, sequential compression devices are placed on the lower extremities and a 7 Fr. internal ureteral stent of appropriate length is inserted. A 16 Fr. Foley catheter and a nasogastric (NG) tube are also placed. The patient is placed with the umbilicus at the level of the table break in a 60-degree lateral decubitus position. An axillary roll is placed beneath the contralateral arm, which is brought out perpendicular to the patient. The ipsilateral arm is positioned across the chest to rest on several stacked pillows, or it can be suspended from an ether screen. In the flank position the contralateral knee is bent, the ipsilateral leg is kept straight, and a pillow is inserted between the two (Fig. 15–2). Sandbags can be placed behind the chest and hips to support the patient's position. A wide cloth tape across the shoulder and hip secures the patient to the table. The entire abdomen and flank from the xiphoid process to the genitalia, including the Foley catheter, is shaved and prepared with povidone-iodine (Betadine) solution. Monitors are positioned at the top of the table.

A Veress needle is introduced into the lower abdomen 1 cm below the level of the umbilicus, lateral to the rectus muscle. The peritoneal cavity is insufflated to a pressure of 20 mm Hg, and a horizontal incision is made 1 cm below the costal margin in the midclavicular line (MCL). A straight clamp is used to spread the subcutaneous tissue overlying the fascia, and a 10-mm trocar is then inserted. The remaining trocars,

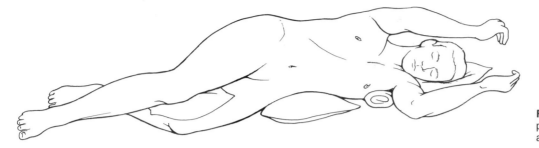

Figure 15–2. The 60-degree flank position used in the laparoscopic approach to the upper ureter.

placed under direct vision, include a 10-mm port at the umbilicus and a 5-mm port in the lower ipsilateral quadrant along the MCL (Fig. 15–3). The primary surgeon operates on the contralateral side of the table through the MCL ports while the first assistant stands on the ipsilateral side and manipulates the camera via the umbilical port. Port sheaths are positioned so that approximately 2 cm of length lies within the peritoneal cavity and is secured to the skin with 2-0 polyglactin suture.

The hydronephrotic kidney can usually be identified bulging lateral to the colon beneath the peritoneum. The peritoneum overlying the kidney is incised from the upper pole to approximately 3 cm below the lower pole (Fig. 15–4). After the peritoneum is incised and the colon retracted medially, one additional 5-mm trocar is inserted in the anterior axillary line (AAL). This trocar allows the first assistant to retract during repair of the UPJ. By following the psoas muscle medially along the lower pole of the kidney, the ureter can be identified; one must be careful not to confuse the gonadal vessels with the ureter. A sweeping motion of the graspers parallel to the ureter and gentle palpation of the indwelling

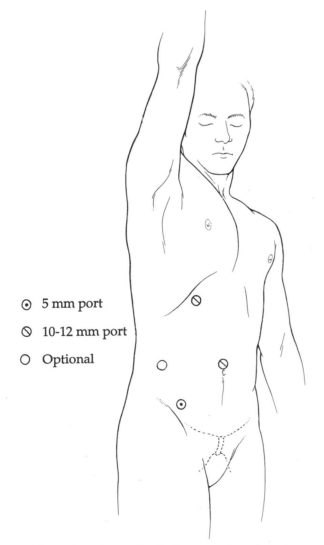

⊙ 5 mm port

⊘ 10-12 mm port

○ Optional

Figure 15–3. Trocar sites for laparoscopic pyeloplasty.

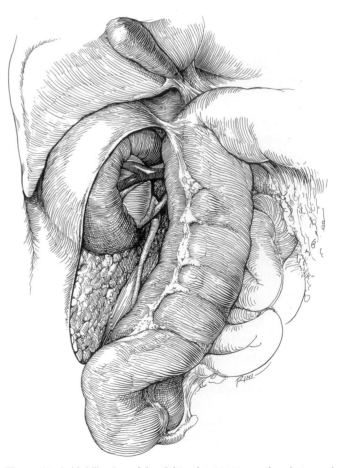

Figure 15–4. Mobilization of the right colon to expose the obstructed ureteropelvic junction (UPJ).

stent are used to bluntly dissect the UPJ and define the location of obstruction. Care is taken to minimize disruption of the ureteral blood supply, and mobilization of the renal pelvis is performed only to the extent necessary for pyeloplasty. Manipulation of the UPJ is made easier by placing a stay suture in the proximal ureter or grasping the renal pelvis with a Babcock clamp.

Articulating scissors are used to transect the UPJ, care being taken not to spiral this incision or cut the proximal ureteral stent. The renal pelvis is first incised above the area of stenosis, the stent is pulled from the pelvis, and the posterior wall is transected. The ureter below the area of obstruction is then cut circumferentially and the ring of ureter is manipulated off the stent. Before closure of the renal pelvis, a stitch is placed at the apex of the spatulated ureter and through the most dependent portion of the cut renal pelvis to guide reconstruction of the UPJ. If a reduction pyeloplasty was performed, the pyelotomy incision is closed with a running 4-0 polyglactin suture on an RB-1 needle. Interrupted sutures may be needed to further tailor the lower anterior segment for anastomosis to the spatulated ureter. All knots are tied intracorporeally to avoid undue stress on the collecting system. A lower pole crossing vessel may be identified as the cause of UPJ obstruction, and this requires transposition of the cut ureter and renal pelvis to a position anterior to the vessel. Care must be taken to prevent inadvertent injury of this vessel, which can result in loss of the lower pole segment.

The anastomosis is continued posteriorly using interrupted 4-0 polyglactin suture on an RB-1 needle cut into 5-inch lengths to optimize knot tying and manipulation. The posterior row is completed with two or three additional interrupted sutures, the proximal stent is fed back into the renal pelvis, and the anterior row is closed with about three additional sutures (Fig. 15–5). Alternatively, an automated suturing device (Endostitch) can be used to perform the anastomosis. Improved laparoscopic suturing, more efficient intracorporeal knot tying, and decreased operative time have been reported with use of this device for laparoscopic pyeloplasty.[11]

A 5-mm suction drain is passed through the lateral 5-mm port and backtunneled in the retroperitoneum to lie posterior to the completed UPJ anastomosis. The colon is replaced in its anatomical position and all ports are removed under direct vision. Interrupted 2-0 polyglactin suture is used to close the abdominal fascia at the 10-mm trocar sites, and the drain is secured with a 3-0 nylon stitch. The pneumoperitoneum is released and all skin incisions are closed with subcuticular 4-0 polyglactin suture and Steri-Strips.

Postoperative Management

The NG tube is removed in the operating room and the Foley catheter is discontinued the next day. The

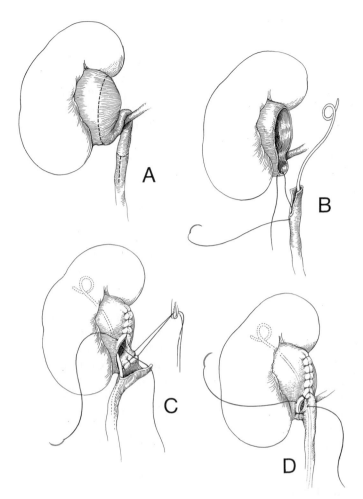

Figure 15–5. Reconstruction of a UPJ obstructed by a lower pole crossing vessel. *A,* Outline of the proposed incisions. *B,* The apex of the spatulated ureter is anastomosed to the dependent cut renal pelvis after transposition in front of the lower pole vessel. *C,* The posterior row is complete and the anterior row is begun. *D,* Completion of the anastomosis.

drain may be removed as soon as drainage is negligible, usually on the second postoperative day. A clear liquid diet is begun the night of surgery and advanced as tolerated. Parenteral antibiotics are continued for 24 hours before switching to an oral agent. The oral antibiotic is continued until the ureteral stent is removed 2 weeks postoperatively. The anastomosis is evaluated with an IVP or retrograde pyelogram 6 weeks after stent removal, and a follow-up nuclear renal scan is obtained 3 months postoperatively.

Results

Schuessler and associates reported their series of five patients who underwent laparoscopic pyeloplasty.[10] Two of these had a large redundant renal pelvis, two had a crossing lower pole vessel, and one had failed a previous open pyeloplasty. Operative time ranged from 3 to 7 hours and mean postoperative stay was 3 days. All patients resumed normal activity within a week and stents were left in place for 6 to 8 weeks. The only reported postoperative complication was a distal ureteral narrowing in one patient, causing severe back pain 24 hours after the ureteral stent was removed. This narrowed area was later balloon dilated and the patient is now doing well. Follow-up radiographs revealed significant radiological improvement in three patients, moderate improvement in one, and minimal improvement in one. All were asymptomatic at 12 months.

Brooks and associates reviewed their experience of 45 patients with UPJ obstruction.[12] Twelve patients underwent laparoscopic pyeloplasty, 13 had antegrade endopyelotomy, nine had Acucise endopyelotomy, and 11 had an open dismembered pyeloplasty. Mean operative time was 6 hours, 2.5 hours, 45 minutes, and 3.8 hours, respectively. The average hospital stay was 1 day for the Acucise patients, 3 days for the laparoscopic and endopyelotomy patients, and more than 7 days for the open pyeloplasty patients. Success rates were 100 percent for laparoscopic and open pyeloplasty, 75 percent for endopyelotomy, and 74 percent for the Acucise balloon. Postoperative complications of laparoscopic pyeloplasty included two cases of anastomotic edema, which resolved after stent placement in one patient and a percutaneous nephrostomy in the other.

URETEROLYSIS

Retroperitoneal fibrosis is an inflammatory condition of the retroperitoneum that occurs either as a primary (idiopathic) process or secondary to conditions such as inflammatory bowel disease, endometriosis, radiation therapy, neoplasm, vascular aneurysms, or drug therapy (e.g., methysergide).[13, 14] The goals of ureterolysis include relief of ureteral entrapment, prevention of recurrent obstruction, preservation of renal function, and diagnosis of possible underlying pathological causes. Kavoussi and associates first reported a laparoscopic technique to dissect and intraperitonealize the ureter of a patient with retroperitoneal fibrosis.[15]

Preoperative Evaluation

An abdominopelvic computed tomographic (CT) scan with oral and intravenous contrast material should be obtained to evaluate the extent of retroperitoneal disease and to look for evidence of occult malignancy. The search for underlying malignant conditions in men over the age of 45 should include digital rectal examination, stool guaiac, and prostate-specific antigen testing. Women in this age range should have a thorough pelvic examination, stool guaiac, breast examination, and mammogram. The

addition of an erythrocyte sedimentation rate test to the routine blood work provides a valuable tool for following the activity of the inflammatory process. An IVP will demonstrate the degree of displacement of the ureters and give an impression of the severity of obstruction. If there is evidence of compromised function on either the IVP or CT scan, a nuclear renal scan should be performed to accurately assess residual function. A retrograde pyelogram is also performed just before laparoscopic intervention to clearly demonstrate the entire course of the ureter and rule out the possibility of stricture.

Technique

After placement of an indwelling ureteral stent, Foley catheter, and NG tube, the patient is prepared and positioned as described for laparoscopic pyeloplasty. A semirecumbent position is used if both collecting systems require treatment. An indwelling ureteral stent may help to identify an encased ureter. The assistant can wiggle the stent while the surgeon observes for motion in the exposed retroperitoneum. Lighted ureteral stents are also available to assist in outlining the course of the involved ureter. After experience has been gained, an indwelling ureteral catheter is usually sufficient.

A pneumoperitoneum is established as previously described and a 10-mm port is placed through a horizontal incision made 2 cm below the costal margin. The remaining ports are placed under direct vision, including a 10-mm port at the umbilicus, a 5-mm port along the AAL at the level of the umbilicus, and a 5-mm trocar in the MCL medial to the anterosuperior iliac spine (Fig. 15–6). The operating surgeon stands on the contralateral side of the table and operates primarily from the two MCL ports. The peritoneal cavity, including all visceral surfaces, should be inspected for any evidence of neoplastic disease before dissection.

The surgeon uses a grasping forceps to retract the colon medially, and the peritoneal reflection is incised across the iliac vessels and MUL. The dissection is then carried proximally to release the hepatic flexure on the right side or the splenic flexure on the left. On the right side the duodenum may need to be kocherized (Fig. 15–7). A medial sweeping motion with the graspers and scissors brings the colon down to expose the psoas muscle. The ureter can usually be identified using a transverse sweeping motion to feel for the stent. If the ureter cannot be located, inspection medial to the MUL near the bladder or proximally near the region of the UPJ will often reveal a segment of ureter uninvolved in the fibrotic process. It is important to remember that the ureter can be retracted medially to the point that it overlies the inferior vena cava or aorta.

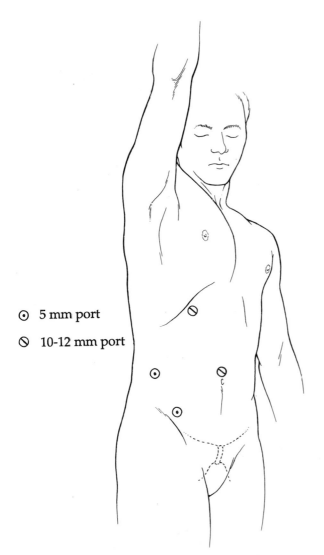

5 mm port

10-12 mm port

Figure 15–6. Trocar sites for laparoscopic ureterolysis.

Once the ureter is identified, the assistant retracts the periureteral tissues laterally while the surgeon develops a window around the ureter. A 4-inch piece of umbilical tape is passed around the freed segment, utilizing grasping forceps. The ends of the tape are fastened together with a single 9-mm clip (Fig. 15–8). This maneuver allows manipulation of the ureter. Multiple biopsies should be taken of the periureteral tissues with laparoscopic biopsy forceps and sent for frozen section.

Ureteral dissection is continued in both a proximal and distal fashion, with the assistant applying lateral traction on the umbilical tape and periureteral tissue while the surgeon provides medial countertraction. A combination of blunt and sharp dissection is used to "shell" the ureter out of the surrounding fibrotic process. Cauterization is kept to a minimum to prevent compromise of the ureteral blood supply. The gonadal vein crosses the ureter on the right side and runs parallel to its course on the left. These vessels can be extensively involved in the inflammatory

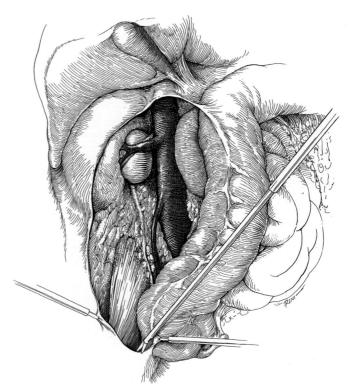

Figure 15–7. Takedown of the right colon and kocherization of the duodenum to reveal the encased right ureter.

process; they need to be dissected off the ureter, clipped, and transected in a controlled fashion. The dissection is continued until the ureter and/or renal pelvis is completely freed from the fibrotic process.

The mobilized ureter is then transposed into the peritoneal cavity by apposing the medial and lateral cut edges of peritoneum behind the ureter. The laparoscopic camera is transferred to the 10-mm UMCL port, and a hernia stapler is passed through the umbilical port to reapproximate the edges of incised peritoneum (Fig. 15–9). If an omental wrap is desired, a GIA stapler can be inserted into the umbilical port and used to split the omentum into an isolated sleeve, which can be positioned around the ureter and secured to itself with 9-mm clips. The ports are then removed and the procedure is concluded.

Postoperative Management

The NG tube is removed before the patient leaves the operating room, and the Foley catheter and pneumatic compression boots are continued until the patient is ambulatory. Parenteral antibiotics are continued for 24 hours and the patient is then switched to a prophylactic oral agent until the ureteral stent is removed. A clear liquid diet is begun the following day and advanced as tolerated. Two weeks postoperatively an IVP is performed; if the ureter remains laterally displaced, the ureteral stent is removed. Follow-up IVPs are performed at 3, 6, and 12 months. Regular activities may be resumed after removal of the stent.

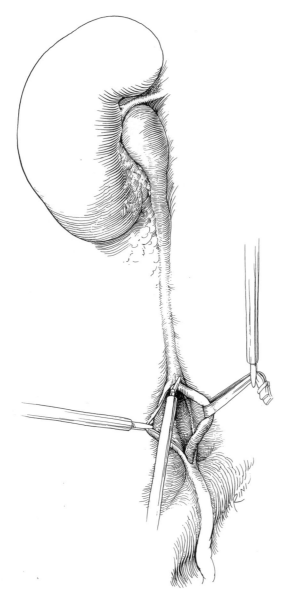

Figure 15–8. A 4-inch piece of umbilical tape is passed around a segment of freed ureter to assist in further manipulations.

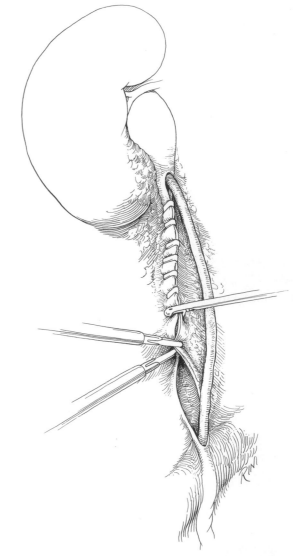

Figure 15–9. The freed ureter is intraperitonealized by reapproximating the cut edges of peritoneum.

Results

A limited number of laparoscopic ureterolysis cases have been performed to date.[15–17] Albala and Kavoussi reported three patients who underwent this procedure: all three required minimal pain medication, were sent home on the third postoperative day, and resumed full activity when the stents were removed 2 weeks postoperatively. At 1-year follow-up, two patients remained unobstructed and the third, who had retroperitoneal fibrosis secondary to a malignancy, experienced recurrence.[16] Puppo and associates performed a case of bilateral laparoscopic ureterolysis that took 10 hours.[17] The patient was discharged home on the second postoperative day and resumed full activity after 2 weeks. An IVP performed at 3 months showed no evidence of recurrence.

URETERECTOMY

A technique for laparoscopic ureterectomy using a combined endoscopic and laparoscopic approach was first described by Figenshau and Clayman.[18] This technique is most frequently performed in conjunction with a laparoscopic nephrectomy for transitional cell carcinoma (TCC) of the renal pelvis or ureter. Other indications include a refluxing ureter with an associated nonfunctioning kidney, a pyoureter from a previous partial or simple nephrectomy, renal tuberculosis, or an ectopic ureterocele.[19]

Preoperative Evaluation

The preoperative evaluation of any patient undergoing a laparoscopic nephroureterectomy for presumed transitional cell malignancy should include a metastatic work-up consisting of a chest radiograph, a nuclear bone scan, and an abdominopelvic CT scan. An IVP is essential for the assessment of a filling defect of the collecting system to establish whether it represents an intrinsic or extrinsic lesion. The diagnosis of TCC of the renal pelvis in a morcellated sample can be difficult and should be performed only when a tissue diagnosis has already been established.

Technique

The patient is placed in a dorsal lithotomy position under a general anesthetic and a cystoscope is used to advance a 0.035 Amplatz Super Stiff wire up the involved ureter. A 7 Fr. ureteral dilating balloon is then inserted over the wire using combined fluoroscopic and cystoscopic guidance until the proximal marking band lies just distal to the ureteral orifice. Dilute Conray contrast is instilled to inflate the balloon to one atmosphere of pressure. This places the submucosal ureteral tunnel on stretch without dilating the intramural ureter. A 24 Fr. resectoscope with a Collings knife is then inserted into the bladder. An unroofing incision is made in the 12 o'clock position from the ureteral orifice to the point where the ureter enters the detrusor muscle. This region appears as a narrowing of the balloon on fluoroscopy. A 1-cm margin is then electrocoagulated around the opened ureteral tunnel to ensure that an adequate cuff of bladder will be taken by the laparoscopic stapler.

The resectoscope and ureteral dilating balloon are removed and a 7.1 Fr. occlusion balloon catheter is inserted over the Super Stiff wire under fluoroscopic control. The balloon is filled with 1 ml of dilute Conray contrast and positioned at the UPJ. If TCC of the renal pelvis is the indication for nephroureterectomy, some authors advocate the instillation of a local chemotherapeutic agent such as thiotepa into the upper tract to kill any free-floating tumor cells.[19] This can be accomplished by backloading the occlusion catheter over a 16 Fr. Councill catheter, removing the Amplatz wire, and fitting the end with a stopcock. Dilute contrast is instilled under fluoroscopic control via the occlusion catheter. Once the renal pelvis is filled, the contrast is removed and replaced with an equal volume of thiotepa (Fig. 15–10). Care should be taken not to spill any of the urine or contrast, which might contain cancer cells. A Tuohy-Bost side-arm adapter is placed onto the end of the occlusion catheter, and the Super Stiff wire is replaced to maintain the local chemotherapeutic agent in the upper tract. The Foley is fixed to a collection bag and placed to gravity drainage.

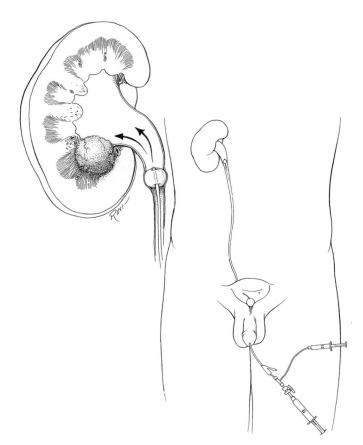

Figure 15–10. Local chemotherapeutic instillation via a ureteral occlusion balloon catheter before nephroureterectomy.

The patient is then placed in a 60-degree lateral decubitus position with the iliac crest placed over the break in the table, and secured as described for laparoscopic pyeloplasty. A lateral insufflation technique is performed with the Veress needle as described earlier, and a total of five trocars are inserted if a concomitant nephrectomy is planned. A horizontal incision is made 2 cm below the rib margins in the MCL and a 12-mm port is introduced. The 10-mm laparoscope is inserted and the remaining trocars are placed under direct vision. A 10-mm trocar is inserted at the umbilicus and an additional 12-mm port in the midline between the umbilicus and pubic symphysis to provide GIA access to the bladder cuff. Two 5-mm trocars are then introduced: one at the AAL 2 cm below the costal margin and a second along the AAL just above the iliac crest (Fig. 15–11). The subcostal 5-mm AAL port can be omitted and the 12-mm MCL port replaced by a 10-mm port if a ureterectomy alone is to be performed.

For patients undergoing laparoscopic nephroureterectomy, the distal ureter is freed first. The peritoneal incision should be extended across the iliac vessels medial to the MUL using the electrocautery scissors. A 5-mm Babcock clamp is placed around the distal ureter via the 12-mm lower midline port to

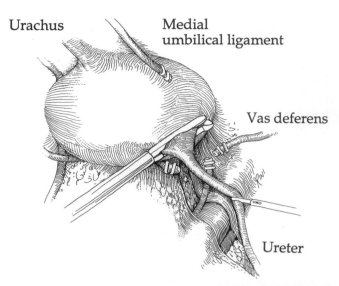

Figure 15–12. After the medial umbilical ligament and vas deferens are transected, the ureterovesical junction is grasped to allow an adequate length of bladder cuff to be obtained with the GIA stapler.

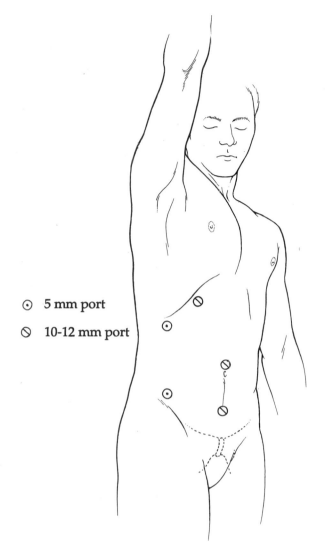

⊙ 5 mm port

⊘ 10-12 mm port

Figure 15–11. Trocar sites for laparoscopic nephroureterectomy.

facilitate retraction and further dissection. A combination of traction and countertraction on the periureteral tissues, while the ureter is elevated in the Babcock clamp, allows dissection of the entire ureter up to the renal pelvis. Careful blunt dissection with parallel sweeping motions is used to elevate the ureter off the iliac vessels. The gonadal vein is encountered as the dissection continues proximally. It is clipped with 9-mm occlusive clips and transected with the electrocautery scissors. Once the kidney is free, the ureter is gently retracted laterally. Care must be taken not to pull too hard on the ureter, or an avulsion can result.

As the dissection continues toward the bladder, the vas deferens in males or the round ligament in females is identified crossing anterior to the ureter. These structures must be dissected free, clipped with 9-mm occlusive clips, and divided to gain access to the distal ureter (Fig. 15–12). To further improve access to the ureterovesical junction (UVJ), the MUL and superior vesical artery may also be divided. A 5-

mm Babcock clamp is used to elevate the distal ureter while the surgeon retracts the bladder medially to expose the UVJ. The dissection is continued to the point where the ureter enters the muscle of the bladder, and a 5-cm area of surrounding perivesical fat is cleared. This step will allow a GIA stapler to be fired cleanly across the base of the bladder to obtain an adequate cuff around the distal ureter. The ureteral occlusion balloon is deflated and removed from the ureter along with the Super Stiff guidewire. A flexible cystoscope is then introduced into the bladder to visualize the ureteral orifice during stapling of the bladder cuff.

The first assistant grasps the ureter just proximal to the UVJ via the lower 5-mm port and retracts cephalad and lateral while the operating surgeon retracts the bladder caudally and medially. A 12-mm laparoscopic GIA tissue stapler is passed through the lower midline port and the jaws are positioned across the desired cuff of bladder (Fig. 15–12). Cystoscopic inspection confirms that all previously fulgurated cuff has been incorporated into the tissue stapler before activating the GIA stapler. After the cuff is transected, the bladder is filled via the cystoscope and inspected from the inside for exposed staples, and from the intraperitoneal surface for leaks. When the surgeon is satisfied that no staples are visible, the cystoscope is removed and the Foley catheter replaced.

When a ureterectomy without associated nephrectomy is being performed, the ureter can be grasped and delivered intact from the abdomen with a pair of grasping forceps inserted through the lower midline port. The nephroureterectomy specimen is delivered in a fashion nearly identical to that described for laparoscopic nephrectomy. The kidney is manipulated into the triangulated entrapment sack, keeping the ureter and attached bladder cuff outside the lip of the bag. The distal ureter is then secured along the inner edge of the sack with a clip applier, and the drawstring is grasped via the lower midline port and delivered through the sheath. A hemostat is used to secure the drawstring, and the port is removed. Gentle pressure is then used to deliver the neck of the sack through the skin incision. This procedure is performed under laparoscopic inspection to ensure that no bowel or omentum is pulled through the fascial defect. If morcellation of the specimen is planned, the longest segment of ureter possible is delivered from the sack, transected, and sent for separate pathological inspection. Morcellation or intact delivery of the kidney is then undertaken and the procedure concluded as described previously.

Postoperative Care

The NG tube is removed at the end of the procedure and the patient may ambulate on the evening of surgery. A clear liquid diet is begun and advanced as tolerated. Parenteral antibiotics are continued for 24 hours, at which time the patient is switched to an oral prophylactic agent for 7 days. A cystogram is performed on the third postoperative day, and if there is no extravasation, the Foley catheter is removed. If extravasation is present, an indwelling catheter is left in place for a full week and radiographical evaluation is repeated.

Results

Clayman and associates reported six patients who underwent laparoscopic nephroureterectomy.[18–20] Operative time averaged 9 hours with a mean hospital stay of 5 days and return to full activity in 4 weeks. Although follow-up data are limited, there have been no reported problems with the stapled bladder closures to date. Animal studies confirm that a GIA stapler can generate a watertight bladder closure, and exposed staples do not show evidence of encrustation at 7 months' follow-up.[21] The first reported patient did have a residual 2-cm refluxing ureteral stump with a single exposed staple that did not show evidence of stone formation at 17 months' follow-up.[19] Clayman also described a successful ureterectomy in a patient who had undergone a previous radical nephrectomy for what later proved to be TCC of the renal pelvis.[19]

URETEROLITHOTOMY

Improvements in extracorporeal shock wave lithotripsy (ESWL) and the development of endoscopic ultrasonic, laser, and electrohydraulic lithotripsy probes have greatly reduced the need for open ureteral stone extractions. There are still a few patients with stones who fail these techniques and may require open incision.[22] A laparoscopic method of ureterolithotomy was first described by Raboy and is now recognized as an acceptable alternative to open stone surgery when endoscopic or ESWL therapy fails.[24]

Preoperative Evaluation

The upper and lower ureteral anatomy must be clearly defined by an IVP before the procedure. If the distal ureter is not visualized adequately, a retrograde pyelogram should be obtained in the operating room to rule out an associated stricture.

Technique

The patient is placed in a supine position under a general anesthetic. An indwelling stent is inserted using a flexible cystoscope to manipulate a 0.035 Bentson floppy-tip or Lubriglide wire past the stone under fluoroscopic guidance. A 7 Fr. double-pigtail stent of appropriate length is passed over the wire and positioned using a metal-tipped pusher and fluoroscopy. An open-ended catheter can be advanced to the level of the stone and used to direct the tip of the wire past a tightly impacted stone. If a wire or stent cannot be passed, an external ureteral stent should be advanced to the level of the stone, brought out through a Councill catheter, and secured via a Tuohy-Bost side-arm adapter.

The patient is then positioned on the operating room table according to the location of the impacted stone. A stone in the upper half of the ureter is approached from a lateral decubitus position with port placement identical to that for ureterolysis (see Fig. 15–6). For lower ureteral stones, the patient is maintained in a supine position; a 10-mm trocar is inserted at the umbilicus for the camera and another is placed lateral to the contralateral rectus at the level of the umbilicus. A 5-mm port is then inserted in each lower quadrant along the MCL (Fig. 15–13). The Veress needle is introduced through the umbilical incision if the patient is in the supine position, or lateral to the rectus muscle if he or she is in a flank position. Carbon dioxide insufflation is carried out to a pressure of 20 mm Hg to facilitate initial trocar placement.

The line of Toldt is taken down as previously described, beginning in a region near the estimated position of the stone. The colon is then reflected medially to expose the retroperitoneal course of the ureter. Gentle grasping or transverse sweeping movements with atraumatic graspers can be used to identify the

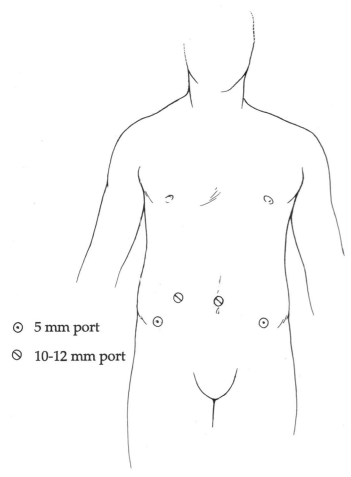

Figure 15–13. Trocar sites for laparoscopic ureterolithotomy performed for a distal left ureteral stone.

⊙ 5 mm port

⊘ 10-12 mm port

position of the ureteral calculus. Dilation of the proximal ureter to the point of stone impaction is not often seen, and spot radiography or fluoroscopy may be needed to localize the stone. Once the stone is located, a longitudinal incision is made in the ureter with articulating scissors. The stone is delivered through the ureterotomy by carefully milking it from the ureter into the jaws of a grasping forceps, or into an organ entrapment sack if it is extremely large (Fig. 15–14A). Every effort should be made to remove the stone intact. The external ureteral stent is then passed into the proximal ureter and exchanged for an indwelling stent.

The ureterotomy is loosely reapproximated over the ureteral catheter using several spaced 4-0 polyglactin sutures cut into 5-inch lengths and mounted on RB-1 needles (Fig. 15–14B). If the incision is small (1 cm or less), it can be left open to heal around the stent. A retroperitoneal drain can be placed and the peritoneal incision closed as described for laparoscopic pyeloplasty. The procedure is then concluded as described previously.

Postoperative Care

The NG tube is discontinued in the operating room and the Foley is removed on the night of surgery. The drain is pulled as soon as collection volumes are negligible. A regular diet may be started on the day of surgery, and parenteral antibiotics are continued for 24 hours before the patient is switched to a prophylactic oral agent. Oral antibiotics are then continued until the stent is removed 6 weeks postoperatively. Follow-up studies include an IVP at 3 months.

Results

Only a few patients have undergone laparoscopic ureterolithotomy to date. Harewood removed ureteral calculi laparoscopically in five patients; all had failed previous endoscopic techniques. These patients required minimal pain medication and were discharged home on the second postoperative day.[23] Raboy and colleagues successfully performed laparoscopic ureterolithotomy in a patient with a distal cystine stone and reported no evidence of obstruction or leak on a 4-week postoperative IVP.[24]

POSTOPERATIVE COMPLICATIONS

The limited number of centers where these procedures are performed makes it difficult to assess the

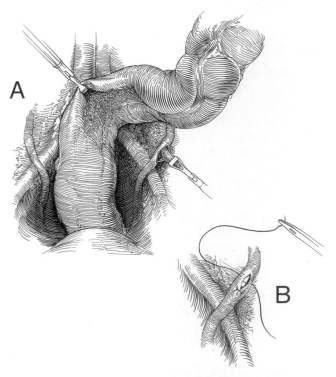

Figure 15–14. *A,* The sigmoid colon is retracted medially to expose the ureterotomy site made at the level of stone impaction. The stone is delivered from the incision. *B,* A ureteral stent is passed proximally, and the ureterotomy is closed with interrupted sutures.

risk percentages associated with laparoscopic ureteral surgery. Possible intraoperative complications include uncontrolled bleeding and injury to visceral organs (i.e., bowel, spleen, pancreas or liver) that might require transfusion, conversion to an open procedure, or both. As with open procedures, potential complications include adhesion formation, incisional hernias or infections, urinoma, fistulous connection between the ureter and skin, and ureteral stricture formation. As these techniques gain appeal and the number of cases increase, an accurate assessment of complication rates will become possible. To date, these risks appear to be low.

THE FUTURE

The current use of laparoscopic methods to treat ureteral pathology already appears to be achieving the desired goals of minimal postoperative pain, decreased length of hospitalization, and shorter duration of convalescence. Animal models and isolated case reports have described the use of laparoscopy for more complex procedures such as ureteral reimplantation, cutaneous ureterostomy, ureteroureterostomy, and creation of a ureteroenteric anastomosis.[25-28] Advances in laparoscopic equipment and improved methods of tissue reconstruction (e.g., tissue welding and automated suture devices) will likely lead to further advances in laparoscopic ureteral surgery in the future.

Editorial Comment
Fray F. Marshall

As laparoscopic techniques improve and more closely approximate open surgery with suturing techniques, these laparoscopic techniques may be used more extensively. I would give one admonition that placement of a double-J catheter for a long time before surgery usually complicates the surgery rather than enhancing it. A ureteral catheter placed at the time of open or laparoscopic surgery may facilitate identification or dissection of the ureter, but if it is placed weeks before surgery it produces an inflammatory reaction that may make surgical dissection and operative repair more difficult. Also, morcellation of a kidney with transitional cell carcinoma makes verification of multicentricity and pathological staging difficult.

REFERENCES

1. Soper NJ, Barteau JA, Clayman RV, et al. Comparison of early postoperative results for laparoscopic versus standard open cholecystectomy. Surg Gynecol Obstet 174:114, 1992.
2. Griffith DP, Schuessler WW, Vancaille TH. Laparoscopic lymphadenectomy: A low morbidity alternative for staging pelvic malignancies. J Endourol 4:S84, 1990.
3. Kelalis PP, Culp OS, Stickler GB, et al. Ureteropelvic junction obstruction in children: Experiences with 109 cases. J Urol 106:418, 1971.
4. Persky L, Krause JR, Boltuch RL, et al. Initial complications and late results in dismembered pyeloplasty. J Urol 118:162, 1977.
5. Wickham JEA, Kellet MJ. Percutaneous pyelolysis. Eur Urol 9:122, 1983.
6. Inglis JA, Tolley DA. Ureteroscopic pyelolysis for pelviureteric junction obstruction. Br J Urol 58:250, 1986.
7. Ramsay JWA, Miller RA, Kellet MJ, et al. Percutaneous pyelolysis: Indications, complications, and results. Br J Urol 56:586, 1984.
8. Meretyk I, Meretyk S, Clayman RV. Endopyelotomy: Comparison of ureteroscopic retrograde and antegrade percutaneous techniques. J Urol 148:775, 1992.
9. Chandhoke PS, Clayman RV, Stone AM, et al. Endopyelotomy and endoureterotomy with the Acucise ureteral cutting balloon device: Preliminary experience. J Endourol 7:45, 1993.
10. Schuessler WW, Grune MT, Tecuanhuey LV, et al. Laparoscopic dismembered pyeloplasty. J Urol 150:1795, 1993.
11. Adams JB, Moore RG, Partin AW, et al. New laparoscopic suture device: Initial clinical experience. Urology (in press).
12. Brooks JD, Preminger GM, Kavoussi LR, et al. Comparison of endourologic approaches to the ureteropelvic junction obstruction. J Urol 151:394A, 1994.
13. Sosa RE, Vaughan ED Jr, Gibbons RP. Retroperitoneal fibrosis. AUA Update Series, Vol 6 (lesson 21), 1987.
14. Lepor H, Walsh PC. Idiopathic retroperitoneal fibrosis. J Urol 122:1, 1979.
15. Kavoussi LR, Clayman RV, Brunt LM, et al. Laparoscopic ureterolysis. J Urol 147:426, 1992.
16. Albala DM, Kavoussi LR. Laparoscopic ureteral surgery. In Das S, Crawford ED, eds. Urologic Laparoscopy. Philadelphia, WB Saunders, 1994, p 151.
17. Puppo P, Carmignani G, Gallucci M, et al. Bilateral laparoscopic ureterolysis. Eur Urol 25:82, 1994.
18. Figenshau RS, Albala DM, Clayman RV, et al. Laparoscopic ureterectomy: Initial laboratory experience. Min Inv Ther 1:93, 1991.
19. Clayman RV. Laparoscopic ureteral surgery. In Clayman RV, McDougall EM, eds. Laparoscopic Urology. St. Louis, Quality Medical Publishing, 1993, p 322.
20. Clayman RV, Kavoussi LR, Figenshau RS, et al. Laparoscopic nephroureterectomy: Initial clinical case report. J Laparoendosc Surg 1:343, 1991.
21. Kerbl K, Chandhoke PS, McDougall E, et al. Laparoscopic staples in the urinary tract: Bladder application. J Endourol 6:S144, 1992.
22. Kachel TA, Vijan SR, Dretler SP. Endourological experience with cystine calculi and a treatment algorithm. J Urol 145:25, 1991.
23. Harewood LM, Webb DR, Pope AJ. Laparoscopic ureterolithotomy: The results of an initial series, and an evaluation of its role in the management of ureteric calculi. Br J Urol 74:170, 1994.
24. Raboy A, Ferzli GS, Ioffreda R, et al. Laparoscopic ureterolithotomy. Urology 39:223, 1992.
25. Clayman RV, McDougall EM, Chandhoke PS, et al. Laparoscopic ureteral reimplantation: Laboratory studies. J Endourol 6:S144, 1992.
26. Goldstein DS, Ho GT, Scott JA, et al. Laparoscopic cutaneous ureterostomy: A porcine model. J Endourol 6:S167, 1992.
27. Nezhat C, Nezhat F, Green B, et al. Laparoscopic ureteroureterostomy. J Endourol 6:143, 1992.
28. Kozminski M. Laparoscopic ileal loop conduit. J Endourol 6:S168, 1992.

Chapter 16

The Laparoscopic Varix Ligation

James F. Donovan, Jr., Eugene D. Kwon, and Jay I. Sandlow

A varix is a dilation of the pampiniform plexus. Many factors have been implicated as a cause of varicocele, including absent or incompetent valves in the spermatic vein, and increased venous pressure due to distal increased hydrostatic pressures within the left renal vein caused by compression between aorta and superior mesenteric artery.[1]

Varices become clinically evident in adolescence and are present in 15 percent of males. Most common on the left side, varices are bilateral in 20 to 50 percent of cases and occur rarely as solitary right lesions. Although the presence of a varicocele does not uniformly produce male infertility, the incidence of varix in patients who present to male infertility clinics is approximately 37 percent.[2, 3] Varicocele is therefore the most common treatable cause of male subfertility. The pathophysiology of varix-induced oligoasthenospermia is not known. Various proximate causes of testicular dysfunction due to varicocele have been invoked, including (but not limited to) the following: increased testicular temperature due to loss of countercurrent heat exchange; exposure of the testicular tissues to increased renal and/or adrenal hormone concentrations due to retrograde venous delivery; and alteration of arterial and/or capillary blood flow, causing reduced oxygen delivery to sensitive tissues.[4–6]

INDICATIONS

Indications for ligation of a clinically palpable varix include (1) male factor subfertility evident in persistent defects of sperm density and/or motility on semen analysis[1, 4]; (2) adolescent testicular growth retardation, defined by enduring failure of the ipsilateral testes to attain the size and consistency of the testes contralateral to the varix[7, 8]; and (3) pain due to the presence of a varix (a diagnosis of exclusion) that is consistent with varix (dull, aching pain that is never present upon awakening and increases during exertion or standing).

CHOICE OF PROCEDURE

Current treatments may be categorized as operative and nonoperative. Nonoperative treatment consists of either transvenous ablation with chemical or physical agents (injection of sclerosing agents or placement of autologous clot or Turcot coils by interventional radiology) or the use of a scrotal hypothermia device.[9, 10] Operative techniques include the inguinal (Ivanissevich), retroperitoneal (Palomo), subinguinal (Marmar, Goldstein), and laparoscopic procedures.[11–18] Although the use of nonoperative treatments obviates the need for general or regional anesthesia and reduces the time to recovery, most urologists treating the infertile male prefer operative intervention because of the surety of treatment: 0.5 to 5 percent varix persistence after operative ligation, compared with a 20 percent recurrence rate after transvenous ablation.[19] The laparoscopic varix ligation offers a minimally invasive procedure, albeit through a transperitoneal approach. Patients are thoroughly informed of the available techniques for varix ablation and the risks and benefits associated with each.[20] In the case of laparoscopy, benefits include rapid return to preoperative levels of activity, low varicocele recurrence/persistence rates, preservation of the spermatic artery in most cases, and the capability of performing both uni- and bilateral varix ligation by means of a three-trocar set-up. Disadvantages include the requisite use of a general anesthetic; the risk of serious complications, including visceral or vascular injury, which would require celiotomy and repair (with prolonged rather than shortened recovery); and the possible need to convert to a traditional approach to varix ligation if exposure of the spermatic vessels cephalad to the internal ring is impeded.

PATIENT PREPARATION

The use of bowel preparation or preoperative antibiotic prophylaxis is left to the discretion of the surgeon. The patient remains NPO status overnight before surgery. General anesthesia is induced. The patient is placed in the supine position with both arms adducted, padded, and tucked. We limit the shave preparation to the abdominal skin between the umbilicus superiorly, the pubic symphysis inferiorly, and the anterior iliac crests bilaterally, but we prepare the entire abdomen and genitals with an aseptic scrub and povidone-iodine paint. The extended abdominal preparation provides sterile access to the abdominal cavity or inguinal region in the event of complication and celiotomy. Access to the genitals permits gentle traction of the spermatic cord, which facilitates identification of the spermatic vascular bundle with laparoscopy. The skin is draped accordingly.

The anesthesiologist may aspirate the gastric contents if distention is evident after induction. At our institution we insert a straight red rubber catheter and empty the bladder, but no longer leave an indwelling Foley catheter during the operative procedure.

EQUIPMENT

Table 16–1 lists the equipment needed for laparoscopic varix ligation. Both uni- and bilateral laparoscopic varix ligation is easily performed using a single video monitor positioned at the foot of the operating table. Use of the Hasson cannula reduces the probability of serious injury; its insertion requires direct exposure of the linea alba, the aponeurosis of the transversus abdominal muscle (i.e., the posterior rectus sheath), and the peritoneal membrane. This somewhat extended dissection appears cumbersome in comparison with Veress needle insertion, but the

TABLE 16–1. Devices and Instruments for Laparoscopic Varix Ligation

	Size (mm)	No.
TV monitor		1
Video camera with coupling device		1
Video recorder		1
Laparoscope	10.5	1
Fiberoptic light source		1
Electrocautery unit with connection and cord		1
Suction/irrigation device	5	1
Hasson cannula	10.5	1
Trocar	10.5	2
Curved scissors	5	1
Curved dissector	5	2
Hemoclip applier (medium clips)	10.5	1
Laparoscopic Doppler probe	5	1

reduced operative complication risk is sufficient to justify open laparoscopy. Furthermore, a comparison of the Hasson cannula and Veress needle in terms of time elapsed between skin incision and insertion of laparoscope has shown no significant difference (average 4.5 minutes).

A curved scissors and curved dissector permit delicate and precise dissection of the spermatic vascular bundle. Electrocautery, usually applied through the curved scissors, is used sparingly during the course of dissection and never in close proximity to the spermatic artery. Hemoclips ligate spermatic veins, which are subsequently divided between clips to provide optimal exposure of the spermatic artery. The laparoscopic Doppler probe expedites identification of the spermatic artery and facilitates preservation. During our initial experience, identification of the spermatic artery relied on visual confirmation of pulsatile movement within the artery. We frequently noted arterial spasm during the course of dissection, making positive identification of the artery impossible, pending resolution of spasm with application of 2 percent lidocaine or papaverine.[17] The Doppler probe is capable of providing immediate localization of the spermatic artery even when blood flow is reduced, and thus proves invaluable in reducing operative time.[21]

OPERATIVE PROCEDURE

After the patient preparation outlined above (induction of anesthesia, skin preparation and draping, bladder emptied by straight catheter), a vertical 1- to 2-cm subumbilical incision is made through the linea alba. Stay sutures of 0 PDS in a horizontal mattress secure either side of the fascial incision. Small S-shaped retractors facilitate exposure. Sharp dissection between the rectus abdominis muscles reveals the posterior rectus sheath, which is incised. The peritoneum may then be punctured bluntly by a small finger or incised by a scalpel. We then insert a finger into the peritoneal cavity and sweep the anterior abdominal wall to identify any adhesions that might interfere with subsequent insertion of trocars. The Hasson cannula is inserted into the abdomen, firmly wedging the cone-shaped olive into the fascial incision. The 0 PDS stay sutures secure the Hasson cannula to the rectus fascia, maintaining an airtight seal.

Carbon dioxide insufflation proceeds at a rate of 6 to 9 L/min to provide an intraperitoneal pressure of 20 mm Hg. At this pressure the abdominal wall is relatively rigid and will accept the insertion of additional trocars with minimal deflection, decreasing the chance of injury to intra-abdominal viscera during trocar insertion. The laparoscope is inserted into the abdominal cavity, and inspection of the abdominal wall and viscera identifies anatomical landmarks for placement of subsequent trocars. We have modified the original array of trocars used in laparoscopic varix ligation and currently place 10.5-mm trocars in each lower quadrant between the umbilicus and anterior iliac crest lateral to the rectus abdominis muscle (Fig. 16–1). Care must be taken to locate the trocars slightly below the umbilicus, not below the iliac crest, to allow sufficient distance between the end of the trocar sheath and the spermatic vessels for complete insertion of the instrument tips to permit appropriate function. When scissors or dissector tips remain within the trocar sheath, proper opening and closing of the instrument may be encumbered by the sheath. The abdominal wall is transilluminated by the laparoscope, and the lateral border of the rectus abdominis muscle is delineated by its silhouette; the operating trocar is positioned lateral to the rectus muscle to avoid injury to the deep inferior epigastric vessels, which adhere to the posterior surface of the muscle. Transillumination also provides an outline of subcutaneous vessels that should be avoided in making 1.0-cm incisions for trocar placement. Through these skin incisions, 10.5-mm trocars are thrust into the abdominal cavity while the trocar tip

piercing the peritoneum is observed on the laparoscope video image. A perpendicular alignment between trocar and abdominal wall during insertion must be maintained. We have observed a tendency to aim the trocar medially during penetration of the abdominal wall, with potential injury of the rectus muscle and underlying deep inferior epigastric vessels, despite proper position of the skin incision lateral to these structures. Once each operating trocar is inserted, a 2-0 silk suture secures the trocar insufflation valve to the skin. The stay suture is placed so as to limit excursion of the trocar, with 1 to 2 cm of trocar sheath remaining within the peritoneal cavity.

With operating trocars inserted and secured, spermatic vessels are identified and isolated. Frequently, the sigmoid colon is adherent to the left lateral pelvic wall and must be mobilized to expose the spermatic vessels above the internal ring. One should incise these peritoneal attachments carefully to avoid entry into the retroperitoneal space. The spermatic vessels are most easily seen just beneath the peritoneal membrane cephalad to the internal ring. In the obese patient, or in the case of adhesions that obscure the pelvic anatomy, traction on the ipsilateral testes resulting in movement of the spermatic vascular bundle in the retroperitoneal space may assist in this process. One must note any collateral vessels that pass through the internal ring to ensure complete ablation of veins that might contribute to the varicocele and testicular dysfunction.

Immediately above the internal ring, a 3- to 5-cm incision is made through the peritoneum lateral and parallel to the spermatic vascular bundle (Figs. 16–2 and 16–3). Small vessels are coagulated with electrocautery. Lifting the medial edge of peritoneum, the spermatic vessels are swept from the overlying peritoneum using the closed curved scissors before incising the medial peritoneal flap perpendicular to the first incision (and to the spermatic vessels) (Fig. 16–4). Retraction of the peritoneal membrane edges exposes the spermatic vessels, which are fixed by the transversalis fascia. The fascia is cut on either side of the spermatic vessels, permitting elevation of the entire spermatic vascular bundle with two curved dissectors. Once the spermatic vessels are freed from the transversalis fascia and the underlying psoas muscle, complete ligation of the spermatic vascular bundle (veins and arteries) is possible. The goal is preservation of the artery, however, and mass ligation with hemoclips should be resorted to only in the event of uncontrolled bleeding (Fig. 16–5).

With only veins or loose adventitial tissue grasped in one curved dissector, the vascular bundle is divided into two packets (medial and lateral) using a combination of traction and blunt dissection with the second curved dissector (Fig. 16–6). The laparoscopic Doppler probe locates the spermatic artery, and the

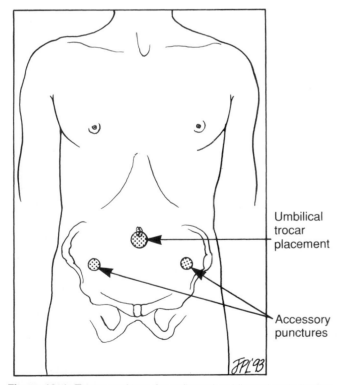

Figure 16–1. Trocar positions for unilateral or bilateral varix ligation. The umbilical trocar is routinely a Hasson type for open laparoscopy. The lower quadrant trocars are 10.5 mm in diameter, thus permitting insertion of the hemoclip applier from either ipsilateral or contralateral ports. (From Winfield HN. Urologic laparoscopic surgery. Atlas Urol Clin North Am 1:17, 1993.)

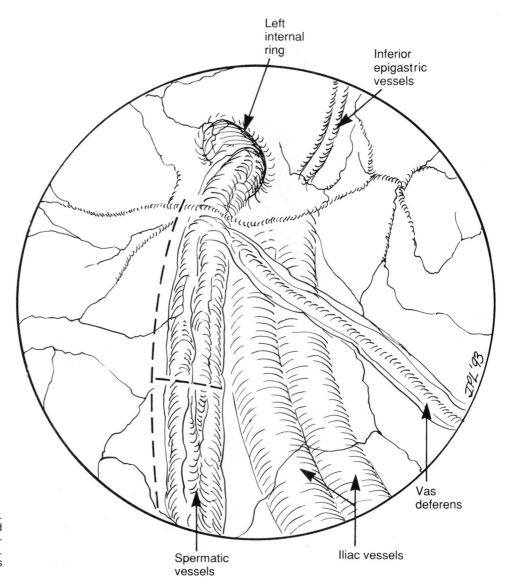

Figure 16–2. Suprainguinal anatomy. The spermatic vessels are depicted above the internal ring and the T incision is indicated. (From Winfield HN. Urologic laparoscopic surgery. Atlas Urol Clin North Am 1:18, 1993.)

nonarterial pack is hemoclip ligated and divided between clips. The remaining vascular bundle is divided, and after confirmation of spermatic artery location, the nonarterial component is similarly clip ligated and divided (Fig. 16–7). This process is repeated until only the spermatic artery remains. Typically, small venules adhere to the spermatic artery and require more delicate dissection to isolate. Having abandoned the 600-μm neodymium:yttrium-aluminum-garnet (Nd:YAG) laser,[22] we currently achieve this separation by gently teasing the artery from the venule with one element of the open dissector. Tenacious veins are separated a sufficient distance from the artery to permit ligation by hemoclip application. Preservation of the spermatic artery requires painstaking and cautious dissection if complete venous ablation is to be achieved. Upon completion of the varix ablation, the Doppler is inserted to document the conservation of arterial flow.

Occasionally, multiple spermatic arteries are identified within the spermatic vascular bundle, making the dissection more tedious.[23, 24] With patience, the spermatic artery/arteries is/are spared in most cases. In cases of spermatic artery spasm, the spermatic artery may be bathed with 2 percent lidocaine either through an irrigation port or via a spinal needle inserted directly through the abdominal wall anterior to the area of dissection. Bleeding from the spermatic artery may respond to topical application of Surgicel or Gelfoam. Despite these maneuvers, when faced with bleeding that cannot be controlled by conservative measures, we have been forced infrequently to purposefully ligate the spermatic artery.

Termination

Before removal of trocars, intra-abdominal pressure is reduced to 6 to 8 mm Hg and any bleeding stopped

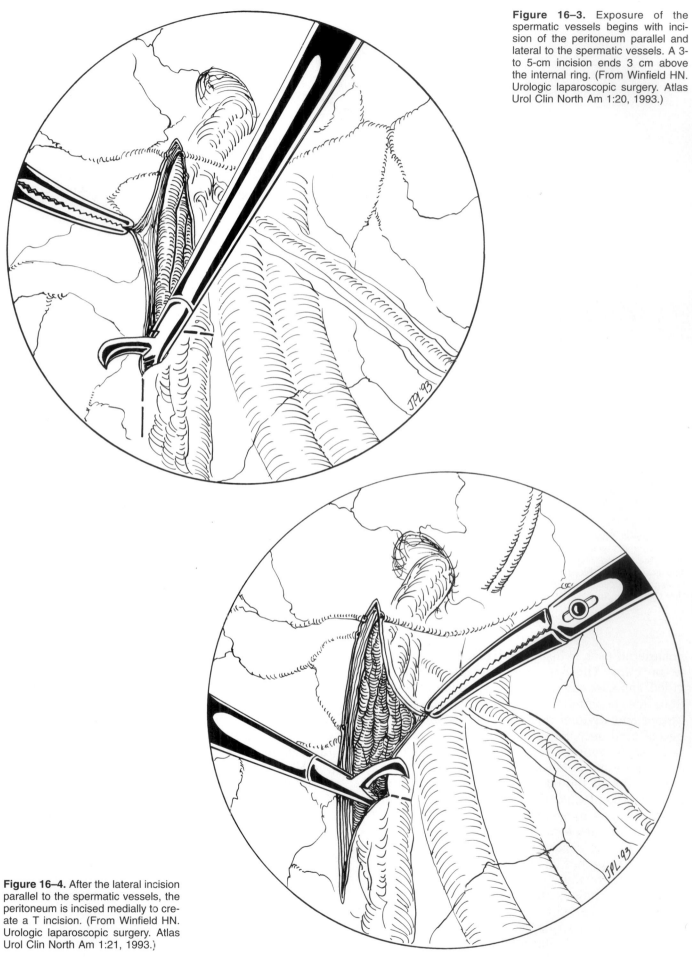

Figure 16–3. Exposure of the spermatic vessels begins with incision of the peritoneum parallel and lateral to the spermatic vessels. A 3- to 5-cm incision ends 3 cm above the internal ring. (From Winfield HN. Urologic laparoscopic surgery. Atlas Urol Clin North Am 1:20, 1993.)

Figure 16–4. After the lateral incision parallel to the spermatic vessels, the peritoneum is incised medially to create a T incision. (From Winfield HN. Urologic laparoscopic surgery. Atlas Urol Clin North Am 1:21, 1993.)

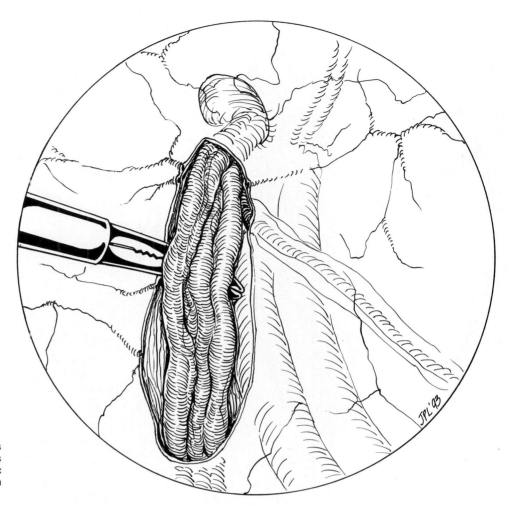

Figure 16–5. The spermatic vessels mobilized from the underlying psoas muscle. (From Winfield HN. Urologic laparoscopic surgery. Atlas Urol Clin North Am 1:24, 1993.)

by electrocoagulation. Any irrigant or blood is aspirated from the peritoneal cavity. The laparoscope is then positioned at the trocar insertion site and the trocar removed. Trocar insertion sites greater than 10.5 mm are inspected during placement of interrupted 2-0 PDS fascial sutures. The Hasson cannula is freed from the stay sutures and removed with the laparoscope in place, acting as an obturator to prevent entrainment of small bowel. Under direct vision, additional fascial sutures are placed in the linea alba above and below the stay sutures, and then all sutures are tied to secure closure of the midline fascia. Subcutaneous sutures are used as needed, and the skin is closed by a subcuticular absorbable suture.

POSTOPERATIVE CARE

All patients resume oral intake after recovery from general anesthesia. Discharged on the day of surgery, patients increase activity ad lib. Oral analgesics suffice to control pain. Typically, patients return for wound inspection 1 week after surgery. For the infertile male, an assessment of response to varix ablation entails a semen analysis 4 and 6 months postoperatively and at 3-month intervals thereafter.

COMPLICATIONS

Serious complications of laparoscopic varix ligation are rare and decrease with experience. We encountered one serious complication in our first 75 patients undergoing laparoscopic varix ligation: 21 days after varicocelectomy a patient required abdominal exploration and ligation of bleeding from the spermatic artery, presumably injured by cautery or the Nd:YAG laser. In reports confined to laparoscopic varix ligation, major complications occur in 0 to 4 percent of patients undergoing laparoscopic varix ligation.[16, 17, 23] The most common intraoperative complication involves abdominal wall injury due to inappropriate location of operating trocars, resulting in injury to deep inferior epigastric artery or veins (14 percent of patients in the series reported by Enquist and colleagues[25]). Use of the open laparoscopy technique with the Hasson cannula reduces the potential for catastrophic injury to vascular structures or abdominal viscera, and care in selection of trocar insertion site with insertion of operating trocars under vision should reduce or eliminate potential abdominal wall complications. Postoperative complications are rare; in our series, wound infection is detected in less than 1 percent and pampiniform phlebitis in 2

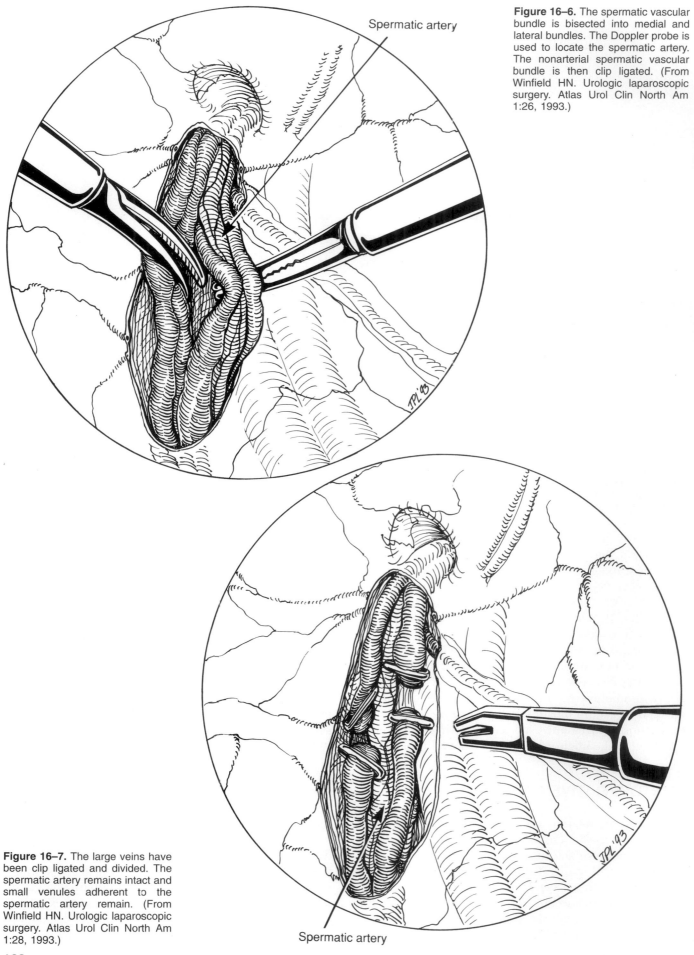

Spermatic artery

Figure 16–6. The spermatic vascular bundle is bisected into medial and lateral bundles. The Doppler probe is used to locate the spermatic artery. The nonarterial spermatic vascular bundle is then clip ligated. (From Winfield HN. Urologic laparoscopic surgery. Atlas Urol Clin North Am 1:26, 1993.)

Figure 16–7. The large veins have been clip ligated and divided. The spermatic artery remains intact and small venules adherent to the spermatic artery remain. (From Winfield HN. Urologic laparoscopic surgery. Atlas Urol Clin North Am 1:28, 1993.)

Spermatic artery

percent. Varicocele persists or recurs in 1.0 to 1.6 percent of patients undergoing laparoscopic varix ligation.[17, 24]

Conclusion

The development of laparoscopic surgical skills requires training in basic laparoscopic techniques and accumulation of operative experience to refine the use of instruments and techniques specific to laparoscopy.[26, 27] Initially, application of laparoscopy to varicocelectomy requires a prolonged operating time. The extended duration of the laparoscopic varix ligation is primarily due to the time devoted to careful dissection and preservation of the spermatic artery. In our initial experience, operating times required for varix ligation were 107 minutes for unilateral (range 50 to 199 minutes) and 164 minutes for bilateral (range 110 to 298 minutes) varicoceles.[28] With experience and the use of the laparoscopic Doppler probe to speed identification of the spermatic arteries, the duration of surgery has been reduced to 60 minutes, a time comparable with that required for microscopical inguinal or subinguinal varix ligation with spermatic artery preservation.

Editorial Comment
Louis Kavoussi

Varicocelectomy represents one the most straightforward laparoscopic procedures to perform. It is a relatively basic operation for urologists to gain experience with interventional laparoscopy. However, the use of laparoscopy to treat a varicocele is controversial among urologists who specialize in infertility. Opponents argue that the length of the procedure, the need for a general anesthetic, and the transperitoneal approach all make it less desirable than open microscopic repair. Advocates argue that with experience time is not a factor and that postoperative recovery is quicker. A prospective randomized study is needed to resolve this debate.

REFERENCES

1. Thomas AJ Jr, Geisinger MA. Current management of varicoceles. Urol Clin North Am 17:893, 1990.
2. Dubin C, Amelar RD. Etiologic factors in 1294 consecutive cases of male infertility. Fertil Steril 22:469, 1971.
3. Cockett ATK, Takihara H, Cosentino MJ. The varicocele. Fertil Steril 41:5, 1984.
4. Pryor JL, Howards SS. Varicocele. Urol Clin North Am 14:499, 1987.
5. Kaufman SL, Kadir S, Barth KH, et al. Mechanisms of recurrent varicocele after balloon occlusion or surgical ligation of the internal spermatic vein. Radiology 147:435, 1983.
6. Zorgniotti AW, Macleod J. Studies in temperature, human semen quality, and varicocele. Fertil Steril 24:854, 1973.
7. Kass EJ, Freitas JE, Bour JB. Adolescent varicocele: Objective indications for treatment. J Urol 142:579, 1989.
8. Belman AB. The dilemma of the adolescent varicocele. Contemp Urol 3:21, 1991.
9. Walsh PC, White RI Jr. Balloon occlusion of the internal spermatic vein for the treatment of varicoceles. JAMA 246:1701, 1981.
10. Salgarello G, Cagossi M, Salgarello TL, et al. Transvenous sclerotherapy of the gonadal veins for treatment of varicocele: Long-term results. Angiology 41:427, 1990.
11. Palomo A. Radical cure of varicocele by a new technique: Preliminary report. J Urol 61:604, 1949.
12. Ivanissevich O. Left varicocele due to reflux: Experience with 4,470 operative cases in forty-two years. J Int Coll Surg 34:742, 1960.
13. Marmar JL, DeBenedictis TJ, Praiss D. The management of varicoceles by microdissection of the spermatic cord at the external inguinal ring. Fertil Steril 43:583, 1985.
14. Goldstein M, Gilbert BR, Dicker AP, et al. Microsurgical inguinal varicocelectomy with delivery of the testis: An artery and lymphatic sparing technique. J Urol 148:1808, 1992.
15. Aaberg RA, Vancaillie TG, Schuessler WW. Laparoscopic varicocele ligation: A new technique. Fertil Steril 56:776, 1991.
16. Hagood PG, Mehan DJ, Worischeck JH, et al. Laparoscopic varicocelectomy: Preliminary report of a new technique. J Urol 147:73, 1992.
17. Donovan JF Jr, Winfield HN. Laparoscopic varix ligation. J Urol 147:77, 1992.
18. Sanchez de Badajoz E, Diaz Ramirez F, Marin Martin J. Tratamiento endoscopico del varicocele. Arch Esp Urol 41:15, 1988.
19. Fisch H. The surety of surgical repair of varicoceles. Contemp Urol 3:68, 1991.
20. Donovan JF Jr. Legal issues in laparoscopy. Contemp Urol 4:74, 1992.
21. Loughlin KR, Brooks DC. The use of a Doppler probe to facilitate laparoscopic varicocele ligation. Surg Gynecol Obstet 174:326, 1992.
22. Donovan JF Jr, Winfield HN. Laparoscopic varix ligation with the Nd:YAG laser. J Endourol 6:165, 1992.
23. Jarow JP. Personal communication, 1991.
24. Jarow JP, Assimos DG, Pittaway DE. Effectiveness of laparoscopic varicocelectomy. Urology 42:544, 1993.
25. Enquist E, Stein BS, Sigman M. Laparoscopic versus subinguinal varicocelectomy: A comparative study. Fertil Steril 61:1092, 1994.
26. See WA, Winfield HN, Fisher RJ, Donovan JF Jr. Laparoscopic surgical training: Effectiveness and impact of urological surgical practice patterns. J Urol 149:1054, 1993.
27. See WA, Cooper CS, Fisher RJ. Predictors of laparoscopic complications after formal training in laparoscopic surgery. JAMA 270:2689, 1993.
28. Donovan JF Jr. Laparoscopic varix ligation. Atlas Urol Clin North Am 1:15, 1993.

Chapter 17

Minilaparotomy Staging Pelvic Lymphadenectomy (Minilap)

Fray F. Marshall, Mitchell S. Steiner, and Alan Partin

PREOPERATIVE EVALUATION

Noninvasive radiological imaging cannot always determine whether there are pelvic lymph node metastases in patients with prostatic cancer. There may be occasional patients with transitional cell carcinoma of the bladder who may also be potential candidates for staging pelvic lymphadenectomy. Treatment may change, depending on the status of lymph node involvement. Prostate cancer patients have a higher risk for positive lymph nodes with such findings as prostate-specific antigens (PSA) over 20 ng/ml, high Gleason grade 8 or 9, or extensive local tumor involvement of the prostate. A staging pelvic lymphadenectomy may then be indicated. In general, a pelvic lymphadenectomy is performed at the time of a radical prostatectomy. If a grossly positive node is found, a prostatectomy is not performed.

The minilaparotomy staging pelvic lymphadenectomy (or minilap) was devised in part as an alternative to a standard pelvic lymphadenectomy or a laparoscopic pelvic lymphadenectomy.[1] All patients were evaluated by digital rectal examination, serum enzymatic prostatic acid phosphatase levels, serum PSA, bone scan, and often computed tomography (CT). All patients were under the age of 70 and had no medical contraindications to surgery.

SURGICAL TECHNIQUE

The patient is placed in the supine position with the umbilicus centered over the kidney rest. The table is flexed so that the distance between the umbilicus and pubic symphysis is increased. The patient is prepared and draped in the usual manner and a 22 Fr. Foley catheter with a 30-ml balloon is passed into the bladder. A midline 5- to 6-cm incision is made 1

to 2 cm above the pubic symphysis (Fig. 17–1). The rectus fascia is sharply divided between the rectus muscles, and the transversalis fascia is incised to provide access to the space of Retzius (Fig. 17–2). A Richardson retractor is used to retract the incision to the right side of the patient. If there were obvious tumor on the left side of the prostate, the initial lymph node dissection would be begun on the left. The retroperitoneal space is developed and the peritoneum is mobilized off the external iliac vessels to the bifurcation of the common iliac arteries. The retractor is hooked under the vas deferens and the peritoneum is mobilized (Figs. 17–3 and 17–4).

The Omni tract retractor with small blades provides excellent exposure. First a small superficial fixed curved blade is used to pull the incision laterally to the side of the pelvic lymphadenectomy (Fig. 17–5). This blade is hooked under the vas deferens and peritoneum. The iliac vessels are carefully avoided. The bladder is retracted medially with a long Harrington (sweetheart) blade (Fig. 17–6). A small Harrington blade can be used to retract the peritoneum superiorly, and additional small blades placed as necessary. If the Omni tract retractor is not available, a combination of Richardson, Harrington, and Deaver retractors can be used to obtain good exposure.

The pelvic lymphadenectomy is performed under direct vision. Tissue over the external iliac vein is divided cephalad to the hypogastric artery and caudally toward the femoral canal. A Gil-Vernet retractor is used to temporarily elevate the external iliac vein. The distal lymphatic package is isolated below the external iliac vein and above the obturator nerve. A metal clip is placed on the distal lymphatic package just proximal to the node of Cloquet, and this lymphatic tissue is incised (Fig. 17–7). Dissection is carried along the obturator nerve and care is taken to

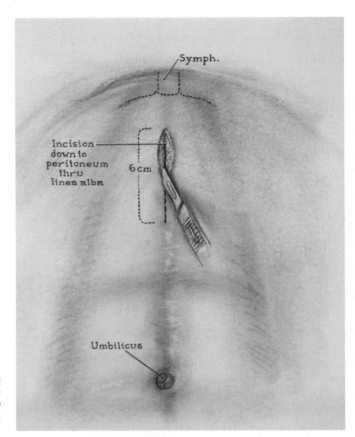

Figure 17–1. A 6-cm lower abdominal incision is made 1 to 2 cm above the pubic symphysis. (From Steiner MS, Marshall FF. Mini-laparotomy staging pelvic lymphadenectomy [minilap]: Alternatives to standard and laparoscopic pelvic lymphadenectomy. Urology 41:202, 1993.)

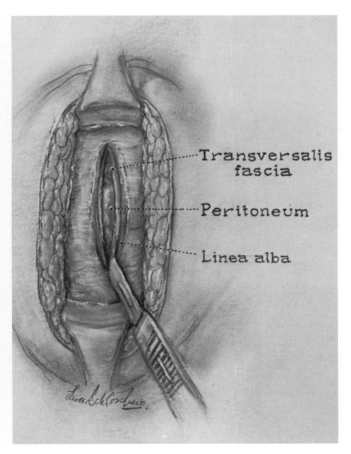

Figure 17–2. The rectus fascia is divided in the midline between the rectus muscles, and the transversalis fascia is sharply incised. (From Steiner MS, Marshall FF. Mini-laparotomy staging pelvic lymphadenectomy [minilap]: Alternatives to standard and laparoscopic pelvic lymphadenectomy. Urology 41:202, 1993.)

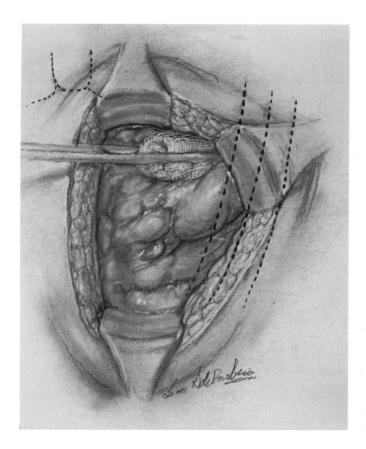

Figure 17–3. The peritoneum is mobilized superiorly and the space of Retzius is developed. (From Steiner MS, Marshall FF. Mini-laparotomy staging pelvic lymphadenectomy [minilap]: Alternatives to standard and laparoscopic pelvic lymphadenectomy. Urology 41:203, 1993.)

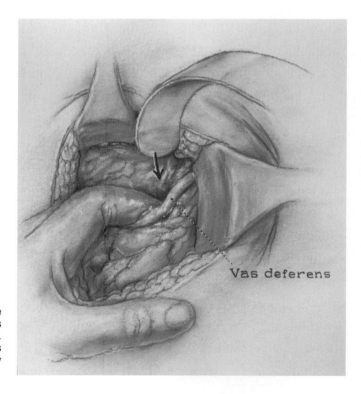

Vas deferens

Figure 17–4. The vas deferens is identified and mobilized with the peritoneum. The Mayo retractor blade is used to retract both the vas deferens and peritoneum laterally. (From Steiner MS, Marshall FF. Mini-laparotomy staging pelvic lymphadenectomy [minilap]: Alternatives to standard and laparoscopic pelvic lymphadenectomy. Urology 41:203, 1993.)

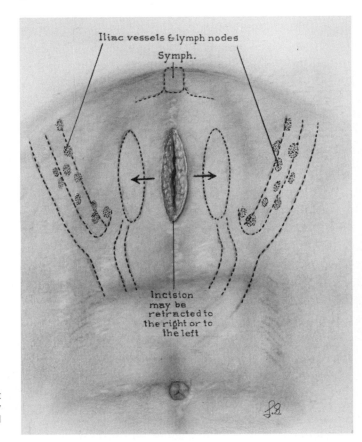

Figure 17–5. The incision may be moved to either side to permit maximal exposure. (From Steiner MS, Marshall FF. Mini-laparotomy staging pelvic lymphadenectomy [minilap]: Alternatives to standard and laparoscopic pelvic lymphadenectomy. Urology 41:203, 1993.)

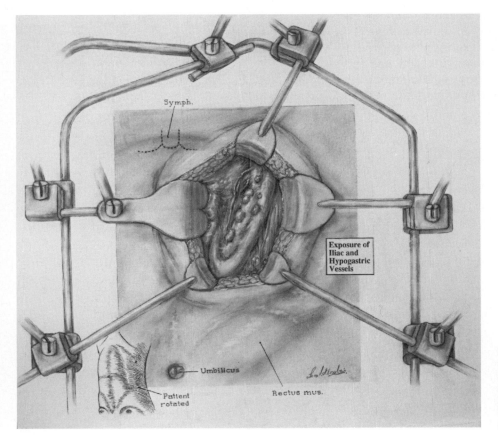

Figure 17–6. The Omni tract retractor provides both superficial and deep exposure. (From Steiner MS, Marshall FF. Mini-laparotomy staging pelvic lymphadenectomy [minilap]: Alternatives to standard and laparoscopic pelvic lymphadenectomy. Urology 41:204, 1993.)

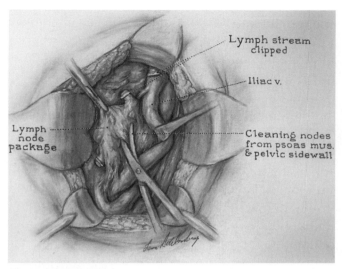

Figure 17–7. The lymph node package is removed from the obturator fossa after the lymphatic package adjacent to the external iliac vein has been clipped. The lymphatic package is mobilized posteriorly and along the obturator nerve. (From Steiner MS, Marshall FF. Minilaparotomy staging pelvic lymphadenectomy [minilap]: Alternatives to standard and laparoscopic pelvic lymphadenectomy. Urology 41:204, 1993.)

avoid lacerating an accessory obturator vein or additional vessels. Clips are placed as needed. Hypogastric nodes can also be dissected and clips placed as necessary. The entire package is removed after it is dissected off the obturator neurovascular bundle and off the lateral pelvic wall.

If the pelvic nodes are suspicious, they are submitted to the pathology department for frozen section. If they are negative by gross examination, they are sent for permanent sections and a radical retropubic prostatectomy is performed. A 5- or 6-cm incision can be utilized for the lymphadenectomy and enlarged slightly to 7 to 8 cm if a radical retropubic prostatec-

tomy is performed. The incision is closed with a No. 1 PDS suture. A small Davol drain can be left for 1 day and removed if there is minimal drainage. In some instances, no drain has been left. Typically, patients can be discharged within 48 hours.

POSTOPERATIVE MANAGEMENT AND COMPLICATIONS

If patients have only a lymphadenectomy, they can be discharged rapidly. Bleeding has not been a major problem and the operation can be performed rapidly without the extensive equipment necessary for the laparoscopic approach. In addition, it is a retroperitoneal procedure. The average intraoperative time is slightly more than 30 minutes once the actual procedure has begun. A recent study that we conducted demonstrated that the number of lymph nodes, the complications, and the degree of continence in patients undergoing a pelvic lymphadenectomy and radical prostatectomy with a minilap incision were similar to those in patients undergoing a standard operation with a symphysis-to-umbilicus incision.

The minilap incision has also been used for other operations, including a distal ureterolithotomy, drainage of lymphocele, and continence surgery in females. It appears to be an attractive alternative for high-risk patients with prostatic cancer who require a staging pelvic lymphadenectomy.

REFERENCE

1. Steiner MS, Marshall FF. Mini-laparotomy staging pelvic lymphadenectomy (minilap): Alternative to standard and laparoscopic pelvic lymphadenectomy. Urology 41:201, 1993.

Chapter 18

Laparoscopic Pelvic Lymph Node Dissection

J. Matthew Glascock and Howard N. Winfield

The excitement accompanying the development of laparoscopic procedures in general surgery gained the attention of the urological community, and the first laparoscopic pelvic lymph node dissection (LPLND) was reported in 1991.[1] It afforded the urologist a minimally invasive technique to assess the pelvic lymph nodes of men with cancer of the prostate. Since that time this operation has been perfected, albeit modified to some extent, and the indications for the procedure have been more clearly defined. An extended LPLND may also be offered to patients with cancer of the bladder, penis, or urethra.

The objectives of this chapter are to (1) describe the indications for LPLND and the appropriate preoperative evaluation of the patient who chooses this procedure, (2) extensively describe the intra- and extraperitoneal approaches, (3) discuss the postoperative management of a patient who has undergone successful LPLND, and (4) review the potential complications that may be encountered during the performance of this technically challenging procedure.

PREOPERATIVE CONSIDERATIONS

The major advantages of laparoscopic intervention over open surgery include a shortened postoperative hospitalization and convalescence, a reduction in postsurgical pain and narcotic requirement, a less intensive nursing requirement, and an improved cosmetic appearance of the abdominal scars. The cosmetic advantage is suggested but not proven to date by means of prospective, randomized studies. Therefore, before offering this type of surgery to patients, the urologist must believe that the information gained by obtaining the lymph nodes will direct subsequent therapeutic decisions. For patients with cancer of the prostate, the discovery of metastatic nodes will obviate radical surgery or radiotherapy. If radical perineal prostatectomy is being considered, a preliminary LPLND is justified although not mandatory in lower-grade (Gleason score) tumors. In patients with bladder cancer, positive pelvic lymph nodes suggest the need for neoadjuvant chemotherapy before cystectomy, whereas in penile or urethral cancer the possibility of achieving a curative radical extirpation of the primary cancer is extremely remote in the presence of pelvic lymphatic metastases. When there is a reasonably good chance of discovering positive lymph nodes by laparoscopically obtaining pelvic lymphatic tissue for histopathological evaluation, the patient may be spared the greater morbidity and longer convalescence associated with an open pelvic lymph node dissection.

Assuming that the staging information attained after LPLND will benefit the patient, each candidate should be considered in light of the absolute and relative contraindications. With experience, the only absolute contraindications include poorly controlled bleeding diatheses, severe chronic obstructive pulmonary disease, generalized peritonitis, abdominal wall infection, and significant intestinal obstruction. However, it is unlikely that one would want to operate on these patients in the first place. Relative contraindications include obesity, severe diverticular disease, previous abdominal surgery, radiotherapy, and/or chemotherapy. The individual surgeon's experience with LPLND will modify the exclusionary potential of each relative contraindication. The absolute and relative contraindications to open surgery with regard to anesthetic risk apply similarly to LPLND candidates.

If LPLND is indicated, the patient must be fully informed of the potential risks as well as the benefits obtained through the election of this procedure. In addition, the complications of this form of surgery, and the ways to deal with these problems should they arise, must be discussed if an informed decision is to be made by the patient. Of particular importance, the possibility of intraoperative misadventure necessitating conversion to an open surgical procedure should be fully understood by the patient. The potential complications one may encounter during laparoscopic pelvic surgery are outlined later in this chapter. Alternative treatment plans, including doing nothing, should also be discussed. Furthermore, the experience of the surgical team should be clarified. After obtaining informed consent, the patient is ready for preoperative evaluation.

Preoperative Evaluation

The standard presurgical evaluation is appropriate for patients who have elected to undergo LPLND. This includes a general screen of blood chemistry and a hemogram as well as an assessment of coagulability. A blood typing and antibody screen is mandatory in case vascular injury necessitates emergency transfusion. A recent chest radiograph is needed, and the patient should be cleared for surgery with regard to any coexistent cardiopulmonary disease.

In the absence of any contraindications, the patient is instructed to self-administer an oral laxative such as GoLYTELY or an enema the night before surgery to decompress the bowel. This is intended to decrease the risk of accidental enterotomy during insufflation, trocar placement, or laparoscopic dissection. The patient is then admitted to the hospital on the morning of surgery. However, if relative contraindications exist, the likelihood of encountering extensive adhesions requiring lysis increases the risk of bowel injury. These patients should be admitted to the hospital the evening before surgery for a thorough mechanical and antibiotic bowel preparation. In addition, if further surgery is planned in case intraoperative pathological evaluation reveals an absence of metastatic disease, the more intensive bowel preparation is indicated.

OPERATIVE PROCEDURE

All patients receive a parenteral broad-spectrum antibiotic on call to the operating room. Upon arrival there, the patient is fitted with pneumatic anti-embolic compression boots. General anesthesia affords the surgeon improved muscle relaxation, positioning, and exposure, but because of its association with visceral distention, the inhalational agent nitrous oxide should be excluded from the anesthetic regimen. After adequate general anesthesia is obtained, the bladder and stomach are decompressed by placement of a Foley catheter and a nasogastric

tube, respectively. With wide adhesive tape across the thighs and chest, the patient is secured to the table in a supine position with arms carefully padded at the sides (Fig. 18–1). The abdomen is then antiseptically prepared and draped in a manner suitable for the performance of a traditional laparotomy. During the surgeon's early experience, the surgical nursing staff should have immediately available a standard laparotomy tray in the operating room in case an emergency laparotomy becomes necessary. The video monitoring equipment should be arranged so as to afford an unobstructed and comfortable view to all members of the surgical team.

Transperitoneal Laparoscopic Pelvic Lymph Node Dissection

After pneumoperitoneum has been obtained, a 10/11-mm trocar-sheath unit is placed through a 2-cm subumbilical incision. A 0-degree telescope is then introduced into the abdominal cavity and a thorough examination made for any injury to the underlying viscera. The remaining working ports are placed under direct laparoscopic visualization to reduce the risk of inadvertently injuring the underlying abdominal contents. The diamond configuration of four laparoscopic ports affords a suitable arrangement for reaching the pelvic lymph nodes laparoscopically (Fig. 18–2). This configuration includes two bilaterally placed 5-mm ports situated along the lateral borders of the rectus muscles at the midpoint of a line connecting the umbilicus and the anterosuperior iliac spines. In addition, a 10-mm trocar-sheath unit is placed 3 to 5 cm superior to the symphysis pubis through the linea alba. Injury to the superficial and inferior epigastric vessels can be avoided by laparoscopic transillumination of the puncture sites during placement. An alternative arrangement resembling an

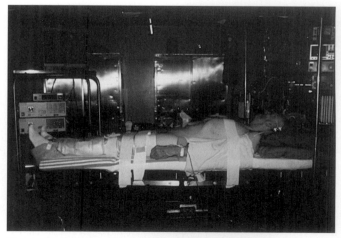

Figure 18–1. Appropriate positioning of the patient in preparation for laparoscopic pelvic lymph node dissection.

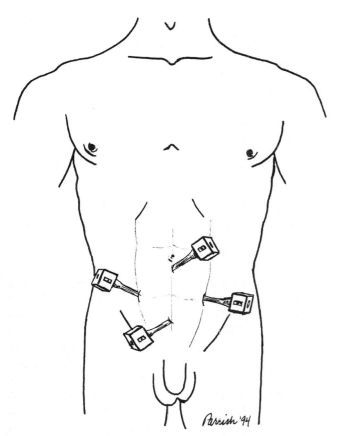

Figure 18–2. Diamond configuration of four laparoscopic ports for pelvic lymph node dissection.

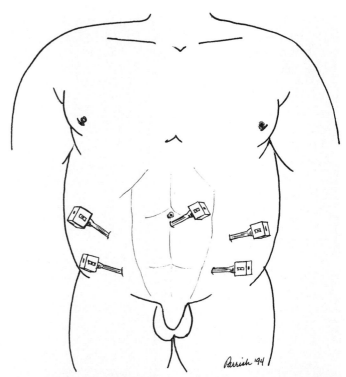

Figure 18–3. Horseshoe configuration of five laparoscopic ports for pelvic lymph node dissection in obese patients.

inverted U or horseshoe has proved advantageous in obese patients in whom an overabundance of urachal fatty tissue impedes access to the pelvic lymph nodes via the standard diamond configuration of port placement (Fig. 18–3).

After the ports have been secured in position, the patient is placed in approximately 30 degrees of Trendelenburg with 15 degrees of lateral rotation contralateral to the field of dissection. This facilitates gravitation of the viscera away from the operative site, thus improving exposure of the obturator fossa. Further mobilization of the bowel may require lysis of adhesions to more clearly expose the operative field. This is particularly true on the left side where diverticular disease is commonly accompanied by extensive adhesions of the sigmoid colon to the pelvic side wall. An incision along the white line of Toldt should release the attachment of the sigmoid colon to the pelvic wall, thereby allowing a clear view of the iliac-obturator region. At this point, it is essential to accurately identify several important anatomical landmarks. The vas deferens and testicular vessels should be appreciated as they enter the pelvis through the internal inguinal ring. The testicular vessels should be visualized as they course cephalad, while the vas deferens continues posteromedially to cross the internal iliac vessels and the obliterated

umbilical artery (ligament) en route to its terminus where it joins the seminal vesicle deep within the pelvis. The obliterated umbilical artery should be traced from its attachment on the anterior abdominal wall to its junction with the internal iliac artery near the bifurcation of the common iliac artery. It must be realized that the most proximal portion of the obliterated umbilical artery near its internal iliac artery branch point remains widely patent and has proved to be the source of laparoscopically intractable hemorrhage. In nonobese patients, pulsation of the external iliac artery may delineate its position beneath the posterior peritoneal membrane (Fig. 18–4).

Obturator Lymph Node Dissection

This procedure is performed primarily for the operative staging of patients with adenocarcinoma of the prostate. The information in Table 18–1, which outlines the current indications for the use of LPLND as a means of pathologically staging adenocarcinoma of the prostate, is based on a review of our series of over 200 procedures. For patients with carcinoma of the prostate, it has been shown that the primary lymph node "landing zone" for early lymphatic dissemination is the obturator lymph node chain in over 85 percent of cases.[2, 3] In addition, the likelihood of metastases bypassing the obturator lymph nodes with subsequent involvement of the more proximal iliac

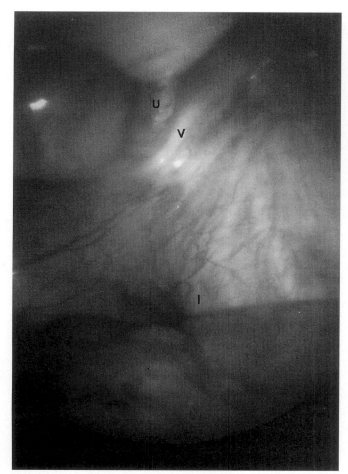

Figure 18–4. Laparoscopic view of the iliac-obturator region. U, obliterated umbilical artery; V, vas deferens; I, iliac vessels. (From Gomella LG, Kozminski M, Winfield HN. Laparoscopic Urologic Surgery. New York, Raven Press, 1994.)

TABLE 18–1. Indications for Laparoscopic Obturator Lymph Node Dissection

1. Stage B2 to D0 cancer of the prostate regardless of the follow-up treatment being considered. It is expected that these patients will have a >25% chance of having lymphatic metastasis. Patients with A2 disease and a Gleason score of ≥6 are also advised to undergo LPLND.
2. Elevated enzymatic assay for prostatic acid phosphatase with a negative bone scan (stage D0 disease).
3. Serum prostate-specific antigen >30 ng/ml. These patients are highly likely to have lymphatic metastasis.
4. Patients choosing transperineal prostatectomy.
5. Patients with A1, A2, or B1 disease with moderately to poorly differentiated histological subtypes (Gleason score ≥6) who have chosen radiotherapy or surgery.

or aortic lymph node regions is only 6 to 14 percent.[3] This has facilitated the establishment of the obturator lymph node dissection as the standard operative staging procedure for the evaluation of patients with adenocarcinoma of the prostate.

The initial incision through the posterior peritoneal membrane originates at a point midway between the obliterated umbilical artery and the internal inguinal ring. The linear incision is continued cephalad just medial to the external iliac artery toward a point near the bifurcation of the common iliac artery. It is extremely important to appreciate the proximity of the ureter to the iliac bifurcation, as an injury to the ureter will at least require stenting and may necessitate open surgical repair. Once the initial incision has been accomplished, the external iliac vein is exposed through a careful dissection of all fibrofatty lymphatic

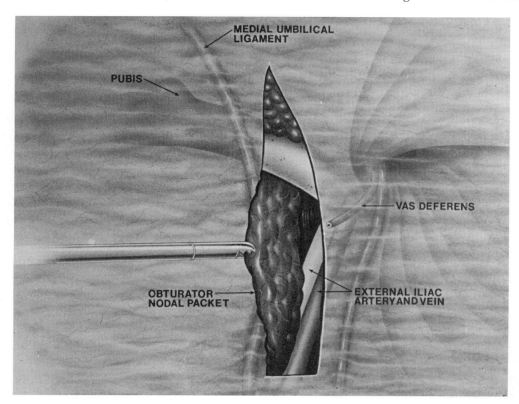

Figure 18–5. Creation of the lateral border of the right obtutator lymph node packet. (From Gomella LG, Kozminski M, Winfield HN. Laparoscopic Urologic Surgery. New York, Raven Press, 1994.)

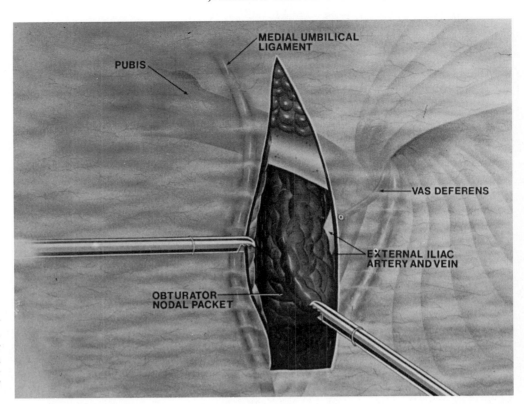

Figure 18–6. Creation of the medial border of the right obturator lymph node packet. (From Gomella LG, Kozminski M, Winfield HN. Laparoscopic Urologic Surgery. New York: Raven Press, 1994.)

tissue medial to the external iliac artery. Through blunt and sharp dissection, the lateral border of the obturator lymph node packet is developed by clearing all of the lymph node–bearing tissue away from the anteromedial aspect of the external iliac vein (Fig. 18–5).

The medial boundary of the dissection is established by gentle medial traction placed on the obliterated umbilical artery. Blunt dissection directed laterally to the obliterated umbilical artery develops this plane inferiorly to the distal apex of the obturator lymph node packet near the pubic bone and Cooper ligament (Fig. 18–6). In this region, venous variations are commonly encountered. Not infrequently, an accessory obturator vein joins the external iliac vein soon after the external iliac vein enters the pelvis through the femoral canal. With careful manipulation, the distal apex of the obturator lymph node packet may be maneuvered out from under this accessory vein. However, sparing of this vessel is not possible in many cases, and its hemoclip ligation and division necessarily precede liberation of the distal extent of the obturator lymph node packet. The distal apex of the dissection is then freed via careful electrocautery. The packet is then grasped at this apex and elevated superiorly while blunt dissection at the base continues to develop the dissection proximally. As this process continues, the underlying obturator nerve and vessels should become clearly visible. Judicious electrocautery should be used to seal any small vessels or lymphatic channels that become apparent

as the dissection progresses. The dissection is carried proximally toward the bifurcation of the common iliac artery. Again, the proximity of the ureter to the proximal extent of the dissection places it in jeopardy of inadvertent injury, so an awareness of this anatomical relationship is essential. When development of the proximal extent of the dissection has been accomplished, electrocautery is used to seal and divide any remaining lymphatic vessels. This should result in a free lymph node packet (Fig. 18–7).

With spoon-shaped or Russian forceps, the free lymph node packet is delivered through the 10/11-mm suprapubic port. By manually holding the flap-valve open and using a gentle twisting motion during the removal of the lymph node packet, the likelihood of shearing off and loss of lymphatic tissue is reduced. If further radical surgery is planned pending a negative histopathological evaluation of the lymphatic tissue, the node packet is sent for immediate intraoperative frozen section analysis. Attention is then turned to the contralateral side. The table is rotated in the opposite direction and a similar dissection proceeds on the contralateral side.

Extended Lymph Node Dissection

In certain clinical situations a more extensive lymphatic dissection is indicated. For patients with carcinoma of the urinary bladder, urethra, or penis, the internal, external, and common iliac lymph node chains responsible for the lymphatic drainage of

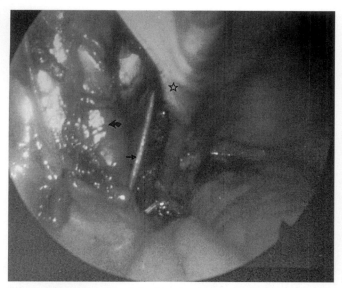

Figure 18–7. Complete left obturator lymph node dissection. The small arrow denotes the obturator nerve; the curved arrow indicates the external iliac vein; the star is situated just lateral to the left obliterated umbilical artery. (From Winfield HN, Donovan JF, See WA, et al. Urologic laparoscopic surgery. J Urol 146:941, 1991.)

these organs are the sites where early metastatic disease will be discovered. In certain instances, when metastatic adenocarcinoma of the prostate is highly suspected on the basis of laboratory and clinical evidence but the obturator lymph nodes are free of metastatic disease, the extended dissection may also be indicated. Table 18–2 summarizes the indications for this extended dissection, which includes the excision of all lymphatic tissue situated within an area bounded by the urinary bladder wall medially, the genitofemoral nerve laterally, and the common iliac artery proximally. Consequently, a more thorough mobilization of the sigmoid colon and cecoappendiceal regions must precede this more extensive operation in order to provide a broader exposure of the operative field. An alternative initial incision intended to provide greater exposure of the iliac region has been described. This "inverted V" peritoneotomy includes the previously described initial incision as well as an additional incision that originates at the same point high over the pubic bone but is instead continued in a more posteromedial direction and equidistant to the initial incision. The peritoneal free

TABLE 18–2. Indications for Extended Laparoscopic Pelvic Lymph Node Dissection

1. Carcinoma of the urinary bladder, urethra, or penis
2. Carcinoma of the prostate in the absence of obturator lymph node positivity in the following situations:
   a. Elevated serum (enzymatic) prostatic acid phosphatase (stage D0)
   b. Prostate-specific antigen elevation >60 ng/ml (Hybritech)
   c. Clinical stage C disease

flap thus formed allows for a greater exposure of the underlying obturator-iliac region when the flap is elevated.[4] By careful medial retraction of the external iliac vessels, access to the underlying lymphatic tissue is possible (Fig. 18–8).

Extraperitoneal Laparoscopic Pelvic Lymph Node Dissection

Throughout the development of any new surgical procedure, extensions, modifications, and different approaches by which the same end result may be obtained are often formulated. The evolution of LPLND offers no exception to this type of progress. Since 1993, select patients at the University of Iowa Hospitals and Clinics have undergone LPLND through an alternative extraperitoneal approach. Although this novel approach is still under investigation, several advantages have become apparent. It is well known that direct instrumentation and manipulation of the intraperitoneal contents constitutes a major stimulus to the development of adhesions. In addition, when the intraperitoneal space is entered, the risks of visceral injury, peritonitis, and the possible spillage of potentially tumor-laden lymphatic tissue become significant. There is a chance of circumventing these complications by maintaining the integrity of the peritoneal membrane.

Creation of the Extraperitoneal Space

Beginning at the inferior crease of the umbilicus, a 3-cm midline incision is deepened to the level of the rectus abdominis fascia. By dividing the rectus abdominis and transversus abdominis fasciae in the

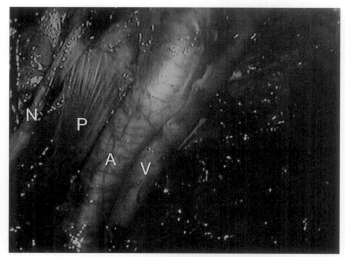

Figure 18–8. Left extended pelvic lymph node dissection for cancer of the bladder, urethra, or penis. V, external iliac vein; A, external iliac artery; P, psoas major muscle; N, genitofemoral nerve.

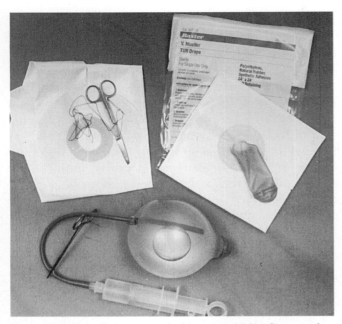

Figure 18–9. Polyethylene natural rubber material (the finger cot from a TUR drape) used as a balloon dilation device for creation of the extraperitoneal space.

midline, the properitoneal space is then entered. Through the use of blunt finger dissection, the properitoneal space is developed to the extent that a balloon dilation device can be introduced. A modified Gaur-type device has proved successful for the development of the properitoneal space.[5] This device features the finger cot of a transurethral resection drape that has been secured to a 20 Fr. red rubber (Robinson) catheter by silk free ties (Fig. 18–9). It was determined through experimenting with several alternative materials that this thicker polyethylene natural rubber material can withstand the pressure exerted by the 800 to 1000 ml of saline needed to dilate the space of Retzius, with a lower risk of balloon rupture than with the alternative materials. After the balloon is placed within the space of Retzius, 800 to 1000 ml of normal saline is slowly injected into the balloon to develop the properitoneal space. In the event of balloon rupture, a thorough search for fragments within the properitoneal space is mandatory.

With successful expansion of the space of Retzius, the pubic bone and external iliac vessels should become clearly visible (Fig. 18–10). A Hasson-type cannula is then secured within the subumbilical incision, and carbon dioxide (CO_2) insufflation commences at 12 to 15 mm Hg. The working ports are then placed in the diamond configuration and lymphadenectomy proceeds as previously described. It is important to avoid traversing the peritoneal membrane during port placement, as this will likely effect an obliteration of the properitoneal space. For this reason, the surgeon must be capable of converting the

ports from an extra- to an intraperitoneal position should the need arise.

Some already recognized advantages of this approach include the elimination of time spent in extensive adhesiolysis and mobilization of the sigmoid colon and cecoappendiceal regions. In addition, the intact peritoneal membrane holds back loops of bowel that tend to interfere with full exposure of the operative field. This may idealize the extraperitoneal approach for obese patients or those in whom the likelihood of encountering extensive adhesions is high.

Conversely, the more confined working space and distortion in the relative positions of the key anatomical landmarks that accompany this approach may pose an obstacle to the inexperienced surgeon. Specifically, the position of the vas deferens is displaced cephalad in the extraperitoneal approach. In addition, any previous lower abdominal or pelvic intra- or extraperitoneal surgery, e.g., inguinal herniorrhaphy, may render impossible an adequate development of the properitoneal space. Also, if radical retropubic prostatectomy is a future consideration, the postsurgical sequelae of scarring and fibrosis after extraperitoneal LPLND may complicate the operation considerably. It is also possible that the development of lymphocele formation after extraperitoneal LPLND exceeds that following its intraperitoneal counterpart. A prospective randomized study at the University of Iowa completed in 1995 sought to further characterize the advantages and disadvantages of this novel approach. Of particular interest was the comparison of CO_2 metabolism between patients undergoing the intra- versus the extraperitoneal approach to LPLND. Findings suggested a more rapid absorption of CO_2

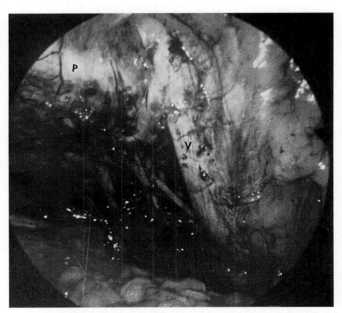

Figure 18–10. Balloon expansion of the extraperitoneal space of Retzius. P, pubic bone; V, external iliac vein.

in patients approached extraperitoneally, and in rare instances the development of iatrogenic hypercapnia was accompanied by significant respiratory acidosis. More expansive subcutaneous emphysema was also noted to attend the extraperitoneal approach.

At the completion of the lymphadenectomy, a thorough and systematic survey of the operative fields is undertaken. As meticulous hemostasis is requisite, generous irrigation and suction should be used to evaluate the obturator fossae. Electrocautery and/or hemoclip ligation of any discovered bleeder is necessary to reduce the risk of significant hematoma formation. Intra-abdominal pressure is then lowered to 5 mm Hg, at which time any venous bleeding formerly tamponaded by the higher intra-abdominal pressures maintained throughout the procedure should be made apparent. The secondary ports are then removed under direct laparoscopic observation to ensure that any lacerated abdominal wall vessels formerly compressed by the trocar-sheath units are detected. The primary port is then removed over the laparoscope. Since the laparoscope is the final instrument to be removed from the intra-abdominal space, a final assessment to ensure the attainment of adequate hemostasis is possible. This sequence of instrument removal guards against accidental herniation of the abdominal contents at the conclusion of the procedure. Digital exploration of all incisions 10 mm or larger is also useful to make certain that herniation has not occurred. Any remaining CO_2 is expressed from the abdominal cavity, and all 10-mm or larger incisions are closed with a single fascial suture of 2-0 polydioxanone. Finally, all incisions are approximated with Steri-Strip closures and are dressed with Tegaderm. Before emergence from the operating room, the nasogastric tube is removed. Routine postanesthesia care is appropriate for the uncomplicated LPLND patient after completion of the operation.

POSTOPERATIVE CONSIDERATIONS

All patients are admitted to the hospital after LPLND and are administered two additional postoperative doses of a parenteral broad-spectrum antibiotic at an 8-hour interval. The diet is advanced as tolerated, and any postsurgical pain should respond to oral analgesics; narcotics are rarely indicated. The Foley catheter should be removed as soon as the patient is alert and oriented. Ambulation should be encouraged on the evening after surgery. As with all postsurgical patients, vital signs should be monitored regularly to detect early postoperative infection. Most patients are discharged from the hospital on the first postoperative day and are able to resume normal activity by the end of the first week after surgery.

PROCEDURAL COMPLICATIONS

General Considerations

As with any invasive procedure, there is a possibility of misadventure resulting in severe morbidity. The nature of laparoscopic surgery necessitates a discussion of its unique potential complications. Although the likelihood of severe complications developing during laparoscopic surgery is greatly reduced by arming oneself with a thorough understanding of and respect for the regional anatomy, a firm academic grasp of the fundamental principles of laparoscopic surgical technique, and the development of a methodical, experienced approach, there remains the possibility of intraoperative complications.[6] The laparoscopic surgeon should become astute at the identification and management of these potential pitfalls in case they occur during the procedure.

Specific Complications of Laparoscopic Pelvic Lymph Node Dissection

A review of the medical records of the more than 200 patients who have elected to undergo LPLND at the University of Iowa Hospitals and Clinics confirms that LPLND is typically a very well tolerated procedure. However, the known potential complications of laparoscopic surgery became clinical reality for several patients in our series. Table 18–3 outlines the complications of LPLND encountered throughout the experience with this technique at the University of Iowa. Any visceral or vascular injury was discovered and remediated intraoperatively. This truly attests to

TABLE 18–3. Complications of Laparoscopic Pelvic Lymph Node Dissection (University of Iowa)*

Hemorrhage	9
Controllable laparoscopically	8
Requiring open repair	1
Injury to external iliac artery	1
Injury to inferior epigastric vessels	6
Bleeding from obliterated umbilical artery	2
Bowel perforation/injury	4
Deep venous thrombosis/pulmonary embolism (after prostatectomy/ radiotherapy)	2
Wound infection/dehiscence	2
Abscess formation	1
Scrotal/suprapubic ecchymosis	3
Unsatisfactory dissection	1
Postoperative ileus	4
Urinary retention	4
Bowel obstruction	1
Obturator nerve neuropraxia, transient	1
Hypercapnia (extraperitoneal approach)	1
Postoperative sedation (anesthesia)	1
Intraoperative ST-segment depression	1

*Based on 195 cases.

TABLE 18-4. Laparoscopic Pelvic Lymph Node Dissection: Etiology of Conversion to Laparotomy

Conversions to open procedure (out of 195 LPLNDs)	9
Contributing factors*	
Obesity	5
Previous abdominopelvic surgery/radiotherapy	4
Bowel injury/enterotomy	2
Vascular injury	1
Unsatisfactory pathological specimen	1
Equipment failure	1

*More than one contributing factor may apply in each case.

the benefit of thoroughly inspecting the intraperitoneal contents, operative fields, and intra-abdominal aspects of the port sites to rule out injury and ensure that meticulous hemostasis has been achieved before closure. If left unnoticed, these complications would have almost invariably necessitated the performance of open laparotomy for repair. It was also noted that most procedures in which complications developed were among the very earliest operations performed. Again, this finding calls to attention the considerable learning curve associated with the mastering of this complicated operation. More recently, through the mastering of advanced laparoscopic techniques, such as laparoscopic suturing, several procedure-aborting complications were repaired intraoperatively.

Throughout the experience with LPLND at the University of Iowa Hospitals and Clinics, complications considered to be laparoscopically insurmountable arose in nine instances. For these intraoperative conversions from laparoscopic to open pelvic lymph node dissection, Table 18–4 summarizes the contributing etiologies. It is important to note that a contributing factor in more than half of the aborted laparoscopic procedures was obesity. Again, these aborted laparoscopic attempts all occurred early in the series.

Summary

At this institution, since May 1990 and for over 200 patients, LPLND has repeatedly proved to be a reliably excellent, minimally invasive staging procedure for the evaluation of men with adenocarcinoma of the prostate. However, many potential applications for laparoscopic surgery demand further characterization. For example, the standardization of extended LPLND for the operative staging of patients with urological pelvic malignancies involving the urinary bladder, urethra, and penis is an ongoing endeavor for many enthusiastic laparoscopic surgeons. In addition, the indications for and advantages and disadvantages of the newly developed extraperitoneal approach to LPLND represent an area worthy of further study. The minimally invasive nature of laparoscopic surgery truly sets it apart from open surgery as the ideal method for obtaining lymphatic tissue for pathological staging of individuals with urological pelvic malignancy—the "gold standard" on which appropriate therapeutic decisions are based.

Finally, the discussion of potential complications, many of which are ominous indeed, needs to be tempered with the understanding that surgical experience and a strict adherence to the basic fundamentals of laparoscopic surgical technique will virtually eliminate the occurrence of the aforementioned intraoperative pitfalls.

REFERENCES

1. Schuessler WW, Vancaillie TG, Reich H, et al. Transperitoneal endosurgical lymphadenectomy in patients with localized prostate cancer. J Urol 145:899, 1991.
2. Winfield HN, Donovan JF, See WA, et al. Laparoscopic pelvic lymph node dissection for genitourinary malignancies: Indications, techniques, and results. J Endourol 6:103, 1992.
3. McLaughlin AP, Salzstein SL, McCollough DL, et al. Prostatic carcinoma: Incidence and location of unsuspected lymphatic metastases. J Urol 115:89, 1976.
4. See WA, Cohen MB, Winfield HN. Inverted V peritoneotomy significantly improves nodal yield in laparoscopic pelvic lymphadenectomy. J Urol 149:772, 1993.
5. Gaur DD, Agarwal DK, Purohit KC. Retroperitoneal laparoscopic nephrectomy: Initial case report. J Urol 149:103, 1993.
6. Kerbel K, Clayman RV. Basic techniques of laparoscopic surgery. Urol Clin North Am 20:361, 1993.

Chapter 19

Laparoscopic Surgery for Stress Incontinence

Laurence M. Harewood

The laparoscope offers a new approach to the bladder neck that may be exploited to provide the results of open surgery for stress urinary incontinence (SUI), with the advantages of a minimally invasive approach. Currently the best results are obtained with either a Burch[1] or a Marshall-Marchetti-Kranz (MMK)[2] procedure. Both, however, are open procedures with concomitant morbidity, postoperative pain, prolonged hospital stay, and extended convalescence. The alternative, less invasive Stamey[3] and Raz[4] procedures also have problems of postoperative pain, plus a short-term failure rate of 5 to 10 percent, postoperative voiding difficulties in up to 50 percent, and a long-term failure rate of 30 to 50 percent.[5]

The fundamental defect in SUI is an instantaneous descent of the bladder neck when the patient coughs or strains. The proximal urethra is carried beyond the zone of transmission of the intra-abdominal pressure, and incontinence ensues. This is a dynamic process. The goal of treatment is to prevent the bladder neck descending. The aim of an ideal procedure should be to:

- Prevent descent of the bladder neck when the patient coughs or strains, rather than pull the bladder neck up. Elevating the bladder neck under tension causes postoperative bladder spasms, pain, failure to void, and cut-through of the sutures through the vaginal wall, leading to failure of the procedure. The correct tension is therefore "no slack and no tension." The sutures should be tied to hold the bladder neck in the rest position. This must be done under vision if slack in the suture is to be avoided, which might cause early recurrence. It is not necessary to pull the bladder neck until it is closed in the rest position, as the neck will close when the patient coughs or strains if it is properly supported.

- Attach the suture to the pectineal ligaments, as these are the most developed structures that can take sutures, and attachment to these does not lead to the postoperative pain seen with sutures tied over the rectus fascia, such as with the Stamey and Raz procedures.

- Produce permanent fixation of the vaginal wall to the pectineal ligament or the lateral pelvic wall. Long-term cut-through of the sutures in the vaginal wall is a cause of late failure.

- Not cause any urethral obstruction.

- Entail minimal dissection of the vaginal and urethral walls to avoid damage to the delicate urethral smooth muscle, which may lead to a type III or intrinsic stress incontinence.

- Use a minimally invasive approach to achieve the least morbidity and hospital stay.

Laparoscopic bladder neck suspension is a versatile, minimally invasive procedure that should not only provide the current results, but be exploited to give better results than open bladder neck suspension.

The first report of a laparoscopic bladder neck suspension was by Vancaillie and Schuessler in 1991,[6, 7] who used a transperitoneal approach and placed a single suture of Ethibond on each side from the vaginal wall to the symphysis pubis. The suture was tied extracorporeally with a Weston knot, thus reproducing a MMK procedure. Liu[8] reported a transperitoneal laparoscopic retropubic colposuspension (Burch procedure) suturing the vaginal wall to the pectineal ligament, using intraperitoneal suturing and knot tying. There are great difficulties inherent in suturing and knot tying laparoscopically, and this is not an easy procedure even for the experienced laparoscopist. An alternative using a clip on the suture simplifies this but still requires placing the sutures laparo-scopically.[9]

In 1993 Harewood[10] reported a laparoscopic needle colposuspension that used the Stamey needle under laparoscopic control to suspend the bladder neck. A heavy Ethibond (Ethicon) suture was introduced on a Stamey needle, a full-thickness double bite of the vaginal wall was taken, and the suture was tied over a silicone button on the anterior rectus fascia. This avoided intraperitoneal suturing and knot tying.

Ou and colleagues[11] in 1993 described a modified laparoscopic Burch procedure in which a 1- by 3-cm piece of Prolene hernia mesh (Ethicon) was stapled to the vaginal wall at the bladder neck, and to the pectineal ligament using titanium staples placed with an endoscopic stapler (Ethicon).

Chapple and Osborne[12] and Raboy and colleagues[13] in 1993 described an extraperitoneal laparoscopic approach to the bladder neck. Both used insufflation of the extraperitoneum with carbon dioxide (CO_2) plus blunt dissection to create a working space. Chapple placed an absorbable suture between the vaginal wall and the rectus fascia using a Bonney-Reverdin needle, allowing extracorporeal suturing and knot tying. Raboy used endoscopic suturing to place a nylon suture in the vaginal wall at the bladder neck, and attached this anteriorly to the pectineal ligament, the pubic symphysis, or the rectus fascia. Riza and Deshmukh[14] in 1994 described placing a helical suture in the vagina, and used an extraperitioneal approach and a special needle to pass the suture to the suprapubic area where it was tied.

Gaur[15] in 1992 developed a method of developing a working space in the retroperitoneum by balloon dilation. He used a surgical glove tied on the end of a catheter as a balloon. This was placed in the retroperitoneum via a small incision, and inflated with air using a pneumatic pump from a blood pressure apparatus. This technique greatly facilitated the extraperitoneal laparoscopic approach. Knapp and associates[16] in 1994 used this technique to create an extraperitoneal space. A vaginal suture was placed, brought into the retropubic space with a Stamey needle, withdrawn into the suprapubic area, and sutured into the fascia at the pubic tubercle.

The procedure described in this chapter makes use of all the advances in laparoscopic stress incontinence surgery to achieve an extraperitoneal laparoscopic Burch colposuspension with extracorporeal suturing and knot tying. It consists of a triple pulley loop of heavy Prolene suture, placed with a Stamey needle, passing between the pectineal ligament and the full thickness of the vaginal wall (Fig. 19–1).

It has the following features:

- An extraperitoneal approach, avoiding the complications associated with transperitoneal access to bowel and vessel injury, adhesions, and hernia formation.
- Anterior placement of the suture through the lacunar ligament and the pectineal ligament in the same manner as the Burch procedure, effectively reproducing a Burch operation.
- Placement of the sutures with a Stamey needle, so that all suturing and knot tying are done extracorporeally, avoiding the problems of laparoscopic suturing and knot tying.
- Placement of the sutures precisely at the bladder neck under direct vision with the laparoscope.
- Tying of the suture under direct vision, allowing suspension of the bladder neck with no tension and no slack.

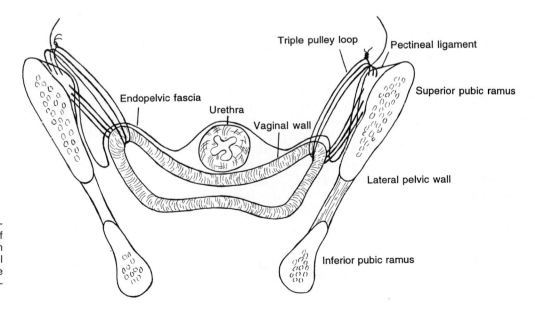

Figure 19–1. Schematic representation showing the triple loop of Prolene suture passing between the pectineal ligament and the full thickness of the vaginal wall. Note that the vaginal wall is pulled laterally toward the lateral pelvic wall.

- A lateral vector of the vaginal wall sutures that places the vaginal wall against the lateral pelvic wall, giving direct tissue apposition and allowing a firm scar attachment of the vaginal wall to the lateral pelvic wall.

The laparoscopic approach is used not just as a minimally invasive approach, but as an opportunity to incorporate a whole philosophy in the surgical management of SUI. It therefore represents a modern version of the classic Burch procedure.

PREOPERATIVE EVALUATION

The patient should be assessed clinically, and urodynamically if necessary, to ensure that she has an anatomically genuine SUI. An intrinsic or type III incontinence is a contraindication. Grades 1 and 2 cystocele will be corrected by the procedure, but a grade 3 cystocele will need additional vaginal surgery. Previous retropubic surgery such as an MMK or Burch procedure may make the extraperitoneal approach difficult. Previous abdominal or vaginal hysterectomy is not a contraindication. A urine culture should be obtained and appropriate antibiotics given if necessary. A cystoscopy should be performed either before or at the time of surgery to exclude any complicating bladder pathology. Preoperative antibiotics are given, e.g., metronidazole for anaerobic bacteria, and either an aminoglycoside or a cephalosporin. It is not necessary to cross-match blood.

Consent should be obtained that recognizes the following factors:

- This is a relatively new procedure for which there is limited follow-up, although it uses a standard surgical method of treatment of SUI.
- There are complications specific to laparoscopic surgery that do not occur in other procedures.
- There are complications specific to insufflation with CO_2.
- It may not be possible to complete the surgery laparoscopically, and the procedure may have to be converted to either an open or some other minimally invasive procedure.

Patients should be specifically warned that they will be given a suprapubic tube, that there may be difficulty voiding postoperatively, and that it may be necessary for them to go home with the suprapubic tube or self-catheterize for a period. They should also be advised that there may be some pain from the laparoscopic ports for a short time postoperatively, and that any preexisting urgency may be made worse for a time after surgery. Also, as this is a procedure to treat stress incontinence specifically, an associated

prolapse may not be fully reduced and an enterocele may ensue.

OPERATIVE TECHNIQUE

The procedure is carried out under general, spinal, or epidural anesthesia. The patient is placed in the low lithotomy position and the abdomen, perineum, and vagina are shaved, prepared with povidone-iodine (Betadine), and draped leaving access to the vagina. A 16 Fr. Foley catheter is passed and the balloon inflated. The labia are sutured laterally to facilitate hand access to the vagina. The surgeon stands on the patient's left side, with the assistant and scrub nurse on the right side. Two monitors are placed, one at each foot, with the insufflator at the patient's right foot so it can be easily seen by the surgeon. The diathermy machine is best located behind the surgeon. A laparoscopic sucker and irrigator should be available. A horizontal 2-cm incision is made at the lower border of the umbilicus and deepened to the rectus fascia (Fig. 19–2). A vertical 2-cm incision just large enough to take an index finger is made in the anterior rectus fascia and deepened to the posterior rectus fascia. An index finger is inserted and a space created between the rectus muscle and the posterior rectus fascia. An extraperitoneal balloon dissector is inserted into the space created. This may be made by cutting the middle finger off a No. 8½ glove and tying it onto the end of a Foley catheter. This is inflated with 1 L of saline by connecting it via a standard irrigation set to a bag of saline. This may run under gravity only or may require a pressure cuff. Alternatively, a commercial device such as an Origin or a Spacemaker balloon may be used. The Origin balloon is inflated with air to a maximum volume of 600 ml (30 pumps) under direct vision using the laparoscope telescope, which allows the space to be observed as it is created. It is very quick to use but is an added expense, and if it ruptures, it theoretically could cause a tear in the peritoneum. This has not been a problem to date, however. The balloon dilation is repeated once or twice until the retropubic space has been dissected. Great care should be taken to avoid causing a tear in the peritoneum, which would produce a pneumoperitoneum and lead to loss of the retropubic space.

If the patient has had previous abdominal surgery such as an abdominal hysterectomy, it will be necessary to avoid the scar by placing the initial incision below it. This may reduce access to the pectineal ligaments and limit space for the working ports, but it is necessary if extraperitoneal access is desired. The alternative is to go transperitoneal. This may entail division of intraperitoneal adhesions. The ret-

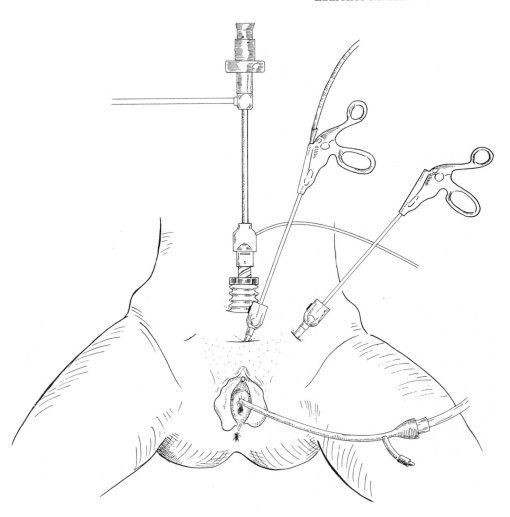

Figure 19–2. An incision 2 cm long is made just below the umbilicus and deepened to the anterior rectus fascia, which is incised. The rectus muscle is retracted and a space is made between the posterior sheath of rectus and the rectus muscle. A catheter, with the finger of a glove tied on the end, is introduced into the extraperitoneal space. It is inflated with 1000 ml saline via an irrigation set, connected to a bag of saline, and pressurized with an anesthetic pressure cuff. The balloon is introduced between the anterior and posterior sheaths of rectus, behind the rectus muscle. This procedure is repeated until the retropubic space is dilated. Alternatively a commercial balloon (Origin, Medsystems Inc., CA) may be used, with the dilation carried out under vision.

ropubic space is entered by dividing the peritoneum transversely above and lateral to the bladder, between the left and right medial umbilical ligaments. Care should be taken not to inadvertently enter the bladder, which should be filled with 300 ml of water to clearly identify it.

If the patient has had previous retropubic surgery such as an MMK vesicourethral suspension, the initial incision should be made just above the symphysis, so that the retropubic space can be created with the index finger. This may necessitate placing a second 10-mm port for the telescope toward the umbilicus to allow visualization of the pectineal ligaments.

A figure-of-eight suture of polyglycolic acid is placed at the upper and lower end of the incision in the rectus fascia, but not tied. A Hasson cannula is sutured into the extraperitoneal space, the space is inflated with CO_2 at 12 to 15 mm Hg, and the telescope is inserted (Fig. 19–3). Two 5-mm working ports are placed under vision, one in the middle halfway between the pubis and the umbilicus, and the other midway between the anterosuperior iliac spine and the umbilicus, taking care to avoid the

inferior epigastric vessels. The space is inspected and the landmarks of the symphysis pubis, superior pubic ramus and bladder containing the Foley catheter, and balloon, are identified. This is assisted by pushing up on the balloon with a hand in the vagina.

A pair of diathermy laparoscopic scissors are placed through the midline port with the diathermy connected to them, and a pair of laparoscopic dissectors are placed through the left lateral port. The transversus fascia is incised, and the urethra and vaginal wall are dissected down to the pelvic floor. This is facilitated by placing the left hand in the vagina and pushing up the vaginal wall. The tips of the scissors may be felt, giving a tactile third dimension. The bladder is filled with 200 ml of water to aid in its identification. The urethra is identified by palpation. The vaginal wall should be cleaned until it is clearly identified. The pectineal ligaments are identified as thick, glistening structures along the margin of the superior pubic ramus. They are cleaned of overlying tissue to expose them clearly. The lacunar ligament and the medial end of the inguinal ligament are also identified and cleaned. The external

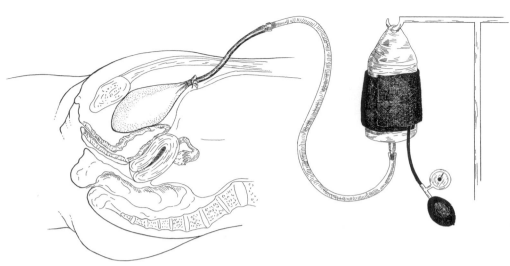

Figure 19–3. A Hasson cannula is sewn into the incision and two 5-mm working ports are placed, one midway between the umbilicus and the symphysis and one in the left iliac fossa. The vaginal wall, symphysis, and lacunar and pectineal ligaments are dissected and the margin of the bladder is identified.

iliac vein and artery are seen laterally as they pass over the pectineal ligaments and deep to the inguinal ligament.

A Stamey needle is loaded with heavy Prolene and a site on the right side chosen for its insertion. This should be about 1 cm above the pectineal ligament just medial to the iliac vein, avoiding the inferior epigastric vessels. A stab incision is made with a No. 15 blade and the Stamey needle passed into the extraperitoneal space (Fig. 19–4). The vaginal wall is pushed up with a finger and the Stamey needle pushed through into the vagina. The initial site should be lateral to the urethra, which is identified by palpation, and distal to the bladder neck. The Prolene suture is retrieved from the needle in the vagina (Fig. 19–5). The needle is then withdrawn into the space almost to the anterior abdominal wall,

taking great care not to withdraw it fully from the abdomen. It is then passed deep to the lacunar ligament, making sure a good bite is obtained (Fig. 19–6). The needle is passed through the vaginal wall again as lateral as possible to the first passage, loaded with the Prolene suture, and withdrawn through the lacunar ligament, but again not fully from the abdomen (Fig. 19–7). The loaded needle is passed through the vaginal wall just proximal to the first suture passage and the procedure repeated, passing the needle through the pectineal ligament, making sure a good bite is obtained by skating the needle along the surface of the superior pubic ramus. A third pass is made, passing the needle more lateral still through the pectineal ligament, giving three full loops of Prolene passing around the pectineal ligament and full thickness through the vaginal wall (Fig. 19–8). The

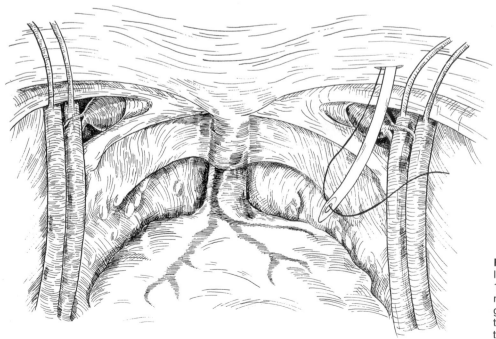

Figure 19–4. The Stamey needle, loaded with heavy Prolene, is brought in 1 cm above the pectineal ligament, just medial to the external iliac vein. The vaginal wall is pushed up with a finger and the needle is pushed through lateral to the urethra, which is easily palpated.

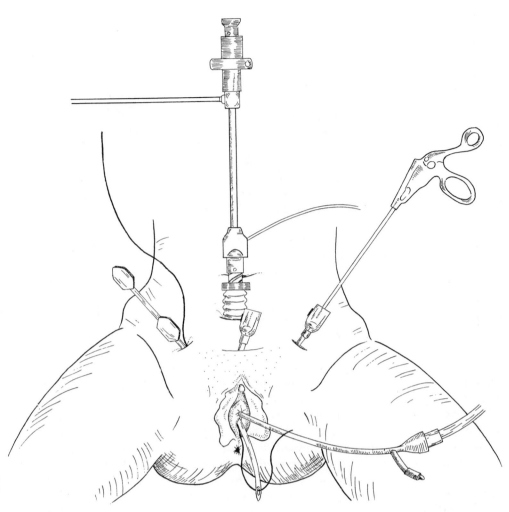

Figure 19–5. The Stamey needle is advanced out of the introitus and the Prolene suture is retrieved.

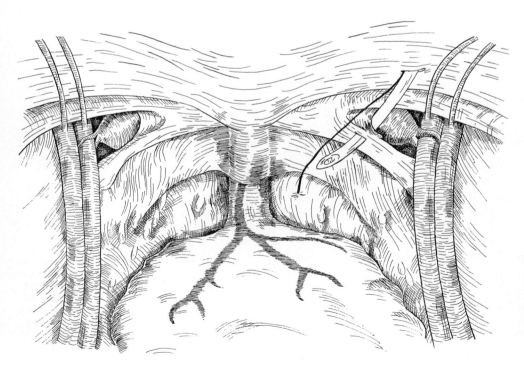

Figure 19–6. The Stamey needle is withdrawn into the retroperitoneal space but not fully from the abdomen. It is passed deep to the lacunar ligament, through the pectineal ligament, and again through the vaginal wall as lateral as possible to obtain as wide a bite as feasible.

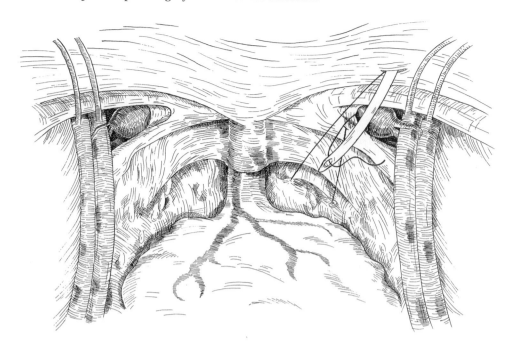

Figure 19–7. The Prolene suture is loaded on the needle in the vagina, and the needle is withdrawn through the pectineal ligament but again not fully from the abdomen. It is passed through the vaginal wall just lateral to the urethra, proximal to the first suture.

Prolene suture quickly buries into the vaginal mucosa, as demonstrated by Gittes and Loughlin.[17]

The Stamey needle is used in a sewing machine manner to place the suture. It is critical that the needle not be accidentally removed from the abdomen; it should ultimately be removed via by same hole through which it was introduced. During passage of the needle through the vaginal wall, the bladder should be clearly visualized. There is often some bleeding from the vaginal wall, which may obscure the view. It is best to place a sucker on the vaginal wall and use this to retract the fluid-filled bladder, so

as to provide adequate vision. Should the needle traverse the bladder at the bladder neck, some fluid will escape, allowing the needle to be removed without ill effect. Alternatively, some blood will be seen in the fluid draining from the urethral catheter. If any doubt exists over whether the needle has passed into the bladder or not, the patient should be panendoscoped.

Finally the Stamey needle is removed, withdrawing the Prolene suture from the abdomen. To determine the correct position of the bladder neck, the suture is pulled up and the bladder neck allowed to

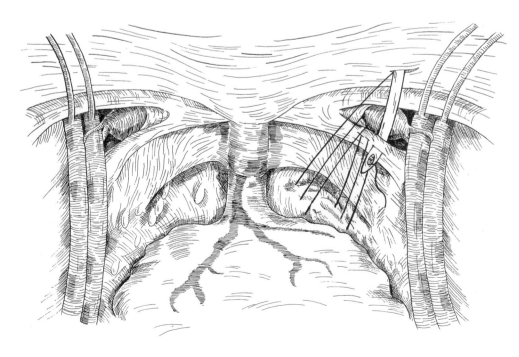

Figure 19–8. The suture is again retrieved from the needle and the same procedure is repeated, using the needle in a sewing machine manner, passing it alternately deep and superficial to the pectineal ligament, and through the vaginal wall into the vagina, until a total of three full loops have been placed, spaced along the pectineal ligament.

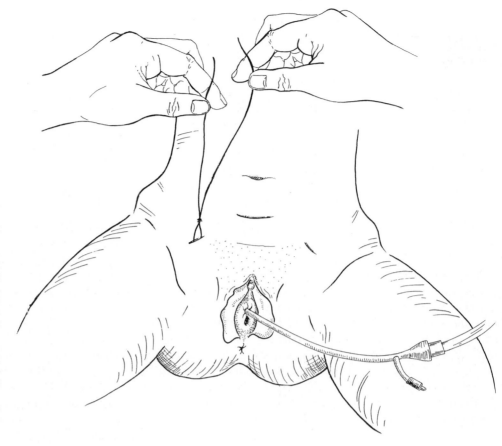

Figure 19–9. The Stamey needle is fully withdrawn from the abdomen through the same hole into which it was originally introduced. The suture is pulled up and the vaginal wall is watched as it is allowed to sink back to its rest position. This is the correct position in which to tie the suture. A single knot is tied in the suture and allowed to pull down onto the pectineal ligament. If there is slack, the knot should be tightened up a little further. If there is no slack, the suture should be pulled up and the knot completed with a further three or four throws, under vision. Care should be taken that the knot is not tightened up further, which would increase the tension. It is essential that the end result be "no slack and no tension."

return to the rest position (Fig. 19–9). A single-throw surgeon's knot is tied and allowed to pull down onto the pectineal ligament. If there is slack, the knot should be tightened up a little further until there is no slack. The bladder neck should be fixed at the point at which it just returns to the rest position after

being pulled up. The knot is then completed under vision and allowed to pull down to sit on the pectineal ligament permanently (Fig. 19–10). It is essential that there be no tension in the suture to avoid postoperative voiding problems. The correct tension is "no slack and no tension."

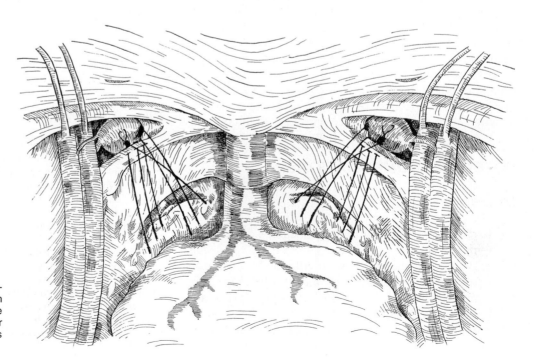

Figure 19–10. Finally the completed knot is allowed to pull down onto the pectineal ligament. The procedure is repeated on the other side and a suprapubic tube is placed.

The triple pulley provides a number of advantages:

- Three bites of the vaginal wall are necessary to prevent cut-through of the suture in the short term.
- The continuous suture spreads the load equally across all three sutures when the patient coughs or strains, and so the suture is less likely to break or cut through.
- The pulley effect allows precise control over the position of the bladder neck. It is, however, a very powerful mechanism, and care should be taken not to pull the bladder neck up to the pectineal ligament, as described by Burch, unless a significant cystocele is present and this can be done without tension.

The procedure is repeated on the left side and a suprapubic tube placed under direct vision after filling the bladder with water. The ports are removed and the rectus fascia is closed with interrupted sutures. If the patient is obese and there has been significant oozing of blood, a suction drain is placed to prevent hematoma formation, which has been a complication under these circumstances. The urethral catheter is removed and the suprapubic tube placed on free drainage.

POSTOPERATIVE MANAGEMENT

Narcotic analgesics may be required for the first 24 hours and parenteral antibiotics are continued for 24 hours, or longer if a fever occurs. The suprapubic tube is clamped on the first postoperative day, and twice-daily residual urine measurements are made until the patient is voiding with residuals of less than 200 ml, when the suprapubic tube is removed. This is usually on the second postoperative day. Most patients void on the first postoperative day, but if they do not they may be sent home with the suprapubic tube, or taught to self-catheterize. Patients may be discharged on the first or second postoperative day, or when they are voiding and ready for discharge.

POTENTIAL COMPLICATIONS

Operative

- Perforation of the bladder with the needle is dealt with above.
- A peritoneal tear may occur during the dilation and allow a pneumoperitoneum to develop. This results in loss of the space, making progress difficult or impossible. If the tear can be seen, it may be closed with clips. The pneumoperitoneum may be decompressed by placing a Veress

needle into the peritoneal cavity, or even a port if necessary.
- The CO_2 may track up to the mediastinum and rupture through into the pleural cavity, creating a tension pneumothorax. This requires immediate drainage and may necessitate termination of the procedure.
- Subcutaneous emphysema may occur but does not require treatment.

Postoperative

- A wound hematoma may occur, particularly in obese patients, and may become infected. A suction drain should be placed if there is considerable bleeding.
- Bleeding may occur into the retropubic space from any small vessels that continue to ooze. Great care should be taken to ensure hemostasis, particularly of the bladder wall.
- Wound infection may occur. Perioperative antibiotics should be used to minimize this possibility.
- Failure to void is a common problem with bladder neck suspension and colposuspension procedures. A suprapubic tube should be placed to facilitate management of this problem. Alternatively, intermittent self-catheterization may be necessary.
- An enterocele or rectocele may be exacerbated by the repair of a cystocele.

Summary

This procedure uses a minimally invasive approach to achieve a Burch procedure by a simple laparoscopic technique. The results to date are very satisfactory and offer good results, with a short hospital stay and a low incidence of voiding problems.

Editorial Comment
Louis R. Kavoussi

Just as there are a multitude of open surgical procedures to treat true urinary stress incontinence, a variety of laparoscopic procedures have recently been developed. The technique described in this chapter is ideal for those with limited laparoscopic experience, as it avoids the need for the technically demanding task of intracorporeal suture tying.

I would caution the reader to maintain a perspective when considering a patient as a candidate for a laparoscopic urethropexy. Although several laparoscopic applications have documented benefits over their traditional open counterparts, the advantages of the laparoscopic bladder suspensions have yet to be proved superior. Long-term follow-up is needed to assess their place in the urological armamentarium.

Editorial Comment

Fray F. Marshall

The laparoscopic approach to stress incontinence is described. It really is a variant of some of the other suspension procedures. This kind of repair can potentially be done without laparoscopy, although laparoscopy provides visualization of suture placement. It may be possible to make a small retroperitoneal suprapubic incision and perform this operation without an intraperitoneal or laparoscopic retroperitoneal approach. Better instrumentation for suturing will allow more standard operating room technique for laparoscopic surgery.

REFERENCES

1. Burch JC. Urethrovaginal fixation to Cooper's ligament for correction of stress incontinence, cystocele, and prolapse. Am J Obstet Gynecol 81:281, 1961.
2. Marshall VF, Marchetti AA, Kranz KE. The correction of stress incontinence by simple vesicourethral suspension. Surg Gynecol Obstet 88:509, 1949.
3. Stamey TA. Endoscopic suspension of the vesical neck for urinary incontinence. Surg Gynecol Obstet 136:547, 1973.
4. Raz S. Modified bladder neck suspension for female stress incontinence. Urology 17:82, 1981.
5. Lam TC, Hadley HR. Surgical procedures for uncomplicated female stress incontinence. Urol Clin North Am 18:327, 1991.
6. Vancaillie TG, Schuessler W. Laparoscopic bladderneck suspension. J Laparoendosc Surg 1:169, 1991.
7. Albala DM, Schuessler W, Vancaillie TG. Laparoscopic bladder neck suspension. J Endourol 6:137, 1992.
8. Liu CY. Laparoscopic retropubic colposuspension (Burch procedure). A review of 58 cases. J Reprod Med 38:526, 1993.
9. McDougall EM, Klutke CG, Clayman RV, et al. Comparative analysis of vaginal (Raz) and laparoscopic bladder neck suspension for type I or II stress urinary incontinence (abstract 1085). J Urol 151:499A, 1994.
10. Harewood LM. Laparoscopic needle colposuspension for genuine stress incontinence. J Endourol 7:319, 1993.
11. Ou CS, Presthus J, Beadle E. Laparoscopic bladder neck suspension using hernia mesh and surgical staples. J Laparoendosc Surg 3:563, 1993.
12. Chapple CR, Osborne JL. Laparoscopic colposuspension—a new procedure. Min Inv Ther 2:59, 1993.
13. Raboy A, Hakim LS, Ferzli G, et al. Extraperitoneal endoscopic vesicourethral suspension. J Laparoendosc Surg 3:505, 1993.
14. Riza ED, Deshmukh MD. A laparoscopic-assisted extraperitoneal bladder neck suspension: An initial experience. J Laparoendoscopic Surg 4:319, 1994.
15. Gaur DD. Laparoscopic operative retroperitoneoscopy: Use of a new device. J Urol 148:1137, 1992.
16. Knapp PM, Siegel YI, Lingeman JE. Laparoscopic retroperitoneal needle suspension urethropexy. J Endourol 8:279, 1994.
17. Gittes RF, Loughlin KR. No-incision pubovaginal suspension for stress incontinence. J Urol 138:568, 1987.

Chapter 20

Laparoscopic Retroperitoneal Lymphadenectomy for Carcinoma of the Testis

Glenn S. Gerber and Daniel B. Rukstalis

Laparoscopic retroperitoneal lymph node dissection (lap RPLND) is a new, investigative procedure that has been reported in only a few patients.[1-3] The role of this technique in men with testicular cancer has not been well defined, but it appears that lap RPLND should currently be considered an extension of the staging evaluation in patients with clinical stage 1 nonseminomatous germ cell tumors. In particular, men with a limited likelihood of harboring metastases in the retroperitoneal lymph nodes may be the most appropriate candidates for lap RPLND. Criteria that suggest the absence of occult stage 2 disease include the lack of vascular or lymphatic invasion in the primary tumor, a limited T stage, the presence of yolk sac and seminomatous elements, and the absence of embryonal cell carcinoma.

PREOPERATIVE EVALUATION

Preoperative evaluation of patients facing lap RPLND should include a complete staging work-up of the testicular malignancy consisting of abdominal and thoracic radiographic studies as well as appropriate serum marker measurements. In general, lap RPLND should be considered only in patients who show no evidence of metastatic disease. In addition, as is true for any transperitoneal laparoscopic procedure, a history of multiple abdominal surgeries, previous episodes of peritonitis, or significant obesity may also be contraindications to lap RPLND. Since most patients with nonseminomatous testicular tumors are young and otherwise healthy, they are usually excellent candidates for a laparoscopic approach to the retroperitoneal lymph nodes.

Patients who are to undergo lap RPLND should have a complete mechanical bowel preparation consisting of oral laxatives and antibiotics. This allows for decompression of the small intestine and also minimizes the risk of complications in the event of an inadvertent bowel injury. Patients should also consider preoperative autologous blood donation, since the risk of significant bleeding appears to be greater with lap RPLND than with a standard open node dissection.[3] Finally, appropriate counseling should be given regarding the experimental nature of lap RPLND as well as the potential risks and benefits.

OPERATIVE TECHNIQUE

Lap RPLND is performed with the patient in a torque position with the ipsilateral side rotated approximately 35 degrees off the table and the pelvis remaining flat (Fig. 20–1). The ipsilateral arm is draped across the chest and suspended on a portable stand or fixed support. Since the operating table will be rotated during the course of the procedure, the patient should be carefully secured to it to prevent injury. A nasogastric tube and Foley catheter are placed before insertion of any laparoscopic instruments to reduce the risk of injury to the stomach and bladder, respectively. As with any laparoscopic procedure, a laparotomy tray should be immediately available in the event of an emergency.

The pneumoperitoneum may be established using a closed (Veress needle) or open (Hasson trocar) technique, most commonly through a small infraumbilical incision. A 10-mm trocar with working sheath is inserted through this site after an intra-abdominal

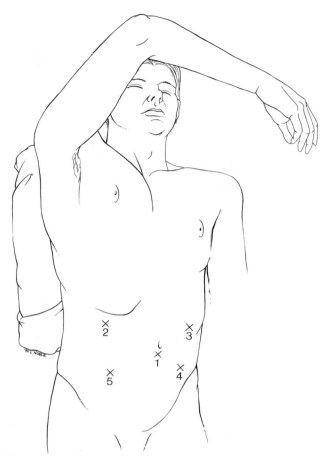

Figure 20–1. Modified right torque position used in patients undergoing right laparoscopic retroperitoneal lymph node dissection.

pressure of 14 mm Hg is achieved. This pressure is maintained throughout the procedure. A 10-mm endoscope with a 0- or 30-degree lens is then inserted. An additional three or four laparoscopic ports are then placed under direct vision as shown in Figure 20–1. For purposes of discussion, the ports will be referred to by the numbers that appear in Figure

20–1. In patients with a right-sided primary testicular tumor, port 4 is optional, although it may be useful at certain points in the procedure as discussed below. It is best to use trocars no smaller than 10 mm at all sites, since this allows for maximal flexibility in moving the endoscope and larger instruments to different ports. In general, a single 12-mm trocar is used at port 5, because there are occasions when a trocar of this size is needed for placement of large grasping forceps or other instruments. After all five laparoscopic ports are placed, the operating table is rolled toward the surgeon, who stands on the contralateral side (right side elevated in a right-sided lap RPLND). If three persons are performing the procedure, the first assistant also stands on the contralateral side of the table, and the second stands on the ipsilateral side and holds the endoscope, which is repositioned through port 2 after trocar placement. The surgeon generally uses instruments placed through ports 1 and 5 and the assistant utilizes ports 3 and 4. If only two surgeons are present, the assistant maintains the endoscope and an instrument in port 3. The surgeon continues to operate from the opposite side of the table using ports 1 and 5. These are only general guidelines, however, and it is important to alternate operating ports, depending on intraoperative assessment of the most appropriate method to perform the dissection.

The limits of a modified retroperitoneal lymphadenectomy are shown in Figure 20–2 and include the renal hilum superiorly, the ureter laterally, the medial aspect of the vena cava or aorta medially (left and right dissection, respectively), and the level of the origin of the inferior mesenteric artery inferiorly. On the ipsilateral side of the dissection, nodal tissue is removed down to the bifurcation of the common iliac vessels, and the stump of the spermatic cord is excised. It should be emphasized that the interaortoca-

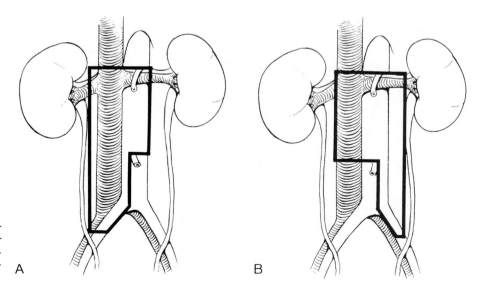

Figure 20–2. Templates for right- and left-sided modified retroperitoneal lymphadenectomy. (From Capelouto CC, Kavoussi LR. Laparoendoscopic surgery of the genital tract. Atlas Urol Clin North Am 1:98, 1993.)

A   B

val nodes are removed while the retrocaval and retroaortic nodes are generally not sampled.

After placement of all operative ports, the endoscope is moved to port 2 and is maintained by the second assistant. The first assistant places a blunt grasping instrument (an endoscopic Babcock clamp) through port 3 or 4 and uses this to pull the right colon toward the left side of the abdomen. The surgeon places a grasping forceps through port 5 and endoscopic scissors through port 1. The first assistant also uses grasping forceps through port 3 or 4. An incision is made lateral to the right colon along the white line of Toldt, and extended inferiorly and superiorly as the bowel is retracted medially (Fig. 20–3). As the right colon is rolled toward the midline, it is important to avoid injury to the undersurface of the colonic mesentery, right ureter, and iliac and gonadal vessels as these structures come into view. It is vital to identify the ureter in order both to define the landmarks for the dissection and to avoid injury to this structure.

Once the colon has been adequately mobilized, the scissors are exchanged for grasping forceps, and blunt dissection is used to identify and free the vascular structures. In some cases, it is necessary for the assistant to continue to retract the colon using an endoscopic Babcock clamp to prevent the operative field from becoming obscured. If active retraction of the colon is not needed, the assistant may use an additional grasping forceps to aid in the dissection. After the ureter is identified, it is traced toward the kidney

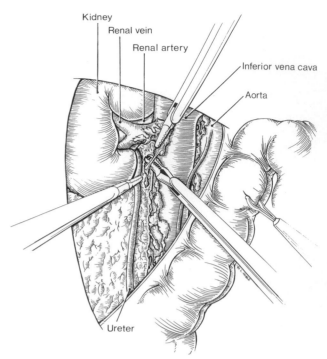

Figure 20–4. Nodal tissue bluntly dissected in the area overlying and adjacent to the IVC.

until the right renal vein comes into view. The inferior and anterior surfaces of the vein are bluntly dissected until the junction with the inferior vena cava (IVC) is noted. The nodal tissue between the ureter and IVC is then removed using blunt dissection (Fig. 20–4). Small lymphatic channels are controlled using electrocautery, and larger pedicles are ligated with an endoscopic clip applier. This dissection is carried out overlying the IVC and is extended inferiorly to the level of the common iliac vessels. The ureter is identified and is also dissected free to this level, with great care taken not to injure this structure. Alternatively, the dissection may be initiated inferiorly along the IVC and then extended superiorly with removal of nodal tissue until the right renal vein is noted.

The dissection is continued by removing the interaortocaval nodes, beginning at the level of the renal hilum (Fig. 20–5). The aorta and IVC are gently retracted laterally using grasping forceps, and blunt dissection is used to free the tissue until the anterior longitudinal (spincus) ligament is clearly visualized. Great care should be taken to avoid injury to an accessory lower pole renal artery, which may be encountered at this position. The interaortocaval nodal tissue is removed to the level of the origin of the inferior mesenteric artery. Lumbar vessels are clipped to prevent tearing and resultant hemorrhage, which may be difficult to control (Fig. 20–6). After the node dissection is completed, the stump of the spermatic cord is excised. The ipsilateral gonadal vessels are generally clipped and ligated during the course of the

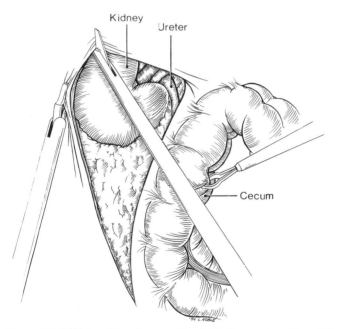

Figure 20–3. Sharp dissection used to divide tissue along the white line of Toldt lateral to the right colon, which is then rolled medially, exposing the ureter and the lateral border of the inferior vena cava (IVC).

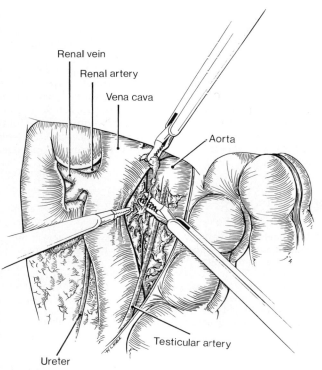

Figure 20–5. Interaortocaval nodes being removed using blunt dissection.

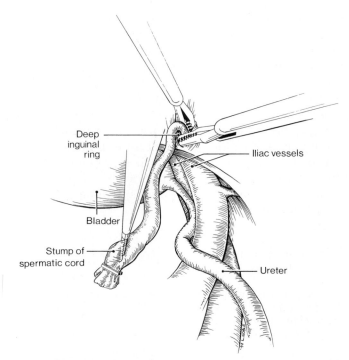

Figure 20–7. Gentle retraction on the stump of the spermatic cord maintained by an assistant as tissue is dissected at the internal inguinal ring to allow removal of the cord remnant.

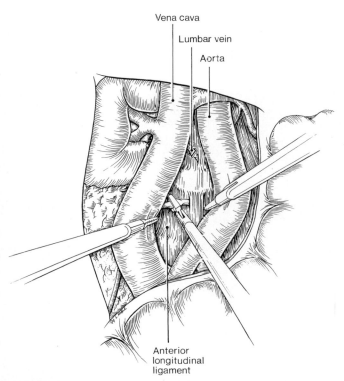

Figure 20–6. Interaortocaval dissection nearly completed with clips noted on the lumbar vein, and the anterior spinous ligament readily visible.

node dissection. The proximal cut ends of the vessels are gently lifted by the assistant as the surgeon uses sharp and blunt dissection in and around the internal inguinal ring until the remnant of the cord is removed (Fig. 20–7). The nodal tissue and excised spermatic cord are then easily removed from the abdomen with grasping forceps.

After completion of the procedure, the bowel is carefully inspected for injury. Intra-abdominal pressure is then lowered to 5 mm Hg to help visualize any sites of venous bleeding. The laparoscopic ports are then removed under direct vision after the pneumoperitoneum has been completely evacuated. The wounds in the anterior abdominal wall are closed with 2-0 absorbable suture on the fascial layer and 4-0 suture for skin reapproximation. The patient is extubated and the nasogastric tube removed.

POSTOPERATIVE CARE

The hematocrit should be evaluated frequently during the first 24 hours postoperatively. Once the patient is ambulatory and close monitoring of urinary output is no longer necessary, the urethral catheter may be removed. A liquid diet may be initiated when there is evidence of return of bowel function, and rapid advancement to a general diet is usually possible. The median length of hospitalization is approximately 3 days, and most men can expect to return to normal activity levels within 2 to 3 weeks.[3] In addition to hemorrhage, other significant complications include a previously undetected bowel injury that may present with unexplained fever, gastrointestinal symptoms, and abdominal tenderness. Delayed bowel perforation may be secondary to injudicious use of the electrocautery, and a high index of suspicion for such an intestinal injury should be maintained in the perioperative period.

Editorial Comment

Louis R. Kavoussi

This group has demonstrated the feasibility of laparoscopic retroperitoneal lymphadenectomy. This procedure is much more technically demanding than the pelvic lymphadenectomy for prostate cancer and should be attempted only by an experienced laparoscopist. Preliminary studies have demonstrated that an equivalent number of nodes can be obtained with less morbidity than with an open node dissection.

One must bear in mind that an open lymphadenectomy performed in patients with localized disease can be curative. Long-term data in patients undergoing laparoscopic lymphadenectomy are not yet available. Until such data are collected, laparoscopic retroperitoneal lymphadenectomy should be considered only a diagnostic procedure. Patients found to have positive nodes should receive postoperative chemotherapy.

REFERENCES

1. Rukstalis DB, Chodak GW. Laparoscopic retroperitoneal lymph node dissection in a patient with stage 1 testicular carcinoma. J Urol 148:1907, 1992.
2. Hulbert JC, Fraley EE. Laparoscopic retroperitoneal lymphadenectomy: New approach to pathologic staging of clinical stage 1 germ cell tumors of the testis. J Endourol 61:123, 1992.
3. Gerber GS, Bissada NK, Hulbert JC, et al. Laparoscopic retroperitoneal lymphadenectomy: Multi-institutional analysis. J Urol 152:1188, 1994.

Chapter 21

Laparoscopic Adrenalectomy

David M. Albala

During the past three decades, accurate diagnosis, precise radiological localization, satisfactory preoperative medical management, appropriate anesthesia, and refined surgical techniques have combined to make surgical management of adrenal abnormalities a safe endeavor with a predictable outcome. Now, the diagnosis and management of disorders of the adrenal gland are among the most challenging and satisfying aspects of general surgical and urological practice.

Laparoscopic surgery has gained increased popularity in the treatment of urological diseases because of its minimal invasiveness and low morbidity.[1, 2] Some events in the recent history of urological laparoscopy have included the localization of undescended testicles in the 1970s and 1980s, with more advanced procedures such as pelvic lymphadenectomy, varix ligation, and nephrectomy gaining interest in the early 1990s. The current applications of laparoscopic adrenalectomy are reviewed in this chapter.

PREOPERATIVE EVALUATION

There is little disagreement that conventional surgical techniques should be used in patients with large (greater than 6-cm) functioning adrenal neoplasms. However, smaller functioning and nonfunctioning masses may be treated with minimally invasive laparoscopic methods that allow their removal. Medical opinion about nonfunctioning tumors is not unanimous since less is known about their natural history. The number of these tumors that have been removed surgically has increased in the 1990s, mainly because of serendipitous detection by computed tomography (CT). CT has similarly contributed to the incidental detection of adrenal cysts, adenomas, and hematomas. Whether small, nonfunctioning tumors should be surgically removed or not is unclear. The current indications for laparoscopic adrenalectomy include nonfunctioning adenomas that are increasing in size or suspected of causing local symptoms, pheochromocytoma, Cushing adenoma, aldosteronomas, angiomyelipomas, and medullary cysts of the adrenal gland.

Laparoscopy should be avoided in patients at high risk for bowel injury and in those who have medical disorders that may be exacerbated by the pneumoperitoneum. This includes patients with a history of peritonitis, sepsis, extensive adhesions from multiple previous surgical procedures, morbid obesity, mechanical and functional bowel obstruction, large intra-abdominal masses, uncorrected coagulopathy, severe cardiopulmonary disease, or hypovolemic shock.

The preoperative management of hormone-producing adrenal tumors is the same as for open surgical adrenalectomy. In patients with pheochromocytoma, blood pressure should be controlled by alpha-adrenergic blockade. In selected patients, beta blockage may be used to help control arrhythmias only after alpha blockage has been established. Patients with primary hyperaldosteronism should be given spironolactone 2 to 3 weeks before surgery. In these patients, potassium levels and blood pressures should be followed. Control of glucose abnormalities as well as glucocorticoid replacement may be necessary in patients with Cushing syndrome.

All patients require full mechanical and antibiotic bowel preparation. This helps decompress the intestines to increase exposure during dissection, and it also allows for conservative repair if inadvertent bowel injury occurs during the procedure. Patients are given broad-spectrum antibiotics before the procedure, and all are typed and cross-matched for 3 units of blood. The management of adrenal disorders calls for a team approach, including experienced endocrinologists, radiologists, anesthesiologists, and urologists or general surgeons.

OPERATIVE TECHNIQUE

A general endotracheal anesthetic is advised for laparoscopic adrenalectomy. Controlled ventilation is necessary to ensure adequate oxygenation and to avoid hypercapnia. Nitrous oxide may cause bowel distention and should be avoided during this procedure. A nasogastric tube is placed to keep the stomach and bowel decompressed, and a Foley catheter is positioned to allow drainage of the bladder before initiating the pneumoperitoneum. Patients are placed in a lateral decubitus position for carbon dioxide (CO_2) insufflation, which is initiated in the subcostal area with a Veress needle. The abdomen is distended to 15 mm Hg pressure.

Left Laparoscopic Adrenalectomy

After adequate insufflation of the abdomen, a 10/11-mm trocar is inserted in the left subcostal area at the level of the anterior axillary line. A 30-degree laparoscope is then inserted through this trocar. Three additional 10/11-mm trocars are inserted under direct vision in the flank (under the twelfth rib) and dorsally (Fig. 21–1). The splenic flexure of the colon is incised with endoscopic scissors to open the retroperitoneal space between the spleen and the lateral portion of the abdominal wall. The patient may also be placed in the Fowler position to permit downward migration of the bowel loops and peritoneal fluid. The upper pole of the left kidney is identified and exposed by freeing the posterolateral attachments of the spleen in the direction of the diaphragm (Fig. 21–2A). The spleen is retracted medially and superiorly with a fan or balloon retractor. This maneuver exposes the adrenal gland and allows the dissection to begin in the correct plane.

The superior aspect of the adrenal gland is dissected first, with the dissection carried medially. Dissection of the inferior portion of the gland should be done last; starting here will lead to retraction of the superior gland and cause unnecessary bleeding. The inferior phrenic arterial branches are ligated with titanium clips after mobilization of the superior pole of the gland. The left adrenal vein is then visualized, dissected free, and ligated with two laparoscopic clips. The inferior portion of the adrenal gland is dissected last, and then the gland is separated from the surrounding tissue. Hemostasis is obtained with an irrigation/aspiration device.

A small entrapment sack is placed through the medial trocar and opened with grasping forceps. The adrenal gland is placed in the entrapment sack under laparoscopic control. The bag is then removed through the most inferior trocar site with minimal spreading of the oblique muscles, using a Kelly clamp. All trocar sites require a fascial closure with 2-0 Vicryl suture before the skin is reapproximated and closed with 4-0 Vicryl.

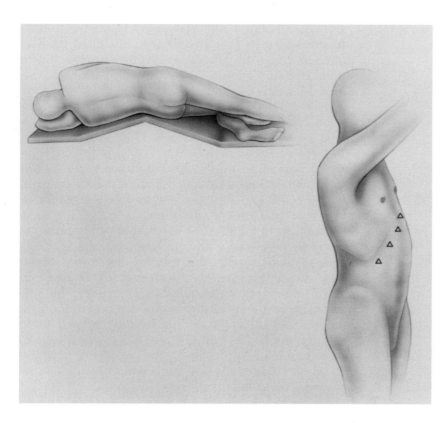

Figure 21–1. Placement of trocars for laparoscopic adrenalectomy. Four trocars are used and placed 2 cm below the costal margin.

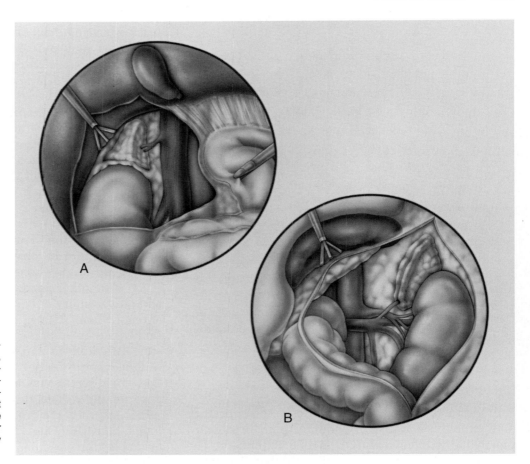

Figure 21–2. *A,* The peritoneal reflection is opened on the right side, exposing the adrenal gland and upper pole of the kidney. A fan retractor is used to elevate the liver superiorly and medially. *B,* The left adrenal gland and upper pole of the kidney are exposed. A fan retractor is used to lift the spleen superiorly and medially.

Right Laparoscopic Adrenalectomy

After adequate insufflation with a Veress needle, the entire abdomen should be tympanic after the pneumoperitoneum surrounds the liver. Care must be taken during lateral insufflation to avoid placement of the Veress needle into the liver parenchyma. A 10/11-mm trocar is inserted in the anterior axillary line and used for passage of the laparoscope. Two additional 10/11-mm trocars are inserted in the right flank under direct vision. The final 10/11-mm trocar is inserted dorsally after the retroperitoneal space has been entered and the kidney identified.

The right triangular ligament of the liver is dissected free with electrocautery scissors, exposing the inferior vena cava (IVC). A fan or balloon retractor is then placed underneath the liver and retracted superiorly and medially (Fig. 21–2B). The upper pole of the kidney is identified, and the perinephric fat is dissected superiorly and close to the IVC to expose the adrenal gland. The dissection begins at the superior and anterior aspect of the right adrenal gland. Small vessels are secured with laparoscopic clips, and a laparoscopic Kitner dissector is used on the medial aspect of the gland. Meticulous dissection

here will prevent tears of the lateral vascular branches of the IVC. The adrenal vein is identified and isolated, and two laparoscopic clips are placed here before the vein is divided between the clips (Fig. 21–3). The inferior pole of the adrenal gland is dissected last and an entrapment sack is used to remove the adrenal gland through the anterior axillary line trocar site. A 2-0 Vicryl suture is used to close the fascia at all trocar sites, and skin edges are reapproximated with 4-0 Vicryl suture.

POSTOPERATIVE MANAGEMENT

The nasogastric tube and Foley catheter may be removed in the recovery room. Sequential stockings are left in place until the patient is ambulatory. All fluids are begun on the day of surgery as tolerated. A parenteral broad-spectrum antibiotic is administered for 24 hours after surgery and an oral antibiotic preparation is given for 3 days. Oral analgesics are administered as needed, but postoperative pain is usually minimal. If a patient needs a significant amount of analgesic postoperatively, a postoperative complication may be suspected. Patients resume their regular

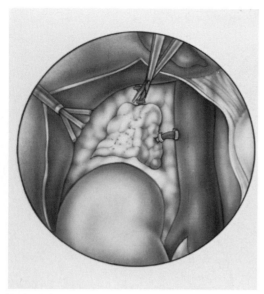

Figure 21–3. The right adrenal gland is first dissected superiorly and medially. Two hemoclips are placed on the adrenal vein before it is divided.

activities as tolerated. They should be told that they may experience transient shoulder pain because of the irritating effects of CO_2 on the diaphragm. The pain is usually described as arthralgic-like discomfort in one or both shoulders. This can usually be prevented by placing the patient in the Trendelenburg position and opening the most superior trocar before removal. The pain usually responds well to oral analgesics and/or anti-inflammatory medications and often resolves spontaneously 24 to 48 hours after surgery. Some adrenal conditions require hormonal support, which is begun in the immediate postoperative period.

POSTOPERATIVE COMPLICATIONS

The first step in minimizing the risk of complications after laparoscopic adrenalectomy is appropriate patient selection. Familiarity with the technical limitations of this procedure, together with an understanding of how intrinsic patient factors may influence the technique, lead to an appropriate matching of patient and procedure. Two points concerning the indications for laparoscopic adrenalectomy should be emphasized: (1) the size of the adrenal lesion and (2) the endocrine disorder of the patient being treated. Tumor size is an important factor in determining the malignant nature of an adrenal mass.[4] The laparoscopic approach for malignant adrenal disease is controversial, but most agree that tumors larger than 6 cm should not be removed in this fashion. Larger

masses have a notably higher risk for malignancy and should be removed via conventional open surgical techniques. Small adrenal lesions, however, are easily localized with laparoscopy because of the magnification effect of the laparoscope.

Insufflation for laparoscopic adrenalectomy is done with the patient in the flank position, shifting the intraperitoneal organs medially. Creation of the pneumoperitoneum in this position can be performed safely, but care should be taken during insufflation on the right to avoid Veress needle placement into the liver parenchyma. After adequate insufflation of the abdominal cavity is achieved, tympany should be noted around the liver. If adequate Veress needle position cannot be obtained in the flank position, a Hasson trocar may be used.

As with other laparoscopic procedures, vascular and bowel injury may occur during dissection of the adrenal gland. If any of these complications arise, immediate open surgical control and repair is necessary. Attempts at laparoscopic control of vascular injuries should be limited to relatively small vessels that are directly visible and accessible and do not pose an immediate threat to the patient's hemodynamic stability. Electrocautery, endoclips, and endoloops constitute the laparoscopic armamentarium available for vascular control. Unfortunately, the rapid accumulation of blood in dependent locations, together with the limited suction capability of the aspiration instruments, limits the attempts at laparoscopic repair to only the most accomplished laparoscopic surgeons.

Complaints of significant abdominal pain in the postoperative period should raise suspicion of an underlying injury. Rectus sheath hematoma may be suspected in any patient with a subcutaneous bulge who complains of severe abdominal pain.

Mechanical intestinal injury, unlike electrocautery injury, usually reveals itself within 48 hours after surgery as patients develop abdominal pain, fever, and signs of peritonitis. Immediate laparotomy is indicated with appropriate repair of the obstruction.

Summary

Laparoscopic adrenalectomy is an advanced procedure that is safe and effective but should be undertaken only by urologists with extensive laparoscopic experience. The transabdominal approach is used most frequently at present. However, as new instruments are developed, the retroperitoneal approach will become possible. Meticulous dissection will allow the adrenal gland to be removed without complication.

Editorial Comment

Louis R. Kavoussi

Several large series have demonstrated the efficacy of this surgical approach in patients with adrenal pathology, including patients with pheochromocytoma. Unlike open adrenalectomy, laparoscopic adrenalectomy is relatively easier to perform than nephrectomy. This procedure should be attempted only by urologists experienced in laparoscopic techniques. The magnification afforded by the laparoscope provides for controlled ligation of the short adrenal vein, while new automated suture devices allow for rapid repair in the event of a caval injury.

REFERENCES

1. McDougall EM, Clayman RV. Advances in laparoscopic urology. Part 1. History and development of procedures. Urology 43:420, 1994.
2. McDougall EM, Clayman RV. Advances in laparoscopic surgery. Part II. Innovations and future implications for urologic surgeons. Urology 43:585, 1994.
3. Hattery RR, Sheedy PF, Stephens DH, van Heerden JA. Computed tomography of the adrenal gland. Semin Roentgenol 16:290, 1981.
4. Aso Y, Homma Y. A survey of incidental adrenal tumors in Japan. J Urol 147:1478, 1992.

Part III

PEDIATRIC ENDOSCOPY AND LAPAROSCOPY

Chapter 22

Endoscopic Surgery in Children

Steven G. Docimo

Ureteroscopy and percutaneous nephroscopy were developed largely for the treatment of urinary calculus disease in the adult. Although considered the standard of care for adult patients with stones, endourological intervention has been adopted somewhat more gradually for children. The introduction of smaller endoscopes has allowed treatment of selected children with stone disease. Other indications for endourological manipulation in children are incision of a ureterocele; resection of posterior urethral valves; biopsy of bladder, ureteral, or renal lesions; treatment of vesicoureteral reflux (VUR); and treatment of ureteral obstruction or stricture. Many of these procedures are covered in other chapters and are only mentioned here.

ANATOMY

The initial obstacle to ureteroscopy in children is the size of the ureter. The average diameter of the distal ureter in a 3-year-old is 3 Fr., of the midureter 10 Fr., and of the ureteropelvic junction (UPJ) 4 Fr.[1] The diameter of the ureter increases with age. Between infancy and the age of 12 years the ureter increases in length from 10 to approximately 25 cm. The proximity of the uterine artery and the vas deferens must be considered, especially when incising distal ureteral strictures. These incisions should never be made anterolaterally because of possible injury to these structures.[2] The diameter of the ureter limits which endoscopes may be used to visualize the upper tract. Another limitation is the size of the urethra. The infant male urethra will generally accept a 9 Fr. endoscope but will only sometimes accept an 11 Fr. instrument. Potential injury and resultant

stricture of the male urethra must be considered when passage of endoscopic instruments appears difficult.

The ureters in children are less fixed in the retroperitoneum than in adults. The ureter is therefore somewhat more mobile and, although smaller, more easily distensible.[2] However, children who develop calculi often have congenitally abnormal ureters, or have undergone previous surgical intervention, which can greatly affect the anatomy and mobility of the ureter. Ureters that have been reimplanted for VUR may have a long intramural tunnel and may have been situated cross-trigonally, making transurethral access difficult.[3] The possibility of creating reflux should be borne in mind during any ureteroscopic procedure, especially if dilation of the ureteral orifice is used.[4]

The mobility of the pediatric kidney with respiration can be problematic during percutaneous access. One must take care in entering the calix not to injure the papilla. The distance to the kidney in small children is significantly less than in adults, and therefore punctures should be relatively shallow.[2]

URETEROSCOPY

Indications and Results

Stone Disease

The most common indication for the use of endourological techniques in children is urinary calculus disease.[5] Ureteroscopy has been used with up to 97 percent success for the removal of lower ureteral calculi in adults.[6] In children, several smaller series have been documented. Caione and associates performed ureteroscopy with an 11.5 Fr. instrument on eight boys, using a hydraulic pump to dilate the orifices, and reported 100 percent success with no residual VUR.[7] In another early series in which an 8.5 Fr. instrument was used to achieve ureteroscopic access in children, there was resultant reflux in one of four patients.[8] More recently, 18 successful ureteroscopic procedures in children were documented.[9] Five patients were treated with the 11.5 Fr. ureteroscope and balloon dilation. The other procedures were carried out with 7.2 or 8.5 Fr. ureteroscopes, and only three children required balloon dilation. Nine of the patients had postoperative cystography, the timing of which was not discussed. One patient had grade III VUR that resolved over 1 year. No significant complications were noted.

As successful as ureteroscopy can be for distal ureteral calculi, there is still debate over whether it should be considered first-line therapy. In a study comparing the cost effectiveness of extracorporeal shock wave lithotripsy (ESWL) and ureteroscopy, ESWL was recommended as the first-line treatment for distal calculi, ureteroscopy being reserved for treatment failures. Once again, this study primarily concerned adult patients.[10]

Endoscopic access to the reconstructed urinary tract may be difficult, especially when performed in retrograde fashion. Despite this, retrograde access to the upper urinary tract can be used as a first approach for stenting or stone removal in patients with conduits. Percutaneous access should be used for large stone burden or ureteral obstruction in association with the stone(s).[11] In children with urinary diversion, the usual paradigm for management of renal or ureteral calculi may need to be altered. For example, the success rate of ESWL in myelomeningocele patients with diverted urinary tracts is lower than in the normal population, and therefore endourological techniques have been recommended as first-line therapy.[12]

Gross Hematuria

The most common indication for diagnostic ureteroscopy in children is benign gross hematuria. Ureteroscopy is indicated when radiological and medical diagnostic techniques have been exhausted and the source of the hematuria remains unknown.

Diagnostic ureteroscopy for hematuria should be performed when the patient is actively bleeding.[2] Cystoscopic examination will exclude a lower tract source of hematuria and should identify which ureter is the source of the hematuria. It has been recommended that the distal ureter be initially examined with the minirigid ureteroscope to avoid iatrogenic lesions caused by the guidewire. After this has been performed, the wire is introduced only as far as the ureter has been examined. A dilating balloon is then used and a flexible ureterorenoscope introduced. If the ureter is free of lesions, the renal pelvis and the upper, middle, and lower calices are carefully inspected. In 50 to 90 percent of patients a source of bleeding will be found.[13–15] Most of these are small vascular abnormalities overlying or adjacent to papillae. Endoscopic fulguration has been successful in causing such hematuria to resolve in most patients, the majority of whom have been adults.

Preoperative Preparation

Preoperative radiological imaging of the pediatric urinary tract is essential for adequate planning and performance of any ureteroscopic procedure. Retrograde pyelography may be performed if there is any doubt as to the anatomy concerned or the position of a presumed ureteral calculus. Intraoperative radiographical visualization is important to the success of endourological procedures. Preoperative bowel preparation can decrease the amount of stool and bowel gas obscuring the retroperitoneal structures.

Grossly infected urine should be sterilized before ureteroscopic manipulation. Preoperative antibiotics should be used routinely. Of patients undergoing percutaneous renal stone removal, 35 percent develop bacteriuria if no prophylaxis is given.[16] Irrigation solutions should be warmed to prevent hypothermia in small children. Saline should be used whenever electrocautery is not being employed, to avoid dilutional hyponatremia in the event of extravasation.

Equipment

The operating table and fluoroscopic equipment should be compatible so as to allow visual monitoring at all times during the procedure. A fluoroscopic monitor with last-image hold and electronic reduction is helpful in order to allow more thorough examination of the radiographical image with decreased radiation exposure to the child.

A great variety of ureteroscopic equipment is available. The minirigid ureteroscopes, using a combination of a rigid sheath and fiberoptic image bundle, are most commonly adaptable to the pediatric patient. The distal tip diameter ranges from 4.5 to 7 Fr. Their design allows some deflection at the tip without distorting the visual image. The endoscopes contain either one or two working channels. There is an advantage to having two working channels, because instruments may be passed without stopping the flow of irrigant. Ureteroscopes with two working channels generally accept instruments up to 3 Fr. There are currently available a number of useful instruments of this size, including laser fibers, electrohydraulic probes, electrocautery probes, grasping forceps, and baskets.[17] Larger rod-lens system ureteroscopes commonly used in adults are available and may occasionally be useful in older children or those with dilated ureters.

Flexible, actively deflectable ureteroscopes are useful when it is difficult to pass a rigid instrument above the pelvic brim.[2] These instruments are generally somewhat larger than the minirigid variety and therefore may not be applicable in the very young child. The light source and visual image are both transmitted along fiberoptic bundles. There is generally one channel for irrigation and passage of instruments. The tip of these ureteroscopes is deflectable, using a mechanism built into the handle. Maximal deflection of these endoscopes is often not possible when an instrument is present in the working channel. Secondary passive deflection of the shaft proximal to the actively deflecting tip is built into some ureteroscopes to allow improved access to the lower calices of the kidney. The flexible, actively deflectable ureteroscopes are passed over the working guidewire. If they cannot be introduced, balloon dilation is performed. If they still cannot be introduced, a 10 to 14 Fr. dilator-sheath system can be introduced into the lower ureter. The endoscope is then introduced over the working wire and through the sheath. The entire intrarenal collecting system can be examined in 65 percent of cases, and in almost all cases more than 75 percent of the collecting system can be seen.[14]

Although not absolutely necessary, an endoscopic video camera and monitor are extremely useful, especially during prolonged endoscopic cases. Such a system allows the surgeon and assistant to monitor the progress of the procedure simultaneously. The assistant is often occupied in manipulating probes or baskets, and the ability to observe the operation enhances the safety of these procedures.

Operative Technique

Proper arrangement in the lithotomy position is essential for potentially prolonged ureteroscopic procedures. In infants and young children, stirrups are usually not necessary. The legs may be positioned over towel rolls at the end of the operating table. Pressure on the lateral calf should be avoided to prevent peroneal nerve injury.[18] The stirrups, if used, should be well padded and adjusted to avoid extreme abduction at the hips.

Ureteroscopy should not be performed without proper safety access to the ureter. A cystoscope is initially introduced into the bladder, and the ureter is negotiated with a floppy-tip guidewire (Bentson

0.035 or 0.038), which is advanced to the renal pelvis. If there is difficulty in negotiating beyond an impacted ureteral calculus, a hydrophilic-coated guidewire with a flexible tip may be useful. Sometimes, a calculus may be successfully bypassed using a combination of a ureteral catheter with a guidewire. Advancing the catheter to the calculus allows the wire more stability and direction and prevents it from turning back on itself. Alternately advancing the wire and the catheter may allow passage. Once the wire has achieved access to the renal pelvis, a second wire is passed using a coaxial 8 Fr./10 Fr. dilator sheath set. After the set is passed over the guidewire, the inner 8 Fr. dilator is removed. The working wire is passed through the 10 Fr. sheath alongside the guidewire, which is then fastened by suturing to either the labium or glans penis.[2]

The minirigid ureteroscopes can often be introduced into the ureter without dilation, especially in older children. For introduction of flexible ureteroscopes, balloon dilation of the ureter is generally necessary. The long-term effects of ureteral dilation in children have not been adequately studied. In the adult population, a 5 to 20 percent incidence of post-procedure VUR has been noted on cystograms taken up to 1 year after ureteroscopy.[4, 19] There are also concerns over ureteral strictures, although probably these are rarely due to balloon dilation. In any case, if dilation is necessary, it should be only sufficient to pass the ureteroscope.[2]

Balloons for ureteral dilation are available with diameters ranging from 3 to 8 mm and lengths ranging from 3 to 10 cm. The dilating balloons have markers to allow accurate positioning under fluoroscopic control. Although used much less commonly, coaxial dilators can be used sequentially to achieve a diameter of the orifice 2 Fr. larger than that of the ureteroscope.[2]

The flexible ureteroscopes can be passed directly into the ureteral orifice, over the working guidewire, or through a flexible plastic ureteral access sheath. A sheath is most useful during procedures that require repeated passage of the endoscope.[2]

Attempts to advance into the upper ureter may be difficult owing to ureteral angulation, edema, or spasm. It is important to remember that the ureteroscope should never be forced, nor should advancement of the ureteroscope take place when the ureteral lumen is not apparent. Visualization can be enhanced by manual or pressure bag pumping of irrigating fluid, in an attempt to maintain a pressure of less than 200 cm H_2O in order to avoid potential renal injury.[20]

If ureteroscopy is being performed for calculus disease, a number of techniques for stone removal can be used. Stones may be removed with either graspers or baskets, taking care that the stone is not large enough to cause a ureteral tear or avulsion. The stone may be fragmented using intracorporeal shock wave lithotripsy (ISWL), from a laser, an ultrasonic, or an electrohydraulic source. The stone may also be manipulated into the renal pelvis in preparation for ESWL. Detailed descriptions of endourological techniques for stone manipulation and the technical aspects of the modalities of lithotripsy are given in Chapters 6 and 8.

The techniques of endourological management of ureteral strictures have been well described in adults. There is limited experience with these techniques in children, and therefore they must not be considered well established. Ureteral strictures can be managed with balloon dilation, incision by cold knife or electrocautery, or both. The narrowed ureteral segment is negotiated with a guidewire. The ureteral wall is incised alongside the wire, usually in a posterolateral direction. If the area is too narrow for an incision to be made in a controlled fashion, initial balloon dilation may be carried out. Results of incision have been good overall, but there is only anecdotal experience in the pediatric population.[21]

At the conclusion of most ureteroscopic procedures, a ureteral stent should be placed because of the possibility of postoperative edema and of known or unknown ureteral tears or perforations. Child-sized double-pigtail catheters are now available from a variety of manufacturers; these may be as small as 3 Fr. and 10 cm in length.[2, 21] The stent may be passed over the working wire at the end of the procedure. Stents can either be removed at a subsequent procedure under anesthesia or a tail of suture may be left on the end of the stent and taped outside the urethral meatus. This suture can then be used to pull the stent in a relatively pain-free manner in an outpatient setting. If a stent is to remain in place for a long time, it is best not to leave a suture, which may at times promote early dislodgment.

Complications

Complications have been reported to occur in approximately 20 percent of ureteroscopic cases.[14] Most of these are minor and involve urinary extravasation, which is usually managed adequately by placement of a ureteral stent. The most significant ureteral injury is avulsion, generally caused during a forceful attempt to extract a calculus. Ureteral avulsion is treated by open repair. Hematuria after ureteroscopic procedures is rarely severe, but if there has been ureteral incision, the risk of significant retroperitoneal bleeding, although rare, should be considered.

Placement of a ureteral stent at the end of a ureteroscopic procedure is for the prevention of transient ureteral obstruction. This is generally due to postoperative edema and will resolve within a few days. Postoperative flank pain may potentially be due to obstruction of the stent, which occasionally will need to be changed. The presence of the stenting catheter can cause flank pain, most commonly during voiding. If there is any question as to the patency of the stent, intravenous urography will document whether the system is obstructed. Cystography is occasionally useful in demonstrating the patency of a stent, but nonvisualization of the upper tract is not sufficient evidence of stent obstruction.

During stone manipulation, fragments of calculus can be pushed through the ureteral wall. Ureteral perforation with retroperitoneal extravasation of stone fragments occurs in less than 2.5 percent of cases. It is recommended that the position of the stone be documented carefully, a stent placed, and perioperative antibiotics administered. Aggressive attempts to retrieve the stone result in injury to the ureter. It seems that the risk after extravasation of known infected stones is small, and the management should therefore be no different.[22] Occasionally, a stone is trapped in a basket and is then found to be too large to be manipulated without ureteral injury. If the basket cannot be removed from the stone, the retraction mechanism of the basket may be disassembled and the ureteroscope backed off the basket wire. The ureteroscope can then be reintroduced alongside the basket wire, and the stone fragmented to free the basket.

Postoperative ureteral stricture formation is rare. This seems to be generally due to previous stone impaction or ureteral perforation and rarely due to balloon or coaxial dilation. Treatment of ureteral stricture may be open or endourological, depending on the location, length, and circumstances of the injury.

NEPHROSCOPY

Indications and Results

Indications for nephroscopy in children are similar to those in adults. The most common indication for percutaneous access to the kidney is stone removal. There are limited data related to percutaneous nephrolithotripsy in children. Woodside and associates reported seven children, all of whom underwent successful stone removal in one stage.[23] No complications were reported. Seven children were reported by Bagli and associates, six of whom experienced complete stone removal.[24] There were no complications except prolonged urinary drainage through nephrostomy sites. Access was maintained with sheaths of 22 to 30 Fr., and the fascial dilating balloons were used to obtain access. Eshghi and associates reported eight patients, the youngest being 16 months of age.[21]

Callaway and associates reported 18 patients under age 16 who underwent percutaneous stone removal.[25] There was 82 percent success in removing the intended stones. Six patients required multiple sessions and four needed blood transfusion. One patient had a significant postoperative infection and one developed UPJ stenosis.

The status of percutaneous stone surgery in children, especially the very young, awaits reports of larger series. In children there is concern over blood loss requiring transfusion, which may be partly preventable through the use of smaller-access cannulas. A reasonable amount of experience with percutaneous renal surgery should be a prerequisite to performing these procedures in children.

Percutaneous access to the renal collecting system has also been used to correct obstructive uropathy. Endourological manipulation of UPJ obstruction and ureteral stricture has been attempted in children. Because of the significantly higher success rates of open pyeloplasties in infants and young children, endourological incision is not recommended as a primary mode of therapy. Shorter recovery time and lower narcotic requirements have been documented for endopyelotomy versus open surgery in adults[26] but not in children, who tend to resume normal activities within 1 week after open surgery. In failed pyeloplasty, however, high success rates for endopyelotomy have been reported, and the success rates and morbidity of open operations argue in favor of an attempt at a percutaneous approach. A stricture 2 cm long or greater is a contraindication to endopyelotomy.[27] In a recent small series, four children underwent endopyelotomy percutaneously for secondary UPJ obstruction after failed pyeloplasty. An electrocautery cutting probe was used to make the incision. A balloon was then inflated to 5 or 6 mm in diameter to calibrate the area of incision. A 3 to 5 Fr. stent was left in place for 3 to 5 weeks. In two children, persistent obstruction was noted at the time of stent removal, and resection of a tissue flap and reincision were performed at that time with good results. All children are well after long-term follow-up (1.5 to 3 years).[28]

In adults, an 85 percent success rate has been reported for endopyelotomy for primary UPJ obstruction.[27, 29] In a series of 17 primary endopyelotomies in children, there were four patients in whom the procedure was technically unsuccessful, and two who demonstrated complete UPJ obstruction at 6 weeks and 6 months, respectively. Four of the patients classified as successes were unchanged radiologically. Radiological success was therefore documented in only seven of the 13 patients who underwent a technically successful procedure.[30] Unfortunately, for congenital UPJ obstruction, the only criteria used for success of endopyelotomy have been stable radiological study results and lack of symptoms. Of 30 patients reported in 1992, only 20 demonstrated radiological improvement.[31]

Caliceal diverticula, renal cysts, and obstructed calices have all been treated by a percutaneous technique. Few such cases have been reported in children, however. As experience is gained with endourological techniques in children, the indications for these procedures will expand, as they have done in the adult population.

Equipment

Percutaneous nephroscopy is equipment intensive. The proper materials must be available, and assistants in the room must be familiar with both the equipment and the techniques. Access to the kidney via a percutaneous technique requires the equipment necessary for puncture into a renal calix. The technique of nephrostomy tube placement is discussed in detail in Chapter 7. In brief, once the nephrostomy tract has been established, a balloon or coaxial dilator is used to create a large enough tract into the kidney for placement of a plastic nephroscopy sheath.[32] The nephroscopes are then introduced through this sheath, which maintains access to the intrarenal collecting system. The presence of a working sheath dramatically decreases working pressures within the renal pelvis as measured manometrically.[33]

Nephroscopes are available in either rigid or actively deflectable configurations. Rigid nephroscopes have an offset lens system that allows the passage of the rigid probes necessary for stone fragmentation and retrieval. The tips of these endoscopes are rounded to decrease the possibility of renal injury. The telescopes come in 0 and 30 degree configurations. The outer diameter of the nephroscopes ranges in size from 17 to 24 Fr.

Flexible nephroscopes were developed in order to reach all the calices of the intrarenal collecting system. These are 15 Fr. actively deflatable endoscopes with a 6 Fr. working channel. These instruments have been specifically manufactured for use in the intrarenal collecting system and have a tip with a very tight turning radius for working in a small space. In addition to the usual 15 Fr. flexible nephroscope, smaller deflectable ureteroscopes can be used to obtain access through narrow infundibula. In addition, if access to a calix can be obtained by wire, a passive, flexible endoscope as small as 5 Fr. can be passed over the wire to visualize the difficult calix.

Accessories for stone fragmentation include ultrasonic probes. These have an advantage for percutaneous work in that the larger probes aspirate stone fragments as they are created. Laser fibers and electrohydraulic probes have been previously described for use through ureteroscopes. These instruments are often useful for passage through a flexible nephroscope. The advantage of a laser fiber or a small electrohydraulic lithotripsy (EHL) probe is that it can be placed through a deflected nephroscope without straightening the tip of the instrument. The application of the coumarin-based pulsed dye laser has allowed the endoscopist to employ more delicate instruments with smaller working channels to treat urinary and biliary calculi.[34] EHL is perhaps the most universally available modality for stone fragmentation. It has been shown by Miller and Wickham that the probes work equally well in normal saline as in water, decreasing the risk from extravasation.[34a] Use under strict visual control has decreased ureteral perforation. EHL is by far the least expensive form of ISWL and is safe and effective under visual control.[35] A new device, the Swiss Lithoclast, consists of a rigid probe that vibrates at a frequency of 12 cycles per second. This instrument acts as a hammer to fragment stones. Probes as small as 3 Fr. are available, and it appears that this device may fragment stones more rapidly and efficiently than ultrasonic lithotripsy.[36]

Instruments for incision of UPJ, or ureteral strictures include cautery probes, laser fibers, small resectoscopes, and visual urethrotomes. A combination dilating balloon and cautery cutting wire has also been used for pediatric endopyelotomy.[37]

Operative Technique

As mentioned under the section on ureteroscopy, fluoroscopic monitoring and a proper fluoroscopic table are essential to the performance of percutaneous renal procedures. Irrigating solutions should be warmed preoperatively to prevent hypothermia in children. Saline should be used whenever electrocautery is not in operation in order to prevent absorption of large amounts of hypotonic solution.

Patient positioning depends somewhat on the procedure being performed, the position of the stone, the location of the kidney, and the anatomy of the intrarenal collecting system. The procedures are performed with the patient in the prone position. Adequate padding, allowing sufficient room for respiration and avoiding pressure points, is essential. A ureteral access catheter placed from below is an important adjunct in obtaining percutaneous access. In children, it is generally necessary to place the catheter with patients in the lithotomy position before turning them to a prone position. In older patients, it may be possible to perform flexible cystoscopy while they are prone in order to place such a catheter. A

Foley catheter should also be inserted before beginning the procedure, to drain the irrigant that may pass down the ureter during nephroscopy.

The ureteral access catheter can be used to instill either contrast or air for visualization of the intrarenal collecting system. The advantage of air is that it outlines first the posterior calices, which are most advantageous for percutaneous procedures. Access to the collecting system can then be obtained by methods previously described. Once an 18-gauge needle has been manipulated into the collecting system, a floppy-tip guidewire is introduced. The needle is then withdrawn and a curved 6 Fr. catheter introduced over the wire. This catheter is then used in an attempt to steer the wire through the UPJ and down the ureter. A second guidewire is placed next, using the 8 Fr./10 Fr. coaxial dilator system. This is passed over the initial wire, and the 8 Fr. catheter is removed. A Super-Stiff guidewire is then passed through the 10 Fr. catheter, which is removed. The safety wire is secured to the skin with a silk suture. Over this working wire, the tract needs to be enlarged to accept a nephroscopy sheath.

A specially designed fascia-incising knife or a No. 11 blade can be used to create a cruciate incision in the fascia. The tract can be dilated with either sequential coaxial dilators or a fascial dilating balloon. The advantage of the dilating balloon is less chance of dislodging the working wire and of injuring the anterior collecting system during overzealous passage of coaxial dilators.

The access obtained should be based on the procedure to be performed. For a caliceal or diverticular calculus, access should be obtained onto the stone. For a stone in the pelvis or at the UPJ, or when an endopyelotomy is planned a middle or upper pole calix provides the best access.

Working sheaths range in size from 18 to 30 Fr., the choice depending on the procedure to be performed and the size of the child, and are matched with dilating balloons of similar size. The sheath is backloaded over the balloon catheter, which is then introduced under fluoroscopic guidance. The balloon is inflated with contrast material until the waist disappears. The sheath is then advanced over the inflated balloon. The balloon is deflated and removed, leaving the working wire in place.

Techniques for stone removal are similar to those described for ureteroscopy. Often, one is dealing with larger calculi, and therefore the advantages of ultrasonic lithotripsy, including rapid stone disintegration and removal of fragments by suction, become important. The ureteral access catheter sometimes prevents small stone fragments from entering the ureter. A balloon catheter can also be used to obstruct the upper ureter and prevent this problem. When calculi do enter the ureter, they are usually small enough to pass on their own.

The performance of endopyelotomy and of incision of a ureteral stricture is similar, and only endopyelotomy will be described. In the technique described by Motola and colleagues, a 6 Fr. catheter is manipulated from below through the UPJ.[27] The patient is turned prone and a percutaneous tract obtained. The stent is pulled out through the flank and a guidewire passed, which is brought out through the urethra. A 16 Fr. fascial dilator is then passed through the UPJ. A ureterotome with cold knife is used to incise posterolaterally in order to avoid renal vessels. A 14 Fr/8.2 Fr endopyelotomy stent is left in place for 6 weeks.[27, 29] Another technique is to splay the UPJ with two guidewires and incise between them posterolaterally. The incision should be calibrated secondarily with a 6-mm balloon.[2] The incision can be made using cold knife, electrocautery,[38] or laser. The endopyelotomy incision has traditionally been stented for 6 weeks; it may be possible to stent for shorter periods with success.[2]

At the end of any percutaneous procedure, it is necessary to leave drainage tubes. It has been recommended that a 5 or 7 Fr. angiographic catheter be placed over the safety wire and into the bladder. Over this, a Councill-tipped Foley catheter is threaded and positioned in the renal pelvis. The purpose of this coaxial system is to minimize the risk of tube dislodgment and allow ready access if the nephrostomy should back out of the collecting system.[2] If the procedure has involved an endoscopic incision, an indwelling stent should be placed under fluoroscopic control. A nephrostomy tube is also left indwelling. Postoperatively, a nephrostogram can be performed, usually within 48 to 72 hours after the procedure. If no extravasation is noted and contrast drains freely down the ureter, the nephrostomy tube can be removed.

Complications

The most distressing complication of percutaneous access to the kidney in the small child is significant bleeding.[25] It is prudent to have at least a type and screen available for any child undergoing percutaneous therapeutic procedures. Bleeding at the time of surgery is managed by tamponade with a large nephrostomy tube or a Kaye tamponade catheter. If this is unsuccessful, arteriography and embolization may be considered. Delayed bleeding after nephrostomy tube removal generally requires angiographic access and embolization.[39] In rare cases, emergency nephrectomy has been necessary for severe bleeding. Patterson and associates outlined recommendations to prevent serious hemorrhage.[39] These include a thorough understanding of the renal vascular anatomy, minimizing the number of percutaneous puncture sites, dilating only as much as is necessary, screening patients for coagulopathy, careful manipulation of instruments, and proper postoperative care of nephrostomy tubes.

Perforation of the collecting system is a common occurrence during these procedures. Tears within the renal pelvis generally heal within 48 hours with adequate drainage of the kidney.[40] Because of the potential extravasation of urine and irrigating fluid that occurs with these perforations, prophylactic antibiotics are recommended. Injury to adjacent organs is occasionally reported and may be especially worrisome in children. The danger of pneumothorax, especially with a supracostal approach, must be considered and chest tube drainage instituted as necessary.[41]

Some complications are relatively specific for endopyelotomy. In a large series, complications included transfusion in two of 212 patients, and ureteral avulsion in one; four patients required ureterocalicostomy and one an ileal interposition, while 18 required open pyeloplasty.[27] One case of necrosis of the ureter after endopyelotomy treated by Boari flap is documented.[42] The complication rate of retrograde (ureteroscopic) endopyelotomy is higher (20 percent ureteral stricture rate) than of percutaneous endopyelotomy.[43]

LOWER URINARY TRACT PROCEDURES

The procedure that may be of most use to the pediatric urologist consists of percutaneous access to the augmented bladder. The incidence of calculi in the augmented bladder has been reported to be as high as 30 percent. Often, there is a delicate continence mechanism such as a Mitrofanoff appendiceal stoma. There is significant risk of disrupting the continence mechanism by attempting to pass large instruments through a catheterizable conduit and remove stone fragments. It has therefore, seemed prudent to reach the bladder via percutaneous techniques.

Generally speaking, the bladder has been fixed to the anterior abdominal wall at the site of the former suprapubic tube. If this site can be identified, this is probably the safest area in which to approach the augmented bladder. It would be useful to confirm from the original operative notes that the bladder was indeed fixed to the anterior abdominal wall at this point, although this can be ascertained by computed tomography or fluoroscopy with contrast.

An 18-gauge, 2-inch needle is introduced into the bladder under cystoscopic guidance. A stiff guidewire is then introduced through this needle, which is removed. The skin and fascia can be incised with a No. 11 blade or a fascial needle as previously described. Coaxial serial dilators are then used with direct visual control from within the bladder to enlarge the tract. Fascial balloon dilators are generally less successful because of the dense scar in the area of the suprapubic site. A percutaneous access sheath such as would be used for nephroscopy is introduced. A full range of instruments may be used, including nephroscopes, cystoscopes, and flexible devices. Often the augmented bladders contain pockets and recesses, and a thorough search, both radiographically and endoscopically, for stone fragments is essential. In the author's experience, patients managed in this way can be treated on an outpatient basis. Intravenous prophylactic antibiotics are essential for these chronically colonized augmented bladders.

Summary

Experience with endourological techniques in children has been significantly smaller than in adults. This is because of the much lower incidence of calculus disease in children. It is, however, becoming apparent that the pediatric urinary tract is amenable to percutaneous and endourological manipulation. Indications for such techniques will increase as experience is broadened. Respect for the differences between the pediatric and adult urinary tracts is essential for the safe performance of these minimally invasive procedures.

REFERENCES

1. Cussen LJ. The morphology of congenital dilatation of the ureter: Intrinsic ureteral lesions. Aust N Z J Surg, 41:185, 1971.
2. Peters CA, Kavoussi LR. Pediatric endourology and laparoscopy. In Walsh PC, Retik AB, Stamey TA, Vaughan ED Jr, eds. Campbell's Urology, 6th ed. Philadelphia, WB Saunders, Update No. 6, 1992, p 1.
3. Santarosa RP, Hensle TW, Shabsigh R. Percutaneous transvesical ureteroscopy for removal of distal ureteral stone in reimplanted ureter. Urology 42:313, 1993.
4. Garvin TJ, Clayman RV. Balloon dilation of the distal ureter to 24F: An effective method for ureteroscopic stone retrieval. J Urol 146:742, 1991.
5. el Damanhoury H, Burger R, Hohenfellner R. Surgical aspects of urolithiasis in children (review). Pediatr Nephrol 5:339, 1991.
6. Blute ML, Segura JW, Patterson DE. Ureteroscopy. J Urol 139:510, 1988.
7. Caione P, De GM, Capozza N, et al. Endoscopic manipulation of ureteral calculi in children by rigid operative ureterorenoscopy. J Urol 144:484, 1990.
8. Hill DE, Segura JW, Patterson DE, et al. Ureteroscopy in children. J Urol 144:481, 1990.
9. Thomas R, Ortenberg J, Lee BR, et al. Safety and efficacy of pediatric ureteroscopy for management of calculous disease. J Urol 149:1082, 1993.
10. Anderson KR, Keetch DW, Albala DM, et al. Optimal therapy for the distal ureteral stone: Extracorporeal shock wave lithotripsy versus ureteroscopy. J Urol 152:62, 1994.
11. Wolf JJ, Stoller ML. Management of upper tract calculi in patients with tubularized urinary diversions. J Urol 145:266, 1991.
12. Cass AS, Lee JY, Aliabadi H. Extracorporeal shock wave lithotripsy and endoscopic management of renal calculi with urinary diversions. J Urol 148:1123, 1992.
13. Patterson DE, Segura JW, Benson RJ, et al. Endoscopic evaluation and treatment of patients with idiopathic gross hematuria. J Urol 132:1199, 1984.
14. Kavoussi L, Clayman RV, Basler J. Flexible, actively deflectable fiberoptic ureteronephroscopy. J Urol 142:949, 1989.
15. Bagley DH, Allen J. Flexible ureteropyeloscopy in the diagnosis of benign essential hematuria. J Urol 143:549, 1990.
16. Charton M, Vallancien G, Veillon B, et al. Urinary tract infection in percutaneous surgery for renal calculi. J Urol 135:15, 1986.
17. Abdel RO, Bagley DH. The 6.9 F semirigid ureteroscope in clinical use. Urology 41:45, 1993.
18. Stiff JL. Respiratory complications and complications of anesthesia. In Marshall FF, ed. Urologic Complications: Medical and Surgical, Adult and Pediatric. St. Louis, Mosby-Year Book, 1990, p 116.
19. Stackl W, Marberger M. Late sequelae of the management of ureteral calculi with the ureterorenoscope. J Urol 136:386, 1986.
20. Eshghi M, Schwalb D, Davidson M. Morphological changes in the urinary tract associated with ureteropyeloscopy: An experimental study. J Urol 141:208A, 1989.
21. Eshghi M, Reda EF, Franco I. Endoscopic surgery of the upper tract in children. In Kelalis PP, King LR, Belman AB, eds. Clinical Pediatric Urology, 3rd ed. Philadelphia, WB Saunders, 1992, p 726.
22. Evans CP, Stoller ML. The fate of the iatrogenic retroperitoneal stone (review). J Urol 150:827, 1993.
23. Woodside JR, Stevens GF, Stark GL, et al. Percutaneous stone removal in children. J Urol 134:1166, 1985.
24. Bagli D, Peters CA, Bauer SB, et al. Endourologic management of pediatric urolithiasis. J Urol 149:314A, 1993.
25. Callaway TW, Lingardh G, Basata S, et al. Percutaneous nephrolithotomy in children. J Urol 148:1067, 1992.
26. Karlin GS, Badlani GH, Smith AD. Endopyelotomy versus open pyeloplasty: Comparison in 88 patients. J Urol 140:476, 1988.
27. Motola JA, Badlani GH, Smith AD. Results of 212 consecutive endopyelotomies: An 8-year followup. J Urol 149:453, 1993.
28. Kavoussi LR, Meretyk S, Dierks SM, et al. Endopyelotomy for secondary ureteropelvic junction obstruction in children. J Urol 145:345, 1991.
29. Lee WJ, Badlani GH, Karlin GS, et al. Treatment of ureteropelvic strictures with percutaneous pyelotomy: Experience in 62 patients. AJR Am J Roentgenol 151:515, 1988.
30. Tan HL, Najmaldin A, Webb DR. Endopyelotomy for pelviureteric junction obstruction in children. Eur Urol 24:84, 1993.
31. Karlin G, Badlani G, Smith AD. Percutaneous pyeloplasty (endopyelotomy) for congenital ureteropelvic junction obstruction. Urology 39:533, 1992.
32. LeRoy AJ, May GR, Segura JW, et al. Rapid dilatation of percutaneous nephrostomy tracks. AJR Am J Roentgenol 142:355, 1984.
33. Saltzman B, Khasidy LR, Smith AD. Measurement of renal pelvis pressures during endourologic procedures. Urology 30:472, 1987.
34. Grasso M, Bagley DH. Endoscopic pulsed-dye laser lithotripsy: 159 consecutive cases. J Endourol 8:25, 1994.
34a. Miller RA, Wickham JEA. Percutaneous nephrolithotomy. Advances in equipment and endoscopic techniques. Urology (Suppl 5) 23:2, 1984.
35. Denstedt JD, Clayman RV. Electrohydraulic lithotripsy of renal and ureteral calculi. J Urol 143:13, 1990.
36. Denstedt JD, Eberwein PM, Singh RR. The Swiss Lithoclast: A new device for intracorporeal lithotripsy. J Urol 148:1088, 1992.
37. Bolton DM, Bogaert GA, Mevorach RA, et al. Pediatric ureteropelvic junction obstruction treated with retrograde endopyelotomy. Urology 44:609, 1994.

38. Figenshau RS, Stone AM, Clayman RV, et al. Endoureterotomy in an animate model: Comparison of electrosurgical, mechanical and balloon treatment modalities. J Urol 147:470A, 1992.

39. Patterson DE, Segura JW, LeRoy AJ, et al. The etiology and treatment of delayed bleeding following percutaneous lithotripsy. J Urol 133:447, 1985.

40. Winfield HW, Clayman RV. Complications of percutaneous removal of renal and ureteral calculi. World Urol Update Series, 1985.

41. Young AT, Hunter DW, Castaneda-Zuniga WR, et al. Percutaneous extraction of urinary calculi: Use of the intercostal approach. Radiology 154:633, 1985.

42. Sutherland RS, Pfister RR, Koyle MA. Endopyelotomy associated ureteral necrosis: Complete ureteral replacement using the Boari flap. J Urol 148:1490, 1992.

43. Meretyk I, Meretyk S, Clayman RV. Endopyelotomy: Comparison of ureteroscopic retrograde and antegrade percutaneous techniques. J Urol 148:775, 1992.

Chapter 23

Laparoscopic Surgery in Children

Steven G. Docimo and Gerald H. Jordan

The use of laparoscopy in urology began in the pediatric population with "exploration" for the non-palpable testis.[1] Laparoscopy in urology was limited because many of the useful applications were pediatric; the existing instrumentation did not lend itself to use in children. After the introduction of laparoscopic cholecystectomy, with the attendant explosion in instrument design and availability, the therapeutic potential of this technology began to be explored in urology. The procedures performed included pelvic lymphadenectomy, nephrectomy, and varicocelectomy. With increasing experience and the introduction of smaller instruments, additional therapeutic applications of laparoscopy became feasible in children. Despite the smaller abdominal cavity, increasing the likelihood of retroperitoneal vascular injury and requiring that procedures be done in cramped quarters,[2] laparoscopic surgery in children is safe and effective in experienced hands.[3] The procedures discussed in this chapter represent the early experience of minimally invasive pediatric urologic surgery. The evolution of these technologies has been and will be exponential over the coming years. The approach and general techniques as applied to the undescended testicle, and a description of the approach to nephrectomy for benign disease, is presented in detail, providing a common foundation for the application of laparoscopy to a variety of conditions.

INDICATIONS

At this time, the most common indication for laparoscopy in the pediatric age group is diagnostic and associated with the evaluation of the nonpalpable testicle. For 20 years the information obtained at laparoscopy was used only to modify the open surgical approach, or avoid open surgery in nearly 40 percent of patients.[1, 3, 4] Now, after the pioneering work of Bloom[5] and Jordan at al,[6] the intra-abdominal testis can be brought to the scrotum using laparoscopic techniques either primarily, or in stages. Examination, biopsy, and/or removal of gonads in intersex states can be readily accomplished laparoscopically, and examination of the pelvic organs can be carried out concurrently.[7-9] Some pediatric surgeons advocate laparoscopic examination of the contralateral inguinal ring at the time of hernia repair as an alternative to open groin exploration. This can be accomplished in a transumbilical fashion, or via the patent processus exposed during open herniorrhaphy.[2, 10]

Since the initial work with the undescended testicle, laparoscopy has been applied to children for a number of extended procedures. Laparoscopic nephrectomy,[11] nephroureterectomy,[12] partial nephrectomy,[13] and renal cyst decortication[14] have all been described anecdotally, representing potential indications for the laparoscopic approach to the upper tract in children. Laparoscopic varicocelectomy[15-18] has gained widespread use, although its advantages over conventional approaches have been questioned.[19, 20] Animal models and clinical experience with laparoscopic extravesical ureteral reimplantation have been explored. Once again, the benefits of this approach in a disease managed well through a small Pfannenstiel incision have yet to be proved. Urinary diversion by ileal conduit has been accomplished laparoscopically in at least two patients.[21] Autoaugmentation of the bladder has been performed laparoscopically,[22] as well as bladder diverticulectomy and simple cystectomy.[23] A laparoscopically assisted appendicovesicostomy has also been described,[24] which could conceivably be combined with techniques for autoaugmentation to create a continent bladder reconstruction in selected patients. In children and adults, pyeloplasty has been performed using laparoscopic suturing techniques.[25, 26] Dismembered pyeloplasty in the very young child has not been accepted because of limitations in the availability of appropriate suture and the difficulty in handling these small sutures with existing laparoscopic instrumentation. Soon, advances in the technology of tissue reapproximation may allow for pyeloplasty in all age groups.

PREOPERATIVE EVALUATION AND ANESTHETIC CONSIDERATIONS

The evaluation of candidates for laparoscopy is similar to that of patients undergoing a similar open operation. The unique aspects of laparoscopy also demand other considerations. Diagnostic and therapeutic laparoscopy will be impeded by extensive intra-abdominal adhesions, and therefore any surgical history or history of peritonitis should be sought. Using open access, previous surgery in general is not a contraindication to the use of laparoscopic techniques. One of the authors (GHJ) recently accomplished laparoscopic orchidopexy in a child born with gastroschisis. Peritoneal or extraperitoneal insufflation with carbon dioxide (CO_2) results in hypercapnia, decreased diaphragmatic excursion, decreased venous return, and increased peripheral vascular resistance.[27, 28] The presence of cardiopulmonary anomalies or diseases might affect the ability to compensate for these changes and should be thoroughly evaluated preoperatively.

The anesthesia team should be well acquainted with the effects of CO_2 pneumoperitoneum. As mentioned, hypercapnia occurs as a result of the absorption of intraperitoneal or extravasated CO_2. Endotracheal intubation is recommended for all laparoscopic procedures in children.[28] Halothane is not recommended as an inhalational agent because of the increased risk of cardiac dysrhythmia, especially in combination with hypercapnia. Nitrous oxide should be avoided because of attendant dilatation of the bowel. The possibility of CO_2 embolus due to intravascular insufflation or rapid absorption of CO_2 can lead to sudden cardiac decompensation. End-tidal CO_2 may be seen to drop rapidly in this situation owing to obstruction of the pulmonary vasculature. The deep left Trendelenburg position, release of the pneumoperitoneum, and aspiration through a central line may all be employed if the diagnosis is suspected.[29] Fluid replacement need not be as vigorous as with open surgery, as third-space losses are less. Urinary output is low during pneumoperitoneum, for reasons that are not clear, and is not a good indicator of hydration status.[28] This finding can be particularly striking in children. In a study of the association with high-pressure pneumoperitoneum, timed insufflation, and effects on end-tidal CO_2, of over 40 cases examined there have been none in which hypercapnia became clinically significant. In all cases, end-tidal CO_2 was maintained with minimal adjustments of respiratory rate and tidal volume.[30]

After taking into account the procedure being performed, the experience of the laparoscopist, and the characteristics of the patient, consideration should be given to having a type and screen in the blood bank.[31] Bowel preparation can improve visibility by decreasing intestinal caliber, and is a necessity if the potential for intestinal injury exists.[31] An enema is suggested as a minimum, with a complete mechanical bowel preparation for cases involving extensive adhesions or the prospect of bowel resection and anastomosis. An intravenous dose of a broad-spectrum antibiotic is recommended before any laparoscopic procedure.[31]

Patients and their parents may be attracted to laparoscopic procedures by the promise of lower morbidity, or simply the supposition that "newer is better." It is incumbent upon practitioners to make clear the potential, albeit small, for serious complications. The possibility of conversion to an open approach if problems arise, or if the laparoscopic approach proves to be less than ideal for the work at hand, should be clearly explained. The need for a change to an open technique must not be viewed by the patient or the surgeon as a failure, but as an expediency. Permission for conversion to an open approach should be included in every consent for operation.

OPERATIVE TECHNIQUE

Pneumoperitoneum

The patient is most commonly in a supine position. The operating table should have the capability of tilting 30 degrees in Trendelenburg, reverse Trendelenburg, and lateral tilt. The patient must be secured to the table to allow manipulation of the table through the extremes without slippage of the patient. General endotracheal anesthesia is used for all pediatric laparoscopic procedures. A nasogastric or orogastric tube should be in good position and on suction before the start of the procedure.[31] A wide antiseptic skin preparation is made to permit placement of trocars laterally if needed, and to allow for wide laparotomy should complications arise. An adhesive plastic film covering the abdomen and securing the drapes is helpful to prevent slipping of the sheets and inadvertent breaks in sterile technique. A Foley catheter is placed in the bladder and gravity drainage instituted to improve exposure and limit the opportunity for bladder injury.[31]

Before a pneumoperitoneum is obtained, the proper equipment should be on the instrument table ready to be used. First, the camera is attached to the laparoscope of choice. Warm irrigant (warmer than body temperature) should be available for warming the lens to prevent early fogging. The insufflation tubing is connected to the automatic insufflator, and the CO_2 tank(s) is/are checked. The light cord and light source are tested. The video camera is white balanced to provide true color definition and focus on the laparoscope checked. It is essential that the system provide a clear view of the abdomen. If a therapeutic procedure is contemplated, an irrigator/aspirator is connected to suction and pressurized irrigation fluid. The irrigation fluid is sometimes heparinized to limit the formation of clots in the abdomen, which are bothersome to break up and remove.[32] A laparotomy set should be open on the back table ready for immediate use.

Access can be obtained by Veress insufflation or open primary cannula placement. In the past, the most anxiety-provoking part of laparoscopy was achieving the initial pneumoperitoneum. If this is accomplished percutaneously, the Veress needle[33] is most often used and is available as a reusable or disposable product. The tip is designed to provide a blunt obturator, which is spring loaded. As the needle passes through the resistance of the posterior fascia and peritoneum, the obturator springs out, presenting a blunt tip to the abdominal contents. If this form of access is chosen, disposable needles are generally preferred in children, because the tip is always sharp, the mechanics are more reliable, and the lumen is always clean.[34, 35] To achieve inflation, an automatic insufflator is employed, with CO_2 most frequently used. A well-calibrated insufflator is essential to avoid the potential complications of overinsufflation, including pneumothorax, pneumomediastinum, pneumopericardium with tamponade, and gas embolus.[27, 36] The automatic insufflator instills gas at a preset rate and automatically arrests flow when a preset intra-abdominal pressure is reached.

The table is positioned in slight (15-degree) Trendelenburg. A nick is made in the skin in the lower portion of the umbilicus, and the Veress needle is inserted. If there is a scar from previous abdominal surgery, a different area for initial puncture should be chosen.[31] Various advice is given about the merits of lifting the abdominal wall at this juncture. This maneuver clearly cannot create an open space in the vacuum of the abdomen, but it does increase the distance to the retroperitoneal vessels, a concern especially in the smaller child. The Veress needle is advanced with a slight tilt into the hollow of the pelvis, thus aiming below the level of the bifurcation of the great vessels. If the angle is too steeply caudal, preperitoneal placement will almost invariably occur. As the needle is advanced, the resistance of the abdominal wall fascia is passed, with an audible click of the spring-loaded obturator.

Correct intraperitoneal placement of the needle tip is essential and must be verified before insufflation. Even a small amount of preperitoneal gas can cause enough emphysema to obscure landmarks and make laparoscopic examination difficult. A large preperitoneal insufflation makes laparoscopy technically almost impossible and may require postponement of the procedure. There are several signs, none of which

is infallible, that intraperitoneal placement has been achieved.[32] First, one should aspirate through the Veress needle. The return of air or succus may indicate intravisceral placement; urine indicates intravesical placement; frank blood suggests placement in a large vessel and should prompt exploration. Holding the needle immobile until exploration has begun can potentially occlude the defect in the wall of the vessel and decrease blood loss. The needle can also be followed to the site of injury.

If aspiration through the Veress needle reveals nothing, irrigation with sterile saline is performed. The saline should instill easily, and on aspiration should not return. On removal of the syringe, the meniscus of saline should immediately drop out of sight if the low-pressure environment of the peritoneal cavity is cannulated. Finally, moving the tip of the needle in a circle to confirm free intraperitoneal placement has been described.[32] This is a subjective test and should not be performed before aspiration and irrigation, in case of intravascular or visceral placement.[34] The authors do not advocate the use of the circle test. The insufflation tubing is then attached and inflation at 1 L/min begun. Opening pressure must be noted and must be less than 5 mm Hg. Maintenance of low intra-abdominal pressure during the early moments of insufflation is the best indicator of intraperitoneal placement. As the pneumoperitoneum progresses, the tympany noted on percussion should be equivalent in all abdominal quadrants. The persistence of liver dullness suggests preperitoneal insufflation.[35]

The insufflation is continued until the intraperitoneal pressure is in the vicinity of 20 mm Hg. In the small infant, this may be achieved with less than 1 L of CO_2, whereas in the older child or adult several liters will be required. The site for placement of the primary-access laparoscopic cannula is chosen. Because of the intra-abdominal location of the bladder in the young infant, a supraumbilical site may be preferred. In older children and adults, an infraumbilical position is adequate. A horizontal incision, appropriately sized for the cannula chosen, is made in the appropriate position. The subcutaneous tissues are spread to the level of fascia. In most series of laparoscopic procedures, a blind percutaneous technique of initial surgical port placement is used. The surgical ports and trocars are either reusable or disposable, but the disposable ones (Fig. 23–1) have more reliable sharpness, and most come with a shield that springs over the blade after the peritoneum has been entered.[35] With a finger alongside the shaft of the trocar/cannula to limit its excursion onto the abdomen, it is introduced with a twisting motion. Once the pneumoperitoneum has been established, the issue of preperitoneal placement is irrelevant, and a more caudal tilt to avoid the retroperitoneal great

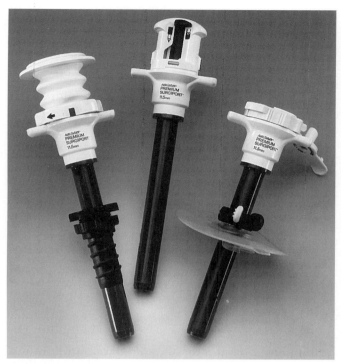

Figure 23–1. Three examples of disposable laparoscopic cannulas. The sheath on the left demonstrates a screw-type device for maintaining the position of the cannula. The middle cannula has an automatically retracting trocar, to prevent injury to intra-abdominal organs. (Courtesy of Auto Suture Company, Norwalk, CT. Copyright © 1995, United States Surgical Corporation. All rights reserved. Reprinted with the permission of United States Surgical Corporation.)

clearly visualized. This technique seems superior to the blind passage of a trocar, but still requires initial insufflation of the abdomen with a Veress needle.

Because of the risks inherent in the percutaneous access to pneumoperitoneum, there are many pediatric laparoscopists who advocate open cannula placement in all situations.[14] Open placement is made by carrying the incision to and through the level of the fascia, exposing and opening the peritoneum. Stay sutures are placed on the fascia on either side of the incision. A cannula with a fixation device is dilated through the opening and secured. Some practitioners note no inherent advantage of the open approach in a previously unoperated abdomen, and difficulty with air leak may be increased with the Hasson cannula.[3] True Hasson-style cannulas do not work well in children as they are bulky, designed for use in adults, and not as effective at maintaining a gastight trocar site. Because the child's abdominal wall is thin, the open access incision can actually be made smaller than the cannula size, and thus screw fixation devices are effective for both air seal and cannula stability. Those who have adopted routine open access find that access can be achieved faster with virtually no anxiety and doubt, and they have found no problems with cannula fixation or gas seal. In a multicenter review of complications of laparoscopic surgery, most were associated with blind primary access or Veress insufflation.[38]

Diagnostic Laparoscopy

With the patient in the Trendelenburg position and the camera in place, the normal anatomy of the pelvis in the child is impressively distinct. The inguinal

vessels should be employed. If a disposable trocar is used, the click of the safety shield will signal entrance into the abdomen. Otherwise, a loss of resistance will be felt. The trocar is removed, and the rush of gas from the side port confirms placement in the insufflated cavity. The laparoscope is immediately inserted to confirm the intraperitoneal position and to examine for intra-abdominal injuries. If injuries are noted, appropriate action must be taken immediately. Veress needle injuries to bowel or bladder can be managed conservatively, but trocar injuries require open or laparoscopic primary repair.[31] Vascular injuries generally necessitate open repair, although injuries to abdominal wall vessels can often be managed percutaneously.[37] Rapid access to the peritoneal cavity can be achieved by levering the laparoscope against the anterior abdominal wall and cutting down onto it.[31]

A new option for initial trocar placement is the use of a direct vision-obturator (Visi-Port) (Fig. 23–2). This is an instrument with a clear lens at the tip through which the laparoscope can view the tissues as the trocar is advanced. A trigger-activated cutting blade incrementally incises the tissue forward of the lens, and the layers of the abdominal wall can be clearly seen as they are traversed. Blood vessels and intra-abdominal structures can be avoided by changing direction, and the passage into the peritoneum is

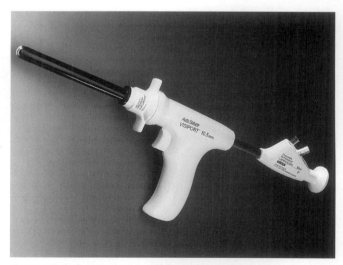

Figure 23–2. System for introduction of the laparoscopic cannula that allows visualization of the layers of the abdominal wall as they are traversed. A blade in the clear plastic lens cuts tissue when the trigger is activated. (Courtesy of Auto Suture Company, Norwalk, CT. Copyright © 1995, United States Surgical Corporation. All rights reserved. Reprinted with the permission of United States Surgical Corporation.)

rings are located just lateral to the medial umbilical ligaments on either side. Examination for the presence of the nonpalpable testis begins by looking at the internal ring on the side of the normal testis (if there is one). The spermatic vessel leash is seen to join the vas deferens, coursing medial to lateral, just before their joint course through the inguinal canal. Traction on the testicle will move the spermatic vessels and vas, making the anatomy more obvious. The affected side is then examined, and one of many possible observations will be made. A review of all the English language reports of laparoscopy for the cryptorchid testis was undertaken by Peters and Kavoussi.[3] On average, in 45 percent of cases, a vas deferens and spermatic vessels are seen to exit the ring into the groin. Pressure can be applied over the internal ring to see if there is a testicle that can be expressed back into the abdomen. If not, exploration for a testicle or testicular nubbin should be undertaken. It has been suggested that in the absence of a patent processus vaginalis, there may be no need for an inguinal exploration.[39] In a prospective study of 104 children, Moore et al found that only 50 percent of viable canalicular or ectopic testes were associated with a patent processus.[40] Passage of a laparoscope or a flexible cystoureteroscope into the patent processus to identify a testicle has been described, and can be helpful if easily accomplished.[32] In most cases, the gonadal remnant can be removed from above using a laparoscopic technique. Since, by definition, nothing is palpable in the groin, the spermatic vessels and/or vas can be grasped and with dissection pulled up into the abdomen. Care must be taken with traction on the vas, as it is easily avulsed. Likewise, one must be careful to cauterize the gubernacular remnants once the testis or end of the cord has been delivered, because they can cause troublesome bleeding if avulsed or divided without electrocautery. Gonadal remnants tethered in the prepubic area cannot be routinely excised from above, but once freed in this way, the remnants can be removed through a 1-cm incision made directly over the gonadal tissue.

In 16 percent of boys with a nonpalpable gonad, blind-ending vas and spermatic vessels will herald the vanishing testis,[3] probably the result of prenatal intra-abdominal testicular torsion. In these cases, no further exploration is warranted. If a blind-ending vas or vas and epididymis is seen, but not vessels, disjunction may have occurred. Further laparoscopic exploration should be carried out to rule out the presence of a gonadal remnant alongside the pericolic gutter or near the lower pole of the kidney. Occasionally, placement of secondary cannulas will assist in this examination by allowing retraction and reflection of the colon. If no testis or testicular vessels are found laparoscopically, it is controversial whether further exploration involving examination of the renal hilum

should be undertaken. The occurrence of a testicle outside the confines of the laparoscopically examinable peritoneal cavity is a rare event, and it is doubtful that such an exploration is warranted.[41] The suggestion has been made that a computed tomographic scan or magnetic resonance image of the upper abdomen can be obtained postoperatively to rule out this possibility.[42]

Finally, in 38 percent of cases, an intra-abdominal testis is found (Fig. 23–3).[3] The position of the testicle in relation to the internal ring should be noted. It has been suggested that any testis more than 1 to 2 cm above the ring will not reach the scrotum without division of the testicular vessels. The appearance of the testis and the epididymis can also be used to decide whether orchiectomy or orchidopexy is the most reasonable procedure to perform. It has been shown that preoperative administration of human chorionic gonadotropin can decrease the need for laparoscopy by rendering more testicles palpable.[43] This is undoubtedly true, but the 40 to 53 percent of children with an absent testis[40, 44] will have received hormonal therapy to no benefit. The rationale for this approach needs to be considered by the individual provider.

If an intra-abdominal testicle is found, one can proceed to open surgery or therapeutic laparoscopy. Three procedures can be performed laparoscopically on the intra-abdominal testis: orchiectomy,[45–48] division of the spermatic vessels as the first stage of a two-stage Fowler-Stephens orchidopexy,[5] or primary orchidopexy maintaining the integrity of the spermatic vessels.[6] The possibility of performing a laparoscopically assisted microvascular orchidopexy has also been proposed.[42] If further laparoscopic manipulation is to be performed, additional cannulas will need to be inserted into the abdomen.

Therapeutic Laparoscopy

Placement of additional trocars should be performed under direct vision from within the abdomen, thus increasing safety. Raising the intra-abdominal pressure to 20 mm Hg facilitates cannula insertion while minimizing the excursion of the abdominal wall.[42] The appropriate site for trocar placement is chosen. Transilluminating the site from within the abdomen allows visualization of larger abdominal wall vessels. An incision large enough to admit the cannula is made along Langer's lines in the skin. The anterior fascia is exposed bluntly. The trocar is inserted with a twisting motion, again limiting its excursion with a finger along the shaft of the cannula. From within the abdomen, the trajectory of the trocar can be monitored until safe placement has been confirmed. The trocar site should be inspected for bleed-

Deep inferior epigastric a.

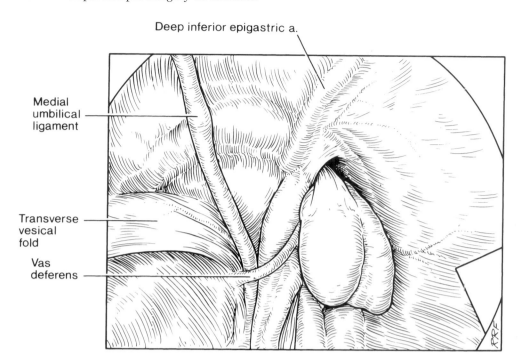

Medial umbilical ligament

Transverse vesical fold

Vas deferens

Figure 23–3. Appearance of the inguinal anatomy in the presence of an intra-abdominal undescended testis. (From Jordan GH, Winslow BH. Laparoscopic single stage and staged orchiopexy. J Urol 152:1249, 1994. Copyright Williams & Wilkins, 1994.)

ing from injury to an abdominal wall vessel. The cannula can be secured after the trocar is removed. Either a screw or balloon device can be used (see Fig. 23–1), or the cannula can be simply fixed to the skin with a suture. These methods prevent inadvertent removal of the cannula as instruments are withdrawn. It is a good idea at this time to move the camera into an accessory cannula to examine the original cannula site for bleeding, and to secure this cannula appropriately.

Cannula placement for laparoscopic orchiectomy or orchidopexy is similar (Fig. 23–4A). The smaller the child, the higher in the abdomen the more cephalad cannulas should be, to allow enough room to work. If there is a patent processus vaginalis associated with the intra-abdominal testis, this can be closed with clips, or a peritoneal incision can be made around the mouth of the sac and the edges pulled together with staples or sutures.[42] The vessels to the testis can be divided using clips, staples, suture, or occasionally electrocautery. The testis, once freed, can usually be brought out of the abdomen through a 10-mm cannula, or withdrawn with the cannula through the incision. A lap sack can be used if the testis is too large to be easily manipulated through the incision. Closure of the abdomen is then carried out as discussed below.

Laparoscopic orchidopexy is an evolving technique that seems to have some surgical advantages over open orchiectomy for the intra-abdominal testicle.[6] Practitioners of this procedure believe they can achieve a more complete dissection of the spermatic vessels laparoscopically than can be accomplished through an inguinal incision.[3] Although the morbid-

ity of open orchidopexy is low in young patients, older children or adolescents may experience significant postoperative pain. The long-term results of laparoscopic orchidopexy are as yet unknown, but early results have been promising. Technically, this is a complicated procedure that should be attempted only in conjunction with persons who have had considerable experience in laparoscopic surgery.

The positioning of cannulas for laparoscopic orchidopexy is illustrated in Figure 23–4A. The peritoneum distal and medial to the patent processus vaginalis (if present) is incised with a scissors (Fig. 23–4B). The incision can be carried proximally along the lateral side of the spermatic vessels. The peritoneum between the vasal and spermatic vessels is left intact if possible, at least until it becomes fairly clear that there will be enough length to reach the scrotum. The anterior wall of the processus vaginalis can then be incised in the midline and retracted into the abdomen, bringing the back wall with the long-looped vas deferens, if present, with it. After the distal extent of the vas is seen, the gubernacular attachments can be divided with electrocautery (Fig. 23–4C), and the remainder of the patent processus allowed to retract into the canal. Traction on the freed testis will then allow an estimate of spermatic leash length. If it seems that there will be enough for scrotal placement of the testis, the peritoneum overlying the vessels is stripped away, increasing significantly the length of the pedicle (Fig. 23–4D). The vessels can be freed to the level of the renal hilum if necessary. Additional mobility can be achieved by dividing the peritoneum distal to the vas overlying the medial umbilical ligament.

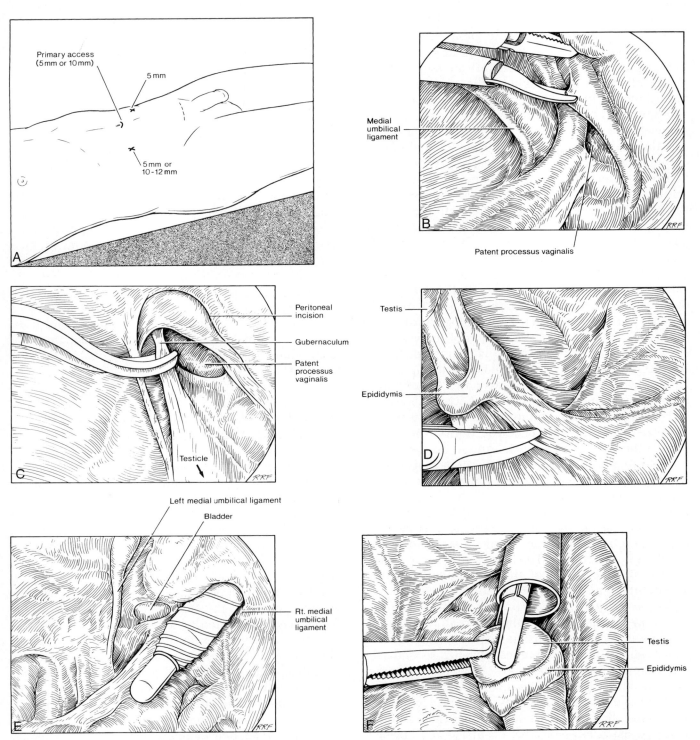

Figure 23–4. *A,* Typical laparoscopic cannula positioning for a laparoscopic orchiopexy or orchiectomy. *B,* The peritoneum distal and lateral to the patent processus vaginalis is incised. The space behind the cord will be developed bluntly to allow traction. *C,* After the distal extent of the vas deferens is ascertained, the gubernaculum is divided. *D,* The peritoneum along the lateral cord is divided to allow a straight course to the inguinal canal. The peritoneum can also be stripped off the anterior cord, further releasing potential vascular length. *E,* A cannula has been introduced via the scrotal incision. *F,* The testis is grasped in preparation for withdrawing through the new internal ring and into the scrotum. (From Jordan GH, Winslow BH. Laparoscopic single stage and staged orchiopexy. J Urol 152:1249, 1994. Copyright Williams & Wilkins, 1994.)

After the testis is dissected free, it should easily reach the opposite internal ring. A horizontal incision is made on the anterior scrotum and a dartos pouch developed as in a routine orchidopexy. With a hemostat, the inguinal canal is developed to, but not into, the peritoneal cavity. To take full advantage of the length of the vascular pedicle, the testis should be passed medial to the lateral umbilical ligament (inferior epigastric pedicle), clearly seen from within the abdomen. To limit the need for mobilization of the vas, the testis is passed medial to the medial umbilical ligament (obliterated umbilical artery). A grasper is passed from within the abdomen out through the scrotal incision. A 10-mm cannula is passed into the abdomen over this grasper, and the grasper is withdrawn. Alternatively, a cannula changer may be passed through the new inguinal canal into the abdomen and, after dilating the canal, a 10-mm trocar placed (Fig. 23–4E). Using atraumatic technique, the substance of the testis is grasped and the testis partially withdrawn into the cannula (Fig. 23–4F). The cannula and testis are then brought together through the scrotal incision. The orientation of the vas deferens and the vessels is examined within the abdomen; it is not uncommon for a twist to occur during testicular passage. The testis is fixed in the dartos pouch in whichever manner is preferred. Care should be exercised not to put undue strain on the testicular vessels, as avulsion has occurred during this procedure. If the testis does not reach the scrotum comfortably at this point, either orchiectomy or inguinal fixation with the idea of a staged approach is a viable option. Microvascular transplantation may also be considered if the time, skill, and equipment are available. Dividing the testicular vessels at this juncture would risk ischemia due to the dissection of the distal peritoneal tissue. The best solution is to realize the insufficient length of the vessels early on and perform the appropriate intervention.

The peritoneal defect remaining at the end of this procedure in the area of the internal ring can be closed with vascular clips, as described by Jordan et al,[6] or can be left open to reperitonealize secondarily. No postoperative hernias have been reported after this procedure thus far. The pressure in the abdomen is decreased to allow venous bleeding, if present, to become more obvious. Meticulous hemostasis is achieved using clips or electrocautery. The bowel is examined for evidence of inadvertent electrocautery or penetrating injury.

Dividing the testicular vessels as the initial step of a staged Fowler-Stephens orchidopexy requires one cannula in addition to the camera port for placement of a clip applier.[5] The clip should be applied across the entire pedicle, which can sometimes be accomplished without incising the peritoneum.

Experience with laparoscopic orchidopexy has identified one situation in which the testicle migrates medial to the ipsilateral medial umbilical ligament. In general, these medial ectopic abdominal testicles are associated with relative shortness of the spermatic vessels, and also the vas is quite short. The appearance can initially be quite confusing, as there is usually no patent processus, and the very prominent gubernacular vessels simulate the spermatic vessel leash. On careful inspection, however, the path of the vas deferens will be noted to track rostrally, away from the anatomical location of the "internal ring," and at that point the displaced gonad will become apparent. Because these gonads are associated with rather short vessels, primary orchidopexy can be difficult. Because the vas is often short or atretic, staged orchidopexy is not a good option either. If there is a normal contralateral testicle, laparoscopic orchiectomy is probably indicated. If not, primary laparoscopic orchidopexy should be performed, with the testicle placed at the base of the scrotum as well as can be accomplished. The dissection associated with these testicles is technically very difficult, and if the surgeon is not well experienced with laparoscopic techniques, open orchidopexy is probably the best choice.[49]

Removal of Laparoscopic Cannulas and Closure of Abdominal Incisions

At the end of any laparoscopic procedure, an orderly and meticulous routine for cannula removal and fascial closure must be followed. If a single cannula is used, a final inspection of the abdomen is made. The abdomen is meticulously purged of CO_2, and the laparoscope is reintroduced to look for pockets of gas that can be aspirated. Remaining CO_2 is a source of postoperative pain due to the conversion to carbonic acid and peritoneal irritation.[31] The cannula is removed over the laparoscope, withdrawing the laparoscope then under vision. This ensures that bowel or omentum is not drawn through the site by the cannula. The anterior fascia is closed with an absorbable suture under direct vision. All cannula sites in children should be closed because of the documented incidence of omental evisceration,[50] even through 4-mm port sites.

If more than one cannula is used, all secondary cannula sites should be inspected, followed by moving the camera to a secondary port to visualize the primary site. The cannulas should then be withdrawn while watching from within to ensure that there is no bleeding that had been tamponaded by the cannula.[31] While observing from within, the sites are closed as described. Another option for fascial closure is the use of a specialized suture-carrying needle (e.g., Auto-Stitch, Auto-Suture), loaded with a fascial stitch through a spring-loaded obturator that is much like a crochet hook. The needle is passed through the fascia and into the abdomen. A grasper is used to withdraw the stitch, and the needle is removed. It is reintroduced on the opposite side of the fascial opening, and the grasper is used to reload the suture. The needle is withdrawn, and the two ends of the suture are available for tying. At this point, the cannula is removed and the suture is tied. In children, these automatic closure devices are seldom required. On removal of the cannula, a Joseph skin hook is introduced through the site, one on each side. The hooks engage the peritoneum, and by definition also elevate the fascia. An absorbable suture on a small half-circle needle can be used to close both fascia and peritoneum, with the path of the needle directly observed from within. This method of closure is very effective, and in cases so closed in which interval repeat laparoscopy has been required, there have not been any adhesions to the cannula sites.[51]

The last cannula is removed in a fashion similar to that described for a single port after all the CO_2 has been evacuated. The skin incisions can be closed with adhesive strips or interrupted subcuticular sutures. Small bandages, Band-Aids, or transparent film generally suffice for a postoperative dressing.

POSTOPERATIVE MANAGEMENT

Most of these patients can be discharged home on the day of the procedure. There is no special precaution to be taken, except for the usual postoperative limitations after orchidopexy, which include no straddle toys, restriction on bathing for 2 to 3 days, and standard wound care. There is sometimes pain postoperatively due to the presence of residual CO_2 in the peritoneal space,[31] although this is unusual in children. This resolves over several hours and is rarely severe enough to require overnight hospitalization. The pain is also very effectively eliminated by using one of the nonsteroidal analgesic agents.

If a pledget or button is used to secure the testicle, this must be removed after 1 week. The position and consistency of the testicle should be noted in the immediate postoperative period, and then again at 3 months and 1 year. The possibility of testicular tumor in the undescended or contralateral testis should be explained, along with a recommendation for testicular self-examination teaching and regular office examinations after puberty. In short, in that laparoscopic surgery is merely "open surgery" accomplished through laparoscopic access, follow-up is identical to that for a standard open operation.

LAPAROSCOPIC NEPHRECTOMY

The indications for laparoscopic nephrectomy or partial nephrectomy in children are most commonly a symptomatic multicystic dysplastic kidney or a nonfunctional hydronephrotic kidney or renal moiety. As in open nephrectomy, patient positioning is important to the ease of operation. To allow intra-abdominal contents to fall away from the kidney, a lateral decubitus position is advantageous. For creating a pneumoperitoneum, placing the patient in a horizontal position is most comfortable for the surgeon. A 30- to 40-degree lateral oblique position on a table that can be tilted 30 degrees in either direction allows both positions to be used as necessary without repositioning the patient on the table.[13] Pneumoperitoneum is achieved as described earlier, and cannulas are placed at the umbilicus and at the ipsilateral anterior axillary line, one just below the costal margin and one in the lower abdominal quadrant. Depending on the procedure being performed, additional cannulas are placed, often laterally in the midaxillary line. The colon is mobilized and reflected. The ureter is identified in the retroperitoneum. This is sometimes made easier by cystoscopic placement of a ureteral catheter. The ureter is used for traction on the kidney, which is bluntly dissected free of fatty attachments to the lower pole. The vessels are identified in the renal hilum using blunt dissection. The vessels can be individually ligated with vascular clips. If the clips are not large enough, the GIA stapler may be advantageous. The vessels in a nonfunctioning kidney are often small, yet hemostasis at the hilum remains of paramount importance. After the hilar vessels are secured, the upper pole is mobilized. The ureter is divided last, using clips. Most dysplastic and nonfunctioning kidneys can be removed intact through the larger incision sites. If not, an impermeable sack (Lapsac) can be used in conjunction with a morcellator to remove the kidney.[11] The renal bed is inspected for hemostasis, reducing the intra-abdominal pressure to unmask venous bleeders. The colon is then reattached laterally, and closure of the trocar sites is undertaken as previously described. In children, vascular anomalies are often associated with nonfunctioning kidneys, as is malrotation. A laparoscopic Doppler is very useful for identifying these anomolously placed vessels, and speeds the dissection in the renal hilum. If upper pole nephroureterectomy is being performed because of complicated duplication anomalies, again the Doppler is invaluable for identifying upper pole vessels and also delineating the tissues containing the main renal vessels, under which the upper pole ureter invariably passes. The pneumodissector, an instrument currently under development, has been successfully used in children and has been found to speed the dissection of the ureter and the renal hilum. Additionally, the dissection of perirenal fat off the renal capsule is effectively accomplished with this new surgical tool. Further evaluation of this technique in laparoscopic surgery is warranted.

Summary

The laparoscopic approach to surgery in children is safe, effective, and probably superior to the open approach for specific applications. As instrumentation improves, the spectrum of disease that can effectively be treated laparoendoscopically will expand to include most of the procedures now performed in an open fashion. Already, safer and more accurate methods of reaching the abdomen are being developed. As surgical experience and instrumentation advance, the advantages of minimally invasive approaches to pediatric problems will become more obvious. The wide surgical field, optical magnification, and decreased postoperative morbidity are having an impact on the way we approach the nonpalpable testis and nonfunctioning kidney. As this science progresses, low-morbidity surgical alternatives to therapy for vesicoureteral reflux, neurogenic bladder, and hydronephrosis may significantly alter our basic approach to these disorders by shifting the balance toward surgical therapy.

REFERENCES

1. Cortesi N, Ferrari P, Zambarda E, et al. Diagnosis of bilateral abdominal cryptorchidism by laparoscopy. Endoscopy 8:33, 1976.
2. Lobe TE. The applications of laparoscopy and lasers in pediatric surgery. Surg Annu 1:175, 1993.
3. Peters CA, Kavoussi LR. Pediatric endourology and laparoscopy. In Walsh PC, Retik AB, Stamey TA, Vaughan ED Jr, eds. Campbell's Urology, 6th ed. Philadelphia, WB Saunders, 1993, p 1.
4. Castilho LN, Ferreira U, Netto NR, et al. Laparoscopic pediatric orchiectomy. J Endourol 6:155, 1992.
5. Bloom DA. Two-step orchiopexy with pelviscopic clip ligation of the spermatic vessels. J Urol 145:1030, 1991.
6. Jordan GH, Robey EL, Winslow BH. Laparoendoscopic surgical management of the abdominal/transinguinal undescended testicle. J Endourol 6:159, 1992.
7. Das S. Laparoscopy in pediatric urology. J Endourol 6:151, 1992.
8. Gu CX, Ge QS, Tang MY, et al. Laparoscopic assessment of gonadal function. Chin Med J (Engl) 99:369, 1986.
9. Droesch K, Droesch J, Chumas J, et al. Laparoscopic gonadectomy for gonadal dysgenesis. Fertil Steril 53:360, 1990.
10. Easter DW. Inguinal hernia in pediatrics: Initial experience with laparoscopic inguinal exploration of the asymptomatic contralateral side (letter; comment). J Laparoendosc Surg 2:361, 1992.
11. Clayman RV, Kavoussi LR, Soper NJ, et al. Laparoscopic nephrectomy: Initial case report. J Urol 146:278, 1991.
12. Figenshau RS, Clayman RV, Kerbl K, et al. Laparoscopic nephroureterectomy in the child: Initial case report. J Urol 151:740, 1994.
13. Jordan GH, Winslow BH. Laparoendoscopic upper pole partial nephrectomy with ureterectomy. J Urol 150:940, 1993.
14. Ehrlich RM, Gershman A, Fuchs G. Laparoscopic renal surgery in children. J Urol 151:735, 1994.
15. Hagood PG, Mehan DJ, Worischeck JH, et al. Laparoscopic varicocelectomy: Preliminary report of a new technique. J Urol 147:73, 1992.
16. Donovan JF, Winfield HN. Laparoscopic varix ligation. J Urol 147:77, 1992.
17. Donovan JF, Winfield HN. Laparoscopic varix ligation with Nd:YAG laser. J Endourol 6:165, 1992.
18. Ralph DJ, Timoney AG, Parker C, et al. Laparoscopic varicocoele ligation. Br J Urol 72:230, 1993.
19. Ross LS, Ruppman N. Varicocele vein ligation in 565 patients under local anesthesia: A long-term review of technique, results and complications in light of proposed management by laparoscopy. J Urol 149:1361, 1993.
20. Clayman RV. Pediatric laparoscopy: Quo vadis? A view from the outside. J Urol 152:730, 1994.
21. Kozminski M, Partamian KO. Case report of laparoscopic ileal loop conduit. J Endourol 6:147, 1992.
22. Ehrlich RM, Gershman A. Laparoscopic seromyotomy (autoaugmentation) for non-neurogenic bladder in a child: Initial case report. Urology 42:175, 1993.
23. Parra RO, Boullier JA. Endocavitary (laparoscopic) bladder surgery. Semin Urol 10:213, 1992.
24. Jordan GH, Winslow BH. Laparoscopically assisted continent catheterizable cutaneous appendicovesicostomy. J Endourol 7:517, 1993.
25. Schuessler WW, Grune MT, Tecuanhuey LV, et al. Laparoscopic dismembered pyeloplasty. J Urol 150:1795, 1993.
26. Kavoussi LR, Peters CA. Laparoscopic pyeloplasty. J Urol 150:1891, 1993.
27. Wolf JS, Stoller ML. The physiology of laparoscopy: Basic principles, complications and other considerations. J Urol 152:294, 1994.
28. Sosa RE, Weingram J, Poppax D, et al. Physiological considerations in laparoscopic surgery. J Endourol 6:85, 1992.
29. Monk TG, Weldon BC. Anesthetic considerations for laparoscopic surgery. J Endourol 6:89, 1992.
30. Jordan GH, Winslow BH. The effects in children of high pressure pneumoperitoneum using CO_2 insufflation on end-tidal CO_2. In preparation, 1995.
31. Kavoussi LR, Sosa RE, Capelouto C. Complications of laparoscopic surgery. J Endourol 6:95, 1992.
32. Winfield HN, Donovan JF, See WA, et al. Urological laparoscopic surgery (review). J Urol 146:941, 1991.
33. Veress J. Neus Instrument zur Ausfuhrung von Brust oder Bachpunktionen und Pneumthorax Behandlung. Dtsch Med Wochenschr 64:1480, 1938.
34. Karatassas A, Walsh D, Hamilton DW. A safe, new approach to establishing a pneumoperitoneum at laparoscopy. Aust N Z J Surg 62:489, 1992.
35. Wolf JS, Carroll PR. Laparoscopic access to and exit from the abdomen. Atlas Urol Clin North Am 1:1, 1993.
36. Evans RM, Reddy PK. Complications of laparoscopy. Semin Urol 10:164, 1992.
37. Green LS, Loughlin KR, Kavoussi LR. Management of epigastric vessel injury during laparoscopy. J Endourol 6:99, 1992.
38. Kavoussi LR, Sosa E, Chandhoke P, et al. Complications of laparoscopic pelvic lymph node dissection. J Urol 149:322, 1993.
39. Weiss RM, Seashore JH. Laparoscopy in the management of the nonpalpable testis. J Urol 138:382, 1987.
40. Moore RG, Peters CA, Bauer SB, et al. Laparoscopic evaluation of the nonpalpable testis: A prospective assessment of accuracy. J Urol 151:728, 1994.
41. Guiney EJ, Corbally M, Malone PS. Laparoscopy and the management of the impalpable testis. Br J Urol 63:313, 1989.
42. Jordan GH. Management of the abdominal nonpalpable undescended testicle. Atlas Urol Clin North Am 1:49, 1993.
43. Naslund MJ, Gearhart JP, Jeffs RD. Laparoscopy: Its selected use in patients with unilateral nonpalpable testis after human chorionic gonadotropin stimulation. J Urol 142:108, 1989.
44. Boddy SA, Corkery JJ, Gornall P. The place of laparoscopy in the management of the impalpable testis. Br J Surg 72:918, 1985.
45. Stewart LH, Heasley RN, Loughridge WG. Laparoscopic removal of intra-abdominal testis. Br J Urol 70:208, 1992.

46. Beck RO, Nicholl P, Hickey NC, et al. Laparoscopic excision of an intra-abdominal testis. Br J Urol 70:105, 1992.

47. O'Donoghue J, Rogers E, Keeling P, et al. Laparoscopic removal of an intra-abdominal seminoma. Br J Urol 71:109, 1993.

48. Pan BS, Ooi LL, Mack PO. Laparoscopic assessment and orchidectomy for the undescended testis. Aust N Z J Surg 64:118, 1994.

49. Jordan GH, Winslow BH. Laparoscopic single stage and staged orchiopexy. J Urol 152:1249, 1994.

50. Bloom DA, Ehrlich RM. Omental evisceration through small laparoscopy port sites. J Endourol 7:31, 1993.

51. Moore RG, Kavoussi LR, Bloom DA, et al. Adhesion formation after urologic laparoscopy in the pediatric population. J Urol 153:792, 1995.

SECTION II

ADULT UROLOGICAL SURGERY

Part I
Surgery of the Kidney

Part II
Renovascular Surgery

Part III
Surgery of the Retroperitoneum and Ureter

Part IV
Surgery of the Bladder

Part V
Urinary Diversion

Part VI
Surgery of the Prostate

Part VII
Surgery of the Seminal Vesicles

Part VIII
Surgery of the Urethra in the Male

Part IX
Surgery of the Scrotum, Testis, and Penis

Part X
Outpatient Surgery

Chapter 24

Adrenal Surgery

E. Darracott Vaughan, Jr.

At the present time, the diagnosis of the major adrenal disorders that require subsequent adrenalectomy is extremely accurate. This precision is due to the development of accurate analytical methods for adrenal hormones and radiographical techniques for localization of specific adrenal lesions.[1, 2]

The major pathological entities that require surgical intervention include primary hyperaldosteronism, Cushing syndrome, adrenocortical carcinoma, pheochromocytoma, and neuroblastoma. Bilateral adrenalectomy is utilized rarely as an ablative treatment for metastatic breast carcinoma.

Primary hyperaldosteronism is characterized by hypertension, hypokalemia, elevated urinary or plasma aldosterone levels when sodium and potassium levels are repleted, and low plasma renin activity when sodium levels are depleted (Fig. 24–1).[3, 4] This syndrome can be due to solitary adenoma (60 percent), a surgical lesion, or bilateral adrenal hyperplasia (40 percent), a medical lesion. Lateralization tests are critical to differentiate between the two entities. Unilateral adrenalectomy is the treatment of choice for a patient with an adenoma. A patient with bilateral hyperplasia is usually treated with spironolactone, 100 to 400 mg/day, and adrenalectomy is avoided except in the unusual case of marked asymmetry of aldosterone production. In this setting, removal of the dominant adrenal gland results in transient or long-term remission of hyperaldosteronism.[4]

Cushing syndrome can be due to central, hypothalamic, or pituitary excess secretion of adrenocorticotropic hormone (ACTH) (Cushing disease); primary adrenal hypercorticalism caused by an adrenal adenoma or carcinoma; or ectopic secretion of ACTH.[5] The steps to accurate diagnosis are shown in Figure 24–2. Cushing disease is currently treated with bilateral adrenalectomy only when transsphenoidal surgery, pituitary irradiation, or both have failed. The major role of surgery lies in the treatment of functional adrenal adenomas or adrenal carcinomas. Uni-

lateral adrenalectomy remains the treatment of choice for patients with localized adrenal disease. At times patients with ectopic ACTH syndrome from unresectable tumors are candidates for bilateral adrenalectomy. There is a reasonable prognosis.

Adrenocortical carcinoma in either adults or children has an extremely poor prognosis; fortunately, the tumor is rare.[6] The tumors can produce a variety of adrenal hormones or may be nonfunctioning. Accordingly, any patient with an adrenal mass needs to be fully evaluated for hormonal activity. Virilization, elevated 17-ketosteroid levels, or elevated dehydroepiandrosterone (DHEA) levels should heighten the clinician's suspicion of carcinoma rather than adenoma. All hormonally active tumors should be removed if surgically possible. Most reported adrenal carcinomas are greater than 5 cm. Currently, all nonfunctioning adrenal tumors found accidentally, "incidentalomas," that are greater than 5 cm should be removed. Smaller nonfunctional lesions may be watched with serial computed tomography (CT) or magnetic resonance imaging (MRI) if the imaging pattern is consistent with an adenoma; i.e., low-signal intensity on MRI. However, if the MRI signal shows a high intensity on a T2 image or is heterogeneous, exploration is indicated.

Pheochromocytomas and neuroblastomas as well as other benign retroperitoneal neural tumors arise from neural crest cells.[7, 8] The presentation varies with the production of active metabolites. Fortunately, accurate assays for catecholamines and metabolites are available (Fig. 24–3). The introduction of metaiodobenzyl guanidine (MIBG) isotopic adrenal medullary scanning coupled with MRI now gives excellent localization of pheochromocytomas, often resulting in unilateral adrenal exploration.

Other indications for adrenalectomy are (1) palliative bilateral excision in metastatic breast cancer, (2) rare solitary metastasis to the adrenal from another primary, (3) some adrenal cysts, and (4) in association with renal cell carcinoma as part of a radical nephrectomy.

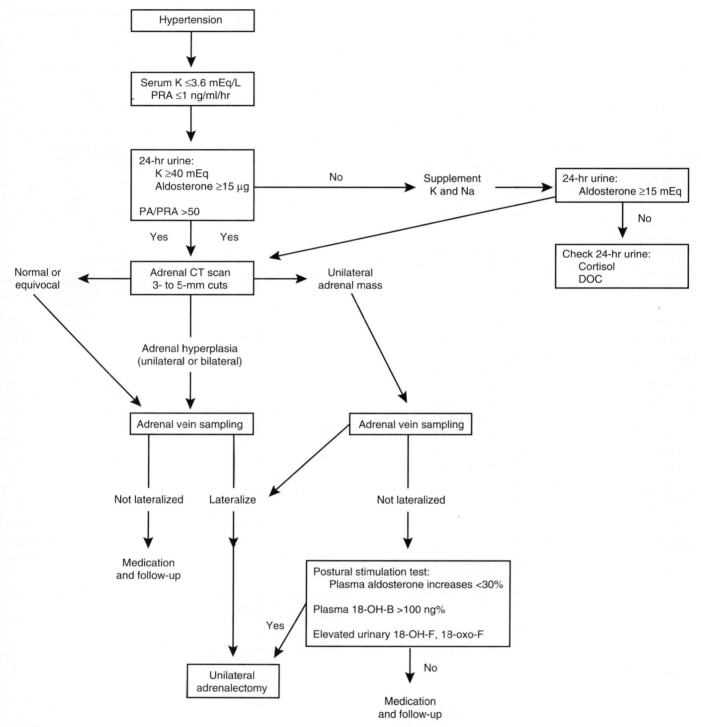

Figure 24–1. Evaluation for surgically treatable primary hyperaldosteronism. (Adapted from Blumenfeld JD, Sealey JE, Schlussel Y, et al. Diagnosis and therapy of primary hyperaldosteronism. Ann Intern Med 121:877, 1994.)

PREOPERATIVE MANAGEMENT

The preoperative management for adrenal surgery is dependent on the primary adrenal lesion. Specific needs are outlined in Table 24–1. Patients with primary hyperaldosteronism are generally otherwise healthy, and spironolactone provides good blood pressure control. Rarely, postoperative potassium re-

tention occurs; therefore, serum potassium levels should be watched closely. Patients with Cushing syndrome have severe systemic effects from the hyperglucocorticoidism. Hence, they are obese, have diabetic tendencies, are poor wound healers, easily sustain bony fractures, and are susceptible to infection. They are thus at high risk for complications.

The major problem for a patient with pheochromo-

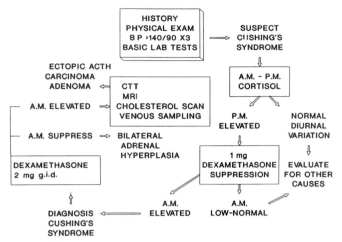

Figure 24–2. Evaluation for Cushing syndrome. (From Vaughan ED Jr. Diagnosis of adrenal disorders in hypertension. World J Urol 7:111, 1989.)

cytoma is obviously cardiovascular lability due to catecholamine secretion. Stability is achieved with preoperative alpha-adrenergic blockade and, if necessary, reduction of catechol production with alpha-methyl tyrosine. It is critical that the anesthesiologists be fully informed about the case. They must also be familiar with the anesthetic management of these particular patients.[7, 9, 10]

The management of patients with adrenal disorders is approached on a team basis, including experienced endocrinologists, radiologists, anesthesiologists, and urologists or general surgeons.

SURGICAL OPTIONS

Numerous approaches can be made to the adrenal gland (Table 24–2). The proper approach depends on

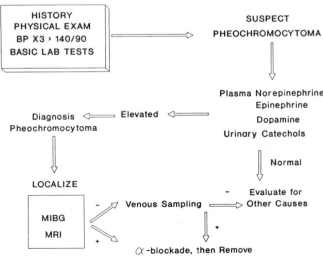

Figure 24–3. Evaluation for pheochromocytoma. (From Vaughan ED Jr. Diagnosis of adrenal disorders in hypertension. World J Urol 7:111, 1989.)

TABLE 24–1. Preoperative Management

	Treatment
Primary hyperaldosteronism	Spironolactone, 100 to 400 mg/day, 2–3 wk Follow K⁺ until normal Blood pressure should fall
Cushing syndrome	Control of glucose abnormalities Documentation of osteoporosis Glucocorticoid replacement (before, during, and after surgery) Perioperative antibiotics

Pheochromocytoma	Adrenergic blockade
	  Phenoxybenzamine (Dibenzyline), 20–160 mg/day
	  Metyrosine (if needed)
	Volume expansion
	  Crystalloid
	Beta blockade if cardiac arrhythmias (only after alpha blockade established)
	Anesthesia consultation

the underlying cause of the adrenal pathology, the size of the adrenal, the side of the lesion, the habitus of the patient, and the experience and preference of the surgeon. In some cases, options are available, and a careful review of all variables is required before a choice is made. Thus, each case should be considered individually, although some approaches are preferred for given diseases. For example, a posterior or modified posterior approach is preferred for small, well-localized lesions, whereas an abdominal approach is preferred for multiple pheochromocytomas. In contrast, a patient with a large adrenal carcinoma may

TABLE 24–2. Surgical Approaches in Adrenal Disorders

	Approach
Primary hyperaldosteronism	Posterior (left or right) Modified posterior (right) 11th rib (left > right) Posterior transthoracic
Cushing adenoma	11th rib (left or right) Thoracoabdominal (large) Posterior (small)
Cushing disease Bilateral hyperplasia	Bilateral posterior Bilateral 11th rib (alternating)
Adrenal carcinoma	Thoracoabdominal 11th rib Transabdominal
Bilateral adrenal ablation	Bilateral posterior
Pheochromocytoma	Transabdominal (chevron) Thoracoabdominal (large, usually right) 11th rib
Neuroblastoma	Transabdominal 11th rib

require a thoracoabdominal approach. A well-localized large pheochromocytoma may best be excised through a similar incision, if nothing suggests multiple lesions.

A number of adrenalectomies utilizing a laparoscopic approach have been performed successfully and reported. This technique is described in Chapter 21.

OPERATIVE TECHNIQUES

Before a description of the specific techniques, some unifying concepts warrant attention. The adrenal glands are posterior or dorsal structures lying against the posterior abdominal musculature and diaphragm. As well as being posteriorly located, they also lie high behind the posterior peritoneum, covered anteriorly by the liver on the right and the pancreas and spleen on the left. The cranial blood supply comes from the phrenic system intimately related to the diaphragm. Inferiorly, the glands sit upon or are molded by the kidneys. The anterior surface drops dorsally to the apex, thereby falling away from the operator using an anterior approach.

Taking these anatomical facts into consideration, several points can be made. Adequate visualization with a headlamp is critical, and hemostasis should be rigorously maintained. The operator should bring the adrenal down by initially exposing the cranial attachments and dividing the rich blood supply between right-angled clips, using forceps cautery for additional control. The blood supply bounds the gland in a stellate fashion. It is often simplest to begin dissection laterally, identifying the vascular supply and working around the cranial edge of the gland. Interestingly, the posterior surface of the adrenal is usually devoid of vasculature. The gland can be drawn caudally with gentle traction on the kidney. The gland is extremely friable and fractures easily, which causes troublesome bleeding. In essence, the patient should be dissected from the tumor, a concept particularly true for a pheochromocytoma, in which the gland should not be manipulated and early venous control is preferred.

Posterior Approach

The posterior approach can be used for either bilateral adrenal exploration or unilateral removal of small tumors (Fig. 24–4). In the past, all patients with primary aldosteronism were explored in this fashion because of inability to localize the lesion. Today, localization is mandatory before exploration is recommended.[4] The bilateral approach is primarily employed for ablative total adrenalectomy. The options

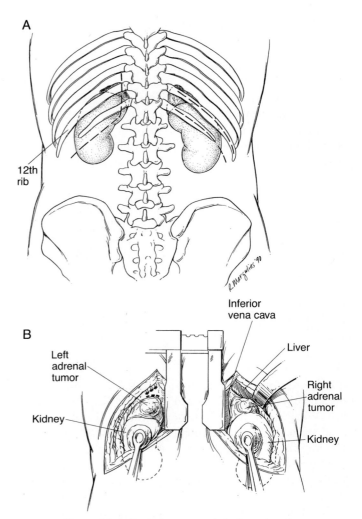

Figure 24–4. Posterior approach to the adrenals.

for incisions are shown; generally, rib resection is preferable to obtain high exposure. After standard subperiosteal rib resection, care should be taken with the diaphragmatic release, the pleura should be avoided, and the diaphragm is swept cranially.

The fibrofatty contents within Gerota's fascia are swept away from the paraspinal musculature, exposing a subdiaphragmatic "open space" that is the apex of the resection. The liver, within the peritoneum, is dissected off the anterior surface of the adrenal. The cranial blood supply is divided. Medially, on the right, the inferior vena cava (IVC) is visualized. The short, high adrenal vein, entering the cava in dorsolateral fashion, is identified and can be clipped or ligated. The adrenal can then be drawn caudally by traction on the kidney. Care must be taken to avoid apical branches of the renal artery. On the left, the approach is similar, with division of the splenorenal ligament giving initial lateral exposure.

The posterior approach can also be modified for a transthoracic adrenal exposure through the diaphragm[11]; however, this more extensive approach is rarely found necessary for small adrenal tumors.

Modified Posterior Approach

Although the posterior approach has the advantage of rapid adrenal exposure and low morbidity, there are definite disadvantages. The jackknife position may impair respiration, the abdominal contents are compressed posteriorly, and the visual field is limited. The advantage of the posterior approach is primarily for control of the short right adrenal vein (Fig. 24–5); therefore, a modified approach for right adrenalectomy has been developed.[12]

The approach is based on the anatomical relationship of the right adrenal, which lies deeply posterior and high in the retroperitoneum behind the liver (Fig. 24–5A). In addition, the short, stubby right adrenal vein enters the IVC posteriorly at the apex of the adrenal. Hence, we utilize an approach that is posterior, but the patient is in a modified position, similar to that used for a Gil-Vernet dorsal lumbotomy incision (Fig. 24–5B).[13] The patient is placed in this position and the eleventh or twelfth rib is resected with care to avoid the pleura. The diaphragm is resected off the underlying peritoneum and liver and should be sharply dissected free to gain mobility. Similarly, the inferior surface of the peritoneum, closely associated with the liver, is sharply dissected from Gerota's fascia, which is gently retracted inferiorly.

The adrenal will become visible in the depth of the incision as the final hepatic attachments are divided. A lateral space can be found, exposing the posterior abdominal musculature. The adrenal lies against the paraspinal muscles. Multiple small adrenal arteries that course behind the IVC and emerge over the paraspinal muscles are clipped and divided (Fig. 24–5C). At this point, the adrenal can usually be moved against the paraspinal musculature, exposing the IVC below the adrenal gland.

The major advantage of this approach is that the adrenal vein is easily identified because it emerges from the segment of the IVC exposed and courses up to the adrenal, which now rises toward the surgeon. In other flank or anterior approaches, the adrenal vein resides in its posterior relationship, requiring caval rotation with the chance of adrenal vein avulsion. After adrenal vein exposure, it is doubly tied and divided or clipped with right-angled clips and divided (Fig. 24–5D).

The adrenal can now be easily retracted inferiorly for division of the remaining arteries and removal. The wound is not drained and is closed with interrupted 0 polydioxanone sutures.

This technique is used for all patients with right adrenal aldosterone-secreting tumors and for other patients with benign adenomas less than 6 cm. I do not recommend the approach for patients with large lesions or malignant adrenal neoplasms.

Flank Approach

The standard extrapleural, extraperitoneal eleventh rib resection is excellent for either left or right adrenalectomy.[14] This approach is described in detail elsewhere; only the adrenal dissection is described here.

After completion of the incision, the lumbocostal arch is utilized as a landmark showing the point of attachment of the posterior diaphragm to the posterior abdominal musculature. Gerota's fascia, containing the adrenal and kidney, can be swept medially and inferiorly, giving exposure to the splenorenal ligament on the left, which should be divided to avoid splenic injury (Fig. 24–6A). Working anteriorly on the left, the spleen and pancreas within the peritoneum can be lifted cranially, exposing the anterior surface of the adrenal gland.

On the right side, a similar maneuver is used to lift the liver within the peritoneum off the anterior surface of the adrenal. Quite often the adrenal gland cannot be identified precisely until these maneuvers are performed. One should not attempt to dissect into the body of the adrenal or to dissect the inferior surface of the adrenal off the kidney. The kidney is useful for retraction. The dissection should continue from lateral to medial along the posterior abdominal and diaphragmatic musculature, with precise ligation or clipping of the small but multiple adrenal arteries (Fig. 24–7A). While the operator clips these arteries with one hand, the opposite hand is employed to retract both adrenal and kidney inferiorly. With release of the superior vasculature, the adrenal becomes easily visualized. On the left medially, the phrenic branch of the venous drainage must be carefully clipped or ligated (Fig. 24–8D). This vessel is not noted in most atlases but can cause troublesome bleeding if divided. The medial dissection along the crus of the diaphragm and aorta will lead to the renal vein; finally, the adrenal vein is controlled, doubly tied, and divided. The adrenal is then removed from the kidney with care to avoid the apical branches of the renal artery (Fig. 24–6B).

On the right side, the dissection is similar. However, after release of the adrenal from the superior vasculature, it is helpful to expose the IVC and divide the medial arterial supply. This maneuver allows mobilization of the cava for better exposure of the high posterior adrenal vein, which is again doubly tied or clipped and divided (Fig. 24–7B). Patients with large adrenal carcinomas may require en bloc resections of the adrenal and kidney following the principles of radical nephrectomy (Fig. 24–7C).

A major deviation from this technique is used in the patient with pheochromocytoma, in whom the initial dissection should be aimed toward early control and division of the main adrenal vein on either

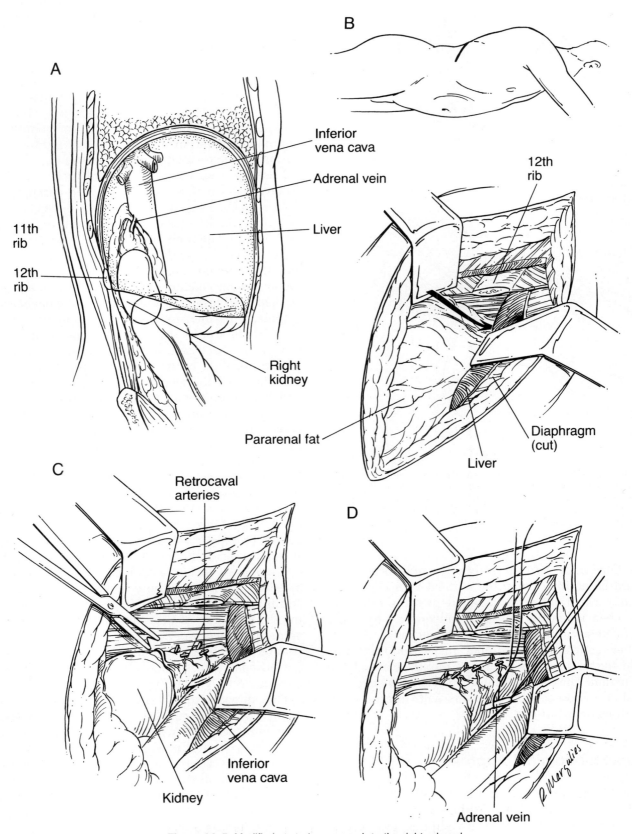

Figure 24–5. Modified posterior approach to the right adrenal.

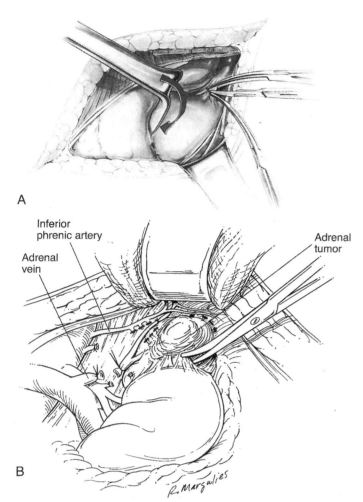

Figure 24–6. Release of the splenorenal ligament early in the exposure of the left adrenal. (Reprinted with permission from Siragy HM, Vaughan ED Jr, Carey RM. Cushing's syndrome. In Vaughan ED Jr, Carey RM, eds. Adrenal Disorders. New York, Thieme, 1989, p 159. Copyright, Thieme Medical Publishers, Inc.)

side. Obviously, in this setting, the anesthesiologist should be notified when the adrenal vein is divided because a marked drop in blood pressure often occurs, even when the patient is adequately hydrated and treated with alpha-adrenergic blockade.

After removal of the adrenal, inspection should be made for any bleeding and for pleural tears of the diaphragm. The kidney should also be inspected. The incision is closed without drains with interrupted 0 polydioxanone sutures.

Thoracoabdominal Approach

The thoracoabdominal ninth or tenth rib approach is utilized for large adenomas; for some large adrenal carcinomas; and for well-localized pheochromocytomas, especially on the right side. The incision and exposure is standard (Fig. 24–8), with a radial incision through the diaphragm and a generous intraperi-

toneal extension. The techniques described for adrenalectomy with the eleventh rib approach are used.

Transabdominal Approach

The transabdominal approach is commonly selected for patients with pheochromocytomas, for children, and for some patients with adrenal carcinomas. The concept is to have the ability for complete abdominal exploration to identify either multiple pheochromocytomas or adrenal metastases.

I use the transverse or chevron incision, which I believe gives better exposure of both adrenal glands than a midline incision. The rectus muscles and lateral abdominal muscles are divided, exposing the peritoneum. Upon entering the peritoneal cavity, the surgeon should gently palpate the para-aortic areas and the adrenal areas. Close attention is given to blood pressure changes in an attempt to identify any unsuspected lesions if the patient has a pheochromocytoma. This maneuver is less important today because there are the excellent localization techniques previously discussed. In fact, with precise preoperative localization of the offending tumor, the chevron incision does not need to be completely symmetrical and can be limited on the contralateral side.

If the patient has a lesion on the right adrenal, the hepatic flexure of the colon is reflected inferiorly. The incision is made in the posterior peritoneum lateral to the kidney and carried superiorly, allowing the liver to be reflected cranially (Fig. 24–9). Incision in the peritoneum is carried downward, exposing the anterior surface of the IVC to the entrance of the right renal vein. Once the cava is cleared, one or two accessory hepatic veins are often encountered, which should be secured (Fig. 24–10). These veins are easily avulsed from the cava and may cause troublesome bleeding. Ligation of these veins gives 1 to 2 cm of additional caval exposure, which is often useful during the exposure of the short posterior right adrenal vein. Small accessory adrenal veins may also be encountered. The cava is then rolled medially, exposing the adrenal vein, which should be doubly tied or clipped and divided (Fig. 24–10C).

The surgeon should inform the anesthesiologist when the vein is ligated in a patient with a pheochromocytoma because a precipitous fall in blood pressure can occur at this point, requiring volume expansion or even vasopressors. After control of the adrenal vein, it is simplest to proceed with the superior dissection, lifting the liver off the adrenal and securing the multiple small adrenal arteries arising from the inferior phrenic artery, which is rarely seen. The adrenal can be drawn inferiorly with retraction on the kidney, and the adrenal arteries traversing to the adrenal from under the cava can be secured with right-

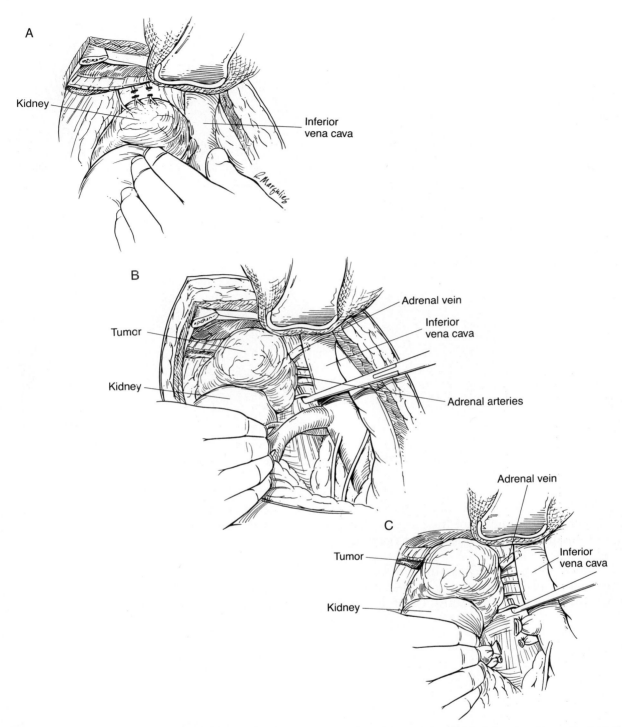

Figure 24–7. Exposure of the right adrenal with and without nephrectomy. *A*, Superior exposure. *B*, Medial and end vessels divided without nephrectomy. *C*, Medial vessels divided with nephrectomy.

angled clips. The final step is removing the adrenal from the kidney.

The left adrenal vein is not as difficult to approach because it lies lower, partially anterior to the upper pole of the kidney, and the adrenal vein empties into the left renal vein. Accordingly, on the left side, the colon is reflected medially, exposing the anterior surface of Gerota's capsule; the initial dissection should involve identification of the renal vein (Fig. 24–9*B*).

In essence, the dissection is the same as for a radical nephrectomy for renal carcinoma. Once the renal vein is exposed, the adrenal vein is identified, doubly ligated, and divided. After this maneuver the pancreas and splenic vasculature are lifted off the anterior surface of the adrenal gland. Because of additional drainage from the adrenal into the phrenic system, I generally continue the medial dissection early to control the phrenic vein. I then work cepha-

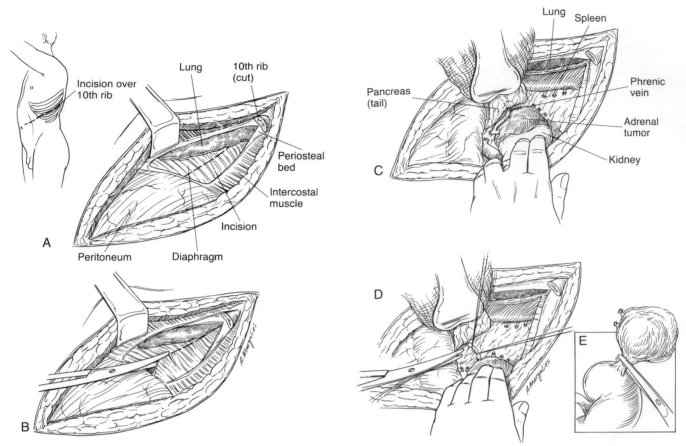

Figure 24–8. Thoracoabdominal approach to the left adrenal.

lad and lateral to release the splenorenal ligament and the superior attachments of the adrenal. The remainder of the dissection is carried out as previously described.

After removal of the tumor, regardless of size, careful inspection is made to ensure hemostasis and the absence of injury to adjacent organs. Careful abdomi-nal exploration is carried out, after which the wound is closed with the suture material of choice. No drains are used.

Patients with multiple endocrine adenopathy or family histories of pheochromocytoma, as well as pediatric patients, should be considered at high risk for multiple lesions. Preoperative evaluation should

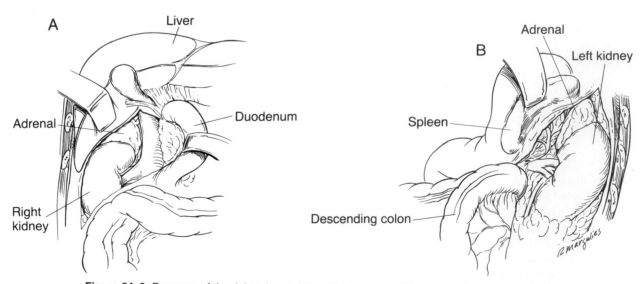

Figure 24–9. Exposure of the right adrenal (A) and left adrenal (B) by a transabdominal approach.

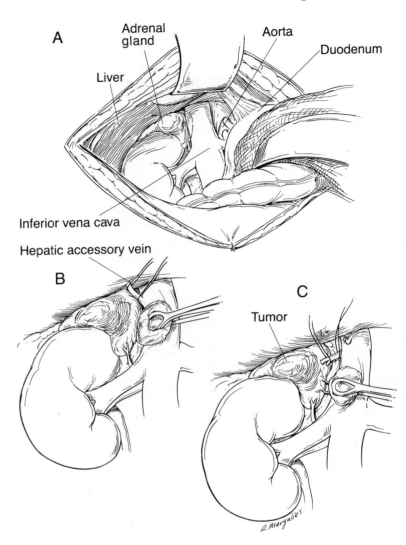

Figure 24–10. Further transabdominal exposure of the right adrenal with ligation of an accessory right hepatic vein.

identify these lesions, but, regardless, a careful abdominal exploration should be carried out.

In patients with suspected malignant pheochromocytomas, en bloc dissections may be necessary to obtain adequate margins, a concept that also applies in patients with adrenal carcinomas. Evaluation with MRI to obtain transverse, coronal, and sagittal images is extremely useful to define clearly the adrenal relationships to the IVC and renal vessels as well as to localize the adrenal vein.

In patients with pheochromocytomas, postoperative management includes maintenance of arterial and venous lines in an intensive care setting until they are stable. Often, 24 to 48 hours is required for the full effect of phenoxybenzamine, the alpha-blocking agent commonly given, to wear off and for normal alpha-receptor activity to be restored.

COMPLICATIONS AND POSTOPERATIVE MANAGEMENT

Complications arising from adrenalectomy can be divided into general perioperative complications as-

sociated with abdominal surgery and specific complications associated with adrenal disorders.

Surgical Complications

The most troublesome surgical complication is damage to the right adrenal vein and IVC. Exposure and meticulous dissection are critical to avoid injury. If injury does occur, it is best to pack the area and to gain additional caval exposure. The cava can be partially occluded with a sponge stick; the adrenal vein stump can be grasped with a vascular clamp or an Allis forceps and suture ligated.

On the left side, care should be taken to avoid the spleen and body or tail of the pancreas. If injury does occur, general surgical consultation is generally obtained for direction. If a pancreatic injury occurs, the incision is drained.

Specific complications are related to the underlying adrenal disorders.[15] Patients with glucocorticoid excess have suppression of contralateral adrenal function and thus require steroid replacement until recovery occurs. The obvious treatment is prevention, and a variety of replacement regimens have been described. I generally utilize 100 mg hydrocortisone intramuscularly or intravenously preoperatively, and 100 mg every 4 to 6 hours postoperatively, until the patient can be given oral replacement. Mineralocorticoid replacement is usually not necessary unless bilateral adrenalectomy has been performed; however, plasma sodium and potassium levels should be monitored.

Patients with Cushing syndrome have protean manifestations of glucocorticoid excess and are at risk for various complications. They are obese and catabolic, and heal poorly. They have muscle wasting, fragile skin, osteoporosis, glucose intolerance, and hypertension. Accordingly, they are at risk for wound infection, thromboembolism, associated cardiovascular disease, and psychological instability. In florid cases, pharmacological blockade with metyrapone, an 11-beta-hydroxylase inhibitor, has been administered to inhibit excess steroid synthesis.

In contrast, patients with primary hyperaldosteronism rarely exhibit any postoperative difficulties. These patients are routinely given spironolactone preoperatively until potassium levels are normal. Occasionally, a patient retains potassium postoperatively and requires treatment.

Preoperative management of patients with pheochromocytomas with alpha-adrenergic blockade is generally recommended to gain blood pressure stability and volume expansion and to decrease the possibility of cardiac arrhythmia. Beta-adrenergic blockade is used only if arrhythmias persist after blood pressure control. Patients also undergo volume expansion with crystalloid preoperatively.

During the procedure, an accomplished anesthesiologist must be present with a full armamentarium of cardiovascular drugs and monitoring devices. Both high and low extremes of blood pressure are not uncommon during the procedure. After tumor removal, I prefer to maintain blood pressure with fluid expansion rather than alpha-adrenergic agonists, if possible. Postoperative intensive care monitoring for 24 to 48 hours is often utilized.

Summary

Adrenal surgery is an extremely satisfying procedure for both physicians and patients. Rarely in medicine do we have a better understanding of the under-lying pathophysiology than with adrenal disorders. Moreover, we have highly sophisticated analytical and radiographical diagnostic techniques that confirm clinical impressions. We have developed elegant surgical approaches to the adrenal that can be individualized for the specific case and can be successfully performed with minimum risk to the patient.

Editorial Comment
Fray F. Marshall

The management of adrenal tumors is well summarized. Physiological as well as surgical considerations are important and vary, depending on the tumor. The surgical approaches also differ. Proceeding with the superior dissection above the adrenal first, with downward traction on the kidney, can facilitate the surgery. Right-angled clips are used, which are easier to apply in this area. The right adrenal vein is always higher and more posterior than expected.

REFERENCES

1. Vaughan ED Jr, Blumenfeld JD. The adrenals. In Walsh PH, Retik AB, Stamey TA, Vaughan ED Jr, eds. Campbell's Urology, 6th ed. Philadelphia, WB Saunders, 1992.
2. Libertino JA, Novick AC, eds: Adrenal surgery. Urol Clin North Am 16:417, 1989.
3. Vaughan ED Jr, Atlas S, Carey RM. Hyperaldosteronism. In Vaughan ED Jr, Carey RM, eds. Adrenal Disorders. New York, Thieme Medical Publishers, 1989.
4. Blumenfeld JD, Sealey JE, Schlussel Y, et al. Diagnosis and therapy of primary hyperaldosteronism. Ann Intern Med 121:877, 1994.
5. Orth D. Cushing's syndrome. N Engl J Med 332:791, 1995.
6. Vaughan ED Jr, Carey RM. Adrenal carcinoma. In Vaughan ED Jr, Carey RM, eds. Adrenal Disorders. New York, Thieme Medical Publishers, 1989.
7. Reckler JM, Vaughan ED Jr, Tjeuw M, Carey RM. Pheochromocytoma. In Vaughan ED Jr, Carey RM, eds. Adrenal Disorders. New York, Thieme Medical Publishers, 1989.
8. Coyle MA. Neuroblastoma. In Vaughan ED Jr, Carey RM, eds. Adrenal Disorders. New York, Thieme Medical Publishers, 1989.
9. Malone MJ, Libertino JA, Tsapatasaris NP, Woods BO. Preoperative and surgical management of pheochromocytoma. Urol Clin North Am 16:567, 1989.
10. Jovenich JJ. Anesthesia in adrenal surgery. Urol Clin North Am 16:583, 1989.
11. Novick AC, Straffon RA, Kaylor W. Posterior transthoracic approach for adrenal surgery. J Urol 141:254, 1989.
12. Vaughan ED Jr, Phillips H. Modified posterior approach for right adrenalectomy. Surg Gynecol Obstet 165:453, 1987.
13. Gil-Vernet J. New surgical concepts in removing renal calculi. Urol Int 20:255, 1965.
14. Riehle RA Jr, Lavengood RW. An extrapleural approach with rib removal for the 11th rib flank incision. Surg Gynecol Obstet 161:276, 1985.
15. Angermeier KW, Montie JE. Perioperative complications of adrenal surgery. Urol Clin North Am 16:597, 1989.

Part I
SURGERY OF THE KIDNEY

Chapter 25

Simple Nephrectomy

Ihor S. Sawczuk, Erik T. Goluboff, and Carl A. Olsson

Although early descriptions of incidental nephrectomies during operations for other lesions have been reported, the first intentional nephrectomy was probably performed in 1869 by Gustav Simon for treatment of a ureterovaginal fistula. With advances in preoperative preparation, antibiotics, and surgical and anesthetic techniques, the indications for simple nephrectomy have broadened while the morbidity and mortality have decreased.[1]

INDICATIONS

In selected instances, simple nephrectomy is indicated in kidneys affected by trauma, hypertension, symptomatic hydronephrosis, infection, or calculous disease.[1,2] Simple nephrectomy is generally not indicated for neoplastic diseases of the kidney. Trauma resulting in an irreparable renal unit or severe renal parenchymal or vascular injury in the presence of other life-threatening injuries warrants nephrectomy. Medically uncontrolled hypertension due to unilateral parenchymal or renovascular disorders not amenable to reconstruction is another indication. In the presence of long-standing hydronephrosis associated with renal parenchymal loss and nonfunction, nephrectomy may also be considered. Renal infectious processes that cannot be controlled with appropriate systemic antibiotic therapy or other forms of management, such as percutaneous drainage, are also indications for simple nephrectomy. Xanthogranulomatous pyelonephritis and, in some instances, nonfunctioning renal tuberculous kidneys may be reasons for nephrectomy. Instances of symptomatic staghorn calculi within nonfunctioning infected kidneys, especially in the elderly, are best handled by nephrectomy.

PREOPERATIVE MANAGEMENT

The patient's presentation is dependent on the cause of the renal disorder necessitating a simple nephrectomy. In emergent instances, such as trauma, a complete preoperative evaluation is impossible. However, in patients with renal injury, the extent of the injury can be evaluated by either computed tomography (CT) or intravenous pyelography (IVP). Even at this rushed time, at least the knowledge of a functioning opposite kidney should be obtained, whenever possible.

A routine preoperative evaluation includes a complete history and physical examination. Because of the special positions required for exposure during renal surgery, attention to cardiac and pulmonary status in the preoperative evaluation takes on some importance. The flank incision in the lateral position can be associated with impaired venous return and pulmonary compromise.[1] Specifically, any history of heart disease, smoking, or respiratory disorders should be elicited, and the patient's functional status optimized before surgery. Evaluation by cardiac and pulmonary function tests as well as appropriate consultation with medical and anesthesia colleagues should be considered. Preoperative incentive spirometry training and smoking cessation are recommended. Any history of bleeding disorders should be elicited. A complete blood count, electrocardiogram, and chest radiograph should be obtained for every patient.

From the history and examination, the etiology may be elucidated and appropriate laboratory studies obtained, including serum creatinine and blood urea nitrogen levels, excretory urogram, and occasionally total creatinine clearance. The contralateral kidney should be evaluated by an excretory urogram, CT scan, or differential function calculated by nuclear

231

renal scan. Preoperative antibiotics, if indicated, may be administered, especially in cases of infected renal units. CT, with its excellent visualization of the retroperitoneum, is recommended in most patients being considered for simple nephrectomy. In patients with elevated serum creatinine levels or contrast allergy, ultrasound examination of the kidneys can be considered. Renal arteriography, to determine the feasibility of vascular reconstruction, may be indicated in the evaluation of patients with medically uncontrolled hypertension due to renovascular disorders. It is rarely indicated in other patients undergoing simple nephrectomy.

OPERATIVE TECHNIQUE

Numerous surgical approaches to the kidney have been described. In general, the surgical approach is determined both by the diagnosis of the problem and by the particular anatomy of the patient. Operative approaches to the kidney include the retroperitoneal flank approach, with or without rib resection; the anterior transabdominal approach, either trans- or extraperitoneal; the thoracoabdominal approach; and the lumbar approach. Each approach has been reported to be associated with various incisions, advantages, and disadvantages.[1, 2] In cases of trauma or renovascular disorders, a transabdominal approach is preferred, allowing early renal pedicle control. Most often, the retroperitoneal flank approach is used via a transcostal, intercostal, or subcostal incision. The choice of incision is also influenced by the anatomy of the patient. For example, an obese patient is best serviced by a flank approach. Our preferred approach is from the flank in most instances. Because of the lower position of the right kidney, a twelfth rib resection or subcostal incision is common. On the left side, an eleventh rib resection or intercostal incision between the eleventh and twelfth ribs is typical.

The patient is placed in the standard flank position (Fig. 25–1). An incision is made on or below the chosen rib extending from the posterior rib angle to the edge of the rectus muscle. In this manner, the

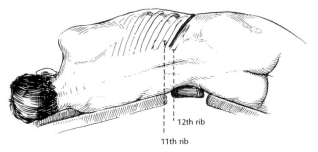

Figure 25–1. The patient is placed in the flank position and an intercostal incision is made. (From Glenn J. Urologic Surgery, 4th ed. Philadelphia, JB Lippincott, 1991, p 75.)

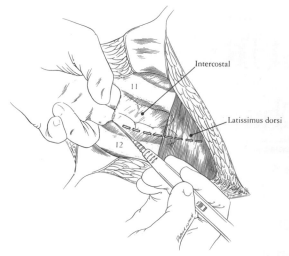

Figure 25–2. The latissimus dorsi and intercostal muscles are divided close to the superior edge of the lower rib. (From Lytton B. Surgery of the kidney. In Walsh PC, Gittes RE, Perlmutter AD, Stamey TA, eds. Campbell's Urology, 5th ed. Philadelphia, WB Saunders, 1986, p 2406.)

rib or its interspace is exposed. For an intercostal approach, the intercostal neurovascular bundle is avoided by keeping the incision close to the upper rib border. The intercostal muscle is divided, exposing the pleura and diaphragm fibers (Fig. 25–2). With a rib-resecting technique, after exposure of the rib, the intercostal muscles are stripped from the upper and lower rib surfaces with an Alexander costal periosteotome.[2] The rib is freed from the periosteum by subperiosteal resection or from the pleura with a periosteal elevator. A Doyen costal elevator is slipped beneath the rib to free it. The proximal and distal portions of the rib are immobilized with Kocher clamps, and the rib is divided proximal to its angle with a right-angled rib cutter. The costal cartilage is cut free with scissors. The cut surface of the rib is inspected for spicules, which are removed with a rongeur.[2] The diaphragmatic fibers are then incised posteriorly, care being taken not to injure the pleura. By dividing the diaphragmatic attachments posteriorly, the pleura can be retracted superiorly and the ribs spread apart to reveal the retroperitoneal space.

The peritoneal border is identified medially and the peritoneum can be separated bluntly from Gerota's fascia, though it need not be for a simple nephrectomy. Once the peritoneal edge is identified, Gerota's fascia is incised posterior to this line (Fig. 25–3). Using blunt and sharp dissection, a plane can be developed along the posterior renal border. Moving inferiorly, the lower pole can also be freed. Whenever a vessel is encountered, it is clipped and transected. Care should be taken to avoid avulsing aberrant renal vessels, especially along the inferior pole. The ureter can be identified at this point, ligated with an absorbable suture, and transected. With the posterior and inferior aspects

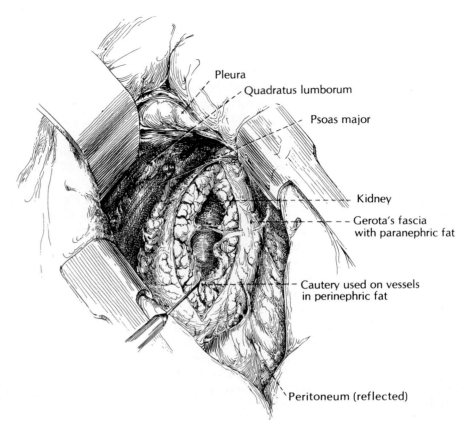

Pleura
Quadratus lumborum
Psoas major
Kidney
Gerota's fascia with paranephric fat
Cautery used on vessels in perinephric fat
Peritoneum (reflected)

Figure 25–3. Gerota's fascia is opened, permitting dissection of the kidney. (From Glenn J. Urologic Surgery, 4th ed. Philadelphia, JB Lippincott, 1991, p 74.)

freed, attention can be turned to the superior pole. With downward traction on the kidney, a plane can usually be developed between the adrenal gland and the kidney, since the adrenal is encompassed in a separate compartment within Gerota's fascia. Sharp dissection and clipping of blood vessels in this region is usually necessary to free the superior pole. At this point, only the anterior renal border and the renal hilar vessels need be identified (Fig. 25–4). Both the vein and artery are identified, separated, ligated, and transected. The artery is taken before the vein, to avoid renal congestion. Both vessels are doubly ligated proximally with 0 silk sutures and distally with one 0 silk suture. Rarely, it may be necessary to ligate both vessels in one ligature.

Once the vessels are transected, the kidney can be removed. If purulence is encountered or in the case of nephrectomy for an active infectious process, a drain may be placed in the retroperitoneal space and brought out through a separate stab wound posteriorly; otherwise, drainage is not required.

Occasionally, the kidney may be adherent to the surrounding tissues because of inflammatory processes, and a subcapsular nephrectomy may be necessary. This is done by making a renal capsular incision and then stripping the capsule from the renal tissue. The capsule is freed up to the renal hilum, where it must be incised to identify, ligate, and resect the renal vessels.

POSTOPERATIVE MANAGEMENT AND COMPLICATIONS

Nephrectomy can be associated with significant alterations in fluid and electrolyte balance, and these should be carefully attended to in the postoperative

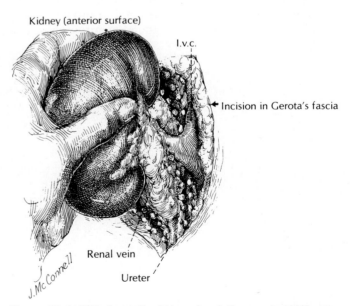

Kidney (anterior surface)
I.v.c.
Incision in Gerota's fascia
Renal vein
Ureter
J. McConnell

Figure 25–4. With the entire kidney freed, the renal vessels may then be exposed. (From Glenn J. Urologic Surgery, 4th ed. Philadelphia, JB Lippincott, 1991, p 74.)

period. Pain control, aggressive pulmonary toilet, and early mobilization are also important to prevent pulmonary and vascular complications. Perioperative antibiotics should usually be stopped within the first 48 hours, unless there was evidence of renal infection preoperatively. After the retroperitoneal flank approach, return of gastrointestinal function should occur in the first 2 or 3 days.

Postoperative complications, including wound infections, pulmonary problems, and cardiovascular and gastrointestinal events, may occur.[3-5] Wound infections, especially in patients with infected renal units, may be common: up to 30 percent in some older series. It is not unusual for these patients to be elderly and have other compromising medical problems, such as diabetes, which can further increase the risk of wound infections. The use of drains in infected cases and the prompt drainage of infected wound sites will help minimize morbidity. Intravenous antibiotics, with selection based on culture results, should be provided when indicated.

It is important to suspect, recognize, and promptly treat atelectasis, occasionally leading to the development of frank pneumonia, and pneumothorax, especially after unrecognized violation of the pleural cavity. We prefer to obtain a portable chest radiograph in the recovery room to guard against unsuspected pneumothorax whenever a rib resection or intercostal approach is used.

Deep venous thrombosis and (rarely) pulmonary embolus may also occur; early mobilization and the use of prophylactic measures such as compression boots, stockings, and sometimes anticoagulation can help prevent these complications. As after any major surgery, myocardial ischemia or infarction needs to be rapidly diagnosed and treated. Ileus occurs more commonly after the transabdominal approach and is usually self-limited; injury to adjacent organs can occur intraoperatively, with the liver and duodenum at most risk during right nephrectomies and the spleen and pancreas during left ones, but these are generally recognized and treated intraoperatively. Finally, and importantly, postoperative bleeding can occur. Serial blood counts and a high index of suspicion should be maintained. Significant blood loss may be hidden from physical examination by the capacious retroperitoneum. Careful attention to control of the renal pedicle as well as any accessory vessels cannot be overemphasized. Mortality, according to surgical series from the 1970s, is generally less than 2 percent and depends on the specific disease etiology necessitating nephrectomy and on concomitant medical problems.

Summary

A simple nephrectomy is indicated in the appropriate circumstances. As with renal surgery in general, adequate exposure and adherence to surgical principles will aid in achieving an uncomplicated postoperative course.

REFERENCES

1. Lytton B. Surgery of the kidney. In Walsh PC, Gittes RE, Perlmutter AD, Stamey TA, eds. Campbell's Urology, Vol 3, 5th ed. Philadelphia, WB Saunders, 1986, p 2406.
2. Crawford ED. Nephrectomy and nephroureterectomy. In Glenn JF, ed. Urologic Surgery, 4th ed. Philadelphia, JB Lippincott, 1991, p 22.
3. Schiff M Jr, Glazier WB. Nephrectomy: Indications and complications in 347 patients. J Urol 118:930, 1977.
4. Gonzalez-Serva L, Weinerth JL, Glenn JF. Minimal mortality of renal surgery. Urology 9:253, 1977.
5. Scott RF, Selzman HM. Complications of nephrectomy: Review of 450 patients and a description of a modification of the transperitoneal approach. J Urol 95:307, 1966.

Chapter 26

Donor Nephrectomy

John M. Barry

Supply and Demand

Although 11,000 kidney transplants were performed in the United States in 1994, there were still 27,000 patients on the United Network for Organ Sharing (UNOS) national waiting list for cadaver kidney grafts early in 1995.[1] The demand for transplantable kidneys far exceeds the supply. About 25 percent of kidney transplants are from living relatives of the recipient. Most of the rest are from cadaver donors, but a few are from unrelated living donors.

Donor Criteria

The basic criteria for a renal donor are no renal disease, no active infection, no transmittable malignancies, ABO blood group compatibility with the recipient, and a negative cross-match between donor lymphocytes and recipient serum. The surgical goals for living or cadaver donor nephrectomy are to eliminate warm ischemia time, preserve anomalous or multiple renal vessels, and preserve ureteral blood supply. An additional goal in the cadaver donor is to remove enough blood, lymph nodes, and splenic tissue for histocompatibility testing, which may include multiple cross-matches locally or remotely, not only for potential cadaver kidney transplant recipients, but also for potential recipients of other organs from the same donor. Cadaver kidney grafts from very young (under 6 years) or old (over 60 years) donors are not always transplanted because graft survivals are significantly worse than cadaver kidney transplants from donors between the ages of 6 and 60 years.[2]

ANATOMICAL CONSIDERATIONS OF THE RENAL VASCULAR PEDICLE

Renal vascular variations important to the renal donor surgeon were illustrated in 16 figures and very well described by Pick and Anson in 1940.[3] More than one renal artery was noted in 32 percent of kidneys, and this occurred with almost equal frequency bilaterally. Two or more renal veins were encountered in 28 percent of right kidneys and only 1 percent of left kidneys. A circumaortic venous ring was described in 17 percent and a single left renal vein coursing dorsal to the aorta in 3 percent of 202 cadaver dissections. The left renal vein communicated with hemizygous and lumbar veins in 60 percent of the specimens. Congenital anomalies of the retroperitoneal venous structures are demonstrated in Figure 26–1.[4]

LIVING DONOR

Preoperative Evaluation

Preoperative living donor evaluation is performed weeks before donor nephrectomy. On the basis of this evaluation, one must be able to assure the donor of near-normal function after unilateral nephrectomy. Potential donors are educated about the risks and benefits of renal donation. Volunteers are then screened for medical history, medication list, social history, and ABO blood type. If there is no evidence of emotional instability, high risk of donor mortality or morbidity, renal disease, significant transmittable disease, or ABO incompatibility, tissue typing and a microcytotoxicity cross-match are performed between donor lymphocytes and recipient serum. If the cross-match is negative, the following examinations and tests are performed: physical examination, stool occult blood examination, PPD, skin test, pelvic examination and Papanicolaou smear (women), pregnancy test (potentially fertile women), complete blood count, at least two serum creatinine levels, fasting blood sugar, serum electrolytes, liver function studies, infectious serologic studies (human immunodeficiency virus [HIV], human T-lymphoproliferative

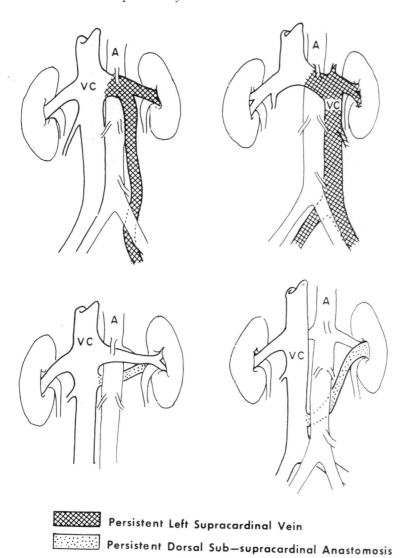

Persistent Left Supracardinal Vein

Persistent Dorsal Sub—supracardinal Anastomosis

Figure 26–1. Congenital anomalies of retroperitoneal venous structures of importance to kidney retrieval surgeons. These are duplication of the inferior vena cava (IVC) *(top left)*, transposition of the IVC *(top right)*, circumaortic left renal vein *(bottom left)*, and retroaortic left renal vein *(bottom right)*. (From Ortenberg J, Novick AC, Stewart BH. Vascular Problems in Urologic Surgery. Philadelphia, WB Saunders, 1982, p 118.)

virus type 1, hepatitis, cytomegalovirus, and syphilis), prothrombin time, activated partial thromboplastin time, urinalysis, urine culture, electrocardiogram (ECG), chest radiograph, mammogram (women over 40), prostate-specific antigens (PSA) (men over 50), and stress cardiac scintigraphy (age over 50, chest pain, or abnormal ECG). If there is still no evidence of emotional instability, unacceptable risk of mortality or morbidity, renal disease, or significant transmittable disease, an excretory urogram or radioisotope renogram is performed. If the results from either of those imaging studies is acceptable, a renal arteriogram or digital subtraction arteriogram is performed. If the results of this test are acceptable, the donor-recipient lymphocyte cross-match is repeated close to the time of renal donation. If that test is negative, donor nephrectomy is performed. If one of the donor's kidneys has a minor abnormality, that kidney is used for transplantation. Because hydronephrosis of pregnancy occurs predominantly in the right kidney, some transplant teams prefer to use that kidney from women who may become pregnant.

Preoperative Preparation

The healthy donor requires no special care. Oral fluids are encouraged until the patient is on NPO status for surgery. Overnight intravenous hydration is unnecessary.

Surgical Technique

Living donor nephrectomy is usually performed through a flank incision. Either a rib-resecting or a supracostal approach provide excellent exposure.[5, 6] After induction of anesthesia, bladder catheterization, and positioning of the patient, intravenous fluids are administered at 1 L/hr to initiate and maintain a diuresis. With the skin incision, 25 gm mannitol is infused over 1 hour. The incision is deepened through the muscular layers, and exposure is maintained with a self-retaining retractor such as a Burford or a jointed Bookwalter that has been modified to fit the flank (Fig. 26–2). The perirenal fascia is opened, and the fat is separated from the kidney to expose

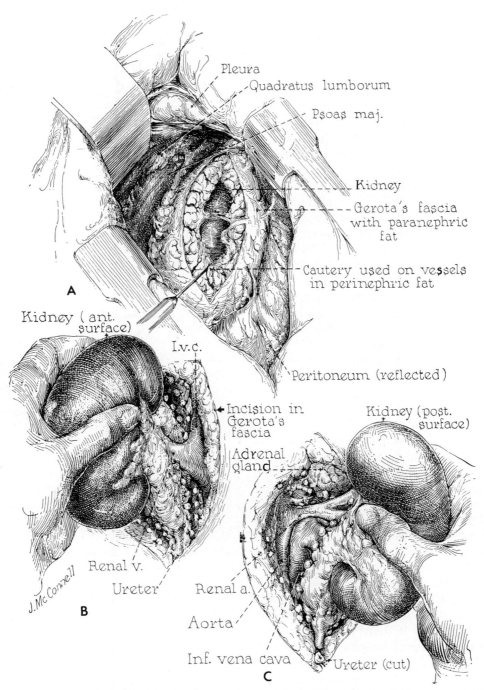

Figure 26–2. Right donor nephrectomy. *A,* Incision of perirenal fascia and fat. *B,* Anterior surface of the kidney with dissection of the IVC to allow placement of two Satinsky clamps. *C,* Posterior surface of the kidney with exposure of the right renal artery in preparation for clamping. The cut end of the ureter is observed to make certain that a diuresis is occurring. (From Marchioro TL, Brittain RS, Hermann G, et al. Use of living donors for renal homotransplantation. Arch Surg 88:711, 1964. Copyright 1964, American Medical Association.)

the renal hilum and the adrenal gland. The peritoneal contents are retracted medially and held in place with a padded retractor.

On the right, the adrenal gland is separated from the kidney, and the right renal vein and lateral inferior vena cava (IVC) are exposed. The medial margin of the gonadal vein is used as a landmark to preserve ureteral blood supply, and the plane between the gonadal vein and the IVC is developed caudally until the gonadal vessels cross the ureter. The gonadal vessels are divided between ligatures lateral to the ureter and at the lateral margin of the IVC. The ureter is then dissected distally to where it crosses the common iliac artery.

The kidney is rotated medially and the renal artery is identified posterior to the IVC. The lymphatic and nervous tissue overlying the renal artery is separated in the longitudinal axis of the renal artery, and the latter is delivered through the opening. The lymphatic and nervous tissue are separated into bundles and divided between ligatures. The kidney is now completely freed from the surrounding structures and tethered only by the main renal vessels and the ureter. The ureter is transected to confirm the presence of a diuresis. If there is no diuresis, the renal artery is examined for vasospasm. If vasospasm is present, it is treated with subadventitial injections of papaverine through a 27- or 30-gauge needle. Furosemide, 10 to 80 mg, or an additional 12.5 gm of mannitol can be administered, if necessary.

Once a diuresis is confirmed, the renal artery is clamped, two Satinsky clamps are applied to the side of the IVC (Fig. 26–3) to provide a cuff of IVC for the renal vein anastomosis in the recipient, and the renal artery and IVC cuff are transected. Administration of heparin to the donor is unnecessary. The kidney is removed and an ice-cold preservation solution such as EuroCollins, Collins 2, or University of Wisconsin solution is infused through the renal artery until the venous effluent is clear. The kidney is then placed in a basin filled with ice-cold preservation solution, covered with a sterile drape, and transported into the recipient's operating room. If there is to be a delay until the time of the recipient operation, the kidney can be packaged in a sterile container, which is then packed in ice until the time of transplantation.

The renal artery is doubly ligated with 0 silk or oversewn with 5-0 vascular suture, the outer Satinsky clamp is removed, the IVC cuff is oversewn with 5-0 vascular suture, and the remaining Satinsky clamp is removed.

The procedure for left donor nephrectomy is nearly the same as for right donor nephrectomy with one exception (Fig. 26–4). The adrenal vein is divided between ligatures at the cephalad border of the left renal vein. Care is taken to determine whether one of the following left renal vein variations is present:

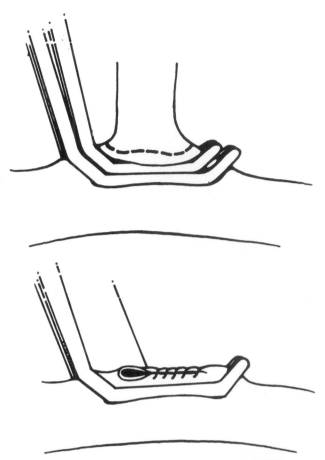

Figure 26–3. Double Satinsky clamp technique for providing an IVC cuff for right renal vein anastomosis in the recipient and for ensuring IVC control during closure.

retroaortic left renal vein, circumaortic left renal vein, lumbar vein draining into the posterior left renal vein, transposition of the IVC, or duplication of the IVC. It is necessary to leave only one major vein to provide adequate drainage for the kidney; the other tributaries are divided between ligatures.

The wound is closed in a standard fashion. If a supracostal approach has been made, a pericostal synthetic absorbable 0 suture can be used to approximate the ribs.[6] Care must be taken to exclude the neurovascular bundles. If a pleural entry has occurred, a small catheter is inserted into the pleural space, the pleura is closed with 5-0 synthetic absorbable suture, the muscle layers are approximated, the end of the pleural catheter is placed under water, the lung is hyperinflated, and the catheter is withdrawn after all the pleural air is evacuated. Drains are generally not used. Skin closure with a running, absorbable subcuticular suture is more comfortable for patients than skin clips or nonabsorbable sutures that require removal. A chest radiograph is taken in the recovery room to make certain that a significant pneumothorax does not exist. If it does, it can be aspirated through the second anterior intercostal space.

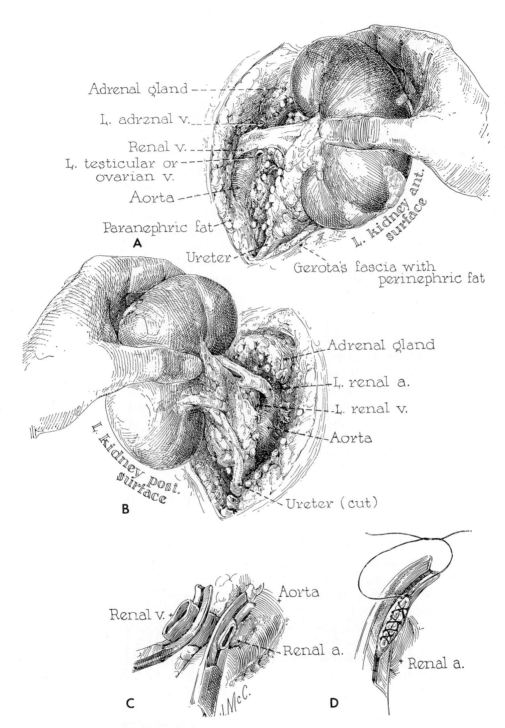

Figure 26–4. Left donor nephrectomy. *A,* Dissection of the left renal vein. Some surgeons do not divide the gonadal vein where it enters the renal vein but divide it after it crosses the ureter inferiorly. *B,* Exposure of the left renal artery. *C,* Clamps on stumps of renal artery and vein. *D,* Suture closure of vascular cuffs. Simple double ligation with 0 silk ligatures is also adequate. (From Marchioro TL, Brittain RS, Hermann G, et al. Use of living donors for renal homotransplantation. Arch Surg 88: 711, 1964. Copyright 1964, American Medical Association.)

Postoperative Care

The urethral catheter is removed a day or two after nephrectomy. Parenteral fluids are administered until gastrointestinal continuity returns in 3 to 5 days, and the patient is discharged 4 to 7 days after surgery. Unless problems occur, usually only one postoperative visit 3 weeks after surgery is needed. At that visit, an interval history, blood pressure determination, limited physical examination, complete blood count, serum creatinine determination, and urinalysis are undertaken. If results are acceptable, future follow-up is with the donor's primary care physician. The donor is advised not to lift anything weighing more than 5 pounds for 6 weeks after surgery, and then nothing weighing more than 20 pounds for a further 6 weeks.

CADAVER MULTIPLE ORGAN DONOR

Preoperative Care

The declaration of brain death is the responsibility of the potential cadaver organ donor's physician. The transplant team is available for consultation but cannot declare brain death and cannot assume care of the donor until brain death has been declared.

The goals of cadaver donor preparation are documentation of the function of transplantable organs, reduction of the risk of transmitting infection or malignancy to potential recipients, restoration of intervascular volume, elimination of vasopressors, and establishment of a diuresis.[7]

The medical history and physical examination provide information that may disqualify the donor or specific organs, and highlight special studies necessary before actual organ procurement proceeds. Required laboratory tests for cadaver organ donors are a complete blood count, serum electrolytes, ABO typing, infectious serologic studies (hepatitis, cytomegalovirus, syphilis, HIV, and human T-lymphoproliferative virus type 1), and blood cultures if they are hospitalized for 72 hours or more. Renal tests are for serum creatinine, blood urea nitrogen, and urinalysis. Specific tests for heart, lung, liver, and pancreas are performed if any of those organs are also to be retrieved.

The initial resuscitation goals are systolic blood pressure of 90 mm Hg and urinary output of 0.5 ml/kg/hr. Secondary goals are hematocrit of 25 or more; normal potassium, calcium, magnesium, phosphorus, and sodium; and normal PO_2 and PCO_2. Central venous pressure measurements or pulmonary capillary wedge pressure monitoring are helpful for managing fluid administration. The prospective donor can be fluid challenged by administration of at least 30 ml/kg/hr of Ringer's lactate solution, and the urinary volume then matched with intravenous Ringer's lactate solution or 0.45 percent sodium chloride solution containing 30 mmol/L potassium phosphate if diabetes insipidus ensues. Serum electrolytes should be checked every 2 to 4 hours to maintain electrolyte balance. If the central venous pressure is greater than 15 cm H_2O and hypotension persists, a dopamine or dobutamine infusion of less than 10 µg/kg/min can be administered without causing renal vasospasm. If bradyarrhythmia does not respond to dopamine, epinephrine up to 0.1 µg/kg/min may be used as long as the urinary output continues, otherwise a temporary pacemaker can be inserted. Tachyarrhythmias usually respond to volume correction and reduction of vasopressors. If urinary output is less than 1.0 ml/kg/hr after correction of hypovolemia and hypotension, furosemide, 1 mg/kg, or mannitol, 0.5 to 1.0 gm/kg, can be infused. Diabetes insipidus with a urinary output greater than 500 ml/hr can be managed by a continuous infusion of aqueous vasopressin (0.5 to 15 units/hr) to reduce urinary output to the range of 2 to 3 ml/kg/hr.

Since hypothermia with temperatures under 28°C can cause cardiac irritability, and under 32°C a coagulopathy, the head can be wrapped, intravenous fluids can be warmed to 37°C, and the body can be placed on a warming blanket. The goal is a temperature of 34°C or more.

A total of 100 ml of blood can be drawn for histocompatibility testing before organ retrieval.

Surgical Technique

The steps in multiple abdominal organ retrieval from a cadaver donor are (1) adequate exposure, (2) control of the great vessels above and below the organs to be removed, (3) initiation of preservation, (4) removal of organs, (5) completion of preservation, (6) collection of histocompatibility specimens, (7) removal of iliac vessels, and (8) organ packaging. An anesthesiologist is essential to maintain artificial respiration, cardiac function, and organ perfusion until the moment of organ retrieval, and hyperreflexia may require the administration of muscle relaxants. The cerebrally dead cadaver organ donor receives at least 30 mg/kg/hr of crystalloid every hour the abdomen is open and a 1 gm/kg mannitol intravenous push with the skin incision. Colloid or blood administration may be necessary to improve organ perfusion. If pancreas retrieval is planned, 500 ml of povidone-iodine solution is infused into the stomach through a nasogastric tube.

The following is a sequence for rapid en bloc removal of the abdominal aorta, IVC, liver, pancreas, kidneys, stomach, and duodenum with or without

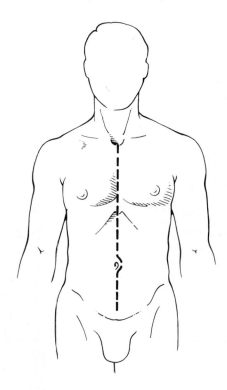

Figure 26–5. A total midline incision exposes all potentially transplantable organs in the chest and abdomen. (From Barry JM. Cadaver donor nephrectomy. In Novick AC, Streem SB, Pontes JE, eds. Stewart's Operative Urology, 2nd ed. Baltimore, Williams & Wilkins, 1989, p 295. Copyright Williams & Wilkins, 1989.)

chest organ retrieval. This technique incorporates principles of multiple organ retrieval developed by several teams.[8–12] A total midline incision is made between the suprasternal notch and the pubis (Fig. 26–5). The sternum is split with a sternal saw or a mallet and Lebsche knife, and self-retaining retractors are placed in the chest and abdomen. The stomach is aspirated and the nasogastric tube removed. While the chest organ retrieval team exposes the heart and lungs, the abdominal organ retrieval team exposes and controls the distal abdominal aorta and IVC (Fig. 26–6). The small bowel is retracted cephalad and to the right. The posterior peritoneum is opened from the hepatic flexure around the cecum, to the ligament of Treitz. This exposes the gonadal vessels, right ureter, IVC, aorta, and inferior mesenteric artery (IMA). The IMA is divided between ligatures of 0 silk, and the distal abdominal aorta and IVC are controlled with No. 1 silk ligatures or umbilical tapes. In preparation for cannulation, each of the great vessels is encircled twice with a No. 1 silk ligature cephalad to the controlling ligatures or tapes. The proximal jejunum can be divided between staples at this time. The small bowel is placed back in its normal position, the left coronary ligament of the liver is incised, the left lobe of the liver is retracted to the right, the distal esophagus is divided between staples, and the aorta is controlled either through the crus of the diaphragm (Fig. 26–7) or in the chest. Care is taken to identify and preserve an aberrant left hepatic artery that may arise from the left gastric artery. The cardiac team provides control of the IVC

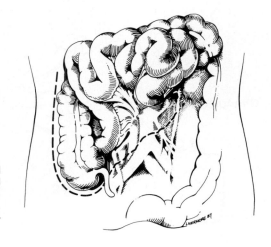

Figure 26–6. Opening the posterior peritoneum from the inferior mesenteric vein around the cecum exposes the great vessels, kidneys, and ureters in the retroperitoneum. Distal control of the aorta and IVC and division of the proximal jejunum can now take place. (From Barry JM. Cadaver donor nephrectomy. In Novick AC, Streem SB, Pontes JE, eds. Stewart's Operative Urology, 2nd ed. Baltimore, Williams & Wilkins, 1989, p 295. Copyright Williams & Wilkins, 1989.)

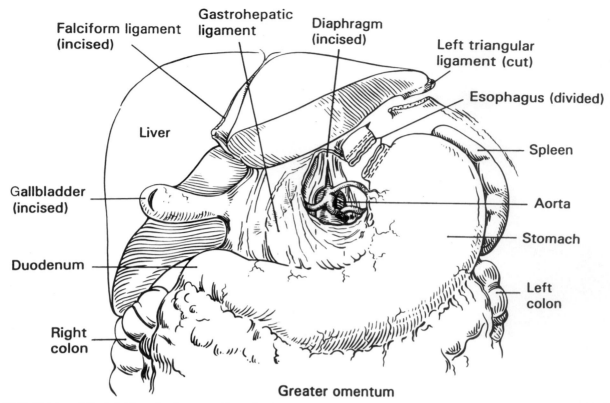

Figure 26–7. Division of the left triangular ligament allows the liver to be retracted to the right for exposure of the gastroesophageal junction and the aortic hiatus. Division of the stapled esophagus and incision of the median arcuate ligament expose the supraceliac aorta, which is encircled with a vascular tape. Watch out for an aberrant left hepatic artery that may arise from the left gastric artery.

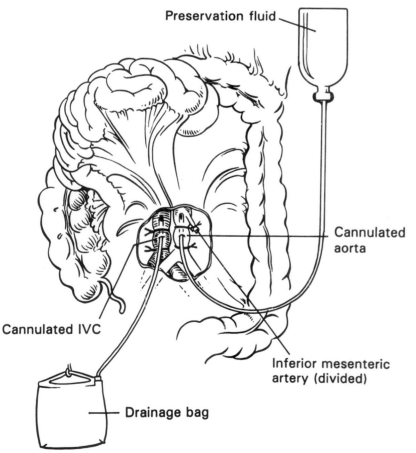

Figure 26–8. After confirmation that the chest team is ready, heparin is administered and the distoral aorta and IVC are cannulated. When the chest team is ready for circulatory arrest, the supraceliac aorta is clamped, the IVC cannula is opened, and ice-cold preservation solution is administered by gravity infusion through the aortic cannula. Saline slush is placed in the abdomen.

TABLE 26–1. Composition of University of Wisconsin Preservation Solution

Substance	Amount in 1 L	Function
KH$_2$PO$_4$	25 mmol	Hydrogen ion buffer, ATP synthesis
MgSO$_4$	5 mmol	To stabilize cell membrane
Adenosine	5 mmol	ATP synthesis during reperfusion
Glutathione	3 mmol	Free radical scavenger
Allopurinol	1 mmol	To inhibit xanthine oxidase and generation of free radicals
Potassium lactobionate	100 mmol	To minimize cellular swelling
Raffinose	30 mmol	To minimize cellular swelling
Hydroxyethyl starch	50 gm	To minimize cellular swelling
Dexamethasone	8 mg	To stabilize cell membrane
Insulin	40 units	

ATP, adenosine triphosphate.

at the heart. The gallbladder is incised, drained, and flushed with a cold preservation solution to prevent autolysis. After coordination with the chest team, 150 to 500 units/kg heparin is administered, the distal aorta and IVC are occluded and cannulated, the proximal aorta is occluded, and the distal aorta is flushed with ice-cold preservation solution (Fig. 26–8). This is usually University of Wisconsin solution (Table 26–1)[13] in the following amounts, based on cadaver donor weight: 4 to 6 L for over 80 kg, 3 to 5 L for 50 to 80 kg, 2 to 3 L for 20 to 50 kg, and 1 to 2 L for under 20 kg. The IVC can be decompressed into the chest, but this results in lukewarm effluent spilling into the abdominal cavity; it is better done via the abdominal IVC cannula. Saline slush is placed in the abdomen. Liver preservation and cooling is achieved via the hepatic artery and portal vein after the preservation solution has washed out the vascular beds of the gastrointestinal tract, spleen, and pancreas. The gastrocolic ligament is divided, the hepatic and splenic flexures of the colon are taken down, the line of Toldt is incised, the transverse mesocolon and small bowel mesentery are opened, and the superior mesenteric artery (SMA) and vein are ligated and divided (Fig. 26–9). The jejunum is divided between staples at the ligament of Treitz if this was not done earlier in the procedure. The right diaphragm is incised and the en bloc organ specimen, including the right kidney, is retracted anteriorly and to the left. The dissection is continued posteriorly, transecting the lumbar veins, lumbar arteries, and distal right ureter. The en bloc specimen is then retracted to the right, and the spleen, stom-

ach, pancreas, and left kidney are elevated. The distal left ureter is cut, the left lumbar arteries and veins are transected, the distal abdominal aorta and IVC are transected, the proximal abdominal aorta is transected, the central diaphragm is divided between the aorta and the IVC, and the en bloc specimen is removed from the cadaver donor (Fig. 26–10). This technique preserves the aberrant right and left hepatic arteries that may arise from the SMA and left gastric artery, respectively. It also prevents portal venous hypertension and pancreas edema.

The organ block is placed face down in a pan of sterile slush, and the posterior abdominal aorta is split between the lumbar arteries (Fig. 26–11). The aorta is transected between the renal arteries and the SMA. The IVC is transected just cephalad to the entrance of the renal veins. The right and left kidneys with their respective adrenal glands are dissected from the posterior surfaces of the liver, duodenum, pancreas, and spleen. These maneuvers separate the kidney block from the other organs. The kidneys are then separated by dividing the anterior aorta between the renal artery ostia. The left renal vein is transected at its entrance into the IVC, and the right renal vein is left with the IVC so that it can be extended, if necessary. The liver is separated from the pancreas, duodenum, and stomach. The pancreas-duodenum segment graft is then prepared. The separated organs are often reflushed with preservation solution: 300 ml for each kidney, 500 ml for the pancreas, and 1000 ml for the liver.[13]

The external iliac veins and the iliac arteries are removed and sent with the liver and pancreas specimens. These vessels can be used for vein extensions and pancreatic or hepatic artery reconstruction before transplantation. It is common to use a Y-graft of iliac arteries to join the splenic artery and SMA stumps of the pancreas-duodenum graft.

Twenty lymph nodes and the spleen are removed for histocompatibility testing. If the number of lymph nodes in the bowel mesentery is inadequate, pelvic, interaortocaval, or renal hilar lymph nodes can be removed.

Technical Variations

Some surgeons prefer to carry out the portal dissection in situ before initiation of preservation, and to initiate hepatic cooling via the portal vein. When the pancreas is not to be retrieved, the splenic, inferior mesenteric, superior mesenteric, or portal vein is ligated caudally, cannulated, and infused with ice-cold preservation solution. When the pancreas is to be retrieved, a cannula is placed in the superior mesenteric vein and passed into the portal vein, where it is held in place with a snare. The portal vein is then partially transected caudal to the snare to allow venous decompression of the pancreas. An alternative technique is to cannulate the portal vein and transect it caudal to the cannula.

When only the kidneys are to be retrieved, the multiple abdominal organ retrieval technique is significantly altered. The distal aorta and IVC are prepared for cannulation. The portal triad structures can be divided between heavy ligatures to expose the SMA and celiac axis, which are divided between ligatures. Heparin is administered, the distal aorta and IVC are cannulated (see Fig. 26–7), and the proximal aortic clamp is applied at the level of the celiac axis. This prevents compromise of the renal artery ostia and inadequate in situ kidney flushing. The distal IVC is vented, the IVC is occluded above the renal veins with a Rumel tourniquet, and the aorta is flushed with a preservation solution through the aortic cannula. When only the kidneys need to be preserved, EuroCollins or Collins 2 solution is often used in place of the more expensive University of Wisconsin solution. The distal aorta and IVC are transected and retracted anteriorly by gentle traction on the cannulas. This exposes the lumbar vessels, which are divided between clips to the level of the proximal aortic clamp and IVC tourniquet. The IVC and aorta are transected and the en bloc specimen, which consists of the kidneys, aorta, and IVC, is removed and taken to the back table where the kidneys are separated, reflushed, and packaged as described below.

Kidney Packaging

After separation and reflushing, the kidneys are packaged according to UNOS guidelines (Fig. 26–12).[13] The organs must be protected by a triple sterile barrier and one rigid container. Each organ package is then placed in a Styrofoam container that is lined with plastic and contains ice. This in turn is placed in a cardboard box with the histocompatibility testing specimens, labeled, and sent to the transplanting center.

Summary

Expected results of renal transplantation based on 40,756 first kidney transplants done between October 1987 and October 1993 at 245 U.S. transplant centers are 1-year graft survivals of 81 percent for cadaver kidney grafts, 90 percent for parental kidney grafts, and 95 percent for HLA-identical sibling kidney grafts. The projected half-lives of those kidney transplants are 9, 12, and 24 years, respectively.[14] Kidney

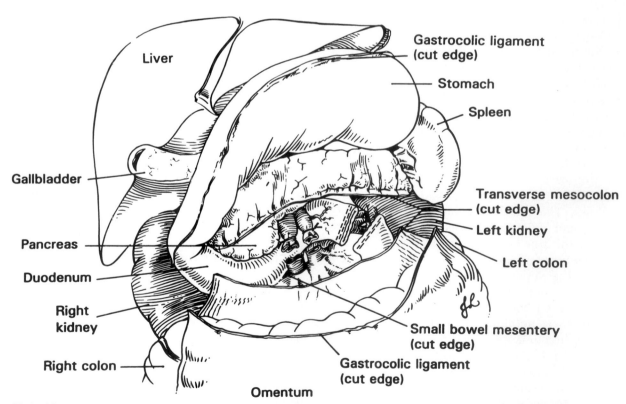

Figure 26–9. After the preservation solution has been infused, the gastrocolic and phrenicocolic ligaments are divided. The transverse mesocolon and small bowel mesentery are incised to expose the superior mesenteric artery (SMA) and vein, which are ligated and divided, as is the inferior mesenteric vein. If not done earlier, the proximal jejunum is divided between staples.

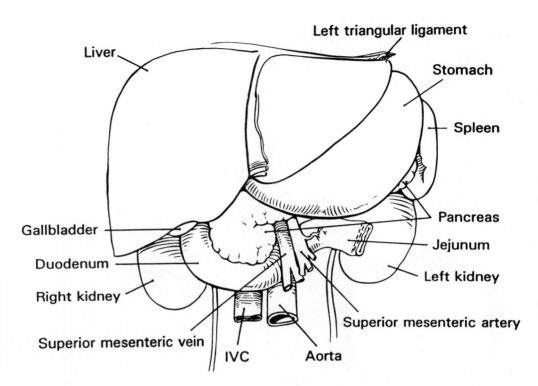

Figure 26–10. Anterior view of the removed en bloc organ specimen. (Modified from Nakazato PZ, Concepcion W, Bry W, et al: Total abdominal evisceration: An en bloc technique for abdominal organ harvesting. Surgery 111: 37, 1992.)

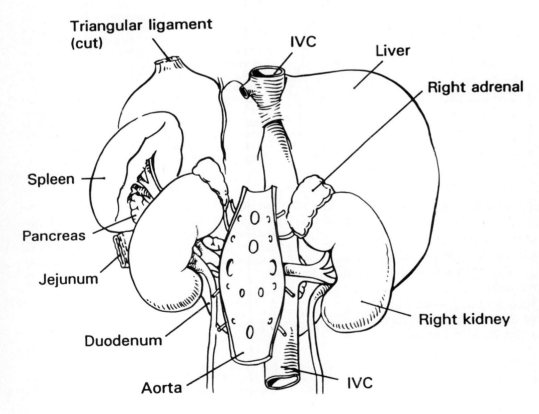

Figure 26–11. Posterior view of the en bloc specimen. The diaphragm segment covering the right lobe of the liver has been removed by the artist to illustrate the IVC. The aorta is split posteriorly between the lumbar arteries to expose the ostia of the celiac axis, SMA, renal arteries, and inferior mesenteric artery. Transection of the aorta between the SMA and the renal arteries, and transection of the IVC just above the entrance of the renal veins, allow separation of the en bloc kidney specimen from the other organs. The kidneys are separated by splitting the anterior surface of the aorta and transecting the left renal vein at its junction with the IVC. (Modified from Nakazato PZ, Concepcion W, Bry W, et al. Total abdominal evisceration: An en bloc technique for abdominal organ harvesting. Surgery 111:37, 1992.)

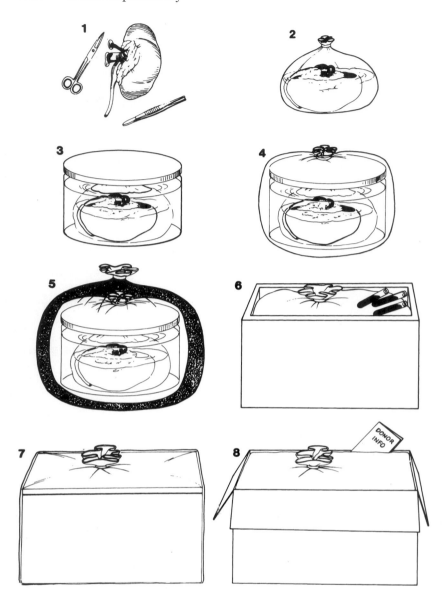

Figure 26–12. Organ packaging according to United Network for Organ Sharing (UNOS) guidelines. The kidney is placed in a sterile, leak-proof plastic bag, which is placed in a sterile, rigid container. The rigid container is then placed in another sterile plastic bag, and this bag is placed into an expanded polystyrene-insulated container lined with a nonsterile plastic bag containing nonsterile ice. Tissue typing containers and a "red top" tube of blood are placed on the ice-filled plastic bag that is in the polystyrene container. A lid is placed on the polystyrene container, which is wrapped in a plastic bag and placed, with the donor information, into a double-strength, wax-impregnated fiber outer container. Labels must be on the outermost surface of each organ specimen container. (From Hoffman RM, Belzer FO. In Phillips MG, ed. UNOS Organ Procurement, Preservation, and Distribution in Transplantation. Richmond, VA, UNOS, 1991, p 118.)

transplants from living donors continue to be an important source of transplantable organs because of the excellent results, the ability to electively schedule the operation, the limitation of the recipient's waiting time on dialysis, and the partial alleviation of the insufficient supply of cadaver kidneys.

The ability to take an organ from one person (especially a cadaver), transplant it into another person, and have it function most of the time is a miracle.

Editorial Comment

Fray F. Marshall

Living related donor kidney transplantation continues to be an option for some patients with renal failure, particularly in view of the difficulty of obtaining cadaveric kidneys. In the near future, magnetic resonance imaging with gadolinium may supplant standard angiography for the evaluation of donors. Typically in the performance of a left donor nephrectomy, the lumbar and ovarian veins, and occasionally the adrenal vein, may all be taken to provide greater length for the left renal vein. The longer vein facilitates the technical ease of renal transplantation. If cadaveric renal transplants are going to be used, it is important to be well versed in the cadaveric multiple organ donor dissections described.

REFERENCES

1. UNOS Update 11:39, 1995.
2. Cecka JM, Terasaki PI. The UNOS Renal Scientific Registry—1990. In Terasaki PI, ed. Clinical Transplants, 1990. Los Angeles, UCLA Tissue Typing Laboratory, 1991, p 5.
3. Pick JW, Anson BJ. The renal vascular pedicle: An anatomical study of 430 body-halves. J Urol 44:411, 1940.
4. Ortenberg J, Novick AC, Stewart BH. Clinical problems involving the inferior vena cava. In Novick AC, Straffon RA, eds. Vascular Problems in Urologic Surgery. Philadelphia, WB Saunders, 1982, p 117.
5. Marchioro TL, Brittain RS, Hermann G, et al. The use of living donors for renal homotransplantation. Arch Surg 88:711, 1964.

6. Barry JM, Hodges CV. The supracostal approach for live donor nephrectomy. Arch Surg 109:448, 1974.
7. Soifer BE, Gelb AW. The multiple organ donor: Identification and management. Ann Intern Med 110:814, 1989.
8. Starzl TE, Iwatsuki S, Shaw BW Jr, Gordon RD. Orthotopic liver transplantation in 1984. Transplant Proc 17:250, 1985.
9. Barry JM. Cadaver donor nephrectomy. In Novick AC, Streem SB, Pontes JE, eds. Stewart's Operative Urology, 2nd ed. Baltimore, Williams & Wilkins, 1989, p 294.
10. deVille deGoyet J, Hausleithner V, Malaise J, et al. Liver procurement without in-situ portal perfusion. Transplantation 57:1328, 1994.
11. Anthuber M, Zuelke C, Forst H, et al. Experiences with a simplified liver harvesting technique—single aorta in-situ flush followed by portal back table flush. Transplant Proc 25:3154, 1993.
12. Nakazato PZ, Concepcion W, Bry W, et al. Total abdominal evisceration: An en bloc technique for abdominal organ harvesting. Surgery 111:37, 1992.
13. Hoffmann RM, Belzer FO. Organ preservation: Kidney, liver, pancreas. In Phillips MG, ed. UNOS Organ Procurement, Preservation, and Distribution in Transplantation. Richmond, VA, UNOS, 1991, p 105.
14. Cecka JM, Terasaki PI. The UNOS Scientific Renal Transplant Registry. In Terasaki PI, ed. Clinical Transplants, 1993. Los Angeles, UCLA Tissue Typing Laboratory, 1994, p 1.

Chapter 27

Radical Nephrectomy: Flank Approaches

Fray F. Marshall

INDICATIONS

Radical nephrectomy is usually performed for carcinoma. Occasionally, benign processes, such as xanthogranulomatous pyelonephritis, in a poorly functioning kidney are best managed by a "radical" nephrectomy (excision of all tissue within Gerota's fascia) because normal tissue planes are disrupted by inflammation or infection. The general principles of radical nephrectomy have included excision of the kidney with early ligation of the renal artery and vein, excision of all perinephric tissue within Gerota's fascia, ipsilateral adrenalectomy, and regional lymph node dissection. Recent data suggest that ipsilateral adrenalectomy may not always be necessary unless there is an upper pole tumor.

PREOPERATIVE MANAGEMENT

The typical patient presents with hematuria and is found to have a renal mass on intravenous pyelography or sonography. Computed tomographic scans of the abdomen and chest are obtained. A digital arteriogram can be obtained from the same study without an arterial puncture. Formal arteriography is performed infrequently and is generally used for partial nephrectomy or other special situations. Magnetic resonance imaging (MRI) has been helpful in the evaluation of the vena cava and regional disease. Occasionally, if movement of the distal thrombus in the vena cava occurs, MRI may not delineate clearly the superior extent of the tumor thrombus.

In the absence of obvious metastatic disease, a radical nephrectomy is planned. Patients can donate several units of their own blood so that autologous transfusions are available. No other evaluations are obtained unless central nervous system or other

symptoms are present. If the alkaline phosphatase is elevated or if bone pain is suspected, a bone scan is ordered. The patient is hydrated with intravenous fluids the night before the operation.

OPERATIVE TECHNIQUE

The basic tenets of radical nephrectomy are followed. An attempt is made to perform early ligation of the renal artery to reduce bleeding and theoretically reduce dissemination of tumor cells. Sometimes, with a large tumor on the left, this ligation can be performed more easily posteriorly. The renal vein is not always ligated at the same time as the renal artery because of possible parasitization of the renal arterial blood supply, and because occasionally a polar renal artery can be missed. Early venous ligation can create venous hypertension and increased bleeding. The most important part of the radical nephrectomy is excision of all perinephric tissue, because many tumors extend through the renal capsule; many of these patients so affected can still be cured.

Although some investigators have suggested that the adrenal gland can remain, Gerota's fascia is violated if the adrenal gland remains (Fig. 27–1). As a result, the adrenal is generally included in the specimen. I have advocated regional lymphadenectomy as well, because adjuvant therapy has not been particularly effective.[1] Patients with bulky nodal metastases have a poor prognosis, but those with microscopic disease fare better. These are precisely the patients who will profit most by regional lymphadenectomy (Figs. 27–1 and 27–2).

The incision should be dictated by the size of the tumor, the body habitus of the patient, and the experience of the surgeon. Although many surgeons prefer an anterior approach, obesity is a common finding in

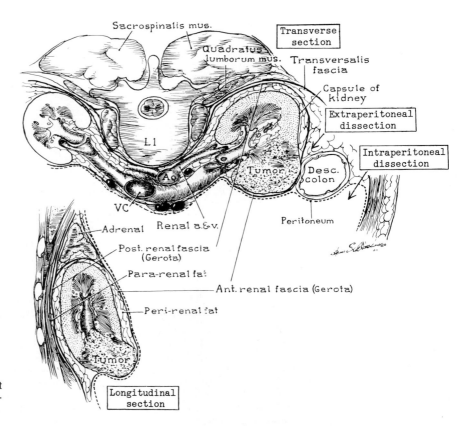

Figure 27–1. Cross-section demonstrating a left renal tumor with the relationships of the peritoneum, Gerota's fascia, colon, and kidney.

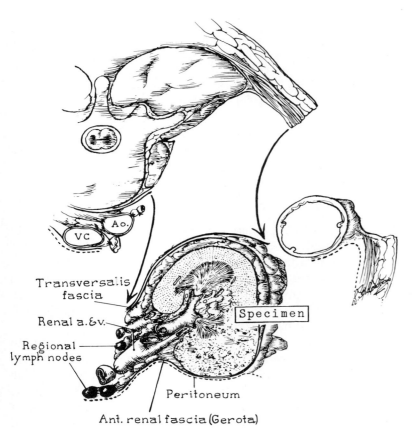

Figure 27–2. Radical nephrectomy specimen indicates excision of the tumor, perinephric tissue, small portion of the peritoneum, regional lymph nodes, and regional fascia.

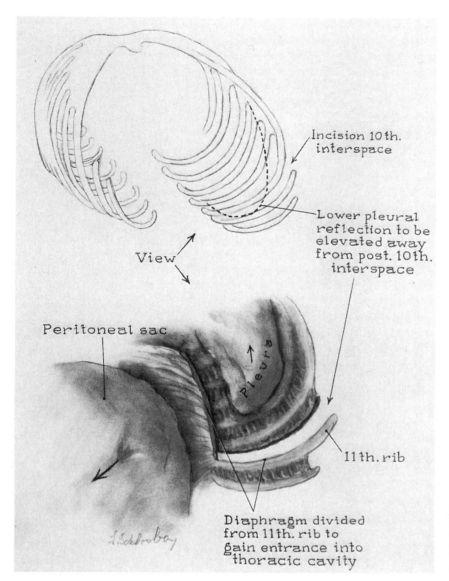

Incision 10th. interspace

Lower pleural reflection to be elevated away from post. 10th. interspace

View

Peritoneal sac

pleura

Pleura

11th. rib

Diaphragm divided from 11th. rib to gain entrance into thoracic cavity

Figure 27–3. The thoracic cage is demonstrated with the lower margin of the pleura extending to the eleventh rib. The pleura is dissected from the inside of the chest wall to allow it to retract superiorly. The peritoneal sac and Gerota's fascia have been mobilized from the diaphragm.

our patient population and an anterior, midline, or subcostal approach can be difficult in such patients. I have preferred the flank approach or, if necessary, a thoracoabdominal approach. If the tumor is small, a supra-twelfth rib (eleventh interspace) incision is made, extending from the edge of the erector spinae musculature in a diagonal fashion to the lateral border of the rectus muscle.

A subperiosteal rib resection can also be performed, but this is not required. An intrathoracic but extrapleural approach can avoid a chest tube in the supra-twelfth rib approach. If the tumor is larger, a supra-eleventh rib, tenth interspace incision can be performed, as this rib is the last without a distal costal attachment to other ribs (Fig. 27–3). This incision usually affords excellent exposure even for sizable lesions.

If the tumor is huge or if vena caval involvement occurs, a fifth or sixth rib incision with a thoracoabdominal approach is performed. In this instance, the

rib is usually excised and the costal cartilage divided. The excision can be extended across the rectus musculature to the midline. The rectus fascia can then be divided in the midline in an inferior, vertical direction or the incision can be extended transversely across the contralateral rectus muscle. Another option in a patient who has a large tumor with caval involvement is an extensive midline incision and a midline sternotomy with extension to the lower abdomen. I have used all of these incisions, but this description focuses on the supra-eleventh rib (tenth interspace) intrathoracic but extrapleural approach to radical nephrectomy.

The patient is placed in the flank position with the table flexed. The kidney rest is usually elevated so that the flank musculature is placed on tension. The patient is not in the straight upright position but is rotated back somewhat to allow a medial extension of the incision, if required. The patient is fixed in position with wide tape across the hip and the shoulder, although an arm rest can be used. A small axillary roll is placed in the dependent axilla. The skin incision is marked and extends from the edge of the erector spinae muscle along the course of the tenth interspace in an oblique fashion to the border of the rectus muscle. The incision should follow the angle of the rib so that intercostal neurovascular bundles are not divided. The external and internal oblique muscles are divided. The retroperitoneal space is entered through the transversalis muscle just off the tip of the eleventh rib to avoid inadvertent division of the peritoneum or pleura (Fig. 27–4).

The peritoneum is mobilized off the posterior aspect of the transversalis muscle and fascia. The peritoneum can be divided and an intraperitoneal inspection made of the liver and abdominal contents. Gerota's fascia is mobilized from the inner side of the diaphragm as well as off the quadratus and psoas musculature (Fig. 27–5). The dissection is carried down along the edge of the rib in the tenth interspace, carefully looking for the plane between the pleura and the chest wall. With the Kitner dissector the pleura can then be dissected off the ribs.

The chest is entered, but the dissection is extrapleural. The diaphragm is dissected off the chest wall and isolated with the pleura free above it and all retroperitoneal tissue removed below it. The diaphragmatic attachments to the chest wall are divided down to its insertion between the quadratus and psoas musculature. Excellent exposure is provided.

The dissection is carried posteriorly along the rib until the intercostal ligament is divided between the ribs, allowing the rib to hinge inferiorly (Fig. 27–6). A chest retractor can then be placed between the tenth and eleventh ribs. Alternatively a subperiosteal rib resection can be performed.

The renal mass can usually be rotated medially and the dissection carried posteriorly with dissection off the quadratus and psoas muscles. The iliohypogastric and ilioinguinal nerves and the twelfth thoracic neurovascular bundle can usually be identified (Fig. 27–7).

On the left side the renal artery can be identified posteriorly, ligated, and divided (Fig. 27–8). On the right side or with larger tumors the aorta can be approached medially and the renal artery ligated from an anterior approach.

The colon is held superiorly and a plane between the colonic mesocolon and Gerota's fascia can be identified (Fig. 27–9). All tissue within Gerota's fascia will rotate laterally and the colon will rotate medially. Occasionally, if there is attachment of the peritoneum over the tumor, the peritoneum can be excised as well (see Figs. 27–1, 27–2, and 27–9).

After dissection across the psoas muscle to the aorta, an en bloc aortic node dissection can be per-

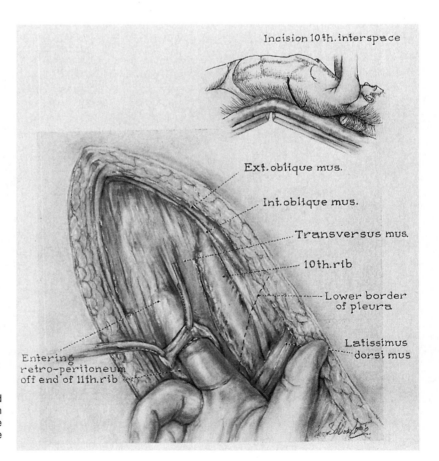

Figure 27–4. The patient is rotated on the table and flexed in the flank position. The incision is made through the transversalis abdominis muscle off the end of the eleventh rib to avoid the pleura and peritoneum. The lower border of the pleura is demonstrated.

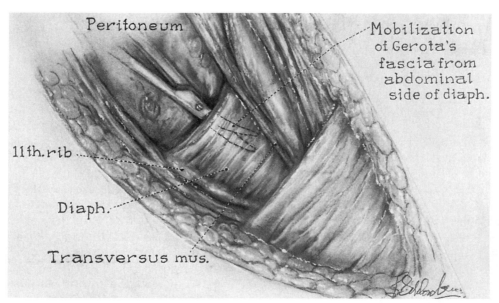

Figure 27–5. As the left radical nephrectomy continues, Gerota's fascia is mobilized off the abdominal side of the diaphragm. The diaphragm can be seen after the transversalis muscle has been divided. Pleura is identified in the space between the transversus abdominis muscle and the diaphragm. It can then be mobilized with the Kitner dissector superiorly.

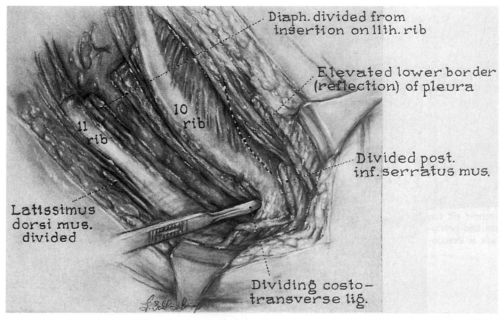

Figure 27–6. The transverse costal (intercostal) ligament is divided after the pleura has been reflected superiorly and the diaphragm has been divided. Division of the intercostal ligament allows the eleventh rib to hinge inferiorly and improves the exposure.

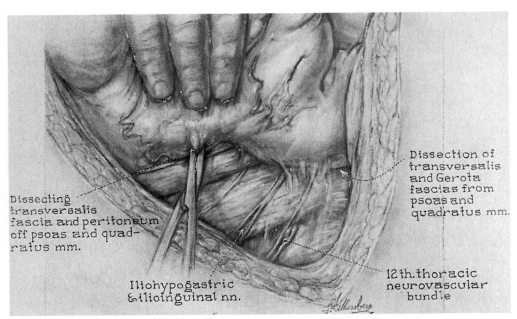

Figure 27–7. The transversalis fascia and Gerota's fascia are mobilized from the psoas and quadratus musculature posteriorly. The iliohypogastric and ilioinguinal nerves and twelfth thoracic neurovascular bundle are seen.

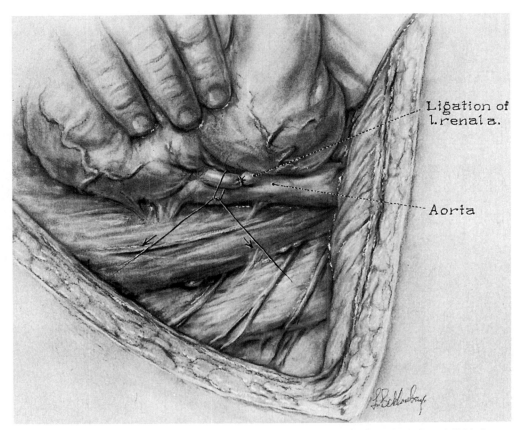

Figure 27–8. The aorta is located and the renal artery can be identified, ligated, and divided.

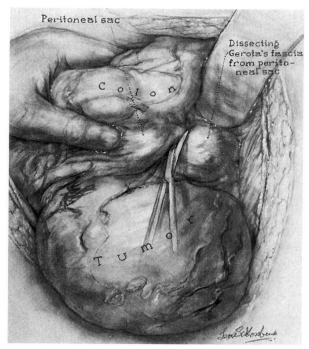

Figure 27–9. The medial dissection includes mobilization of the colon and mesocolon from Gerota's fascia. Gerota's fascia remains with the specimen. The aorta is identified and an en bloc periaortic node dissection begun. Care is taken not to injure the femoral branch of the genitofemoral nerve on the psoas muscle.

formed. The gonadal vessels and ureter are ligated and divided as dissection ascends the aorta. The en bloc node dissection is continued and the inferior mesenteric artery is usually left in place (Figs. 27–10 and 27–11). The renal vein is encountered as it courses over the aorta; this vein is ligated and divided (Fig. 27–12). Some small adrenal arteries and an inferior phrenic arterial branch may be seen just along the crus of the diaphragm. Superiorly the adrenal is removed and other vascular branches along the diaphragm are ligated or clipped. The specimen is removed, including the ipsilateral adrenal gland and

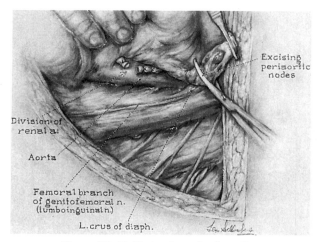

Figure 27–10. Periaortic node dissection.

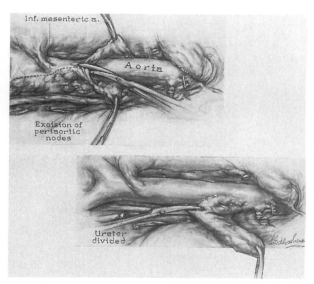

Figure 27–11. The node dissection is completed.

all tissue within Gerota's fascia; an en bloc regional lymphadenectomy is performed (Fig. 27–13).

On the right side the regional nodal drainage includes interaortocaval nodes.[1] I have not always performed the interaortocaval dissection, especially in older patients or in patients with small tumors. A periaortic or perivena caval dissection is routine.

The diaphragm is not repaired if only the lateral attachments have been taken down and the pleura remains intact. If the standard thoracoabdominal approach is performed, the diaphragm is closed with 2–0 or 3–0 sutures and a chest tube is left in place. Sometimes, during the intrathoracic but extrapleural approach, the chest is entered.

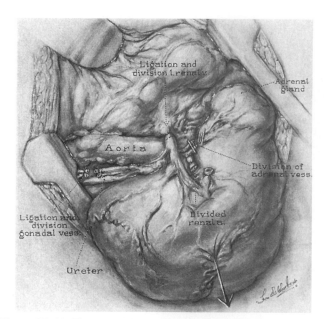

Figure 27–12. The gonadal vessels and ureter are ligated inferiorly. The regional node dissection is carried along the aorta, and the renal vein is ligated and divided. Additional vessels to the adrenal gland are ligated and divided.

If a small pleurotomy is found, the air can be bubbled out with a temporary small chest tube and removed after the skin closure. If there is any doubt, a small chest tube is left in place. The wound is usually irrigated with an antibiotic solution. Hemostasis is verified, and any small holes in the peritoneum and pleura are closed.

The kidney rest is lowered. The first closing fascial suture is usually placed off the end of the rib in the middle of the incision to keep the incision symmetrical, after changing the position of the patient on the table.

The incision is closed with figure-of-eight interrupted absorbable sutures encompassing both the transversalis and internal oblique muscles as a single layer. The external oblique is closed with a running absorbable suture. The subcutaneous tissue is closed, and the skin is closed with clips. If a chest tube is placed, it is usually removed after 1 to 2 days.

POSTOPERATIVE MANAGEMENT AND COMPLICATIONS

The supra-eleventh rib incision, intrathoracic, extrapleural approach has provided excellent exposure for many patients undergoing radical nephrectomies. Pulmonary toilet is very important in these patients, as some patients can have a 30 percent reduction in vital capacity in the immediate postoperative period from the incision alone. I have utilized a chronic thoracic epidural catheter for pain relief. It works well. The incision is usually well tolerated. Other short-term potential complications include wound infection and bleeding. Usually, bleeding is a rare postoperative complication if good hemostasis is observed during the procedure.

Later complications have included the "flank sag." If more than one intercostal nerve is divided, a flank sag can sometimes occur, so an attempt is made to avoid division of more than one intercostal nerve. When the genitofemoral nerve is divided, an area of

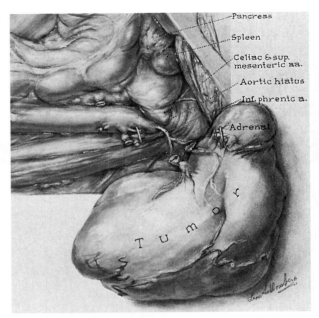

Figure 27–13. Additional vessels superiorly, especially the adrenal and inferior phrenic vessels, are ligated. Dissection is then completed along the diaphragm and the specimen is removed.

anesthesia may occur on the anterior part of the thigh. Blunting of the costophrenic angle may be observed on a postoperative chest radiograph, but this finding is usually of little significance.

RESULTS

When a complete radical nephrectomy is performed, the local disease recurrence rate has been very low. There has been local recurrence when extensive venous invasion or nodal disease is noted.

REFERENCE

1. Marshall FF, Powell KC. Lymphadenectomy for renal cell carcinoma: Anatomical and therapeutic considerations. J Urol 128:677, 1982.

Chapter 28

Radical Nephrectomy: Anterior Approach

Andrew C. Novick

INDICATIONS AND EVALUATION

Radical nephrectomy is the treatment of choice for patients with localized renal cell carcinoma.[1, 2] The preoperative evaluation of patients with renal cell carcinoma has changed considerably in recent years because of the advent of new imaging modalities such as ultrasonography, computed tomography, (CT), and magnetic resonance imaging (MRI). In many patients a complete preliminary evaluation can be performed employing noninvasive modalities. Renal arteriography is no longer routinely necessary before a radical nephrectomy. All patients should undergo a metastatic evaluation, including chest radiography, abdominal CT scanning, and occasionally a bone scan. A bone scan is necessary only in patients with bone pain or an elevated serum alkaline phosphatase level. Radical nephrectomy is occasionally performed in patients with metastatic disease to palliate severe associated local symptoms, to allow entry into a biological response modifier protocol, or concomitant with resection of a solitary metastatic lesion.

Renal cell carcinoma involving the inferior vena cava (IVC) should be suspected in patients who have lower extremity edema, a varicocele, dilated superficial abdominal veins, proteinuria, pulmonary embolism, a right atrial mass, or nonfunction of the involved kidney. Currently, MRI is the preferred diagnostic study for demonstrating both the present and distal extent of IVC involvement.[3] Contrast inferior venacavography is reserved for patients in whom MRI is either nondiagnostic or contraindicated. The approach to patients with renal cell carcinoma involving the IVC is reviewed in detail elsewhere in Chapter 27.

Radical nephrectomy encompasses the basic principles of early ligation of the renal artery and vein, removal of the kidney outside Gerota's fascia, removal of the ipsilateral adrenal gland, and performance of a complete regional lymphadenectomy from the crus of the diaphragm to the aortic bifurcation.[1] Perhaps the most important aspect of radical nephrectomy is removal of the kidney outside Gerota's fascia, because capsular invasion with perinephric fat involvement occurs in 25 percent of patients. Studies suggest that removal of the ipsilateral adrenal gland is not routinely necessary unless the malignancy either extensively involves the kidney or is located in the upper portion of the kidney.[4] Although lymphadenectomy allows for more accurate pathological staging, its therapeutic value remains controversial.[5] A study by Giuliani and associates suggests that a subset of patients with micrometastatic lymph node involvement may benefit from a lymphadenectomy.[6] At the present time, the need for routine performance of a complete lymphadenectomy in all cases is unresolved, and there remains a divergence of clinical practice among urologists with respect to this aspect of radical nephrectomy.

SURGICAL ANATOMY

The anatomical relationship of the kidneys to surrounding structures is illustrated in Figure 28–1. The kidneys are located on either side of the vertebral column in the lumbar fossa of the retroperitoneal space. Each kidney is surrounded by a layer of perinephric fat, which in turn is covered by a distinct fascial layer termed Gerota's fascia. Posteriorly, both kidneys lie on the psoas major and quadratus lumborum muscles. Posteriorly and superiorly, the upper pole of each kidney is in contact with the diaphragm.

A small segment of the anterior medial surface of the right kidney is in contact with the right adrenal gland. However, the major anterior relationships of

256

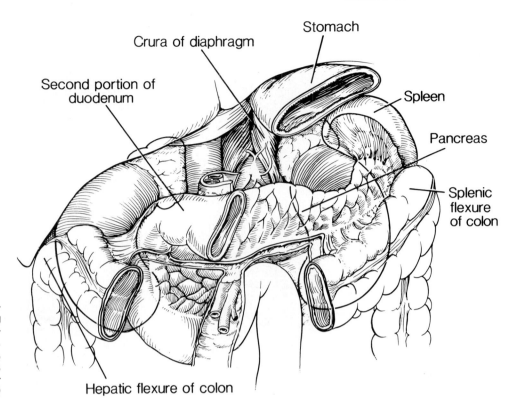

Figure 28–1. The anatomical relationship of the kidneys to the surrounding structures. The liver is retracted superiorly. (From Novick AC, Streem SB. Surgery of the kidney. In Walsh PC, Retik AB, Stamey TA, Vaughan ED Jr, eds. Campbell's Urology, 6th ed. Philadelphia, WB Saunders, 1992, p 2414.)

the right kidney are the liver, which overlies the upper two thirds of the anterior surface, and the hepatic flexure of the colon, which overlies the lower one third. The second portion of the duodenum covers the right renal hilum.

A small segment of the anterior medial surface of the left kidney is also covered by the left adrenal gland. The major anterior relationships of the left kidney are the spleen, body of the pancreas, stomach, and splenic flexure of the colon.

SURGICAL INCISIONS

The surgical approach for radial nephrectomy is determined by the size and location of the tumor as well as the habitus of the patient.[7] The operation is usually performed through a transperitoneal incision to allow abdominal exploration for metastatic disease and early access to the renal vessels with minimal manipulation of the tumor. Occasionally, an extraperitoneal flank incision is employed in elderly patients or in patients with small tumors who are also classified as poor risks.

The author prefers an extended subcostal or a bilateral subcostal incision for most patients undergoing radical nephrectomy (Fig. 28–2). This incision provides better access to the lateral and superior portion of the kidney than a midline abdominal incision. When an anterior subcostal incision is used, the patient is in the supine position with a rolled sheet

beneath the upper lumbar spine. The incision begins approximately 1 to 2 fingerbreadths below the costal margin in the anterior axillary line and then extends with a gentle curve across the midline, ending at the midportion of the opposite rectus muscle. The incision is carried through the subcutaneous tissues to the anterior fascia, which is divided in the direction of the incision. In the lateral aspect of the inci-

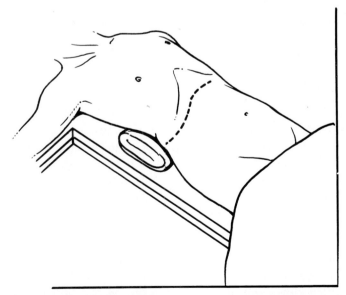

Figure 28–2. Patient positioning for anterior subcostal transperitoneal incision. (From Novick AC, Streem SB. Surgery of the kidney. In Walsh PC, Retik AB, Stamey TA, Vaughan ED Jr, eds. Campbell's Urology, 6th ed. Philadelphia, WB Saunders, 1992, p 2425.)

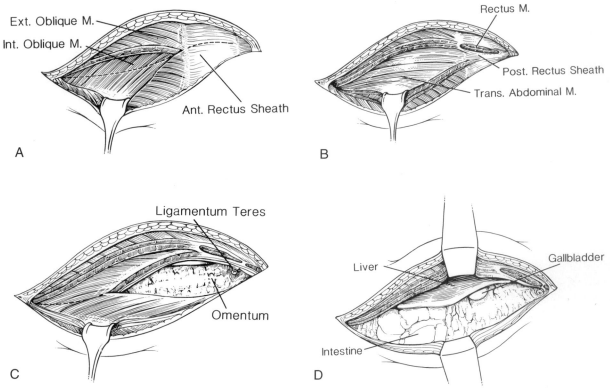

Figure 28–3. *A* to *D,* The various steps in performing an anterior subcostal transperitoneal incision (see accompanying text). (From Novick AC, Streem SB. Surgery of the kidney. In Walsh PC, Retik AB, Stamey TA, Vaughan ED Jr, eds. Campbell's Urology, 6th ed. Philadelphia, WB Saunders, 1992, p 2425.)

sion, a portion of the latissimus dorsi muscle is divided. The external oblique muscle is divided, exposing the fibers of the internal oblique muscle (Fig. 28–3*A*). The rectus, internal oblique, and transversus abdominis muscles are divided along with the posterior rectus sheath (Fig. 28–3*B* and *C*). The peritoneal cavity is entered in the midline and the ligamentum teres is divided (Fig. 28–3*D*).

The thoracoabdominal approach is preferable for performing radical nephrectomy in patients with large tumors involving the upper portion of the kidney (Fig. 28–4). It is particularly advantageous on the right side, where the liver and its venous drainage into the upper vena cava can limit exposure and impair vascular control as the tumor mass is being removed. There is less need for a thoracoabdominal incision on the left side, because the spleen and pancreas can usually be readily elevated away from the tumor mass. The patient is placed in a semioblique position, with a rolled sheet placed longitudinally beneath the flank. The incision is begun in the eighth intercostal space, near the angle of the rib, and is carried across the costal margin to the midpoint of the opposite rectus muscle, above the umbilicus. The latissimus dorsi, external oblique, rectus, and intercostal muscles are divided in the direction of the incision (Fig. 28–5*A*). The costal cartilage between the tips of the adjacent ribs is divided (Fig. 28–5*B*)

and the pleura is then opened to obtain complete exposure of the diaphragm (Fig. 28–5*C*).

The diaphragmatic incision is made at the periphery about 2 cm inside its attachment to the chest wall, with the incision carried around circumferentially to

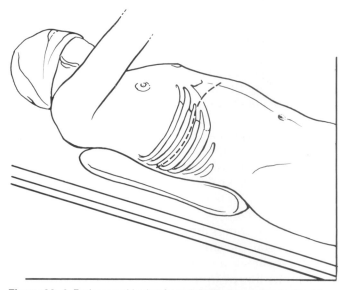

Figure 28–4. Patient positioning for a right thoracoabdominal incision. (From Novick AC, Streem SB. Surgery of the kidney. In Walsh PC, Retik AB, Stamey TA, Vaughan ED Jr, eds. Campbell's Urology, 6th ed. Philadelphia, WB Saunders, 1992, p 2429.)

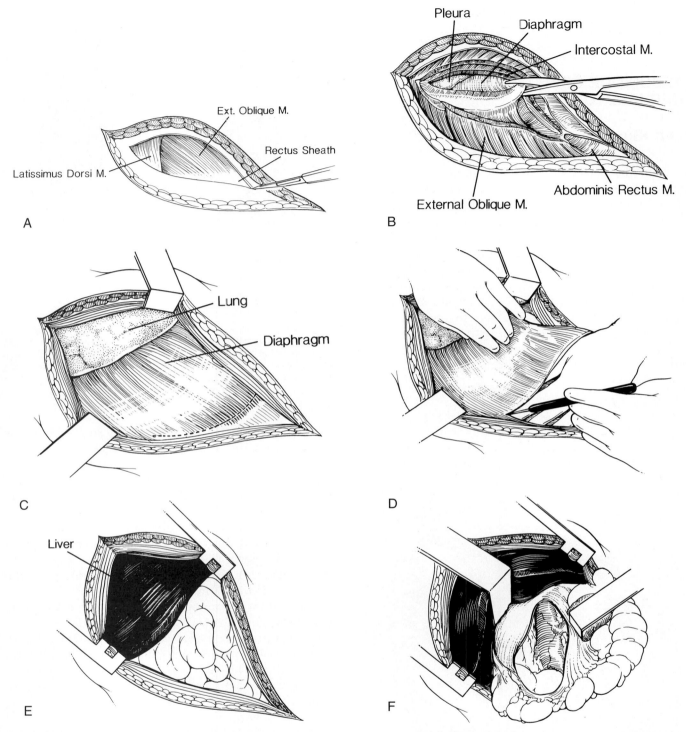

A

B

C

D

E

F

Figure 28–5. *A* to *F,* The various steps in performing a thoracoabdominal incision (see accompanying text). (From Novick AC, Streem SB. Surgery of the kidney. In Walsh PC, Retik AB, Stamey TA, Vaughan ED Jr, eds. Campbell's Urology, 6th ed. Philadelphia, WB Saunders, 1992, p 2429–2430.)

the posterior aspect of the diaphragm (Fig. 28–5*D*). Circumferential incision of the diaphragm obviates damage to the phrenic nerve and also creates a diaphragmatic flap, which can be pushed into the chest to provide complete exposure of the liver, which is then retracted upward (Fig. 28–5*E*). If further mobilization of the liver is needed, the right triangular and

coronary ligaments can be incised to mobilize the entire right lobe of the liver upward. This maneuver provides excellent additional exposure of the suprarenal vena cava. Medial to the ribs, the internal oblique and transversus abdominis muscles are divided, and the peritoneal cavity is entered. The kidney and great vessels may then be exposed by upward retraction of the liver and medial visceral mobilization (Fig. 28–5*F*).

TECHNIQUE OF RADICAL NEPHRECTOMY

Left Kidney

After the peritoneal cavity is entered, a thorough exploration is made to rule out metastatic disease. The posterior peritoneum lateral to the left colon is incised vertically and the incision carried upward to divide the lienorenal ligament. Care must be taken to avoid tearing the delicate capsule of the spleen. The plane between the kidney and adrenal gland posteriorly, and the pancreas and spleen anteriorly, is developed by blunt dissection. The left colon and duodenum are reflected medially, and the pancreas and spleen are reflected cephalad, with care taken not to injure the spleen or the pancreas (Fig. 28–6). When adequate exposure of the kidney and great vessels

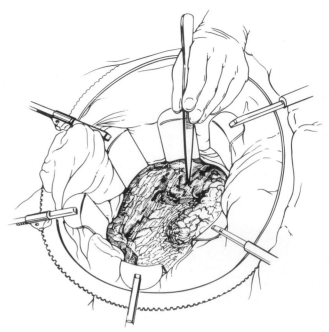

Figure 28–7. A self-retaining ring retractor is inserted to maintain exposure of the operative field. (From Novick AC, senior ed. Stewart's Operative Urology. Baltimore, Williams & Wilkins, 1989. Copyright Williams & Wilkins, 1989.)

has been obtained, a self-retaining ring retractor is inserted to maintain the operative field (Fig. 28–7).

The operation is initiated with dissection of the renal pedicle. The left renal vein is quite long as it passes over the aorta. The vein is mobilized completely by ligating and dividing gonadal, adrenal, and lumbar tributaries. The vein can be retracted to expose the artery posteriorly, which is then mobilized toward the aorta (Fig. 28–8). The renal artery is ligated with 2-0 silk ligatures and divided, and the renal vein is then similarly managed.

The kidney is mobilized outside Gerota's fascia with blunt and sharp dissection as needed (Fig. 28–9). Remaining vascular attachments are secured with nonabsorbable sutures or metal clips. Visualization of the upper vascular attachments is facilitated by downward retraction of the kidney. The ureter is then ligated and divided to complete the removal of the kidney and adrenal gland (Fig. 28–10).

The classical description of radical nephrectomy includes the performance of a complete regional lymphadenectomy. The lymph nodes can be removed en bloc with the kidney and adrenal gland or separately, after the nephrectomy. The lymph node dissection is begun at the crura of the diaphragm just below the origin of the superior mesenteric artery. A readily definable periadventitial plane is seen close to the aorta that can be entered. The dissection may then be carried along the aorta and onto the origin of the major vessels, to remove all the periaortic lymphatic tissue. Care must be taken to avoid injury to the

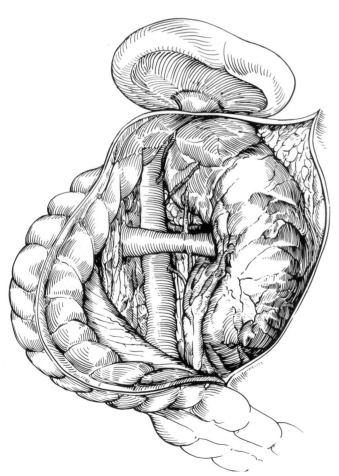

Figure 28–6. After entering the peritoneal cavity, the colon is reflected medially to expose the left kidney and great vessels. (From Novick AC, senior ed. Stewart's Operative Urology. Baltimore, Williams & Wilkins, 1989. Copyright Williams & Wilkins, 1989.)

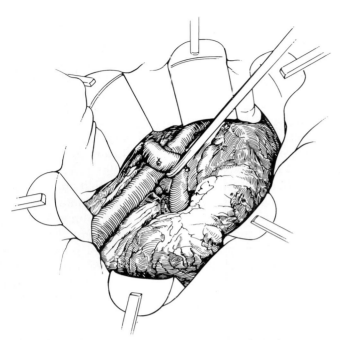

Figure 28–8. The left renal vein is mobilized by ligating its major branches to expose the artery posteriorly. (From Novick AC, senior ed. Stewart's Operative Urology. Baltimore, Williams & Wilkins, 1989. Copyright Williams & Wilkins, 1989.)

origins of the celiac and superior mesenteric arteries superiorly, as they arise from the anterior surface of the aorta. The dissection of the periaortic and pericaval lymph nodes is then carried downward en bloc to the origin of the inferior mesenteric artery. The sympathetic ganglia and nerves are removed together with the lymphatic tissue. The cisterna chyli is identified medial to the right crus. Entering lymphatic

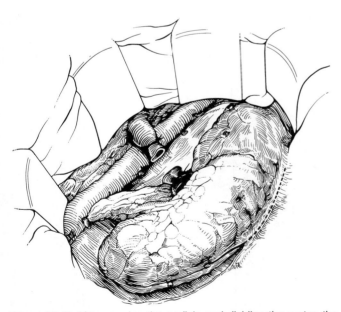

Figure 28–9. After securing the pedicle and dividing the ureter, the kidney is mobilized outside Gerota's fascia. (From Novick AC, senior ed. Stewart's Operative Urology. Baltimore, Williams & Wilkins, 1989. Copyright Williams & Wilkins, 1989.)

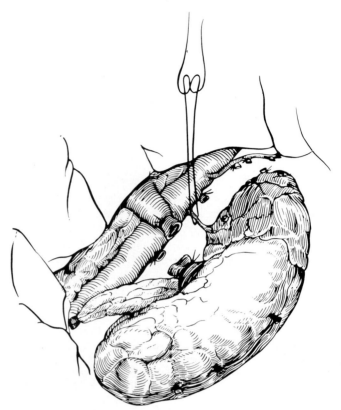

Figure 28–10. Remaining medial vascular attachments are secured and divided to complete the nephrectomy. (From Novick AC, senior ed. Stewart's Operative Urology. Baltimore, Williams & Wilkins, 1989. Copyright Williams & Wilkins, 1989.)

vessels are secured to prevent the development of chylous ascites.

Right Kidney

On the right side, after the peritoneal cavity is entered, the posterior peritoneum lateral to the right colon is incised vertically and the incision carried high up along the vena cava to the level of the hepatic veins. The right colon and duodenum are reflected medially, and the liver and gallbladder are retracted upward (Fig. 28–11). Care is taken to avoid trauma to the delicate hepatic veins, which may enter the vena cava at this level. When adequate exposure of the kidney and adrenal gland is obtained, a self-retaining ring retractor is inserted to maintain the operative field.

The vena cava and renal vein are retracted medially and downward to expose the right renal artery. Alternatively, with a large medial tumor, the renal artery may be exposed between the vena cava and the aorta (Fig. 28–12). Ligation of the renal artery and vein is performed with 2-0 silk ligatures as described for the left side. Since the right renal vein is usually short, ligation should take place at the level of its entrance to the vena cava. The remainder of the radical ne-

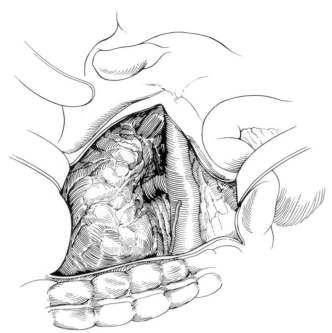

Figure 28–11. After entering the peritoneal cavity, the right colon and duodenum are reflected medially to expose the right kidney and great vessels. (From Novick AC, senior ed. Stewart's Operative Urology. Baltimore, Williams & Wilkins, 1989. Copyright Williams & Wilkins, 1989.)

phrectomy is performed as described for left-sided tumors.

POSTOPERATIVE COMPLICATIONS

After radical nephrectomy, postoperative complications occur in approximately 20 percent of patients, and the operative mortality rate is approximately 2 percent.[8] Systemic complications may occur after any surgical procedure, including myocardial infarction, cerebrovascular accident, congestive heart failure, pulmonary embolism, atelectasis, pneumonia, and thrombophlebitis. The incidence of these problems can be reduced by adequate preoperative preparation, avoidance of intraoperative hypotension, appropriate blood and fluid replacement, postoperative breathing exercises, early mobilization, and elastic support of the legs both during and after surgery.

An intraoperative gastrointestinal injury should always be checked for during the procedure, and lacerations repaired and drained. Tears of the liver may be repaired with mattress sutures. Splenic injuries usually require splenectomy, although small lacerations may be managed by application of Avitene or Oxycel. Injuries to the tail of the pancreas, which may occur with left radical nephrectomy, are best managed by partial amputation.

A particularly distressing postoperative complication is the development of a pancreatic fistula due to unrecognized intraoperative injury to the pancreas. This complication is usually manifested in the immediate postoperative period with signs and symptoms of acute pancreatitis and drainage of alkaline fluid from the incision. Treatment involves either percutaneous or surgical drainage of the fluid collection to avoid the development of a pancreatic pseudocyst or abscess. Most fistulas close spontaneously with adequate drainage, and surgical closure is only occasionally necessary.

Another gastrointestinal problem that may occur consists of a generalized ileus or a functional obstruction caused by a localized ileus of the colon overlying the operated renal fossa. Oral feedings should not be given until adequate bowel sounds are present and the patient has flatus. Nasogastric suction is given in more severe cases. When a prolonged period of ileus is anticipated, or when the patient is in a poor nutritional state, parenteral hyperalimentation should be instituted.

Secondary hemorrhage may occur after radical nephrectomy and is manifested by pain, signs of shock, abdominal or flank swelling, and drainage of blood through the incision. Bleeding may be from the kidney or renal pedicle but is occasionally from an unrecognized injury to a neighboring structure, such as the spleen, the liver, or a mesenteric vessel. Patients should be given blood and fluid replacement as needed. In most cases, it is best to reopen the wound, evacuate the hematoma, and secure the bleeding point. In the event of diffuse bleeding from a clotting

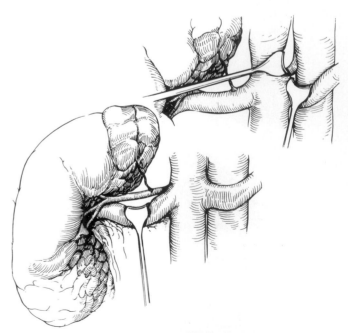

Figure 28–12. The right renal artery may be mobilized either lateral to the vena cava (*below*) or between the vena cava and the aorta (*above*). (From Novick AC, senior ed. Stewart's Operative Urology. Baltimore, Williams & Wilkins, 1989. Copyright Williams & Wilkins, 1989.)

disorder, it may be necessary to temporarily pack the wound with gauze, which can be gradually removed after 24 to 48 hours.

Pneumothorax may occur after a thoracoabdominal incision. Before complete closure of the incision, a red rubber catheter is inserted into the pleural cavity and a pursestring suture tied around the catheter. The anesthesiologist is then asked to hyperinflate the patient's lungs. With hyperinflation and suction on the catheter, air and fluid in the hemithorax are forced out through the red rubber catheter, which is then removed. The pursestring suture is secured. An alternative method is to place the distal end of the catheter in a basin of water. As the anesthesiologist hyperinflates the lung, air and fluid are forced out of the pleural cavity through the red rubber catheter and into the basin of water. When the pleura is entered, a chest radiograph should be obtained in the recovery room to ensure adequate re-expansion of the lung. A pneumothorax greater than 10 percent, a tension pneumothorax, or one causing respiratory distress requires insertion of a chest tube.

Postoperative atelectasis is common after radial nephrectomy and is probably caused by the positioning of the patient during the procedure. This complication is a common cause of fever postoperatively and may be effectively treated with pulmonary physiotherapy, including deep breathing, coughing, and incentive spirometry.

Infection is another common postoperative complication. Superficial wound infections are best managed by removal of skin sutures or staples to allow for drainage. Deeper infections must be treated by the establishment of adequate drainage and administration of appropriate antibiotics for systemic manifestations of the infection. Accumulations of lymph or serous fluid in the renal fossa or pleura are best managed expectantly, unless there are associated symptoms.

Editorial Comment
Fray F. Marshall

The anterior approach of radical nephrectomy is described very lucidly. In some obese patients an anterior approach may be more difficult. We have been inclined to perform a flank approach more often. The anterior approach often allows earlier ligation of the renal artery. Knowledge of different approaches is important so that the incision can be tailored to each specific patient.

REFERENCES

1. Robson CJ, Churchill BM, Anderson W. The results of radical nephrectomy for renal cell carcinoma. J Urol 101:297, 1969.
2. Skinner DG, Colvin RB, Vermillion CD, et al. Diagnosis and management of renal cell carcinoma: A clinical and pathological study of 309 cases. Cancer 28:1165, 1971.
3. Goldfarb DA, Novick AC, Lorgi R, et al. Magnetic resonance imaging for assessment of vena caval tumor thrombi: A comparative study with vena cavography and CT scanning. J Urol 144:1110, 1990.
4. Sagalowaky AI, Kadesky KT, Ewalt DM, Kennedy TJ. Factors influencing adrenal metastasis in renal cell carcinoma. J Urol 151:1181, 1994.
5. Marshall FF, Powell KC. Lymphadenectomy for renal cell carcinoma: Anatomical and therapeutic considerations. J Urol 128:677, 1982.
6. Giuliani L, Giberti C, Martorama G, Rovida S. Radical extensive surgery for renal cell carcinoma. J Urol 143:468, 1990.
7. Novick AC, Streem SB. Surgery of the kidney. In Walsh PC, Retik AB, Stamey TA, Vaughan ED Jr, eds. Campbell's Urology, 6th ed. Philadelphia, WB Saunders 1992, 2413.
8. Swanson DA, Borges PM. Complications of transabdominal radical nephrectomy for renal cell carcinoma. J Urol 129:704, 1983.

Chapter 29

Radical Nephrectomy with Excision of Vena Caval Tumor Thrombus

Fray F. Marshall and Bruce A. Reitz

Renal cell adenocarcinoma has a propensity for venous invasion. Between 4 and 10 percent of patients with renal cell adenocarcinoma will have neoplastic extensions into the vena cava. This intracaval neoplastic extension can ascend through the intrahepatic portion of the vena cava into the heart.

Surgical problems may increase when caval extension occurs. If there is only a small projection from the renal vein into the cava, a vascular clamp can be placed on the side wall of the cava and surgical excision can be accomplished without undue difficulty. If the tumor thrombus is larger, control of the cava above and below the tumor thrombus as well as the contralateral renal vein can allow successful removal of all the tumor. Alternatively, when the tumor thrombus extends into the liver or above, isolation of the cava becomes much more difficult. A variety of techniques have been used, including Foley and Fogarty catheters and clamping of the aorta and porta hepatis. Total control of bleeding often has not been accomplished.

This chapter describes our systematic approach to the larger vena caval tumor thrombus generally extending at least into the liver. There is now significant experience with vena caval tumor thrombi that extend into the liver or above.[1-4]

PREOPERATIVE EVALUATION AND MANAGEMENT

All patients are carefully evaluated for metastatic disease. This generally includes computed tomographic (CT) scans of the chest and abdomen, bone scan, magnetic resonance imaging (MRI), and stan-

dard blood work. We have used both MRI and inferior venacavography. For total occlusion of the vena cava, MRI has sometimes provided a very clear picture of the superior aspect of the tumor thrombus. In comparison, if the tumor thrombus moves significantly in the vena cava, MRI may not delineate clearly the superior aspect of the intracaval neoplastic extension. In some instances, we have continued to use inferior venacavography, but MRI usually suffices.

Renal cell carcinoma can metastasize to unusual places. If any other symptoms are reported, they should be investigated carefully. If any metastatic disease is demonstrated, we have not performed radical nephrectomy, particularly involving cardiopulmonary bypass (CPB). There is good evidence that the prognosis is very poor and is not altered by nephrectomy in the presence of metastatic disease. As adjuvant chemotherapy and immunotherapy become more effective, some of these high-risk patients may become candidates for nephrectomy and removal of caval tumor thrombus.

The general medical status of the patient is evaluated, an anesthesia consultation is obtained, and any other medical problems are addressed carefully. Some groups have performed additional cardiac vascular surgery in conjunction with radical nephrectomy and removal of the tumor thrombus. If the patient is generally asymptomatic, the addition of a coronary artery graft or carotid surgery would seem to be inappropriate.

Preoperative medication is usually restricted to short-acting narcotics. Antibiotic coverage is provided with a cephalosporin. A hypothermic blanket is utilized on the operating room table. Standard monitoring procedures are carried out, including

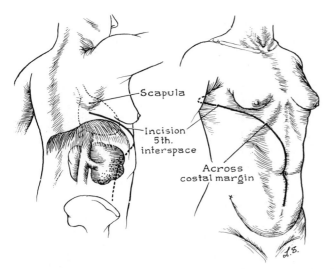

Figure 29–1. Thoracoabdominal incision extending from the tip of the scapula across the costal margin to the midline halfway between the umbilicus and xyphoid process of the sternum. The shoulder is rotated, but the pelvis is flat.

pressures in the radial artery; central venous pressure; pulmonary arterial wedge pressure; urinary output; esophageal and rectal temperatures; and electrocardiographic, O_2, and CO_2 measurements.

OPERATIVE TECHNIQUE

Anesthesia is usually induced with meperidine (Demerol), 3 to 9 mg/kg, or fentanyl, 6 mg/kg, and pancuronium, 1.3 mg/kg, and is maintained with nitrous oxide. Thiopental, 30 mg/kg, on intravenous drip for 30 to 90 minutes is given for possible protective effects on the central nervous system.

After induction of anesthesia, the skin incision can vary significantly (Figs. 29–1 and 29–2). The thoracoabdominal incision can extend from the tip of the scapula across the costal margin to the midline of the abdomen approximately halfway between the umbilicus and the xyphoid. An incision can then be carried inferiorly past the umbilicus to the lower abdomen in the midline. To make this incision, the shoulder is rotated toward the contralateral side and the table is flexed slightly. The hips remain almost flat on the table. This incision provides access to both chest and abdomen. It is often easier to dissect the primary tumor through this incision.

Dissection is easier for the urologist, particularly posteriorly under the diaphragm. The disadvantage of this incision lies in the difficulty of cannulating the aortic arch for CPB. In addition, abundant musculature is divided.

We now usually employ a midline sternotomy (Fig. 29–2), which can be extended inferiorly as a single incision, especially in someone who is rather thin. In a heavier patient a chevron incision can be made as an alternative. In some patients this variation may provide improved exposure. In this incision the rectus muscles are divided on each side, as each wing of the incision extends in a transverse direction.

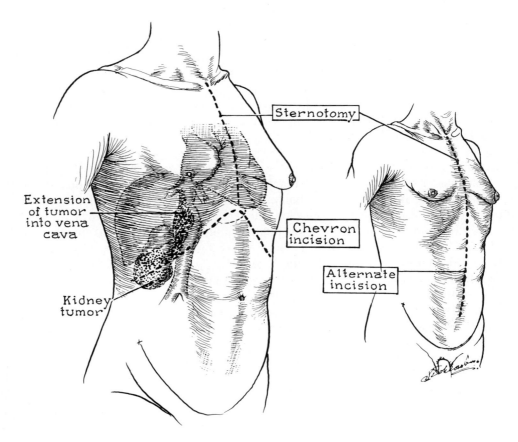

Figure 29–2. A midline sternotomy can be performed with a straight vertical incision or with a chevron incision extending laterally. The choice depends on the body habitus of the patient.

We make the entire incision initially rather than only a portion of it, because exposure is better with a larger incision. After the initial incision is made, the abdominal contents are inspected. If obvious significant metastatic disease is present, the operation may be stopped, as longevity is not greatly improved by the procedure. In two patients, we found very small nodules in the lung or metastatic lymph nodes after initiation of the procedure. We have generally completed the operation in that situation if it appears technically feasible. We are adding gene therapy (immunotherapy) with some of these more extensive caval cases because our longer-term initial experience has demonstrated metastases that occur frequently even after 3 or 4 years.

In dissection of the right kidney, the right colon is mobilized with a peritoneal incision around the inferior aspect of the cecum and extension superiorly up to the ligament of Treitz. The bowel contents can then be put in a bowel bag and placed on the chest. An effort is made to ligate the renal artery before any extensive dissection, to reduce blood loss. As the peritoneum is incised over the aorta, the renal artery can usually be identified. The right renal artery, for example, can be identified under the left renal vein. This incision is often too large for any standard ring retractor, but retractors are available (Omni-Tract) that can be mounted on the operating room table and work well. Otherwise, a very large Balfour retractor may suffice.

Once the renal artery is ligated, the dissection proceeds posteriorly along the quadratus and psoas muscles. Usually, Gerota's fascia can be elevated from these muscles quite easily. Occasionally, some small perforating veins occur in this area. Dissection can then be carried out superiorly along the diaphragm. From the anterior approach, the diaphragm can be taken down as well to facilitate dissection. From the thoracoabdominal approach, dividing the diaphragm posteriorly usually provides excellent access to the superior aspect of a large tumor.

The posterior attachments of the liver can be divided and the liver rotated medially. The dissection can then be carried down right on the vena cava. The adrenal vein needs to be identified, ligated, and divided. The medial dissection is facilitated by identifying the large bowel and finding a plane between Gerota's fascia and the mesocolon. Occasionally, if the peritoneum is directly involved, this area should be excised. Otherwise, the space between Gerota's fascia and the colon is identified. This plane brings the surgeon's position onto the cava in a right dissection. The duodenum is identified and reflected. Inferiorly the ureter, the gonadal vessels, and any other prominent vasculature are divided.

The specimen resides on a stalk of renal vein with tumor thrombus in it. The vena cava is then isolated with careful dissection. The cava is dissected below the renal vein (Fig. 29–3). Sometimes, blood thrombus can be seen in this segment of the vena cava. The vena cava is isolated, with control obtained of the proximal vena cava below the tumor thrombus and the contralateral renal vein. The dissection is then carried superiorly to the level of the caudate lobe. The venous drainage of the caudate lobe is highly variable. We have seen two or three large veins or seven or eight small perforating veins entering the caudate lobe. Sometimes these veins are short and require suture ligatures, particularly in the hepatic segment. If control of the cava can be obtained above the tumor thrombus, bypass is not necessary. An elliptical incision can be made around the ostium of the renal vein, the cava opened, and the tumor thrombus removed. The cava can then be oversewn. It is important to be sure that all lumbar veins are also ligated, as one patent lumbar vein may provide significant bleeding.

CARDIOPULMONARY BYPASS, HYPOTHERMIA, AND TEMPORARY CARDIAC ARREST

After the standard median sternotomy incision is made and after careful inspection of the abdomen, the intra-abdominal, retroperitoneal dissection is performed first. Once the kidney and the tumor on its pedicle are isolated, the thoracic dissection is initiated. The pericardium is opened and retracted with stay sutures, and systemic heparinization is initiated. Cannulas are inserted in both the ascending aorta and right atrial appendage. Usually a 22 Fr. Bardic cannula is inserted in the aorta and a 32 Fr. venous cannula through the right atrial appendage.

Flow is initiated through the bypass machine, and flow rates are kept between 2.5 and 3.5 L/min (approximately 55 ml/kg/min). The gas flow consists of a mixture of 95 percent O_2 and 5 percent CO_2 at 1 L/min and 100 percent O_2 at 1 L/min, as dictated by the blood gas results. With pulsatile flow the rectal temperature of 18° to 20°C is usually reached after about 30 minutes. The bypass hematocrit is usually kept at 18 to 20 volume percent. If any left ventricular distention occurs, a vent is placed. In general, a gradient of 8° to 10°C is maintained between the perfusion and the patient's core temperature. Once a temperature of approximately 20°C is attained, an aortic cross-clamp is applied, and 500 ml of cold crystalloid cardioplegic solution will achieve cardiac arrest. The bypass machine is stopped. The venous line is left open and the patient temporarily exsanguinated into the oxygen reservoir. Ice bags are placed around the patient's head to prevent any rewarming of the brain.

At this time there is no anesthesia, ventilation,

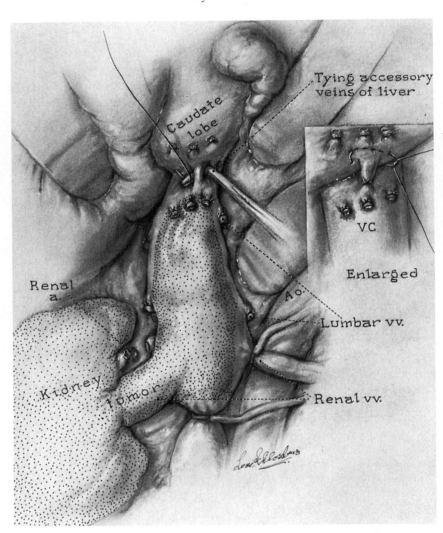

Figure 29–3. After dissection of the renal tumor, the vena cava is isolated and multiple venous branches to the hepatic caudate lobe are identified and divided. Control of the vena cava can then be accomplished above the tumor thrombus. (From Marshall FF, Dietrick DD, Baumgartner WA, Reitz BA. Surgical management of renal cell carcinoma with intracaval neoplastic extension above the hepatic veins. J Urol 139:1169, 1988.)

or circulation. Approximately 45 to 60 minutes of circulatory arrest time are available for dissection, although we have generally tried to keep the arrest time under 45 minutes (Fig. 29–4). The only patient who had massive coagulopathy was a man whose CPB time was very long, with a total arrest time exceeding 1 hour.

Dissection can now be performed with excellent vision within the heart and vena cava. An elliptical incision is made around the ostium of the renal vein. Frequently, invasion of the wall of the vena cava occurs, requiring excision. In some cases, excision of the entire vena cava below the hepatic veins may be performed.

A left-sided tumor with tumor thrombus extending well into the intrahepatic cava calls for a more difficult dissection (Figs. 29–5 and 29–6). An anterior midline incision is required, as this dissection has to be performed in both the left and right sides of the abdomen and retroperitoneum. The left colon is reflected and the tumor dissected free again, isolating it on its renal venous extension to the vena cava (Fig. 29–5).

A similar dissection is performed on the right with mobilization of the right colon as well as the duodenum so that the area of the vena cava around the left renal vein ostium is carefully dissected free. At that time the patient is placed on bypass after all the renal dissection is completed. It is emphasized that the bypass should be reserved until after most of the dissection has been performed. In several patients we have initiated bypass with low flow because of extensive bleeding, and this helped control the dissection. Under ordinary circumstances the entire dissection of the tumor is performed before bypass.

Thrombus has been seen extending from the iliac veins to the right ventricle. In general, all thrombus is blood thrombus below the renal veins (Fig. 29–7). We have removed tumor thrombus from the contralateral renal vein, lumbar veins, hepatic veins, right atrium, and right ventricle. We have seen adherence of the tumor thrombus even within the heart. Therefore, tumor thrombus even at that level is not entirely free at times. CPB with temporary exsanguination and cardiac arrest with associated hypothermia allows careful inspection of the interior of the heart and cava.

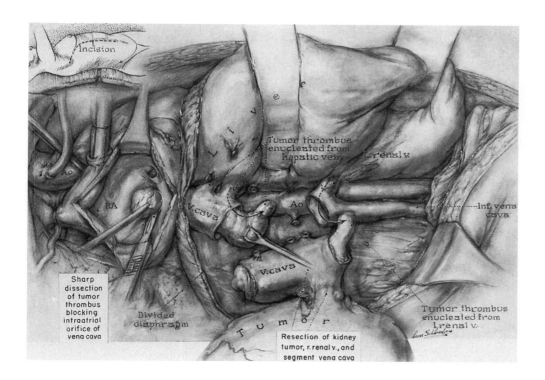

Figure 29–4. A right thoracoabdominal incision is made. The cannulas can be identified in the aortic arch and the right atrial appendage. After institution of bypass and hypothermia, exsanguination is performed. Under cardiac arrest a dissection is performed within the atrium, and the infrahepatic vena cava is excised. Tumor thrombus is extracted from the contralateral renal vein as well as the hepatic veins. (From Marshall FF, Reitz BA, Diamond DA. A new technique for management of renal cell carcinoma involving the right atrium: Hypothermia and cardiac arrest. J Urol 131:104, 1984.)

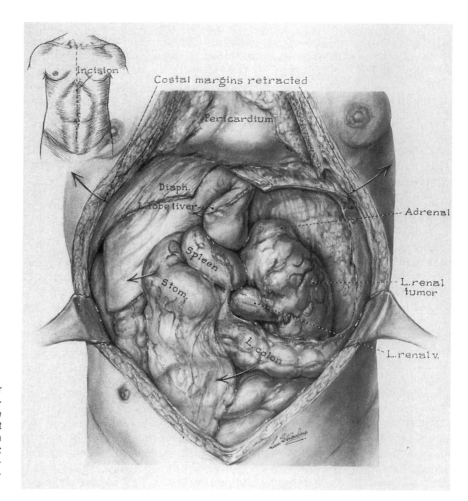

Figure 29–5. The patient with a left-sided tumor thrombus has a midline incision through the sternum extending well below the umbilicus and the abdomen. The left colon is reflected and the left renal tumor is dissected free while remaining on its renal venous pedicle. (From Marshall FF, Reitz BA. Technique for removal of renal cell carcinoma with suprahepatic vena caval tumor thrombus. Urol Clin North Am 13:551, 1986.)

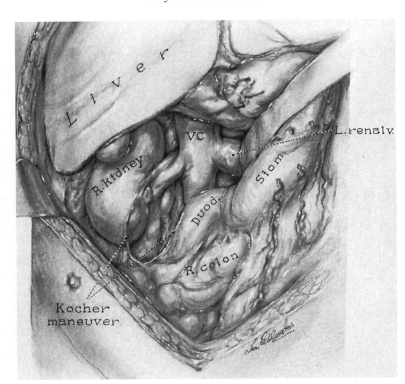

Figure 29–6. The right colon is reflected, as is the duodenum, and the cava is isolated. Cardiopulmonary bypass and hypothermia can then be initiated (From Marshall FF, Reitz BA. Technique for removal of renal cell carcinoma with suprahepatic vena caval tumor thrombus. Urol Clin North Am 13:551, 1986.)

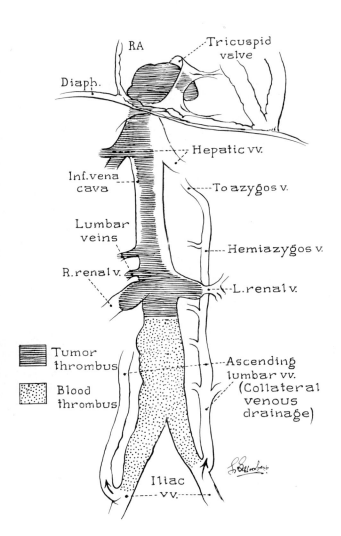

Figure 29–7. The vena cava can have thrombus throughout its entire extent. Below the renal vein ostia, this is generally a blood thrombus. From the level of the renal veins above, it is a tumor thrombus. We have extracted tumor thrombi from the contralateral renal vein, lumbar veins, hepatic veins, right atrium, and right ventricle. (From Marshall FF, Reitz BA. Technique for removal of renal cell carcinoma with suprahepatic vena caval tumor thrombus. Urol Clin North Am 13:551, 1986.)

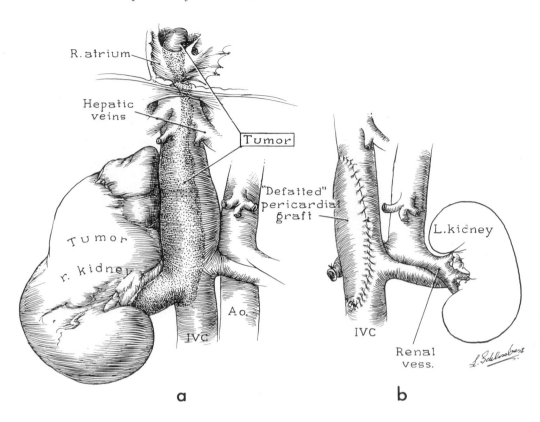

a   b

Figure 29–8. To avoid compromise of the vena caval lumen and to ensure venous patency, a defatted pericardial graft is placed within the vena cava. This is an effort to maintain venous drainage, not only of the contralateral kidney but also of the lower torso and extremities. (From Marshall FF, Reitz BA. Supradiaphragmatic renal cell carcinoma tumor thrombus: Indications for vena caval reconstruction with pericardium. J Urol 133:267, 1985.)

Once the main thrombus has been removed, inspection of the interior of the cava and heart can be accomplished. Any additional adherent thrombus can be "endarterectomized" from the interior of the vena cava. The cava is then reconstructed with 4–0 or 5–0 cardiovascular polypropylene sutures. In several patients who required excision of a major segment of the vena cava, the cava was reconstructed with a pericardial graft (Fig. 29–8).[5] Venous collateral circulation is not always fully developed in the absence of total occlusion of the vena cava. With excision of the caval wall, compromise of the lumen of the cava can occur and caval thrombosis can result.

The contralateral kidney can be at risk. We have had experience with patients who required renal dialysis postoperatively. For this reason, if the lumen of the cava is compromised by more than 50 percent, caval reconstruction with a pericardial graft can be considered in an effort to ensure venous drainage. In total occlusion of the vena cava, good collateral circulation is generally present. If a left-sided tumor exists, venous drainage of the right kidney must be preserved or it will undergo venous infarction. A pericardial graft might be utilized in special circumstances, with excision of a portion of the cava for a left-sided lesion. In our experience with left-sided lesions, massive dilation of the cava is usually observed and enough cava has been present without direct invasion to provide for continuity, at least to the hepatic vena caval segment. Venous drainage could also be reconstructed through the portal circulation.

After completion of the nephrectomy, CPB is reinstituted. The blanket is turned on and set 10°C warmer than the patient's core temperature. The heat exchanger circulation is also kept 10°C warmer than the patient to a maximum of 41°C. Any higher temperature gradient creates the possibility of thermal damage to the blood or gas embolism. The heat exchanger is placed on the venous side, and any bubbles are trapped in the oxygenator. Rectal and nasopharyngeal temperatures are monitored regularly along with arterial and venous blood gas values. Mannitol, 12.5 gm, is given every hour on bypass. Heparin is given to keep the activated clotting time at more than 450 seconds. Potassium supplement is provided as necessary. Calcium chloride (1 gm) is given as the nasopharyngeal temperature reaches 25°C.

Sometimes the heart starts beating spontaneously, but occasionally electrical defibrillation is necessary with an internal countershock of 10 to 15 watt seconds. After defibrillation, blood is gradually returned to the patient from the oxygen reservoir. Once the heart's ejection is effective, pulsatile bypass is stopped. Rewarming usually takes at least 1 hour. Thermal blankets and placement of warm saline within the chest and abdomen also facilitate warming of the patient.

Heparin is neutralized with protamine, usually 1½ times the total heparin dose. Further doses of protamine are given according to the activated clotting time.

POSTOPERATIVE MANAGEMENT AND COMPLICATIONS

Excessive bleeding is potentially a dangerous complication of bypass and hypothermia. Routinely, 6 units of platelets and 4 units of fresh frozen plasma are given. Factor 9 concentrate and cryoprecipitate are sometimes required. Additional calcium chloride may be needed to improve cardiac function. Furosemide is given if urinary output is low. Elastic bandages are applied on the lower extremities to decrease venous stasis. The temperature usually stabilizes at normothermia within 3 to 5 hours.

Other than minor standard postoperative problems, one major complication has been renal failure. Several patients have required dialysis. This problem has prompted the use of the pericardial patch for caval reconstruction in an effort to reduce venous hypertension and improve venous drainage from the remaining contralateral kidney. Coagulopathy occurred only in patients with a very long bypass and complete arrest times.

RESULTS

Patients with significant lymphadenopathy may not be good candidates, and their prognoses are poor.

Although some long-term survivors are known, many patients have developed metastatic disease, even 3 to 4 years after operation. In our experience the tumor is rarely confined within the renal capsule pathologically. Obviously, these patients have extensive regional disease and sometimes occult metastatic disease. The feasibility of this operation has been clearly demonstrated. Undoubtedly, with increased efficacy of chemotherapy and immunotherapy, patients will continue to be candidates for this operation. It may also be utilized in patients with tumors involving the liver, adrenal, and retroperitoneum as well as the kidney.

REFERENCES

1. Marshall FF, Reitz BA, Diamond DA. A new technique for management of renal cell carcinoma involving the right atrium: Hypothermia and cardiac arrest. J Urol 131:103, 1984.
2. Marshall FF, Dietrick DD, Baumgartner WA, Reitz BA. Surgical management of renal cell carcinoma with intracaval neoplastic extension above the hepatic veins. J Urol 139:1166, 1988.
3. Marshall FF, Reitz BA. Technique for removal of renal cell carcinoma with suprahepatic vena caval tumor thrombus. Urol Clin North Am 13:551, 1986.
4. Novick AC, Kaye MC, Cosgrove DM, et al. Experience with cardiopulmonary bypass and deep hypothermic circulatory arrest in the management of retroperitoneal tumors with large vena caval thrombi. Ann Surg 212:472, 1990.
5. Marshall FF, Reitz BA. Supradiaphragmatic renal cell carcinoma tumor thrombus: Indications for vena caval reconstruction with pericardium. J Urol 133:266, 1985.

Chapter 30

Partial Nephrectomy

Fray F. Marshall

INDICATIONS

Surgical excision remains the primary treatment of renal cell carcinoma. Although radical nephrectomy has been recommended and carries a good survival rate,[1] preservation of renal tissue is indicated in certain patients. Many groups of patients are candidates for partial nephrectomy: those with nephrectomy for previous tumor, calculus disease, or infection; those with renal agenesis, which occurs in 1 in 500 people; those (2 to 4 percent) with bilateral renal cell carcinomas[2]; those with multifocal renal carcinomas, which can occur in conditions such as von Hippel-Lindau disease[3]; and those with familial inherited renal cell carcinoma.[4] Other tumors, such as angiomyolipomas or oncocytomas, can be confused with renal cell carcinomas, and a partial nephrectomy can still preserve renal tissue in these patients. In an aging population, compromised renal function increasingly is another indication for preservation of renal tissue. Diagnostic dilemmas may occur. Unusual cystic lesions and focal xanthogranulomatous pyelonephritis may mimic renal cell carcinoma.[5] Partial nephrectomy can provide tissue for diagnosis. If an occult malignancy is found, it can be totally excised with a partial nephrectomy. More recently, partial nephrectomy is being performed for smaller, serendipitous tumors even if the contralateral kidney is normal.[6]

PREOPERATIVE MANAGEMENT

The patient usually presents with hematuria or other signs and symptoms suggestive of carcinoma. A mass is appreciated on intravenous pyelography (IVP) or sonography and verified on computed tomography (CT). Magnetic resonance imaging (MRI) has also been employed to evaluate mass lesions in the kidney. If there is compromised renal function with both kidneys, a renal scan may indicate the contribution of each renal unit. Although angiography is not routinely performed for radical nephrectomy, it can be considered if a partial nephrectomy is planned for a larger tumor. Oblique selective renal arteriograms will help demonstrate the anterior and posterior branches of the main renal artery and allow the surgeon to plan the partial nephrectomy preoperatively. Arteriography is used less frequently now.

The work-up for metastatic disease includes a CT scan of the chest and often a bone scan. Although sonography can evaluate the vena cava, MRI also provides good imaging of the cava without the need for contrast material.

Any other medical problems should be carefully evaluated preoperatively. If there is any possibility that the patient might lose all remaining renal parenchyma, a nephrologist should be consulted and plans for possible dialysis made. I have had experience with patients who required dialysis postoperatively after removal of all renal tissue. They all had extensive or multifocal tumors managed by total nephrectomy.

The night before surgery, intravenous fluids are given to maintain good hydration. In general, no antibiotics are given unless there is a well-documented previous infection.

SURGICAL OPTIONS

Surgical options include radical nephrectomy and dialysis, surgical enucleation, partial nephrectomy, and bench surgery and autotransplantation. Total nephrectomy should always be anticipated but is not usually necessary. If all renal tissue is removed, renal transplantation can be considered later if the patient survives more than 1 or 2 years without any evidence of metastatic disease.

Although bench surgery with possible autotransplantation is an option,[7] most of these operations can be performed in situ without bench surgery.

Partial nephrectomy remains the best surgical op-

272

tion if feasible. There is often a pseudocapsule around the lesions, so that removal of a rim of normal parenchyma is preferable to enucleation.[8] Enucleation may leave tumor in the presence of venous invasion, multiple tumor nodules, occult disease in lymph nodes, or extrinsic spread through the renal capsule.

OPERATIVE TECHNIQUE

Although some urologists prefer a transabdominal or subcostal approach, obesity and previous abdominal surgery in the general American population frequently make the anterior approach more difficult. The thoracoabdominal approach has generally been preferred (Fig. 30–1). It is important that the incision be made high enough for easy access to the renal hilum and the renal vasculature. The peritoneum is usually mobilized away from Gerota's fascia. Gerota's fascia and perinephric tissue are left adherent to the kidney over the tumor, but the remainder of the kidney is dissected on the renal capsule. During the dissection the main renal vasculature is identified. Mannitol, 12.5 gm, is given before any manipulation of the renal vasculature in order to provide diuresis. If fluids and mannitol are not successful in producing diuresis, furosemide is added and usually increases urinary output. Anticoagulation and heparinization have not been used routinely.

An intestinal bowel bag is placed around the kidney and a small hole made at the bottom of the bag so that the kidney can be brought through it. Intraoperative ultrasonography can be very helpful in delineating the tumor, especially when it is hard to see from the exterior of the kidney.[9] Ringer's lactate slush is placed around the kidney to cool it after the renal vasculature is occluded (Fig. 30–2). Vascular clamps are usually placed across both the artery and vein, because venous back bleeding can occur, espe-

cially on the right side (Fig. 30–2). If the vascular clamp is placed on both vessels, the vessels are not skeletonized and a tissue "cushion" exists around the vessels.

After the vascular supply is occluded and the kidney cooled, the renal artery is carefully dissected. The branches of the renal artery to the tumor are divided as previously determined on the renal arteriogram. The renal capsule is incised sharply with 1.0 cm of normal renal tissue (Fig. 30–3). The renal parenchyma can then be divided bluntly either with the back hand of the knife handle or with a neurosurgical brain elevator. Perinephric tissue remains over the tumor. Any significant intraparenchymal vessels are identified and ligated individually. The collecting system is divided and oversewn when encountered.

Frozen sections from the surface of the remaining kidney are obtained to verify that the pathological margin is adequate. To verify that no urine is leaking, a small vessel loop is placed around the ureter to occlude it and the renal pelvis is injected with a dilute solution of methylene blue. Any defects in the collecting system are oversewn with absorbable sutures (Fig. 30–4). The renal vascular clamp is usually removed briefly to identify any obvious nonligated arterial or major venous branches. The argon beam coagulator is used for hemostasis, and collagen (Avitene) is placed on the surface of the kidney (Fig. 30–5). Avitene has been very helpful in maintaining hemostasis. If feasible, 2-0 chromic sutures are placed to appose the remaining renal tissue. Perinephric fat can sometimes be incorporated in the closure. The vascular clamps are removed, and the kidney is compressed manually for at least 5 minutes. The kidney is usually fixed to the psoas muscle.

A drain is brought through Gerota's fascia and a separate stab wound. The remaining Gerota's fascia is reapproximated anatomically. Double-J catheters are generally not used.

This operation has also been performed for transitional cell carcinomas in a few patients,[10] but most patients have had renal cell adenocarcinomas.

POSTOPERATIVE MANAGEMENT AND COMPLICATIONS

Most patients have had few immediate postoperative complications. Even azotemic patients with diabetes or renal vascular disease have usually maintained stable serum creatinine levels in spite of extensive surgery on the kidney.

Postoperative complications initially involve anesthesia, with the typical problems of atelectasis and pneumonia. Postoperative bleeding has not been a significant problem when the previously outlined protocol has been followed. In one large series, hem-

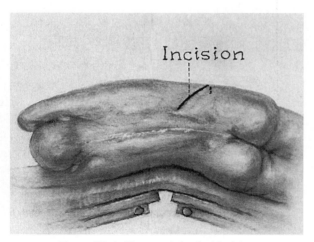

Figure 30–1. Thoracoabdominal incision.

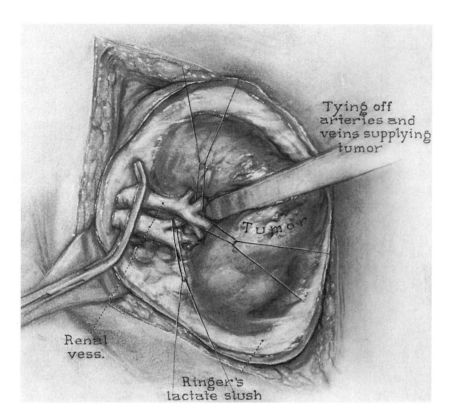

Figure 30–2. The kidney has been dissected. An intestinal bag has been placed and filled with Ringer's lactate slush. Vessels that supply the tumor are divided. The main renal vasculature has already been occluded.

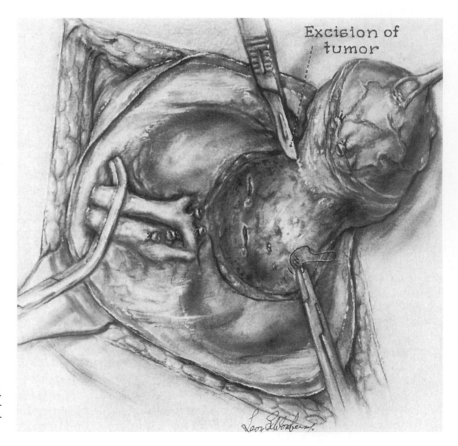

Figure 30–3. The renal capsule is divided sharply. Vessels are ligated or oversewn as they are encountered when the parenchyma is divided delicately.

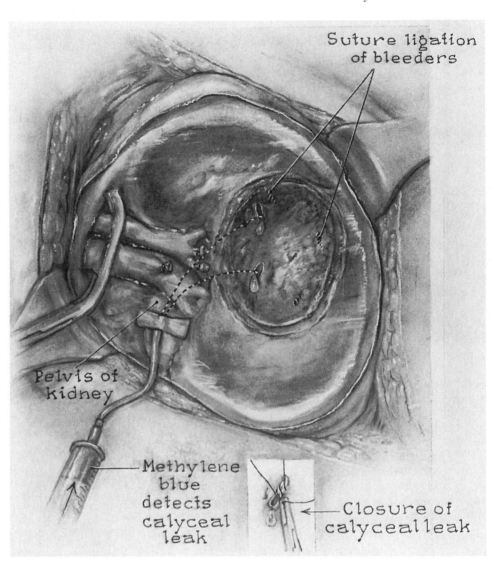

Suture ligation of bleeders

Pelvis of kidney

Methylene blue detects calyceal leak

Closure of calyceal leak

Figure 30–4. Methylene blue is injected into the renal pelvis after occlusion of the ureter with a vessel loop. Any leaks in the collecting system are oversewn.

orrhage occurred in only a few patients; there was one splenectomy.[11] Some wound or urinary infections have occurred, particularly when there was prolonged urinary extravasation. Urine leaks have usually closed spontaneously and have not required any further manipulation. If methylene blue is used and the collecting system closed meticulously, a leak should be infrequent. If there is continued urinary leakage, placement of a retrograde catheter or a double-J catheter as a stent may help.

If there are bilateral renal tumors, we have usually not operated on both kidneys simultaneously. In general, I operate on the healthier kidney first to verify that it is functioning well before operating on the second kidney. Often a radical nephrectomy has been necessary on the contralateral side, and the possibility of temporary dialysis is lessened. On the other hand, if one tumor is quite large and the contralateral tumor is small, it may sometimes be more appropriate to perform an initial radical nephrectomy for the more dangerous, larger tumor.

With partial nephrectomy, local control of tumor has been good. Recurrence has usually been noted with distant metastatic disease. A number of patients with elevated serum creatinine levels have maintained stable renal function postoperatively for years.

Although there are other techniques, including the laser[12] and ultrasonic aspirator,[13] the described operative approach works very well. It is not clear that the laser will coagulate large vessels, and the ultrasonic aspirator is slow and cumbersome.

Summary

In properly selected patients, partial nephrectomy can provide good local control of renal tumors with preservation of functioning renal parenchyma. An increasingly older population with compromised renal function may require this operation more often. Many patients with small serendipitous tumors are also candidates for partial nephrectomy. When effec-

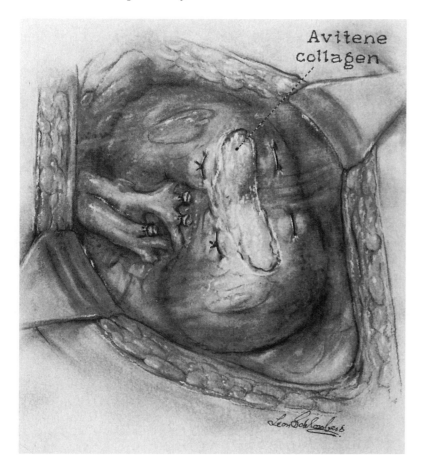

Figure 30–5. Collagen (Avitene) is placed for hemostasis, and several 2-0 chromic catgut sutures are placed to partially reapproximate renal parenchyma.

tive adjuvant chemotherapy becomes available, partial nephrectomy will remain an important operation, especially if the chemotherapy is nephrotoxic.

REFERENCES

1. Robson CJ, Churchill BM, Anderson W. The results of radical nephrectomy for renal cell carcinoma. J Urol 101:297, 1969.
2. Vermillion CD, Skinner DG, Pfister RC. Bilateral renal cell carcinoma. J Urol 108:219, 1972.
3. Pearson JC, Weiss J, Tanagho EA. A plea for conservation of kidney in renal cell adenocarcinoma associated with von Hippel-Lindau disease. J Urol 124:910, 1980.
4. Pathak S, Strong LC, Ferrell RE, Trindade A. Familial renal cell carcinoma with a 3:11 chromosome translocation limited to tumor cells. Science 217:939, 1982.
5. Elder JS, Marshall FF. Focal xanthogranulomatous pyelonephritis in adulthood. Johns Hopkins Med J 146:141, 1980.
6. Steinbach F, Stöckle MJ, Müller SC, et al. Conservative surgery of renal tumors in 140 patients: 21 years of experience J Urol 148:24, 1992.
7. Gittes RF, McCullough DL. Bench surgery for tumor in a solitary kidney. J Urol 113:12, 1975.
8. Marshall FF, Taxy JB, Fishman EK, Chang R. The feasibility of surgical enucleation for renal cell carcinoma. J Urol 135:231, 1986.
9. Marshall FF, Holdford SS, Hamper UM. Intraoperative sonography of renal tumors. J Urol 148:1393, 1992.
10. Marshall FF, Walsh PC. In situ management of renal tumors: Renal cell carcinoma and transitional cell carcinoma. J Urol 131:1045, 1984.
11. Bazeed MA, Scharfe T, Becht E, et al. Conservative surgery of renal cell carcinoma. Eur Urol 12:238, 1986.
12. Malloy TR, Schultz RE, Wein AJ, Carpiniello VL. Renal preservation utilizing neodymium:YAG laser. Urology 27:99, 1986.
13. Chopp RI, Shah BB, Addonizio JC. Use of ultrasonic surgical aspirator in renal surgery. Urology 22:157, 1983.

Chapter 31

Nephroureterectomy for Carcinoma of Renal Pelvis and Ureter

Jerome P. Richie

Carcinoma of the renal pelvis, a relatively rare tumor, comprises approximately 7 percent of all renal neoplasms and less than 1 percent of all genitourinary tumors. The incidence of renal tumors is often expressed in relation to the number of tumors in the urinary bladder. In a 20-year study, the ratio of tumors of the bladder, renal pelvis, and ureter was 51:3:1.[1] Tumors of the renal pelvis are more frequent in men than in women in a ratio of 2:1. The peak incidence is in the fifth and sixth decades of life, with a progressive increase in incidence with age. Ureteral tumors have a propensity for the lower third of the ureter. No predilection for laterality is observed for either renal pelvic or ureteral tumors. Bilateral tumors are distinctly uncommon.

Most of these neoplasms are of urothelial origin, and most represent transitional cell tumors. Squamous cell carcinoma and adenocarcinoma, usually associated with chronic infection or stones, are relatively uncommon. Squamous cell cancer constitutes about 10 percent of all tumors of the upper collecting system, and adenocarcinoma is extremely rare.

PREOPERATIVE EVALUATION

Careful evaluation must be carried out in a patient with a diagnosis of renal pelvic or ureteral tumors to exclude multiplicity of tumors as well as distant metastases. Grabstald and associates[2] reported that approximately half the patients with renal tumors had associated tumors in the bladder, ureter, or both. In view of the likelihood of multiplicity, it is essential that the entire urinary tract, including the urethra and bladder mucosae, be visualized by either radio-graphical or endoscopic procedures. If an intravenous pyelogram is not adequate to reveal the entire surface, a retrograde pyelogram should be used.

Staging procedures, in addition to assessment of the urothelium, should include chest radiography, radionuclide bone scan, and serum multichannel analysis. Liver scans or computed tomographic (CT) scans of the liver should not be utilized in the absence of abnormal liver profile results. Ultrasonography or CT may be of some benefit in assessing the presence or absence of retroperitoneal lymphadenopathy. Magnetic resonance imaging (MRI) has not proved beneficial.

The difficulty in establishing the diagnosis, as well as the limited accuracy of available staging procedures, has precluded the development of a clinical staging system. Instead, classification of renal pelvic tumors is based on pathological findings. Grabstald and associates,[2] after studying 70 patients with renal pelvic tumors, proposed a classification system based on tumor stage and grade. A modification of this system, proposed by Batata and associates,[3] is illustrated in Figure 31–1. This system, similar to the Jewett-Marshall-Strong system for bladder cancer, employs letters to indicate depth of invasion.[3] Stage 0 neoplasms are confined to the mucosa, stage A tumors invade the lamina propria, stage B tumors invade the muscle, stage C tumors extend into the peripelvic fat or renal parenchyma, and stage D represents metastatic disease.

Transitional cell carcinoma may spread by direct extension or metastasis via hematogenous or lymphatic routes. Regional lymph nodes are commonly involved before other sites of metastases. Therefore, surgical therapy should include regional lymphade-

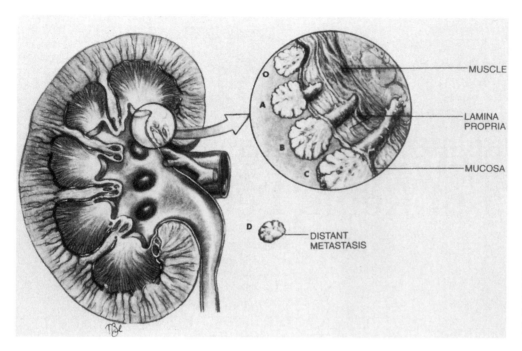

Figure 31–1. Staging system for renal pelvic tumors. (Modified from Batata MA, Whitmore WF, Hilaris BS, et al. Primary carcinoma of the ureter: A prognostic study. Cancer 35:1626, 1975.)

nectomy. Almost any organ may receive metastases from transitional cell tumors of the upper urinary tract.

INDICATIONS

The classical management of renal pelvic or ureteral tumors is nephroureterectomy with excision of a cuff of bladder and bladder mucosa. Although nephroureterectomy has traditionally been considered the treatment of choice, advocates of less radical procedures have continued to increase in numbers and now represent a strong minority. Proponents of radical nephroureterectomy with removal of a cuff of bladder emphasize the difficulty both in distinguishing histological grade of the tumor and in accurate preoperative estimation of stage. Half of all cases of ureteral tumor involve at least the musculature and may have lymphatic involvement. The high incidence of multiple ipsilateral lesions, both overt and in situ, makes removal of the entire ureteral segment in general preferable to partial ureterectomy for adequate tumor surgery. The well-known phenomenon of recurrence of tumor in the remaining ureteral stump has been reported in more than 30 percent of patients treated by nephrectomy and partial ureterectomy.[4] Laparoscopic ureterectomy or nephroureterectomy remains an experimental approach.[5, 6]

Advocates of conservative surgical intervention for renal pelvic or ureteral tumors stress the poor prognosis associated with advanced lesions, regardless of the form of surgical therapy, and the higher mortality rate occurring with more radical procedures. Studies by Cummings,[7] Gittes,[8] and McCarron and associates[9]

illustrate the difficulties in choosing between radical and conservative therapy for patients with tumors of the upper urinary collecting system.

The likelihood of implantation, especially with tumors of higher grades, must be considered an increased risk for kidney-sparing procedures as opposed to kidney-sacrificing procedures. Analogous experiences with open bladder surgery would indicate a higher likelihood of implantation.

Local recurrence and follow-up remain major problems for patients who undergo kidney-sparing procedures. Because the major site of recurrence in a patient with kidney-sparing procedures is the ipsilateral system, nephroureterectomy obviates the need for follow-up of the initially involved upper system, which is the main thrust of the follow-up for a patient receiving a conservative procedure. Nocks and associates[10] reported a high incidence of associated severe dysplasia or carcinoma in situ associated with high-grade, high-stage tumors. They concluded that nephroureterectomy was preferable to conservative procedures in a patient with carcinoma of the renal pelvis.

In light of these considerations, my personal preference remains, in general, nephroureterectomy with excision of a cuff of bladder for most patients with renal pelvic or ureteral tumors. However, several exceptions are readily apparent. In the patient with a solitary kidney, compromised renal function, bilateral lesions, or endemic nephropathy, conservation is essential. The preferred treatment would be local excision of a renal pelvic lesion with or without partial nephrectomy or, in the case of ureteral tumor, ureteral excision or ureterectomy with replacement by ileum. Local excision and reanastomosis should be limited to a patient with a localized filling defect, usually when tumors are polypoid, low grade, and presumably low stage. In such a patient, local excision with adequate margins may be the preferred treatment.

For patients with apparent solitary tumors of the lower third of the ureter, especially low-grade tumors, distal ureterectomy with regional lymphadenectomy and reimplantation of the ureter with a psoas hitch represents a reasonable alternative. In the patient with a lesion of higher grade or higher stage, the likelihood of coexistent upper tract lesions or compromise to the renal parenchyma would still favor nephroureterectomy. Tumors of the middle or upper third of the ureter are generally best treated by nephroureterectomy, unless cytological and brush biopsy specimens demonstrate a low-grade and presumably low-stage tumor. In such an instance, excisional biopsy with ureteroureterostomy can be considered.

Selected lesions in the renal pelvis and caliceal system may also be considered for conservative treatment, provided that the cytological results show less than a high-grade lesion, and brushing specimens or endoscopic biopsy specimens demonstrate a low-grade transitional cell tumor. In such an instance, ureteroscopy is helpful to make certain that the tumor is not of a more extensive nature and that the offending collecting system can be walled off and removed by partial nephrectomy. Gerber and Lyon have categorized percutaneous and endoscopic techniques for management with laser photocoagulation and supplemental chemotherapy.[11]

OPERATIVE TECHNIQUE

I prefer a one-incision technique with the patient in a torque-like or semiflank position and the table flexed, similar to the position for radical retroperitoneal lymphadenectomy for testicular tumor (Fig. 31–2). The distal aspect of the incision is continued as a paramedian incision down to the symphysis pubis, allowing adequate exposure for removal of the distal ureter and a cuff of bladder. The peritoneal envelope is mobilized completely across the midline, allowing complete exposure of the entire course of the ureter for resection and for lymphadenectomy. With this approach, the disadvantages of the two-incision technique are eliminated.

In a patient with a low-lying kidney or without obvious invasion into the renal parenchyma, a simple nephrectomy rather than radical nephrectomy can be performed. Gerota's fascia may be entered and the kidney removed without the entire envelope of this fascia and the ipsilateral adrenal gland. The additional buffer of the kidney provides protection against metastasis and local invasion. This maneuver allows

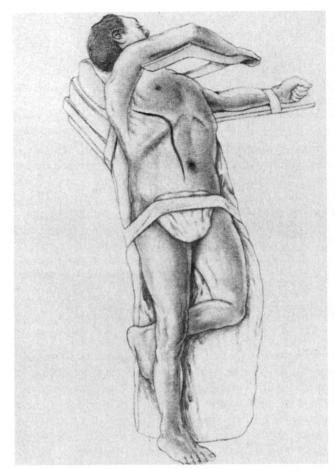

Figure 31–2. Proper positioning of the patient for thoracoabdominal single-incision approach to nephroureterectomy. The pelvis is nearly supine and the ipsilateral shoulder is angulated approximately 50 degrees. The abdominal portion of the incision extends inferiorly as a paramedian incision. (From Richie JP. Carcinoma of the renal pelvis and ureter. In Skinner DG, Lieskovsky G, eds. Diagnosis and Management of Genitourinary Cancer. Philadelphia, WB Saunders, 1988, p 332.)

an incision to be made off the tip of the twelfth rib or between the eleventh and twelfth ribs in an extrapleural fashion as opposed to a thoracoabdominal incision, which is usually not necessary.

The addition of lymphadenectomy allows for more accurate staging and may have therapeutic implications, since the regional nodes appear to be the first and most common site of metastatic spread. Batata and associates[3] reported that 22 of their patients had initial or subsequent metastases, 17 involving the regional nodes and five involving distant sites. Lymphatic metastases were ipsilateral in 90 percent of the cases with involved para-aortic nodes. This high incidence of predominantly ipsilateral regional lymphatic involvement in invasive tumors makes extensive lymphadenectomy a logical extension of the therapeutic surgical approach.

Regardless of the choice of incision, the bladder should be opened and the ureter removed intra- as well as extravesically (Fig. 31–3). Attempts to extricate the distal ureter extravesically are fraught with failure. Strong and Pearse[4] reported nine cases in which the procedure was described by the surgeon as a "complete nephroureterectomy" by tenting up the distal ureter. On subsequent cystoscopy and retrograde ureterography, all nine patients were noted to have a ureteral orifice and an intramural ureter remaining on that side. In two of the nine patients, there was subsequent recurrence of tumor in the ureteral stump. The cuff of bladder should include a 1-cm circumferential margin around the ureteral orifice. An anterior cystotomy allows visualization of the trigone and contralateral ureteral orifice (Fig. 31–3). A two-layer closure of the bladder is effected after dissection.

RESULTS

The rate of survival is influenced by the grade and stage of the tumor. Overall survival rates are approximately 40 percent, with a 5-year survival rate for a well-differentiated malignancy of 56 percent, as opposed to 16 percent for poorly differentiated lesions (Table 31–1). Of patients with noninvasive disease, 60 percent survive 5 years, compared with 25 percent of those with invasive disease. Flow cytometry may provide useful prognostic information, especially with high-grade malignancies.[13]

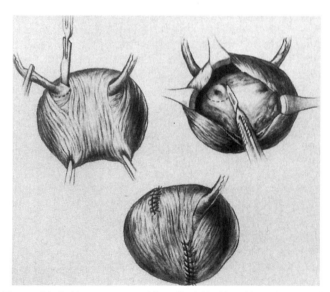

Figure 31–3. Ureterectomy with cuff of bladder. Note that anterior cystotomy permits visualization of the trigone and contralateral ureter and minimizes the risk of injury. This portion of the procedure can be approached through the thoracoabdominal incision as described in Figure 31–2. (From Richie JP. Carcinoma of the renal pelvis and ureter. In Skinner DG, Lieskovsky G, eds. Diagnosis and Management of Genitourinary Cancer. Philadelphia, WB Saunders, 1988, p 333.)

TABLE 31–1. Correlation of 5-Year Survival Rate (%) with Pathological Characteristics

	Bloom et al (1970) (54 Patients)	Batata et al (1975) (41 Patients)
Histologic grade		
I	83.0	78.0
II	52.0	50.0
III	18.0	0
IV	12.0	0
Pathological Stage		
0, A	62.0	91.0
B	50.0	43.0
C	33.3	23.0
D	0	0

Editorial Comment

Fray F. Marshall

Nephroureterectomy remains the classic treatment for upper urinary tract transitional cell carcinoma. Lesions that are higher grade or multiple are generally best managed by total excision of the ipsilateral urinary tract. This operation can be done as described with a single or double incision. We have often used the supra-twelfth rib or eleventh interspace incision. The adrenal gland is often left in place with a transitional cell tumor as opposed to a renal cell adenocarcinoma. The ureter and periureteral tissue are dissected down to the level of the bladder, but an extravesical dissection usually does not remove the entire intramural ureter. We have usually opened the bladder through a separate incision after closing the flank incision.

With an apparent solitary, low-grade, papillary lesion in the distal ureter, ureteroscopy may be a reasonable alternative, especially in higher-risk patients. Alternatively, upper urinary tract transitional cell carcinoma is usually a "field-change" disease with great potential for multicentricity, so that careful evaluation of the entire upper urinary tract is essential.

We have even preserved renal tissue in six patients with renal pelvic transitional cell carcinomas with excision of either a majority of the pelvis or a portion of the kidney. Although these patients have generally done well for several years, the potential for recurrence still exists in either the upper urinary tract or bladder.

REFERENCES

1. Williams CB, Mitchell JP. Carcinoma of the ureter—a review of 54 cases. Br J Urol 45:377, 1973.
2. Grabstald H, Whitmore WF Jr, Melamed MR. Renal pelvic tumors. JAMA 281:845, 1971.
3. Batata MA, Whitmore WF, Hilaris BS, et al. Primary carcinoma of the ureter: A prognostic study. Cancer 35:1626, 1975.
4. Strong DW, Pearse HD. Recurrent urothelial tumors following surgery for transitional cell carcinoma of the upper urinary tract. Cancer 38:2173, 1976.
5. Chandhoke PS, Clayman RV, Kerbl K, et al. Laparoscopic ureterectomy: Initial clinical experience. J Urol 149:992, 1993.
6. Kerbl K, Clayman RV, McDougall EM, et al. Laparoscopic nephroureterectomy: Evaluation of first clinical series. Eur Urol 23:431, 1993.
7. Cummings KB. Nephroureter: Rationale in the management of transitional cell carcinoma of the upper urinary tract. Urol Clin North Am 7:569, 1980.

8. Gittes RR. Management of transitional cell carcinoma of the upper tract: Case for conservative local excision. Urol Clin North Am 7:559, 1980.

9. McCarron JP, Mills C, Vaughn ED Jr. Tumors of the renal pelvis and ureter: Current concepts and management. Semin Urol 1:75, 1983.

10. Nocks BN, Heney NM, Daly J, et al. Transitional cell carcinoma of renal pelvis. Urology 19:472, 1982.

11. Gerber GS, Lyon ES. Endourological management of upper tract urothelial tumors. J Urol 150:2, 1993.

12. Bloom NA, Vidone RA, Lytton B. Primary carcinoma of the ureter: A report of 102 new cases. J Urol 103:590, 1970.

13. Miyakawa A, Tachibana M, Nakashima J, et al. Flow cytometric bromodeoxyuridine/deoxyribonucleic acid bivariate analysis for predicting tumor invasiveness of upper tract urothelial cancer. J Urol 152:76, 1994.

Chapter 32

Pyelonephrolithotomy

Martin I. Resnick

INDICATIONS

Pyelonephrolithotomy is primarily indicated for removal of large intrarenal calculi in the renal pelvis and lower pole collecting system. When these are associated with scarred and strictured infundibula or when fragmentation is believed to be difficult to accomplish because of stone size, composition, and location, pyelonephrolithotomy can often be used to accomplish complete stone removal. The procedure is particularly useful for a small intrarenal pelvis and, in contrast to a lower pole nephrectomy, preserves functioning renal parenchyma.

PREOPERATIVE MANAGEMENT

Before surgical removal of the calculus, a metabolic evaluation should be performed on all stable patients to identify predisposing factors related to stone formation. Although most large-volume stones form as a result of chronic infection, approximately 50 percent of patients so affected demonstrate a metabolic disorder that results in initial stone formation. Hypercalciuria, hyperparathyroidism, hyperuricuria, hypocitruria, cystinuria, and renal tubular acidosis have all been shown to be associated with the formation of these large stones. Preoperative renal function should be determined by measuring serum creatinine levels. Measurements of serum and urine calcium, phosphate, oxalate, and uric acid concentrations should be obtained. Infection stones occur in the presence of urea-splitting bacteria, especially *Proteus mirabilis, Providencia, Klebsiella,* and occasionally *Pseudomonas. Pseudomonas* infections are often difficult to treat and are associated with the highest incidence of recurrent stone formation.

A complete and thorough radiological evaluation of the urinary tract is indicated before surgical intervention. Many stones are poorly mineralized and relatively nonopaque on routine radiographical examination. Plain nephrotomograms obtained before the

injection of contrast material often help to detect small fragments that otherwise might have gone undetected. Excretory urography with tomograms and oblique views are essential to evaluation of the intrarenal anatomy and assessment of the contralateral kidney. Retrograde pyelograms are also indicated when the kidney is functioning poorly or when better visualization of the intrarenal collecting system is desired. Often this study allows for better delineation of strictured infundibula and the detection of other intrarenal anatomical abnormalities. Other imaging studies, particularly angiography, are not considered necessary.

Appropriate antibiotics based on culture and sensitivity results should be initiated preoperatively and continued postoperatively. A variety of new, safe, non-nephrotoxic agents are available that are most effective in treating many of the bacterial infections associated with stone formation.

An understanding and appreciation of the anatomical relationship of the intrarenal vasculature to the collecting system is essential when contemplating open surgery for removal of renal calculi, particularly pyelonephrolithotomy.[1] Important concepts have been well emphasized in the descriptions of anatrophic nephrolithotomy, but they apply to other operative procedures as well. Posterior nephrotomies along the inferior aspect of the kidney permit ready access to the lower pole infundibulum, thus providing adequate exposure for removal of stones in this region (Fig. 32–1). Because of the distribution of the renal vessels in this portion of the kidney, damage to major segmental arteries is unlikely, hemostasis is relatively easy to maintain, and renal pedicle clamp with organ hypothermia is often not required. It is important to avoid parenchymal incisions in the midportion of the kidney overlying the renal pelvis so as to prevent injury of the posterior segmental artery.

SURGICAL OPTIONS

With the advent of percutaneous techniques and extracorporeal shock wave lithotripsy (ESWL), the

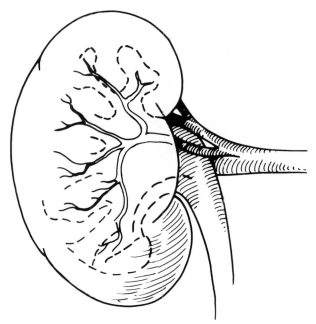

Figure 32–1. The relationship of the posterior segmented artery to the lower pole infundibulum and calices is demonstrated.

need for open surgical procedures to remove renal stones has been markedly diminished. Although controversial, open surgical procedures continue to be performed in selected instances on the basis of such factors as stone size; composition; location; the presence of strictures or scarring of the intrarenal collecting system, or both; and the presence of anatomical abnormalities that require repair (e.g., ureteropelvic junction obstruction).[2, 3] For instance, uric acid stones can often be dissolved by systemic alkalinization, and magnesium ammonium phosphate (struvite) stones usually respond satisfactorily to ESWL, especially when present in a nondilated collecting system. Calcium oxalate calculi, particularly the monohydrate type, do not fragment well and are best treated by either a percutaneous or an open surgical approach. If a stone is large (greater than 3 or 4 cm) or associated with intrarenal abnormalities, some surgeons prefer to remove the stone and repair the kidney with an open procedure. In patients who have not responded to less invasive approaches or who have residual stone fragments, an open surgical procedure may be required to resolve a particular problem.[4] Experience has indicated that stone-free rates for lower pole calculi are less with ESWL than with percutaneous nephrostolithotomy (59 versus 90 percent in one study), and the effectiveness of ESWL is inversely correlated to stone burden.[5]

OPERATIVE TECHNIQUE

Once the patient has been anesthetized and placed in a flank position, a Foley catheter is inserted in the bladder and an incision is made over the eleventh or twelfth rib, which is usually satisfactory for exposing the kidney. After all muscles are incised and Gerota's fascia has been identified, it is preferable to incise this fascial plane in a cephalad-caudal direction. This maneuver preserves the structure to which the kidney should be returned after completion of the nephrotomy. The fatty layer overlying the kidney is sharply dissected from the renal capsule, and the kidney is suspended with 1-inch umbilical tapes.

After complete exposure of the kidney it is useful to identify the main renal artery and if possible its divisions, particularly the posterior branch. Control of the pedicle with a vessel loop is important, but clamping of the main renal artery with the use of hypothermia is not necessary. The renal pelvis is identified and the kidney positioned so that the entire renal pelvis and posterior surface of the kidney are in the operative field.

A pyelotomy is then made and directed so that it will extend in the direction of the lower pole infundibulum (Fig. 32–2). It is useful to direct the more distal portion of the pyelotomy away from the ureteropelvic junction so that if tears occur during stone extraction they will not extend into this region. The nephrotomy is made along the renal tissue overlying the lower pole infundibulum. Incisions in this region avoid injury to the posterior segmental artery. Initially the renal capsule is incised sharply, but the

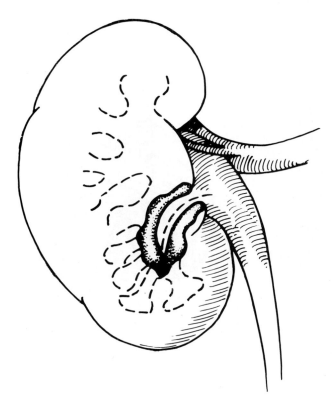

Figure 32–2. The pyelotomy incision is positioned so that it will extend into the lower pole infundibulum.

renal parenchyma is separated by blunt dissection, usually with the back of the scalpel handle. This step minimizes injury to the intralobular arteries that lie near the infundibulum. Small vessels are usually readily identified, are ligated with 5-0 or 6-0 catgut suture, and transected. The incision should extend into the lower pole infundibulum and associated calices (Fig. 32–3). With appropriate exposure the calculus lying within the lower pole can be extracted. If caliceal extensions exist, these should be opened individually before stone manipulation. When the stone has been removed, each calix should be examined and irrigated to ensure complete removal of all fragments. If scarred infundibulum or calices are noted, reconstruction can be carried out at this time. Similarly, if caliceal diverticula are encountered, these too can be excised.

Nonreactive double-J stents are used and typically are passed from the renal pelvis into the bladder early in the procedure. This prevents migration of stone fragments down the ureter and provides good drainage postoperatively. The incidence of postoperative urinary extravasation is thus minimized.

Intraoperative radiographs are important to ensure complete stone removal. An important step in the procedure is to obtain an intraoperative plain radiograph before performing the nephrotomy. A radiograph should be obtained routinely before renal closure to document removal of all fragments. All fragments must be removed if urinary tract infection

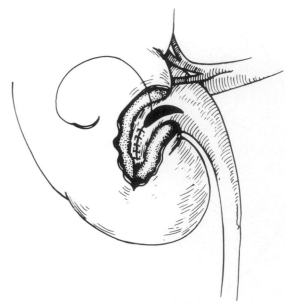

Figure 32–4. The renal pelvis and lower pole infundibulum are closed with running 6-0 chromic catgut.

is to be eradicated and recurrent stone formation prevented. Intraoperative ultrasonography with high-frequency transducers is also useful in locating the "wayward" stone fragment. Fragments as small as 2 mm can be detected and, once localized, removed with grasping forceps or through a separate nephrotomy, which is usually easily accomplished.[6, 7]

After removal of all stones the renal pelvis and lower pole infundibulum are closed with a running 6-0 chromic catgut suture (Fig. 32–4). A running 4-0 chromic catgut suture is used to close the renal capsule (Fig. 32–5). Parenchymal renal veins should be

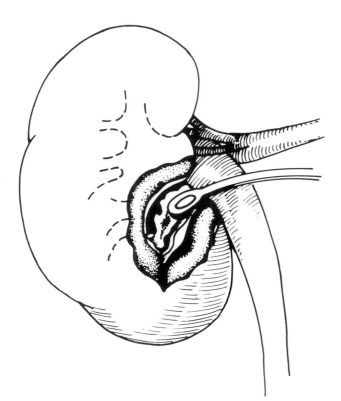

Figure 32–3. The nephrotomy is made along the renal tissue overlying the lower pole infundibulum.

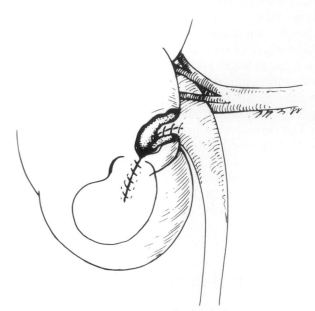

Figure 32–5. The renal capsule is closed with a running 4-0 chromic catgut suture.

suture ligated, and hemostasis should be ensured after suturing the renal capsule and before wound closure. No mattress-type sutures are used because they are likely to result in tissue ischemia and eventual hemorrhage.

At the completion of the procedure the vessel loop is removed and the kidney returned to Gerota's fascia, which is closed with an interrupted chromic catgut suture. The lower pole of the kidney and upper ureter are also covered with perirenal fat. By surrounding the kidney and upper ureter with fat, the risk of adhesion formation and perirenal scarring is reduced. If Gerota's fascia has been obliterated because of chronic inflammation from previous surgical procedures, an omental flap is mobilized to cover the kidney and upper ureter. The flank wound is closed with layers of interrupted chromic catgut sutures. A small Penrose drain or suction drain is left within Gerota's fascia and brought out through a separate stab incision to provide a drainage tract for fluid collections. The drain is left in place until all drainage subsides.

POSTOPERATIVE MANAGEMENT AND COMPLICATIONS

The general principles of postoperative care apply as for other patients who undergo renal surgery. Patients are maintained on intravenous fluids and are generally allowed to begin oral fluids on the first or second postoperative day. Antibiotics are administered on the basis of previous cultures and are continued for 5 to 7 days. The Foley catheter is usually removed the first postoperative day, and the Penrose drain is removed within 48 hours, being left in place longer only if urinary drainage is present. The ureteral stent is removed cystoscopically 2 to 3 weeks after surgery. Urine cultures are obtained 72 hours postoperatively, and if findings are positive, appropriate alternative antibacterial agents are instituted.

Postoperative complications vary.[8] Pulmonary dysfunction is probably the most common, occurring in 5 to 10 percent of all patients who undergo open renal surgery. The lateral flank position creates a 14 percent decrease in total volume in the anesthetized patient because of restriction of the chest wall in all directions.[9] Deep breathing and coughing are extremely important during the postoperative period. If necessary, pulmonary physiotherapy should be instituted and continued well into the postoperative period. Routine inspiratory spirometry and aerosols also appear to be of value.

Pneumothorax occurs in less than 5 percent of patients who undergo open surgery for removal of renal stones. Patients who have had previous renal surgery and those with a history of pyelonephritis are at higher risk for pneumothorax. When these patients are identified intraoperatively, repair should be carried out. Portable chest radiographs should be obtained in the recovery room if pleural repair has been performed or if pneumothorax is suspected. If pneumothorax is confirmed, a chest tube should be inserted. Follow-up chest radiographs are essential.

Pulmonary emboli can occur after any surgical procedure, and specific techniques to prevent them are controversial. Early ambulation is important, and perhaps thigh-high elastic stockings or sequential venous compression stockings should be considered in high-risk patients.

In addition to pulmonary complications, cardiovascular changes should be considered. In the flank position, decreased venous return can be a problem, and hypotension may be encountered intraoperatively. It is therefore important to gradually add flexion and raise the "kidney rest" while continuing to monitor blood pressure.

Significant postoperative renal hemorrhage occurs in less than 10 percent of renal surgical procedures. When bleeding is encountered, it frequently occurs spontaneously 1 to 2 weeks postoperatively. The bleeding often results from inadequately closed intrarenal vessels, and expectant treatment is generally sufficient. Blood transfusions, intravenous fluids, and bed rest often stabilize the patient. The administration of aminocaproic acid (Amicar) is recommended if hemorrhage does not subside.

Stone migration during intraoperative manipulation of the kidney, with the resultant inability to localize, is a serious problem when encountered. The placement of a double-J stent often obviates the passage of fragments down the ureter. Additional aids to stone localization and subsequent removal include intraoperative ultrasonography, intrarenal inspection with a nephroscope, and ample irrigation.[7] Associated with this problem is that of retained stone fragments. Retained stones represent a major concern and are reported to have an incidence of 5 to 30 percent. Residual stone fragments are probably of less concern with calcium oxalate, cystine, and uric acid stones than with struvite stones. Stones of the first three types may grow in size but are influenced by the amount and concentration of those products in urine that influence crystal nucleation, aggregation, and growth (e.g., calcium, oxalate, citrate). Sleith and Wickham reported that 70 percent of retained infected stones increased in size, but only 30 percent of noninfected stones did so.[10]

The potential for developing or aggravating preexisting hypertension is of concern with any procedure performed on the kidney. This complication appears unusual. Boyce reviewed over 900 patients undergoing anatrophic nephrolithotomy and noted that postoperative hypertension was unusual.[11] Whether hypertension is directly related to the surgical procedure rather than a spontaneous occurrence obviously is debatable. By carefully dissecting the renal artery and accurately performing and repairing the nephrotomy, ischemia of the kidney can be minimized.

Despite following all the techniques to preserve renal function, damage to the renal parenchyma can occur. Some patients demonstrate diminished renal function postoperatively. Boyce and Elkins noted that of 100 patients undergoing anatrophic nephrolithotomy, only two had a decrease in renal function postoperatively; one of these two subsequently required a nephrectomy.[12] Experience with anatrophic nephrolithotomy in patients with a solitary kidney also revealed that the average preoperative renal function equaled the average postoperative function.[13] Although diminution in function occurred in some patients, marked improvement was noted in others. In this last group the relief of obstruction and resolution of infection associated with stone removal likely contributed to this result.

After eradication of all stone fragments, subsequent stone recurrence is a potential problem for all patients. The recurrence rate has been reported to be 20 to 30 percent over a period of 6 to 10 years after anatrophic nephrolithotomy.[14, 15] No data are available for pyelonephrolithotomy. Russell and colleagues noted that the recurrence rate was only 9 percent in females but 43 percent in males.[15] Better control of urinary tract infection, particularly the *Pseudomonas* strain, with the more recently available broad-spectrum antibiotics may be expected to help lower the recurrent stone rate. Appropriate use of suppressive antibiotics in patients with recurrent urinary tract infections may also be of benefit in reducing stone recurrence. Acetohydroxamic acid, a urease inhibitor, may also be of benefit in slowing infection, stone growth, and possible recurrence. Probably the most important aspect in reducing this recurrence rate lies in identifying and treating metabolic problems as they relate to stone formation.

Pyelocutaneous fistula after prolonged urinary leakage represents another complication associated with renal stone surgery. Distal ureteral obstruction or infection, or both, are the main causes and generally resolve spontaneously within 2 or 3 weeks postoperatively. Intervention is rarely required, but when necessary placement of an indwelling ureteral stent often suffices. Routine placement of a double-J ureteral stent after pyelonephrolithotomy is suggested. Urinoma formation is a rare complication resulting from premature removal of operative drains. Placement of the ureteral stent can help manage this problem, but percutaneous or open surgical drainage may be required.

If metabolic disorders contributing to stone formation are discovered in the preoperative evaluation, corrective medical therapy should begin to prevent stone recurrence. Long-term follow-up includes periodic urine cultures and treatment of all urinary infections. Repeat 24-hour urine collections are also required because, with the clearing of urinary obstruction and infection, abnormalities of excessive calcium excretion may become evident postoperatively. If metabolic problems are diagnosed during this period, they should be treated appropriately. Intravenous urography, including nephrotomography, without injection of contrast agents is performed 3 months postoperatively and repeated if clinically indicated. These patients require many years of follow-up to both prevent and detect the development of recurrent disease.

Summary

With the advent of ESWL and percutaneous nephrostolithotomy, the need for open surgical procedures to remove large stones has markedly diminished. If especially hard stones are present or if associated intrarenal anatomical disorders require repair, an open surgical procedure is often needed. The choice of approach is often based on the ability and experience of the surgeon in consultation with the patient.

Editorial Comment
Fray F. Marshall

Inability to find a residual calculus can be a perplexing problem in a pyelonephrolithotomy. Intraoperative radiography and ultrasonography can be most helpful. In particular, ultrasound with a high-frequency probe can localize even 1- to 2-mm calculus fragments.[1]

Although there is less indication for operative stone surgery, anatomical obstruction associated with stones often mandates open operative intervention.

Unless there is documented fibrinolysin activity, the use of aminocaproic acid (Amicar) for bleeding may sometimes be deleterious, because very tenacious clots are created and it does not always stop bleeding.

1. Marshall FF, Smith NA, Murphy JC, et al. A comparison of ultrasonography and radiography in the localization of renal calculi: Experimental and operative experience. J Urol 126:576, 1981.

REFERENCES

1. Resnick MI. Pyelonephrolithotomy for removal of calculi from the inferior renal pole. Urol Clin North Am 8:585, 1981.
2. Resnick MI, Boyce WH. Bilateral staghorn calculi: Patient evaluation and management. J Urol 123:338, 1980.
3. Smith MJV, Boyce WH. Anatrophic nephrotomy and plastic calyrhaphy. Trans Am Assoc Genitourin Surg 59:18, 1967.
4. Assimos DG, Boyce WH, Harrison LH, et al. The role of open stone surgery since extracorporeal shock wave lithotripsy. J Urol 142:263, 1989.
5. Lingeman JE, Siegel YI, Steele B, et al. Management of lower pole nephrolithiasis: A critical analysis. J Urol 151:663, 1994.

6. Marshall FF, Smith NA, Murphy JC, et al. A comparison of ultrasonography and radiography in the localization of renal calculi: Experimental and operative experience. J Urol 126:576, 1981.

7. Pahira JJ, Elyanderani MK. Intraoperative localization of renal calculi. Urol Clin North Am 12:787, 1985.

8. Bodner DR, Resnick MI. Complications of surgery for removal of renal and ureteral stones. In Marshall FF, ed. Urologic Complications: Medical and Surgical, Adult and Pediatric, 2nd ed. St. Louis, Mosby-Year Book, 1990.

9. Birch AA, Mims GR. Anesthesia consideration during nephrolithotomy with slush. J Urol 113:433, 1975.

10. Sleith MW, Wickham JEA. Long-term follow-up of 100 cases of renal calculi. Br J Urol 49:601, 1977.

11. Boyce WH. Surgery of urinary calculi in perspective. Urol Clin North Am 10:585, 1983.

12. Boyce WB, Elkins EB. Reconstructive renal surgery following anatrophic nephrolithotomy: Follow-up of 100 consecutive patients. J Urol 111:307, 1974.

13. Stubbs AJ, Resnick MI, Boyce WH. Anatrophic nephrolithotomy in the solitary kidney. J Urol 119:457, 1968.

14. Griffith DP. Infection induced stones. In Coe FL, ed. Nephrolithiasis: Pathogenesis and Treatment. Chicago, Year Book, 1978.

15. Russell JM, Webb RT, Harrison LH, Boyce WH. Long-term follow-up of 100 anatrophic nephrolithotomies with calyceal reconstruction. In Backus JG, Finlayson B, eds. Urinary Calculus. Littleton, MA, PSG Publ., 1981.

Chapter 33

Surgery for Renal Cysts and Renal Abscesses

Charles Lee Jackson and James E. Montie

Renal Cysts

Most renal cysts are benign cortical fluid collections that rarely require surgical exploration or management. Surgical management is indicated for renal cysts that are infected, cause pain, obstruct the collecting system, bleed, or are associated with renal neoplasm. The need to distinguish simple renal cysts from cystic renal neoplasm dominates most evaluations for renal cystic disease and represents the most common indication for surgical exploration. Surgical exploration is also frequently required for evaluation of cystic conditions such as von Hippel-Lindau disease (Figs. 33–1 and 33–2), adult polycystic disease, and acquired cystic disease of end-stage renal disease that are commonly associated with neoplasms.

PREOPERATIVE EVALUATION

Renal cysts associated with neoplasms have a reported incidence of 2.3 to 7 percent.[1] An evaluation to distinguish a simple renal cyst from a complex cystic neoplasm typically begins with renal sonography, abdominal computed tomographic (CT) scanning, or both. The diagnosis of a benign renal cyst can be made with a high degree of certainty on the basis of radiographic features that include a sharply defined wall, absent internal echoes, and a round or oval shape. Those cystic masses with internal echoes, septa, solid components, thickened capsules, or calcifications are considered suspicious for associated neoplasia and should be further evaluated (Figs. 33–3A and 33–4).

Evaluation may include percutaneous cyst puncture with fluid aspiration for histochemical and cytological examination and radiographical examination of the cyst cavity with contrast material (Fig. 33–5). Cyst puncture may also document the clinical significance of those cysts thought to be causing pain or intrarenal urinary obstruction.

Magnetic resonance imaging (MRI) has demonstrated an ability to help differentiate hemorrhagic cysts from simple cysts and may therefore lead to early surgical intervention.[2] In general, however, MRI adds little to the evaluation of complex cystic renal masses.

Renal angiography is also not very helpful in the differential diagnosis because most cystic renal neoplasms are hypovascular. However, epinephrine augmentation may help distinguish neoplastic vessels from normal vessels, and a knowledge of the renal vascular supply helps in planning surgical exploration for possible excisional biopsy or extended hilar dissection.

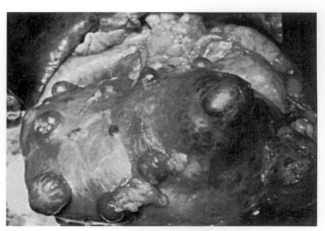

Figure 33–1. Multiple solid and cystic neoplasms on the surface of the kidney in a patient with von Hippel-Lindau disease.

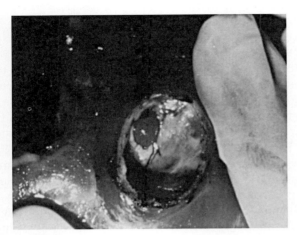

Figure 33–2. Small neoplasm seen at the base of an unroofed cyst in von Hippel-Lindau disease.

The sequential application of these studies will provide an accurate diagnosis for 97 percent of renal cystic masses. Surgical exploration will be required in the remaining 2 to 3 percent.[3] This is especially true of hemorrhagic cysts and the complex cystic lesions found in von Hippel-Lindau disease, adult polycystic kidney disease, and the acquired cystic disease of end-stage renal disease.

SURGICAL OPTIONS

The surgical options for management of renal cysts include percutaneous aspiration with injection of sclerosants, percutaneous resection and fulguration, retrograde ureteronephroscopic marsupialization, laparoscopic cyst ablation, open excisional biopsy, partial nephrectomy, and radical nephrectomy.

Percutaneous aspiration with injection of sclerosants for benign simple cysts is easy to perform and provides fluid for cytological examination. However, the rate of cyst recurrence is high and complications have been reported in approximately 10 percent.[4]

Percutaneous resection with fulguration allows visual inspection of the cyst interior and provides cyst

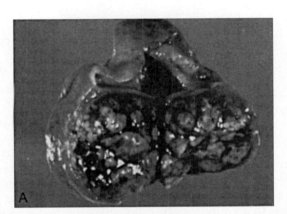

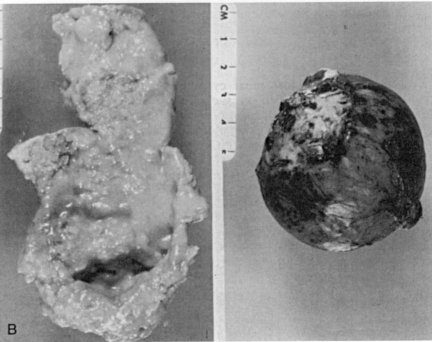

Figure 33–3. *A,* Neoplasm in a hemorrhagic cyst. Aspirated fluid was only blood tinged. *B,* Excised cyst. Aspiration findings are negative. The cyst wall is benign with an organized hematoma.

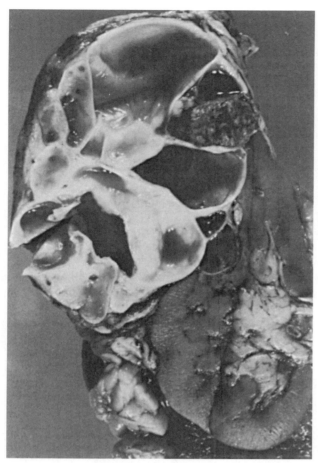

Figure 33–4. Neoplasm as seen in a multiloculated cyst.

wall biopsy material for pathological examination.[5] This procedure, however, is technically difficult and requires a large nephrostomy tract through which access is limited to a solitary cyst.

Retrograde ureteronephroscopic cyst marsupialization is similarly limited to treatment of obstructing peripelvic cysts.[6]

Laparoscopic cyst ablation, on the other hand, is applicable to multiple cysts, including peripheral and

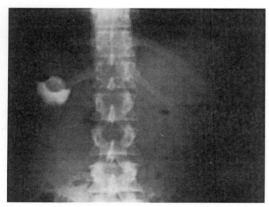

Figure 33–5. Percutaneous contrast in this cyst shows a filling defect consistent with neoplasm.

peripelvic cysts. It is best applied to cysts that are refractory to percutaneous aspiration and sclerosis. It should be limited to radiographically benign cysts with cytologically benign aspirated fluid to avoid unroofing a cystic neoplasm.[7] Early detection of an unsuspected neoplasm may occur, however, because of the opportunity for magnified visual inspection of the cyst interior, excision of the cyst wall, and biopsy of the cyst base. This may lead to early surgical management and possible cure. The theoretical risk of tumor implantation and the long-term efficacy of laparoscopic cyst ablation are presently unknown.

Suspicious cysts such as multilocular, hemorrhagic, or calcified cysts with increased risk of associated neoplasia should be approached by open flank exploration. The kidney should be mobilized outside Gerota's fascia with early isolation and clamping of the renal artery. Intravenous infusion of mannitol and in situ surface cooling of the kidney are carried out, and the suspicious cyst is excised and examined (Figs. 33–3B, 33–6, and 33–7). Partial or radical nephrectomy is then carried out as indicated by the pathological condition and clinical situation (Fig. 33–7).

OPERATIVE TECHNIQUES

The laparoscopic approach to renal cysts is similar to other laparoscopic procedures and may be trans- or retroperitoneal.[8] Technical aspects specific to laparoscopic evaluation and ablation of renal cysts include leaving the cyst distended to assist visual inspection of the cyst margins before cyst wall puncture and resection.[9] The base of the cyst should be cauterized with electrocautery or an argon beam laser to provide hemostasis and prevent cyst recurrence.

For open surgical management of suspicious cysts, a standard flank approach is recommended. Entry through the eleventh or twelfth rib bed may be required to ensure that the incision is sufficiently cephalad to allow access to the renal pedicle. The peritoneum is swept medially, separating it from Gerota's fascia. The latter is then opened, exposing the cyst and normal parenchyma adjacent to it. The tissue surrounding the cyst is packed off to prevent contamination, and the cyst wall is excised and sent for pathological examination (Fig. 33–8). Care is taken not to excise the cyst wall too close to normal parenchyma to avoid unnecessary bleeding. The base of the cyst is then examined and biopsied cautiously to prevent entry into the intrarenal veins, which if entered may bleed profusely and require figure-of-eight suture ligation with 4-0 chromic catgut. Bleeding from the edge of the cyst wall can be controlled with electrocautery or a running 3-0 chromic catgut suture around the periphery of the cyst. The perinephric fat may then be brought in to fill the cyst basin, and fixed with a few interrupted 3-0 chromic catgut sutures. If the collect-

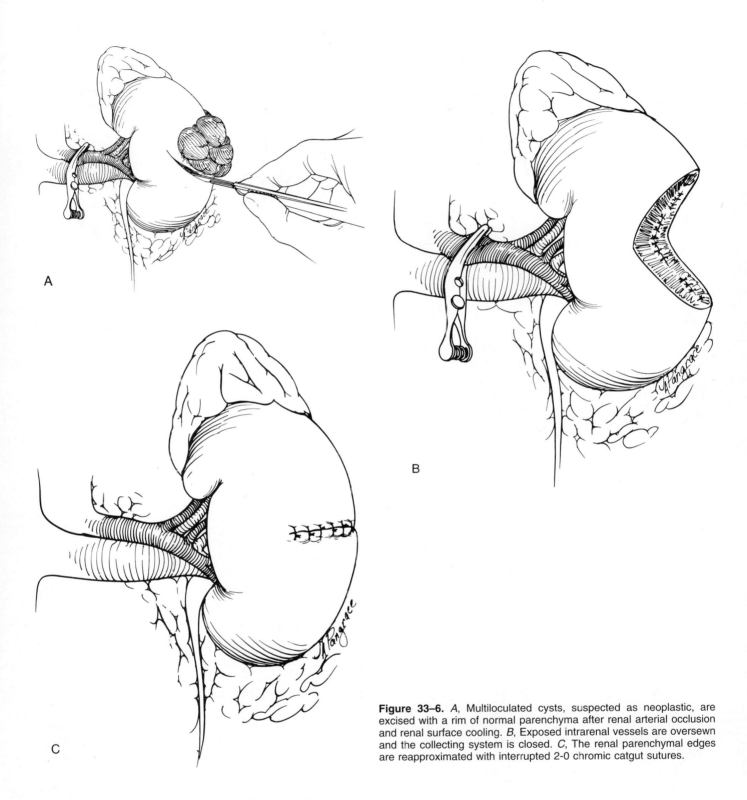

Figure 33–6. *A*, Multiloculated cysts, suspected as neoplastic, are excised with a rim of normal parenchyma after renal arterial occlusion and renal surface cooling. *B*, Exposed intrarenal vessels are oversewn and the collecting system is closed. *C*, The renal parenchymal edges are reapproximated with interrupted 2-0 chromic catgut sutures.

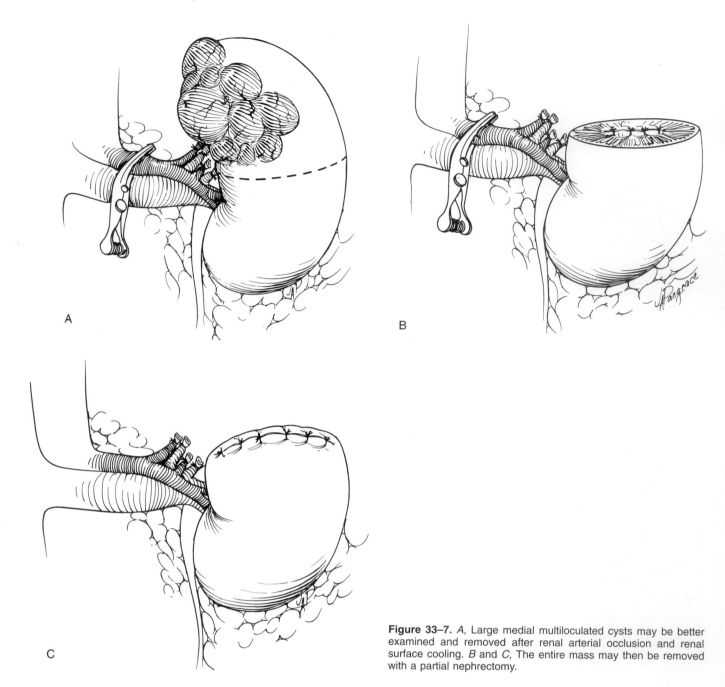

A

B

C

Figure 33–7. *A,* Large medial multiloculated cysts may be better examined and removed after renal arterial occlusion and renal surface cooling. *B* and *C,* The entire mass may then be removed with a partial nephrectomy.

ing system is entered or if cyst fluid is infected, a Penrose or a soft, flat, closed suction drain may be placed and brought through a separate stab incision. The wound is then closed in a standard fashion.

For an obstructed peripelvic cyst, the renal pedicle should be isolated early and clamped (see Figs. 33–6 and 33–7). Intravenous mannitol infusion and in situ surface cooling of the kidney is carried out as described for partial nephrectomy. This reduces the size of the hilar tissue, facilitates hilar dissection, and provides improved visualization to avoid injury to the collecting system and intrarenal arteries. The cyst is then excised as previously described.

POSTOPERATIVE MANAGEMENT

The goals of postoperative management for open surgery are to treat pulmonary atelectasis produced by the flank position and anesthesia, and to observe for bleeding. If a drain is placed, it is typically removed over a period of 48 hours between the fifth and seventh postoperative days.

Postoperative management after laparoscopic cyst ablation includes the patient resuming a regular diet and ambulation on the first postoperative morning and returning to normal activity within 2 weeks. The risks of complications from laparoscopic renal cyst ablation

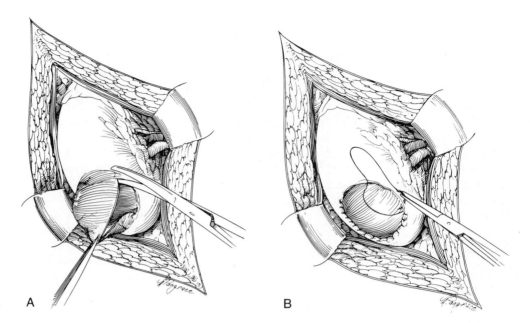

Figure 33–8. *A*, The cyst wall is excised and sent to the pathology laboratory for examination. *B*, The edge of the cyst wall is controlled with a running 3-0 chromic catgut suture.

A

B

are similar to those from other laparoscopic procedures and include bowel injury and hemorrhage.

Summary

Most renal cysts are benign and can be clearly identified as such by radiographical evaluation. Symptomatic, benign cysts refractory to percutaneous aspiration may be managed laparoscopically. Complex cysts (e.g., hemorrhagic or calcified) must be surgically explored to diagnose and treat possible neoplasm. Evaluation of the complex cyst and the operative approach should prepare one for the possibility of partial or radical nephrectomy if neoplasm is discovered. Preoperative evaluation should therefore include the function of the contralateral kidney and renal vasculature. The flank approach allows management of the whole spectrum of disease from simple cyst exploration and excision to partial nephrectomy, and has the advantage of confining the operation to the retroperitoneum.

Renal Abscess

Renal abscess is a rare disease with potentially life-threatening consequences. It is estimated to account for 0.9 to 4.0 cases in 10,000 hospital admissions.[10]

Mortality rates as high as 33 to 50 percent have been reported in the past. Early diagnosis, improved antibiotics, and early surgical drainage have reduced these rates dramatically.

The spectrum of disease ranges from small, isolated intrarenal abscesses to large, solid, infectious tumefactions completely replacing functioning renal tissue. Surgical management is tailored to the amount of disease present. Making the diagnosis and characterizing the disease remain difficult in spite of improved imaging techniques.

PREOPERATIVE EVALUATION

The goal of the initial evaluation is early distinction between pyelonephritis and abscess, with identification of the precise anatomical location of the process. Patients with either diagnosis typically present with fever, flank and abdominal pain, chills, and dysuria. The symptoms have usually been noted for more than 5 days at the time of presentation in patients with renal abscess. An abscess is also more likely to occur in patients with diabetes, those with spinal cord injury, immunocompromised patients, and patients with renal calculi.

A complete blood count, electrolyte determinations, creatinine concentrations, urinalysis, and blood and urine cultures are obtained. The patient is immediately provided with broad-spectrum parenteral antibiotics designed to cover common urinary pathogens. A renal abscess is more commonly caused by ascending ureteral or lymphangitic spread from lower urinary tract organisms, such as *Escherichia coli* and *Proteus*, than by hematogenous spread of staphylococcal skin infections as seen in the past.[11]

An intravenous pyelogram may be normal up to 20 percent of the time or may reveal a variety of subtle abnormalities. The most reliable sign of abnormality is decreased renal motion with respiration due to renal fixation to surrounding tissue by the inflammatory process. Renal function versus nonfunction of the affected side can also be appreciated. Verification of the suspected abscess is best obtained with CT, which can distinguish between a segmental bacterial nephritis and a true abscess. Scanning will also show the relationship of the mass to the collecting system and contiguous structures, thus providing guidance for needle aspiration.

SURGICAL OPTIONS

All management options assume the administration of broad-spectrum antibiotics. Observation, percutaneous needle aspiration, percutaneous catheter drainage, and open surgical drainage with concomitant or delayed nephrectomy have all been employed successfully when applied to the appropriate situation.

Small, isolated intrarenal abscesses may be observed in patients clinically responding to antibiotics alone. Serial imaging is required to document resolution of the collection.

Isolated intrarenal abscesses that do not respond to antibiotics alone should be percutaneously aspirated with radiographical guidance. Aspiration of purulent fluid with microbiological examination can confirm the diagnosis and guide antibiotic therapy. The tract may be dilated with fascial dilators to allow definitive catheter drainage of simple unilocular intrarenal abscesses. Serial CT examination is required to document therapeutic progress.

Multilocular complex perirenal abscesses require standard open surgical drainage (Fig. 33–9). If preoperative studies indicate decreased or absent ipsilateral renal function, it is advisable to limit the initial procedure to incision and drainage of the abscess. It is not uncommon for renal function to recover after adequate treatment of the abscess. Nephrectomy should be delayed until subsequent re-evaluation demonstrates persistently absent renal function. If renal function does not recover, a delayed nephrectomy may then be performed, with a lower mortality rate than that associated with immediate nephrectomy. Abscess drainage with immediate nephrectomy may be required, however, in cases of solid infectious renal replacement, such as xanthogranulomatous pyelonephritis. These cases are commonly associated with an irrevocable loss of renal function and obstructing renal calculi.

OPERATIVE TECHNIQUE

Surgical drainage is achieved by a standard extraperitoneal flank approach to prevent peritoneal con-

tamination. An incision is made off the tip of the twelfth rib and carried down to the lumbar dorsal fascia. This is carefully incised and the peritoneum swept away medially. Gerota's fascia is opened, entering the perirenal space, and the abscess cavity is evacuated. Specimens are obtained for Gram stain and culture. Loculations are broken up with blunt finger dissection (Fig. 33–9). Extensive retroperitoneal debridement may be required for abscesses down the psoas or along the spermatic cord. The flank is copiously irrigated with antibiotic solution to lessen the remaining bacterial burden. Several closed suction drains are placed and brought out through separate stab incisions. The muscle and fascial layers may be left open and packed with povidone-iodine (Betadine)-soaked gauze or closed primarily with monofilament sutures. The subcutaneous muscle and skin are packed and left open to heal by secondary intention.

POSTOPERATIVE MANAGEMENT

The goals of postoperative management are to promote wound healing, restore nutritional balance, and

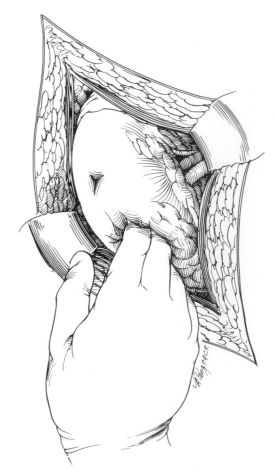

Figure 33–9. Large multiloculated abscesses require operative drainage and interruption of loculation with blunt finger dissection. Secondary nephrectomy may be required if renal function does not return, but it is often safer to perform as a separate procedure after initial abscess drainage.

avoid pulmonary complications. The wound is inspected and packed daily. Parenteral antibiotics are continued for a minimum of 3 to 5 days or until the patient has been afebrile for at least 24 hours. Oral antibiotics are then provided.

Consideration may be given to total parenteral nutrition in a patient who has been severely debilitated by a prolonged course of inflammatory disease. The drains are advanced and removed over a period of 48 to 72 hours approximately 7 to 10 days postoperatively. Urinary drainage from the wound should suggest distal obstruction of the collecting system, most probably by stone. Routine chest physiotherapy should be encouraged, and any evidence of persistent fever should prompt CT examination of the abdomen, retroperitoneum, and thoracic cavity. Violation of the pleura at the time of percutaneous procedures or operative drainage may result in effusion or emphysema and requires drainage.

Summary

Improved antibiotics and imaging studies have greatly assisted in the management of the subtle and often lethal condition of renal abscess. In spite of these advantages, however, renal abscess remains an aggressive process that demands aggressive therapy. The patient is often ill and debilitated and at great risk of dying unless a correct diagnosis is made early, followed by immediate administration of antibiotics and drainage. Drainage may be achieved percutaneously in a few cases, but most often formal operative drainage confined to the retroperitoneum is required.[12]

Editorial Comment
Fray F. Marshall

Ambiguous renal cysts remain a diagnostic dilemma. Imaging has improved in the past decade so that fewer explorations are made for suspicious renal masses. Some patients, however, still require exploration.

Some renal abscesses can be treated with parenteral antibiotics, but drainage of liquefied or localized abscesses is still indicated. Chronic infection can produce xanthogranulomatous pyelonephritis. This can occur on a focal basis and not necessarily involve the entire kidney.[1] If emphysematous pyelonephritis with gas is seen within the renal parenchyma, a nephrectomy is generally indicated, as these patients have a high mortality rate.

Although radiological techniques, including sonography, CT, and MRI, have improved, ambiguous renal cystic lesions remain and sometimes require surgical exploration. Total excision with partial nephrectomy is often the currently preferred management. If the pathology report reveals cancer, then all obvious tumor has been removed. If the lesion is benign, the kidney has been preserved.

1. Elder JS, Marshall FF. Focal xanthogranulomatous pyelonephritis in adulthood. Johns Hopkins Med J 146:141, 1980.

REFERENCES

1. Ambrose SS, Lewis EL, O'Brien DP, et al. Unsuspected renal tumors associated with renal cysts. J Urol 117:704, 1977.
2. Murray J, Eustace S, Breatnach E. MR diagnosis of hemorrhagic cystic renal cell carcinoma. J Comput Assist Tomogr 18:68, 1994.
3. Marshall FF. The role of selective exploration and ambiguous renal cystic lesions. Urol Clin North Am 7:689, 1980.
4. Holmberg G, Hietala SO. Treatment of simple renal cysts by percutaneous puncture and installation of bismuth-phosphate. Scand J Urol Nephrol 23:207, 1989.
5. Hulbert JC, Hunter D, Young AT, Castaneda-Zuniga W. Percutaneous intrarenal marsupialization of a perirenal cystic collection—endocystolysis. J Urol 139:1039, 1988.
6. Kavoussi L, Clayman R, Mikelsen D. Ureteronephroscopic marsupialization of obstructing peripelvic renal cyst. J Urol 148:411, 1991.
7. Hulbert JC. Laparoscopic management of renal cystic disease. Semin Urol 6:239, 1992.
8. Munch L, Gill I, McRoberts W. Laparoscopic retroperitoneal renal cystectomy. J Urol 151:135, 1994.
9. Rubenstein S, Hulbert JC, Pharand D. Laparoscopic ablation of symptomatic renal cysts. J Urol 150:1103, 1993.
10. Sheinfeld J, Erturk E, Spataro RF, Cockett ATK. Perinephric abscess: Current concepts. J Urol 137:191, 1987.
11. Malgieri JJ, Kirsch ED, Persky L. The changing clinical pathology of abscesses in or adjacent to the kidney. J Urol 118:230, 1977.
12. Fowler J, Perkins T. Presentation, diagnosis, and treatment of renal abscesses: 1972–1988. J Urol 151:847, 1994.

Chapter 34

The Lumbodorsal Approach to the Kidney

S. Vaidyanathan and Mani Menon

The kidney can be approached by several surgical routes. The flank approach is used most frequently for renal access; its main drawback is postoperative pain that occurs from muscle transection. The anterior transabdominal approach, classically indicated for oncological surgery because of the ease of early vascular control, provides excellent exposure of the kidney. However, the length of convalescence with this approach is prolonged and the morbidity is increased. The posterior lumbodorsal approach to the kidney provides good exposure, causes less postoperative pain, and offers the advantages of decreased hospitalization time and more rapid return to normal daily activities. No muscles are transsected and the incision is easier to close. This approach provides a strong wound closure and obviates the anterolateral bulging of the abdomen that commonly results from flank incisions. Despite these obvious benefits, this approach has never been popular among urologists. The major criticisms of the lumbodorsal approach are that the surgical exposure is limited and vascular control may prove difficult if required.

Of historical interest, the first planned nephrectomy was performed through a lumbodorsal incision by Simon in 1870.[1] Modifications of this initial technique have been reported by Guyon, Rosenstein, Lurz, Gil-Vernet, and Andaloro and Lilien, and by others more recently.[1-7] Variations deal primarily with patient positioning and skin incision. Despite various modifications in technique and later attempts to resurrect the technique, the lumbodorsal approach to the kidney is still not included in the armamentarium of most urologists. In 1992, Sheldon and associates presented the evolution in the management of infant pyeloplasty and observed a change in the type of surgical approach used with changing time in their practice.[8] Whereas between 1973 and 1984 the flank incision was by far the most prevalent approach, in

more recent years there has been a significant decline in the use of this exposure in favor of the dorsal lumbotomy technique.

The dorsal lumbotomy incision is a useful approach for removal of a small kidney, bilateral nephrectomy in the patient with end-stage renal disease, open renal biopsy, pyeloplasty, pyelolithotomy, and upper ureterolithotomy when the stone is firmly impacted. These have been safely performed in both children and adults.[1-11] Relative contraindications to this approach include patients with (1) renal malrotation or nonrotation; (2) renal fusion anomalies; (3) renal ectopia; (4) long-segment ureteral strictures, or strictures distal to the ureteropelvic junction; (5) repeat pyeloplasty; (6) severe spinothoracic deformities limiting access, as is commonly found in spina bifida patients; (7) malignancy (the 10-year survival rate for patients with tumor stage T1 to T2 renal carcinoma undergoing radical nephrectomy varied significantly according to the approach: thoracoabdominal [100 percent], lumbotomy [60 percent][12]); (8) extreme obesity; (9) caliceal stones behind stenotic infundibula, and (10) staghorn calculi. In fact, for oncological surgery, the transabdominal approach affords the best exposure of the great vessels and allows simultaneous bilateral dissection for staging and tumor removal.[7] We believe, however, that the standard lumbodorsal incision can be modified so that extended exposure can be obtained to allow safe performance of difficult procedures as well, such as anatrophic nephrolithotomy, renovascular surgery, complex renal reconstruction, and adrenal surgery.

To become more comfortable with this technique, an understanding of the anatomy of the lumbodorsal region is critical. The lumbodorsal region is located between the twelfth rib above, the iliac crest below, the spinous processes of the vertebral column dorsally, and an imaginary line connecting the costal

296

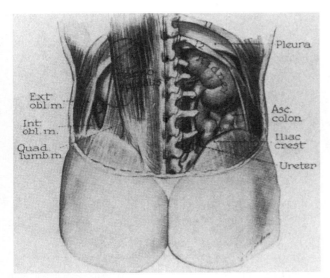

Figure 34–1. The lumbodorsal region. (From Thorek P. Anatomy in Surgery, 2nd ed. Philadelphia, JB Lippincott, 1962.)

muscle in the posterior wall is the quadratus lumborum, which lies beneath the sacrospinalis and is contained within a fascial sheath created by the middle and ventral layers of the lumbodorsal fascia (Fig. 34–3). The ilioinguinal and iliohypogastric nerves course along the inner aspect of the quadratus.

OPERATIVE TECHNIQUE

Positioning

The patient is positioned in the lateral decubitus position with the involved side upward and is tilted 45 degrees forward. The table is not flexed, as this places the muscles on stretch and impedes their retraction (Fig. 34–4). The abdomen is allowed to fall forward, away from the operative site. The surgeon should stand on the side of the table corresponding to the side of the kidney to be exposed.

Incisions

A variety of incisions have been reported.[3, 7, 9] We use an incision that begins 2 to 3 fingerbreadths lateral to the spine and extends from the eleventh rib to the sacroiliac joint with a slight hockey-stick curvature at the lower end (Fig. 34–5). The incision is made over the prominent belly of the sacrospinalis muscle. The subcutaneous tissue is divided along the length of the incision, and the lumbodorsal fascia is identified at the middle and lower part of the incision. This fascia encloses the sacrospinalis muscle and must be incised sharply so that it can be reapproximated at closure (Fig. 34–6).

margin to the anterosuperior iliac spine anteriorly (Fig. 34–1). The first layer of muscles encountered in this area are the sacrospinalis (medially), latissimus dorsi (posteriorly), and external oblique (laterally). The internal oblique muscle lies deep to the external oblique and crosses it anteriorly and superiorly. In the same plane as the internal oblique are the sacrospinalis and serratus posterior inferior. The sacrospinalis is adjacent to the spinous processes of the vertebral column and is encased in a fascial sheath created by the posterior and middle layers of the lumbodorsal fascia (Fig. 34–2). The serratus posterior inferior overlies the inferior costovertebral ligament, which is in close proximity to the underlying pleura. The deepest

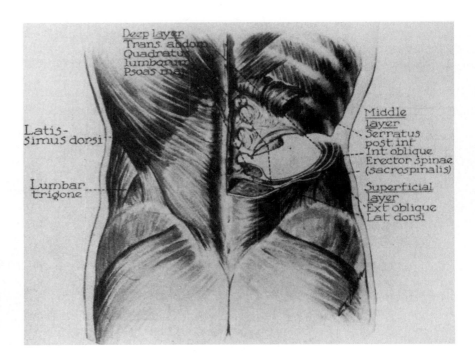

Figure 34–2. Posterolateral abdominal wall muscular attachments. The fascial sheaths that encase the sacrospinalis and quadratus lumborum muscles are depected. (From Thorek P. Anatomy in Surgery, 2nd ed. Philadelphia, JB Lippincott, 1962.)

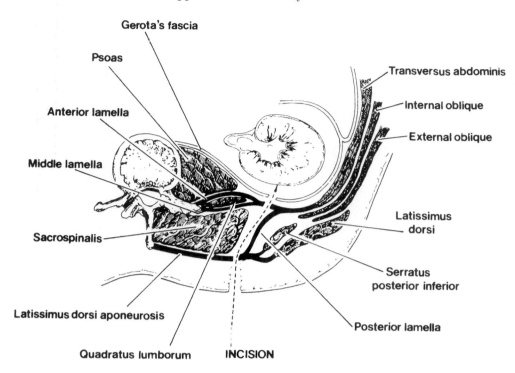

Figure 34–3. Cross-sectional anatomy of the lumbodorsal region demonstrates the course of the incision. (From Orland SM, Snyder HM, Duckett JW. The dorsal lumbotomy incision in pediatric urological surgery. J Urol 138:963, 1987.)

The lumbodorsal fascia thins out superiorly over the eleventh and twelfth ribs where fibers of the latissimus dorsi, serratus posterior inferior, and trapezius are intertwined. After the lumbodorsal fascia is incised, the sacrospinalis muscle is dissected from its undersurface. Tendinous insertions of the sacrospinalis to the eleventh and twelfth ribs are sharply incised 5 mm away from the inferior aspect of these ribs to avoid the intercostal neurovascular bundle. Retracting the sacrospinalis muscle, the quadratus lumborum can be seen at the lower aspect of the incision under the middle layer of the lumbodorsal fascia. Lateral to the quadratus lumborum, the middle and anterior layers of the lumbodorsal fascia are fused. This fused layer of fascia is incised along the length of the incision, which allows the quadratus lumborum to be retracted medially (Fig. 34–7). Care must be taken to avoid injury to the iliohypogastric nerve that runs at right angles across the line of incision. After medial retraction of the quadratus, the fused layer of transversalis fascia and Gerota's fascia is encountered (Fig. 34–8).

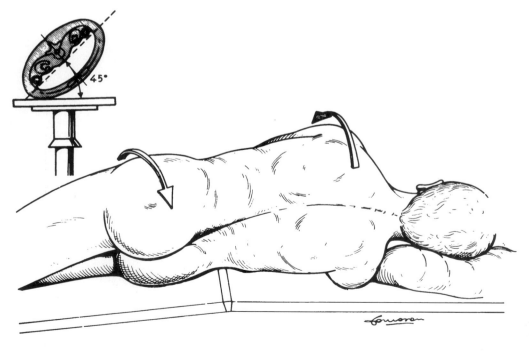

Figure 34–4. Position of the patient on the operating table, tilted forward 45 degrees toward the operating surgeon. (From Pansadoro V. The posterior lumbotomy. Urol Clin North Am 10:573, 1983.)

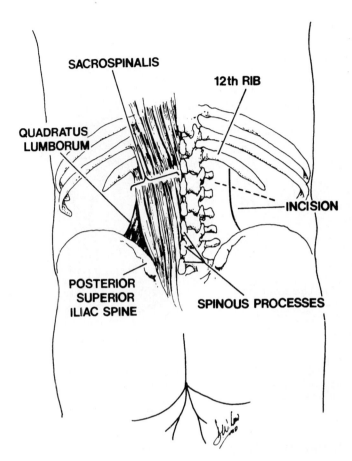

Figure 34–5. The lumbotomy skin incision, showing the hockey-stick curvature of the inferior aspect. (From Orland SM, Snyder HM, Duckett JW. The dorsal lumbotomy incision in pediatric urological surgery. J Urol 138:963, 1987.)

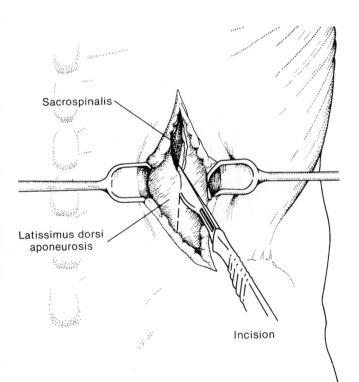

Figure 34–6. Incision through the posterior layer of lumbodorsal fascia. This layer will be reapproximated at closure. (From Orland SM, Snyder HM, Duckett JW. The dorsal lumbotomy incision in pediatric urological surgery. J Urol 138:963, 1987.)

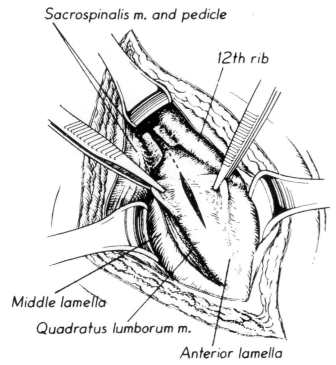

Figure 34–7. The middle and anterior layers of lumbodorsal fascia are fused. Incision through this fused layer allows entry into the retroperitoneal space. (From Freed SZ. Bilateral nephrectomy in transplant recipients. Urology 10:16, 1977.)

Extended Dorsal Lumbotomy

At this stage, without any muscles having been transected, the exposure should be adequate to permit the safe performance of simple upper urinary tract procedures. In some patients, exposure may be limited by the twelfth rib superiorly and iliac crest inferiorly. To obtain optimal exposure for extensive renal surgery, the standard lumbodorsal approach must be modified. The initial step to improve exposure is to transect the costovertebral ligament; with detachment of the costovertebral ligament, the twelfth rib can be retracted superiorly and laterally, rendering resection of the rib unnecessary. In case the exposure is still inadequate, a 2-cm segment of the twelfth rib is next removed posterior to its angle. By excising the posterior rather than the anterior rib segment, more exposure can be obtained. It is important not to injure the subcostal nerve and vessels during this maneuver.

Once this segment of rib is removed, the origin of the diaphragm can be identified and incised to the level of the eleventh rib. The pleura extends close to the ribs this far posteriorly and can be dissected away bluntly or opened along the line of incision. These extra steps effectively double the surgical exposure (Fig. 34–9).

The iliohypogastric and subcostal nerves can be seen traversing the incision and must be skeletonized and preserved. Injury to these can produce varying degrees of analgesia and muscle weakness. Occasionally the subcostal nerve cannot be preserved and can be sacrificed. The iliohypogastric nerve, however, should be preserved in all cases.

A self-retaining retractor can now be inserted into the wound. Gerota's fascia will be apparent and can

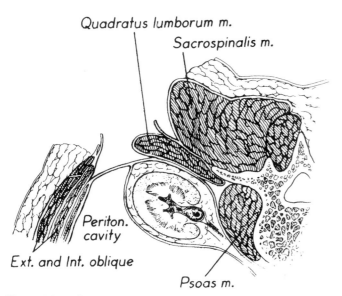

Figure 34–8. Cross-sectional anatomy demonstrates the exposure obtained after all layers of the lumbodorsal fascia are incised. (From Freed SZ. Bilateral nephrectomy in transplant recipients. Urology 10:16, 1977.)

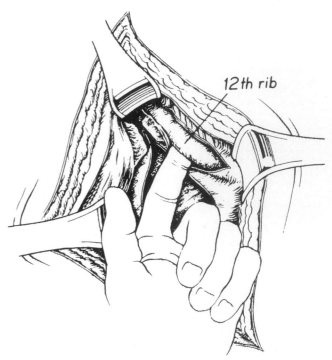

Figure 34–9. To improve exposure, a posterior twelfth rib segment is excised. The pleura can be dissected away bluntly along the line of the incision. (From Freed SZ. Bilateral nephrectomy in transplant recipients. Urology 10:16, 1977.)

be opened in the line of the incision. The underlying kidney can be identified under perinephric fat. The kidney can be completely mobilized, and the planned surgical procedure performed. Bilateral lumbotomy incisions have been carried out for bilateral nephrectomy before transplantation, bilateral renal pelvic stones, or impacted upper ureteral stones and for transureteropyelostomy for ureteral necrosis after a Mainz continent umbilical urinary diversion.[13]

Closure

To close the incision, initial attention is directed toward the diaphragm. If the pleural cavity has been entered, a 14 Fr. red rubber catheter is placed in this cavity and one end brought out through the incision. It is not necessary to close the pleura. All that is rrequired is to reapproximate the diaphragm to the intercostal muscles with running absorbable sutures, thus obliterating the dead space. It is not necessary to reapproximate the incised fused anterior and middle layers of the lumbodorsal fascia. The strength of the closure lies in reapproximating the dorsal layer of lumbodorsal fascia. This step is done with a single layer of interrupted or continuous nonabsorbable sutures. Once this layer is closed securely, the lung is hyperinflated by the anesthesiologist while the red rubber catheter's end is placed into a water basin. During lung hyperinflation, air will bubble through the water. The tube may be clamped and removed at peak inspiration when bubbles are no longer seen. The skin and subcutaneous tissue can then be closed in routine fashion.

POSTOPERATIVE MANAGEMENT AND COMPLICATIONS

Postoperative care of the patient depends on the procedure performed. No specific care is required of the lumbodorsal incision.

Complications in our patients were related to the procedure performed and not to the incision or exposure. Similar findings have been reported by others using this technique.[1, 5–11] In our experience with the lumbodorsal approach in 52 patients, no operation had to be abandoned and no incision had to be extended in a T fashion because of poor exposure or inability to perform the desired procedure. However, the exposure of the great vessels and renal artery and vein is limited with the standard dorsal lumbotomy (although *not* with the extended dorsal lumbotomy), and it may be difficult to control inadvertent damage to these vessels, which may result in significant hemorrhage. There have been instances in which it has been necessary to securely pack the wound posteri-

orly and to immediately turn the patient over for exploration either through the flank or transabdominally to gain control of the hemorrhage sites.[14] Although we have no personal experience with such a complication, we would suggest simply extending the incision, rather than repositioning the patient.

RESULTS

The results of the lumbodorsal approach to the kidney have been examined in terms of operative time, postoperative analgesic requirements, and duration of hospitalization. In comparison with the standard flank incision, the lumbodorsal approach results in quicker mobilization, less postoperative analgesic requirements, less postoperative ileus, and shortened hospital stay. In addition, shorter operating times have been demonstrated with the lumbodorsal incision than with the flank incision.[10, 11]

Summary

The lumbodorsal approach to the kidney can be safely used for both simple and extensive upper urinary tract procedures. Excellent exposure can be obtained and the success of the procedure will not be jeopardized. This technique makes for "very comfortable and grateful patients"[11] who exhibit rapid recovery with little postoperative morbidity, spend less time in the hospital, and have an overall more pleasant operative experience.

Editorial Comment
Fray F. Marshall

This procedure produces less pain and is well tolerated by most patients. Its principal deficiency relates to operative exposure. I have not always rotated the patient forward 45 degrees, but somewhat less, because in some patients the kidney falls away from the surgical incision if they are rotated too far forward.

REFERENCES

1. Hudnall CH, Kirk JF, Radwin HM. The role of posterior lumbotomy in the management of surgical stone disease. J Urol 139:704, 1988.
2. Gil-Vernet J. New surgical concepts in removing renal calculi. Urol Int 20:255, 1965.
3. Andaloro VA, Lilien DM. Posterior approach to the kidney. Urology 5:600, 1975.
4. Novick AC. Posterior surgical approach to the kidney and ureter. J Urol 124:192, 1980.
5. Pansadoro V. The posterior lumbotomy. Urol Clin North Am 10:573, 1983.
6. Gittes RF, Belldegrun A. Posterior lumbotomy: Surgery for upper tract calculi. Urol Clin North Am 10:625, 1983.

7. Orland SM, Snyder HM, Duckett JW. The dorsal lumbotomy incision in pediatric urological surgery. J Urol 138:963, 1987.

8. Sheldon CA, Duckett JW, Snyder HM. Evolution in the management of infant pyeloplasty. J Pediatr Surg 27:501, 1992.

9. Das S, Harris CJ, Amar AD, Egan RM. Dorsovertical lumbotomy approach for surgery of upper urinary tract calculi. J Urol 129:266, 1983.

10. Freiha F, Zeineh S. Dorsal approach to upper urinary tract. Urology 21:15, 1983.

11. Gardiner RA, Naunton-Morgan TC, Whitfield HN, et al. The modified lumbotomy versus the oblique loin incision for renal surgery. Br J Urol 51:256, 1979.

12. Banos GJL, Gomez FJM, Garcia MB, et al. Does the surgical approach used for radical nephrectomy change the prognosis of renal carcinoma? Arch Esp Urol 45:429, 1992.

13. Van Poppel H, Baert L. Transuretero-pyelostomy for ureteral necrosis following a Mainz continent umbilical urinary diversion. Acta Urol Belg 59:17, 1991.

14. Smith RB. Complications of renal surgery. In Smith RB, Ehrlich RM, eds. Complications of Urologic Surgery, 2nd ed. Philadelphia, WB Saunders, 1990, p 128.

Chapter 35

Nephrostomy and Renal Biopsy

Mani Menon and S. Vaidyanathan

NEPHROSTOMY

Surgical creation of a nephrostomy is a distinctly uncommon operation these days with the advent of minimally invasive percutaneous techniques.

Indications

An open operation may be indicated in the following situations: (1) difficulty in establishing a percutaneous nephrostomy because of altered anatomy or lack of expertise and facilities for endourology, a situation commonly encountered in developing nations; (2) a minimally dilated upper urinary tract; and (3) as a procedure complementary to reconstructive surgery of the upper urinary tract, e.g., pyeloplasty and ureterocalicostomy.

Patient Preparation

Before nephrostomy drainage is performed, the urine should be sterile. However, in emergency situations in which such drainage is being carried out for relief of obstructive anuria or for drainage of pyonephrosis, sterile urine cannot be achieved. In such cases, prophylactic administration of a broad-spectrum parenteral antibiotic before the nephrostomy procedure is recommended. Further, patients with obstructive anuria may require preliminary dialysis if the clinical condition warrants it. Any bleeding diathesis or uncontrolled hypertension must be corrected before nephrostomy drainage if time permits.

Surgical Approach

Many techniques have been described for nephrostomy. They can be divided into two groups: (1) those using a pyelostomy to allow internal identification of the collecting system and (2) those using an external or trocar approach to the collecting system. In our experience, we have limited the trocar nephrostomy technique, which involves using a Campbell trocar and introducing a 14 or 16 Fr. Foley catheter into the hugely dilated pelvicaliceal system, to selected patients with giant hydronephrosis or pyonephrosis. A pyelostomy reduces the risk of improper placement of the catheter and should be the method of choice for most cases. Nephrostomy tube insertion is generally performed through an extraperitoneal flank incision or a dorsal lumbotomy.

Patient Positioning

Depending on the surgical approach, the patient is placed either in the flank position with the table flexed to extend the lumbar region, or in the prone position with the table flexed to increase the distance between the twelfth rib and the iliac crest. We use the latter position when performing bilateral nephrostomy for obstructive anuria, a flank approach for a unilateral nephrostomy, and an anterior approach if a simultaneous intra-abdominal operation is being carried out.

Surgical Technique

Either through a subcostal incision or through a vertical lumbar incision, the kidney is mobilized, and the renal pelvis exposed (Fig. 35–1). Two 4-0 Vicryl sutures are placed in the renal pelvis well away from the ureteropelvic junction, and a 1.5-cm incision parallel to the border of the hilum is made with the hooked knife blade. In patients with obstructive anuria, there may be extensive tissue edema and congestion. The renal pelvis can look bluish from venous congestion and may be confused with a venous structure on a limited approach. Care must be taken not

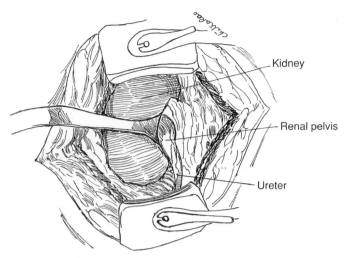

Figure 35–1. The kidney is mobilized and the renal pelvis exposed.

to injure the posterior branch of the renal artery, which proceeds posterior to the renal pelvis to supply a large posterior segment of the kidney. A 22 or 24 Fr. catheter is used for nephrostomy drainage in cases of pyonephrosis; a smaller catheter may be used for simple drainage of a hydronephrotic kidney. A Malecot catheter may be used for nephrostomy drainage, as it has certain advantages over the Foley catheter in that its lumen is larger for a given external diameter and is maintained in position without the need for a balloon. A whistle-tip Foley catheter allows a guidewire to be passed through it and down the ureter to make catheter changes much easier. The Cummings rat-tailed catheter with a 10-cm extension down the ureter may be preferable when nephrostomy is performed at the end of a procedure such as pyeloplasty. When a Malecot catheter is used, it is desirable to cut off two of the four wings to lessen their irritation of the renal pelvis. The disadvantage of the Malecot catheter is that it is more difficult to change than a Foley. Choice of the size and type of catheter used for nephrostomy depends not only on the preference of the urologist but also on the configuration of the renal pelvis. In patients with a small renal pelvis, a Foley catheter should not be used because the balloon may obstruct the ureteropelvic junction or the other calices.

The catheter chosen for nephrostomy drainage is prepared by transfixing the tip with a 1-0 silk suture. A long curved clamp, a malleable probe, or a Randall stone forceps with a suitable curvature is introduced into a lower calix through the pyelostomy (Fig. 35–2). The nephrostomy tube should emerge from the convex border of the kidney and not in the anterior or posterior surface of the kidney. The site of exit of the nephrostomy tube should be in a dependent portion of the kidney, with the calix having the least amount of overlying cortex. The tip of the Randall stone forceps or the malleable probe is pressed firmly into the

convex border of the kidney, and the tip is palpated from outside. The renal capsule is incised in a radial direction over the tip of the clamp. It is opened slightly to dilate the tract. The silk suture on the tip of the Malecot catheter is grasped with the forceps (Fig. 35–3). While the assistant firmly holds the kidney, the Malecot catheter is stretched by pulling on the clamp with one hand and the catheter with the other hand. By moving both hands in concert, the stretched Malecot catheter is introduced into the renal pelvis (Fig. 35–4) and the silk suture is cut. The catheter is withdrawn slowly until it fits snugly in the lower calix (Fig. 35–5). The nephrostomy tube is secured to the renal capsule with a 3-0 absorbable pursestring or figure-of-eight suture.

The pyelostomy is closed with a running or interrupted 4-0 Vicryl suture. The Malecot catheter is brought out through a separate stab wound, ensuring that the catheter tract is straight and the catheter is not kinked as it passes from the kidney to the exterior. The nephrostomy tube is secured to the skin with a 2-0 silk suture to prevent inadvertent dislodgment of the tube. A Penrose drain is placed near the pyelostomy, the perirenal fat is replaced, and the Gerota's fascia is approximated with interrupted absorbable sutures. The drain is brought out through a separate stab wound, and the loin incision is closed in layers. For permanent nephrostomy, horizontal mattress sutures of 2-0 chromic catgut are placed on each side of the nephrostomy. The kidney is mobi-

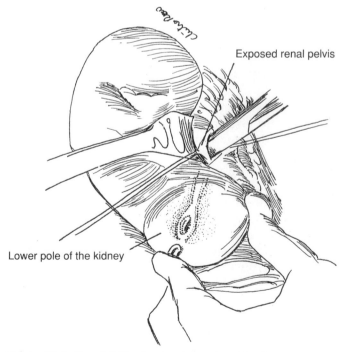

Figure 35–2. Two 4-0 Vicryl sutures are placed in the renal pelvis well away from the ureteropelvic junction, and a 1.5-cm long incision is made parallel to the border of the hilum. A long curved clamp is introduced into a lower calix through the pyelostomy.

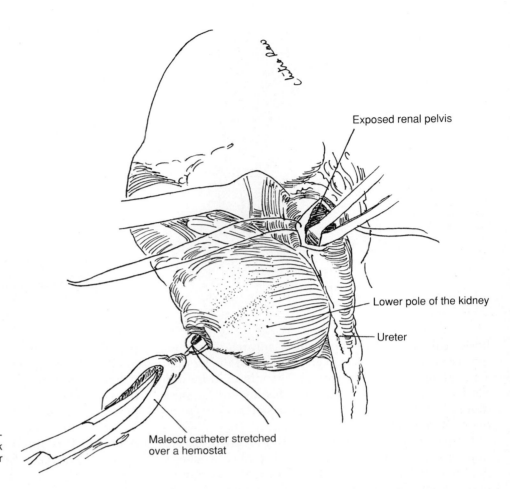

Exposed renal pelvis

Lower pole of the kidney

Ureter

Malecot catheter stretched
over a hemostat

Figure 35–3. The renal capsule is incised over the tip of the clamp. The silk suture on the tip of the Malecot catheter is grasped with the forceps.

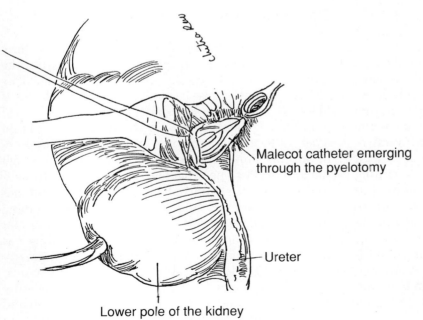

Malecot catheter emerging
through the pyelotomy

Ureter

Lower pole of the kidney

Figure 35–4. As the curved clamp is withdrawn, the stretched Malecot catheter is introduced into the renal pelvis.

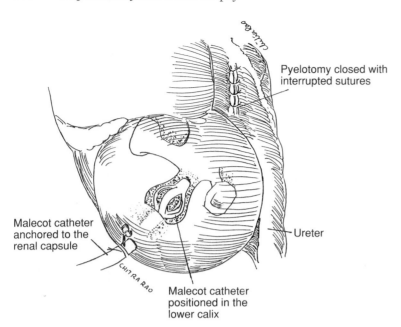

Pyelotomy closed with interrupted sutures

Malecot catheter anchored to the renal capsule

Ureter

Malecot catheter positioned in the lower calix

Figure 35–5. The silk suture is cut and the Malecot catheter positioned in the lower calix. It is secured to the renal capsule with a 3-0 absorbable suture. The pyelostomy is closed with interrupted 4-0 Vicryl sutures.

lized sufficiently to enable these sutures to anchor the lower pole to the fascia and muscle of the wound. This maneuver of fixing the lower pole of kidney to the lateral abdominal wall provides a short, straight drainage tract and thus makes it easier to change the nephrostomy tube.

King and Belman[1] described the following technique for nephrostomy in the absence of calicectasis. A radial pyelostomy is made, opening the extrarenal pelvis from a point a few centimeters above the ureteropelvic junction to the edge of the renal parenchyma. When no extrarenal pelvis is present, the uppermost ureter is incised along its long axis. We have also resorted to incising the uppermost ureter in patients with an intrarenal pelvis and did not encounter any long-term sequelae to this particular operative step.

A curved, blunt-tipped clamp is passed through the pyelostomy/ureterotomy, which should emerge through the inferior calix onto the renal capsule. As the jaws of the clamp are gently opened, the overlying renal capsule is incised. The clamp then grasps the end of a length of umbilical tape and is withdrawn, the tape trailing. The end of the tape is drawn through the pyelostomy and threaded on a cutting needle with a large eye. The tape is then sutured to the de Pezzer or Malecot catheter, the distal end of which has been transected obliquely to achieve a tapering end. Alternatively, a vertical slit is made in the distal end of the Malecot catheter, and the umbilical tape is brought through the slit and tied (Fig. 35–6). The umbilical tape guides retrograde insertion of the catheter through the pyelostomy and then through the incision in the parenchyma.

The above technique is a reliable, relatively atraumatic means of establishing nephrostomy drainage in patients in whom hydronephrosis is absent. Loop nephrostomy drainage has also been recommended when a small intrarenal pelvis is encountered, when there is severe inflammatory reaction at the ureteropelvic junction, or when irrigation of the renal pelvis is required to remove calculus fragments or debris.[2] Although it is important that the nephrostomy tube emerge from the renal parenchyma in a straight line onto the skin, the tube should be brought out as far anteriorly as possible so that patients can lie on their back comfortably and the tube is not compressed while they are lying supine.

Complications

If significant bleeding occurs during the procedure, it can be controlled by manually compressing the kidney at the site of the nephrostomy tract. This almost always stops intraoperative hemorrhage. If bleeding continues, horizontal mattress sutures of 2-0 chromic catgut on atraumatic needles are placed adjacent to the nephrostomy and tied over a buttress of fat; this prevents the suture from tearing through the kidney. Postoperative hemorrhage is usually self-limiting, but if significant hematuria occurs the nephrostomy catheter should be clamped. By clamping the tube, the pelvis fills with blood, forming a clot that acts as a tamponade. When active bleeding has ceased, the tube is unclamped and left to gravity drainage. The clots that form do not require removal by irrigation, as the production of urokinase generally results in dissolution of these clots. Alagaratnam and Leong[3] reported the formation of a false aneurysm in a kidney after nephrostomy for pyonephrosis that was successfully managed by ligating the feeding ar-

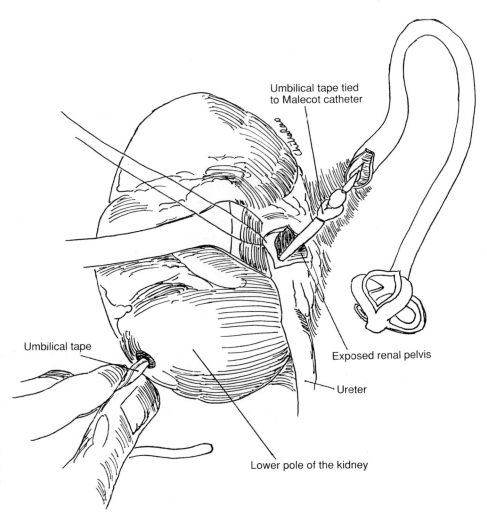

Umbilical tape tied to Malecot catheter

Umbilical tape

Exposed renal pelvis

Ureter

Lower pole of the kidney

Figure 35–6. In the technique described by King and Belman,[1] a curved, blunt-tipped clamp is passed through the pyelostomy/ureterotomy and should emerge through the inferior calix of the kidney. The clamp grasps the end of an umbilical tape and the clamp is withdrawn, the tape trailing. The end of the umbilical tape is tied to the distal end of the Malecot catheter. The tape is withdrawn slowly, and the Malecot catheter is introduced through the pyelostomy and then through the incision in the renal parenchyma. This retrograde insertion of the Malecot catheter is a reliable method of establishing nephrostomy in patients in whom hydronephrosis is absent.

tery and excising the false aneurysm. If a nephrostomy tube fails to drain in the immediate postoperative period, the tube should be carefully inspected for kinks and straightened if necessary. If no kinks are found, the tube should be gently irrigated with sterile saline. If the tube cannot be irrigated freely, an antegrade nephrostogram under gravity should be promptly obtained to check proper positioning of the tube and to determine whether there are clots in the renal pelvis causing the drainage problems. If the nephrostomy tube is in the collecting system, it is probable that the kidney is not producing a normal amount of urine, and the patient is accordingly given appropriate fluid and electrolyte therapy. If the tube is not in the collecting system, it may be repositioned via the established tract under ultrasonographic control, but this may be difficult.

Postoperative Management

Initial change of an established nephrostomy is usually performed under fluoroscopic control. If an established tube becomes dislodged, it is essential

that the patient report immediately for a replacement, since the nephrostomy tract can rapidly decrease in size, and any delay can make tube replacement much more difficult. The patient should bring the dislodged tube at the time of the visit, as an established tube undergoes color change at the skin level that gives some idea of its length from the skin level to the renal pelvis. The corresponding length should be marked on the new catheter to help with depth control during replacement. It may be desirable to replace the Malecot catheter with a Foley at this time. If the tube appears to be in the correct position, a gentle gravity nephrostogram should be performed to ensure its proper positioning within the renal pelvis and to find out whether there is any extravasation of contrast material. Positive urine cultures may be obtained from the nephrostomy tube drainage; antimicrobial therapy is not warranted unless the patient is symptomatic. Long-term, low-dose suppressive antimicrobial therapy is of questionable value. Stone formation may occur if the tube is not changed at regular intervals, or if the urine is infected with urea-splitting organisms. A persistent urinary leak after removal of the nephrostomy tube indicates an obstructive lesion in the collecting system that needs to be treated. We have seen perinephric abscess associated with untreated distal obstruction and continued urinary extravasation after premature removal of the nephrostomy tube.

OPEN RENAL BIOPSY

Bolton and Vaughan[4] compared percutaneous renal biopsy performed in 171 patients with open renal biopsy performed in 100 patients during the same interval at the University of Virginia School of Medicine in Charlottesville. Patients who underwent an open biopsy had more severe renal dysfunction and hypertension than those who had a percutaneous renal biopsy. Open renal biopsy in a high-risk population was associated with a high yield of tissue adequate for diagnosis, with no increase in complications.

Indications

Bolton and Vaughan[4] listed the following circumstances in which open renal biopsy is indicated: (1) antihypertensive therapy that is unsuccessful in lowering diastolic pressure consistently to less than 110 mm Hg without severe postural signs; (2) uremic patients; (3) patients with massive obesity; (4) an anticipated skip or focal lesion; (5) patients who are unable to cooperate for percutaneous renal biopsy or who refused a percutaneous biopsy; and (6) a unilateral, ectopic, or horseshoe kidney. These authors demonstrated that open renal biopsy is a safe procedure, even in patients with medical contraindications to closed renal biopsy. An open renal biopsy was also performed in patients in whom percutaneous renal biopsy had failed. Cosgrove[5] recommended open surgical biopsy for pregnant patients and for those with solitary, horseshoe, or very small kidneys; hydronephrosis; renal mass lesions; severe hypotension; or coagulation difficulties. Poor-risk patients were invariably selected for open renal biopsy.

Preoperative Preparation

Patients undergoing open renal biopsy should, as far as possible, be in good fluid and electrolyte balance, have any anemia and coagulation abnormalities corrected, and have optimal cardiopulmonary status. We do not routinely cross-match blood for this procedure. When there is no preference for performing biopsy on the right or left kidney, we choose the lower pole of the right kidney, as it is more easily accessible than the left kidney. It is mandatory to

determine preoperatively the number of kidneys present and their precise location, size, and relative function. Cosgrove[5] advocates biopsy of the larger, more accessible, and better functioning kidney. Anesthesia is necessary for open renal biopsy. With the advances made in anesthesiology, we prefer to use general anesthesia for this procedure. However, Gonick and Grau[6] infiltrate 10 ml of 1 percent lidocaine over the line of subcostal incision in addition to another 5 to 10 ml injected below the eleventh and twelfth rib margins, just distal to the angle of the rib. As the incision is deepened, the muscles are infiltrated with additional local anesthetic. The only complication attributable to the local anesthetic technique during 205 biopsies in 202 patients was the development of pneumothorax in a 63-year-old man that might have been produced by the local anesthetic injection of the eleventh subcostal nerve.

Surgical Technique

The patient is placed in the flank position with the kidney bridge raised. A 3-inch subcostal incision is made 1 cm below the tip of the twelfth rib. The muscles are split in the line of their fibers. Gerota's fascia is incised and the lower pole of the kidney cleared of all fat and fascia. We do not mobilize the entire kidney for this procedure. It is ensured that the vials for specimen collection for histopathology, electron microscopy, and immunological studies are ready. A 3-0 Vicryl suture is kept ready as well as a piece of Gelfoam. With a scalpel, an elliptical wedge of renal cortex measuring 1 × 0.5 cm is excised (Fig. 35–7). The biopsy specimen should not be held with

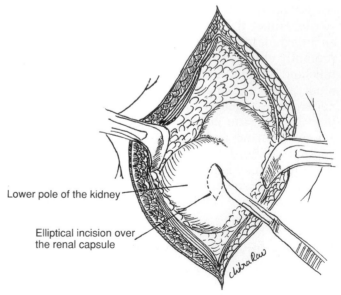

Lower pole of the kidney

Elliptical incision over the renal capsule

Figure 35–7. The lower pole of the kidney is exposed. With a scalpel, an elliptical wedge of renal cortex measuring 1 × 0.5 cm is excised.

a forceps, as the tissue may be crushed; we prefer to lever it out with the blades of a scissor (Fig. 35–8). In some patients with end-stage kidney disease or in those with obstructive uropathy, there can be extensive perirenal fibrosis because of previous episodes of urinary extravasation, and we ensure that we have taken an adequate amount of renocortical tissue by performing frozen section studies on the excised biopsy specimen. Rarely, the initial wedge biopsy in such cases contained only fibrous tissue, and frozen section studies guided us to perform another biopsy to include renal cortex.

We close the defect in renal cortex with interrupted 3-0 Vicryl sutures tied over a piece of Oxycel (Fig. 35–9). If there is an arterial bleeder, it is ligated separately with a figure-of-eight suture. When hemostasis is secure, the perirenal fat is replaced and Gerota's fascia approximated with interrupted 3-0 chromic catgut sutures. We close the flank incision in layers with 2-0 Vicryl after leaving a Penrose drain at the site of renal biopsy. The drain is generally removed after 48 hours. Sometimes, in patients with very thin renal parenchyma, we have inadvertently opened the collecting system while taking the renal biopsy. However, this should be immediately recognized and the defect in the collecting system closed with 4-0 Vicryl. When performing such a corrective step, we did not encounter any case of urinary leak. Our retrieval rate of diagnostic quality tissue was 100 percent.

With this technique of open renal biopsy, no special instruments are required; there is no x-ray exposure to patient or physician. The technique can be carried out in most hospitals of developing nations where facilities for imaging may not be available for

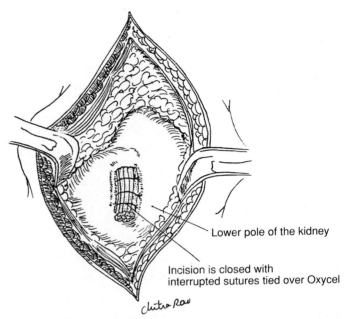

Figure 35–9. The defect in the renal cortex is closed with interrupted 3-0 Vicryl sutures tied over a piece of Oxycel.

percutaneous renal biopsy or for performing selective renal artery embolization for post–needle biopsy bleeding.

Gillenwater[7] recommends the use of an Allis clamp to pull the biopsy specimen out of the incision. He closes the biopsy site with a horizontal mattress suture of 3-0 or 4-0 chromic catgut tied over a piece of fat on each side to prevent tearing out of the suture. Gillenwater[7] and Hinman[8] advocate taking a wedge biopsy of the renal cortex as well as a needle biopsy specimen under direct vision to obtain material from the deep cortical and juxtamedullary levels. Burrington[9] described a technique of open renal biopsy in children in which the child was placed prone over the kidney bar of the operating table, which was then elevated. The kidney was exposed by a dorsal lumbotomy. Two or three cores of tissue were removed using a disposable biopsy needle. The biopsies were taken 1 cm from the lower edge of the kidney, because biopsy near the inferior pole gave a maximal number of glomeruli with minimal risk of injury to the calices, renal pelvis, or major blood vessels. The biopsy sites were gently compressed until all bleeding stopped. Rarely, a hemostatic suture in the capsule was necessary. Almkuist and Buckalew[10] stated that an open needle biopsy, although it might provide deeper tissue through a smaller incision, might cause occult hemorrhage and caliceal tears if directed incorrectly. The wedge biopsy allowed better hemostasis and provided a larger sample, which was particularly helpful in focal lesions, but it might allow juxtamedullary abnormalities to be missed unless a deep wedge was excised. Our preference is for wedge biopsy, and we have not encountered any case

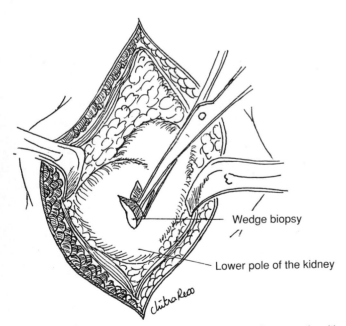

Figure 35–8. The renal biopsy specimen is levered out gently with the blades of a scissor.

of primary or secondary hemorrhage with the technique described above.

Postoperative Management

Very rarely, in hypertensive patients, those with coagulation problems, and patients undergoing hemodialysis, a retroperitoneal hematoma or a wound hematoma may form. Wound infection is uncommon. In uremic patients the skin sutures are not removed until the eighth day.

Editorial Comment
Fray F. Marshall

When performing an open nephrostomy tube insertion, it is often less traumatic to place the tube retrograde or from inside out. We have utilized a malleable probe with a hollow end that allows placement of the suture through the nephrostomy tube and through the probe to secure it as it is pulled through the kidney. It is important to create a short, straight nephrostomy tube tract to allow easier tube placement in the future if the nephrostomy tube requires changing. At the present time, there are relatively few indications for loop nephrostomy.

Two small points warrant mention. First, the body does not like silk suture, so nylon is used for suturing any drain into the skin. Second, we have more often relied on closed drainage such as with a soft Jackson-Pratt or Davol drain than on a Penrose drain, but the closed drainage systems cost more.

REFERENCES

1. King LR, Belman AB. A technique for nephrostomy in the absence of calicectasis. J Urol 108:518, 1972.
2. Hawtrey CE, Boatman DL, Brown RG, Schnidt JD. Clinical experience with loop nephrostomy for urinary diversion. J Urol 112:36, 1974.
3. Alagaratnam TT, Leong CH. An iatrogenic complication of nephrostomy. J Urol 113:286, 1975.
4. Bolton WK, Vaughan ED Jr. A comparative study of open surgical and percutaneous renal biopsies. J Urol 117:696, 1977.
5. Cosgrove MD. Commentary: Percutaneous vs. open renal biopsy. In Whitehead ED, Leiter E, eds. Current Operative Urology, 2nd ed. Philadelphia, Harper & Row, 1984, p 297.
6. Gonick P, Grau J. Open renal biopsy technique: Results in 202 patients. Urology 11:568, 1978.
7. Gillenwater JY. Commentary on open renal biopsy. In Hinman F Jr, ed. Atlas of Urologic Surgery. Philadelphia, WB Saunders, 1989, p 840.
8. Hinman F Jr. Open renal biopsy. In Hinman F Jr, ed. Atlas of Urologic Surgery. Philadelphia, WB Saunders, 1989, p 839.
9. Burrington JD. Technique and results of fifty-five open renal biopsies in children. Surg Gynecol Obstet 140:613, 1975.
10. Almkuist RD, Buckalew UM. Techniques of renal biopsy. Urol Clin North Am 6:503, 1979.

Part II

RENOVASCULAR SURGERY

Chapter 36

Renal Arterial Grafts and Renal Bench Surgery

Andrew C. Novick

Revascularization of the kidney is indicated in order to treat renovascular hypertension; to preserve renal function that is threatened by advanced vascular disease; or, occasionally, to prevent rupture of an arterial aneurysm. Most revascularization operations involve bypass with an interpositional graft from a healthy donor's artery to the distal disease-free portion of the renal artery. The donor artery may comprise the aortic, hepatic, splenic, mesenteric, or iliac vessels. Notwithstanding the variety of techniques available for treating patients with renal artery disease, aortorenal bypass remains the preferred method in the absence of significant aortic disease. In this chapter the different types of renal artery bypass grafts are reviewed and the technique of aortorenal bypass is described.

Extracorporeal renal surgery and autotransplantation have become the treatments of choice for selected patients with complex branch renal artery disease or extensive malignancy. The operative techniques for renal bench surgery in such cases are also described in this chapter.

The earliest materials to be used as bypass grafts were prepared arterial homografts and synthetic prostheses. As the inherent advantages of nonantigenic autogenous tissue grafts were recognized, these materials were used increasingly and currently represent the optimal bypass grafts for renal artery replacement.

The largest collective experience with autogenous vascular grafts has been accumulated with the saphenous vein, and excellent results have been reported in the treatment of renal artery disease.[1] This vessel is generally free of disease and may be obtained readily in almost any desired length. The saphenous vein is easy to work with, is similar in caliber to the renal artery, and may be utilized to bypass most renal

arterial lesions. Long-term studies of aortorenal saphenous vein grafts have shown a large number of dilated grafts on follow-up angiography.[2, 3] This has been observed more frequently in children and may reflect an enhanced susceptibility to mural ischemia of vein segments procured from children. This concept is compatible with studies on the changes that occur in the nutrient blood supply of veins before adulthood. The clinical significance of these abnormal-appearing vein grafts is uncertain because most patients remain normotensive with excellent renal function.[4] The saphenous vein graft remains a very satisfactory material for renal artery replacement in adults. However, for reasons stated, its use in the prepubertal child is best avoided.

Arterial autografts are theoretically advantageous for renal artery bypass surgery. The viscoelastic properties of arterial grafts match those of the renal artery, and postoperative graft dilation has not been observed. Free grafts of either the hypogastric or splenic artery may be used for aortorenal bypass with excellent results.[5, 6] The hypogastric artery is generally a short vessel best suited for bypass of proximal or left renal artery lesions. Hypogastric aortorenal bypass is particularly advantageous as a means of renal revascularization in children. The splenic artery provides a longer graft but is more difficult to procure and is not suitable for use in children. In a patient over 50 years of age, either of these arterial grafts may be precluded by atherosclerotic involvement. In such a case, a saphenous vein graft is used. The spermatic or ovarian veins should never be employed as bypass grafts. These veins are extremely friable and may either rupture or undergo severe dilation postoperatively.

Synthetic vascular grafts are indicated only when autogenous vascular grafts are not available. Dacron

311

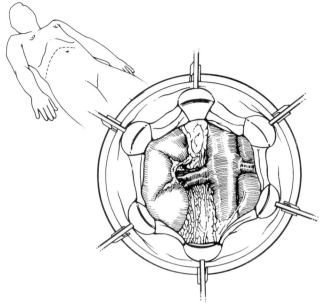

Figure 36–1. Aortorenal bypass is performed through a subcostal transperitoneal incision. A self-retaining ring retractor is used to maintain exposure. (From Novick AC, et al, eds. Stewart's Operative Urology. Baltimore, Williams & Wilkins, 1989.)

grafts were employed initially; however, a 15 to 35 percent incidence of early postoperative thrombosis and graft failure was observed. Polytetrafluoroethylene (PTFE) has emerged as the preferred material when a synthetic graft is necessary.[7] The preference for PTFE is based on a low rate of infection, a reduced incidence of thrombosis, and an elimination of true and false aneurysm formation. The graft is light and pliable and requires no preclotting; problems related to angulation or kinking have not been encountered. Only monofilament suture material should be used in performing vascular anastomoses with PTFE.

AORTORENAL BYPASS

The performance of an aortorenal bypass for right renal revascularization is illustrated in Figure 36–1. However, the approach is analogous on the left side. A transperitoneal subcostal incision is made, the medial end of which is curved across the midline. The kidney is exposed by reflecting the ascending colon medially; the Kocher maneuver is performed on the duodenum. Exposure of the renal vessels, inferior vena cava, and aorta is thereby obtained. The Buckwalter self-retaining ring retractor is inserted to maintain exposure. Gerota's fascia is opened laterally to expose the surface of the kidney so that its color and consistency may be observed throughout the revascularization procedure.

The aorta is exposed from the level of the left renal vein to the inferior mesenteric artery, ligating overlying lymphatic vessels and lumbar segmental branches as necessary to gain exposure. An end-to-side anastomosis of the bypass graft to the aorta is done first to minimize the time of renal ischemia. A DeBakey clamp is placed to occlude the aorta, care being taken to avoid compression of the mesenteric and contralateral renal arteries. In most cases the lateral aortic wall is only partially occluded, thereby preserving distal aortic flow and obviating the need for systemic heparinization. An oval aortotomy is made on the anterolateral wall of the aorta for an end-to-side anastomosis with the spatulated bypass graft. This anastomosis is performed with interrupted 6-0 vascular sutures (Fig. 36–2).

After completion of the proximal anastomosis, the graft is occluded beyond its origin with a bulldog clamp, and the aortic clamp is gently released. The

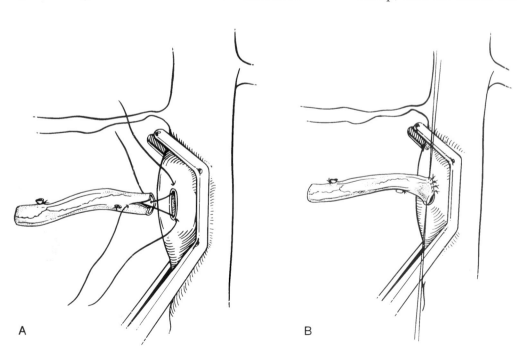

A   B

Figure 36–2. *A,* The aortic wall is partially occluded with a DeBakey clamp, and an oval aortotomy is made for end-to-side anastomosis with the spatulated bypass graft. *B,* The proximal anastomosis is performed with interrupted vascular sutures. (From Novick AC, et al, eds. Stewart's Operative Urology. Baltimore, Williams & Wilkins, 1989.)

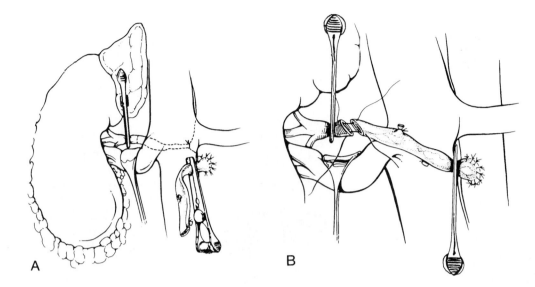

Figure 36–3. *A,* After completion of the proximal anastomosis, the renal artery is mobilized and prepared. *B,* End-to-end anastomosis of the spatulated graft and distal renal artery is performed. (From Novick AC, et al, eds Stewart's Operative Urology. Baltimore, Williams & Wilkins, 1989.)

main renal artery is then mobilized in its entirety. The renal artery is ligated proximally, the bulldog clamp is placed distally, and the diseased arterial segment is excised and sent for pathological examination. Before the distal anastomosis is performed, 10 ml of dilute heparin solution is instilled into the distal renal artery. End-to-end anastomosis of the spatulated graft and distal renal artery is performed with interrupted 6-0 vascular sutures (Fig. 36–3). An end-to-end anastomosis of the graft to the renal artery is preferred to an end-to-side technique because the former provides better flow rates, is easier to perform, and allows removal of the diseased renal arterial segment for pathological study.

The completed aortorenal bypass operation and a postoperative angiogram are depicted in Figure 36–4. When performing aortorenal bypass on the right side, it is important to bring the graft off the anterolateral aspect of the aortic wall to avoid kinking of the proximal anastomosis as the graft passes in front of the vena cava. If the aortotomy is made too far anteriorly or posteriorly, the graft may kink, with subsequent development of stenosis or thrombosis (Fig. 36–5). The graft should follow a direct course from the aorta to the renal artery with no acute angulation or torsion, which can also predispose the patient to stenosis or thrombosis (Fig. 36–6).

Surgical revascularization is more complicated

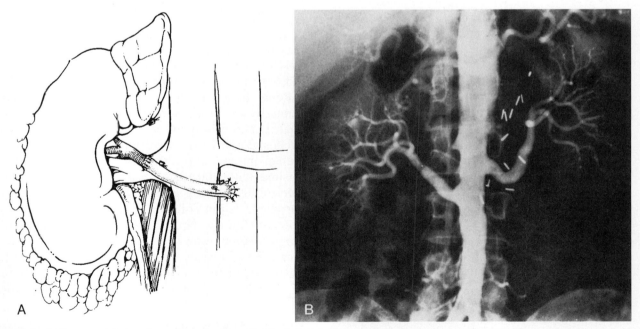

Figure 36–4. *A,* The completed aortorenal bypass operation is depicted. (From Novick AC, et al, eds. Stewart's Operative Urology. Baltimore, Williams & Wilkins, 1989.) *B,* Aortogram. 7 years after bilateral aortorenal saphenous vein bypass, shows patient grafts to both kidneys. (From Novick AC. Complications of renovascular surgery. In Ehrlich RM, Smith RB, eds. Complications in Urologic Surgery. Philadelphia, WB Saunders, 1988.)

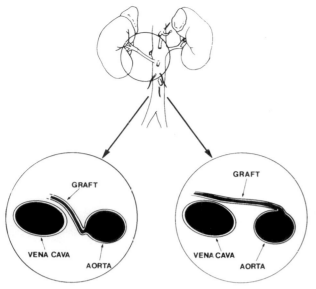

Figure 36–5. On the right side, if the aortotomy is made too far anteriorly or posteriorly, the graft will kink and may subsequently occlude. (From Novick AC. Complications of renovascular surgery and percutaneous transluminal angioplasty. In Marshall FF, ed. Urological Complications. Chicago, Year Book, 1986.)

when the disease extends into branches of the renal artery or when vascular reconstruction is required for a kidney supplied by multiple arteries. When disease-free distal arterial branches occur outside the renal hilus, an aortorenal bypass operation can often be done in situ. Aortorenal bypass with a branched vascular graft provides the most useful and versatile technique for in situ vascular reconstruction of two or more diseased renal arteries.[8, 9] Although the hypo-

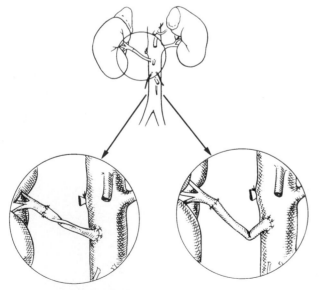

Figure 36–6. The bypass graft must be placed to avoid angulation *(right)* or torsion *(left)*, which can cause postoperative obstruction. (From Novick AC. Complications of renovascular surgery and percutaneous transluminal angioplasty. In Marshall FF, ed. Urological Complications. Chicago, Year Book, 1986.)

gastric artery may be removed intact with its branches, this type of graft is invariably too short to reach from the aorta to the renal artery branches. In these cases, a branched saphenous vein graft is fashioned by attaching one or more side arms of vein to the main graft. These end-to-side anastomoses are made with interrupted 7-0 vascular sutures and lead to creation of a multibranched graft that can replace several diseased renal artery branches. After insertion of the proximal graft into the aorta, direct end-to-end anastomosis of each graft branch to a renal artery branch is performed. During performance of each individual branch anastomosis, the remainder of the kidney continues to be perfused, and overall renal ischemia is thus limited to the time required for completion of a single end-to-end anastomosis (approximately 15 to 20 minutes), which is an important advantage (Fig. 36–7).

RENAL BENCH SURGERY

Extracorporeal or renal bench surgery with auto-transplantation has become the treatment of choice for complex branch renal artery disease and occasionally for extensive renal malignancy.[9–13] In evaluating patients for this approach, preoperative renal and pelvic arteriography should be performed to define renal arterial anatomy; to ensure relatively disease-free iliac vessels; and, in patients with branch renal arterial lesions, to assess the hypogastric artery and its branches for their usefulness as a reconstructive graft. Autotransplantation of kidneys with severe parenchymal disease should be avoided. Such kidneys generally flush poorly after removal, which may result in irreversible ischemic damage with lack of postoperative function. Also, autotransplantation may not be possible when severe atherosclerotic disease renders the iliac arteries unsuitable for anastomosis to the renal artery.

Renal bench surgery and autotransplantation are generally performed through a midline transperitoneal incision; in heavyset or obese patients, separate subcostal and lower quadrant incisions may be preferable. Immediately after its removal, the kidney is flushed with 500 ml of chilled Collins intracellular electrolyte solution and is then placed in a basin of ice slush saline solution for hypothermic preservation outside the body.[14] When the kidney is ready, autotransplantation is always performed into the prepared iliac fossa using the same vascular techniques as described for renal allotransplantation (see Chap. 37, Renal Transplantation and Autotransplantation).

Branch Renal Artery Disease

Vascular disease involving the branches of the renal artery is most often caused by one of the fibrous

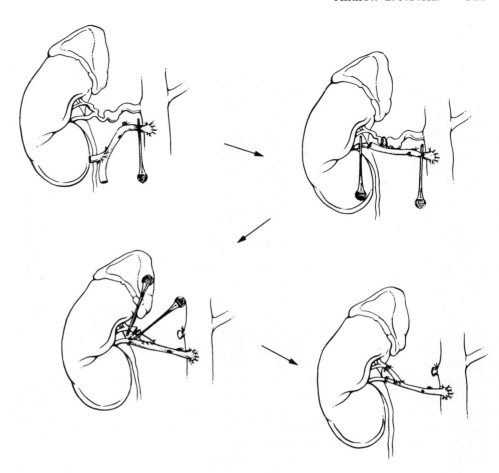

Figure 36–7. Sequential vascular anastomoses involved in performing aortorenal bypass with a double-armed, branched saphenous vein graft. (From Novick AC, et al, eds. Stewart's Operative Urology. Baltimore, Williams & Wilkins, 1989.)

dysplasias: intimal, medial, or perimedial fibroplasia. Other causes of branch disease include arterial aneurysm, arteriovenous malformation, Takayasu's arteritis, neurofibromatosis, trauma, and (rarely) atherosclerosis. In such cases the task of renovascular reconstruction is considerably more complicated, since it necessitates multiple vascular anastomoses to renal arterial branches that may be difficult to expose and are small in caliber. Before the advent of renal bench surgery, many patients in this category were considered inoperable or candidates for total or partial nephrectomy.

Extracorporeal branch arterial repair and autotransplantation are indicated primarily when preoperative arteriography with oblique views demonstrates intrarenal extension of renovascular disease. Patients with dissecting fibrous lesions, previous renovascular operations, or calcified aneurysms may have diseased renal vessels that are difficult to mobilize in situ because of intense surrounding fibrotic reaction and adherence to adjacent hilar structures. Some of these patients may be more safely and effectively managed with extracorporeal revascularization.

The advantages of renal bench surgery include optimal exposure and illumination, a bloodless surgical field, greater protection of the kidney from ischemia, and less complex microvascular techniques and opti-

cal magnification. Removing and flushing the kidney also cause it to contract, thereby enabling more peripheral dissection in the renal sinus for the mobilization of distal arterial branches. The completed branch anastomoses can be tested for patency and integrity prior to autotransplantation.

Extracorporeal renal revascularization may be carried out on the abdominal wall with the ureter attached or, alternatively, on a separate workbench after division of the ureter. I prefer the latter, since this method provides better exposure for the extracorporeal operation and allows a second surgical team to simultaneously prepare the iliac fossa. Renal preservation during extracorporeal revascularization can be simply and effectively achieved with simple cold storage. After removal and flushing of the kidney (Fig. 36–8), the organ is placed in a basin of ice slush saline solution. Under surface hypothermia, the renal artery branches are mobilized distally in the renal sinus beyond the area of vascular disease (Fig. 36–9), and extracorporeal revascularization is performed.

The optimal method for extracorporeal branch renal arterial repair involves a branched autogenous vascular graft.[15, 16] This technique permits separate end-to-end microvascular anastomosis of each graft branch to a distal renal artery branch. A hypogastric arterial autograft is the preferred material for vascular

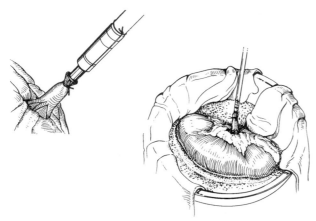

Figure 36–8. The removed kidney is flushed intra-arterially with a cold electrolyte solution and placed in a basin of ice and saline slush to maintain hypothermia. (From Novick AC, et al, eds. Stewart's Operative Urology. Baltimore, Williams & Wilkins, 1989.)

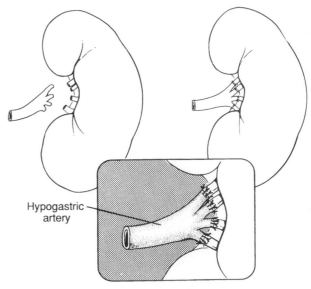

Figure 36–10. Extracorporeal repair with a branched hypogastric arterial autograft. (From Novick AC, et al, eds. Stewart's Operative Urology. Baltimore, Williams & Wilkins, 1989.)

reconstruction because the hypogastric artery may be obtained intact with several of its branches (Fig. 36–10).

Occasionally, the hypogastric artery is not suitable as a reconstructive graft because of atherosclerotic degeneration. In this case, a long segment of saphenous vein graft can be harvested and, employing sequential end-to-side microvascular anastomoses, a branched graft fashioned. This branched graft is then used in a similar manner to achieve reconstruction of the diseased renal artery branches (Fig. 36–11).

Branched grafts of the hypogastric artery and saphenous vein occasionally may prove too large for anastomosis to small secondary or tertiary renal arterial branches. In these cases, the inferior epigastric artery provides an excellent alternative free graft for extracorporeal microvascular repair. This artery measures 1.5 to 2.0 mm in diameter, is rarely diseased, and coapts closely in caliber and thickness to small renal artery branches. The inferior epigastric artery may be employed as a branched graft either by itself or in conjunction with a segment of saphenous vein (Fig. 36–12).

Although a branched autogenous vascular graft provides a simple, versatile, and effective method for renal arterial reconstruction, other techniques occasionally are preferable, depending on the extent of

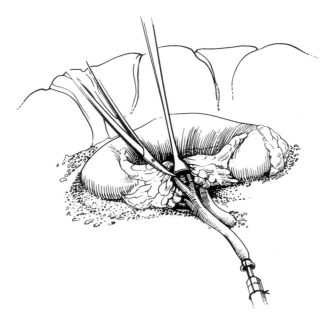

Figure 36–9. The diseased renal artery branches are mobilized in the renal sinus while under surface hypothermia. (From Novick AC, et al, eds. Stewart's Operative Urology. Baltimore, Williams & Wilkins, 1989.)

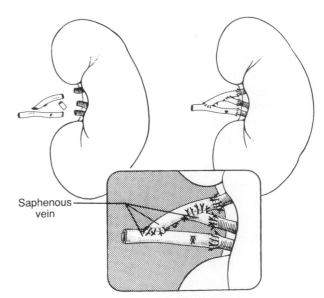

Figure 36–11. Extracorporeal repair with a prefashioned, branched saphenous vein graft. (From Novick AC, et al, eds. Stewart's Operative Urology. Baltimore, Williams & Wilkins, 1989.)

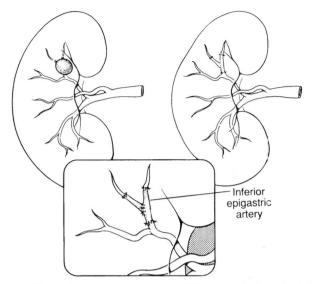

Figure 36–12. Extracorporeal repair with a branched graft of the inferior epigastric artery. (From Novick AC, et al, eds. Stewart's Operative Urology. Baltimore, Williams & Wilkins, 1989.)

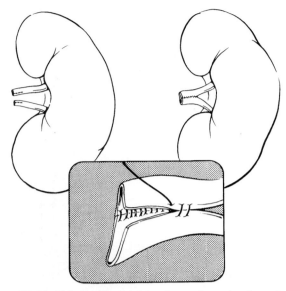

Figure 36–14. Side-to-side (conjoined) anastomosis of renal artery branches of equal caliber.

vascular disease. In some patients with localized segmental intrarenal branch lesions, other arterial branches may be uninvolved or may have more proximally located vascular disease. Such branches with longer disease-free distal segments may be anastomosed end to side either into a larger arterial branch or into a reconstructive vascular graft (Fig. 36–13). Occasionally, two distal arterial branches of similar diameter and free of disease are found adjacent to one another. These two adjacent branches can be conjoined and then anastomosed end to end to a single limb of the branched graft (Fig. 36–14).

Renal artery aneurysms have variable presentations, and the method of extracorporeal repair is de-

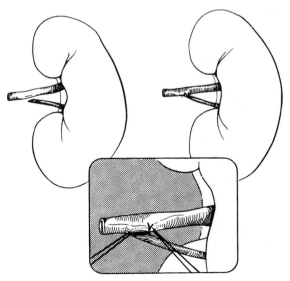

Figure 36–13. End-to-side reimplantation of a small renal artery branch into a larger one. (From Novick AC, et al, eds. Stewart's Operative Urology. Baltimore, Williams & Wilkins, 1989.)

termined by whether renovascular involvement is focal or diffuse (Fig. 36–15). If the renal artery wall at the base of an aneurysm is intact, aneurysmectomy with patch angioplasty can be performed. Aneurysms with short focal involvement of renal artery branches may also be simply resected with end-to-end branch reanastomosis or end-to-side reimplantation into an adjacent branch. In other cases with more extensive vascular disease, aneurysmectomy and revascularization with a branched autogenous graft are indicated.

These extracorporeal vascular techniques are all performed with interrupted sutures, except for the conjoined anastomosis where a continuous suture is used. When revascularizing multiple arterial branches, one must anticipate the position that the various branches will assume in relation to one another upon completion of the repair. Individual branch anastomoses are then performed with careful attention to avoid subsequent malrotation, angulation, and tension. In all cases, extracorporeal repair leads to creation of a single main renal artery so that autotransplantation may be performed with one arterial anastomosis and no increase in revascularization time. When extracorporeal revascularization has been completed, the kidney may be placed on the hypothermic pulsatile perfusion unit to verify the patency and integrity of the repaired branches. Alternatively, this assessment can be made by gravity reflushing of the kidney. Renal autotransplantation into the iliac fossa is then performed with anastomosis of the renal vessels to the iliac vessels and restoration of urinary continuity by ureteroneocystostomy.

Renal Malignancy

Extracorporeal partial nephrectomy and autotransplantation have been employed in the management

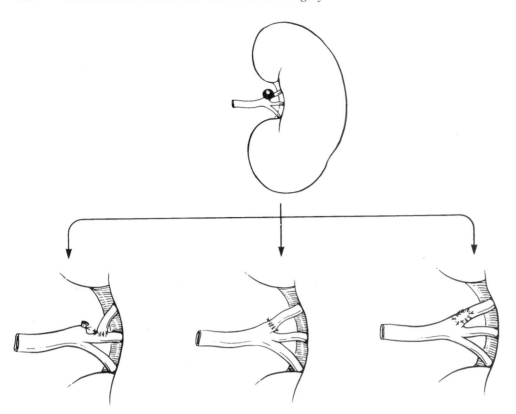

Figure 36–15. Techniques for renal artery aneurysmectomy with patch angioplasty *(right)*, resection and re-anastomosis *(middle)*, and end-to-side reimplantation *(left)*. (From Novick AC, et al, eds. Stewart's Operative Urology. Baltimore, Williams & Wilkins, 1989.)

of selected patients with renal cell carcinoma, Wilms tumor, or renal pelvic transitional cell carcinoma when a nephron-sparing operation is indicated.[12] In most patients who undergo nephron-sparing surgery for renal malignancy, partial nephrectomy can be successfully carried out in situ.[13] Renal bench surgery and autotransplantation are required only in the patient with an exceptionally large, hypervascular, and central tumor that would otherwise be considered inoperable. The advantages of an extracorporeal approach in such a case include improved exposure, ability to carry out a more precise operation with maximal conservation of renal parenchyma, and greater protection of the kidney from prolonged ischemia.

The technique of extracorporeal partial nephrectomy is depicted in Figure 36–16. The kidney is mobilized and removed outside Gerota's fascia, with ligation and division of the renal artery and vein as the last steps in the operation. A regional lymphadenectomy may be carried out. Immediately after dividing the renal vessels, the removed kidney is flushed and submerged in a basin of ice slush saline solution. If possible, it is best to leave the ureter attached in such a case to preserve its distal collateral vascular supply, particularly with large hilar or lower renal tumors in which complete excision may unavoidably compromise the blood supply to the pelvis, ureter, or both. In this situation, the extracorporeal operation is done on the abdominal wall of the patient. If the ureter is left attached, it must be temporarily oc-

cluded to prevent retrograde blood flow to the kidney while it is outside the body. Often, unless the patient is thin, working on the abdominal wall with the ureter attached is cumbersome because of the tethering and restricted movement of the kidney. If this problem is observed, the ureter should be divided and the kidney placed on a separate workbench to improve the exposure. If concern exists over the adequacy of ureteral blood supply, the risk of postoperative urinary extravasation can be diminished by restoring urinary continuity through direct anastomosis of the renal pelvis to the retained distal ureter.

The removed kidney is divested of all perinephric fat to appreciate the full extent of the neoplasm. Because such tumors are usually centrally located, dissection is begun in the renal hilus with identification of major segmental arterial and venous branches. Vessels clearly directed toward the neoplasm are secured and divided; those vessels supplying uninvolved renal parenchyma are preserved. The tumor is then removed by incising the capsule and parenchyma to preserve a 1- to 2-cm surrounding margin of normal renal tissue. Transected blood vessels on the renal surface are secured and the collecting system is closed.

After completion of the resection, tumor-free margins are verified by frozen-section histopathology. The renal remnant is then placed on the pulsatile perfusion unit to facilitate identification and suture ligation of any remaining potential bleeding points. The kidney is alternately perfused through the renal

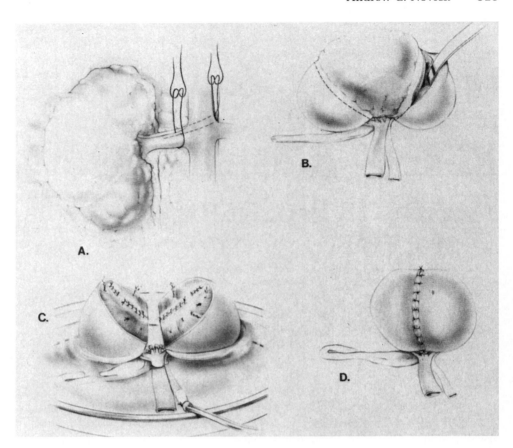

Figure 36–16. Technique of extracorporeal partial nephrectomy for a large central malignancy. *A,* The kidney is removed outside Gerota's fascia. *B,* The tumor is excised extracorporeally while preserving the vascular branches to uninvolved parenchyma. *C,* Pulsatile perfusion is used to identify transected blood vessels. *D,* The kidney is closed upon itself. (From Novick AC. Partial nephrectomy for renal cell carcinoma. Urol Clin North Am 14:419, 1987.)

artery and vein to ensure both arterial and venous hemostasis. Because the perfusate lacks clotting ability, some parenchymal oozing may continue, which can safely be ignored. If possible, the defect created by the partial nephrectomy is closed by suturing the kidney upon itself to further ensure a watertight repair. Autotransplantation into the iliac fossa is then effected with urinary continuity restored by ureteroneocystostomy or pyeloureterostomy.

Editorial Comment
Fray F. Marshall

This chapter beautifully summarizes the multitude of options available for renal or renal arterial reconstruction. In general, autologous material is preferred. Consideration of the use of the epigastric vessels is a helpful addition to the reconstruction of very small renal arterial branches.

REFERENCES

1. Straffon RA, Siegel DF. Saphenous vein bypass graft in the treatment of renovascular hypertension. Urol Clin North Am 2:337, 1975.
2. Dean RH, Wilson JP, Burko H, et al. Saphenous vein aortorenal bypass grafts: Serial arteriography study. Ann Surg 80:469, 1974.
3. Ernst CB, Stanley JC, Marshall FF, Fry WJ. Autogenous saphenous vein aortorenal grafts: A 10-year experience. Arch Surg 105:855, 1972.
4. Novick AC, Ziegelbaum M, Vidt DG, et al. Trends in surgical revascularization for renal artery disease: Ten years' experience. JAMA 257:498, 1987.
5. Novick AC, Stewart BH, Straffon RA. Autogenous arterial grafts in the treatment of renal artery stenosis. J Urol 118:919, 1977.
6. Wylie EJ. Endarterectomy and autogenous arterial grafts in the surgical treatment of stenosing lesions of the renal artery. Urol Clin North Am 2:351, 1975.
7. Khauli RB, Novick AC, Coseriu GV. Renal revascularization with polytetrafluoroethylene graft. Cleve Clin Q 51:365, 1984.
8. Streem SB, Novick AC. Aortorenal bypass with a branched saphenous vein graft for in situ repair of multiple segmental renal arteries. Surg Gynecol Obstet 155:855, 1982.
9. Novick AC. Microvascular reconstruction of complex branch renal artery disease. Urol Clin North Am 11:465, 1984.
10. Kaufman JJ. Renal autotransplantation and ex vivo surgery for renovascular hypertension. Urol Clin North Am 6:295, 1979.
11. Salvatierra O, Olcott C, Stoney RJ. Ex vivo renal artery reconstruction using perfusion preservation. J Urol 119:16, 1978.
12. Novick AC. Partial nephrectomy for renal cell carcinoma. Urol Clin North Am 14:419, 1987.
13. Novick AC, Streem SB, Montie JE, et al. Conservative surgery for renal cell carcinoma: A single center experience in 100 patients. J Urol 141:835, 1989.
14. Novick AC. Renal hypothermia: In vivo and ex vivo. Urol Clin North Am 10:637, 1983.
15. Novick AC. Management of intrarenal branch arterial lesions with extracorporeal microvascular reconstruction and autotransplantation. J Urol 126:150, 1981.
16. Novick AC. Use of inferior epigastric artery for extracorporeal microvascular branch renal artery reconstruction. Surgery 89:513, 1981.

Chapter 37

Renal Transplantation and Autotransplantation

Arthur I. Sagalowsky

Renal Transplantation

INDICATIONS

Currently, over 80,000 people in the United States are enrolled in the end-stage renal disease (ESRD) program. Dialysis and renal transplantation are the two forms of renal replacement therapy. The major causes of renal failure are glomerulonephritis, hypertension, and diabetes mellitus; obstructive uropathy, ureterovesical reflux, and congenital renal disorders are also important.[1] Early transplantation is considered in some diabetic or pediatric patients with severe renal insufficiency prior to actual ESRD.

Renal transplantation offers optimal management of ESRD with regard to the degree of renal function, patient rehabilitation, and quality of life. For pediatric patients with renal failure, growth potential is better with transplantation than with dialysis. Patient survival is higher for diabetics after successful renal transplantation compared with dialysis. Overall patient survival for ESRD patients is at least equivalent for transplantation and dialysis, as the morbidity and mortality rates of renal transplantation have declined.

PREOPERATIVE MANAGEMENT

The extensive ongoing management problems of patients with ESRD are beyond the scope of this chapter. The causes of renal failure directly or indirectly produce chronic volume overload, hypertension, anemia, and secondary hyperparathyroidism as renal function deteriorates. Diabetic or uremic neuropathy are also often present. Patients with renal failure have a high incidence of cardiovascular and peripheral vascular disease. Optimal management of

each of these problems by the nephrologist renders the patient a safer candidate for transplantation. Age alone and diabetes mellitus are no longer exclusions. Infants and patients 60 years of age and over may undergo transplantation with acceptable risks and good results. Although diabetics suffer lower graft survival than nondiabetics, patient survival remains similar and is superior to that of diabetics who remain on dialysis.

Active acid-peptic disease of the gastrointestinal tract must be treated or excluded to minimize risks of ulceration and bleeding after transplantation. Current immunosuppressive regimens utilizing cyclosporine and lower doses of corticosteroids are decreasing the risk from peptic ulcer disease in transplantation.

Patients with angina, and all diabetic patients, would benefit from formal cardiology consultation as part of the pretransplant work-up. There is no agreement on the optimal use of treadmill and thallium scan stress tests, or coronary angiography, for patients who are awaiting transplantation.

The status of the urinary tract demands special attention. Most patients with ESRD do not require bilateral nephrectomy before transplantation. The kidneys provide some degree of volume control and erythropoietin production, which lessens the anemia of chronic renal failure. Uncontrollable malignant hypertension, marked ureteral reflux and urinary infection, and massive polycystic kidneys that have recurring hemorrhage into the cysts or that physically fill the iliac fossa are all infrequent reasons for pretransplant bilateral nephrectomy. Patients with hematuria from the upper tract and with acquired cystic renal disease should undergo nephrectomy because of the risk of renal cell carcinoma developing in these end-stage kidneys. Laparoscopic nephrectomy is possible in some cases. Small end-stage kidneys resulting from glomerulonephritis are particularly well suited to a laparoscopic or retroperitoneal endoscopic approach. The availability of recombinant erythropoietin lessens the consequences of bilateral nephrectomy. Bladder function should be evaluated with a voiding cystourethrogram. Knowledge of bladder function and rehabilitation allows for renal transplantation with urinary drainage into the bladder in nearly all cases.

Cadaver renal transplantation, unlike living renal donor transplantation, is invariably an unscheduled event dependent on organ availability. However, one should not lose sight of the concept that even cadaveric renal replacement (unlike liver or heart transplantation, which is lifesaving and without back-up) is an elective or semielective procedure. Although minimal renal preservation time is desirable, some prolongation is tolerable if it allows stabilization (e.g., dialysis) of the recipient before surgery. Cadaver recipient evaluation just before transplantation is quite simple if careful pretransplant procedures are followed. The patient's cardiopulmonary status, fluid volume, serum potassium level, blood count, and liver enzyme concentrations should all be stable. The presence of any active infection must be excluded before transplantation. A central venous catheter is placed in all patients for pressure monitoring of fluid status. Diabetic recipients receive a continuous glucose infusion and an adjustable insulin infusion, described in detail elsewhere, to maintain steady serum glucose levels perioperatively.[1] Preoperative parenteral broad-spectrum antibiotics are given for gram-positive and gram-negative coverage.

TREATMENT OPTIONS

The major options concern immunosuppressive strategies for recipient preparation and postoperative management. The roles of recipient blood transfusions, histocompatibility testing between donor and recipient, and various combinations and sequences of the immunosuppressive drugs cyclosporine, azathioprine, antithymocyte preparations (polyclonal ATG, monoclonal OKT), and prednisone have been reviewed.[1] New agents with specific immunosuppressive actions on the cellular and/or humeral components of the immune response and antigen recognition complex are in various stages of preclinical and clinical testing. Rapamycin (Sirolimus), brequinar, anti-Cd45 monoclonal antibody, and a mycophenolic acid derivative RS-61445 are but a few of these newer agents. Another important option is the choice between a living donor source (related or unrelated) and a cadaveric source of the kidney. Improved results for cadaveric renal transplantation have renewed the

philosophical and ethical issues regarding donor nephrectomy from a healthy individual. However, the long-term safety and very low morbidity of donor nephrectomy remains intact. Moreover, the graft survival for living donor transplants continues to exceed that of cadaveric allografts. The increasing demand for transplantation makes cadaveric kidneys an ever more scarce resource. The growing disparity between cadaver kidney availability and the size of the transplant waiting list are cause for a broader interest in living unrelated kidney donation from a so-called "emotionally related" donor. The donor safety record and the high transplant success rate in these cases justifies this approach in fully informed individuals.

OPERATIVE TECHNIQUE

The patient is positioned supine with slight table flexion to aid the exposure of the iliac fossa (Fig. 37–1A). A straight or curved skin incision is made in either lower quadrant. The external oblique, internal oblique, and transversalis muscle layers are incised. A portion of the rectus muscle and fascia is incised to release tension medially and allow access to the bladder. A 3- to 4-cm division of external oblique muscle at the upper end of the incision is generally adequate. The entire incision may be extended to the tip of the twelfth rib when necessary. The muscles should be divided at least 2 fingerbreadths above the iliac crest to avoid difficulty in closing the lower edge of the wound over the allograft. The inferior epigastric vessels are ligated and divided, as is the round ligament in women. In men the spermatic cord is mobilized and preserved unless previous surgery and scarring hinder exposure and require division of this structure. The peritoneum is mobilized superomedially to complete the exposure of the iliac fossa. With a Bookwalter retractor the peritoneal contents, bladder, and abdominal wall may be retracted as shown, leaving the surgeon's and assistant's hands completely free (Figs. 37–1 and 37–2).

A small hole cut in the center of a laparotomy pad allows the renal artery and vein to be exposed while the kidney remains packed in ice slush (not shown). The renal vein is anastomosed end to side to the external iliac vein with running 5-0 vascular Prolene suture (Fig. 37–3A). With a single renal artery and a healthy recipient hypogastric artery, an end-to-end spatulated anastomosis is performed with running 6-0 vascular Prolene suture (Fig. 37–3B and C). If the donor renal artery is small, if the two renal arteries are close together, or if the recipient hypogastric artery is unsuitable, arterial anastomosis of a Carrel patch of donor aorta end to side to the external or common iliac artery is performed (Fig. 37–4A). Alternatively, multiple renal arteries may be joined side to

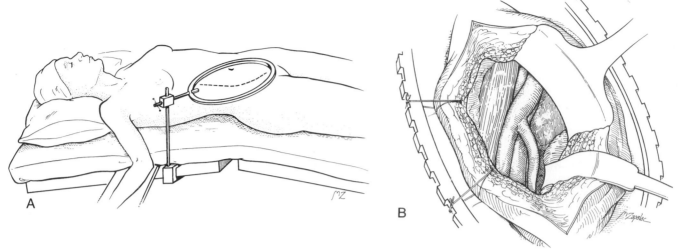

Figure 37–1. *A*, The patient is positioned with the iliac crest just below the break in the table so that table flexion aids exposure during placement of the kidney, and returning the table to a neutral position aids wound closure. *B*, Generally a broad malleable blade and a deeper Harrington blade for the Bookwalter retractor are adequate to retract the peritoneum and bladder, respectively. The lateral body wall is sutured to the ring retractor to complete the exposure. Avoiding the use of retractor blades laterally prevents possible traction injury to the pelvic nerves and facilitates performing the vascular anastomoses.

side to form one common lumen (Fig. 37–4*B*), or the smaller renal artery may be anastomosed end to side into the larger renal artery (not shown).

The ureter is sewn to the bladder via a tunneled, nonrefluxing anastomosis with 4-0 and 5-0 chromic sutures. An intravesical technique allows a tunneled reimplant along the bladder floor with the orifice situated near the trigone (Fig. 37–5). The anterior cystotomy is closed in three layers with 4-0 chromic suture on the mucosa and 3-0 chromic suture on the muscular and seromuscular layers.

Many transplant surgeons prefer an extravesical approach to ureteral reimplantation (Fig. 37–6). Barry and Hatch[2] modified this approach by creating a tunnel that connects two parallel incisions through bladder serosa and muscularis rather than making a longitudinal trough. After considerable experience with both intra- and extravesical techniques, I believe the

Figure 37–2. View into the right iliac fossa after exposure is completed. No hand-held retraction is necessary. The vessel loop is around the external iliac artery, and the bulldog clamp is on the divided internal iliac artery. The external iliac vein is deeper and medial to the external iliac artery.

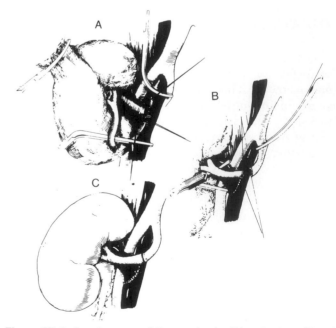

Figure 37–3. Anastomoses of the renal vein *(A)* and artery *(B and C)* are shown.

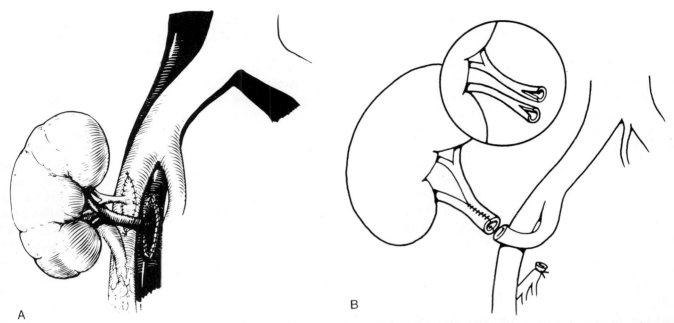

Figure 37–4. *A,* A patch of donor aorta is used for end-to-side arterial anastomosis. When possible the arterial and venous anastomoses should be separated rather than overlying one another. *B,* The side-to-side method of joining double renal arteries.

extravesical trough technique shown in Figure 37–6 is at least equally successful, quicker, and easier and is accompanied by less postoperative hematuria and bladder discomfort than is seen with the intravesical implant. The extravesical reimplant is also ideal when only a short length of ureter is available.

At the completion of all the anastomoses, the kidney is positioned in the iliac fossa so that neither the vessels nor the ureter is twisted. The table is returned to a flat position to release tension on the wound edges. The muscle layers are closed with running 0 polydioxanone (PDS) suture. The subcutaneous tissue is approximated with polyglycolic acid suture and the skin closed with staples. Drains are not used routinely. If required, a closed suction drain is brought through a separate stab wound.

Close communication between the anesthesiologist and transplant surgeon is mandatory during the procedure. Large doses of muscle relaxants for the necessary operative exposure are not required. Atracurium (Tracrium), a nondepolarizing muscle relaxant that hydrolyzes over 30 to 45 minutes independent of renal function, is the agent of choice for a patient with renal failure. Nevertheless, the recipient is invariably hypothermic (from ice slush in the wound) and acidotic at the conclusion of the procedure. Extu-

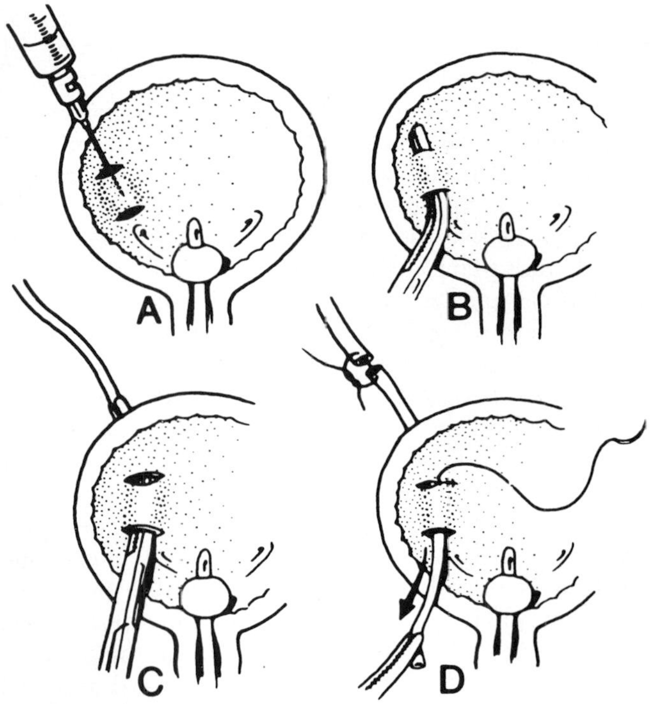

Figure 37–5. *A* to *D,* A modified Leadbetter-Politano intravesical ureteral reimplant may be performed.

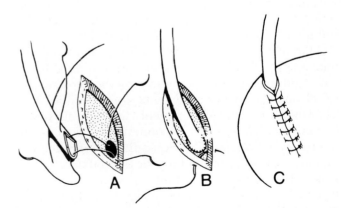

Figure 37–6. *A* to *C,* An extravesical, tunneled, nonrefluxing ureteral reimplant is performed most often.

bation should be performed cautiously and only after the patient exhibits sustained neuromuscular control for several minutes. Central venous pressure (CVP) monitoring is helpful in assessing the large intraoperative fluid needs.

The usual fluid replacement during renal transplantation includes 40 to 50 ml/kg of crystalloids and 1.0 to 1.5 gm/kg of albumin. Blood transfusion is used more selectively than in the past owing to better baseline hematocrit levels in renal failure patients taking erythropoietin, concerns over inducing recipient sensitization, and the risks of transmissible infectious diseases. The typical replacement volumes in a 70-kg patient are 2 units of packed red blood cells, 3500 to 4000 ml of crystalloids, 70 to 95 gm of albumin, and 25 gm of mannitol. In studies at our institution, Dawidson and coworkers[3] showed that liberal colloid and crystalloid replacement, as described, results in the highest immediate graft function rates and correlates with the ultimate graft and patient survival.

In diabetic patients the glucose-insulin infusion described above greatly stabilizes the perioperative course. However, insulin infusion in an unconscious patient requires careful serial monitoring of blood glucose levels. The glucose-insulin infusions should be separate from the main intravenous access for blood and fluid administration and CVP monitoring to minimize the chances of error.

POSTOPERATIVE MANAGEMENT AND COMPLICATIONS

This discussion considers only those events directly related to the surgical procedure and immediate postoperative care. Patients are ambulatory within 1 day of surgery and are able to resume oral intake as soon as they feel able, also generally within 1 day. In diabetic recipients the glucose-insulin infusions are continued until they take their usual daily insulin dose and eat a meal. The bladder catheter is removed within 36 to 48 hours in patients with intravesical reimplants, or in 7 days in patients with extravesical reimplants or marked bladder abnormalities.

Significant perioperative bleeding requires a systematic approach. Clinical monitoring of blood pressure and pulse rate, palpation of the wound, and serial hematocrit measurements are the initial steps as in any postoperative patient. Inability to sustain hemodynamics and blood counts with transfusions, or obvious evidence of an expanding wound, requires urgent re-exploration. Venous or arterial anastomotic leak is the first consideration. Bleeding from uncontrolled hilar vessels may occur as the kidney warms and renal vascular resistance decreases, even though the kidney may have appeared hemostatic at the time

of wound closure. Sudden hemorrhage from a renal allograft rupture may occur rarely as a result of swelling from hyperacute or acute rejection or from acute tubular necrosis.

Venous complications of anastomotic bleeding or thrombosis are rare. Arterial anastomotic bleeding 1 to 2 weeks postoperatively almost always represents infection of the suture line. Although resection and reanastomosis may succeed, nephrectomy is the safest course. Transplant renal artery stenosis should be considered in patients with severe hypertension or declining allograft function that is not explained by rejection. Transplant renal artery stenosis has been the subject of a comprehensive review.[4] Transplant renal artery stenosis is usually due to postanastomotic narrowing from chronic rejection rather than to faulty suture technique at the anastomosis. The preferred management is percutaneous dilation, with surgery reserved for the failures with this approach.

Wound infections fortunately are very rare in renal transplant recipients when preoperative antibiotics are given; drains are not used routinely. Superficial wound infections respond to prompt drainage, wound care, and antibiotics. However, subfascial infections in the immunocompromised renal transplant recipient may require nephrectomy or carry a significant mortality risk.

Urinary complications after transplantation can be divided into leaks, obstructions, and infections. Urinary leak is the most serious problem and requires urgent treatment. Swelling over the scrotum or labia on the side of the allograft, and a complaint by the patient of a burning or tearing sensation along the groin with urination, are valuable clinical signs of urinary leak. Sonography allows early detection of fluid around the kidney.

Bladder leak along the cystotomy is confirmed by cystography. It should be very rare in the absence of severe infection, but when it occurs it is best treated by prompt re-exploration and repair.

Ureteral leak at the site of anastomosis in an extravesical reimplant usually responds to prolonged bladder catheterization. A ureteral leak above the level of either type of reimplant is a much more serious problem, usually resulting from ischemic necrosis of a segment of ureter. In my experience, prompt exploration, ureteral debridement with proximal closure, and nephrostomy drainage allow the patient to stabilize. Secondary ureteropyelostomy connecting the native ureter to the allograft renal pelvis is the definitive repair of choice. Ureteral obstruction is usually due to ischemic fibrosis of the distal reimplant. Retrograde pyelography and placement of a ureteral stent are diagnostic and therapeutic when possible. More often, however, ureteral obstruction is diagnosed on ultrasonography and treated initially by percutaneous nephrostomy. Balloon dilation, prolonged double-J catheter drainage, and open repair are also options for correction of a transplant ureteral stenosis.

Lymphocele may occur from disrupted lymphatics along the iliac vessels. A small lymphocele is quite commonly detected on ultrasonography and requires no treatment. Symptomatic lymphoceles (not necessarily larger) may produce ureteral obstruction, extrinsic compression of the iliac vein, and ipsilateral lymphedema of the lower extremity. Infection may complicate a lymphocele acutely or chronically. Lymphocele is confirmed and distinguished from uri-

nary leak by needle aspiration and measurement of fluid urea, creatinine, and potassium content compared with serum content. Percutaneous catheter drainage is the preferred initial treatment. Persisting or recurrent lymphocele requires more definitive treatment. Surgical creation of a large window between the lymphocele wall and the peritoneal cavity is the technique of choice. In recent years this procedure has been accomplished by laparoscopic rather than open surgery. External surgical drainage is usually reserved for patients with an infected lymphocele.

Renal Autotransplantation

INDICATIONS

Renal cell carcinoma (RCC) in patients with bilateral tumors (Fig. 37–7), tumor in a solitary kidney (Fig. 37–8A), or tumor with a poorly functioning contralateral kidney are the main indications for radical nephrectomy, bench surgery tumor excision, and remnant renal autotransplantation. Transitional cell carcinoma (TCC) of the upper urinary tract or complex ureteral strictures may be rare indications for the procedure. The procedure is formidable and should be performed only when in situ treatment is impossible. Increased understanding of the requisites for hypothermic renal preservation and refined surgical techniques allow an increasing number of such

tumors to be managed in situ. Thus, the actual number of cases treated by autotransplantation should be few.

PREOPERATIVE MANAGEMENT

The most important aspect of preoperative management for renal autotransplantation is a thorough discussion of the procedure. First, the physician must know the relative risk of the procedure, the natural history of the disease, and the dialysis-related risks. For example, in an elderly patient with extensive low-grade TCC of the renal pelvis that has been present for years in a solitary kidney, the risks of total nephrectomy and chronic dialysis may exceed the risk of no treatment. The unknown factor is when or if the tumor may spread. Such thinking is difficult for surgeons and patients alike. Patients must be made aware of the risk of tumor spillage or recurrence in the renal remnant. They must be prepared for the possibility that intraoperative hemorrhage may require permanent nephrectomy and long-term dialysis. Permanent dialysis must be psychologically acceptable to the patient before any of the surgical alternatives are attempted. Renal autotransplantation often requires temporary dialysis until the kidney resumes function. Therefore, a preoperative nephrology consultation is wise.

The mandatory imaging studies are computed tomography (CT) or magnetic resonance imaging (MRI) and angiography. CT or MRI reveals the true intrarenal depth and extent of the tumor. Deep tumor penetration near the hilum of the kidney is what ultimately requires bench surgery rather than in situ partial nephrectomy (Figs. 37–7 and 37–8A). Large tumors near the surface of the kidney may be treated by in situ partial nephrectomy. However, in situ re-

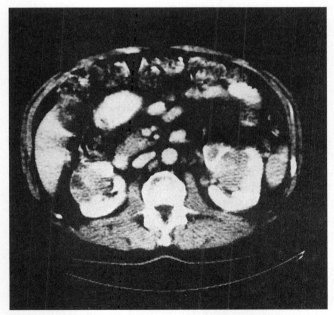

Figure 37–7. Contrast-enhanced computed tomographic scan of a patient with large bilateral renal cell carcinomas. Note the deep penetration by the tumors near the renal hilum.

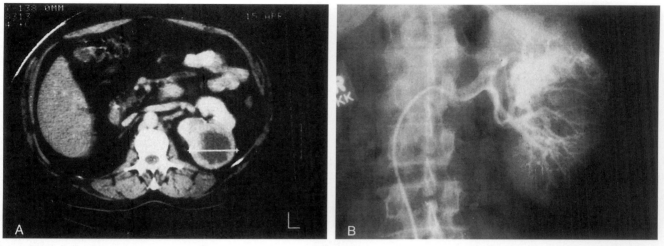

Figure 37–8. *A,* A large renal tumor penetrates deep into the renal hilum in a patient with a solitary kidney. *B,* Arteriogram demonstrates extreme tumor hypervascularity with upper and lower renal artery branches feeding the tumor.

pair of the multitude of divided veins near the center of the kidney may not be possible in a small but deep tumor. Neither an excretory urogram nor an angiogram provides this three-dimensional information. Angiography reveals the number of renal arteries and the extent of tumor supply by arterial branches (Fig. 37–8*B*). Preoperative knowledge of the number of renal arteries is essential for rapid clamping and kidney removal and cooling as in donor nephrectomy.

The serum creatinine level in these patients, after the necessary contrast-enhanced imaging studies, should be at or near baseline values before proceeding with surgery. Preoperative volume expansion with intravenous fluids and mannitol are given the night before surgery. The option for autologous blood storage is discussed in advance with the patient.

SURGICAL OPTIONS

The point needs repeating that any lesion amenable to in situ repair should not be considered for autotransplantation. For RCC, radical nephrectomy and long-term dialysis or subsequent renal transplantation are options. The overall annual patient mortality risk for hemodialysis is 10 to 15 percent. The risk of activating micrometastases with immunosuppression for transplantation is real but unquantified. The risk of unrecognized residual tumor in the kidney is approximately 8 percent. The risk of multiple tumor recurrences after partial nephrectomy for familial RCC in von Hippel-Lindau disease is higher than previously recognized. Many of these patients are better served by total nephrectomy.

For TCC of the renal pelvis, endourological percutaneous tumor resection and nephrostomy instillation of chemotherapy are other options besides open surgical excision and autotransplantation. Here the risks of tumor spillage and wound implantation should be very real in view of historical experience of wound implantation after open surgery. However, endourological treatment of TCC in solitary kidneys is increasingly popular at this time.

Ileal ureteral interposition is preferable to autotransplantation for most complex ureteral strictures that cannot be repaired by lesser procedures.

OPERATIVE TECHNIQUE

The patient is positioned supine with the break in the table just below the lower edge of the rib cage (Fig. 37–9). Elevation of the kidney rest and table flexion allow increased exposure. An anterior subcostal incision extending 4 to 5 cm beyond the midline provides excellent exposure for the nephrectomy. The incision may be extended to a full chevron if necessary. In a thin individual the upper transverse incision may also provide exposure into the iliac fossa for the autotransplantation. Usually, however, a lower quadrant standard transplant incision is made. A single vertical midline incision from xyphoid to pubis is rapid but is less than ideal for either nephrectomy or autotransplantation. The two-incision approach allows extraperitoneal placement of the autotransplant and provides a degree of tamponade to localize and minimize postoperative bleeding from the kidney.

The kidney is approached just as in a live donor nephrectomy, except that all of Gerota's fascia and the perinephric fat are removed as in a radical nephrectomy. The adrenal gland may be preserved if the contralateral adrenal gland is absent. During the dissection, rotational torque of the kidney should be avoided to prevent intrarenal vasospasm and mini-

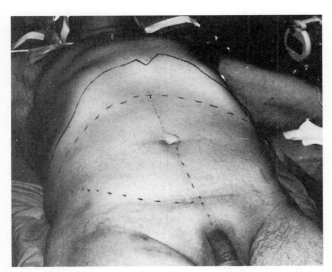

Figure 37–9. The patient is supine and the table is flexed after the kidney rest is elevated. The rib margin and xyphoid are shown by the solid line. An extended subcostal or chevron incision provides excellent exposure for the nephrectomy. When necessary the autotransplant is performed through a separate lower quadrant, standard transplant incision. Alternatively, the entire procedure may be performed through a midline incision.

mize the risk of tumor dissemination. The renal vessels are isolated with vessel loops and dissected free of adjacent tissue. The patient is systemically heparinized after the kidney is entirely mobilized and the renal vessels are isolated.

The ureter and gonadal vessels are ligated and divided in the pelvis below the level of the iliac artery bifurcation. A maximal length of renal artery and vein should be included with the specimen to facilitate autotransplantation. The renal artery is ligated near its origin from the aorta with two 0 silk ties. The renal vein is occluded with a Satinsky vascular clamp placed on the lateral vena cava for right-sided tumors, or across the renal vein distal to the insertion of the inferior adrenal vein for left-sided tumors. If the renal vein is simply ligated, the vein ends pucker and the length of renal vein left with the specimen will be less than anticipated.

As soon as the renal vessels are divided, the kidney is removed and placed promptly into ice slush (Fig. 37–10). Next, the renal vein stump is closed with running 5-0 vascular Prolene suture. An assistant closes the upper abdominal wound while the surgeon perfuses the kidney on the back table.

The kidney remains packed in slush the entire duration of the ex vivo dissection. First, all remaining blood is flushed out by instilling chilled intracellular- or extracellular-type electrolyte solution via a cannula in the renal artery. For the relatively short time of ex vivo preservation, extracellular fluids are adequate, unlike the case in cadaveric organ storage.

Gerota's fascia and perinephric fat are stripped away from the renal capsule from the normal portion of the kidney and are left attached to the tumor-bearing portion. Uninvolved areas of Gerota's fascia and perinephric fat are preserved with the kidney to aid hemostasis and renal closure. A circumferential incision through the renal capsule is made with a scalpel blade, leaving a 4- to 5-mm rim of normal renal parenchyma around the tumor. The blunt end of the scalpel handle is used to dissect through the parenchyma. The fibrous pseudocapsule characteristic of RCC facilitates complete removal of the intact tumor. Frozen-section examination of the surgical margins is obtained to exclude residual tumor.

Major intrarenal vessels are ligated with 4-0 chromic suture as they are encountered during the dissection (Fig. 37–11A). Early intrarenal venous tumor thrombi may be seen and extracted in continuity with the tumor (Fig. 37–11B). Openings in the collecting system are closed with running 4-0 chromic suture. The time-consuming portion of the surgery involves securing hemostasis by suture ligating severed intrarenal vessels with figure of-eight sutures of 4-0 chromic suture on an RB-1 needle (Fig. 37–12A). Continued perfusion through a renal artery cannula is extremely helpful in identifying major leak points in a controlled bloodless field. After maximal intrarenal hemostasis is achieved, the parenchyma is folded on itself and the edges of the renal capsule are closed with running 3-0 chromic suture (Fig. 37–12B). This step is crucial in limiting blood loss and is far more effective than placing perinephric fat into the parenchymal defect. The argon beam laser may be used for the intrarenal dissection and to assist with hemostasis. However, this technique is very slow and prolongs the preservation time. The laser should be

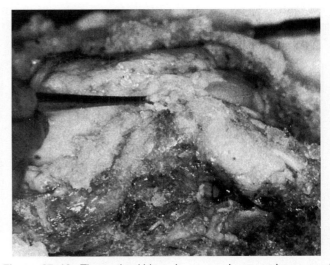

Figure 37–10. The entire kidney is removed, preserving a good length of renal artery and renal vein, as in donor nephrectomy, and Gerota's fascia and all the perinephric fat attached, as in radical nephrectomy. The adrenal is preserved unless it is grossly involved with tumor. The forceps points to the tumor. Gerota's fascia and perinephric fat remain attached during tumor excision.

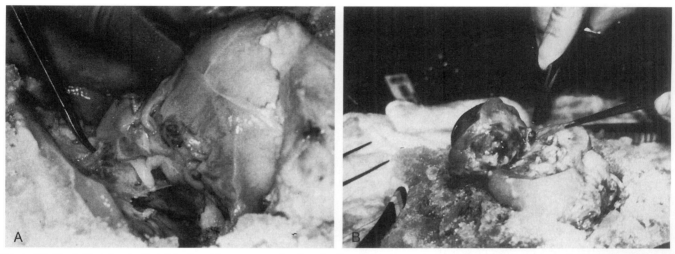

Figure 37–11. *A,* Bleeding is diminished and the process of suture ligating divided vessels minimized if major intrarenal vascular branches are secured when encountered. *B,* Occasionally an intrarenal venous tumor thrombus is encountered and removed without difficulty.

viewed as a supplement but not a replacement for meticulous suturing technique as described above.

Next, the renal vessels are prepared for autotransplantation (Fig. 37–13). The patient remains systemically heparinized during this portion of the surgery. The renal vein is anastomosed end to side to the external iliac vein with running 5-0 Prolene suture (Fig. 37–14*A*). The renal artery is anastomosed end to side to the external or common iliac artery with running or interrupted 5-0 or 6-0 Prolene suture (Fig. 37–14*B*). Compression is held over the kidney, and the venous and arterial clamps are released. The patient's blood pressure and volume status are crucial at this time. Once the need for reclamping is excluded, the patient receives protamine sulfate intravenously for 5 to 10 minutes to reverse anticoagulation. When hemostasis is adequate, end-to-end ureteroureterostomy with 5-0 chromic suture over a soft, double-J indwelling stent is performed. A flat suction drain is placed in the iliac fossa and brought out through a separate stab wound. The wound is closed in layers with 0 PDS suture.

POSTOPERATIVE MANAGEMENT AND COMPLICATIONS

These procedures are often 8 to 12 hours in duration. Intraoperative blood and fluid requirements may be large. At the same time, the patient must be considered functionally anephric. Careful hemodynamic and laboratory monitoring is therefore essential during and after surgery. The large, raw parenchymal surface may hemorrhage in the early postoperative period. Serial renal ultrasound and radionuclide scans are helpful in confirming renal blood flow, assessing excretory function, and following the extent of any bleeding. Patients often require hemodialysis

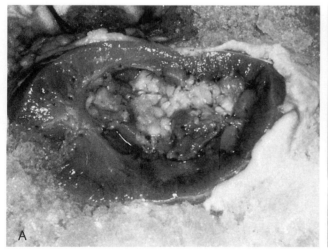
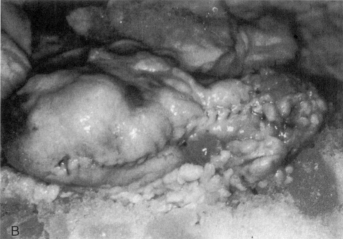

Figure 37–12. *A,* After the tumor is excised the collecting system and the multitude of divided vessels must be secured with absorbable sutures. *B,* Next the parenchymal edges are folded and the renal capsule is closed as completely as possible.

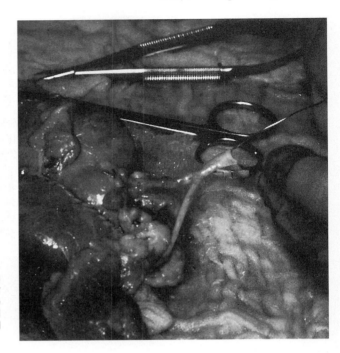

Figure 37–13. The renal vessels are prepared for reanastomosis. In this patient the lower pole renal artery was too far from the main renal artery and the discrepancy in size too great for side-to-side reconstruction. The small, lower pole artery was anastomosed end to side to the main renal artery with interrupted 6-0 and 7-0 vascular Prolene sutures with the aid of loupe magnification.

for several weeks after renal autotransplantation. A Quinton subclavian dual-access catheter provides temporary vascular access. The drain is removed as soon as perioperative bleeding subsides and provided that no evidence of urinary extravasation is found. The ureteral stent is removed cystoscopically 6 weeks after surgery.

Summary

Renal transplantation offers the best available treatment of ESRD in an increasing number of patients. The surgical technique is standardized and has low complication rates. Allograft and patient survival are improving steadily with modern immuno-suppressive regimens. Renal autotransplantation is a formidable procedure that offers renal-sparing tumor surgery for a highly selected group of patients with compromised overall renal function.

Editorial Comment
Fray F. Marshall

As the population in the United States ages, patients with renal failure will become more numerous. Dramatically improved quality of life is possible with a successful renal transplantation as opposed to dialysis. The question of pretransplant nephrectomy in chronic renal failure often arises. Acquired renal cystic disease with the potential for associated renal cell carcinoma is being recognized with greater frequency. This disease appears to be partly a function of time on dialysis, so that careful investigation of all patients before transplantation is important.

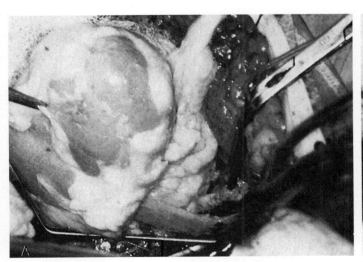

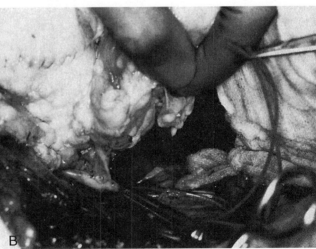

Figure 37–14. The renal vein *(A)* and renal artery *(B)* are anastomosed to the external iliac vessels.

Later renal artery stenosis is associated with chronic rejection. I have often thought that late stenosis of the ureter may also be associated with chronic rejection because the distal end of the ureter may be most susceptible to microvascular injury from the effects of this rejection. If operative repair is required, ureteropyelostomy is frequently an excellent solution.

Bench surgery and renal autotransplantation have been used less often in recent years. An extensive intrarenal dissection can sometimes be performed in situ, but there still may be times when renovascular reconstructions or other extenuating circumstances warrant autotransplantation. As pointed out, the argon beam may be helpful for small vessel bleeding but should not be used to control bleeding from larger vessels. MRI or spiral CT can sometimes demonstrate the proximal renal arterial tree but do not provide sufficient detail for intrarenal surgery.

REFERENCES

1. Sagalowsky AI, Helderman JH, Peters PC. Renal transplantation. In Gillenwater J, ed. Adult and Pediatric Urology, 2nd ed. Chicago, Year Book, 1991, pp 815–852.
2. Barry J, Hatch DA. Parallel incision, unstented extravesical ureteroneocystostomy: Follow-up of 203 kidney transplants. J Urol 134:249, 1985.
3. Dawidson I, Sagalowsky A, Peters P, Reisch J. Intraoperative colloid infusion affects the outcome after cadaveric kidney transplantation. Presented at the Fourth World Congress for Microcirculation, Japanese Society for Microcirculation, Tokyo, Japan, July 26–Aug 2, 1987.
4. Sagalowsky AI, McQuitty DM. The assessment and management of renal vascular hypertension following kidney transplantation. Semin Urol 12:211, 1994.

Chapter 38

Celiac Axis for Renal Revascularization: Splenorenal and Hepatorenal Arterial Bypass Procedures

John A. Libertino

The original description of the hepatic artery[1] for renal revascularization and the notion of alternative forms of renal revascularization[2] were received with skepticism when originally described by the author in the mid-1970s and early 1980s. These were originally conceived as alternative or bail-out procedures in atherosclerotic patients with a troublesome aorta: an alternative to the gold standard, the aortorenal saphenous vein bypass graft. Although the use of these procedures was initially very controversial, today the use of the celiac axis for renal revascularization is so successful on a global basis that it has replaced the standard aortorenal saphenous vein bypass graft. Currently the hepatorenal and splenorenal bypass grafts have emerged as the bypass procedures of choice for atherosclerotic patients requiring renal revascularization.[3-6]

INDICATIONS

Generally, corrective surgery for renovascular hypertension should be considered in a patient who has significant diastolic hypertension secondary to a functionally significant renal artery lesion and who is a reasonable surgical risk. Specifically, patients with the following manifestations of renovascular hypertension are clearly candidates for surgical intervention: (1) poor control of hypertension after aggressive antihypertensive therapy, (2) poor compliance, (3) total renal artery occlusion or dissection, (4) deterioration of renal function as manifested by an ele-

vation of either blood urea nitrogen or creatinine concentration, (5) pyelographic evidence of renal parenchymal loss, (6) angiographic evidence of progressive renal artery disease, (7) severely symptomatic or accelerated hypertension, (8) anuria from arterial occlusion in a solitary kidney, or (9) any combination of these factors.[1]

The type of pathologic entity and its natural history also influence my judgment as to the indication for operation. Because of the natural history of atherosclerosis, it seems advisable to operate on patients who are good risks and who have recent onset of hypertension and a functionally significant unilateral lesion. Patients with long-standing hypertension, evidence of disseminated atherosclerosis, and bilateral disease are poor risks. Surgery should be advised only when uncontrollable hypertension persists, arterial obstruction progresses, or renal function deteriorates.

The celiac axis as an arterial inflow source is especially useful in patients with diffuse aortic atherosclerotic disease.

In patients with mural dysplasia, balloon angioplasty is the first order of treatment. Those who fail to respond to balloon angioplasty are candidates for renal revascularization.

PREOPERATIVE AND INTRAOPERATIVE MANAGEMENT

Patients with renovascular hypertension may present with the complex problems of systemic atherosclerosis and the widespread effects of hypertension on the vasculature of other organs. Careful preoperative recording of all distal arterial pulses and bruits in all extremities and in the neck should be performed to obtain baseline values. If cerebrovascular or cardiac disease is suspected or if there is a history of stroke, transient ischemic episode, or angina, cerebral or coronary angiography should be undertaken. Significant obstructive lesions should be repaired before a major renal arterial reconstructive procedure is attempted. The perfusion pressure of the heart and brain may be reduced significantly after successful renal revascularization, with decreased blood pressure possibly resulting in stroke or myocardial injury.[7]

Antihypertensive drugs infrequently used now, such as guanethidine sulfate (Ismelin) and reserpine, which deplete catecholamine stores in the nerve end plates, are discontinued 2 weeks before surgery to avoid hypotensive episodes during the operative procedure. Hypokalemia from secondary hyperaldosteronism or long-term diuretic use should be corrected before operation to avoid the potentiating effects of anesthetic agents. Urinary tract infections should be resolved completely before surgery. An episode of acute pyelonephritis should be treated for a minimum of 3 weeks before any major surgical procedure is considered. Patients with severe hypertension are given an effective, safe, short-acting drug up until the time of operation, because such agents usually do not deplete the epinephrine or norepinephrine content of the nerve end plates.

To protect the already somewhat impaired renal parenchyma from the effects of ischemia, dopamine, mannitol, or furosemide (Lasix) is given approximately 2 hours before the renal vessels are clamped. Mannitol or renal-dose dopamine is continued throughout the procedure, during which the urinary output and central venous pressures are monitored every 15 minutes. Systemic anticoagulation is carried out routinely. Doses of 3000 to 5000 U heparin are administered intravenously 30 minutes before clamping of the renal vessels, celiac vessels, or aorta. Without heparinization, thrombi may form proximal to the vascular clamps, with possible embolization to the kidneys or lower extremities when the clamps are removed. Thromboembolism is even more critical when microvascular surgery is performed on 2- to 3-mm secondary to tertiary branch arteries, in which anastomotic patency is even more dependent on adequate heparinization.

Many individuals with renovascular hypertension present with complex problems and often are older, high-risk surgical patients who require intraoperative monitoring of cardiac output and pulmonary artery and wedge pressures. Therefore, these patients require preoperative placement of a Swan-Ganz catheter in addition to central venous pressure monitoring.

SURGICAL EXPOSURE OF RENAL VESSELS

The patient is placed in the supine position with the arms at the sides. A Foley catheter is introduced into the bladder to monitor urinary output. The skin of the chest, abdomen, and legs is prepared and draped so that both lower extremities, as well as the abdomen and lower part of the chest, are exposed. This method of draping also provides a field for saphenous vein procurement. The feet are wrapped in sterile Lahey intestinal bags so that they can be observed carefully during the procedure. This permits access to the lower arterial tree so that the color of the leg and distal pulses can be assessed during operation if embolization of the atherosclerotic plaque should occur. I have also employed Doppler monitoring to evaluate pedal pulses intraoperatively and postoperatively.

The type of incision used to approach the renal vasculature is of great importance in safely facilitating dissection and subsequent technical maneuvers. Although a midline vertical incision may be useful in some situations, it is not, in my opinion, the best incision for renal artery exposure. A transverse upper abdominal incision from the lateral border of the contralateral rectus muscle, extending across the midline into the ipsilateral flank between the eleventh and twelfth ribs, provides more adequate access to the high-lying retroperitoneal aortorenal junctions and their covering veins, and greater technical freedom (Fig. 38–1).

After the abdominal cavity is investigated carefully and all adhesions are lysed, the small intestine is packed in a Lahey bag or in a warm, moist pad and retracted away from the site of the repair. The renal vessels are best exposed by reflection of the colon. The right colon is mobilized by entering the retroperitoneal space through an incision in the lateral peritoneal gutter along the white line of Toldt. The peritoneum is incised around the cecum up to the ligament of Treitz. The hepatic flexure and proximal transverse colon are detached from the hepatic peritoneal ligaments.

The avascular space between the colonic mesentery and the anterior surface of Gerota's fascia is entered without opening the fascia. The lateral duodenal attachments are incised and the second and third portions of the duodenum mobilized. The right renal vein and inferior vena cava are exposed. The right colon, small bowel, and duodenum are retracted upward and medially, permitting an approach to both renal veins, the aorta, and the infrahepatic portion of

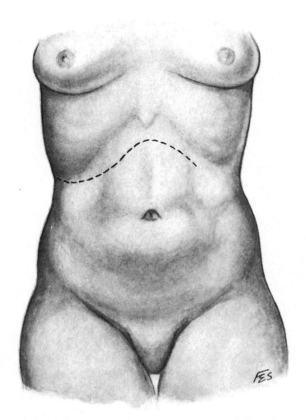

Figure 38–1. Transverse incision for adequate exposure of right renal vasculature from the tip of the eleventh rib to the lateral border of the left rectus muscle. (From Zinman L, Libertino JA. Renovascular hypertension. In Libertino JA, Zinman L, eds. Reconstructive Urologic Surgery: Pediatric and Adult. Baltimore, Williams & Wilkins, 1977.)

spleen, because splenectomy and its attendant rise in platelet count may cause hypercoagulability.

The extent of dissection depends largely on the type of reconstructive procedure selected. A bypass technique requires less exposure of the more hazardous suprarenal portion of the aorta, whereas transaortic endarterectomy requires control of the suprarenal aorta. The renal veins and inferior vena cava are the first structures to be mobilized for exposure of the renal artery. The adrenal and gonadal veins are divided and ligated on the left side, along with any posterior lumbar tributaries. Two or three pairs of posterior lumbar veins and the right gonadal veins are divided to facilitate mobilization of the vena cava and exposure of the right renal artery. The vena cava is retracted laterally and the left renal vein upward to expose the origin of the right renal artery (Fig. 38–4). Arterial tapes are placed around the renal veins so that they can be retracted into optimal positions for access to the proximal and distal main renal arterial circulation. The artery can be localized by palpation after the vein is retracted. The renal artery should be dissected out by incising the enveloping nerves and lymphatics and very gently retracting the renal vein with smooth Silastic vessel loops to prevent spasm and injury to the fragile thin wall of the vein.

the inferior vena cava (Fig. 38–2). This maneuver may also be performed initially when bilateral renal artery lesions are repaired, because it permits wide exposure of the origin of both renal arteries. However, there are few indications for bilateral repair. In general, it is neither advisable nor my practice to carry out simultaneous bilateral renal artery reconstructions because of the higher morbidity and mortality associated with these procedures.

For dissection of the left renal vasculature, left descending colon, splenic flexure, and distal half of the transverse colon are mobilized by first incising the peritoneal reflection along the lateral descending colon (Fig. 38–3A). The spleen is protected by first dividing the gastrocolic ligament and extending the incision laterally into the avascular space toward the splenocolic attachments, which are divided last. The splenic flexure is retracted downward and medially, exposing the left renal vein, perihilar fat, adrenal gland, and distal portion of the pancreas (Fig. 38–3B). The spleen is retracted with a covering protective abdominal pad. The kidney is not mobilized from its bed in order that collateral circulation, which affords protection during long ischemic clamping time, is not disturbed. Great care is taken not to injure the

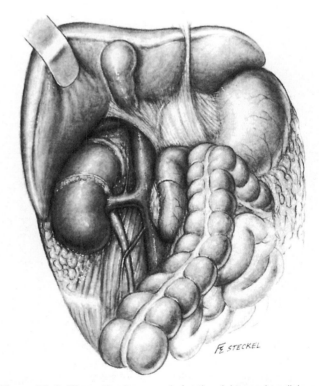

Figure 38–2. The optimal approach for the right renal pedicle and aorta is the paracolic exposure with medical retraction of the right colon, duodenum, and small bowel. (From Zinman L, Libertino JA. Renovascular hypertension. In Libertino JA, Zinman L, eds. Reconstructive Urologic Surgery: Pediatric and Adult. Baltimore, Williams & Wilkins, 1977.)

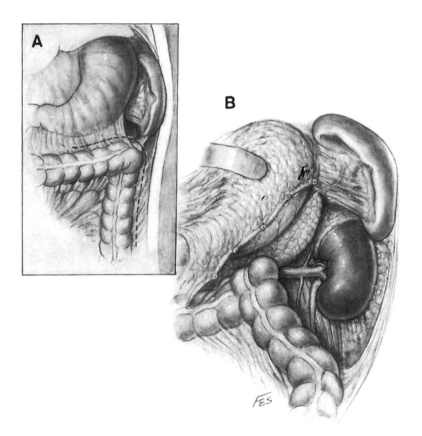

Figure 38–3. *A,* The left gastrocolic, phrenocolic, and lateral peritoneal attachments are divided to release and retract the splenic flexure and descending colon to expose the left renal vein and underlying renal artery. *B,* The stomach, pancreas, and spleen are gently retracted upward without mobilizing the kidney. (From Zinman L, Libertino JA. Renovascular hypertension. In Libertino JA, Zinman L, eds. Reconstructive Urologic Surgery: Pediatric and Adult. Baltimore, Williams & Wilkins, 1977.)

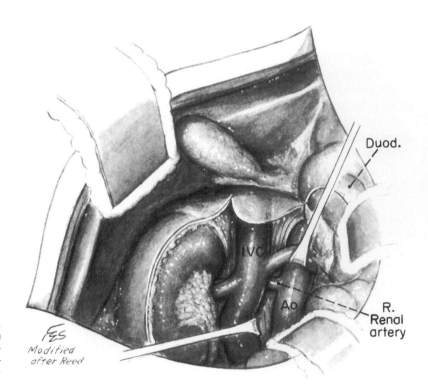

Figure 38–4. Surgical exposure of the right renal artery. Note the retrocaval course of the right renal artery. (From Libertino JA, Zinman L. Surgery for renovascular hypertension. In Breslin JA, Swinton NW Jr, Libertino JA, Zinman L, eds. Renovascular Hypertension. Baltimore, Williams & Wilkins, 1982.)

Splenorenal Arterial Bypass

In a patient who has stenosis of the left renal artery, the use of splenorenal arterial bypass as a substitute for aortorenal saphenous vein bypass is associated with many desirable features. This technique is particularly well suited to patients who have diffuse atherosclerosis or thrombosis of the aortic lumen and to patients who have undergone previous difficult reconstructive operations on the aorta.[2] The splenic artery has the advantage of being an autogenous artery that has not been separated from its nutrient vasa vasorum, is exposed easily by a relatively uncomplicated anatomical dissection, and requires only one vascular anastomosis.

Carefully monitored oblique and lateral angiography of the celiac axis is required to help determine the patency of the splenic artery, because atherosclerosis can affect the lumen early in a patient's life. Surgical exploration and intraoperative evaluation by palpation and measurement of the splenic blood flow are needed to establish the suitability of the splenic artery for renal revascularization. If the blood flow is diminished, the splenic artery should not be used as a source for renal bypass.

The splenic artery is exposed through a routine transverse incision with extension into the distal portion of the eleventh rib after the posterior rib cage is elevated 10 degrees off the operating table, or through a supracostal eleventh rib flank approach (Fig. 38–5). The splenic flexure and upper descending colon are mobilized and retracted medially. The renal vein is identified, the gonadal and adrenal branches are ligated and divided, and the renal vein is retracted caudally (Fig. 38–6). The renal artery is exposed and tapes are placed proximally and distally. The lesser sac is exposed widely by separating the gastrocolic omentum to the point of the midtransverse colon. The splenic artery can be identified by palpation and dissection at the superior border of the tail of the pancreas. The pancreas is retracted upward, and the splenic artery is mobilized and encircled with Silastic tape. Through careful dissection, the entire extrapancreatic portion of the artery is mobilized. To avoid traumatic or ischemic injury to the pancreatic tail, several of the pancreatic branches of the splenic artery are preserved.

Blood flow is measured with an electromagnetic flowmeter. The artery is divided just proximal to its primary division in the hilum of the spleen after a Lorenz vascular clamp is applied to the proximal portion. Removal of the spleen is not necessary, because adequate blood flow continues to reach it from the short gastric arteries. The pulsating full splenic artery with its distal clamp is brought under the pancreas to the renal artery and is measured so that the exact position and appropriate length for anastomosis can be determined.

Some anatomical variations in the position of the pancreas and splenic vessels have been observed. The splenic artery may be located directly anterior or parallel to the renal vessels or even caudal to the midportion of the kidney. This location makes the anastomosis less difficult to perform. The position of the splenic artery may occasionally be more cephalad and require more dissection from the pancreas than is usually necessary to obtain proper arterial length. The end of the splenic artery is divided. The renal

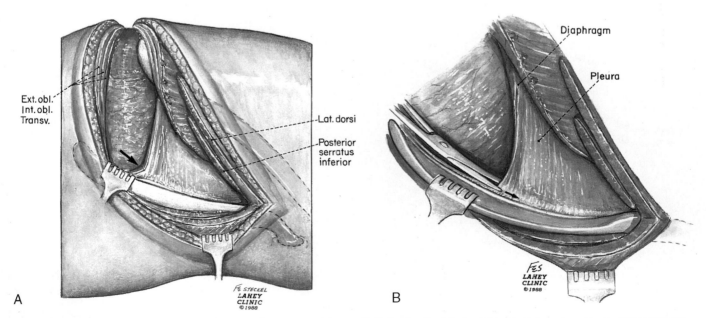

Figure 38–5. *A,* Relationship of flank musculature to the supracostal area. *B,* Following the intercostal nerve to remain extrapleural back to the intercostal ligament. (Courtesy of the Lahey Clinic, 1988.)

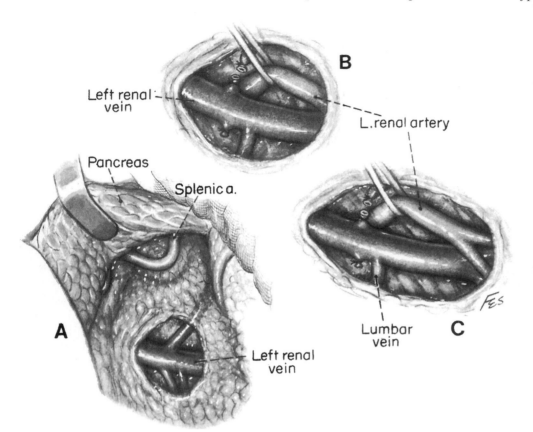

Figure 38–6. *A*, Dissection of the left renal vessels and identification of the splenic artery inferior to the tail of the pancreas for splenorenal arterial bypass. *B* and *C*, Gonadal and adrenal veins are divided to allow retraction of the left renal vein for exposure of the renal artery. (From Zinman L, Libertino JA. Renovascular hypertension. In Libertino JA, Zinman L, eds. Reconstructive Urologic Surgery: Pediatric and Adult. Baltimore, Williams & Wilkins, 1977.)

artery is divided and an end-to-end anastomosis carried out (Fig. 38–7). In certain situations, such as a patient undergoing reoperation, an end-to-side anastomosis from the splenic to the renal artery may be more appropriate. The decision to perform either an end-to-side or an end-to-end anastomosis depends on the anatomical situation the surgeon is presented with at the time of the procedure.

If sufficient arterial length has not been achieved, an interpositional saphenous vein graft with an end-to-end renal artery anastomosis is performed after the kidney is completely mobilized. This maneuver usually permits the surgeon to perform splenorenal arterial bypass without tension on the suture line. When the pancreas is dissected extensively or when injury to the tail of the pancreas is suspected, the

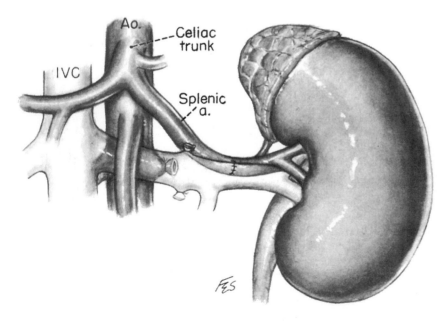

Figure 38–7. Completed end-to-end splenorenal anastomosis. (From Libertino JA, Zinman L. Surgery for renovascular hypertension. In Breslin JA, Swinton NW Jr, Libertino JA, Zinman L, eds. Renovascular Hypertension. Baltimore, Williams & Wilkins, 1982.)

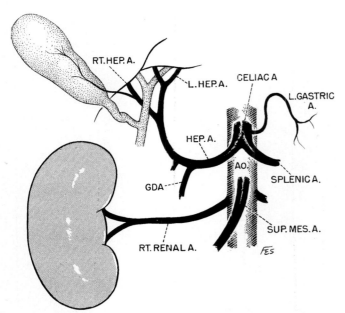

Figure 38–8. The most common pattern of hepatic artery circulation, with the common hepatic dividing into the right and left hepatic arteries, which supply the corresponding lobes of the liver. GDA, gastroduodenal artery.

retroperitoneal space is drained for 10 days to prevent the serious complications of pancreatic leakage. Some surgeons prefer to resect the distal end of the pancreas when ischemic or traumatic injury is suspected.

Splenic artery disease, an inherent risk of pancreatitis, and formation of a pancreatic pseudocyst are some of the limitations that have restricted the use of the splenic artery for left renal artery revascularization.

Hepatorenal Arterial Bypass

Previous aortic surgery, extensive atherosclerosis, and complete thrombosis of the aorta may preclude the use of aortorenal bypass for the treatment of renovascular hypertension. When the surgeon is confronted with stenosis or occlusion of the right renal artery in association with these pathological limitations of the aorta, a hepatorenal saphenous vein bypass procedure can be utilized.[1] In our extensive series of surgically treated patients at Lahey Clinic, I have had to resort to this procedure in approximately 75 patients.

The hepatic artery arises from the celiac axis and courses along the upper border of the pancreas. When it reaches the portal vein, it divides into an ascending and a descending limb. The ascending limb is a continuation of the main artery upward within the lesser omentum, and lies in front of the portal vein and to the left of the biliary tree. The descending limb forms the gastroduodenal artery. In the porta hepatis the

hepatic artery ends by dividing into the right and left hepatic arteries, which supply the corresponding lobes of the liver (Fig. 38–8).

The anatomical variations of the hepatic circulation should be appreciated before this procedure is employed. The right hepatic artery is more variable than the left. It may be anterior (24 percent) or posterior (9 percent) to the portal vein. In addition, the left hepatic artery arises from the left gastric artery in 11.5 percent of patients (Fig. 38–9).

Hepatorenal arterial bypass requires careful dissection of the porta hepatis with exposure of the common hepatic, gastroduodenal, and right and left hepatic arteries before any anastomotic procedure is attempted. Arterial tapes are placed around each of these vessels, and the common bile duct and portal vein are identified. After careful dissection and mobilization of the right renal artery, a Lorenz clamp is placed on the proximal portion of the common hepatic artery and its distal branches. The gastroduodenal artery is divided and ligated (Fig. 38–10). An arteriotomy 10 to 12 mm in length is made at the site of the origin of the gastroduodenal artery. A reverse saphenous vein graft is inserted end to side to the hepatic arteriotomy with 6-0 continuous Prolene sutures.

When this anastomosis is completed, a microvascular clamp is placed on the vein graft after filling it with heparin and obtaining the proper alignment and length for the renal artery anastomosis. The Lorenz clamps are then removed from the hepatic artery and one clamp is placed on the distal end of the renal artery. The origin of the renal artery is ligated and

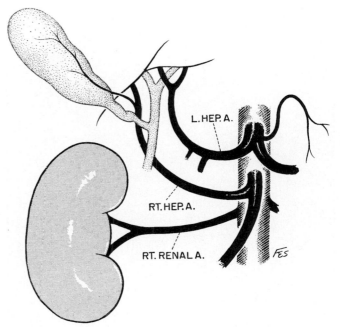

Figure 38–9. The most common variation in the hepatic circulation is to have the right hepatic artery arise from the superior artery.

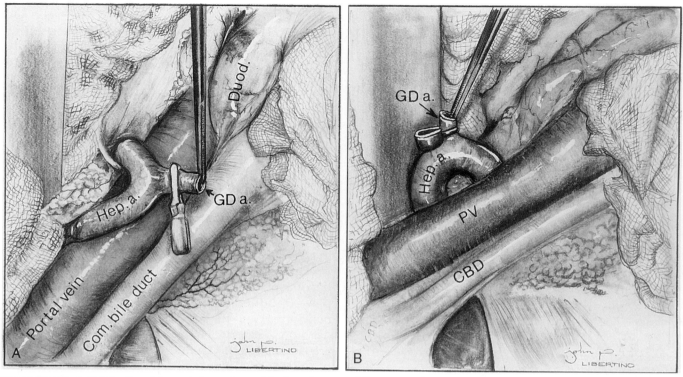

Figure 38–10. *A,* Mobilization of the anterior surface of the hepatic artery. GD a., gastroduodenal artery. *B,* Mobilization of the posterior surface of the common hepatic artery. PV, portal vein; CBD, common bile duct.

the vein graft is anastomosed to the renal artery end to end, again using interrupted 6-0 Prolene sutures (Fig. 38–11). On rare occasions, an end-to-side anastomosis to the renal artery may be performed instead of a direct end-to-end anastomosis (Fig. 38–12).

The hepatic circulation is unique in that it is a portal system with portal venous and hepatic arterial inflow. The liver receives approximately 28 percent of the cardiac output (1500 ml/min) in resting adults, 80 percent through the portal vein and 20 percent

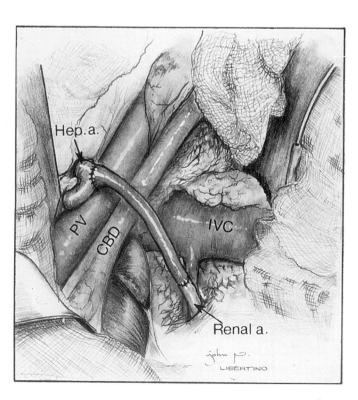

Figure 38–11. Hepatic-to-renal artery saphenous vein bypass graft. IVC, inferior vena cava.

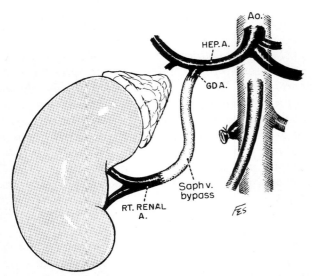

Figure 38–12. End-to-side gastroduodenal renal bypass graft. (From Libertino JA, Zinman L. Surgery for renovascular hypertension. In Breslin JA, Swinton NW Jr, Libertino JA, Zinman L, eds. Renovascular Hypertension. Baltimore, Williams & Wilkins, 1982.)

through the hepatic artery. The flow through the hepatic artery averages approximately 300 ml/min, an amount certainly sufficient to maintain renal circulation adequately. In fact, the mean pressure in the hepatic artery branches as they converge on the liver is approximately 90 mm Hg. According to the curve that describes renal circulatory autoregulation, when the kidney is perfused at pressures of 90 to 250 mm Hg, the renal vascular resistance varies with pressure so that a relatively constant renal blood flow is maintained. Therefore, the hepatic circulation has the proper flow and pressure profile to maintain renal circulation adequately.

In addition, the hepatic circulation has the added benefit of a vast collateral circulation, which protects the liver from injury should the bypass graft thrombose and the clot propagate into the hepatic circulation. The saphenous vein graft has occluded several times in my experience without retrograde clotting of the hepatic circulation. Total hepatic artery ligation is not only compatible with life but is also commonly used in conjunction with chemotherapy to treat hepatic malignant disease. Hepatic arterial collateral circulation follows four major pathways: intercalary arteries, translobar collateral arteries, inferior phrenic arteries, and gastric and pancreaticoduodenal collateral arteries.[8]

Hepatic arterial flow may be reconstituted safely distal to a ligated hepatic artery up to 10 hours after interruption of blood flow. When the right or left hepatic artery adjacent to the liver is interrupted, the translobar collateral vessels will reconstitute flow. When the common hepatic artery is ligated, the major rearterialization channels are the inferior phrenic and the gastroduodenal arteries. Because intrahepatic ar-

teries are not end arteries and interruption of the arterial flow to the liver is followed by rapid rearterialization of the lobe or segment, the hepatic circulation is uniquely qualified for this bypass procedure. Postoperative angiography in patients who have undergone hepatorenal arterial bypass has demonstrated the absence of a renal hepatic steal syndrome, and liver function has not been compromised in any of my patients to date.

POSTOPERATIVE MANAGEMENT AND COMPLICATIONS

Thrombosis and hemorrhage are the two potential problems inherent in any vascular procedure. Serious bleeding from a disrupted anastomosis is fortunately a rare event and is usually associated with approximation of diseased vessels and errors in surgical technique. Polypropylene sutures in renal and aortic anastomoses have helped to avoid bleeding at the suture line in the presence of systemic heparinization.

Bleeding may occur during the first 24 hours from perihilar collateral vessels, which attain significant size with high-grade renal artery stenosis. Unrecognized venous bleeding from adrenal vessels can also occur during and after a difficult left renal artery dissection, because the adrenal gland may be adherent to the anterior portion of the renal vein, renal artery, and perihilar tissue. In my experience, this bleeding has occurred on two occasions and demands gentle handling of adrenal vessels with compulsory hemostasis during dissection.

False aneurysms may also occur in any vascular anastomosis, including the renal arteries.[9] These sometimes result in intermittent delayed bleeding into the gastrointestinal tract or the retroperitoneal space. This complication is minimized by paying meticulous attention to anastomotic details, avoiding silk sutures, and using an end-to-end or end-to-side tension-free graft to normal undiseased parts of the renal artery.

Late bleeding from an aortoduodenal erosion fistula after a prosthetic bypass graft has been reported.[10] Intestinal hemorrhage is more common with prosthetic replacements when silk sutures have been selected for the anastomosis. Delayed bleeding with erosion of the third portion of the duodenum has accounted for most of these instances, and has been reduced with the use of autogenous graft material and synthetic sutures and interposition of peritoneum or omentum between the graft and duodenum.

The most prevalent postoperative complication of renal artery surgery is graft or renal artery thrombosis. This is more common after renal artery bypass with a Dacron prosthesis or renal endarterectomy. Thrombosis usually occurs early in the postoperative period and may be difficult to detect in an end-to-side anastomosis when the kidney is perfused through its primary vessel. Factors that may predispose the patient to thrombosis are porous Dacron grafts of small caliber; atrophy of the kidney with a thin-walled, diseased main renal artery and high intrarenal resistance; coincidental splenectomy with hypercoagulable sequelae; and any significant hypotension or hypovolemia in the postoperative period. Normal rapid-sequence intravenous pyelography cannot ensure a patent graft. Therefore, when severe unexplained hypertension persists after operation, digital subtraction angiography is required to determine the patency of the graft.

If the celiac axis is not usable, aortic thrombosis and distal extremity embolization from aortic plaque dislodgment and cholesterol microembolization are uncommon but extremely ominous complications that may occur at the time of aortic clamping or unclamping. Systemic heparinization will aid in prevention, but the groin and lower extremities should be prepared and in the operative field of view so that the color of the lower legs and distal pulses can be assessed after aortic unclamping.

The surgeon should be more acutely aware of the possibility of this complication when operating on a patient with a diffusely atherosclerotic aorta and a compromised iliofemoral circulation. When this event is suspected, aortic thromboendarterectomy and femoral artery embolectomy should be performed, followed by careful, monitored heparinization. In patients who experience cholesterol microemboli, papaverine hydrochloride, systemic heparinization, and fasciotomy may be of help. When small vessels such as digital arteries are involved, amputation may be required. These complications are usually avoided by use of the celiac axis for renal revascularization.

Aneurysmal dilation of the autogenous saphenous vein graft and internal iliac artery bypass graft has been shown to occur on late angiographic follow-up studies.[11] Most of these studies demonstrate a uniform increase in the diameter throughout the entire length of the graft, with a few frank aneurysms noted. Several patients have been referred to me with vein graft dilations. Re-evaluation with posterior and oblique angiography showed narrowing of the distal renal artery anastomoses. Although this is speculative, the stenosis of the renal suture line may cause aneurysmal dilation of the graft proximal to the stenosis because of high-pressure aortic inflow. No one as yet has reported the rupture of such a vein graft, and patients thus far have remained normotensive with good renal function. Autologous hypogastric artery appears to be superior in this respect, with less dilation seen on long-term study.

Summary

At the Lahey Clinic we have performed nearly 500 surgical procedures for the treatment of renovascular hypertension. More than 250 of these revascularization procedures were accomplished using the celiac axis, i.e., the splenic or hepatic arterial bypass procedure as the arterial inflow source for renal revascularization. Seventy-five patients underwent hepatic-to–right renal artery bypass procedures, and 175 patients splenorenal arterial bypasses, for left renal artery stenosis or occlusion. The operative mortality rate was 2.8 percent. Six postoperative graft thromboses (5.5 percent) occurred.

Using the criteria described by Kaufman,[12] an analysis was made of patients who underwent these procedures for the treatment of hypertension and who were followed for a minimum of 1 year. The cure and improvement rate was 86.3 percent. Only 13.7 percent of patients failed to obtain any benefit from renal artery revascularization.

I believe these results demonstrate that, when surgeons are confronted with difficult or troublesome aortas, the use of the celiac axis is preferable to an aortorenal bypass graft for the treatment of renovascular hypertension and the stabilization of deteriorating renal function resulting from renal artery stenosis or occlusion in the atherosclerotic patient population.

Editorial Comment
Fray F. Marshall

This chapter accurately describes the primary use of autogenous vessels in reconstruction of the right renal artery (hepatorenal arterial reconstruction) and left renal artery (splenorenal arterial reconstruction). Although these patients are not commonly seen by most urologists, Dr. Libertino's excellent results confirm his careful, technical approach to such high-risk patients.

REFERENCES

1. Libertino JA, Zinman L, Breslin DJ, Swinton NW Jr. Hepatorenal artery bypass in the management of renovascular hypertension. J Urol 115:369, 1976.
2. Libertino JA, Selman FJ Jr. Alternatives to aortorenal revascularization. J Cardiovasc Surg 23:318, 1982.
3. Libertino JA. Renovascular surgery. In Walsh PC, Retik AB, Stamey TA, Vaughan ED Jr, eds. Campbell's Urology, 6th ed. Philadelphia, WB Saunders, 1992, p 2521.
4. Chibaro EA, Libertino JA, Novick AC. Use of the hepatic circulation for renal revascularization. Ann Surg 199:406, 1984.
5. Libertino JA, Lagneau P. A new method of revascularization of the right renal artery by the gastroduodenal artery. Surg Gynecol Obstet 156:220, 1983.
6. Libertino JA, Flam TA, Zinman L. Changing concepts in the surgical management of renovascular hypertension. Arch Intern Med 148:357, 1988.
7. Javid H, Ostermiller WE, Hengesh JW, et al. Carotid endarterectomy for asymptomatic patients. Arch Surg 102:389, 1979.

8. Mays ET, Wheeler CS. Demonstration of collateral arterial flow after interruption of hepatic arteries in man. N Engl J Med 290:993, 1974.

9. Nerstrom B, Engell HC. Operative treatment of renovascular hypertension: A study of 60 consecutive patients with followup findings between 1 and 7 years postoperatively. Ann Surg 176:590, 1972.

10. Cerny JC, Fry WJ, Gambee J, Koyangyi T. Aortoduodenal fistula. J Urol 107:12, 1972.

11. Stanley JC, Ernst CB, Fry WJ. Fate of 100 aortorenal vein grafts: Characteristics of late graft expansion, aneurysmal dilatation, and stenosis. Surgery 74:931, 1973.

12. Kaufman JJ. Long-term results of aortorenal Dacron grafts in the treatment of renal artery stenosis. J Urol 111:298, 1974.

Part III

SURGERY OF THE RETROPERITONEUM AND URETER

Chapter 39

Idiopathic Retroperitoneal Fibrosis: Ureterolysis

Herbert Lepor

Idiopathic retroperitoneal fibrosis (IRPF) describes a fibrotic process of unknown etiology that is commonly associated with ureteral obstruction.[1] Retroperitoneal fibrosis is usually limited to the region between the renal hilus and sacral promontory. IRPF has been reported in patients ranging in age between 5 and 85 years,[2] and it most commonly occurs in the fifth and sixth decades of life. The male-to-female incidence ratio is approximately 3:1.

The symptoms commonly associated with IRPF are nonspecific. Pain is a presenting complaint in approximately 80 percent of cases,[2] usually localized to the abdomen, back, or flank. The pain is usually insidious at onset, commonly dull, and noncolicky. Other associated presenting symptoms include weight loss, nonspecific gastrointestinal symptoms, anorexia, fever, and anuria. The physical examination is usually unrevealing.

Retroperitoneal fibrosis has been associated with primary and metastatic malignancies; retroperitoneal injury secondary to hemorrhage, trauma, and radiation; regional enteritis and diverticulitis; infectious agents of urinary tract infection and histoplasmosis; and drugs, most notably methysergide.[2] The diagnosis of IRPF implies the absence of these processes. The preoperative assessment is designed to identify any malignant process, define the extent of the fibrosis, and assess renal function. The primary objectives of surgical intervention are establishing the cause of the fibrosis and relieving the ureteral obstruction.

Every effort should be made to preserve renal parenchyma, because IRPF has the propensity to be bilateral and progressive.

PREOPERATIVE MANAGEMENT

A patient with IRPF may present with this condition in association with anuria, chronic renal insufficiency, and severe anemia. Anemia, renal insufficiency, and electrolyte imbalance should be corrected preoperatively.

Compromised renal function and nonspecific abdominal, back, or flank pain are the features of IRPF that lead to a radiographical evaluation of the urinary tract. The renal function should be assessed before obtaining any imaging studies requiring the administration of iodinated contrast agents. A renal sonogram is the preferred imaging study in the presence of renal compromise. An intravenous pyelogram may reveal the classical findings of retroperitoneal fibrosis that include bilateral ureteral narrowing at the level of the fourth and fifth lumbar vertebrae in approximately 74 percent of cases.[3] An abdominal computed tomographic (CT) scan should be obtained to further evaluate the findings of hydroureteronephrosis demonstrated on renal ultrasonography or intravenous pyelography. The extent of the retroperitoneal fibrosis is accurately assessed by the abdominal CT scan.[4] Bilateral retrograde pyelograms are obtained to fur-

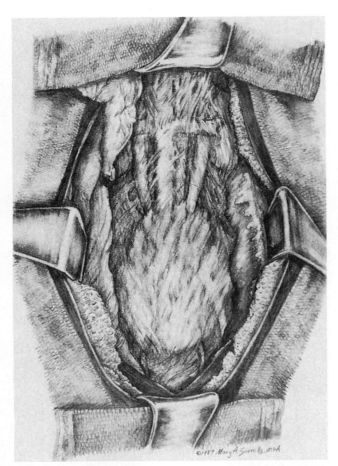

Figure 39–1. The retroperitoneum is exposed through a midline incision extending from the xyphoid to the pubic symphysis. The ileum is packed, out of the operative field, and exposure is facilitated by use of a ring retractor. The fibrotic process commonly involves the distal aorta, vena cava, iliac vessels, and midportions of the ureters. Fibrosis appears as a glistening, grayish-white, woody-hard fibrous plaque.

ther assess the extent of ureteral involvement and exclude the possibility of an intrinsic obstruction. A renal radionuclide scan may be useful for assessing relative renal function.

Retroperitoneal fibrosis has been associated with retroperitoneal lymphomas, sarcomas, and metastatic carcinomas of the breast, colon, pancreas, stomach, lung, and kidney, and with carcinoid tumor.[2] The preoperative assessment should be directed toward the exclusion of these processes.

Surgical exploration should be temporarily deferred if there is evidence of reversible renal insufficiency. Renal insufficiency may resolve after administration of high doses of steroids.[5] Renal function is likely to improve after placement of indwelling double-J ureteral stenting catheters. A nonfunctioning kidney associated with a thin rim of renal cortex should be temporarily decompressed with a nephrostomy tube. The return of renal function can be assessed by measuring the differential creatinine clearance rates. A nephrectomy may be considered if the

creatinine clearance after decompression remains less than 5 to 10 ml/min.

OPERATIVE TECHNIQUE

The patient should be brought to the operating room well hydrated. A formal bowel preparation is usually not performed. Preoperative antibiotics are administered according to the personal preferences of the physician.

General endotracheal anesthesia is employed, and a Foley catheter and nasogastric tube are placed. Ureteral stents are usually placed immediately before the abdominal exploration, because the catheters may facilitate identification of the ureters.

The patient is placed in the supine position and a midline incision made from the xyphoid to the pubic symphysis. The rectus fascia is incised in the midline and the peritoneum is entered. The intra-abdominal viscera are systematically inspected to identify any unsuspected malignant process. Exposure may be facilitated with a Wilkinson ring retractor. The right and left colon are mobilized and retracted medially if the retroperitoneal process is extensive. The ileum is packed out of the operative field (Fig. 39–1). The fibrosis is usually limited to the region between the renal hilus of the kidney and the sacral promontory. The aorta, vena cava, iliac vessels, and ureters are enveloped by the fibrous plaque.

The posterior peritoneum is incised over the dilated ureter as it enters the retroperitoneal process (Fig. 39–2). The incision in the posterior peritoneum is extended inferiorly along the course of the ureter. Several deep biopsy specimens are obtained from the fibrotic process and sent immediately for frozen-section diagnosis. The operative procedure continues, provided that no malignancy is encountered.

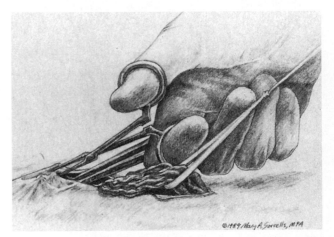

Figure 39–2. The posterior peritoneum is incised over the dilated ureter as it enters the retroperitoneal fibrotic process. The incision in the posterior peritoneum is extended inferiorly along the course of the ureter. The ureter is mobilized with sharp and blunt dissection.

The ureter proximal to the fibrotic process is isolated and encircled with a vessel loop. Mobilization of the ureter may be performed using blunt dissection with a right-angled hemostat. The plane between the ureteral adventitia and fibrotic process should develop relatively easily because the fibrotic process rarely invades the ureteral wall. The right-angled hemostat is inserted along the ureteral adventitia and the fibrotic plaque is sharply incised. The periureteral tissue is sent as another frozen-section specimen.

The lysed ureters may be intraperitonealized by reapproximating the incised posterior peritoneum behind the ureter (Fig. 39–3). The primary complication of this approach is ureteral angulation and obstruction. Alternatively, the ureter may be transposed laterally and anteriorly, interposing retroperitoneal fat

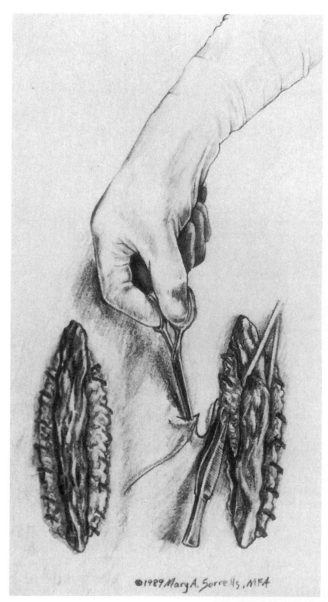

Figure 39–4. Alternatively, the ureter may be transposed laterally and anteriorly, interposing retroperitoneal fat between the ureter and the fibrotic process.

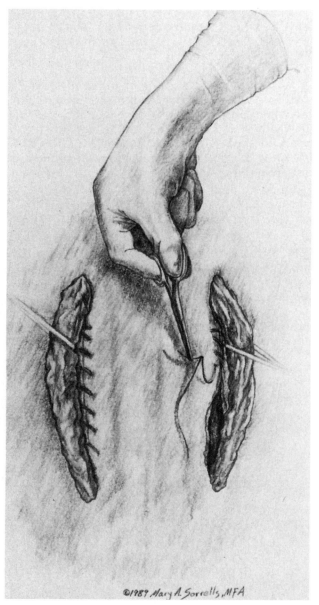

Figure 39–3. The lysed ureters may be intraperitonealized by reapproximating the incised posterior peritoneum behind the ureter.

between the ureter and the fibrotic process (Fig. 39–4). The retroperitoneal fat is sutured to the edges of the posterior peritoneum.

The best safeguard against recurrence of ureteral obstruction is to envelop the ureters in omentum. The omentum is separated from the transverse colon by sharply incising the relatively avascular connections between these structures. It is separated from the greater curvature of the stomach by dividing the short gastric vessels with 2-0 silk suture ligatures (Fig. 39–5). The omentum is divided in the midline, taking care not to ligate the gastroepiploic vessels in the middle of the arch. The two long flaps of omentum are wrapped around the ureters (Fig. 39–6) and the omentum is secured with absorbable sutures.

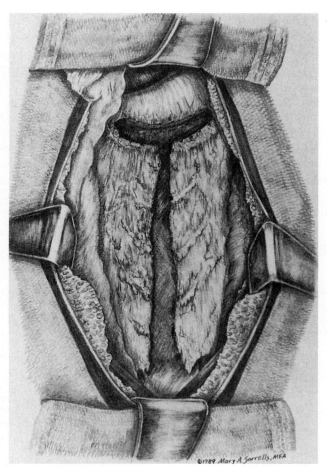

Figure 39–5. The omentum is separated from the greater curvature of the stomach by dividing the short gastric vessels. The omentum is divided in the midline.

The abdomen is closed in routine fashion. The nasogastric tube is removed after the return of bowel sounds; the Foley catheter is removed when the patient is hemodynamically stable. The ureteral stents are removed at the end of the procedure, provided that the ureter has not been inadvertently injured.

It is conceivable that the preoperative assessment did not identify an occult malignancy. An intraoperative consultation should be obtained with a medical oncologist and general surgeon if the frozen-section diagnosis reveals a malignant process. This consultation will ensure the appropriate surgical management of a nonurological malignancy. Several malignant processes are very responsive to radiation or chemotherapy. It may be inadvisable to perform a ureterolysis in a patient with such a malignancy. Ureterolysis may be the optimal management for a malignant process that is not sensitive to radiation therapy or chemotherapy.

Most cases of ureteral obstruction secondary to IRPF are managed by ureterolysis alone. Mikkelsen and Lepor reported the use of bilateral psoas hitch reimplantations and dismembered pyeloplasty for two atypical cases of IRPF.[6] Extensive IRPF may be treated with ureteral substitution using bowel segments or renal autotransplantation.[7]

STEROID THERAPY

The role of steroids in the management of IRPF is controversial, and IRPF represents an acute and a chronic inflammatory process. The acute inflammatory process appears to respond favorably to steroids. Ureteral obstruction has been observed to markedly diminish after preoperative administration of steroids.[5] Steroid therapy is not an acceptable substitute for abdominal exploration and ureterolysis because the presence or absence of a malignant process must be determined unequivocally. Steroids may be effective for stabilizing renal function, or as definitive treatment for elderly and debilitated patients who are not surgical candidates. Steroids may also be administered if the erythrocyte sedimentation rate (ESR) does not return to a normal level after ureterolysis. A persistently elevated ESR suggests that the inflammatory process is active.

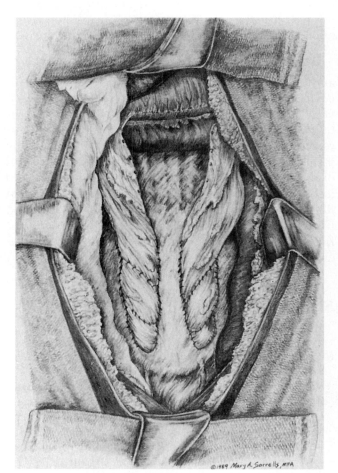

Figure 39–6. The two long flaps of omentum are wrapped around the ureters. The omentum is secured to the posterior peritoneum.

POSTOPERATIVE MANAGEMENT AND COMPLICATIONS

The ureter may be inadvertently injured during ureterolysis. A small ureteral laceration should be reapproximated with interrupted 5-0 chromic sutures. A ureteral stenting catheter should be left indwelling for approximately 10 to 14 days. A complete transection of the ureter can be managed by performing a spatulated reanastomosis with a running 5-0 chromic suture. A ureteral stenting catheter should be left indwelling approximately 14 to 21 days. The retroperitoneum is drained with a Penrose drain.

The inadvertent excision of a large segment of ureter poses a very challenging surgical dilemma. A ureteral reimplantation coupled with a psoas hitch or Boari flap may allow for a tension-free anastomosis if the ureteral injury is below the level of the bifurcation of the iliac vessels. A major ureteral injury may be managed with renal autotransplantation or substitution of the ureter with an ileal segment.

The aorta, vena cava, and iliac vessels are usually enveloped in the retroperitoneal fibrotic process. Extensive blood loss may be minimized if the proximal dilated ureter is identified and the ureterolysis performed directly over the course of the ureter. Every effort should be made to avoid dissecting in the area of the great vessels.

Early complications after abdominal exploration and ureterolysis include wound infection, ileus, atelectasis, pneumonia, pulmonary embolus, and deep vein thrombosis. Ureterolysis, with or without omental wrapping, is associated with successful long-term resolution of ureteral obstruction in approximately 90 percent of cases.[8, 9] The development of ureteral obstruction after ureterolysis may be secondary to ischemia of the ureter or progressive retroperitoneal fibrosis. A long ureteral stricture may be managed using ureteral reimplantation with a psoas hitch or Boari flap, ureteral substitution with ileum, or renal autotransplantation.

Summary

Ureterolysis, with or without omental wrapping, is the accepted treatment for ureteral obstruction secondary to IRPF. It proceeds quite uneventfully, provided that the plane between the ureteral adventitia and fibrotic process is identified. Meticulous care should be taken to preserve the blood supply to the ureter. An omental wrapping of the ureter should be performed if such a maneuver is technically feasible. Ureterolysis, with or without an omental wrap, is associated with successful long-term resolution of ureteral obstruction in approximately 90 percent of cases. Steroid therapy is not an acceptable alternative for abdominal exploration and ureterolysis because the presence or absence of a malignant process must be determined unequivocally.

Editorial Comment
Fray F. Marshall

As Dr. Lepor has emphasized, pathological diagnosis is generally indicated rather than primary treatment with steroids, as some have suggested. Omental wraps are also very helpful.

ACKNOWLEDGMENTS

The author wishes to thank Ms. Karon Hertlein for providing editorial assistance and Ms. Mary Sorrells for illustrating the operative procedure.

REFERENCES

1. Ormond JK. Bilateral ureteral obstruction due to envelopment and compression by an inflammatory retroperitoneal process. J Urol 59:1072, 1948.
2. Lepor H, Walsh PC. Idiopathic retroperitoneal fibrosis. J Urol 122:1, 1979.
3. Wagenknecht LV, Auvert J. Symptoms and diagnosis of retroperitoneal fibrosis. Analysis of 31 cases. Urol Int 26:185, 1971.
4. Krinsky S, Zieverink SE, Peterson GH, Abaskaron M. Computed tomographic diagnosis of retroperitoneal fibrosis. South Med J 76:517, 1983.
5. Arap S, Denes FT, deGroes GM. Steroid therapy in idiopathic retroperitoneal fibrosis: Report of two successful cases. Eur Urol 11:352, 1985.
6. Mikkelsen D, Lepor H. Innovative surgical management of idiopathic retroperitoneal fibrosis. J Urol 141:1192, 1989.
7. Rose MC, Novick AC, Rybka SJ. Renal autotransplantation in patients with retroperitoneal fibrosis. Cleve Clin Q 51:357, 1984.
8. Kerr WS Jr, Suby HI, Vickery J, Fraley E. Idiopathic retroperitoneal fibrosis: Clinical experiences with 15 cases, 1956–1967. J Urol 99:575, 1968.
9. Tiptaft RC, Costello AJ, Paris AMI, Blandy JP. The long-term follow-up of idiopathic retroperitoneal fibrosis. Br J Urol 54:620, 1982.

Chapter 40

Ureterocalicostomy

W. Scott McDougal

INDICATIONS

Ureterocalicostomy was first described by Neuwirt in 1947.[1] Subsequent reports by Couvelaire and associates[2] and others[3, 4] established this technique as a viable procedure for the relief of very specific types of ureteropelvic junction obstruction. A modification of the procedure has also been used as a method of exposure and repair after renal stone surgery.[5] The most common indication for ureterocalicostomy is a failed pyeloplasty associated with a small extrarenal pelvis and severe peripelvic and periureteral fibrosis. It has been my observation that a failed pyeloplasty is often associated with a rather desmoplastic peripelvic fibrotic process.[6] Urinary extravasation and urinoma formation may be etiological in the fibrotic process, but the reason for the failure of the pyeloplasty often cannot be ascertained.

There are, however, identifiable causes that result in obliteration of the proximal ureter and extrarenal pelvis. Previous stone surgery, trauma with unrecognized avulsion of the ureteropelvic junction, delayed repair of renal injuries, tuberculosis, and renal transplantation associated with ureteropelvic ischemia are a few of the disorders that may result in an obstruction at the ureteropelvic junction, which is not amenable to the standard type of repair and can be relieved only by a special type of operative technique such as ureterocalicostomy.[7, 8] This procedure may also be indicated as a primary repair for obstructed small intrarenal pelves, long proximal segment ureteral strictures with severe peripelvic fibrosis, and ureteropelvic junction obstructions in horseshoe kidneys.[9, 10]

The advantages of ureterocalicostomy are that it affords absolute dependent drainage; eliminates a large, redundant floppy pelvis, which may have poor tonus; avoids the need for isthmectomy in a horseshoe kidney, in order to obtain dependent drainage; and obviates the need for troublesome dissection around the hilum of kidneys in which extensive perirenal fibrosis has occurred. Dissection is simplified since only the lower pole needs to be free, and dissection in this area is usually accomplished without undue risk to vital structures.

PREOPERATIVE MANAGEMENT AND OPERATIVE TECHNIQUES

Preoperatively, all patients should have the urine sterilized and a mechanical bowel preparation performed. If a possibility exists of using bowel in the repair, an antibiotic bowel preparation should be added. The incision may be either flank or transabdominal. The latter is preferred if a segment of bowel is to be used. The lower pole of the kidney is mobilized. However, occasionally the length of the ureteral stricture makes it necessary to mobilize the entire kidney in order to move it caudad to juxtapose normal ureter to calix. In situations in which this maneuver is neither advisable nor possible, a segment of bowel may be used to bridge the gap between calix and ureter.

The renal capsule is incised at the inferiormost margin of the kidney and stripped back both anteriorly and posteriorly. If the pelvis can be approached, a probe is placed in the pelvis along the lower pole infundibula and out the end of its calix (Fig. 40–1). This step allows identification of the parenchyma overlying the infundibula, which is to be used for the anastomosis. It is this parenchyma that must be removed. If the incision is made along the plane of the infundibula, the lower pole segment will be resected without transection of major vessels (Fig. 40–2).

It is important to remove an adequate amount of renal parenchyma. One may occlude the main renal artery and vein during parenchymal removal; however, this is not necessary. This portion of the procedure can usually be done by careful dissection with individual ligation of vessels as they are encountered.

347

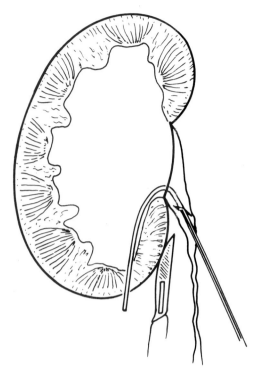

Figure 40–1. Exposure of the lower pole collecting system is facilitated by passing a probe along the lower pole infundibulum and out the parenchyma. This probe serves as a guide for parenchymal excision.

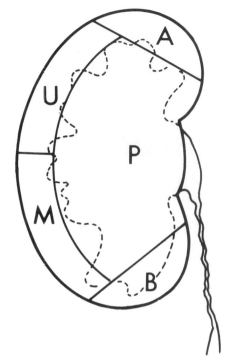

Figure 40–2. Segmental anatomy of the hydronephrotic kidney. Notice that removal of the lower pole segment exposes the calix and infundibulum without violating major vascular structures. A, apical; U, upper; P, pelvis; M, middle; B, basilar.

The plane of dissection is kept along the plane of the infundibula. The amount of parenchyma removed must be sufficient so that the ureterocaliceal anastomosis will not be engulfed by parenchymal tissue. If the amount of parenchyma removed is not sufficient, extensive scar formation and fibrosis will inevitably result in a stricture at the anastomotic line. A minimal amount of tissue is the amount that results in exposure of an area with a diameter of approximately 2 cm. The parenchyma should be resected so that the calix protrudes out from its margin. The calix and infundibula are opened and the ureter is spatulated, being careful to preserve its blood supply (Fig. 40–3).

The anastomosis should be approximately 1.5 to 2 cm in diameter. The capsule is laid over the parenchyma and sutured to the more distal portion of the infundibula. Often the calix is relatively fragile and dissection more distally will afford stronger tissue. If the sutures do not hold to the urothelium, the renal capsule, collecting system, and ureter can be incorporated into a common suture to give added strength to the anastomosis (Fig. 40–4).[11] It is exceedingly important not to close parenchyma over the suture line; when this has been done, an anastomotic stricture has occurred.[12] The anastomosis must be without tension and without angulation. It should be watertight, completely dependent, and adequate in size.

A nephrostomy tube is placed before completing the anastomosis, and a soft Silastic nonocclusive

stent is placed through the anastomosis into the ureter (Fig. 40–5). The anastomosis is drained with a flat Jackson-Pratt drain. If the ureter cannot be mobilized sufficiently to reach the infundibula without jeopar-

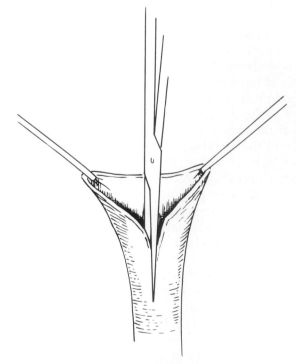

Figure 40–3. Viable nonscarred ureter is spatulated laterally.

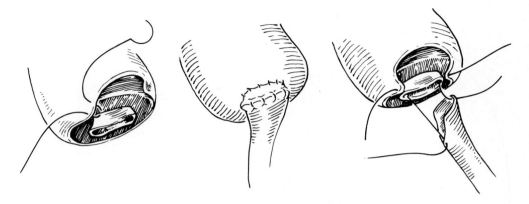

Figure 40–4. The renal capsule is sutured to the exposed collecting system proximal to its severed end, covering the raw parenchymal surface, which aids in hemostasis. The ureter is then sewn to the collecting system. If the tissues of the collecting system are tenuous, the renal capsule, collecting system, and ureter are incorporated into a common suture for added strength.

dizing the blood supply, the appendix may be used, when the lesion is on the right side, or a segment of small bowel may be used (Fig. 40–6). Utilization of the appendix has not been as successful as that of the small bowel because stricture formation is more common with the appendix.[2, 13]

The lower pole of the kidney may require removal because of (1) a lesion confined to it, (2) establishment of dependent drainage for a patient with recurrent stones, and (3) the need to visualize the intrarenal collecting system. After lower pole nephrectomy, the kidney may be rotated into the wound, and the entire collecting system may be visualized without optics. Closure of the exposed collecting system may

be accomplished by incorporating the renal pelvis into the infundibulum (Fig. 40–7). Absolute dependent drainage of the entire renal collecting system is accomplished by this closure.

POSTOPERATIVE MANAGEMENT AND COMPLICATIONS

The stent and nephrostomy are left in place until all drainage from the flank drain ceases or after 3

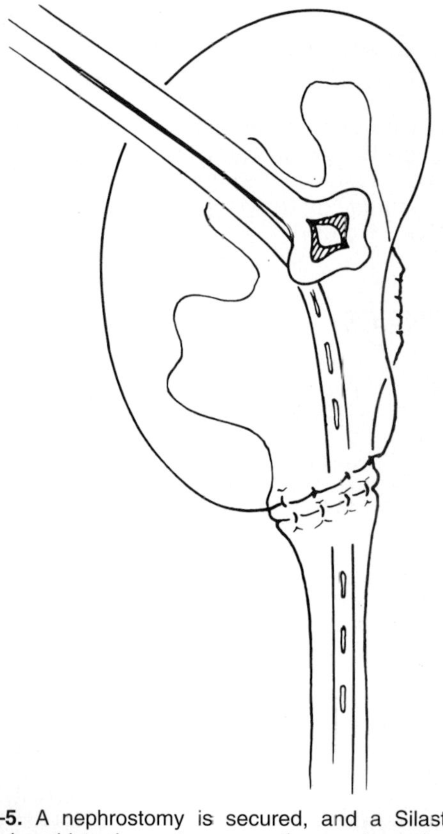

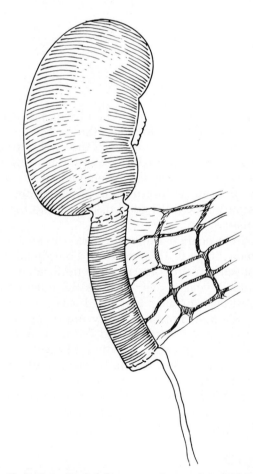

Figure 40–5. A nephrostomy is secured, and a Silastic stenting catheter is placed into the ureter across the anastomosis.

Figure 40–6. A portion of ileum may be used to bridge the gap between the renal collecting system and ureter. The ileum is sutured proximally to the exposed lower pole of the collecting system and sutured distally end to end to the normal spatulated ureter or bladder.

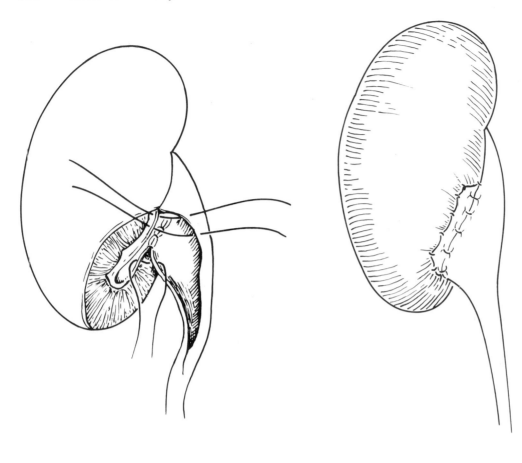

A   B

Figure 40–7. *A,* To achieve dependent drainage or to close the collecting system after a lower pole nephrectomy, the pelvis may be sutured to the lower pole infundibulum. *B,* After closure the entire drainage of the kidney is dependent.

weeks, whichever is longer. When the nephrostogram confirms a secure anastomosis, the stent is removed and the nephrostomy clamped. If the patient tolerates clamping of the nephrostomy for the ensuing week, it is removed. Occasionally, edema about the anastomosis will require intermittent unclamping of the nephrostomy tube until good drainage into the ureter is established.

With ureterocaliceal anastomoses, the success rate is between 50 and 75 percent.[14] Complications are more common if this procedure is performed in children under 1 year of age. Perhaps the most common complication is urinary leakage. However, a leaking anastomosis does not necessarily imply an increased rate of subsequent stenosis and failure of the procedure. A stenting catheter often allows persistent drainage to cease. Occasionally, persistent drainage and urinary sepsis result in the necessity for a nephrectomy.[9] Pyelonephritis, recurrent stricture, hematuria, hypertension, and fecal fistula[13] have also been reported as complications.

RESULTS

In properly selected patients, this procedure has a reasonable degree of success and allows salvage of kidneys that otherwise might require nephrectomy.

Editorial Comment
Fray F. Marshall, M.D.

Ureterocalicostomy is a relatively uncommon operation but can be very useful, particularly if there is a scarred intrarenal pelvis with associated ureteral injury. Resection of scar and renal tissue at the lower pole is important to prevent postoperative stricture.

REFERENCES

1. Neuwirt K. Implantation of the ureter into the lower calyx of the renal pelvis. VII. Congrès de la Société International d'Urologie 2:253, 1947.
2. Couvelaire R, Auvert J, Moulonguet A, et al. Implantations et anastomoses uretero-calicielles: Techniques et midications. J Urol (Paris) 70:437, 1964.
3. Hawthorne NJ, Zincke H, Kelalis PP. Ureterocalicostomy: An alternative to nephrectomy. J Urol 115:583, 1976.
4. Duckett JW, Pfister RR. Ureterocalicostomy for renal salvage. J Urol 128:98, 1982.
5. Turner-Warwick RT. Lower pole pyelo-calyotomy, retrograde partial nephrectomy, and uretero-calycostomy. Br J Urol 37:673, 1965.
6. Persky L, McDougal WS, Kedia K. Management of initial pyeloplasty failure. J Urol 125:695, 1981.
7. Moloney GE. Avulsion of the renal pelvis treated by ureterocalycostomy. J Urol 42:519, 1970.
8. Jarowenko MV, Flechner SM. Recipient ureterocalycostomy in a renal allograft: Case report of a transplant salvage. J Urol 133:844, 1985.

9. Mollard P, Braun P. Primary ureterocalycostomy for severe hydronephrosis in children. J Pediatr Surg 15:87, 1980.
10. Mesrobian HJ, Kelalis PP. Ureterocalicostomy, indications and results in 21 patients. J Urol 142:1285, 1989.
11. Michalowski VE, Modelski W, Kmak A. Die End-zu-End Anastomose zwischen dem unteren Nierenkelch und Harnleiter (Ureterocalicostomie). Z Urol Nephrol 63:1, 1970.
12. Jameson SG, McKinney JS, Rushton JF. Ureterocalicostomy: A new surgical procedure for correction of ureteropelvic stricture associated with an intrarenal pelvis. J Urol 77:135, 1957.
13. Wesalowski S. Uretero-calicostomy. Eur Urol 1:18, 1975.
14. Levitt SB, Nabizadek I, Javaid M, et al. Primary calycoureterostomy for pelvicoureteral junction obstructions. J Urol 126:382, 1981.

Chapter 41

Ureterolithotomy

H. Ballentine Carter

A number of significant advances occurred in the 1980s with respect to the management of patients with stone disease. The development of small ureteroscopes and the introduction and routine use of contact (electrohydraulic, laser, ultrasonic) and noncontact (extracorporeal shock wave) lithotripsy (ESWL) has resulted in less invasive approaches (endourologic) to the treatment of ureteral stones, while maintaining high treatment success rates with minimal morbidity. As a result, a patient presenting with a ureteral stone is unlikely to require ureterolithotomy. It is estimated that less than 2 percent of patients with primary ureteric calculi will require ureterolithotomy for stone removal. Nevertheless, the urologist caring for patients with stone disease should be familiar with the different surgical approaches to the ureter and be capable of performing ureterolithotomy, since indications for the procedure remain. In some cases ureterolithotomy may be underutilized today in our zeal to prevent an incision at all cost. The patient who undergoes repeated ureteral manipulation from above and below after failed ESWL may have ultimately been best served by a small incision for stone removal.

INDICATIONS

Ureteral stones most likely to require ureterolithotomy are dense on radiographs with respect to bone, are greater than 10 mm, and have associated hydronephrosis. The patient who has a ureteral stone that is refractory to in situ ESWL and refractory to attempts to bypass the stone (in preparation for ESWL with stent or an endoscopic approach from above or below) is a candidate for ureterolithotomy. Also candidates are patients with stones that do not disintegrate with contact lithotripsy after bypass and cannot be removed endoscopically. If a ureteral stone exists together with a ureteral stricture, ureterolithotomy and repair of the stricture should be performed together.

Emergency ureterolithotomy and repair would be indicated for the severe ureteral injury that can occur during ureteroscopy.

The patient requiring ureterolithotomy in the endourological era has most often failed repeated attempts at stone disintegration and usually has a hard stone that may be impacted in the ureteral wall. In addition, some of these patients will have undergone ureteroscopic procedures that resulted in injury or perforation of the ureter. Thus, when performing ureterolithotomy in the endourological era, one should adhere to principles that maximize the chances of preserving ureteral blood supply in an attempt to prevent subsequent fibrosis and stricture.

PREOPERATIVE EVALUATION

The possibility of urinary tract infection should be excluded before performing ureterolithotomy. If the urine is infected, adequate treatment before ureterolithotomy is recommended to prevent septic complications. The presence of all stones should be well documented by thorough evaluation of the entire urinary tract before surgery. In the past it was emphasized that the location of the ureteral stone should be confirmed on the morning of surgery or in the operating room before surgery because of the possibility of stone migration. Given that most patients undergoing ureterolithotomy in the present era have stones that are impacted and refractory to other forms of treatment (i.e., manipulation), the chance of spontaneous stone migration is less likely. However, it is prudent to have a recent radiograph to document the location of the stone before surgery.

OPERATIVE TECHNIQUE

Incisions

The incision chosen for ureterolithotomy depends on the location of the stone. The ureter can be divided into proximal, middle, and distal segments for purposes of describing stone location. The proximal ureter extends from the ureteropelvic junction to L5, the midureter overlies the sacrum, and the distal ureter extends from the ureterovesical junction to the sacrum. Options for access to stones above the iliac crest (i.e., proximal ureteral stones) include (1) a subcostal flank incision (Fig. 41–1A), (2) a Foley incision (Fig. 41–1B), and (3) a dorsal lumbotomy incision. For midureteral stones overlying the sacrum, an extended McBurney incision is useful (Fig. 41–1C). For distal ureteral calculi, options include (1) a Gibson incision (Fig. 41–1D), (2) a lower midline incision, (3) a Pfannenstiel incision (Fig. 41–1E), and (4) in females a vaginal incision (Fig. 41–1F). Stones impacted in the intramural ureter should be approached through an incision that allows the option of direct intravesical access and access to the ureterovesical junction.

Upper Ureteral Stones

The *subcostal flank incision* allows direct access to the lower pole of the kidney and the upper ureter

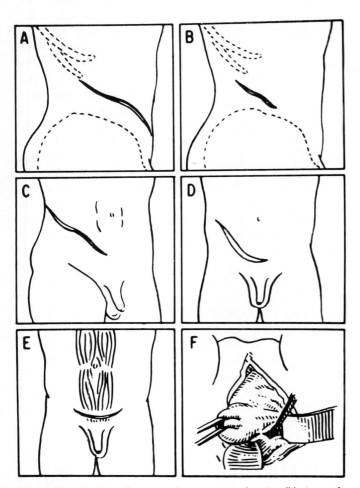

Figure 41–1. Incisions for ureteral exposure and ureterolithotomy. *A,* Subcostal flank. *B,* Foley. *C,* Extended McBurney. *D,* Gibson. *E,* Pfannennstiel. *F,* Vaginal. (From Anderson EE. Ureterolithotomy. In Glenn JF, ed. Urologic Surgery, 4th ed. Philadelphia, JB Lippincott, 1991, p 278.)

(Fig. 41–1A). With the patient in the flank position and the table hyperextended, exposure of the involved lumbar area between the twelfth rib and iliac crest is optimal. The skin incision, 1 cm below the twelfth rib, can be extended posteriorly or anteriorly and inferiorly, depending on the exact location of the stone in the upper ureter (i.e., more posterior for stones closer to the ureteropelvic junction and more anterior for stones closer to L5). After incision of the skin and subcutaneous tissue, the latissimus dorsi muscle posteriorly and the external and internal oblique muscles anteriorly are incised. The twelfth nerve is retracted and the lumbodorsal fascia beneath the latissimus dorsi muscle is incised in the posterior portion of the wound. The transversus abdominis muscle is separated in the anterior portion of the wound, which allows access to the retroperitoneal space. The peritoneum is bluntly dissected off the posterior surface of the transversus abdominis muscle and pushed medially. In the retroperitoneal space, one encounters the psoas muscle posteriorly and the lower pole of the kidney and proximal ureter anteriorly.

The *Foley incision* can be used to gain access to the proximal ureter through the lumbar (Petit) triangle (Fig. 41–2). Since no muscle is incised, postoperative recovery is excellent. A skin incision is made from the middle of the twelfth rib and angled down anteriorly and inferiorly toward the anterosuperior iliac spine, with the patient in the flank position as for a subcostal incision (see Fig. 41–1A). Incision of skin and subcutaneous tissue exposes the lumbar triangle formed by separation of the latissimus dorsi and external oblique muscles where they attach to the iliac crest (Fig. 41–2). This space allows access to the retroperitoneum without muscle incision. The triangle is formed by the free edge of the external oblique muscle medially and the latissimus dorsi muscle laterally. The base of the triangle is formed by the iliac crest inferiorly; the apex, by the convergence of latissimus and external oblique muscles superiorly; and the floor of the triangle, by the internal oblique and transversus abdominis muscles. The external and internal oblique muscles are retracted medially and the latissimus dorsi muscle laterally. The transversus abdominis muscle is separated and the lumbodorsal fascia incised for exposure of the retroperitoneal space and proximal ureter.

The *dorsal lumbotomy incision* (described in Chapter 33) allows good access to the most proximal ureter but more limited access to the lower part of the proximal ureter nearest the iliac crest. This incision would not be indicated for stones near and below the iliac crest, in which exposure would be more difficult.

Midureteral Stones

An extension of the *McBurney incision* provides exposure of the midureter overlying the iliac crest

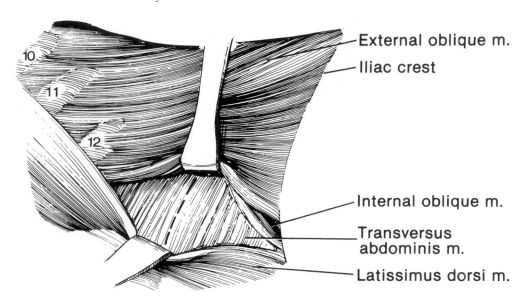

External oblique m.

Iliac crest

Internal oblique m.

Transversus
abdominis m.

Latissimus dorsi m.

Figure 41–2. Lumbar (Petit) triangle as seen with the Foley incision. The base of the triangle is formed by the iliac crest; the apex by convergence of the external oblique muscle medially and the latissimus dorsi muscle laterally. (From Hinman F Jr. Atlas of Urosurgical Anatomy. Philadelphia, WB Saunders, 1993, p 154.)

(see Fig. 41–1C). The patient is positioned by placing rolls underneath the involved lumbar area (30-degree rotation) and extending the table, with the patient's umbilicus over the break. The skin incision is oblique and parallel to the inguinal ligament from the anterior axillary line to the anterior iliac crest at a level one third of the way between the anterosuperior iliac spine and umbilicus. The external and internal oblique muscles are opened in line with the fibers, and the transversus abdominis muscle is separated in line with the fibers. Blunt dissection of the peritoneum medially from the undersurface of the transversus abdominis muscle provides access to the retroperitoneum overlying the sacrum.

Lower Ureteral Stones

A *Gibson incision* runs oblique and parallel to the inguinal fold, extending from 2 fingerbreadths above the anterosuperior iliac spine to 2 fingerbreadths above the symphysis pubis, ending at the border of the rectus muscle (see Fig. 41–1D). The skin incision is made with the patient supine and the table extended, with the patient's umbilicus over the break. The external and internal oblique muscles are opened in line with their fibers, and the transversus abdominis muscle is separated. The transversalis fascia is incised, and the peritoneum is swept anteromedially by first freeing up the peritoneum where it is attached at the internal inguinal ring and then the lateral peritoneum. This maneuver exposes the iliac vessels and the ureter underneath the peritoneal surface. The attachments of the rectus muscle to the symphysis pubis can be divided, with control of the inferior epigastric vessels if more medial exposure is needed.

A *lower midline incision* between the umbilicus and symphysis pubis provides excellent exposure of both ureters from the level of the iliac vessels to the

ureterovesical junction, and equally good exposure of the bladder for access to the intramural ureter. Patient positioning is the same as for the Gibson incision, to extend the space between the pubis and umbilicus. After incision of the skin and subcutaneous tissues between the pubis and umbilicus, the rectus muscles are separated in the midline and the transversalis fascia is incised. Mobilization of the peritoneum anteriorly as with a Gibson incision provides exposure of the iliac vessels and the ureter. A Balfour retractor can be placed for exposure.

The *Pfannenstiel* (suprapubic) *incision* provides good access to the bladder and ureterovesical junction (see Fig. 41–1E). Patient positioning is the same as for the Gibson and lower midline incisions. A curvilinear incision is made 1 fingerbreadth above the pubic symphysis and carried down to expose the anterior rectus sheath. After incision of the rectus sheath and mobilization of the rectus muscle superiorly and inferiorly off the rectus sheath, the rectus muscle can be separated in the midline. The transversalis fascia is incised, exposing the bladder surface.

The rare lower ureteral stone that is easily palpable on bimanual examination in a female can be approached via a *vaginal incision* (see Fig. 41–1F). With the patient in the dorsolithotomy position and a weighted speculum in the vagina, the cervix is grasped with a tenaculum and retracted to the contralateral side. An incision is made in the vaginal wall overlying the palpable stone to expose the ureter after infiltration of the vaginal wall with 1:200,000 phenylephrine.

OPERATIVE TECHNIQUE

Stone Extraction

Through the appropriate incision the ureter is identified and the stone palpated gently. The ureter is mobilized only to the extent necessary for an incision overlying the stone in order to preserve the ureteral blood supply. With a hooked blade knife, an incision is made longitudinally through the ureteral wall overlying the stone. The incision in the ureter is extended with Potts scissors if necessary so that the incision encompasses the length of the stone. The stone is extracted with forceps, and patency of the ureter is confirmed by passing a small feeding tube proximally and distally. The ureterotomy is closed by approximating the adventitia with 4-0 chromic suture.

For stones at the ureterovesical junction, division of the superior vesicle pedicle and uterine artery in the female provides exposure of the distal ureter. A transvesical approach is useful for stones in the intramural ureter. An incision is made above the ureteral orifice overlying the intramural ureter, and the ureter is mobilized enough to expose the stone for extraction.

Ureteral stenting is prudent if multiple previous ureteral manipulations have resulted in marked edema and inflammation of the ureter. The ureter should be stented after extraction of stones at the ureterovesical junction and below because of the propensity for prolonged drainage after ureterotomy in this area. Fat or omentum should be placed around the ureter if there has been ureteral trauma from previous manipulation. A drain is routinely placed around the operative site.

POSTOPERATIVE COMPLICATIONS

Early postoperative complications include urinary leakage and urinoma formation. Persistent urinary leakage for more than 7 to 10 days postoperatively can be the result of (1) a drain lying in close proximity to the ureterotomy, (2) sloughing of the ureter due to vascular compromise, or (3) distal obstruction (i.e., unrecognized stone or stricture). If advancement of the drain fails to result in resolution of the urinary leak, radiographic imaging of the ureter with retrograde pyelography is suggested, with placement of a ureteral stent if possible. If this cannot be accomplished from below, an antegrade approach should be used. Failure to stent the ureter will require re-exploration. A urinoma manifested by fever can result from early removal of a drain. Percutaneous drainage of the urine collection and ureteral stenting are appropriate treatments.

Ureteral stricture is usually a late complication resulting from fibrosis and scarring caused by vascular compromise of the ureter. A short ureteral stricture may be managed successfully by balloon dilation and stenting. Longer strictures require open repair with excision of the fibrotic segment and most often either ureteroureterostomy or ureteroneocystomy.

Editorial Comment
Fray F. Marshall

Ureterolithotomy can still be considered for the occasional patient. A large impacted stone in the midureter may be more easily removed through a small surgical incision than with ESWL or ureteroscopic manipulation. Incisions generally should be made where they can be extended if the stone should happen to move. As a result, it is often reasonable to consider an incision following under the course of the twelfth intercostal nerve. A smaller incision can be made with easy stone removal.

Chapter 42

Extended Psoas Hitch

Francesco Pagano and Agostino Meneghini

Surgical repair of extensive ureteral lesions can be most complex. Their causes may be varied. In recent years trauma to the ureter secondary to urological and endourological procedures, frequently involving the iliac and lumbar ureter, has become more common, and extensive lesions due to gynecological surgery are less common.[1] The diagnostic work-up should be meticulous and complete to locate the injury and evaluate its length and associated tissue injury. The diagnostic evaluation is of paramount importance to determine the most appropriate surgical strategy for ureteral reconstruction.

A technical variation to the classic Boari flap[2] has been developed that allows reconstruction of an extensive ureteral gap up to 7 cm long. The ureteral reimplant is performed via an antireflux technique, even in extended lesions of the lumbar and iliac ureter.[3] The anatomical basis of this technique is derived from an anatomical work on cadaver bladder blood supply[4]; a similar bladder flap study on sheep has been reported.[5]

PREOPERATIVE EVALUATION

Iatrogenic ureteral injuries, like endourological injuries, are usually intraoperative. Sometimes the event is not evident at surgery but becomes manifest in the immediate postoperative period when fever, flank pain, and urinary leakage appear. The first step in the diagnostic evaluation of an ureteral lesion should be intravenous urography, which first of all verifies the condition of the contralateral kidney. In the case of a unilateral lesion the most common findings are hydronephrosis secondary to ureteral stenosis, a nonfunctioning kidney, and retroperitoneal urinary leakage in a case of complete section or avulsion of the ureter. A percutaneous nephrostomy tube should be immediately positioned to restore normal renal function and to enable a more accurate radiological evaluation to be made. A combined nephros-

togram and retrograde ureterogram is probably the best way to determine the exact extent and location of the ureteral injury. If an extended psoas hitch is a possible surgical option, a cystogram is recommended to evaluate bladder wall compliance and capacity. At the induction of anesthesia a broad-spectrum antibiotic is administered, and subsequent antimicrobial prophylaxis is continued until the removal of all catheters or stents.

OPERATIVE TECHNIQUE

Preservation of renal function, ureteral restoration, elimination of underlying causes of obstruction, and prevention of vesicoureteral reflux and recurrent stenosis are the objects of this operation. Complete isolation of the damaged ureter, excision of nonviable tissue, and a tension-free ureterovesical anastomosis are the technical principles necessary for good long-term results. A wide abdominal incision exposing the whole excretory tract is the preferred surgical approach. A thick scar, often secondary to previous treatment and leakage, can cause difficult surgical exposure of the ureter. In order not to damage the delicate vascular network around the ureter,[6] skeletonization of the healthy ureter should be avoided. It is advisable to manipulate the ureter with very delicate clamps, avoiding direct manipulation. The entire stenotic ureter needs to be dissected free and excised. On the other hand, all viable normal ureter should be preserved to avoid further extension of the ureteral defect. The actual length of the ureteral gap can be exactly determined only after complete bladder mobilization, particularly on lateral and posterior walls, and bilateral umbilical artery ligation. Preservation of at least one of the main trunks of bladder arterial pedicle is advisable so as not to jeopardize blood supply to the flap, although an anatomical study[4] demonstrated that it is very difficult to compromise the vascular supply of the flap owing to the very rich anastomotic network of the blood supply. After the bladder is filled with saline via a Foley catheter, a U-shaped incision on the anterior bladder wall—partially extended to the lateral wall, opposite to the ureteral lesion—is performed to obtain the flap (Fig. 42–1). After having verified the extent of cranial elevation of the flap, two full-thickness incisions at different heights—one on the medial, the other on the lateral border of the flap—are made (Fig. 42–2) to move the top of the flap as high as possible. Three stitches of 3-0 absorbable suture hitch the apex of the flap to the psoas muscle. Usually, at the end of the procedure, the ureter is located in a submucosal tunnel that runs just above the psoas hitch sutures. A totally tension-free ureterovesical reimplant is accomplished with antireflux technique (Fig. 42–3). A ureteral stent is optional. The flap is closed with running watertight, double-layer sutures of 5-0 and 3-0 absorbable catgut. Because of the two previous incisions that are sutured in a Z-plasty, the sutured bladder will result in a more conical than spherical shape (Fig. 42–4). A Couvelaire 22 Fr. urethral catheter is left in place. Drainage is ensured by two drains,

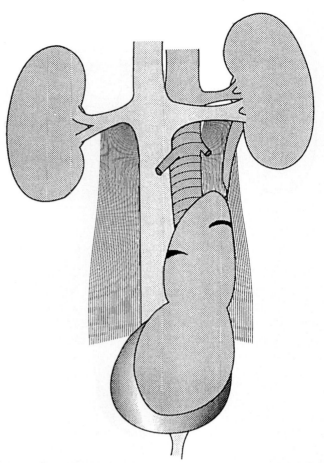

Figure 42–2. Lateral and medial incisions are made at different heights to obtain further elevation. (From Passerini-Glazel G, Meneghini A, Aragona F, et al. Technical options in complex ureteral lesions: "Ureter-sparing" surgery. Eur Urol 2:273, 1994. With permission from S. Karger AG, Basel, Switzerland.)

one near the ureterovesical anastomosis and the other in the space of Retzius.

POSTOPERATIVE MANAGEMENT

Patients should receive adequate antithrombotic prophylaxis, since it is advisable to keep them flat with half-flexed legs for 5 days. On the fourteenth postoperative day a nephrostogram is performed, and if no leakage is evident the ureteral catheter can be removed. Among seven patients treated with extended bladder psoas hitch, one persistent vesical leakage was observed in a young patient operated on after multiple failed attempts at ureteral reimplantation. The leakage spontaneously ceased after 7 days of conservative management. One case of later mild ureterovesical stenosis occurred in an asymptomatic patient with sterile urine.

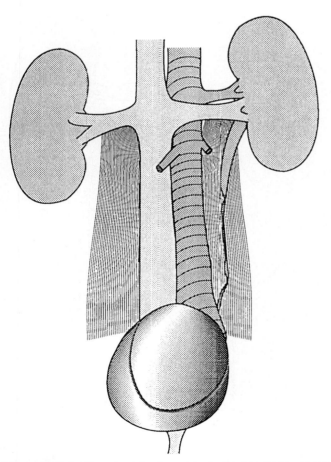

Figure 42–1. A wide anterolateral semicircular bladder flap has been obtained. (From Passerini-Glazel G, Meneghini A, Aragona F, et al. Technical options in complex ureteral lesions: "Ureter-sparing" surgery. Eur Urol 2:273, 1994. With permission from S. Karger AG, Basel, Switzerland.)

Conclusion

Extended psoas hitch represents an additional surgical option in the repair of a complex ureteral lesion.

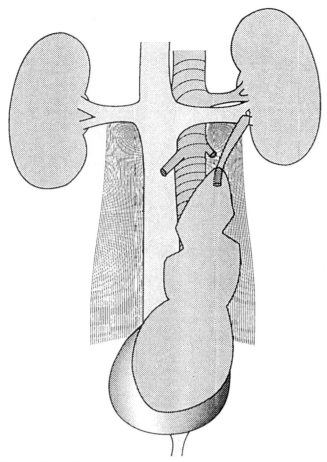

Figure 42–3. After anchoring the flap to the psoas muscle, an antireflux ureteral reimplantation is carried out. (From Passerini-Glazel G, Meneghini A, Aragona F, et al. Technical options in complex ureteral lesions: "Ureter-sparing" surgery. Eur Urol 2:273, 1994. With permission from S. Karger AG, Basel, Switzerland.)

The original work includes the century-old paper of Boari.[2] In more recent years Olsson and Norlen,[7] Hensle and colleagues,[8] and Benson and associates[9] have produced important contributions. Very extensive ureteral defects were bridged in these experiences, but no antireflux ureteral reimplant was reported. The Boari flap modified by Kuss[10] is much more similar to the extended psoas hitch, but the present option allows additional bladder elevation because of the use of a wider flap. This allows additional lengthening after the lateral and medial incisions and subsequent Z-plasty.

For illustration, a case of a 55-year-old man with extensive ureteral injury secondary to multiple failed ureteral reimplantations is presented (Fig. 42–5A). The postoperative nephrostogram (Fig. 42–5B) demonstrates the new vesical configuration. In the early convalescence period a reduction of bladder capacity is frequently observed. Anticholinergic medications can be useful to reduce symptoms. In about 3 months, normal bladder structure is resumed. Urinary frequency and bladder instability spontaneously sub-

side. Cystography and intravenous pyelography were performed 1 year after the procedure (Fig. 42–5C and D).

Surgical repair of complex ureteral lesions is demanding. Different techniques are available, but tailoring the appropriate approach to the patient requires broad clinical and surgical experience. This surgery should be reserved for experienced urologists.[3]

Editorial Comment
Fray F. Marshall

It is generally preferable to try and achieve ureteral reconstruction with the urinary tract rather than resort to insertion of intestine. The extended psoas hitch allows reconstruction of the ureter even when there is more extensive injury to the ureter. Vesical and renal mobilization can often achieve almost the same result. On the other hand, if additional ureteral length is needed, techniques described in this chapter may be helpful. It is important not to make the Boari flap too small or narrow: a generous flap needs to be constructed as outlined.

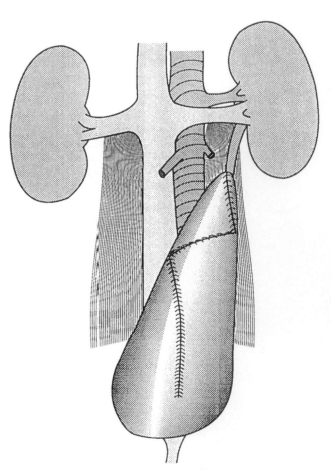

Figure 42–4. Bladder closure in a Z-plasty fashion produces a conical shape of the bladder. (From Passerini-Glazel G, Meneghini A, Aragona F, et al. Technical options in complex ureteral lesions: "Ureter-sparing" surgery. Eur Urol 2:273, 1994. With permission from S. Karger AG, Basel, Switzerland.)

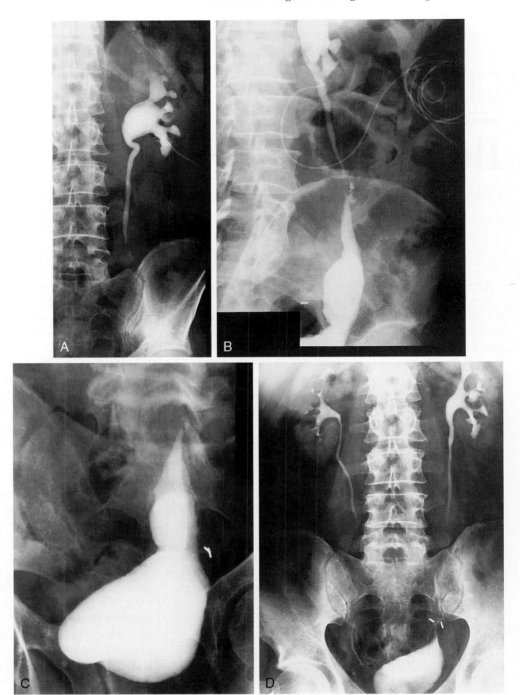

Figure 42–5. *A,* Nephrostogram showing an extensive lesion of the left ureter after two failed attempts at ureteral reimplantation. *B,* Nephrostogram after surgery. The elevated and elongated bladder is brought up to the level of the iliac crest. *C,* Voiding cystourethrogram and *D,* intravenous pyelogram 12 months after surgery. (From Passerini-Glazel G, Meneghini A, Aragona F, et al. Technical options in complex ureteral lesions: "Ureter-sparing" surgery. Eur Urol 2:273, 1994. With permission from S. Karger AG, Basel, Switzerland.)

REFERENCES

1. Patterson LC, Assimos DG. Changing incidence and etiology of iatrogenic ureteral injuries linked to ureteroscopy and laparoscopy. AUA Today 5:1, 1992.
2. Boari A, Casati A. Contributo sperimentale alla plastica dell'uretere. Atti Accad Sci Med e Nat in Ferrara 68:149, 1894.
3. Passerini Glazel G, Meneghini A, Aragona F, et al. Technical options in complex ureteral lesions: The "ureter-sparing" surgery. Eur Urol 25:273, 1994.
4. Aragona F, De Caro R, Munari PF, et al. Premesse anatomochirurgiche all'impiego di lembi vescicali peduncolati. Acta Urol Ital 4 (Suppl 1):529, 1989.
5. Cormio L, Crovace A, Lacalandra G, et al. Bladder Z-plasty for the repair of ureteric injuries. Br J Urol 71:667, 1993.
6. Pagano F, Graziotti P, Lembo A, et al. Terapia ricostruttiva delle alte vie escretrici superiori. Proceedings 58° SIU Meeting: 3, 1985.
7. Olsson CA, Norlen CJ. Combined Boari bladder flap and psoas bladder hitch procedure in ureteral replacement. Scand J Urol Nephrol 20:279, 1986.
8. Hensle TW, Burbige KA, Levin RK. Management of the short ureter in urinary tract reconstruction. J Urol 137:707, 1987.
9. Benson MC, Ring RS, Olsson CA. Ureteral reconstruction and bypass: Experience with ileal interposition, the Boari flap-psoas hitch and renal autotransplantation. J Urol 143:20, 1990.
10. Kuss R. Ureteroplastie per lambeau vesical: à propos de 38 cas personneles. Urol Int 3:175, 1956.

Chapter 43

Ileal Ureter

William J. Aronson, Robert B. Smith, and Jean B. deKernion

The small intestine has been used for partial or complete replacement of a diseased or injured ureter for 90 years. In 1906, Shoemaker performed the first replacement of the ureter by small intestine in an 18-year-old girl. Some 60 years later, Goodwin and associates described the technique of ileal ureter and expanded the indications to include treatment for multiple recurrent calculi. Since 1970, more than 200 ileal ureters have been performed at UCLA.

INDICATIONS

Ileal interposition is a safe and effective technique for repairing extensive ureteral defects that cannot be repaired by other procedures such as ureteroureterostomy, transureteroureterostomy, vesico-psoas hitch, Boari bladder flap, and downward renal mobilization. Frequently these long ureteral defects result from iatrogenic injury after previous attempts at ureteral reconstruction have failed. Ileal ureter is also indicated for recurrent stone formers with difficult ureteral stone passage who are refractory to extracorporeal shock wave lithotripsy and medical and endourological treatments. Other indications include retroperitoneal fibrosis involving the ureter and not amenable to standard medical and surgical treatments, transitional cell carcinoma involving the ureter, and various congenital anomalies in children.

PREOPERATIVE EVALUATION

Careful preoperative planning and evaluation are paramount to the success of ileal interposition. It is important to be aware of any history of previous bowel surgery or abdominal radiation, since the success of the procedure depends on accessible, healthy small bowel. Before an ileal ureter is created or ureteral surgery of any kind is performed, the renal and ureteral anatomy and the functional status of both

kidneys should be studied. The preoperative serum creatinine levels should be less than 2.2 mg/dl (with good ipsilateral renal function) to avoid significant alterations of serum electrolytes and progressive renal impairment.[1] If the ipsilateral renal function is less than 15 or 20 percent of total renal function or if the patient is elderly and chronically ill, nephrectomy should be considered. In addition, there must be adequate bladder emptying without bladder outlet obstruction for the ileal ureter to function properly and to avoid obstruction from mucus produced by the ileum.

Preoperatively, one should treat any urinary tract infection and place a ureteral stent to aid identification of the ureter during the operation. It is necessary to type and cross 4 units of blood, as there can be significant hemorrhage during dissection of the renal pelvis if there is inflammation or retroperitoneal fibrosis. The patient should be hydrated overnight and bowel preparation performed. We start the patients on a full liquid diet 5 days before the operation and convert this to a clear liquid diet 3 days before the procedure. Oral erythromycin and neomycin are also given. With this preparation, the bowel is sufficiently sterilized and decompressed.

OPERATIVE TECHNIQUE

Incision

Position the patient in a torqued flank position with the table flexed to open the space between the costal margin and the pelvis. After prepping and draping the patient, place a Foley catheter to allow distention and identification of the bladder intraoperatively. If there is an indwelling percutaneous nephrostomy tube, it should be prepped into the field in case percutaneous access is needed during the procedure.

Start the incision at the tip of the eleventh or

twelfth rib, carrying it across the rectus muscle and then down the midline to the pubis. Consider resecting the eleventh rib or performing a higher thoracoabdominal incision if renal mobilization will be difficult because of inflammation or scarring. Divide the external and internal oblique and transversus abdominis muscles and fascia, and divide the ipsilateral rectus muscle and fascia. Divide the midline fascia and enter the peritoneal cavity.

Mobilization of Renal Pelvis

Mobilize the ascending or descending colon (depending on which kidney is being exposed) by incising along the white line of Toldt and reflecting the colon medially to expose the kidney. Enter Gerota's fascia and identify the renal pelvis. If this is not possible owing to inflammation and scarring, identify the upper ureter and trace it upward to the pelvis. Free the renal pelvis anteriorly off the renal vessels and then bluntly dissect the renal pelvis circumferentially from the renal parenchyma to enter the renal sinus (Fig. 43–1). This dissection allows access to the lower pole infundibula and calix for the anastomosis. Avoid injuring any lower pole vessels originating from the renal artery or originating separately from the aorta. For patients with recurrent stones, attempt

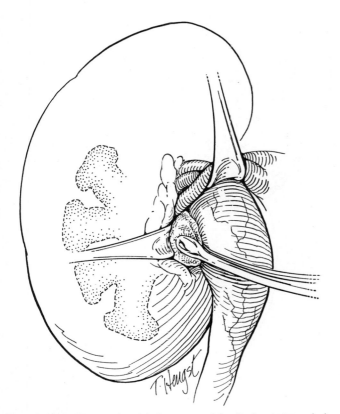

Figure 43–1. The renal pelvis is prepared for ileal anastomosis by bluntly dissecting the pelvis circumferentially from the parenchyma to enter the renal sinus.

ureterolysis, perform ureterolithotomy for ureteral stones, and place a ureteral stent; the ureter is left in situ in case retrograde access is needed in the future.

Comment   If perirenal inflammation and fibrosis prevent identification of the pelvis and ureter, and if there is a large-bore indwelling nephrostomy tube, a curved stone clamp passed through the nephrostomy tract and directed to the lower pole and pelvis may be the only way of identifying the renal pelvis and collecting system. The tissue overlying the clamp is then incised until the clamp is exposed to gain access to the pelvis and lower pole collecting system for the proximal ileal anastomosis.

Ileal Segment

Select a segment of distal ileum 20 to 30 cm in length, with the distal end at least 10 cm from the ileocecal valve, to leave adequate distal ileum for the bowel anastomosis. Make sure there is a good vascular arcade supplying the segment to be used. Anticipate that this mesentery will need to be divided deeply for adequate mobilization of the ileum. Ensure that the proximal portion of the segment reaches the renal pelvis without tension and that the distal portion will reach the bladder. At this time, divide the peritoneal attachments to the bladder and perform an anterior cystotomy; assess the upward mobility of the bladder to minimize the length of the ileal segment. Divide the ileum and its mesentery proximally and distally, using standard techniques, and mark the distal end of the ileal segment with a silk tie to ensure that it remains isoperistaltic. Allow the ileal segment to fall posteriorly and reanastomose the ileum anterior to this segment. Close the mesenteric defect with interrupted 4-0 silk sutures to prevent internal herniation. Bring the ileal segment through the colonic mesentery to the retroperitoneum and orient it in an isoperistaltic fashion (Fig. 43–2). Irrigate the segment internally with saline.

Proximal Anastomosis

For cases in which the ileal anastomosis will be to the proximal ureter, perform this in an end-to-side fashion as in the Bricker procedure using interrupted 4-0 chromic sutures (see Chapter 54). If there is a large extrarenal pelvis, the ileum can be anastomosed directly to the pelvis with running or interrupted 2-0 chromic sutures. If the renal pelvis is small, anastomose the ileum to the lower pole calix, infundibulum, and pelvis. To accomplish this, open the pelvis on its inferior lateral aspect and advance a large-angled Randall forceps to the lower pole calix (Fig. 43–3). Extend the incision in the pelvis into the renal sinus to the lower pole infundibulum and calix, using the Randall forceps as a guide. Bivalve the medial

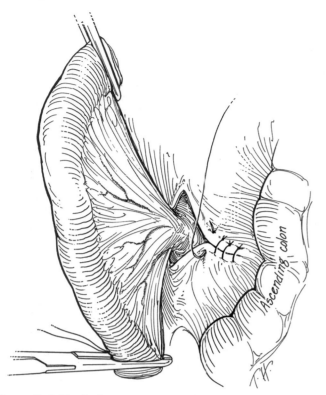

Figure 43–2. The ileal segment is oriented in an isoperistaltic fashion and brought through the colonic mesentery to the retroperitoneum. The colonic mesenteric defect is closed to prevent internal herniation.

lower pole parenchyma over the infundibulum and calix, and gently oversew bleeding vessels with fig-ure-of-eight 4-0 chromic sutures. Hemorrhage coming from the parenchyma adjacent to the collecting sys-tem will be controlled from the ileal anastomosis sutures. Remove any renal stones and consider plac-ing a nephrostomy tube for proximal urine diversion during healing if problems with the proximal anasto-mosis are anticipated.

Spatulate the proximal ileum at its antimesenteric border so that the ileum opening fits the pelvic defect. Place two 2-0 chromic sutures on ⅝-needles at the extreme distal aspect of the lower pole calix, incorpo-rating some adjacent parenchyma, and oppose this with the extreme lateral border of the spatulated bowel. Have your assistant hold the proximal ileum next to the pelvis so that there is no tension during the anastomosis. Perform the posterior portion of the anastomosis by running the 2-0 chromic suture from the calix to the infundibulum and pelvis, and place a hemostat on this suture (Fig. 43–4). Run the other 2-0 chromic suture from the calix to the infundibu-lum and pelvis to complete the anterior portion of the anastomosis, and tie the two sutures. The sutures placed in the collecting system should include paren-chyma and must be placed gently and following the curve of the needle to prevent tearing. We advance a 22 or 24 Fr. red rubber catheter across the anastomo-

sis before running the anterior suture line to avoid suturing the back wall.

Comment   For patients with recurrent stones, always anastomose the ileum to the pelvis or to the lower pole calix, infundibulum, and pelvis. Never anastomose the il-eum to the ureter, even if it is dilated, because once the ureter is decompressed, stones may have difficulty passing.

Distal Anastomosis

Perform a vesico-psoas hitch to minimize the length of ileum needed (see Chapter 41). Resect any redundant distal ileum and mesentery to keep the segment as short as possible but without tension. In rare cases in which the ileum is redundant but the mesentery has no mobility, we resect a middle por-tion of the ileum and reanastomose the ends with a running 2-0 chromic suture and interrupted seromus-cular 3-0 silk sutures. Make a patulous opening in the posterior bladder wall by perforating and stretch-ing with a tonsil clamp. Anastomose the ileum to the posterior bladder wall from within the bladder with

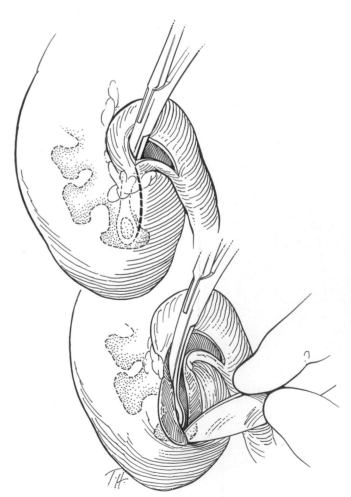

Figure 43–3. To prepare the renal pelvis for ileal anastomosis, the lower pole parenchyma is bivalved over the lower pole calix and infundibulum.

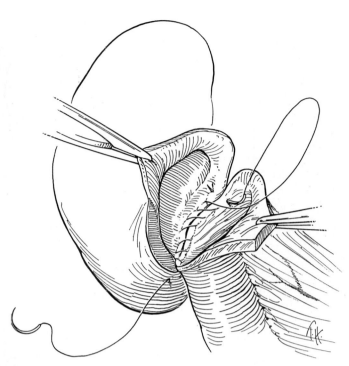

Figure 43–4. To anastomose the ileum to the pelvis, the posterior portion of the anastomosis is first performed by running a 2-0 chromic suture from the calix to the infundibulum and pelvis. The other 2-0 chromic suture is run anteriorly from the calix to the infundibulum and pelvis to complete the anastomosis.

a running 2-0 chromic on a ⅝-needle (Fig. 43–5). In adults, we always make this anastomosis freely refluxing. In pediatric patients, taper the ileum and create a submucosal bladder tunnel to prevent reflux.[2]

Advance a 22 or 24 Fr. red rubber catheter up the ileum and across the proximal anastomosis, and secure it to the bladder with a 2-0 chromic suture. Bring the opposite end of the catheter through the bladder and out from a suprapubic stab wound. We believe that this maneuver prevents kinking of the ileal ureter, allowing it to heal in a straight fashion and facilitating internal drainage during healing. Instill saline into this catheter and oversew sites of leakage. Place a 24 Fr. suprapubic tube and close the bladder.

Close the colonic mesenteric defect around the ileal mesentery with interrupted 4-0 silk sutures to prevent internal herniation and to keep the ileal segment retroperitoneal. Place drains at the proximal and distal anastomoses.

Bilateral Ileal Ureter

For cases requiring a bilateral ileal ureter, two adjacent segments of distal ileum are used. The most distal segment is used to create a left ileal ureter as previously described. The second more proximal ileal segment is anastomosed to the right renal pelvis,

brought through a window in the descending colon mesentery, and anastomosed to the left ileal ureter (Fig. 43–6A). Both ileal segments must be isoperistaltic. In our experience, this Y configuration for bilateral ileal ureter drains the right kidney better than the 7 configuration (Fig. 43–6B).

POSTOPERATIVE MANAGEMENT

Postoperatively, repeatedly irrigate all catheters with normal saline to clear the mucus and prevent obstruction. This procedure should be taught to the patient and continued after discharge.

Remove the urethral catheter and red rubber catheter on the tenth postoperative day if there is minimal drainage. If drainage persists, perform a retrograde pyelogram through the red rubber tube, or a nephrostogram if a nephrostomy tube is in place, before re-

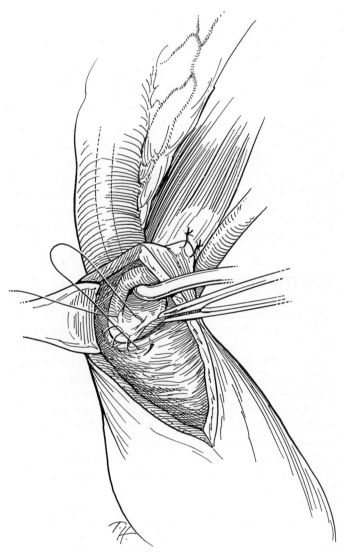

Figure 43–5. After performance of a psoas hitch, the ileum is anastomosed to the bladder with a running 2-0 chromic suture. This is readily done from within the bladder.

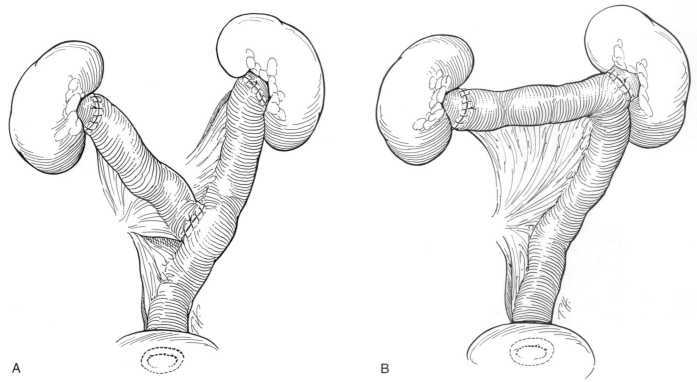

Figure 43–6. *A,* A bilateral ileal ureter that has been fashioned in a Y configuration. Both segments are isoperistaltic. The Y configuration drains the right kidney better than the 7 configuration illustrated in *B.*

moving the catheter. Send the patient home with the suprapubic tube in place, and clamp the suprapubic tube 2 weeks after surgery. Two days later, if the postvoid residual is low, perform a cystogram and remove the suprapubic tube. If a nephrostomy tube is present, clamp it for 48 hours before removing it. Follow up with periodic intravenous urograms. Monitor urine cultures and electrolytes.

POSTOPERATIVE COMPLICATIONS

Urinary leakage across the anastomoses is commonly seen postoperatively and generally resolves if internal and external drainage is adequate. If the leakage is persistent, perform contrast studies to rule out obstruction. Consider placing a percutaneous nephrostomy tube if this was not done previously.

Hyperchloremic metabolic acidosis can also occur and is seen more frequently in patients with a preoperative creatinine level greater than 2.2 mg/dl. With chronic acidosis, osteomalacia and growth retardation have been reported in children. Treat with alkali replacement. Other complications include anastomotic stricture and urinary tract infection. If a stricture occurs at the ileal bladder or the ileal pelvis

anastomosis, revision can be performed. Patients must also be monitored closely and treated for any bladder outlet obstruction to prevent chronic distention of the ileal ureter.

Editorial Comment
Fray F. Marshall

Long ureteral defects can still be bridged with extensive mobilization of the kidney, a psoas hitch, or a Boari flap. If these maneuvers are not feasible, an ileal ureter can be considered. It is also possible to taper the distal ileum and reimplant it so that there is not a freely refluxing ileovesical junction. Excessive ureteral tapering may cause strictures, so care must be taken to preserve the blood supply and handle the tissue delicately. In select circumstances the ileal ureter may be helpful, but it also has a semipermeable mucosal membrane, which may lead to electrolyte abnormalities.

REFERENCES

1. Boxer RJ, Fritzcshe P, Skinner DG, et al. Replacement of the ureter by small intestine: Clinical application and results of ileal ureter in 89 patients. J Urol 121:728, 1979.
2. Hendren WH. Tapered bowel segment for ureteral replacement. Urol Clin North Am 5:607, 1978.

Chapter 44

Retroperitoneal Lymphadenectomy

Richard S. Foster, John P. Donohue, and Richard Bihrle

INDICATIONS

Retroperitoneal lymphadenectomy for carcinoma of the testis is performed for low-stage nonseminomatous disease and high-stage postchemotherapy nonseminomatous and seminomatous disease. The controversy over the appropriate management of patients who have nonseminomatous disease and are clinical stage I will not be addressed specifically in this chapter. Rather, the indications, operative technique, and postoperative care for treatment of low- and high-stage disease are discussed.

Clinical staging of nonseminomatous testis cancer includes serum alpha-fetoprotein (AFP) and beta-human chorionic gonadotropin (hCG) determination, abdominal computed tomography (CT), and chest evaluation with either CT or chest radiography. Patients believed on the basis of radiography to have no or minimal disease in the abdomen and no disease in the chest are eligible for retroperitoneal lymph node dissection (RPLND) for low-stage disease. The discovery of chest disease mandates immediate chemotherapy, as does high-volume abdominal or visceral disease.

After radical orchiectomy, approximately 30 to 35 percent of patients without radiographic evidence of abdominal disease will be found to have metastasis in the retroperitoneum if RPLND is performed. Therefore, retroperitoneal lymphadenectomy provides accurate staging information. Additionally, surgical removal of low-volume retroperitoneal disease yields an approximate 50 to 70 percent chance of cure without the need for adjuvant or subsequent therapeutic chemotherapy.[1] Hence, lymphadenectomy in low-volume disease serves two purposes: staging of the retroperitoneum and therapy if retroperitoneal disease exists.

Approximately 70 percent of patients who receive primary chemotherapy for either high-volume abdominal or chest and abdominal disease will obtain a complete clinical remission.[2] A complete remission consists of normalization of the chest and abdominal CT findings along with normalization of serum AFP and beta-hCG. The remaining 30 percent of patients characteristically show normalization of serum markers but have persistent radiographic disease. These patients therefore undergo postchemotherapy resection of the residual radiographic disease. After primary chemotherapy, this resection will yield teratoma pathologically in about 45 percent of cases, necrosis in about 45 percent, and persistent cancer in about 10 percent. Removal of residual teratoma and cancer serves both a staging and a therapeutic purpose; the finding of necrosis after primary chemotherapy is indicative of an adequate chemotherapeutic dose and response.

The final indication for postchemotherapy RPLND involves only a minority of patients. Some patients with chemoresistant disease have exhibited evidence of that disease in one location (the retroperitoneum) throughout their clinical course. Patients who have evidence of persistent cancer, as shown by elevation in serum markers, are candidates for "desperation" RPLND. Removal of this chemoresistant disease offers an approximately 33 percent chance of cure in this situation.[3] It should be stressed, however, that this group of patients represent a very small minority of all those who undergo postchemotherapy RPLND.

PREOPERATIVE MANAGEMENT

Historically, patients presenting for RPLND for low-stage disease were admitted the night before surgery and hydrated with saline overnight. With the changing health care environment, it became apparent that these patients could be admitted the morning of surgery and, because they were generally young and healthy, did not need overnight intravenous hydration. A type and screen is routinely obtained, since transfusion is extremely rare in this group of patients. Prophylactic antibiotics are not routinely administered.

Postchemotherapy patients presenting for RPLND are managed differently. These individuals are approximately 4 to 6 weeks out from completion of chemotherapy and, in terms of their general medical condition, are not as healthy as patients presenting for low-stage RPLND. Because respiratory distress syndrome can occur after previous administration of bleomycin (and because of the resultant pulmonary morbidity), these patients are admitted the day before surgery and are cautiously hydrated with a colloid solution overnight.[4] Although respiratory failure after postchemotherapy RPLND is rare, it can be devastating, especially since most of these patients experience a good outcome. Hence, overnight hydration is given to avoid the rapid intravenous infusion of fluids necessary if a patient is NPO status overnight without being hydrated intravenously. A type and cross-match is obtained, because these postchemotherapy dissections are sometimes very tedious and complex. Prophylactic antibiotics are not routinely administered.

OPERATIVE TECHNIQUES

The anatomical approach to the retroperitoneum may be through a transabdominal or thoracoabdominal incision. The former is characteristically used for low- and high-stage disease and the latter for more extensive high-stage disease. The transabdominal approach offers an advantage in that excellent bilateral exposure and control is obtained. The thoracoabdominal approach yields excellent exposure of the suprahilar and retrocrural areas and may be necessary in difficult patients for early control of the great vessels.

Technique for Low-Stage Disease

Traditionally, a full bilateral RPLND was performed for low-stage disease.[5] It is now recognized that this is too extensive an operation for patients in this particular stage. However, these full bilateral RPLNDs allowed mapping studies to be performed, which showed that patients with minimal retroperitoneal disease characteristically do not have bilateral retroperitoneal disease.[6] It became apparent that the site of metastasis in the retroperitoneum could be predicted on the basis of the site of the primary tumor

and the amount of retroperitoneal disease. This allowed the development of more limited templates for low-stage disease.

Initially, these more limited templates enabled the therapeutic and staging aspect of the procedure to be maintained but decreased the morbidity, since emission and ejaculation were preserved in some of these patients. Using the so-called modified templates, one third to two thirds of patients who were subjected to modified RPLND maintained the ability to ejaculate. Subsequently, even more limited templates have increased the ejaculation rate to approximately 90 percent.[7]

Since the modified templates maintained the staging and therapeutic aspects of the procedure and showed promise in terms of preserving emission and ejaculation, a more refined approach was developed to increase the postoperative ejaculation rate to close to 100 percent. With increasing knowledge of the anatomy of the retroperitoneal sympathetic fibers, it became clear that these fibers could be dissected prospectively before the modified en bloc dissections. Hence, the nerve-sparing RPLND was developed,[8, 9] which employs two basic aspects: (1) the prospective dissection of retroperitoneal sympathetic fibers and (2) en bloc modified lymphadenectomy.

Transabdominal exposure of the retroperitoneum in low-stage disease is carried out through a midline incision from xyphoid to pubis. A self-retaining ring retractor affixed to the table affords excellent exposure. Initially, palpation of the retroperitoneum is performed to confirm that clinical staging was indeed correct. A finding of more extensive bilateral disease at initial laparotomy mandates abandonment of the nerve-sparing modified dissection. However, it is now clear in this situation that nerve-sparing techniques can indeed be used effectively if a full bilateral dissection is performed.[9, 10]

If palpation of the retroperitoneum at laparotomy reveals no or minimal disease, the nerve-sparing dissection is performed. For a right-sided dissection an incision is made in the posterior peritoneum from the cecum to the ligament of Treitz (Fig. 44–1). The root of the small bowel is dissected off the retroperitoneum, and the inferior mesenteric vein is divided between silk ties. Self-retaining retractors are used to obtain exposure. The split-and-roll technique is then undertaken. Initially the split maneuver is carried out from the left renal vein to the origin of the inferior mesenteric artery over the anterior surface of the aorta. The interaortocaval tissue is then rolled medially to determine whether any lower pole precaval right renal arteries exist. Next, the split maneuver is carried out over the anterior surface of the vena cava, and the origin of the right spermatic vein is identified and divided between silk ties. The lymphatic tissue is then rolled medially off the medial aspect of the

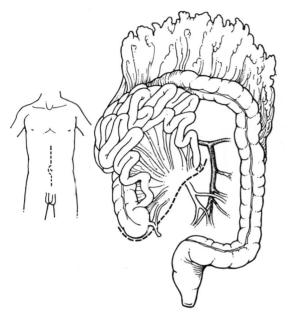

Figure 44–1. Posterior peritoneal incision for right nerve-sparing modified retroperitoneal lymph node dissection (RPLND). (Courtesy of the Medical Illustrations Dept., Indiana University School of Medicine, Indianapolis.)

to injure sympathetic fibers in the process. Lumbar arteries on the medial aspect of the aorta are also divided. Thus, the dissection has effectively freed the sympathetic fibers, the aorta, and the vena cava. The only remaining portion of the procedure is to dissect the interaortocaval and right paracaval lymphatic tissue up off the posterior body wall, taking care to clip lumbar arteries and veins as they pass into the posterior body wall. Finally, the right gonadal vein is dissected distally to the internal ring and passed off as specimen (Fig. 44–3).

For a left-sided dissection the posterior peritoneum lateral to the left colon is incised, and the left colon and mesocolon are elevated off the retroperitoneum and retracted medially. This provides good exposure of the left periaortic, preaortic, and upper interaortocaval zones. Care must be taken to divide the splenocolic ligament in order to avoid injury to the spleen. This initial exposure is very similar to the technique for transabdominal radical nephrectomy.

The next step is to identify the left-sided efferent sympathetic fibers. Two basic techniques can facilitate this identification. The first is to dissect in the area of the left common iliac artery, at which point a condensation of these fibers is usually seen as they pass into the interiliac zone. It is at approximately this point that the right and left sympathetic fibers coalesce before proceeding into the pelvis. These fibers are then looped as they pass over the left common iliac artery and dissected proximally. The origin of the left gonadal vein is then identified, divided from the left renal vein, and dissected distally to the internal ring, at which point it is passed off as

vena cava, revealing lumbar veins passing from the posterior surface of the vena cava to the posterior body wall (Fig. 44–2). Characteristically the retroperitoneal efferent sympathetic fibers pass superior to these veins behind the vena cava to the sympathetic chain. These fibers are dissected and placed in vessel loops. All lumbar veins passing from the vena cava to the posterior body wall are divided, taking care not

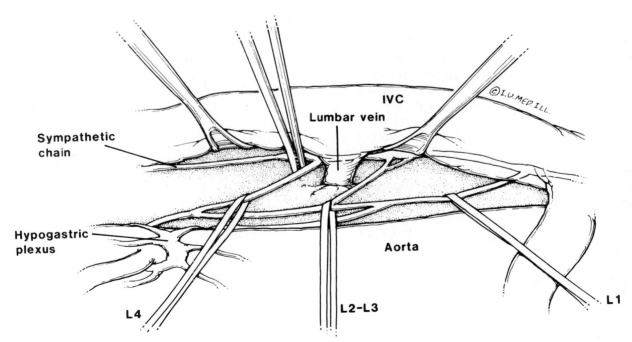

Figure 44–2. The path of sympathetic efferents posterior to the vena cava. Note the passage of the efferent fibers superior to the lumbar veins. IVC, inferior vena cava.

It should be stressed that these procedures are not "node pluckings." The technique of nerve-sparing RPLND has been refined and is reproducible. Results have shown that nerve-sparing RPLND indeed preserves the staging and therapeutic aspects of the procedure and preserves ejaculation at the 99 percent level.[8] Furthermore, nerve-sparing RPLND is worthwhile since a reasonable percentage of these patients are potentially fertile.[11] Finally, it is now known that the morbidity of this procedure is extremely low.[12] The only significant short-term morbidity is wound infection, and the only significant long-term morbidity is an approximately 1 percent risk of developing a small bowel obstruction.

Technique for Postchemotherapy Dissection

As previously discussed, about 30 percent of patients presenting with high-stage testicular cancer experience a partial remission after initial primary chemotherapy. These patients have normalization of serum markers but show persistent retroperitoneal,

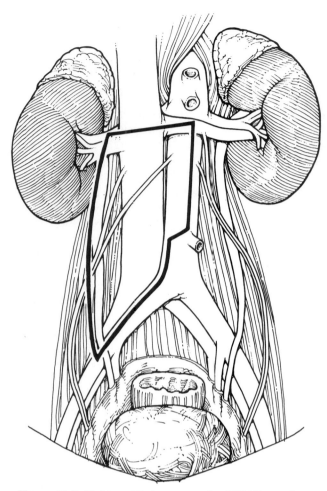

Figure 44–3. Right modified nerve-sparing RPLND template.

specimen. The lateral border of the dissection is then defined by the ureter; therefore, the lymphatic tissue is dissected free of the ureter medial to the ureter. Care must be taken in performing this dissection not to injure a lower pole left renal artery. This lymphatic tissue can then be dissected up off the psoas muscle, exposing the left-sided sympathetic chain. Hence, the efferent fibers have been defined as they pass over the left common iliac artery. In addition, the left sympathetic chain has been defined. The remaining portion of the dissection involves dissecting these efferent fibers completely free, after which all left-sided lumbar arteries passing between the aorta and the posterior body wall are divided before the removal of lymphatic tissue. Care must also be taken to divide the lumbar vein that passes from the left renal vein posteriorly to the body wall. The renal artery is also defined. Finally, lymphatic tissue is removed from the posterior body wall and left psoas muscle. Next, a small amount of upper preaortic lymphatic tissue and interaortocaval tissue is taken to complete the dissection (Fig. 44–4). Care must be taken not to injure right-sided sympathetic efferents in taking this upper interaortocaval tissue.

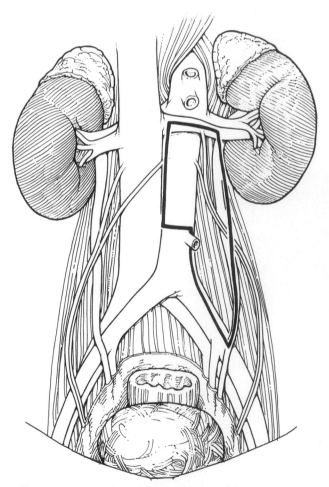

Figure 44–4. Left modified nerve-sparing RPLND template.

retrocrural, mediastinal, thoracic, or neck disease. The surgical approach to each of these areas is dictated by the site and amount of disease. For instance, low- or moderate-volume retroperitoneal disease is approached via a midline incision; retrocrural disease through a midline incision, a thoracoabdominal incision, or thoracotomy; mediastinal disease via sternotomy, thoracotomy, or a thoracoabdominal incision; and neck disease by neck dissections. Visceral disease may exist, and at the time of the operation various ancillary procedures such as partial hepatectomy, pancreatectomy, colectomy, or nephrectomy are sometimes required.

For the standard patient with postchemotherapy retroperitoneal disease, a full bilateral dissection is recommended (Fig. 44–5). This is because mapping studies have previously shown that patients with higher-volume retroperitoneal disease are more likely to have bilateral disease. However, it is well recognized that highly selected patients may undergo modified postchemotherapy or nerve-sparing RPLNDs to preserve ejaculatory competence.[10]

For a standard transabdominal full bilateral post-

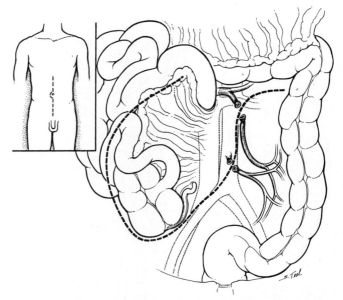

Figure 44–6. Posterior peritoneal incision for full bilateral dissection with mobilization of the root of the small bowel onto the patient's chest. (Courtesy of the Medical Illustrations Dept., Indiana University School of Medicine, Indianapolis.)

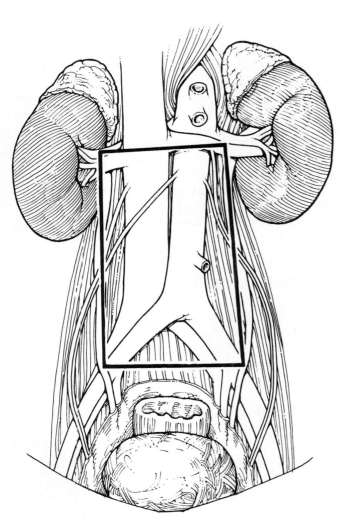

Figure 44–5. Template for full bilateral RPLND.

chemotherapy RPLND, a generous xyphoid-to-pubis incision is performed. A plastic wound protector is placed, and the abdomen is retracted with a self-retaining ring retractor affixed to the table. An incision is then made in the posterior peritoneum from the foramen of Winslow distally around the cecum cephalad to the ligament of Treitz, with division of the inferior mesenteric vein (Fig. 44–6). The root of the small bowel and right colon, along with the head of the pancreas and duodenum, are mobilized off the retroperitoneum, placed in a bowel bag, and retracted onto the patient's chest.

The split-and-roll maneuver is then begun (Fig. 44–7). Initially the split maneuver is carried out over the anterior surface of the aorta to define both the arterial anatomy to the kidneys and the origin of the inferior mesenteric artery. The latter is divided between silk ties and the left mesocolon is retracted to the patient's left, thus giving excellent exposure of the entire retroperitoneum. The standard boundaries of a full bilateral dissection are the crura of the diaphragm superiorly, the bifurcation of the common iliac arteries inferiorly, and the ureters laterally. The split maneuver begun over the aorta is thus carried distally onto the common iliac arteries. Lymphatic tissue and tumor are then rolled medially and laterally off the aorta, giving exposure of the lumbar arteries posteriorly. These arteries, which are usually paired, are exposed and divided between silk ties. Similarly, the renal arteries are dissected free of lymphatic and tumoral tissue. Care must be taken to divide the previously mentioned lumbar vein passing posteriorly from the left renal vein to the posterior

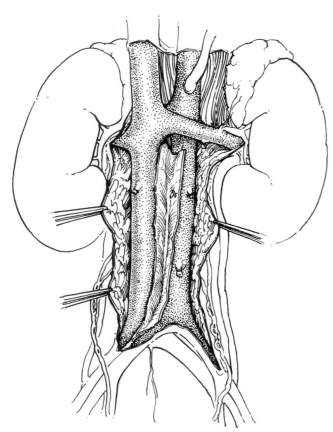

Figure 44–7. Anterior split of the nodal package.

body wall. The aorta has now been effectively freed from surrounding tumor, lymphatic tissue, and the posterior body wall, and attention is turned to the vena cava. The split maneuver is carried out over the vena cava, and the origin of the right spermatic vein is divided. Lymphatic and tumoral tissue is then rolled medially and laterally off the vena cava and the common iliacs, exposing the lumbar veins passing into the posterior body wall. These veins are highly variable in position and structure and are by and large more difficult to dissect in the postchemotherapy patient than are the lumbar arteries. They are identified and divided between silk ties, thus freeing the vena cava and common iliacs from the posterior body wall and tumoral tissue. Attention is then turned to the ureters, which are freed on their medial aspect from the tissue to be removed and are retracted laterally. Hence, four zones of tissue remain to be resected: the right paracaval, interaortocaval, left periaortic, and interiliac specimens. At this point in the procedure, the only remaining attachment is the posterior body wall. These zones are next dissected off the posterior body wall, taking care to clip lumbar arteries and veins as they pass into the latter. This completes postchemotherapy RPLND.

Other specialized surgical techniques are required for resection of retrocrural or posterior mediastinal disease. A thoracoabdominal approach is usually performed for high-volume retrocrural or mediastinal disease. Depending on the side of the lesion, the spleen and tail of the pancreas can be mobilized off the diaphragm and retroperitoneum and mobilized medially to expose the left crus, or the liver can be mobilized from its diaphragmatic attachments and rolled medially to expose the right crus (Fig. 44–8). The crus is then incised, after which the tumor can be removed from its attachments to the aorta medially and the vertebral column posteriorly. If a thoracoabdominal incision is used, this tissue can be approached through the crus or through the chest above the crus.

Surgeons who embark on postchemotherapy RPLND must be committed to a thorough and complete procedure. It is extremely difficult to predict the amount of effort and time required for an individual postchemotherapy procedure, since it is impossible clinically to determine how adherent the tumor will be to great vessels and other retroperitoneal structures. Care must be taken in dealing with the great vessels not to dissect in the subadventitial plane. If this plane is used and repair of an aortic or caval laceration is necessary, the thinned aorta or vena cava sometimes does not hold sutures well. Dissecting in a plane outside the adventitia preserves this strengthening aspect of the great vessels and allows subsequent sutures to hold well.

RPLND for low-stage disease and postchemotherapy RPLND are both vascular procedures. Conceptually, important structures such as the vena cava, aorta, renal vessels, and sympathetic fibers are removed from the tumor mass, after which the tumor mass is removed from the posterior body wall. RPLND is not a haphazard tour of the retroperitoneum. Rather, certain well-defined steps and principles must be used to facilitate an effective and safe procedure.

POSTOPERATIVE COMPLICATIONS

The complications of RPLND for low-stage disease differ dramatically from those presenting after postchemotherapy RPLND for high-stage disease. They will therefore be discussed separately.

After Surgery for Low-Stage Disease

In experienced hands, nerve-sparing RPLND is a procedure accompanied by very low morbidity.[12] As previously noted, the most common short-term morbidity is wound infection (less than 5 percent of patients) and the only significant long-term complication the risk of developing a small bowel obstruction

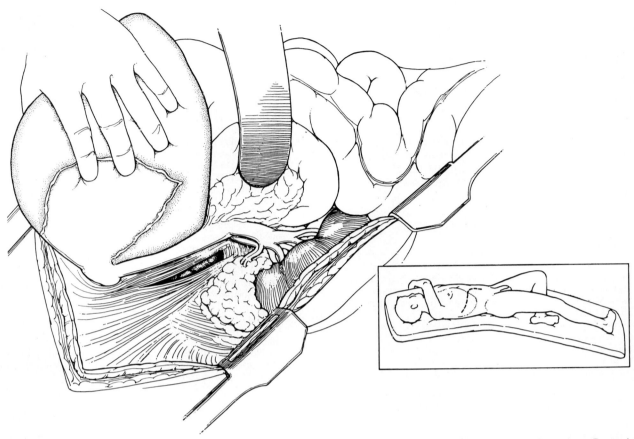

Figure 44–8. Thoracoabdominal exposure for resection of right retrocrural disease. (Courtesy of the Medical Illustrations Dept., Indiana University School of Medicine, Indianapolis.)

(1 percent). Transfusion is not required and hospitalization averages 4 to 5 days. Formerly, nasogastric decompression was used postoperatively; the current practice is to place an oral gastric tube during the procedure, empty the stomach at its completion, and dispense with nasogastric decompression postoperatively.

At one time the major source of morbidity after RPLND was loss of emission and ejaculation. Nerve-sparing RPLND effectively eliminates this problem and allows this group of patients to retain the potential to father children. Thus, one of the major arguments against the use of RPLND for low-stage disease has been eliminated.

After Surgery for High-Stage Disease

The morbidity associated with RPLND for high-stage disease is significantly different from that for RPLND for low-stage disease.[13] A review of 603 patients from Indiana University who underwent postchemotherapy RPLND revealed a 20.7 percent rate of complications. Operative mortality was approximately 1 percent. A major source of morbidity was the lungs, which probably relates to bleomycin-in-duced pulmonary toxicity and prolonged operative procedures required to resect high-volume postchemotherapy disease. There were five deaths in this series, including two patients who died of adult respiratory distress syndrome. The average hospital stay for patients undergoing uncomplicated postchemotherapy RPLND was 7.5 days, and for those with major complications, 19.9 days.

Chylous ascites has also been reported after postchemotherapy RPLND.[14] It is now clear that resection of a previously patent vena cava is a risk factor for development of chylous ascites.

Summary

There is a clear rationale for retroperitoneal lymph node dissection in both low- and high-stage disease. The technique has been clearly elucidated for both stages and is reproducible. Surgeons embarking on nerve-sparing or postchemotherapy RPLND must be thoroughly versed in techniques of vascular control and repair. RPLND for both low- and high-stage disease is a vascular procedure. Finally, the technique and complication rate of nerve-sparing RPLND for low-stage disease is clearly different from those of postchemotherapy RPLND. Fortunately, proper and judicious use of this procedure has afforded an excellent chance for cure with minimal morbidity in patients with testicular cancer.

Editorial Comment
Fray F. Marshall

Nerve-sparing technique can be applied to retroperitoneal lymphadenectomy. As a result, the loss of emission or ejaculation can be avoided. Depending on the clinical stage of the patient, the precise outlines of the dissection are also defined in this chapter.

REFERENCES

1. Donohue JP, Thornhill JA, Foster RS, et al. Retroperitoneal lymphadenectomy for clinical stage A testis cancer (1965–1989): Modifications of technique and impact on ejaculation. J Urol 149:237, 1993.
2. Einhorn LH, Donohue JP. Cis-diamminedichloroplatinum, vinblastine, and bleomycin combination chemotherapy in disseminated testicular cancer. Ann Intern Med 87:293, 1977.
3. Murphy BR, Breeden ES, Donohue JP, et al. Surgical salvage of chemorefractory germ cell tumors. J Clin Oncol 11:324, 1993.
4. Goldiner PL, Schweizer O. The hazards of anesthesia and surgery in bleomycin-treated patients. Semin Oncol 6:121, 1979.
5. Donohue JP. Retroperitoneal lymphadenectomy: The anterior approach including bilateral suprarenal-hilar dissection. Urol Clin North Am 4:509, 1977.
6. Donohue JP, Zachary JM, Maynard BR. Distribution of nodal metastases in nonseminomatous testis cancer. J Urol 128:315, 1982.
7. Richie JP. Clinical stage I testicular cancer: The role of modified retroperitoneal lymphadenectomy. J Urol 144:1160, 1990.
8. Donohue JP, Foster RS, Rowland RG, et al. Nerve-sparing retroperitoneal lymphadenectomy with preservation of ejaculation. J Urol 144:287, 1990.
9. Jewett MA, Kong YS, Goldberg SD, et al. Retroperitoneal lymphadenectomy for testis tumor with nerve sparing for ejaculation. J Urol 139:1220, 1988.
10. Wahle GR, Foster RS, Bihrle R, et al. Nerve-sparing retroperitoneal lymphadenectomy after primary chemotherapy for metastatic testicular carcinoma. J Urol 152:428, 1994.
11. Foster RS, McNulty A, Rubin LR, et al. The fertility of patients with clinical stage I testis cancer managed by nerve-sparing RPLND. J Urol 152:1139, 1994.
12. Baniel J, Foster RS, Rowland RG, et al. Complications of primary retroperitoneal lymph node dissection. J Urol 152:424, 1994.
13. Baniel J, Foster RS, Rowland RG, et al. Complications of post chemotherapy retroperitoneal lymph node dissection. J Urol 153:976, 1995.
14. Baniel J, Foster RS, Rowland RG, et al. Management of chylous ascites after retroperitoneal lymph node dissection for testicular cancer. J Urol 150:1422, 1993.

Chapter 45

Surgery of the Kidney and Ureter in Pregnancy

Jacek L. Mostwin

Decisions regarding surgery of the kidney and ureter during pregnancy can be based on an understanding of the normal anatomical and physiological changes that may occur at this time, and an anticipation of likely complications, which may require surgical intervention. Elective surgery can often be postponed, but emergencies, including the possibility of tumor, cannot and should not. Calculi and hydronephrosis are the most commonly encountered urological surgical conditions during pregnancy, and the use of percutaneous drainage techniques has simplified the management of these conditions. Sonography has become a major imaging technique, replacing conventional radiography in many cases. Other complications, such as benign and malignant tumors, advanced obstruction, and perforation of the urinary tract, are less common; information regarding these complications is scattered in case reports and reviews. Several excellent reviews of more common problems have appeared.[1-4] Some of the highlights of these reviews are presented in this chapter along with information gathered from many case reports found throughout the world's literature. Older reviews may be of historical interest.[5, 3]

RELEVANT PHYSIOLOGICAL AND ANATOMICAL CHANGES

Physiological hydronephrosis of pregnancy is the change with which most urologists are familiar. However, several other physiological and anatomical changes are important in the evaluation of the effect of pregnancy on urological pathology and the suitability of the patient to undergo anesthesia and surgery.[7, 8] Very early in pregnancy, increases occur in total body water, cardiac output, renal blood flow,

and glomerular filtration rate. As a result, nocturia is one of the earliest symptoms of normal pregnancy.

An increase in red blood cell mass occurs, but because of an increase in total body water, dilutional physiological anemia of pregnancy develops. The hematocrit value may drop as low as 30 percent. Clotting factors increase, predisposing the patient to hypercoagulability and thromboembolism. As pregnancy develops, pelvic vascular engorgement, venous stasis, and hypercoagulability increase the risk of thromboembolism during surgery or bed rest. The enlarging uterus compresses the vena cava and aorta, decreasing blood pressure and venous return to the heart.

The enlarging uterus restricts ventilatory movements, reducing arterial PO_2 in the supine position. Tidal volume increases and functional residual capacity decreases in this position, further affecting intra- and postoperative ventilatory movements. Decreased gastrointestinal motility and reduced esophageal sphincteric pressures predispose the patient to gastroesophageal reflux, increasing the risk of postoperative aspiration.

The shape of the bladder and trigone is changed during pregnancy. As the uterus enlarges and rises out of the pelvis, the bladder is elevated with it. The posterior wall becomes more convex until most of the urine-storing capacity of the bladder is laterally displaced. The trigone is stretched both superiorly and laterally by the enlarging cervix, making cystoscopic identification and successful catheterization of the ureteral orifices more difficult.[2]

PHYSIOLOGICAL HYDRONEPHROSIS OF PREGNANCY

Physiological hydronephrosis of pregnancy is a well-recognized condition that has been extensively

373

reviewed.[9, 10] Although both hormonal and mechanical factors have been implicated in the development of urinary tract dilation during pregnancy, most data favor the conclusion that right-sided hydronephrosis is probably due to mechanical compression of the ureter at the pelvic brim by the enlarging uterus.

Schulman and Herlinger[11] reviewed 220 excretory urograms performed during pregnancy in patients with clinically normal urinary tracts. Dilation of the urinary tract was rarely found before midterm. After midterm the right side was found to be dilated in 75 percent of cases and the left in 33 percent. In 86 percent of all cases, the right side was more dilated than the left. Severe dilation was not frequent. The dilation was never found to extend below the brim of the true pelvis. No association was found between the degree of dilation and the position of the fetus, the number of pregnancies, or the presence of urinary infection.

Manometric studies of intraureteral pressure have found normal peristaltic activity of the ureters in pregnancy. Dure-Smith[12] observed notching of the right ureter as it crosses over the iliac artery along its course into the pelvis. At this point the dilated ureter narrows to normal size, implying obstruction at this point. This investigator interpreted these findings to show that the right ureter courses much more acutely over the right iliac artery, whereas the left ureter passes more nearly parallel to the left iliac artery.

The observation that hydronephrosis can often be relieved when the gravid patient assumes the knee-chest position or lateral recumbent position further suggests mechanical obstruction. Additional protection to the left ureter is thought to be provided by the sigmoid colon. Hydronephrosis rapidly resolves after delivery, often within 24 hours.

ACUTE ABDOMEN IN PREGNANCY

Because the possibility of a urological condition may first be raised in the clinical setting of abdominal pain, nausea, or vomiting, the urologist should be familiar with the differential diagnosis of acute abdomen during pregnancy. The topic has been reviewed by Silen[13] in *Cope's Early Diagnosis of the Acute Abdomen*. Several points are worth noting. During the second and third months of pregnancy physiological nausea and vomiting, often in the morning, are to be expected. These may sometimes be more persistent and may give rise to consideration of an acute abdomen. The pain of acute appendicitis may mimic acute right-sided pyelonephritis. The appendix is displaced cephalad in later pregnancy by the enlarging uterus, and the pain may be localized more to the right upper quadrant, mimicking acute cholecystitis and resembling the pain of pyelonephritis. Pyelone-

phritis, however, has a more abrupt onset with high fever and rigors, whereas appendicitis develops more slowly, fever being a late manifestation.

Other acute abdominal conditions occurring during pregnancy include ectopic pregnancy, threatened abortion, retroverted gravid uterus, sepsis after attempted abortion, degeneration of a fibroid, torsion of an ovarian cyst, pedunculated fibroid or normal ovary, perforated gastric ulcer, and peritonitis. The clinical setting and findings at ovarian surgery during pregnancy have been reviewed.[14, 15]

RADIOGRAPHICAL IMAGING

Radiographical imaging has been reviewed by Brendler[16] in *Campbell's Urology*. General agreement exists that exposure below 5 to 10 rad is well tolerated in all trimesters of pregnancy. In the first trimester, during the period of organogenesis, significant radiation will most likely result in spontaneous abortion rather than birth defects. In children born after intrauterine exposure to radiation, the risk of developing a significant birth defect based on this exposure has been calculated to be far smaller than the risk of spontaneous mutation.[17, 18]

Because a complete excretory urogram exposes the patient to less than 1.5 rad, it should be safely tolerated in all trimesters. By shielding the abdomen, collimating screens, and using limited exposure, a functional excretory urogram can be obtained with less than 1.5 rad. Therefore, in the presence of acute urological symptoms, such as flank pain, with or without fever, or hematuria, pregnancy should not be considered a contraindication to obtaining a limited excretory urogram.[19]

Ultrasonography has been utilized extensively throughout all trimesters of pregnancy. No increased risk to fetus or mother has been identified. Although ultrasonography of the kidneys does not provide functional information regarding the urinary tract, it can safely be chosen as the imaging study of first choice.

Radionuclide imaging has been employed in pregnancy, but most radioactive tracers cross the placental barrier and their long-term effect on the fetus is unknown. Although the half-life of many of these substances is quite long, and no safe dosage or technique has been established, no birth defects have been reported.[20, 21] In general, radionuclide imaging during pregnancy has been discouraged.

Computed tomography may be necessary to evaluate a renal mass discovered during pregnancy for the possibility of cancer. A complete study with and without contrast material provides a dose in excess of 5 rad, a level thought to exceed the safe range. A limited study, however, supervised by a radiologist, can be performed using less than 1 rad. Magnetic resonance imaging standards for pregnancy have not been established, although isolated reports utilizing the technique for preoperative staging of tumor have appeared.[22] Harmful effects have not yet been reported.

ANESTHETICS AND ANTIBIOTICS

General drug considerations have been reviewed by Niebyl[23] and antibiotic usage by Hamod and Khouzami.[24] The penicillins are the most widely administered class of drugs during pregnancy and have been found to be safe. Sulfonamides are safe but can cause kernicterus in the newborn. Aminoglycosides have failed to show teratogenetic effects in animal studies. Serum levels may be lower in pregnancy because of increased glomerular filtration rate and should be monitored. Cephalosporins are given extensively in obstetrical practice, although there is still insufficient information to definitely establish their safety. Clindamycin should be restricted to those infections thought to be caused by anaerobic bacteria, because of the risk of pseudomembranous colitis in the mother.

Of these antibiotics, metronidazole is one that has been associated with increased mutagenesis in animal studies. In human studies, however, no significant increase has been reported in congenital defects among newborns and mothers treated with metronidazole. Trimethoprim has also been associated with congenital defects in animal studies. However, in human studies the combined use of sulfa with trimethoprim has not shown increased risk.

In summary, most antibiotics likely to be used in association with urinary tract surgery, for either prophylaxis or treatment of infection, have been shown to be safe during pregnancy. Blood levels of these drugs appear to be even lower in pregnancy than in the nonpregnant state because of greater renal excretion.

Many of the commonly employed inhalational anesthetics, including halothane, nitrous oxide, methoxyflurane, diethyl ether, cyclopropane, and fluroxene, have been studied for teratogenicity in animal models. Evidence of intrauterine death and abnormality has been detected. However, most of these studies have involved long-term exposure to large doses of these agents. Studies of pregnant operating personnel exposed to long-term doses of inhalational agents, as well as studies that have critically evaluated the incidence of birth defects in women receiving general or regional anesthesia during pregnancy, have failed to disclose any significant relationship between clinical exposure to anesthetic agents and birth defects. Morphine and meperidine are commonly employed analgesics that appear to be safe when administered for short periods.[8]

COMPLICATIONS OF URINARY TRACT DILATION AND ENGORGEMENT

Physiological hydronephrosis of pregnancy can progress to unilateral or bilateral obstruction with associated flank pain. This complication may respond to a simple change in position, such as assuming the recumbent position on the side opposite the affected side. However, the placement of ureteral catheters may be necessary.

Spontaneous rupture of the collecting system with urinoma formation has been reported.[25-29] This has been treated by exploration and drainage of the urinoma or by a temporary indwelling ureteral catheter.[30]

Because of increased cardiac output, patients with preexisting arteriovenous malformations or renal artery aneurysms[31] may suffer rupture with severe hemorrhage either retro- or intraperitoneally. Hematuria from bleeding into the collecting system may be seen. Other organs, including the liver, may spontaneously rupture.[32] Dilated urethral veins have been reported as a cause of hemorrhage.[33] Postpartum hematuria attributable to sudden decompression of an engorged pyelovenous system has been reported and has ceased without treatment,[34] but catheter drainage may be required because of clot formation.

OVARIAN VEIN SYNDROME

The ovarian vein syndrome is a condition of right-sided middle or proximal ureteral obstruction caused by aberrant ovarian veins,[35] often found coursing in a common sheath with the ureter.[36] The condition may sometimes become evident during pregnancy, and temporary drainage by ureteral catheter has been recommended.[37] More commonly the condition appears in the postpartum period as acute right flank pain or pyelonephritis.[37a] Right ureteral obstruction may be identified by excretory urography or retrograde pyelography. Electromyography of the ureter has even been used to demonstrate obstruction.[38]

Surgical relief of the obstruction is usually required. In many reports the ureter and vein are described as running in a common sheath.[39, 40] The vein may be phlebitic. Ureterolysis, sometimes accompanied by excision of the dilated or phlebitic vein, is required to free the structure.[41]

RENAL CALCULI

The management of stones during pregnancy has been well reviewed.[42, 43] In a series of 20 of their own patients and a review of the literature, Maikranz and co-workers[44] did not find a higher incidence of stone formation during pregnancy. Renal colic was found to be the most common nonobstetrical cause of abdominal pain that required hospitalization during pregnancy. Most stones were diagnosed during the second and third trimesters. Stones were found equally on the right and the left sides. Usually, 50 percent of stones passed spontaneously. No fetal or maternal complications were reported in this review to be caused by any of the surgical procedures performed for stone management. These investigators concluded that pregnancy has no effect on stone disease.

Premature labor from renal colic may occur but has responded well to beta$_2$-agonist tocolytic therapy.[45] Most instances of premature labor have ceased after removal or passage of the stones.[46]

Modern endoscopic techniques have not greatly affected the management of stone disease in pregnancy, primarily because extracorporeal shock wave lithotripsy and percutaneous surgery, the two major innovations, rely so heavily on fluoroscopy. Ultrasonically guided placement of percutaneous nephrostomy catheters for severe pain or obstruction is a safe and conservative approach to the management of most obstructing calculi. Definitive treatment can be delayed until after delivery.

Ureteroscopic and nephroscopic procedures cannot be advocated because of the high level of radiation involved. The risk of injury to the engorged softened urinary tract may lead to easier perforation than might be expected during normal endoscopy or stone manipulation. Blind ureteroscopy has been reported, but it is unlikely that this technique will be widely accepted. Clayman[47] has managed obstructing stones by percutaneous nephrostomy, delaying definitive procedure until delivery. Lyon reported the use of sonography to guide catheter manipulation of calculi during pregnancy.[48] Bagley reported similar procedures.[49]

In summary, in half the cases, renal calculi identified during pregnancy pass spontaneously. The other half may require instrumentation, but this should be limited to temporary drainage by percutaneous or indwelling double-J catheters. Double-J catheters have been tolerated well throughout the final trimester and through delivery. The risk of perforation of the urinary tract in the placement of retrograde catheters, as well as the increased risk of transmitting infected urine to the obstructed renal pelvis and upper ureter, must be considered. For this reason, percutaneous nephrostomy performed under sonographic control may well be the safest procedure for the expectant mother who requires relief of obstruction or infection from stone.

RENAL AND BLADDER TUMORS

Urological cancer in pregnancy is extremely uncommon. The general topic of cancer in pregnancy was reviewed by Williams and Bitran,[50] who reported the incidence of malignancy in pregnancy to be approximately 1 in 1000. Neoplasms of the breasts and the female genital tract, including cervical, vulvar, vaginal, ovarian, and endometrial carcinomas, were the most common. Leukemia, lymphoma, malignant melanoma, thyroid cancer, and gastrointestinal cancer have been reported and were reviewed by these investigators. Urological cancers were not listed among the tumors reviewed, suggesting that their incidence was very low. Regarding the relative risks of the usual methods of cancer management during pregnancy, these investigators concluded that those from surgery are probably less than those from adjuvant radiation or chemotherapy.

Benign and malignant tumors of the bladder and kidney have been reported during pregnancy, and surgical management has usually been required. Patients with these tumors have presented with palpable masses or spontaneous hemorrhage, occurring intra- or retroperitoneally, or as hematuria from bleeding into the collecting system.[51] Renal cell carcinoma is the most common malignant renal neoplasm of pregnancy but is still rare. Walker and Knight[52] reviewed the literature in 1986 and found only 71 cases, although one must allow for unreported cases.

The mother should always be offered the immediate benefit of surgery upon recognition of the tumor. Numerous case reports and reviews have illustrated the use of selective radiography and surgery for renal cell carcinoma, often with a successful outcome for both mother and fetus.[53–62]

Other benign and malignant tumors of the kidney include Wilms tumor,[63] tubular adenoma,[64] sarcoma,[65] metastatic trophoblastic disease,[66–69] and angiomyolipomas.[70–79] All have been reported and have been successfully removed during pregnancy in all three trimesters without loss of the fetus. When such surgery is contemplated in the third trimester, it may be advisable to perform simultaneous cesarean section if the fetus is sufficiently mature, to prevent inadvertent intrauterine death during or immediately after surgery. A surgically trained obstetrician should therefore be available for consultation. Tocolytic therapy should be on hand if needed.

Pheochromocytoma, if discovered early in pregnancy, can be successfully removed. In the third trimester the risk of premature labor during surgery increases, and delay with drug therapy for the catecholamine excess has been advised.[80, 81]

Low-grade transitional cell carcinomas of the bladder have been reported and have been removed by transurethral resection.[82–87] Squamous cell carcinoma of the bladder in association with schistosomiasis has been reported, requiring cystectomy during pregnancy. The outcome for this particular condition was often poor for both fetus and mother,[88] probably because of advanced local disease at the time of diagnosis.

ECTOPIC KIDNEY AND PREVIOUS UROLOGICAL SURGERY

Abnormalities of renal position have not been associated with difficult labor or delivery. The presence of horseshoe, ectopic, or malrotated kidney does not require special intervention or delivery by cesarean section. Even a pelvic kidney usually rests outside the true pelvis and does not generally interfere with normal labor.

Patients may be managed conservatively who have previously undergone urological diversion or intra-abdominal reconstructive urinary tract surgery. Cesarean section in these patients can be complicated by (1) the presence of previous abdominal adhesions, (2) the distorted urinary tract anatomy created by pregnancy, and (3) uncertainty in regard to the relationship of the ureters and reconstructed bladder or internal reservoir to the enlarged uterus. For these reasons, vaginal delivery is preferable.

In women who have undergone genital reconstruction, e.g., for exstrophy or epispadias, vaginal delivery has been successfully accomplished. These patients may have an increased tendency to miscarriage because of the pubic diastasis.

PREGNANCY AFTER RENAL TRANSPLANTATION

After renal transplantation, ovulation may unexpectedly resume in a patient who had stopped ovulating before this procedure. A patient who is sexually active may then become pregnant. In patients with functioning transplants in whom renal function has been restored, pregnancy can be successfully managed and carried to term. As in ectopic kidney, the location of the kidney in the iliac fossa does not interfere with the normal enlargement of the uterus or the potential for vaginal delivery. Cesarean section should not be necessary.

Summary

Calculi and hydronephrosis are the most commonly encountered urological conditions during pregnancy and can usually be managed conservatively with sonographically guided percutaneous or retrograde catheters. Open surgery is usually reserved for spontaneous rupture or hemorrhage from the urinary tract or the discovery of cancer during the pregnancy, all of which are extremely rare. All sonographic techniques and most radiographical techniques that limit exposure to less than 5 rad are considered safe. Most antibiotics and anesthetic agents are safe during pregnancy. Previous urological surgery, including renal transplantation, should encourage the attending obstetrician and consulting urologist to advise vaginal delivery rather than cesarean section. Despite the anxiety produced by unexpected urological difficulties during pregnancy, the outcome for both mother and fetus is usually favorable.

Editorial Comment
Fray F. Marshall

Urological problems can arise frequently in the pregnant patient. This topic has not been covered extensively in the urological literature. As Dr. Mostwin has indicated, antibiotics and radiography can be employed judiciously with relatively few side effects. Surgery is sometimes required in the pregnant woman. During the second trimester, surgery can usually be accomplished without initiation of labor. Toward the end of pregnancy, especially in the third trimester, labor can often be initiated by surgery. We have performed several nephrectomies in pregnant patients for renal cell carcinomas and have removed a pelvic kidney with a large angiomyolipoma in a young pregnant patient. In general, the patients and children have done well.

Ovarian vein syndrome probably does not occur very often. When it does, I suspect it may be related to septic phlebitis of the ovarian vein with resultant fibrosis.

REFERENCES

1. Buchsbaum HJ, Schmidt JD. Gynecologic and Obstetric Urology, 3rd ed. Philadelphia, WB Saunders, 1993.
2. Freed SZ, Herzig N, eds. Urology in Pregnancy. Baltimore, Williams & Wilkins, 1982.
3. Meares EM. Urologic surgery during pregnancy. Clin Obstet Gynecol 21:7, 1978.
4. Stanton SL. Clinical Gynecologic Urology. St. Louis, CV Mosby, 1984.
5. Crabtree EG. Urological Disease of Pregnancy. Boston, Little, Brown, 1942.
6. Everett HS. Gynecological and Obstetrical Urology. Baltimore, Williams & Wilkins, 1947.
7. Barron WM. Medical evaluation of the pregnant patient requiring nonobstetric surgery. Clin Perinatol 12:481, 1985.
8. Kammerer WS. Nonobstetric surgery in pregnancy. Med Clin North Am 71:551, 1987.
9. Rasmussen RE, Nielsen FR. Hydronephrosis during pregnancy: A literature survey. Eur J Obstet Gynecol Reprod Biol 27:249, 1988.
10. Beydoun SN. Morphological changes in the renal tract in pregnancy. Clin Obstet Gynecol 28:249, 1985.
11. Schulman A, Herlinger H. Urinary tract dilatation in pregnancy. Br J Radiol 48:638, 1975.
12. Dure-Smith P. Pregnancy dilatation of the urinary tract: The iliac sign and its significance. Radiology 96:545, 1970.

13. Silen W. Cope's Early Diagnosis of the Acute Abdomen. New York, Oxford University Press, 1983.
14. Hill LM, Johnson CE, Lee RA. Ovarian surgery in pregnancy. Am J Obstet Gynecol 122:565, 1975.
15. Johnson TRB, Woodruff JD. Surgical emergencies of the uterine adnexae during pregnancy. Int J Gynecol Obstet 24:331, 1986.
16. Brendler CB. Perioperative care. In Walsh PC, Retik AB, Stamey TA, Vaughan ED Jr, eds. Campbell's Urology, 6th. Philadelphia, WB Saunders, 1992, p 2315.
17. Brent RL. The effects of embryonic and fetal exposure to x-ray, microwaves and ultrasound. Clin Perinatol 13:615, 1986.
18. Mole RH. Radiation effects on prenatal development and their radiological significance. Br J Radiol 52:89, 1979.
19. Mossman KL, Hill TH. Radiation risks in pregnancy. Obstet Gynecol 60:237, 1982.
20. Baker J, Ali A, Groch MW, et al. Bone scanning in pregnant patients with breast carcinoma. Clin Nucl Med 12:519, 1987.
21. Zaltsman S, Baron J, Werner A, Chaichik S. Exposure to radio-iodine in the preconception and conception periods. A case report. Isr J Med Sci 16:856, 1980.
22. Greenberg M, Moawad AH, Wieties BM, et al. Extra-adrenal pheochromocytoma: Detection during pregnancy using MR imaging. Radiology 161:475, 1986.
23. Niebyl JR. Drug Use in Pregnancy. Philadelphia, Lea & Febiger, 1988.
24. Hamod KA, Khouzami VA. Antibiotics in pregnancy. In Niebyl JR, ed. Drug Use in Pregnancy. Philadelphia, Lea & Febiger, 1988.
25. Bruce AW, Awad SA. Spontaneous rupture of the kidney in pregnancy. J Urol 95:5, 1966.
26. Cohen SG, Pearlman CK. Spontaneous rupture of the kidney in pregnancy. J Urol 100:365, 1968.
27. Eaton A, Martin PA. Ruptured ureter in pregnancy—a unique case? Br J Urol 53:78, 1981.
28. Kramer RL. Urinoma in pregnancy. Obstet Gynecol 62:27S, 1983.
29. Maresca L, Koucky CJ. Spontaneous rupture of the renal pelvis during pregnancy presenting as acute abdomen. Obstet Gynecol 58:745, 1981.
30. Oesterling JE, Besinger RE, Brendler CB. Spontaneous rupture of the renal collecting system during pregnancy: Successful management with a temporary ureteral catheter. J Urol 140:188, 1988.
31. Cohen SG, Cashdan A, Burger R. Spontaneous rupture of a renal artery aneurysm during pregnancy. Obstet Gynecol 39:897, 1972.
32. Baumwol M, Park W. An acute abdomen: Spontaneous rupture of liver during pregnancy. Br J Surg 63:718, 1976.
33. Prater JM, Warrington P. Urethral varices as an unusual cause of third trimester bleeding. A case report. J Reprod Med 33:664, 1988.
34. Kiracofe HL, Peterson N. Massive postpartum right renal hemorrhage. J Urol 113:747, 1975.
35. Clark JC. The right ovarian vein syndrome. In Emmett JL, ed. Clinical Urography, Vol 2. Philadelphia, WB Saunders, 1964.
36. Derrick FC Jr, Turner WR, House EE, Stresing HA. Incidence of right ovarian vein syndrome in pregnant females. Obstet Gynecol 35:37, 1970.
37. Arvis G. Le syndrome de la veine ovarienne droite. Ann Urol 19:65, 1985.
37a. Yoffa DE. Proceedings: The ovarian vein syndrome. Br J Urol 46:115, 1974.
38. Mortensen SO, Djurhuus JC. Right ovarian vein syndrome. A case with pre- and perioperative electromyographic registration of ureteral activity. Acta Chir Scand Suppl 472:91, 1976.
39. Dykhuizen RF, Roberts JA. The ovarian vein syndrome. Surg Gynecol Obstet 130:443, 1970.
40. Reynolds SRM. Right ovarian vein syndrome. Obstet Gynecol 37:308, 1971.
41. Otnes B, Enge I, Mathisen W. The ovarian vein syndrome: A cause of ureteral obstruction. Scand J Urol Nephrol 6:206, 1972.
42. Horowitz E, Schmidt J. Renal calculi in pregnancy. Clin Obstet Gynecol 28:324, 1985.
43. Rodriguez PN, Klein AS. Management of urolithiasis during pregnancy. Surg Gynecol Obstet 166:103, 1988.
44. Maikranz P, Coe FL, Parks J, Lindheimer MD. Nephrolithiasis in pregnancy. Am J Kidney Dis 9:354, 1987.
45. Colombo PA, Pittino R, Pascalino MC, Quaranta S. Control of uterine contraction with tocolytic agents (ritodrine) 2. Use in case of threatened abortion, cervical incontinence and gynecological surgery in pregnancy. Ann Obstet Gynecol Med Perinatol 102:431, 1981.
46. Broaddus SB, Catalono PM, Leadbetter GW Jr, Mann LI. Cessation of premature labor following removal of distal ureteral calculus. Am J Obstet Gynecol 143:846, 1982.
47. Clayman R. Personal communication, 1989.
48. Blix G, Lyon ES. Management of symptomatic urolithiasis during pregnancy. Presented at the AUA North Central Section Meeting, Orlando, FL, 1988.
49. Rittenberg MH, Bagley DH. Ureteroscopic diagnosis and treatment of urinary calculi during pregnancy. Urology 32:427, 1988.
50. Williams SF, Bitran JD. Cancer and pregnancy. Clin Perinatol 12:609, 1985.
51. Mastrodomenico L, Korobkin M, Silverman PM, Dunnick NR. Perinephric hemorrhage from metastatic carcinoma to the kidney. J Comput Assist Tomogr 7:727, 1983.
52. Walker JL, Knight EL. Renal cell carcinoma in pregnancy. Cancer 58:2343, 1986.
53. Anderson MF, Atkinson DW. Renal carcinoma in pregnancy. Br J Urol 45:270, 1973.
54. Chesley LC. Renal carcinoma and possible renovascular hypertension in a primigravida. Obstet Gynecol 34:231, 1969.
55. Dumas JP, Colombeau P, Steiner E, Jouvie J. Tumors of the kidney and pregnancy. Ann Urol (Paris) 18:339, 1984.
56. Klein VR, Laifer S, Timoll EA, Repke JT. Renal cell carcinoma in pregnancy. Obstet Gynecol 69:531, 1987.
57. Lukomski L, Lukomska K. Ruptured kidney neoplasm as a cause of hemorrhage in puerperium. Ginekol Pol 42:1235, 1971.
58. Ohba S, Moriguchi H, Tanaka S, et al. A case of renal cell carcinoma during pregnancy. Hinyokika Kiyo (Acta Urol Jpn) 32:751, 1986.
59. Ojo OA, Aimakhu VE, Ogunbode O, Wilde HA. Hypernephroma complicating pregnancy. Am J Obstet Gynecol 109:950, 1971.
60. Pelosi M, Hung CT, Langer A, et al. Renal carcinoma in pregnancy. Obstet Gynecol 45:463, 1975.
61. Podluzhnyi GA, Braganets AM. Spontaneous rupture of a nephrocarcinoma in a full-term pregnancy. Akush-Ginekol (Mosk) 6:67, 1987.
62. Stroup RF, Shearer JK, Traurig AR, Lytton B. Bilateral adenocarcinoma of the kidney treated by nephrectomy. J Urol 111:272, 1974.
63. Borisova-Khromenko VM, Maletin AG, Sukovatitsin AM. Wilms' tumor in pregnant women. Akush-Ginekol (Mosk) 1:55, 1981.
64. Ney C, Posner AC, Ehrlich JC. Tubular adenoma of the kidney during pregnancy. Obstet Gynecol 37:267, 1971.
65. Panisic D, Zivkovic J. Surgery of renal angiosarcoma in a woman during the puerperium. Med Pregl 28:221, 1975.
66. Jarrett DD, Prat-Thomas HR. Metastatic choriocarcinoma appearing as a unilateral renal mass. Arch Pathol Lab Med 108:356, 1984.
67. Kumar AB, Chakera TM. Bilateral renal enlargement secondary to metastatic infiltration from choriocarcinoma. Australas Radiol 26:264, 1982.
68. Patrick CE, Norton JH, Dacso MR. Choriocarcinoma in kidney: Case report. J Urol 97:444, 1967.
69. Soper JT, Mutch DG, Chin N, et al. Renal metastases of gestational trophoblastic disease: A report of eight cases. Obstet Gynecol 72:796, 1988.
70. Atalla A, Page IJ, Young KY, et al. Rupture of angiomyolipoma of the kidney presenting as puerperal collapse. J R Army Med Corps 133:166, 1987.
71. Aubert J, Dore B, Orget J. Management of isolated angiomyolipoma of the kidney. J Urol (Paris) 91:575, 1985.
72. Drips RC, Taylor GJ, Valaske MJ, Cowen ML. Symptomatic angiomyolipoma associated with pregnancy. Obstet Gynecol 31:411, 1968.
73. Gallagher JC, Gallagher DJ. Renal hamartoma (angiomyoli-

poma) with spontaneous rupture during pregnancy. Obstet Gynecol 52:481, 1978.

74. Lipman JC, Loughlin K, Tumeh SS. Bilateral renal masses in a pregnant patient with tuberous sclerosis. Invest Radiol 22:912, 1987.

75. Malone MJ, Johnson PR, Jumper BM, et al: Renal angiomyolipoma: 6 case reports and literature review. J Urol 135:349, 1986.

76. Rattan PK, Knuppel RA, Scerbo JC, Foster G. Tuberous sclerosis in pregnancy. Obstet Gynecol 62:21S, 1983.

77. Shinoda I, Takeuchi T, Fujimoto Y, et al. A case of postpartum spontaneous rupture of an angiomyolipoma. Hinyokika Kiyo (Acta Urol Jpn) 31:1027, 1985.

78. Snoddy WM, Nelson RP, Nyberg LM Jr, et al. Symptomatic renal mass in a patient with a positive pregnancy test. J Urol 133:1015, 1985.

79. Sunanta A. Renal hamartoma (angiomyolipoma) with spontaneous massive hemorrhage in sixteen weeks' pregnancy: A case report. J Med Assoc Thai 66:251, 1983.

80. Coombes GB. Phaeochromocytoma presenting in pregnancy. Proc R Soc Med 69:224, 1976.

81. Schenker JG, Granat M. Pheochromocytoma and pregnancy—an updated appraisal. Aust NZ J Obstet Gynaecol 22:1, 1982.

82. Bendsen J, Muller EK, Povey G. Bladder tumor as apparent cause of vaginal bleeding in pregnancy. Acta Obstet Gynecol Scand 64:329, 1985.

83. Cruickshank SH, McNellis TM. Carcinoma of the bladder in pregnancy. Am J Obstet Gynecol 15:145, 1983.

84. Fehrenbaker LG, Rhoads JC, Derby DR. Transitional cell carcinoma of the bladder during pregnancy. Case report. J Urol 108:419, 1972.

85. Hansen JH, Asmussen M. Acute urinary retention in first trimester of pregnancy. Acta Obstet Gynecol Scand 64:279, 1985.

86. Keegan GT, Forkowitz MJ. Transitional cell carcinoma of the bladder during pregnancy: A case report. Tex Med 78:44, 1982.

87. Saeki H, Miura K, Igarashi N. Pheochromocytoma and pregnancy—an updated appraisal. Aust NZ J Obstet Gynaecol 22:1, 1982.

88. Karim M, Ammar R, Dadawy S. Carcinoma of the bladder with pregnancy. J Egypt Med Assoc 51:1037, 1968.

Chapter 46

Preperitoneal Hernia Repair During Urological Surgery

Peter N. Schlegel and Patrick C. Walsh

Inguinal hernias are reported to be present in 5 to 12 percent of patients in those age groups who develop common urological problems, such as clinically detected prostatic cancer, bladder cancer, and benign prostatic hyperplasia. Complications of inguinofemoral hernias may present significant problems in terms of morbidity, and up to a 14 percent mortality rate is noted for emergency operations on strangulated hernias.[1] Any abdominal incision will tend to weaken the abdominal wall and predispose the patient to the development of hernial defects.[2]

Preperitoneal repair of inguinofemoral hernias was first reported by Annandale.[3] Benefits of the preperitoneal approach include ease of exposure and accurate closure of hernial defects with identification of adjacent vascular structures. The indications for the procedure were expanded to include patients with strangulated bowel in whom intestinal resection may be necessary as well as other high-risk patients.[4] Large series have reported recurrence rates as low as 3 percent for indirect hernias and 6 percent for direct hernias repaired by the preperitoneal approach, with a 5-year follow-up.[3]

We have routinely performed preperitoneal hernia repairs in all patients with symptomatic or incidentally discovered inguinal hernias who were undergoing pelvic urological surgery, including radical retropubic prostatectomy and radical cystoprostatectomy. Combined hernia repair and open prostatectomy for benign disease has proved efficacious and reliable, with patient recovery rates and complications comparable with those from simple open prostatectomy.[1, 5–7] Patients are therefore saved an additional anesthetic exposure. We are able to perform simultaneous preperitoneal hernia repair during radical pelvic surgery with excellent results, without a significant increase in operating time or complications.

PREOPERATIVE MANAGEMENT

Patients found to have inguinofemoral hernias on routine physical examinations are re-examined intraoperatively to confirm the presence of the hernial defects and to identify any concomitant hernial defects in the direct or indirect inguinal regions as well as the femoral canal. All defects are repaired. Routine preoperative prophylactic antibiotics are not given; however, patients with evidence of urinary tract infections on routine urinalysis and those with urinary retention and indwelling catheters are treated with appropriate preoperative parenteral antibiotics.

OPERATIVE TECHNIQUE

The patient is placed supine on the operating table with hyperextension of the hips and in slight Trendelenburg position. A median longitudinal incision is made. Hernia repair is performed after prostatectomy[8] or cystectomy[9] to prevent inadvertent disruption of the hernia repair by retraction of the abdominal wall during the pelvic procedure. While awaiting results of the frozen-section analysis of the lymph nodes, the surgeon stands on the contralateral side of the hernia to be repaired. The self-retaining Balfour retractor is removed, and the rectus fascia and anterior abdominal wall are retracted laterally and away from the operating surface with a Richardson retractor by the assistant. The spermatic cord structures are identified and isolated. Excess preperitoneal fat is removed to identify the pertinent structures in the inguinal region, and the hernial defect is confirmed.

An inguinal hernia refers to a defect in the transversalis fascia through which the abdominal contents may protrude. The preperitoneal approach allows ex-

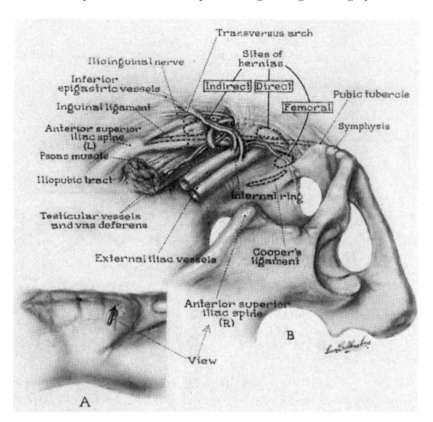

Figure 46–1. *A,* Position of the patient in relation to the surgeon. *B,* Anatomic structures important to the preperitoneal repair of inguinal hernias as viewed with the orientation in *A.* The location of each of the three types of inguinal hernias is also demonstrated. (From Schlegel PN, Walsh PC. J Urol 137:1180, 1987.)

cellent visualization of the anatomy of the inguinal region, especially the transversalis fascia. The spermatic cord structures (testicular vessels and vas deferens) are seen to exit the internal ring lateral to the inferior epigastric vessels (Fig. 46–1). The internal ring is bounded by the transversalis fascia. Superiorly the ring is formed by a double fold of fascia referred to as the transversus arch, which courses medially to form a sling and becomes confluent with the iliopubic tract inferiorly. The iliopubic tract is the thickest portion of the transversalis fascia. This strong fascial band of the transversalis fascia originates laterally along the crest of the ilium and inserts into the superior pubic ramus in a fanlike fashion, forming the medial surface of the femoral ring. The iliopubic tract follows a course parallel to but medial and completely separate from the inguinal (Poupart's) ligament. Understanding and identification of the iliopubic tract are fundamental to the repair of inguinal hernias from the preperitoneal approach, because the tract forms one margin of the defect in each of the common groin hernias (Fig. 46–1).

Indirect hernias result from a defect of the transversalis fascia in the region of the internal ring, lateral to the inferior epigastric vessels and bounded by the iliopubic tract and transversus arch. Direct hernias result from a weakness of the transversalis fascia medial to the inferior epigastric vessels. Direct hernias are located superior to the iliopubic tract and inferior to the transversus arch. Repair of an inguinal hernia

depends on re-establishment of the anatomical integrity of the transversalis fascia.

The technique described by Nyhus is used for the repair of direct and indirect hernias.[3] Epigastric vessels are preserved. Direct hernias are addressed after identification of the transversus arch and iliopubic tract. The hernia sac is reduced, if it was not previously retracted during blunt dissection of the retropubic space prior to the pelvic lymph node dissection. It is usually neither necessary nor advisable to open or excise the direct hernia sac, because part of the wall may be adherent to the bladder. The transversus arch is approximated to the iliopubic tract with interrupted figure-of-eight 2-0 polypropylene sutures, starting at the medial aspect of the hernia. The initial sutures are usually placed down to Cooper's ligament, as they are during a femoral hernia repair, to close the femoral canal region and prevent a potential recurrence in that area. Laterally, sutures are placed from the transversus arch to the iliopubic tract as diagrammed (Fig. 46–2). Each suture is tested as it is placed to ascertain the integrity of the tissues used.

If tissue is found to be inadequate, Cooper's ligament is used instead of the iliopubic tract for the repair. The repair is continued laterally until adequate closure of the defect is obtained. A relaxing incision is made in the ipsilateral posterior surface of the medial rectus fascia for larger hernias to allow adequate release of the tension that may result during closure of the abdominal wound.

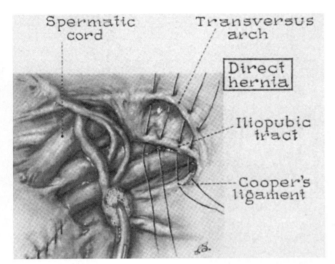

Figure 46–2. Preperitoneal approach to repair of a direct inguinal hernia. (From Schlegel PN, Walsh PC. J Urol 137:1180, 1987.)

entire sac to prevent hydrocele formation from the retained distal sac,[3] and extensive dissection may be harmful to cord structures. The spermatic cord is retracted medially. The transversus arch is approximated to the iliopubic tract with interrupted 2-0 polypropylene figure-of-eight sutures (Fig. 46–4). With small defects, only one or two sutures are necessary to close the internal ring. The excellent exposure provided with this technique easily allows the operator to identify and preserve vascular structures in the region as well as to prevent impingement on cord or vascular structures as a result of the repair.

The operator may then proceed with abdominal wound closure, for which no special precautions are taken.

RESULTS

Indirect hernias are repaired by mobilizing the spermatic cord, which is then isolated with a Penrose drain. Excess adipose tissue, including lipomas of the cord, is dissected free. The hernia sac is identified on the anteromedial portion of the spermatic cord and dissected free. It is sometimes necessary to open the hernia sac to allow placement of one finger into it to help direct dissection of the sac off the cord structures (Fig. 46–3). It is not necessary to remove the

All patients in this series underwent radical retropubic prostatectomy for stage A or B prostate cancer, simple prostatectomy for benign prostatic hypertrophy, or radical cystoprostatectomy for invasive transitional cell carcinoma of the bladder.

During these pelvic urological procedures, 61 hernias were repaired in 50 patients ranging in age from 47 to 69 years. Of these, 35 indirect hernias, 24 direct hernias, and two femoral hernias were repaired.

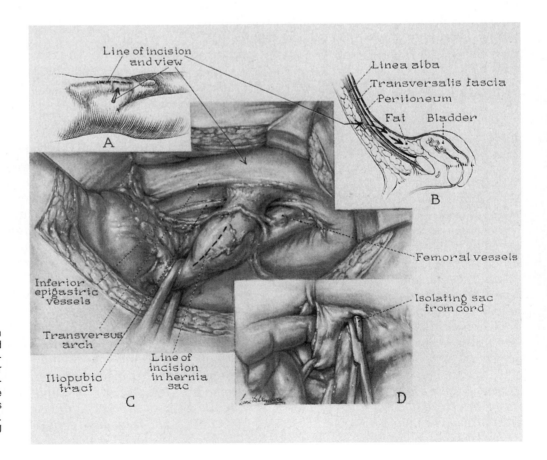

Figure 46–3. *A* and *B,* Orientation of the incision and view for *C* and *D. C,* Demonstration of the preperitoneal approach to the repair of indirect inguinal hernia. *D,* Dissection of the hernia sac from the spermatic cord with the surgeon's finger in the opened hernia sac. (From Schlegel PN, Walsh PC. J Urol 137:1180, 1987.)

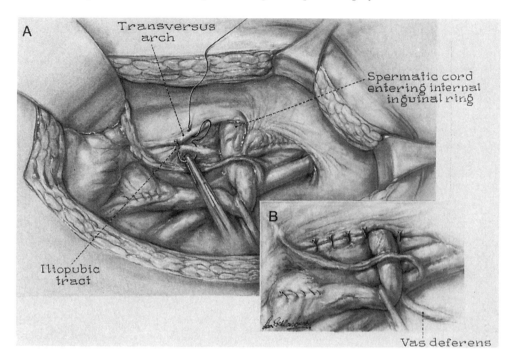

Figure 46–4. *A,* Repair of an indirect inguinal hernia defect. *B,* Completed appearance of the preperitoneal repair of an indirect hernia. (From Schlegel PN, Walsh PC. J Urol 137:1180, 1987.)

Seven of the patients had a history of a previous attempt at repair of the hernia. The only postoperative complication associated with the hernia repairs was the development of an incisional hernia in the inferior portion of the abdominal incision after bilateral direct inguinal hernia repair in two patients. Two patients developed direct inguinal hernias after preperitoneal repair of an ipsilateral indirect inguinal hernia. The follow-up periods were 9 months to 10 years (mean of 5.9 years).

Summary

Riba and Mehn[10] reported the combination of preperitoneal repair with prostatectomy for benign disease. Subsequent series of up to 131 inguinal hernia repairs combined with simple retropubic prostatectomy have demonstrated the efficacy of this simultaneous approach with no complications and low recurrence rate (4.9 percent) for hernias in patients with benign disease.[7] We presented further follow-up of the first series of radical pelvic surgery with simultaneous preperitoneal hernia repair.[11]

Many surgeons have avoided simultaneous hernia repair because of concerns of infection, recurrence of hernia defect, extension of the length of anesthetic time, and unfamiliarity with the technique of repair. Concern over performing a procedure usually done by general surgeons is a factor.

We use nonabsorbable monofilament polypropylene suture because of its low propensity to perpetuate infection or stimulate an inflammatory response, despite urinary contamination, and because of its ability to keep tissues approximated until full healing

has occurred. We have seen no infections in this series of patients attributable to the hernia repair. Although several series have reported high recurrence rates (17 to 35 percent) in preperitoneal repair of direct hernias, Nyhus reported 1200 patients who underwent repair of primary direct hernias with only a 6 percent recurrence rate. We have found that the performance of hernia repair during radical cystectomy or prostatectomy does not prolong the operation significantly. The repair itself rarely takes more than a few minutes. Urological surgeons are the specialists most comfortable with the anatomy of the preperitoneal region of the inguinal canal. The excellent exposure afforded by this technique facilitates performance of the repair.

Follow-up to date has shown low recurrence rates. In addition, most recurrences occur early. Our excellent results portend a low long-term complication rate. We have found the simultaneous repair of preperitoneal hernias during radical pelvic operations to be a safe, efficacious procedure to perform that can avoid a future operation as well as the potential complications of unrepaired hernias.

We advocate careful evaluation of all patients for the presence of symptomatic or incidentally discovered hernias before pelvic surgery, including urological procedures. During the time of this study, six men who were not found to have hernias preoperatively developed symptomatic inguinal hernias that required repair within 6 months of their radical prostatectomy. It is possible that these additional surgical procedures could have been avoided if these patients had been more carefully examined pre- or intraoperatively for incipient hernia defects. We advocate simul-

taneous repair of hernias found in patients undergoing pelvic urological procedures for malignant as well as benign disease.

Editorial Comment

Fray F. Marshall

A significant number of patients have hernias present at the time of pelvic surgery, particularly radical prostatectomy or cystoprostatectomy. Once the surgeon recognizes the hernia and becomes familiar with the technique, closure of a direct or an indirect hernia from the inside is straightforward, avoids further surgery, and should be considered.

We have continued to perform concomitant radical prostatectomy and inguinal herniorrhaphy even with the "minilap" incision.

REFERENCES

1. Jasper WS. Combined open prostatectomy and herniorrhaphy. J Urol 111:370, 1974.

2. Scott J. Development of inguinal hernia following appendectomy. Ill Med J 133:344, 1960.

3. Nyhus LM. The preperitoneal approach and iliopubic tract repair of inguinal hernia. In Nyhus LM, Condon RE, eds. Hernia. Philadelphia, JB Lippincott, 1978.

4. Greenberg AG, Saik RP, Peskin GW. Expanded indications for preperitoneal hernia repair: The high risk patient. Am J Surg 138:149, 1979.

5. Esho JO, Ntia IO, Kuwong MP. Synchronous suprapubic prostatectomy and inguinal herniorrhaphy. Eur Urol 14:96, 1988.

6. Kursh ED, Persky L. Preperitoneal herniorrhaphy: Adjunct to prostatic surgery. Urology 5:322, 1975.

7. Abarbanel J, Kimche D. Combined retropubic prostatectomy and preperitoneal inguinal herniorrhaphy. J Urol 140:1442, 1988.

8. Walsh PC. Radical retropubic prostatectomy. In Walsh PC, Retik AB, Stamey TA, Vaughan ED Jr, eds. Campbell's Urology, 6th ed. Philadelphia, WB Saunders, 1992.

9. Schlegel PN, Walsh PC. Neuroanatomical approach to radical cystoprostatectomy with preservation of sexual function. J Urol 138:1402, 1987.

10. Riba LW, Mehn WH. Combined inguinal hernia repair and retropubic prostatectomy. Q Bull Northw Univ Med Sch 25:62, 1951.

11. Schlegel PN, Walsh PC. Simultaneous preperitoneal hernia repair during radical pelvic surgery. J Urol 137:1180, 1987.

Part IV

SURGERY OF THE BLADDER

Chapter 47

Vesical Diverticulectomy

Charles B. Brendler

Vesical diverticula result from herniation of bladder mucosa through the muscular wall. Diverticula consist of bladder mucosa occasionally surrounded by a small amount of smooth muscle encased in a fibrous pseudocapsule, which results from inflammation. Bladder diverticula occur in about 12 percent of patients with obstructive lesions of the lower urinary tract, most often in older men.[1] Primary or congenital diverticula are less common. Most diverticula arise immediately anterolateral to a ureteral orifice. This is believed to occur because of the attenuation of muscle fibers of the bladder wall by the distal ureteral tunnel.

Diverticula are usually seen in association with bladder outlet obstruction or persistent infection. Complications of bladder diverticula and, therefore, indications for removal include persistent infection (13 to 73 percent),[2, 3] stone formation (5 to 16 percent),[2, 3] ureteral obstruction (8 percent),[2, 3] malignant transformation (4 to 11 percent),[4–6] and urinary retention.[7–9] Demonstration of incomplete emptying is the usual indication for removal of a bladder diverticulum, the underlying cause of most of the aforementioned complications.

PREOPERATIVE MANAGEMENT

Preoperative evaluation should include an intravenous pyelogram to evaluate the upper tracts and, in particular, to verify that the diverticulum is not producing any obstruction or deviation of the ipsilateral ureter. A voiding cystourethrogram is recommended to assess the size of the diverticulum, to evaluate for possible vesicoureteral reflux, and to identify other diverticula that may not be recognized on an intravenous pyelogram. Cystourethroscopy is advisable to determine whether the ureteral orifice is

involved with the diverticulum, which may necessitate ureteral reimplantation at the time of diverticulectomy.

OPERATIVE TECHNIQUES

Techniques of bladder diverticulectomy fall into three categories: intravesical, extravesical, and transurethral. In the extravesical approach (Fig. 47–1), the diverticulum is isolated and excised entirely and the bladder is closed. This approach is performed without difficulty on anterior wall vesical diverticula. It can be exceedingly difficult to perform when the diverticulum is large and located posterior to the bladder. In this situation the risk of injury to adjacent organs such as the rectum can be high with this approach. Because most bladder diverticula arise

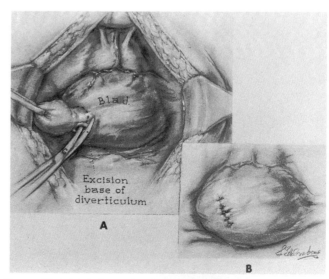

Figure 47–1. Technique of extravesical diverticulectomy. *A,* The diverticulum is isolated and excised. *B,* The bladder is closed.

from the posterolateral wall of the bladder, the surgeon usually is confronted with the more difficult situation.

The intravesical approach to bladder diverticula was first described by Young in 1906.[10] He demonstrated that the mucosal lining of the diverticulum could be removed without having to excise the entire investing fibrous pseudocapsule. The intravesical approach is appropriate for wide-mouthed diverticula located away from the trigone (Fig. 47–2). However, a large, narrow-mouthed diverticulum can be exceedingly difficult to excise with this technique. It is not the wide-mouthed diverticula that cause significant problems but, rather, the narrow-mouthed diverticula, which drain poorly and often require treatment.

The optimal surgical technique for most vesical diverticula combines an intra- and extravesical approach with removal of only the mucosal lining of the diverticulum. This technique was originally described by Barnes[11] and Peirson,[12] but the procedure received little attention in subsequent urological literature until relatively recently.[9]

The operation is performed through a suprapubic approach with either a lower abdominal midline or Pfannenstiel incision (Fig. 47–3, inset). The bladder is opened in the midline, whereupon the mouth of

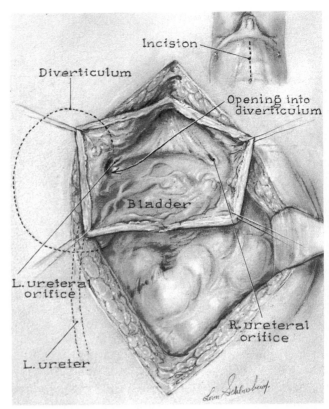

Figure 47–3. After a midline abdominal incision is made, the bladder is opened in the midline, exposing the mouth of the diverticulum and, in this case, the left ureteral orifice.

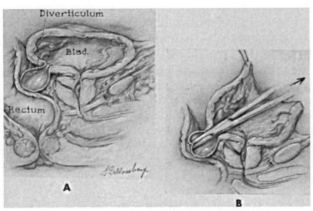

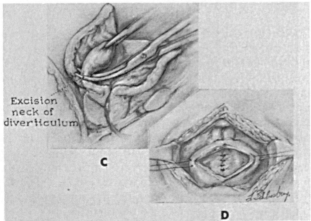

Figure 47–2. Technique of intravesical diverticulectomy. The mucosa of the diverticulum *(A)* is grasped with a clamp *(B)* and excised *(C)*, and the neck of the diverticulum is oversewn *(D)*.

the diverticulum as well as the ureteral orifices can be visualized (Fig. 47–3). At this point the involvement of the ureter by the diverticulum can be assessed and a decision made as to whether ureteroneocystostomy is required.

A finger is then passed into the diverticulum to assess its size and extent as well as possible peritoneal attachments. The peritoneum is freed from the diverticulum with blunt dissection. A separate incision is made laterally in the bladder toward the diverticulum; exposure is facilitated by retracting the bladder to the contralateral side (Fig. 47–4A). The bladder mucosa is incised circumferentially around the opening of the diverticulum to facilitate subsequent dissection from the bladder wall (Fig. 47–4B). Once the orifice has been circumscribed, the diverticulum is opened by extending the lateral incision in the bladder onto the anterolateral surface of the diverticulum (Fig. 47–5).

Dissection of the mucosal lining from the fibrous pseudocapsule of the diverticulum is initiated sharply with scissors, while traction is maintained on the diverticulum to facilitate exposure (Fig. 47–6A). Once the proper plane is achieved, it can be developed easily by blunt dissection alone. Dissection is continued to the base of the diverticulum and the previously circumscribed diverticular opening into the

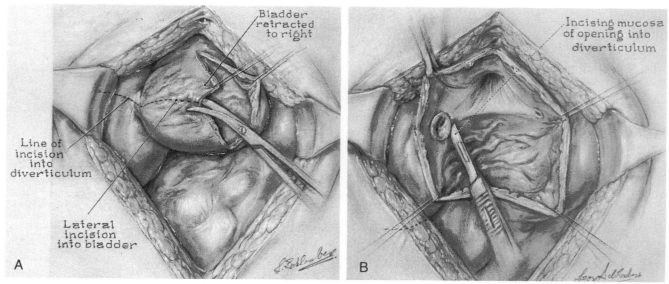

Figure 47–4. *A*, The bladder is retracted to the contralateral side and a separate incision is made laterally toward the diverticulum. *B*, The bladder mucosa is incised around the opening of the diverticulum.

bladder, and the mucosa of the diverticulum is removed intact (Fig. 47–6*B*). After the mucosal lining has been excised completely, the bladder is closed with absorbable sutures starting at the lower end of the lateral incision. A closed suction drain is inserted into the fibrous pseudocapsule and brought out through a separate stab wound (Fig. 47–7). The bladder is drained with either a suprapubic or urethral catheter. A follow-up radiographical study of the pseudocapsule through the drain usually demonstrates complete collapse and obliteration of the cavity within 2 weeks.

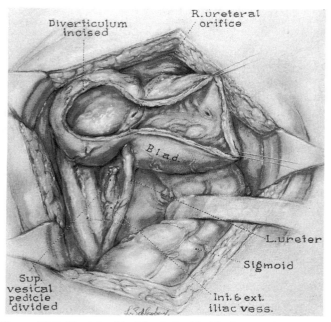

Figure 47–5. The lateral incision in the bladder is extended onto the anterolateral surface of the diverticulum. The superior vesical pedicle has been divided to facilitate exposure.

This combined intra- and extravesical approach offers several advantages in the management of larger posterior-based diverticula over either approach alone. Intravesical exposure allows for identification of both ureters and prevents inadvertent injury. Extravesical exposure facilitates complete removal of the mucosal lining. Since only the mucosal lining is excised, the extravesical dissection can be limited to the anterolateral portion of the diverticulum, thus avoiding inadvertent injury to adjacent organs.

Two transurethral techniques have also been described for the management of bladder diverticula. One is transurethral resection of the diverticular neck, which was described many years ago but has never been accepted widely because of the fear of bladder perforation.[13] The technique was further evaluated and no cases of perforation or extravasation were reported.[14] The other transurethral technique is fulguration of the diverticulum itself. Orandi reported that thorough fulguration of the diverticular surface with a wide loop electrode results in shrinkage or disappearance of the diverticulum.[15] Clayman and associates[16] used a combination of transurethral fulguration of the diverticular mucosa and incision of the diverticular neck to treat 11 patients. Electrohydraulic lithotripsy of bladder stones and transurethral prostatic resection were performed simultaneously when indicated. Postoperative cystograms revealed no cases of bladder perforation and a 75 to 100 percent reduction in size of all diverticula treated. This technique would seem to merit further evaluation.

POSTOPERATIVE MANAGEMENT AND COMPLICATIONS

Proper drainage is essential after open vesical diverticulectomy to prevent urinoma and subsequent

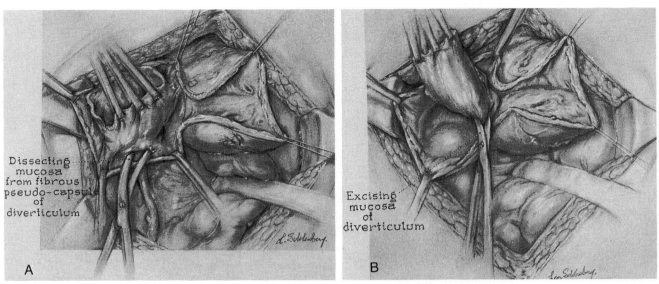

Figure 47–6. *A,* The mucosal lining of the diverticulum is dissected sharply from the fibrous pseudocapsule surrounding it. *B,* The dissection continues to the previously circumscribed opening of the diverticulum, and the mucosa of the diverticulum is removed intact.

infection. If the fibrous pseudocapsule is drained properly, the cavity closes promptly and causes no further difficulty. In removing a posterior diverticulum, it is important to identify the ipsilateral ureteral orifice. If necessary, a ureteral catheter should be passed up the ureter as the dissection is being done. When the ureter is involved in the wall of the diverticulum, the ureter should be transected and reimplanted into the bladder, usually in combination with a psoas hitch. The major risk of transurethral diverticulectomy is bladder perforation with resultant extravasation of urine.

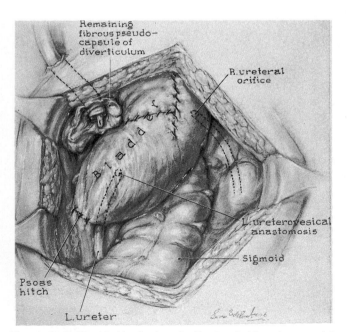

Figure 47–7. The bladder is closed with absorbable sutures and, in this case, after the left ureteroneocystostomy with psoas hitch. A drain is placed in the fibrous pseudocapsule of the diverticulum.

Summary

Bladder diverticula usually result from bladder outlet obstruction and are most commonly located on the posterolateral aspect of the bladder. The surgical technique appropriate for most diverticula involves a combined intra- and extravesical approach with removal of only the mucosal lining. With careful preoperative evaluation, intraoperative dissection, and postoperative drainage, bladder diverticula can be removed safely without serious complications. Transurethral techniques deserve further evaluation.

Editorial Comment
Fray F. Marshall

The presence of a vesical diverticulum is not an indication for operation. As Dr. Brendler indicates, persistent infections, stones, and malignancy are among the more common indications for diverticulectomy. Transurethral surgery for diverticulectomy would appear to be generally inappropriate because the mouth of the diverticulum is never closed. I have resected tumors from diverticula in older patients. This resection can be done, if it is done carefully and if the tumor appears superficial.

If the obstruction that caused the diverticulum is remedied surgically, it may be unnecessary to remove the diverticulum. If the diverticulum is posterior, the dissection can be difficult, and in some instances the overall bladder volume may be reduced significantly.

REFERENCES

1. Winsbury-White HP. Vesical diverticula. Proc R Soc Med 42:553, 1949.
2. Fox M, Power RF, Bruce AW. Diverticulum of the bladder—presentation and evaluation of treatment of 115 cases. Br J Urol 34:286, 1962.

3. McLean P, Kelalis PP. Bladder diverticulum in the male. Br J Urol 40:321, 1968.

4. Piconi JR, Henry SC, Walsh PC. Rapid development of carcinoma in diverticulum of bladder: A pitfall in conservative management. Urology 2:676, 1973.

5. Montague DK, Boltuch RL. Primary neoplasms in vesical diverticula: Report of 10 cases. J Urol 116:41, 1976.

6. Melekos MD, Asbach HW, Barbalias GA. Vesical diverticula: Etiology, diagnosis, tumorigenesis, and treatment. Urology 30:453, 1987.

7. Shah KJ. Bladder diverticulum: An uncommon cause of acute retention of urine in a male child. Br J Radiol 52:504, 1979.

8. Schulze S, Hald T. Voiding inability after transurethral resection of a bladder diverticulum. Scand J Urol Nephrol 17:377, 1983.

9. Jarow JP, Brendler CB. Urinary retention caused by a large bladder diverticulum: A simple method of diverticulectomy. J Urol 139:1260, 1988.

10. Young HH. The operative treatment of vesical diverticulum with report of four cases. Johns Hopkins Hosp Rep 13:411, 1906.

11. Barnes RW. Surgical treatment of large vesical diverticula. Presentation of a new technique. J Urol 42:794, 1939.

12. Peirson EL. An easy method of removing large diverticula of the bladder. J Urol 43:686, 1940.

13. Hartung W, Flocks RH. Diverticulum of the bladder. A method of roentgen examination and the roentgen and clinical findings in 200 cases. Radiology 41:363, 1943.

14. Vitale PJ, Woodside JR. Management of bladder diverticula by transurethral resection: Re-evaluation of an old technique. J Urol 122:744, 1979.

15. Orandi A. Transurethral fulguration of bladder diverticulum. New procedure. Urology 10:30, 1977.

16. Clayman RV, Shahin S, Reddy P, Fraley EE. Transurethral treatment of bladder diverticula. Urology 13:573, 1984.

Chapter 48

Partial and Simple Cystectomy

Charles B. Brendler

Partial Cystectomy

Partial cystectomy, first used in the treatment of bladder cancer in 1884, became popular during the 1950s, at which time it was thought that 20 to 50 percent of patients with bladder cancer might be candidates for this operation.[1] Partial cystectomy subsequently declined in popularity for two reasons. First, improved transurethral instrumentation made it possible to resect large, relatively inaccessible tumors. Second, a better understanding of the pathogenesis of this disease led to the realization that bladder cancer is usually a generalized urothelial condition. Indeed, about 50 percent of patients who undergo partial cystectomy will develop recurrent bladder tumors.[2]

INDICATIONS

Although infrequently indicated, partial cystectomy remains an effective technique for cancer management in appropriately selected patients. Candidates for partial cystectomy ideally should have primary, solitary tumors located in a mobile portion of the bladder away from the bladder neck. Partial cystectomy may also be indicated for tumors on the anterior wall or within a diverticulum that are inaccessible to adequate transurethral resection. Patients who would ordinarily be treated by radical cystectomy but who are too ill for this procedure because of other medical considerations may also be candidates for partial cystectomy.

Contraindications to partial cystectomy include (1) recurrent or multiple tumors occurring at variable sites within the bladder, (2) flat carcinomas in situ (CIS), and (3) tumors involving the bladder neck or posterior urethra.

Controversial Issues

Four controversial issues arise regarding the indications for partial cystectomy. The first is tumor size. A tumor greater than 5 cm in diameter has been regarded as a contraindication to partial cystectomy. Lindahl and associates[2] found, however, that tumor size influenced prognosis only when the diameter was less than 1 cm, patients with such lesions having a better 10-year survival rate than patients with larger tumors. Most of the bladder can be removed if necessary to excise a large tumor. If enough vesical tissue remains to close over a 5-ml catheter balloon, the bladder will usually re-expand to an adequate volume postoperatively.[3]

A second controversy regarding partial cystectomy concerns tumor grade. As with any treatment modality for bladder cancer, recurrence rates are higher and survival rates lower with high-grade tumors. Nevertheless, Cummings and associates,[4] along with others, recommended that patients who otherwise meet the requirements for partial cystectomy should not be excluded on the basis of tumor grade alone, and most results support this recommendation. Peress and associates[5] reported that seven of 13 patients (54 percent) who underwent partial cystectomy for high-grade tumors developed wound recurrence, but this has not been the experience of others.[6]

A third controversy involves the issue of whether partial cystectomy can be performed safely in conjunction with radiation therapy. Whereas the therapeutic benefit of preoperative radiation has not been clearly established, it appears that partial cystectomy is associated with minimal morbidity after both planned preoperative and failed definitive external beam radiation. Ojeda and Johnson[1] reported that only three of 16 patients who received radiotherapy in conjunction with partial cystectomy had a decrease in bladder capacity, and in only one patient was this clinically significant. Matthews and coworkers[7] reported successful results with partial cystectomy in patients who had failed radical radiotherapy. Of their 17 patients, 13 also underwent augmentation enterocystoplasty to restore satisfactory bladder function with minimal morbidity.[7]

A fourth and final controversy regarding partial cystectomy is the location of the tumor and whether patients with trigonal lesions are suitable candidates. Although ideally indicated for tumors of the dome and contraindicated for tumors of the bladder neck or posterior urethra, it appears that partial cystectomy can be performed safely for tumors on the trigone, provided that an adequate (2-cm) margin can be obtained. Several series have reported successful results with partial cystectomy for tumors that required excision of the trigone and ureteroneocystostomy.[8, 9]

PREOPERATIVE MANAGEMENT

Before consideration of partial cystectomy, a urinary cytology study should be undertaken. The tumor should be examined utilizing biopsy and anesthesia to determine grade and stage. Positive cytology findings in association with a low-grade tumor suggest the presence of flat CIS. Random cold cup biopsy specimens should be obtained from other areas within the bladder and, in males, the prostatic urethra. A careful bimanual examination should be made with anesthesia to determine the mobility of the tumor. Tumors amenable to partial cystectomy are frequently located in the dome of the bladder and are not palpable on bimanual examination. An intravenous urogram should be performed to evaluate the upper urinary tract. A metastatic evaluation should include computed tomographic (CT) scans of the pelvis, abdomen, and chest, and possibly a radionuclide bone scan.

OPERATIVE TECHNIQUE

The patient is placed in the supine position, and the table tilted so that the patient is in the mild Trendelenburg position to allow displacement of the peritoneal contents cephalad. The abdomen and genitalia are prepared and draped as a sterile field. A catheter is inserted to empty the bladder and connected to closed drainage. The catheter should be attached to a drainage bag before insertion to avoid spillage of urine, possibly contaminated with tumor cells, into the operative field.

A midline lower abdominal incision is made from the umbilicus to the symphysis pubis. Once the anterior rectus fascia has been incised and the rectus muscles have been separated in the midline, the transversalis fascia is incised sharply and the space of Retzius developed bluntly. The peritoneum is mobilized cephalad on each side of the bladder. At this time, it is important to palpate for possible pelvic lymph node metastases and to ascertain the mobility of the tumor.

The peritoneal cavity is then opened just below the umbilicus. The peritoneal incision is carried laterally on each side toward the bifurcation of the common iliac vessels. The peritoneum overlying the bladder is left intact. Although the value of pelvic lymphadenectomy has not been established in a patient who is undergoing partial cystectomy, it seems advisable to perform at least a unilateral lymph node dissection for staging, as it may determine the need for subsequent adjuvant therapy. The lymphadenectomy is similar to the dissection described for radical cystectomy in Chapter 49.

Once the pelvic lymphadenectomy has been completed, stay sutures are placed in the bladder at the site of proposed entry. The bladder is opened well away from the tumor. A circumferential incision is then made, making sure to excise at least a 2-cm cuff of normal tissue around the entire tumor (Fig. 48–1A). Bleeding can be brisk during this part of the dissection. Allis clamps can be applied to the cut edges of the bladder to obtain hemostasis (Fig. 48–1B). Alternatively, one can use the cautery to incise the bladder, which greatly reduces blood loss. Once the tumor has been excised with adjacent healthy bladder tissue, multiple frozen sections should be obtained from the margins of resection to ensure that all the tumor has been excised.

If the tumor is close to the trigone, it may be necessary to excise the ipsilateral ureteral orifice and perform a ureteroneocystostomy and possible psoas hitch. In men with large obstructing prostates, it is also possible to perform simultaneous prostatic enucleation.[8]

The bladder is closed in two continuous layers with absorbable sutures (Fig. 48–1C). I prefer to close the mucosa and superficial muscularis with a 3-0 polyglycolic acid suture followed by a 2-0 polyglycolic acid suture for the deeper muscle and serosa. The bladder is drained with a urethral catheter. A suprapubic catheter is unnecessary and contraindicated because of the risk of wound contamination with tumor. A closed drain is left in the space of Retzius and removed when the drainage has ceased. The wound is irrigated copiously with sterile water with the thought of lysing any tumor cells, and the incision is then closed in standard fashion. The urethral catheter is left in place for 7 days.

POSTOPERATIVE MANAGEMENT AND COMPLICATIONS

The frequency of tumor recurrence in the bladder after partial cystectomy ranges from 30 to 78 percent,

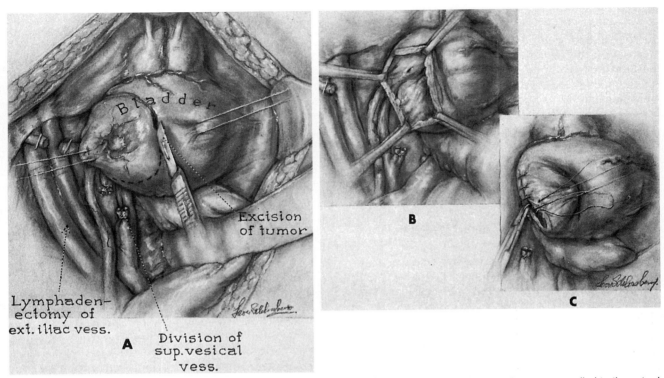

Figure 48–1. *A,* Circumferential incision around the tumor, leaving a 2-cm margin of normal tissue. *B,* Allis clamps are applied to the cut edges of the bladder to control bleeding. *C,* Closure of the bladder in two layers with absorbable continuous suture.

with most series reporting rates slightly above 50 percent.[2, 9–12] The risk of recurrent tumor can be lessened by reserving partial cystectomy for patients with appropriate indications as previously outlined. Kaneti[9] observed a 38 percent recurrence rate in selected patients, whereas Pontes and Lopez[13] reported a 68 percent local recurrence rate in patients who were not carefully screened. Recurrent tumors after partial cystectomy can usually be managed transurethrally.[9] The need for more aggressive therapy, including radiation, total cystectomy, or both, is dependent on initial patient selection and varies from 18[2] to 66 percent.[13]

Incisional recurrence of tumor after partial cystectomy is infrequent. Except for the series of Peress and associates[5] previously mentioned, the frequency of wound recurrence after partial cystectomy appears to be about 1 percent. Merrell[6] and Brannan[8] and their associates had no cases of wound recurrence in a total of 99 patients. Pontes and Lopez[13] reported a wound recurrence rate of 4.2 percent in unselected patients undergoing this procedure. Some workers have recommended that preoperative radiotherapy be administered before partial cystectomy to decrease wound seeding, but, as with radical cystectomy, the value of preoperative radiation in decreasing local recurrence has not been established in controlled trials.

Other complications after partial cystectomy include prolonged urinary drainage from the bladder, which occurs infrequently even in the setting of pre-vious radiation therapy, provided that the bladder is closed and drained properly.[1] Wound infection can develop, but the frequency can be minimized by obtaining thorough hemostasis, providing systemic antibiotic prophylaxis in patients who have infected urine, irrigating the wound postoperatively before closure, and maintaining appropriate drainage.

POSTOPERATIVE EVALUATION

Patients who have undergone partial cystectomy should have follow-up cystoscopy and urine cytology examination every 3 months for 2 years, then every 6 months for 2 years, and then yearly thereafter provided that no evidence of recurrence is found. Because effective multiagent platinum-based chemotherapy is now available for metastatic disease, it would seem advisable to obtain CT scans of the pelvis, abdomen, and chest every 6 months for 2 years to facilitate administration of chemotherapy at the earliest sign of recurrence.

RESULTS

In appropriately selected patients, partial cystectomy appears to yield survival rates equivalent to those of radical cystectomy and urinary diversion. Brannan and associates[8] reported an overall 5-year survival rate of 58 percent and a 10-year survival rate of 32 percent after partial cystectomy. Merrell and colleagues[6] reported the following survival rates by pathological stage: T2 of 67 percent, T3A of 37.5 percent, and T3B of 25 percent. In a later series, Kaneti[9] reported an overall 5-year survival of 50 percent, including 40 percent in T2-T3A tumors and 33 percent in T3B. In contrast, Pontes and Lopez,[13] in a series of patients not carefully selected for partial cystectomy, reported a 5-year survival rate of only 24 percent.

Summary

Partial cystectomy is infrequently indicated in the treatment of bladder cancer. To be effective, partial cystectomy must be reserved for patients who meet the appropriate indications. With this caveat, partial cystectomy appears to yield results equivalent to those of radical cystectomy in the management of this disease.

Simple Cystectomy

Simple cystectomy involves removal of the bladder only, without removal of the prostate and urethra in the male or the urethra and genital organs in the female. A pelvic lymphadenectomy is not done. The indications for simple cystectomy are (1) inflammatory disease induced usually by radiation or previous chemotherapy, most notably cyclophosphamide (Cytoxan); (2) irreparable vesicovaginal or vesicorectal fistula; and (3) palliation for patients with inoperable bladder cancer.

PREOPERATIVE MANAGEMENT

The evaluation of a patient undergoing simple cystectomy for bladder cancer should include a metastatic evaluation with CT scans of the pelvis, abdomen, and chest, and possibly a bone scan. Patients with presumed inflammatory conditions of the bladder should nevertheless receive a urinary cytology examination and multiple bladder biopsies to exclude the possibility of malignancy. Before surgery, patients need a bowel preparation if undergoing simultaneous urinary diversion. In patients with inflammatory disease, it is advisable to administer prophylactic systemic antibiotics and to irrigate the bladder with antibiotic solution preoperatively.

OPERATIVE TECHNIQUE

The technique of simple cystectomy is very similar to that of radical cystectomy. The ureters are transected below the pelvic brim, and the superior vesical pedicles are divided bilaterally. The peritoneum is then incised in the cul-de-sac and a plane developed between the bladder and rectum in the male or between the bladder and vagina or rectum in the female. The lateral pedicles are controlled with ligatures or hemoclips. Once the bladder has been freed posteri-

orly, it is transected at the level of the bladder neck. The remaining vascular pedicles to the bladder are controlled with ligatures. If the posterior wall of the bladder is fixed to the vagina or rectum because of previous radiation, it is preferable to leave a strip of bladder muscle rather than risk injuring these adjacent organs. Once the bladder has been removed, the prostatic urethra is oversewn with a 0 polyglycolic acid suture. In females the urethra is closed with a 2-0 polyglycolic acid suture. The wound is irrigated copiously with an antibiotic solution to minimize the risk of wound infection, and a closed drain is left in place for 48 to 72 hours postoperatively.

POSTOPERATIVE MANAGEMENT AND COMPLICATIONS

The complications of simple cystectomy are as follows:

1. Risk of injury to adjacent organs due to tumor extension or inflammatory reaction. This risk can be minimized by dissecting close to the bladder, leaving a fragment of the bladder wall behind if it is fixed to adjacent structures.
2. Increased risk of infection in previously radiated or otherwise inflamed tissues.
3. Risk of intestinal or urinary fistulas if the patient undergoes a simultaneous urinary diversion. In this regard, if the patient has received high-dose radiation (>6000 rad), it is probably advisable to transect the ureters above the pelvic brim and reimplant them into a transverse colon conduit, because the terminal ileum may have been damaged by previous radiation and therefore may not heal properly.

Editorial Comment
Fray F. Marshall

Although partial and simple cystectomies are not performed very often, these operations have their places. A urachal adenocarcinoma and a transitional cell carcinoma confined to the dome without field change disease are two examples of when partial cystectomy may be indicated.

The surgeon and the patient are often tempted to consider partial cystectomy. It is first appropriate to obtain multiple biopsies of the bladder and prostatic urethra to pathologically verify the extent of the transitional cell carcinoma. If the tumor is involving the trigone and a ureteral reimplant is required for partial cystectomy, it is not a wise idea to consider a partial cystectomy.

REFERENCES

1. Ojeda L, Johnson DE. Partial cystectomy: Can it be incorporated into integrated therapy program? Urology 22:115, 1978.
2. Lindahl F, Jorgensen D, Egvad K. Partial cystectomy for transitional cell carcinoma of the bladder. Scand J Urol Nephrol 18:125, 1984.
3. Baker R, Kelly T, Tehan T, et al. Subtotal cystectomy and total bladder regeneration in treatment of bladder cancer. JAMA 168:1178, 1958.
4. Cummings KB, Mason JT, Correa RJ Jr, Gibbons RP. Segmental resection in the management of bladder carcinoma. J Urol 119:56, 1978.
5. Peress JA, Waterhouse K, Cole AT. Complications of partial cystectomy in patients with high-grade bladder carcinoma. J Urol 118:761, 1977.
6. Merrell RW, Brown HE, Rose JF. Bladder carcinoma treated by partial cystectomy: A review of 54 cases. J Urol 122:471, 1979.
7. Matthews PN, Minton MJ, Haw M, Philip PF. The role of partial cystectomy in the treatment of recurrent invasive bladder cancer following radiotherapy. Br J Urol 60:132, 1987.
8. Brannan W, Ochsner MG, Fuselier HA Jr, Landry GR. Partial cystectomy in the treatment of transitional cell carcinoma of the bladder. J Urol 119:213, 1978.
9. Kaneti J. Partial cystectomy in the management of bladder carcinoma. Eur Urol 12:249, 1986.
10. Novick AC, Stewart BH. Partial cystectomy in the treatment of primary and secondary carcinoma of the bladder. J Urol 116:570, 1976.
11. Schoborg TW, Sapolsky JL, Lewis CW Jr. Carcinoma of the bladder treated by segmental resection. J Urol 122:473, 1979.
12. Utz DC, Schmitz SE, Fugelso PD, Farrow GM. A clinicopathologic evaluation of partial cystectomy for carcinoma of the urinary bladder. Cancer 32:1075, 1973.
13. Pontes JE, Lopez R. Tumor recurrence following partial cystectomy. In Bladder Cancer. Part A: Pathology, Diagnosis, and Surgery. New York, Alan R. Liss, 1984.

Chapter 49

Technique of Radical Cystectomy in the Male

James E. Montie

Radical cystectomy is used primarily for treatment of recalcitrant or locally advanced carcinoma of the bladder. Indications are listed in Table 49–1. Progress in cancer care is dependent not only on development of new strategies for care but also on improved delivery of existing treatment. There is little doubt that there has been continuous improvement in the delivery of radical cystectomy over the last 40 years. Radical cystectomy remains the most effective means of local control of invasive bladder cancer.[1] While research in methods of bladder preservation using a combination of chemotherapy and radiation therapy is desirable, encouraging results have been limited to selected patients with low-volume disease. Concurrently, improvement in patient rehabilitation is noteworthy through better enterostomal therapy support, continent cutaneous diversions, and continent orthotopic neobladders. In this context, there must remain continued emphasis on refining the surgical technique of cystectomy and urinary diversion to provide the utmost safety for the patient.

ASSESSMENT AND PREPARATION

Radical cystectomy has been assessed the highest relative value in terms of difficulty of the surgery for any procedure in urology. The risk of cystectomy is based not only on the technical challenges of the procedure but also on the nature of the patients needing a cystectomy. The incidence of bladder cancer increases continually with advancing age; thus, the responsibility of proving optimal surgical therapy for an elderly and possibly frail patient is common among urologists.[2] Cigarette smoking, one of the most common causes of bladder cancer, is also associated with cardiopulmonary and vascular diseases that contribute to the danger of the operation.[3] Unfortu-

nately, other potentially effective therapies carry morbidity as well; thus, the urologist and patient may face the need for a long, tedious operation in an individual in compromised medical condition.

Preoperative assessment of the overall care and condition of the patient before cystectomy is listed in Table 49–2.

Age

The incidence of bladder cancer increases with age, cresting at a rate of 317 per 100,000 at age 85 years and older, compared with a rate of 110 at age 65.[2, 3] Similarly, mortality in bladder cancer increases with age: 83 percent of men and 87 percent of women dying from bladder cancer are over 65 years of age.[2] In clinical practice, there is no defined upper age limit that precludes a necessary cystectomy. Obviously, the older the patient, the less may be the benefit compared with the increased risk of the operation. However, if a patient is elderly but otherwise in reasonable health, a cystectomy should not be withheld purely on the basis of chronological age.[4–6] One hopes to avoid the dilemma of an elderly patient in good health receiving less than optimal local therapy initially but requiring a cystectomy 1 or 2 years later because of continued local progression or intractable symptoms.[7] In this situation, the danger of the opera-

---

TABLE 49–1. Indications for Radical Cystectomy for Carcinoma of the Bladder

1. Muscle invading cancer (T2–T4)
2. Recurrent or selected cases with invasion of lamina propria (T1)
3. Recurrent noninvasive cancers (Ta or TIS) resistant to endoscopic management and intravesical treatment

---

TABLE 49–2. Risk Assessment and Care in Preparation for Radical Cystectomy

1. Age
2. Pulmonary status
3. Cardiovascular disease
4. Nutrition
5. Obesity
6. Perioperative infection prophylaxis

tion persists and the opportunity for a favorable outcome of the treatment only diminishes. In elderly patients with invasive bladder cancer but otherwise in reasonable health, the greatest risk in the short term is from the bladder cancer, not from their age. Clearly, the margin for safety in the operation on the elderly is diminished because less physiological reserve is present in essentially all organ systems if a complication should develop.[8] A treatable complication in a younger patient may become a catastrophic event in an older one.

Pulmonary Status

Extensive pulmonary disease is frequent in bladder cancer patients owing to the common etiological agent, cigarette smoking. Preoperative assessment is valuable in judging the extent of pulmonary compromise and in planning perioperative supportive care.[9] Retention of carbon dioxide correlates well with the need for postoperative ventilatory support. Preoperative spirometry, before and after bronchodilation, provides an estimate of the reversibility of bronchospasm, and therapy with bronchodilator agents can be valuable in optimizing pulmonary status before surgery. Clearly, specific internal medicine or pulmonary consultation is commonly warranted.

Cardiovascular Disease

Because of the pervasive nature of atherosclerosis in Western society and the association of both bladder cancer and atherosclerosis with cigarette smoking, prevention of cardiovascular morbidity after cystectomy is paramount. Preoperative assessment, in addition to a history and physical examination, may include dynamic stress testing and occasionally coronary arteriography.[10–12] Invasive perioperative monitoring with a pulmonary artery catheter (Swan-Ganz) is necessary in some patients and can be extremely helpful in assessing their response to intravascular volume shifts. A brisk rise in levels of antidiuretic hormone (ADH) after cystectomy has been documented.[13] Hemodynamic monitoring and judicious use of diuretics to counteract the elevated ADH and large amount of fluid often administered during the procedure may prevent complications of congestive heart failure, arrhythmias, myocardial infarction, and renal hypoperfusion.

Nutrition

A substantial advance in surgical therapy over the last two decades is the integration of appropriate pre- and postoperative nutritional care.[14] Patients who have significant malnutrition identified by weight loss and hypoalbuminemia have a substantial increased risk for perioperative complications. If the patient provides a history of weight loss or hypoalbuminemia before the procedure, a formal nutritional assessment is performed preoperatively and nutritional support strongly considered. However, the ability of preoperative nutritional therapy to abrogate the increased risk of complications caused by malnutrition is controversial. As a personal observation, preoperative malnutrition is the most worrisome of all factors influencing surgical risk. Routine perioperative hyperalimentation for the healthy patient is not used in most large centers.

Obesity

Morbid obesity (weight over 100 pounds more than ideal weight) is associated with increased risk of wound infection, dehiscence, and hernias in addition to difficulties encountered with stomal complications.[9] There is no practical way to lessen the risk other than meticulous attention to detail during surgery and a high index of suspicion for potential problems.

Perioperative Infection Prophylaxis

Both a mechanical and antibiotic bowel preparation are performed before cystectomy and urinary diversion.[15, 16] Current practice uses a 1-day bowel preparation consisting of clear liquids; 3 to 4 L of a lavage solution (GoLYTELY or Colyte); and either oral nonabsorbable antibiotics such as neomycin, erythromycin, or metronidazole or broad-spectrum intravenous antibiotics. Wound infection rates have decreased substantially in recent years and now are in the range of 1 to 3 percent.

ANESTHESIA MONITORING

Clear advances are evident in the intraoperative care of the surgical patient.[10] There is continuous monitoring of arterial blood pressure and central venous pressure during cystectomy. Access for rapid infusion of blood or other volume products is necessary. Ventilation and perfusion are more precisely monitored now with improvements in technology. As discussed earlier, invasive monitoring of a high-risk patient with a pulmonary artery catheter can be beneficial.

The need for good communication between the anesthesia and surgical teams during the operation is important. Most bleeding in the pelvis is venous and can be controlled with manual pressure, and therefore if a transient episode of hypotension does occur, immediate communication between anesthesiology team and surgeon allows tamponade of the bleeding, prompt correction of the volume status, and attainment of hemostasis in a more controlled fashion.

OPERATIVE TECHNIQUE

STEP 1: POSITIONING (Fig. 49–1). Two positions are used for cystectomy. The most widely used is a supine position with the table bent in the center, increasing the distance between the pubis and umbilicus and providing additional exposure deep into the pelvis. This is essentially the same position used for radical prostatectomy. One must be careful not to flex the table excessively and risk stretching of pelvic nerves. Preexisting lower back osteoarthritic symptoms can be aggravated by this positioning.

The second option is a modified lithotomy position that allows access to the perineum and rectum should this be necessary. This position is useful if an en bloc urethrectomy is performed. If a urethrectomy is needed at the time of cystectomy, it is possible to complete the cystectomy and diversion using the supine position and then reposition the patient in an exaggerated lithotomy to perform the urethrectomy through the perineum. While this approach provides better exposure for the dissection of the proximal urethra, additional time is added to the procedure by the repositioning and draping.

STEP 2: INCISION (Fig. 49–2). A vertical midline incision that curves around the umbilicus away from the stoma site is generally used. One of the more important aspects of the incision is consideration of the stoma site, regardless of whether a planned cutaneous or orthotopic diversion is being performed. In an uncommon circumstance, a planned orthotopic diversion may not be feasible and the surgeon must fall back upon a second choice of a cutaneous diversion with a stoma. It is important to have the patient evaluated by an enterostomal therapist before the operation to mark the ideal site for the stoma. An otherwise entirely successful operation can turn into a

nightmare for the patient if the collection appliance on the stoma functions poorly because of a faulty stoma location.

STEP 3: PERITONEAL INCISION (Fig. 49–3). After the fascia is divided in the midline, the suprapubic space is entered inferiorly. The suprapubic space is bluntly developed, similar to a radical prostatectomy, sweeping the peritoneum superiorly. The abdominal cavity is then opened at the superior aspect of the incision, and the urachal remnant is identified and divided. With the peritoneum swept off the anterior abdominal wall and pelvic structures, the landmarks used for the incision of the peritoneum can be easily visualized. The peritoneum is incised along the lateral umbilical ligaments, using the urachal remnant as a convenient means of traction.

STEP 4: PERITONEAL INCISION (Fig. 49–4). The incision of the peritoneum is carried down along the lateral umbilical ligament until the vas deferens is encountered. Each vas is clipped and divided; the incision is then carried down a few centimeters more until the anterior surface of the ureter is identified.

STEP 5: PERITONEAL INCISION (Fig. 49–5). Blunt dissection mobilizes the peritoneum in a cephalad direction. On the right side, this is continued to the base of the cecum, exposing the anterior surface of the ureter proximally. On the left side, there are commonly adhesions from the sigmoid colon to the lateral peritoneum; these must be incised before mobilizing the peritoneum in a cephalad direction. The left colon is mobilized medially for a short distance to allow exposure of the ureter just above the pelvic vessels.

STEP 6: MOBILIZATION OF URETER AND ISOLATION OF LATERAL PEDICLE (Fig. 49–6). The ureter is mobilized with a large amount of periureteral adventitial tissue. This is accomplished under direct vision using small clips or cautery to control small vessels coursing to the ureter. The mobilization of the ureter is the same as that done for a donor nephrectomy, preserving as much periureteral blood supply as possible. The ureter is mobilized bluntly down to the bladder. Medial traction on the ureter and bladder allows development of a plane just medial to the lateral vascular pedicle to the bladder. This pedicle is defined superiorly by the superior vesical artery and inferiorly by several smaller branches that course to the bladder to a level just above the endopelvic fascia.

STEP 7: DIVISION OF LATERAL PEDICLE (Fig. 49–7). A convenient landmark for the inferior extent of the lateral pedicle is an ill-defined wad of tissue termed the "pararectal fat pad." This pad has a somewhat characteristic appearance different from peri-

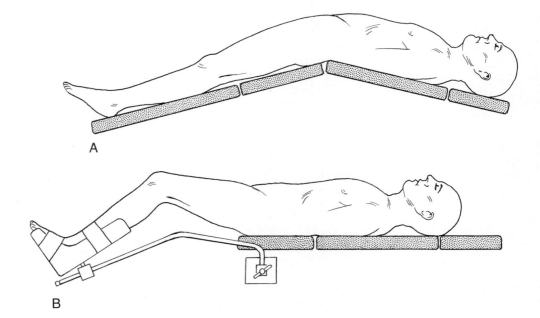

Figure 49–1. Positioning the patient for cystectomy. *A,* Supine position with the table bent in the center, increasing exposure in the pelvis. *B,* Modified lithotomy position with the patient's legs suspended in stirrups to provide adequate support of the lower extremities. Proper padding to avoid vascular or neurological compression of the lower legs is essential.

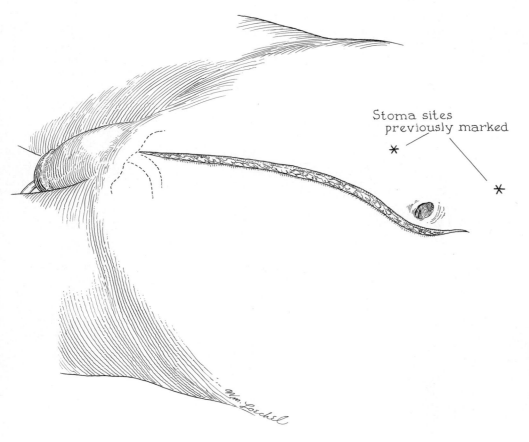

Figure 49–2. A midline incision is made, curving to the opposite side of the umbilicus from the previously marked stoma site. The stoma can be placed in any of the four quadrants, depending on previous surgery and abdominal scarring. The preferred and commonly used site is the right lower quadrant.

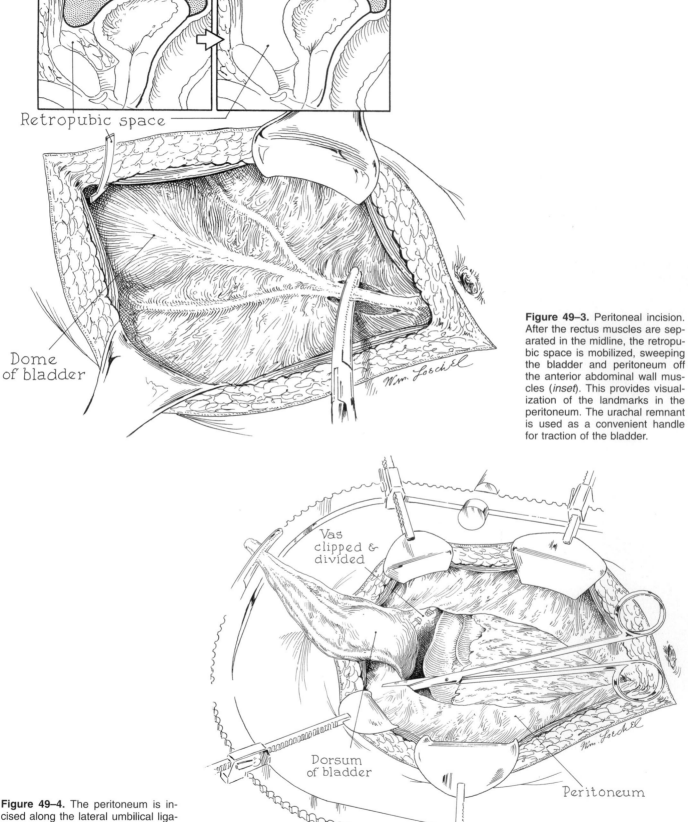

Retropubic space

Dome of bladder

Figure 49–3. Peritoneal incision. After the rectus muscles are separated in the midline, the retropubic space is mobilized, sweeping the bladder and peritoneum off the anterior abdominal wall muscles (*inset*). This provides visualization of the landmarks in the peritoneum. The urachal remnant is used as a convenient handle for traction of the bladder.

Vas clipped & divided

Dorsum of bladder

Peritoneum

Figure 49–4. The peritoneum is incised along the lateral umbilical ligaments; each vas deferens is clipped and divided. A self-retaining retractor is placed to provide constant and untiring exposure. A Bookwalter self-retaining retractor is shown.

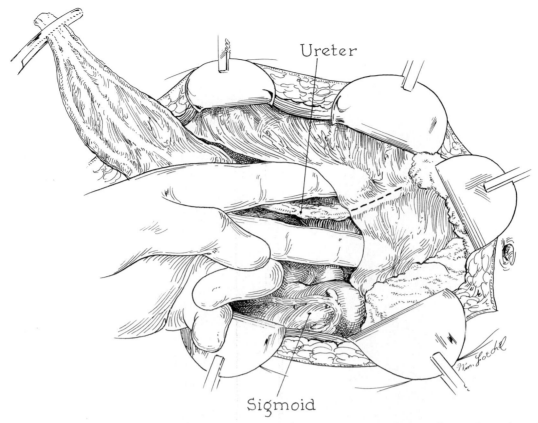

Figure 49–5. The peritoneum is mobilized bluntly in a cephalad direction and then incised to expose the anterior surface of the ureters.

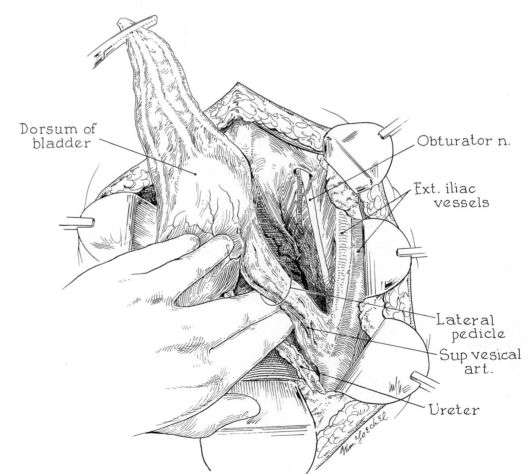

Figure 49–6. The ureters are mobilized with a large amount of periureteral adventitia after incising the peritoneum in a cephalad direction on both the right and left sides. A plane is established between the ureter and the lateral pedicle to the bladder. As the ureter and bladder are retracted medially, the lateral pedicle is exposed. The most cephalad aspect of the pedicle is defined by the superior vesical artery.

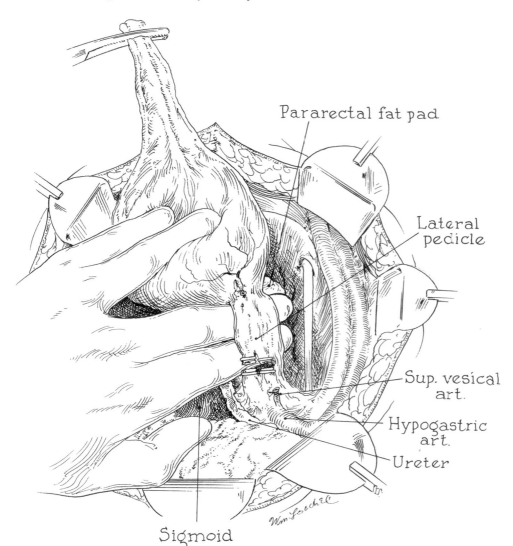

Pararectal fat pad

Lateral pedicle

Sup. vesical art.

Hypogastric art.

Ureter

Sigmoid

Wm Loechel

Figure 49–7. Medial traction on the ureter and bladder with the surgeon's left hand allows division of the lateral pedicle under direct vision. Large clips are usually sufficient for hemostasis.

vesical fat, is lateral to the rectum, and defines the bottom extent of the lateral pedicle above the endopelvic fascia. The important maneuver to provide exposure of the lateral pedicle is medial traction on the bladder with the left hand as described in Figure 49–6. The superior vesical artery is the largest vessel and is individually ligated at its origin and clipped distally. The smaller vessels in this lateral pedicle are controlled with clips and then divided under direct vision. This maneuver should not be done blindly; unexpected bleeding can be controlled under direct vision. If a nerve-sparing dissection is to be performed, the lateral pedicle is not divided in this fashion. Only the superior vesical artery is identified and divided; the remainder of the lateral pedicle is divided closer to the bladder later in the dissection.

STEP 8: ENTRY INTO RECTOVESICAL CUL-DE-SAC (Fig. 49–8). After completion of the division of the lateral pedicle on each side, an incision is made in the peritoneum down to the rectovesical cul-de-sac. If a nerve-sparing dissection is performed, the

incision in the peritoneum is made higher on the base of the bladder, in the region of the tip of the seminal vesicles (Fig. 49–8A). This allows a dissection to expose the posterior aspect of the seminal vesicles and dissection closer to the bladder. For a classical radical cystectomy providing a wider margin of soft tissue around the bladder, the incision of the peritoneum is made on the most dependent portion of the rectovesical cul-de-sac (Fig. 49–8B). A plane is then established bluntly between the posterior aspect of the bladder and prostate and the anterior surface of the rectum. In this classical dissection, the seminal vesicles are neither visualized nor dissected directly. The plane of the dissection always remains behind all layers of Denonvilliers' fascia. As Denonvilliers' fascia merges with the base of the prostate, a plane opens between the apex of the prostate and the anterior rectal surface. If a nerve-sparing dissection is performed, the seminal vesicles are visualized and the dissection is close to the seminal vesicles and inside Denonvilliers' fascia. The seminal

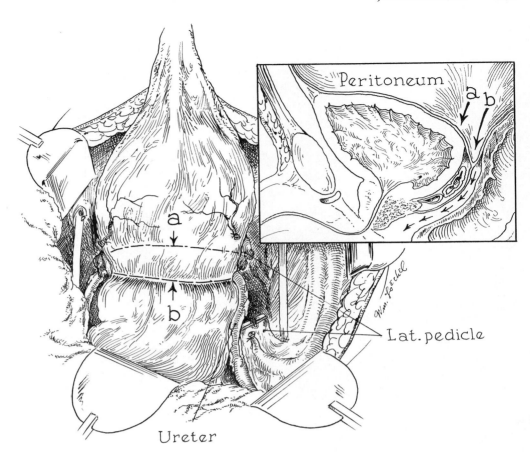

Figure 49–8. An incision is made in the rectovesical cul-de-sac. *A,* For a nerve-sparing dissection the incision is made higher on the base of the bladder to allow visualization of the tip of the seminal vesicles. *B,* With a classical dissection the incision is made at the deepest portion of the reflection of the peritoneum in the cul-de-sac.

vesicles are used as a guide for the dissection, similar to a dissection performed during a radical prostatectomy.

STEP 9: DIVISION OF ANTERIOR VENOUS PLEXUS (Fig. 49–9). Attention is then turned anteriorly. The endopelvic fascia is incised on each side and both puboprostatic ligaments are skeletonized and divided. The venous plexus is controlled using either a ligature or sutures, depending on the surgeon's preference. This dissection is the same as that performed during a radical prostatectomy. After the venous complex is divided, the anterior surface of the urethra is visualized. If the urethra is not to be used, the membranous urethra is mobilized distally as much as possible to remove as much urethra as easily feasible. If an orthotopic reservoir is planned, the dissection must be performed carefully, as in a radical prostatectomy. There is no mobilization of the urethra or periurethral tissue in order to avoid injury to the fragile circular muscular fibers around the urethra.

STEP 10: DIVISION OF URETHRA AND PROSTATIC DISSECTION (Figs. 49–10 and 49–11). The anterior surface of the urethra is divided sharply at the prostatourethral junction; the catheter is used as gentle, cephalad traction and the remainder of the urethra is divided. A retrograde dissection is performed either with or without a nerve-sparing dissection, exactly as done with the radical prostatectomy. A wider excision of the neurovascular bundles does allow easier hemostasis. In Figure 49–10 the small dotted line indicates the site of dissection during a nerve-sparing procedure; the larger dotted line indicates a wider excision of the neurovascular bundle done with a classical wide excision. This posterior pedicle coursing from the middle hemorrhoidal vessels to the base of the prostate and bladder can be visualized from both above and below at this stage in the dissection.

After complete division of the urethra, the plane between the posterior aspect of the prostate and the rectum is generally established easily. If the patient has had a previous transurethral resection or pelvic radiation therapy, it may not be easy to mobilize this plane bluntly. One of the more common causes of injury to the rectum occurs at this stage when the surgeon persists in blunt dissection in an area where normal tissue planes have been obliterated. In this circumstance, it is necessary to perform dissection sharply, under direct vision. Hugging the posterior aspect of the prostate allows dissection to be accomplished with much more safety, decreasing the potential for rectal injury.

STEP 11: DIVISION OF POSTERIOR PEDICLE (Fig. 49–11). The posterior pedicle coursing to the

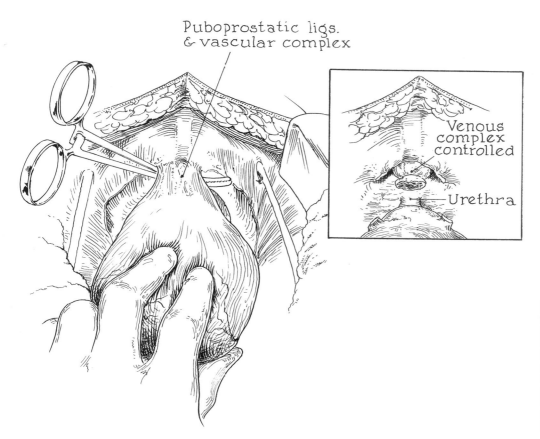

Puboprostatic ligs. & vascular complex

Venous complex controlled

Urethra

Figure 49–9. Division of the anterior venous plexus. Attention is next turned anteriorly to perform the anterior dissection of the prostate. The endopelvic fascia is incised, each puboprostatic ligament divided, and the venous plexus controlled and then divided. The anterior surface of the urethra is exposed, but there is no mobilization of the urethra.

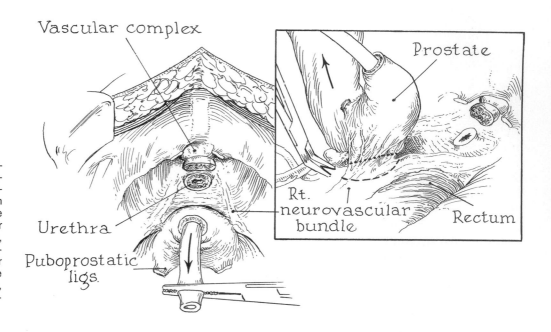

Vascular complex

Prostate

Urethra

Puboprostatic ligs.

Rt. neurovascular bundle

Rectum

Figure 49–10. Division of the urethra and dissection of the prostate. The urethra is divided without any manipulation if an orthotopic neobladder is to be created. The catheter is used for traction in a cephalad direction, similar to that done with a radical prostatectomy. Neurovascular bundles are divided either close to the prostate or more laterally, depending on whether a nerve-sparing dissection is used.

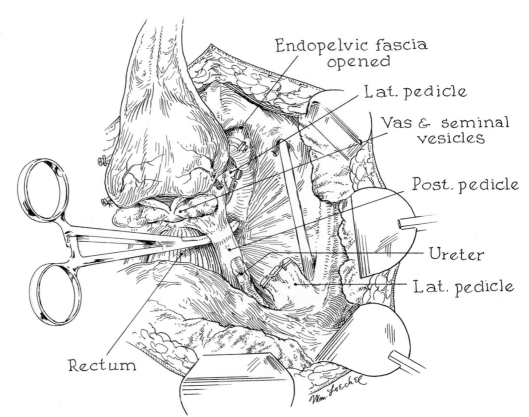

Figure 49–11. The posterior pedicle to the prostate courses from alongside the rectum to the prostate and dependent portion of the bladder. This can be divided either alongside the rectum, as done with a classical dissection, or directly adjacent to the prostate and seminal vesicles for nerve-sparing dissection. The pedicle can be approached from above or below, depending on the exposure.

base of the prostate and bladder neck is divided very close to the seminal vesicles and prostate if a nerve-sparing dissection is performed. In a classical dissection these vessels are divided laterally along the rectum to provide a larger amount of soft tissue. Care must be taken that the rectum is swept down laterally, not tented up and included with the tissue of the pedicle.

After the bladder has been removed entirely, hemostasis is ensured. Common sites of minor bleeding are from periurethral tissue and the venous plexus of Santorini, the neurovascular bundles along the prostate, and the posterior pedicle coursing alongside the rectum. Suture ligatures or cautery are used for additional hemostasis. The pelvis is thoroughly irrigated and packed out of the field while the urinary diversion is performed.

INTRAOPERATIVE COMPLICATIONS

Several intraoperative complications are worthy of specific discussion.

Rectal Injury

Rectal injuries generally occur at one of two sites. The first is during dissection from above, during attempts to establish the plane behind the bladder,

seminal vesicle, and prostate. When the proper plane behind all layers of Denonvilliers' fascia is not entered, excessive pressure with a finger can lead to perforation of the rectum. If the plane is not established, *stop* and proceed anteriorly with subsequent retrograde dissection of the prostate. The second mechanism for injury is an inability to establish a proper plane behind the apex of the prostate. As discussed earlier, sharp, rather than blunt, dissection can provide a much safer mobilization of the prostate off the rectum.

If a rectal injury does occur, primary closure in layers is sufficient unless there has been previous substantial surgery or radiation. If possible, a special attempt should be made to interpose omentum in the pelvis over the site of injury. If the patient has had previous radiation therapy, a similar closure is made, but consideration should be given to a temporary colostomy. One should not hesitate to obtain an intraoperative consultation from a general or colorectal surgeon for an additional opinion.

Vascular Injury

Most bleeding in the pelvis is venous and can be controlled with tamponade. Occasionally, there may be an injury to the external iliac artery, external iliac vein, or internal iliac vein. By far the most difficult of these to control is an injury to the internal iliac vein, often with exposure compromised. The placement of large clamps blindly into the pelvis is rarely successful in controlling the bleeding and often serves only to enlarge the laceration in the vessel. If an injury is noted in a larger vessel, the anesthesia team should be alerted and the bleeding tamponaded with manual pressure until all components of the surgical and anesthesia teams are prepared to deal with the blood loss. The site of injury must be directly visualized and can sometimes be controlled with an Allis clamp. The laceration should be directly oversewn with vascular suture, avoiding, if possible, any further injury to surrounding tissue. This is particularly important for injuries to the external iliac artery or vein in which compromise of the lumen of the vessel can cause substantial postoperative complications. Intraoperative consultation with a vascular surgeon (someone who deals with a similar problem on a daily basis) should be encouraged. A precipitous repair that compromises the lumen may lead to an ischemic extremity or a deep venous thrombosis, increasing the risk of the operation and potentially causing long-term morbidity. The most opportune time to correctly repair the vessel and minimize the risk of further complications is the time of the injury. Reconstruction of the vessel may be necessary in rare cases.

POSTOPERATIVE COMPLICATIONS

The risk of cystectomy has decreased substantially in the last 40 years.[17-19] In a personal series of 341 radical cystectomies for bladder cancer extending from 1979 to 1994, there have been three perioperative deaths (0.9 percent) (Table 49–3). All the patients had significant risk factors and were operated on because of persistent heavy hematuria. Two patients had severe preoperative malnutrition. For the generally healthy patient undergoing an elective cystectomy, the operative risk should not be substantially

higher than that from other major abdominal procedures.

The above discussion should not be interpreted as minimizing the impact of a cystectomy on a patient. The return to normal activities takes 6 to 12 weeks; patients commonly lose 5 to 15 pounds in the postoperative period, and the return of a normal appetite can be protracted. It is not known whether better perioperative nutrition might make the recovery easier even if specific complications are not prevented.

Complications related to urinary diversion are an integral part of the risk of cystectomy. It is beyond the scope of this chapter to delve into complications from various types of diversions. Many life-threatening complications after a cystectomy are related to the diversion itself. Earlier studies of a two-stage cystectomy and diversion have not demonstrated any decrease in risk compared with a single-stage procedure.

Editorial Comment
Fray F. Marshall

Medical evaluation of the cystectomy patient is most important, because bladder cancer typically occurs in older, often debilitated patients. The nutritional aspects are often overlooked, and if the patient is hypoalbuminemic, clearly hyperalimentation should be considered.

It is important to be careful of patients' legs if the lithotomy position is considered during a cystectomy. We have seen problems with anterior compartment syndrome and peroneal nerve palsy when patients' legs are left suspended for the long time required for the cystectomy. With improvements in medical management, anesthesia, and overall operative technique, it is possible to perform cystectomy with a low mortality risk.

REFERENCES

1. Montie JE. High-stage bladder cancer: Bladder preservation or reconstruction? Cleve Clin J Med 57:280, 1990.
2. Yancik R, Ries LA. Cancer in older persons. Magnitude of the problem—how do we apply what we know? Cancer 74:1995, 1994.
3. Smart CR. Bladder cancer survival statistics. J Occup Med 32:926, 1990.
4. Zincke H. Cystectomy and urinary diversion in patients eighty years of age or older. Urology 19:139, 1982.
5. Skinner EC, Lieskovsky G, Skinner DG. Radical cystectomy in the elderly patient. J Urol 131:1065, 1984.
6. Wood DP Jr, Montie JE, Maatman TJ, Beck GJ. Radical cystectomy for carcinoma of the bladder in the elderly patient. J Urol 138:46, 1987.
7. Berkman B, Rohan B, Sampson S. Myths and biases related to cancer in the elderly. Cancer 74:2004, 1994.
8. Harris JE. The treatment of cancer in an aging population. JAMA 268:96, 1992.
9. Whitmore DW, Brennan MF, Harken AH, et al, eds. Care of the Surgical Patient, Vol 2. New York, Scientific American, 1988.
10. Killip T. Anesthesia and major noncardiac surgery. JAMA 268:252, 1992.

TABLE 49–3. Operative Mortality After Radical Cystectomy for Cancer of the Bladder (341 Cases)

Age of Patient (yr)	
77	Salvage after radiation therapy; intractable hematuria; documented inoperable coronary disease; left nephrectomy, cystectomy, urethrectomy
82	Salvage after radiation therapy; intractable hematuria; preoperative malnutrition
61	Emergency cystectomy for severe hematuria; preoperative malnutrition, metastases
Mortality rate:	3 in 341 = 0.9%

11. Fleischer LA, Rosenbaum SH, Nelson AH, Barash PG. The predictive value of preoperative silent ischemia for postoperative ischemic cardiac events in vascular and nonvascular surgery patients. Am Heart J 122:980, 1991.

12. DelGuerico LRM, Savino JM, Morgan JC. Physiologic assessment of surgical diagnosis-related groups. Ann Surg 202:519, 1985.

13. Zabbo A, Montie JE, Orlowski JP. Excessive antidiuretic hormone secretion after radical cystectomy. J Urol 133:789, 1985.

14. Roy LB, Edwards PA, Barr LH. The value of nutritional assessment in the surgical patient. J Parent Ent Nutr 9:170, 1985.

15. Frazee RC, Roberts J, Symmonds R, et al. Prospective, randomized trial of inpatient vs. outpatient bowel preparation for elective colorectal surgery. Dis Colon Rectum 35:223, 1992.

16. Wolff BG, Beart RW Jr, Dozios RR, et al. A new bowel preparation for elective colon and rectal surgery. A prospective, randomized clinical trial. Arch Surg 123:895, 1988.

17. Montie JE, Wood DP Jr. The risk of radical cystectomy. Br J Urol 63:483, 1989.

18. Skinner DG, Lieskovsky G, Boyd SD. Continent urinary diversion. A 5½ year experience. Ann Surg 208:337, 1988.

19. Frazier HA, Robert JE, Paulson DF. Complications of radical cystectomy and urinary diversion: A retrospective review of 675 cases in 2 decades. J Urol 148:1401, 1992.

Chapter 50

Radical Cystectomy (Anterior Exenteration) in the Female

Fray F. Marshall

Transitional cell carcinoma of the bladder is the most common indication for radical cystectomy or anterior exenteration in the female. This operation typically includes a simultaneous pelvic lymphadenectomy, cystectomy, urethrectomy, hysterectomy, salpingo-oophorectomy, and partial vaginectomy. Although various approaches have been described, including a vaginal one,[1, 2] an anterior approach generally provides a better overall exposure.[3, 4] The additional tissue in an anterior exenteration is resected in order to remove adjacent organs that may be at risk for regional spread of transitional cell carcinoma. One ovary can be left if preservation of hormonal function is to be achieved in younger patients. The vagina can also be reconstructed to provide for continued sexual activity postoperatively. Significant recurrence rates of 15 to 28 percent have been reported in the vagina, so a strip of anterior vaginal wall is typically resected en bloc with the specimen.[5] Recently, it has been suggested that the urethra and bladder neck in selected patients may be preserved. However, in one study, 36 percent of patients with transitional cell carcinoma had urethral involvement.[6] Initially a pelvic lymphadenectomy is performed, because if there are grossly positive lymph nodes the exenteration might be deferred or additional adjuvant chemotherapy might be considered postoperatively.

PREOPERATIVE EVALUATION

Patients with transitional cell carcinoma of the bladder typically are older and often have medical problems. These patients deserve a careful medical evaluation before operation. Cystoscopy and pelvic and bimanual examination can be very informative and can identify tumor extending toward the pelvic side wall. Metastatic evaluation is completed with computed tomographic scans of the chest and abdomen. An extensive bowel preparation is typically given with polyethylene glycol electrolyte solution (GoLYTELY). Erythromycin and neomycin are given orally. Intravenous fluids are administered the night before surgery to maintain hydration. A potential stoma site is marked so that it is not placed within a skin crease. Other sites include the umbilicus or even an orthotopic position in the vagina if a continent diversion is contemplated.

OPERATIVE TECHNIQUE

A split-leg fluoroscopy table is used to position the patient so that the legs can be abducted to facilitate a later vaginal dissection. Initially the legs are left together after the vagina is prepared; later they can be separated and the vaginal dissection initiated. This approach is preferred to stirrups or other devices that elevate the legs throughout the procedure, because of the potential complications of peroneal nerve palsy or anterior fascial compartment syndrome with muscular necrosis. These complications are well recognized in patients who have had their legs suspended for extended periods during a cystectomy.

In addition, the patient is placed with the umbilicus at the level of the break in the table so that the table can be flexed. This improves abdominal and pelvic exposure. The vagina is prepared, a Foley catheter left in place, and a midline incision made. If a continent diversion is performed, the incision is often made around the left side of the umbilicus. If an ileal conduit is to be performed, the incision is made only to the level of the umbilicus, but additional exposure can always be gained by increasing the length of the incision. The retroperitoneal space is entered and the peritoneum mobilized laterally off the transversalis

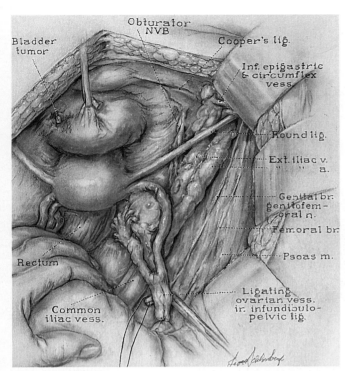

Figure 50–1. General exposure after initial division of the umbilical ligaments and peritoneum. The sigmoid colon has also been dissected free. A moist towel has been placed up each colic gutter to provide exposure. Initial ligation and division of the ovarian vessels is performed. (From Marshall FF, Treiger BF. Radical cystectomy (anterior exenteration) in the female patient. Urol Clin North Am 18:765, 1991.)

fascia. The median and two lateral umbilical ligaments are ligated and divided. Any adhesions within the peritoneal cavity are taken down, and the sigmoid colon may need to be freed from adjacent bowel. Initial inspection of the intraperitoneal contents is made and special attention paid to the liver and para-aortic area to be sure there is no obvious metastatic disease.

The peritoneum lateral to the bladder is divided, as is the round ligament. The ovarian vessels are ligated and divided and the remainder of the peritoneal contents are packed off from the pelvis to provide good exposure (Fig. 50–1). The Omni tract retractor is used to provide good fixed superficial and deep exposure. The end of a moist towel may be placed up each colic gutter and helps prevent the intrusion of small bowel and intraperitoneal contents.

To initiate a pelvic lymphadenectomy, the external iliac vessels are identified and the pelvic lymphadenectomy is started with a dissection lateral to the external iliac artery. The genitofemoral nerve coursing on the psoas muscle should be identified so that it is not injured during initiation of this dissection (Fig. 50–2). This dissection is started above the hypogastric artery and continues along the external iliac artery. It is often possible to dissect initially down

the pelvic side wall. The tissues over the external iliac artery and vein are divided and the dissection is carried down to the obturator fossa. The obturator nerve and neurovascular bundle are identified, and the lymphatic package is divided as it coalesces in the angle between Cooper's ligament and the inferior aspect of the iliac vein. A clip is applied here to reduce the likelihood of a lymphocele (Fig. 50–3).

The lymphatic package can be dissected from the pelvic side wall and is freed from the undersurface of the iliac artery and vein; a Gil-Vernet retractor helps provide superior retraction of the iliac vein (Fig. 50–4A). Once this tissue is freed, it is usually easy to dissect along the obturator nerve and neurovascular bundle. If the nerve is dissected on its lateral aspect initially, there is a decreased risk of tearing into small perforating vessels (Fig. 50–4B). The dissection is then continued superiorly up to the angle of the hypogastric artery, and the lymphatic package is clipped at this juncture as well.

During this dissection the hypogastric artery is dissected carefully and vessels to the pelvic viscera are individually identified, ligated, and divided. Typically we use absorbable 2-0 ties for these ligations (Fig. 50–5). The initial arterial branch is usually the superior vesical artery. The middle vesical, inferior vesical, and uterine arteries are also divided; associated veins are also taken. In general, Kelly clamps with large suture ligatures and extensive clips are avoided in this dissection.

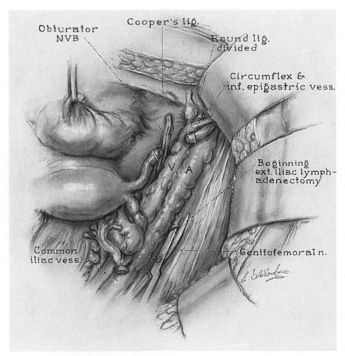

Figure 50–2. Pelvic lymphadenectomy. The dissection is initiated lateral to the external iliac artery. The genitofemoral nerve is avoided. NVB, neurovascular bundle. (From Marshall FF, Treiger BF. Radical cystectomy (anterior exenteration) in the female patient. Urol Clin North Am 18:765, 1991.)

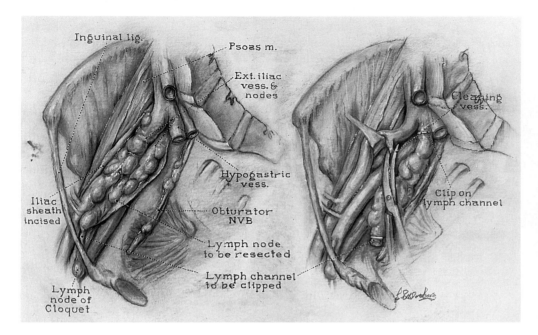

Figure 50–3. The lymphatic tissue is dissected from the iliac artery and vein. A clip is placed on the coalescence of the lymphatic package in the angle between the iliac vein and Cooper's ligament. (From Marshall FF, Treiger BF. Radical cystectomy (anterior exenteration) in the female patient. Urol Clin North Am 18:765, 1991.)

Dissection is carried down to the ureters, which are identified as they insert into the bladder. The ureter is then divided and a frozen section obtained to be sure there is no carcinoma in situ or significant atypia. If there is even atypia, an additional segment of ureter is resected and sent for repeat frozen section. The ureter is typically spatulated at 6 o'clock and a small feeding tube sutured in place to allow easy manipulation of the ureter without injuring it. This feeding tube will later function as a stent (Fig. 50–6). The suture holding the feeding tube is divided and removed at the end of the operation.

To obtain exposure for an incision in the cul-de-sac, traction is applied on the uterus in an anterior direction, with concomitant posterior and superior traction on the rectosigmoid colon. The peritoneum

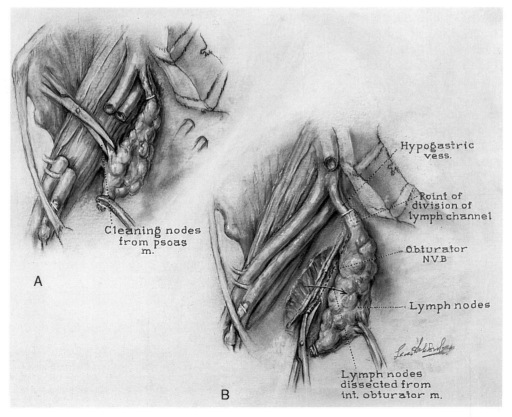

Figure 50–4. Pelvic lymphadenectomy. *A,* The lymphatic package is dissected from underneath the iliac vessels. *B,* The package is rotated medially. The obturator neurovascular bundle can easily be dissected superiorly, where the lymphatics are again clipped. (From Marshall FF, Treiger BF. Radical cystectomy (anterior exenteration) in the female patient. Urol Clin North Am 18:765, 1991.)

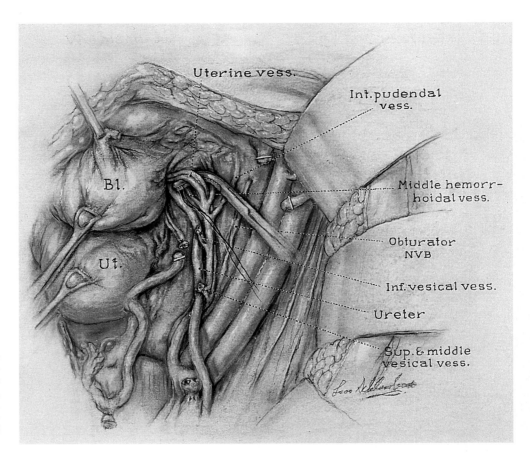

Figure 50–5. Dissection of the hypogastric artery. Superior and inferior divisions of the vesical artery are ligated with individual ties. (From Marshall FF, Treiger BF. Radical cystectomy (anterior exenteration) in the female patient. Urol Clin North Am 18:765, 1991.)

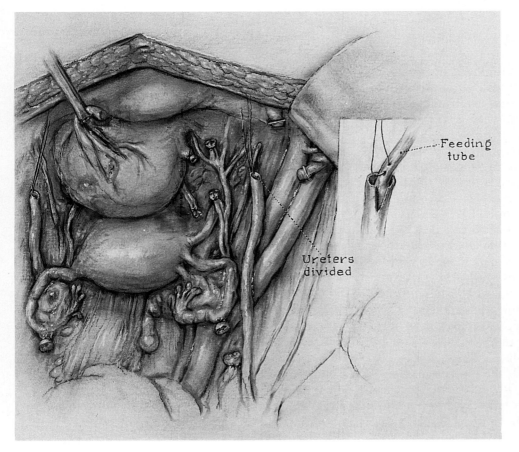

Figure 50–6. The ureters are divided. After a frozen section is obtained, a feeding tube is sutured in place once the ureter is spatulated. This maneuver allows easy atraumatic manipulation of the ureter. (From Marshall FF, Treiger BF. Radical cystectomy (anterior exenteration) in the female patient. Urol Clin North Am 18:765, 1991.)

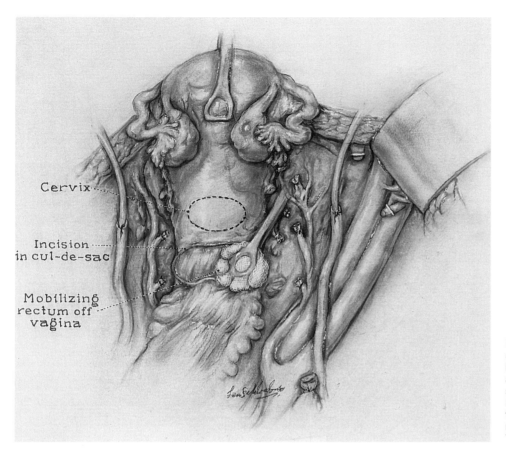

Cervix

Incision
in cul-de-sac

Mobilizing
rectum off
vagina

Figure 50–7. Dissection of the cul-de-sac. Traction is maintained superiorly on both the uterus and the rectosigmoid to allow easy identification of the cul-de-sac and palpation of the cervix. (From Marshall FF, Treiger BF. Radical cystectomy (anterior exenteration) in the female patient. Urol Clin North Am 18: 765, 1991.)

is then incised and the vaginal wall mobilized off of the rectosigmoid (Fig. 50–7). This mobilization allows easier identification of the cervix and posterior vagina. To identify the vaginal wall more precisely, a portion of the cardinal ligament is ligated and divided laterally (Fig. 50–8). The vessels to the vagina run in this rather thick ligament.

A sponge stick in the vagina can help provide significant orientation. With this in place, an incision with the cautery is made directly under the cervix into the vagina. Stay sutures are placed in the thick vaginal wall to provide not only traction but also hemostasis in a well-vascularized organ (Fig. 50–9). Additional division of the cardinal ligament will require ligation, and the cautery can then be used to continue to divide the vaginal wall. The stage and grade of bladder tumor, the age of the patient, and her sexual inclinations should all be considered at this point, because it is very easy to take a large segment of the vagina that may make subsequent vaginal reconstruction difficult. A portion of the anterior vaginal wall remains with the cystectomy specimen. Additional sutures are placed for hemostasis. At this point the specimen is left with only anterior attachments of the urethra, the anterior fascia, and a small portion of the vagina.

Once most of this posterior dissection is com-

pleted, the anterior dissection is initiated and is similar to the anterior dissection made in the male. The endopelvic fascia is divided (Fig. 50–10), as are the pubourethral ligaments. These ligaments are analogous to the puboprostatic ligaments in the male. Division of this tissue allows the urethra and bladder to drop inferiorly. The dorsal vein of the clitoris is ligated and divided in a manner similar to that performed in the dorsal vein of the penis (Fig. 50–10). Typically these veins are present but less prominent than in the male. The urethra can then be dissected under the dorsal vein complex toward the urethral meatus. The only remaining attachments of the specimen are the urethral meatus and a small portion of the vagina (Fig. 50–11).

Vaginal dissection is then started by spreading the legs of the patient and elevating them slightly. A Gelpi retractor is used to spread the labia, although the labia can be sutured for temporary exposure. The cautery is then used to circumscribe the urethral meatus. In general, a minimal amount of dissection is required to free the meatus and urethra, and the specimen is removed. The vagina can then be reconstructed either with closure from posterior to anterior or vertically, depending on the availability of vaginal tissue. A povidone-iodine (Betadine) pack can be left within the vagina (Fig. 50–12). Hemovac drains are

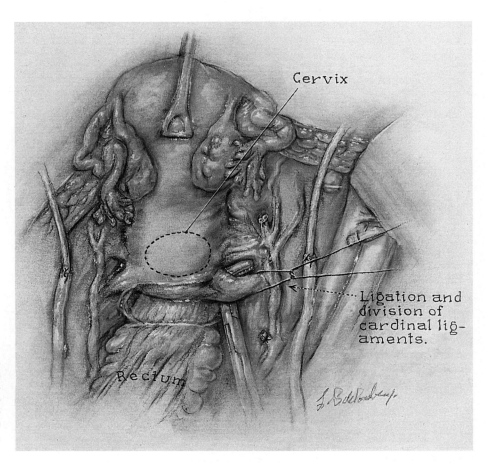

Figure 50–8. The vasculature within the cardinal ligament is ligated and divided to allow exposure of the vagina after the vagina has been mobilized off the rectosigmoid. (From Marshall FF, Treiger BF. Radical cystectomy (anterior exenteration) in the female patient. Urol Clin North Am 18:765, 1991.)

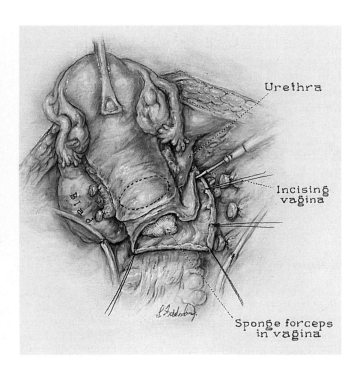

Figure 50–9. A sponge stick is placed in the vagina, and the cautery is used to incise the vagina directly. Stay sutures facilitate the dissection and improve hemostasis. (From Marshall FF, Treiger BF. Radical cystectomy (anterior exenteration) in the female patient. Urol Clin North Am 18:765, 1991.)

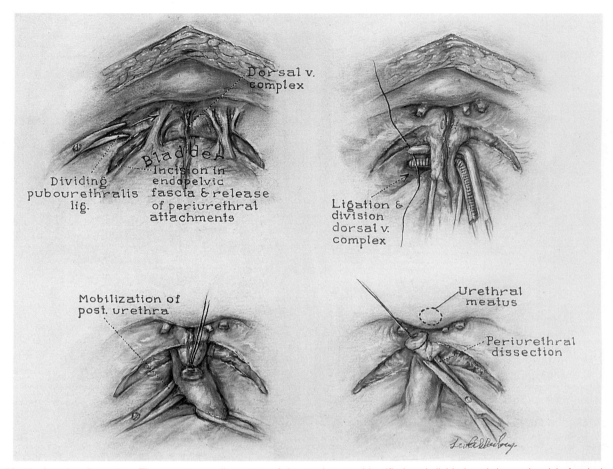

Figure 50–10. Anterior dissection. The suspensory ligaments of the urethra are identified and divided and the endopelvic fascia is incised. This allows inferior displacement of the urethra. The dorsal vein of the clitoris is ligated and divided and the urethra is then mobilized. Dissection can be carried out underneath the dorsal vein complex toward the urethral meatus. (From Marshall FF, Treiger BF. Radical cystectomy (anterior exenteration) in the female patient. Urol Clin North Am 18:765, 1991.)

placed and urinary diversion is then performed. The incision is usually closed with a running No. 1 PDS suture. Occasionally a gastrostomy may be performed to avoid the use of a nasogastric tube, but with lower abdominal incisions it may be difficult to reach the stomach easily for placement of a gastric tube.

POSTOPERATIVE MANAGEMENT AND COMPLICATIONS

The Betadine pack is removed after 48 hours. Hemovac drains are removed after the urinary tract is verified radiographically to be intact. The type of urinary diversion will dictate much of the postoperative management. Stents are usually removed after 1 week. Radiographical studies are obtained. If a continent urinary diversion has been performed, the patient is sent home with a suprapubic tube for 1 month and then returns for tube removal.

Postoperative complications include the usual pulmonary, phlebitis, or wound complications. Abscess may be of more concern in the female patient because of the vaginal dissection. Extensive intraoperative irrigation with antibiotic solution is always performed. The bowel preparation is very important to also reduce postoperative infection.

Later complications include bowel obstruction, urinary tract infection, and ureteral obstruction at the intestinal anastomotic site. Sexual function can frequently be maintained if attention is paid to vaginal reconstruction.[7]

Summary

The operation is performed with a disciplined anatomical approach. A pelvic lymphadenectomy provides excellent staging for carcinoma. Excision of the uterus, vagina, and urethra reduces the potential for pelvic recurrence. Vaginal reconstruction and continent urinary diversion improve later quality of life.

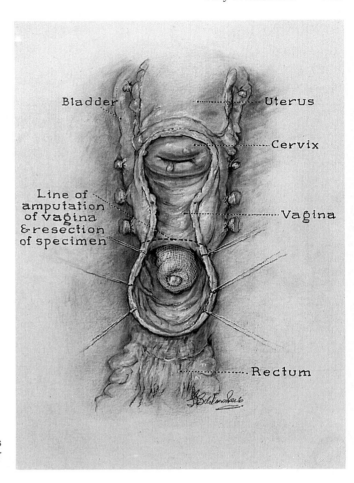

Figure 50–11. Only the vaginal wall and urethra remain. The vagina is amputated. (From Marshall FF, Treiger BF. Radical cystectomy (anterior exenteration) in the female patient. Urol Clin North Am 18:765, 1991.)

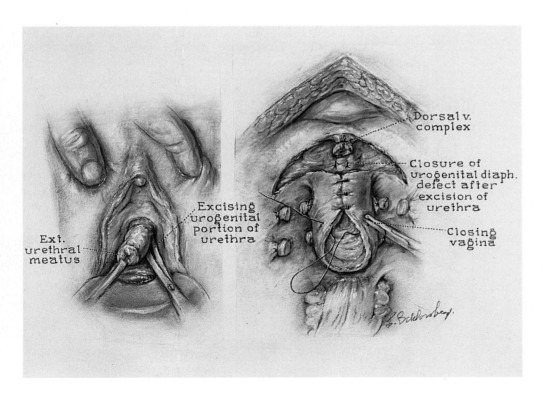

Figure 50–12. The vaginal dissection completes the operation with a circumscribed incision around the urethral meatus. The specimen can then be removed. The vagina is reconstructed. (From Marshall FF, Treiger BF. Radical cystectomy (anterior exenteration) in the female patient. Urol Clin North Am 18:765, 1991.)

REFERENCES

1. Marshall VF, Schnittman M. Vaginal cystectomy. J Urol 57:848, 1947.
2. San Felippo CJ, Kessler R. Vaginal cystectomy. Urology 12:542, 1978.
3. Babaian RJ. Radical cystectomy: Female. In Johnson DE, Boileau MA, eds. Genitourinary Tumors: Fundamental Principles and Surgical Techniques. New York, Grune & Stratton, 1982, p 477.
4. Montie JE. Technique of radical cystectomy. Semin Urol 1:42, 1983.
5. Chin JL, Wolf RM, Huben RP, et al. Vaginal recurrence after cystectomy for bladder cancer. J Urol 134:58, 1985.
6. Paepe ME, Rubin A, Mahadevia P. Urethral involvement in female patients with bladder cancer. Cancer 65:1237, 1990.
7. Schover LR, von Eschenbach AC. Sexual function and female radical cystectomy: A case series. J Urol 134:465, 1985.

Chapter 51

Total Pelvic Exenteration in the Male

W. Scott McDougal

Total pelvic exenteration in the male is a major undertaking that is indicated only in highly selected patients. It may be used to eradicate disease or improve the patient's quality of life.[1] The procedure includes excision of the anus, rectum, prostate, bladder, and pelvic lymph nodes. In some cases, removal of the urethra, corporeal bodies, testes, and perineum is also required (Fig. 51–1). If large portions of the perineum are removed, tissue transfer techniques may be needed to close the defect.

The operation is ideally suited for a patient in whom the disease or tumors are locally extensive, the propensity for distant metastases is low, and the tumors cannot be adequately treated by any other means.[2] Tumors that may demonstrate these characteristics include squamous cell cancer of the urethra; sarcoma of the prostate, seminal vesicles, and bladder; adenocarcinoma of the rectum and seminal vesicles; and squamous cell cancer of the rectum. The operation may also be indicated for local palliation in patients who have complications of pelvic irradiation or tumor necrosis. These complications include pelvic pain; chronic infection; sepsis; fistulas from bowel, bladder, or both; hemorrhage; and urinary-fecal incontinence. In some of these patients, the procedure may not prolong life but rather improve the quality of life.[3]

The operation carries with it a significant morbidity and a 5 to 10 percent mortality. The mortality and morbidity rates are greater in patients who have had previous pelvic irradiation and in those who are advanced in age. Even so, in certain selected patients the procedure will eradicate cancer, and in others bring great relief by removing a necrotic and infected mass that is painful, the source of sepsis, or the cause of the debilitating condition.

The colonic abdominal perineal portion of the operation was originally introduced in 1907 by Miles

and is combined with an anterior exenteration to include prostate and bladder. In some cases, removal of the urethra, corporeal bodies, and major portions of the perineum is also required.

Those who are medically capable of tolerating a major operative procedure must be evaluated for resectability. An examination under anesthesia and a pelvic computed tomographic scan are required for the initial assessment. Not infrequently, however, resectability can be determined only at the time of

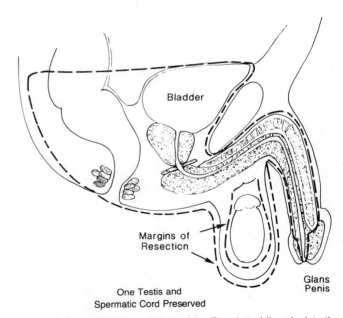

Figure 51–1. Sagittal view of the pelvis. The dotted line depicts the extent of the dissection for a total pelvic exenteration including perineal tissues. The tissue removed for a standard exenteration includes the rectosigmoid colon, prostate, seminal vesicles, and bladder. If the tumor involves the perineum, scrotum, testes, or urethra, each of these structures may be removed en bloc with the rectum, prostate, seminal vesicles, and bladder as illustrated. A bilateral pelvic lymph node dissection is performed; if at this time the lesion is deemed resectable, the exenteration proceeds.

exploratory laparotomy. A patient should not be denied an exploration solely on the basis of radiographical findings or equivocal findings at the time of examination under anesthesia.

PREOPERATIVE MANAGEMENT

The preoperative preparation begins with an antibiotic and a mechanical bowel preparation. The last enema should be given no later than the night before surgery. Broad-spectrum antibiotics are administered 12 hours before surgery as well as intraoperatively. The patient is begun on incentive spirometry and intravenous fluids. A central line for intravenous access and an arterial line for blood pressure monitoring are placed. A Swan-Ganz catheter may be required, depending on the medical and cardiac condition of the patient.

OPERATIVE TECHNIQUE

The patient is placed in the lithotomy position, the legs supported by St. Mark stirrups, and the table is adjusted so that he is in a slight Trendelenburg position. The sacrum is elevated off the table with a sand bag. The abdomen and perineum are prepared with an iodophor. A Steri-Drape is placed on the abdominal portion, and surgical towels are sutured or stapled to the skin to drape the perineal portion.

A midline abdominal incision is made extending from the pubis to well above the umbilicus. The peritoneal cavity is explored. The colon must be thoroughly inspected, as 5 percent of patients with adenocarcinoma of the rectum have another tumor in another portion of the colon. If there are no contraindications to proceeding, the distal ileum and cecum

are mobilized and displaced cephalad. The left colon, beginning at about its midportion, is mobilized by incising the white line of Toldt opposite the left colic artery. A fixed table retractor is placed. The small bowel and cecum are packed cephalad while retained with Mikulicz pads and a moist towel.

If the patient has not received large doses of pelvic irradiation, a bilateral pelvic lymphadenectomy is performed. This extends from the bifurcation of the aorta cephalad to Cooper's ligament caudad, and from the iliac vein anteriorly to the lateral pelvic side wall adjacent to the rectum posteriorly. The tissue around the external iliac arteries is preserved to lessen postoperative leg edema. All pelvic lymphatics are ligated with 4-0 silk suture.

If the patient has received large doses of pelvic irradiation, the area of the obturator fossa and lateral pelvic side wall is inspected for evidence of obvious nodal involvement and, if this is found, biopsied. Usually, this area is so severely sclerosed because of the radiation that the desmoplastic tissue reaction does not allow for identification of any obvious metastases. Moreover, resection of this sclerosed tissue will markedly increase morbidity and significantly increase blood loss. At this point, resectability is determined. If the mass is movable and not invading the pelvic side wall, it can be resected even if it extends into the coccyx, for the latter can be removed. If possible, the hypogastric arteries just proximal to the superior vesicle artery are encircled and bulldog clamps placed bilaterally. The superior vesical artery and obliterated umbilical artery are ligated at their origin from the hypogastric artery and severed.

For mobilization of the colon, the posterior parietal peritoneum is incised on either side of the rectosigmoid colon extending anteriorly to the lateral aspects of the bladder (Fig. 51–2). The left colic artery is

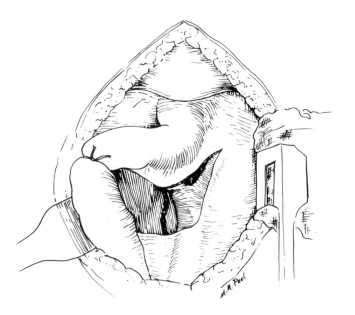

Figure 51–2. The posterior parietal peritoneum is incised on either side of the sigmoid colon. An umbilical tape is placed around the sigmoid and tied to occlude the bowel lumen, and the bowel will be transected cephalad to this tie. The peritoneal incisions are extended anteriorly along the lateral aspects of the bladder.

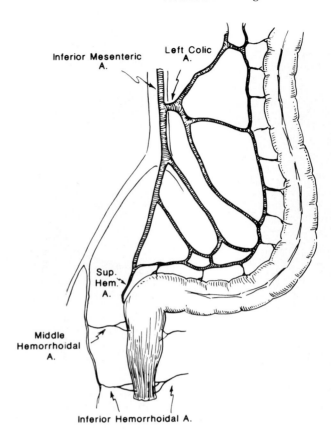

Figure 51–3. The vascular supply of the rectosigmoid colon is illustrated. The inferior mesenteric vessels are transected immediately distal to the origin of the left colic artery.

identified at the point where it branches from the inferior mesenteric artery. Just distal to this point, the inferior mesenteric artery and vein are ligated so that the left colic artery is preserved (Fig. 51–3). The sigmoid mesentery is ligated along the promontory of the sacrum, sweeping the nodes and the hypogastric plexus with the surgical specimen. The left ureter is identified and swept away from the mesentery, as is the right ureter.

The sigmoid colon is transected at least 8 cm above the mass and at a convenient point so that its proximal arterial supply is preserved. Transection can be performed and the end secured either with staples or with three Martel or Zachary-Cope clamps. A hand is placed behind the sigmoid in the midline along the curve of the sacrum and gently passed caudad (Fig. 51–4). The rectum should lift away from the sacrum easily. If fibrous attachments bind it to the sacrum, they should be sharply incised; if they are torn loose, troublesome bleeding will ensue.

The ureters, having been identified, are now traced caudad as far as possible and transected at a convenient level so as not to include any tumor in the distal end of the ureter. Distal ends of the ureter are sent for frozen-section analysis to confirm the absence of tumor. The peritoneum is incised along the lateral borders of the bladder.

Attention is now turned to the space of Retzius where the puboprostatic ligaments and endopelvic fascia are incised. The dorsal vein complex is encircled, ligated, and transected. If the urethra is to be included in the specimen, further distal dissection is performed from the perineal incision. If the urethra is not to be resected, it is transected at the apex of the prostate (Fig. 51–5).

The prostatic pedicles and lateral bladder pedicles are ligated by placing a finger along the course of the ureter entering cephalad, which meets the finger passed along the lateral course of the prostatic pedicles. These are clamped with right-angled clamps and ligated with 2-0 silk sutures and severed (Fig. 51–6). Both the prostatic pedicles and lateral bladder pedicles are suture ligated close to the lateral pelvic side wall.

Attention is then turned to the rectum, where the lateral rectal pedicles are sharply incised close to the pelvic side walls. The middle hemorrhoidal vessels must be identified and ligated. If they are inadvertently cut before being secured, they can be easily grasped and ligated.

After the rectum has been mobilized from the sacrum to the level of the levators and after the lateral rectal, bladder, and prostate pedicles have been ligated, attention is turned to the perineum. The extent of the perineal incision depends on the tumor involvement (Fig. 51–7). If the tumor does not involve the perineum, only the rectum need be circumscribed. The rectum is sutured closed and the skin

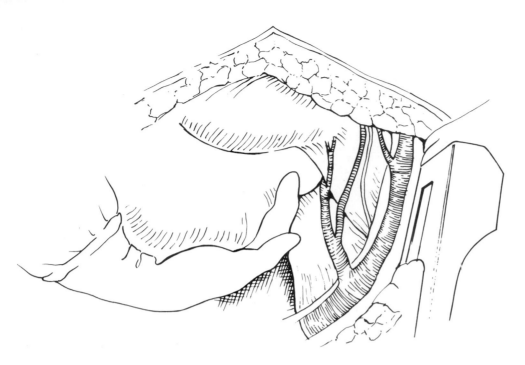

Figure 51–4. The rectum is mobilized from the sacrum. Areas of adherence are sharply incised. By placing the hand in the hollow of the sacrum, the rectum is mobilized anteriorly.

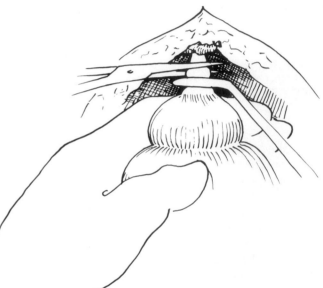

Figure 51–5. The puboprostatic ligaments are severed, and the endopelvic fascia is incised. The dorsal vein complex is encircled with a suture ligature and severed. If the urethra is to be included in the specimen, the urethra is not transected at this point. If, however, the tumor does not involve the urethra, it is transected at this time.

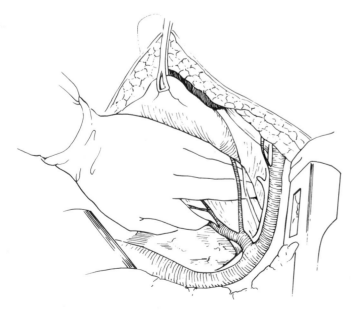

Figure 51–6. The lateral bladder and prostate pedicles are isolated by placing a finger cephalad along the course of the ureter, and placing a finger caudad from the opposite hand adjacent to the rectum through the incised endopelvic fascia, until both fingers meet. The pedicles are suture ligated and severed close to the lateral pelvic side wall. Note that the posterior bladder pedicle is left intact.

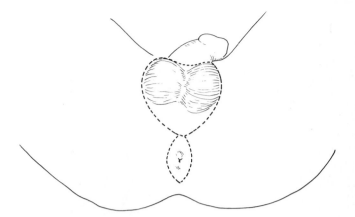

Figure 51–7. The skin incisions are depicted. If the tumor does not involve the perineum or the distal urethra, the perirectal incision is all that is required. If the tumor involves the urethra and perineum, the rectum, perineal area, and involved scrotum are included in the incision.

incision extended through the subcutaneous tissue to expose the distalmost portion of the anus (Fig. 51–8). The posterior central tendon is incised and the distal rectum mobilized (Fig. 51–9). A rubber glove is then placed over the end of the rectum and tied securely with umbilical tape. The iliococcygeal muscles are incised laterally, thus exposing Waldeyer's fascia, which must also be sharply incised (Fig. 51–10). Tearing it risks tearing the middle sacral artery and causing troublesome bleeding. If the tumor is adherent to the coccyx, the coccyx is pushed cephalad and disarticulated, leaving it with the specimen.[4]

The anterior central tendon is cut (Fig. 51–11), exposing the pubococcygeus. The pubococcygeus is cut laterally, thus extending the incision in the levators (Figs. 51–12 and 51–13). If the urethra and corporeal bodies are to be taken, they are isolated in the perineum and removed by retrograde dissection. The bulbar arteries are identified and ligated individually.

Utilizing the electrocautery unit and a penile inversion technique, the corporeal bodies and urethra are removed to the level of the glans. Generally, the glans is preserved, as is the skin of the penile shaft (Fig. 51–14). This maneuver allows for translocation of a testicle into the skin tube, thereby preserving the cosmetic appearance of the penis.[5]

If the urethra is not to be removed, the dissection is continued along the ventral aspect of the rectum until the transected urethra and apex of the prostate are encountered. The levators must be removed laterally to prevent local recurrences. The posterior lateral rectal pedicles are identified distally and incised (Fig. 51–15). The rectum, bladder, and prostate (with urethra and perineum) are then removed. The perineal defect, if small, can be closed primarily. A subcutaneous drain is left in place and a pelvic suction drain brought out anteriorly. If the defect cannot be closed,

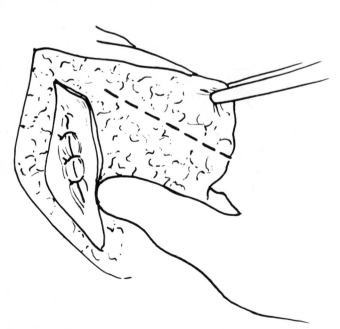

Figure 51–8. The perirectal fat is incised, which exposes the levator ani muscles.

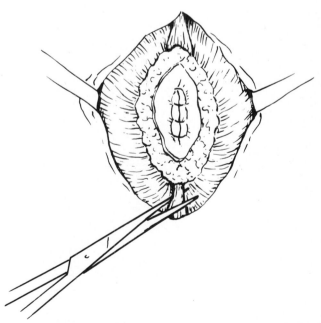

Figure 51–9. The posterior central tendon is incised. If the tumor involves the coccyx, this tendon is left intact and a plane of dissection is developed posterior to the coccyx.

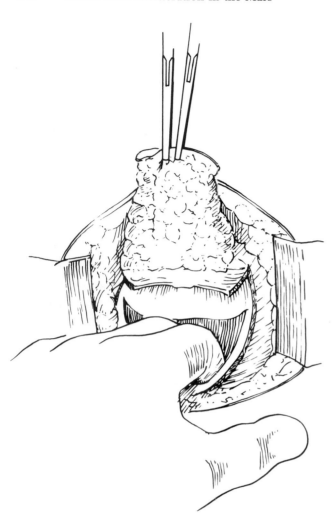

Figure 51–10. The iliococcygeal muscles are incised laterally, exposing Waldeyer's fascia, which is also sharply incised. By placing the surgeon's hand in the hollow of the coccyx and sacrum, the posterior tissue is bluntly and sharply dissected from the coccyx and sacrum. At this point, the hand may be placed from the abdomen into the hollow of the sacrum to meet the other hand placed from the perineum into the hollow of the sacrum. The distalmost portion of the posterior lateral rectal pedicles is still intact, however.

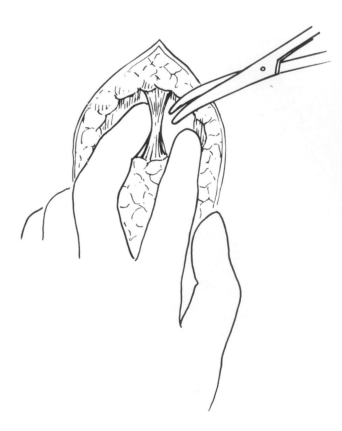

Figure 51–11. If the perineum and scrotum are not to be excised, the anterior central tendon is cut immediately anterior to the rectum, exposing the pubococcygeal muscle.

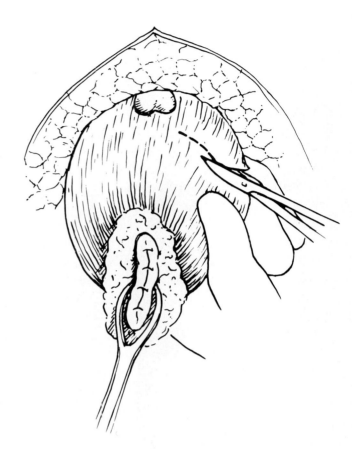

Figure 51–12. The incision in the ileococcygeal muscle is extended anteriorly to the pubococcygeal muscle. Notice the bulb of the urethra.

Urethra

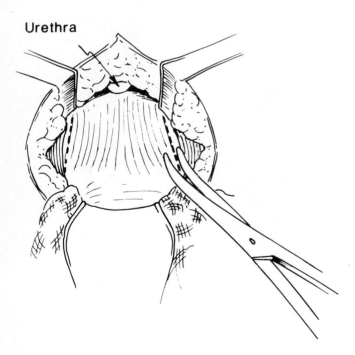

Figure 51–13. The incision in the pubococcygeal muscle is extended anteriorly on both sides of the rectourethral muscle, which is left intact.

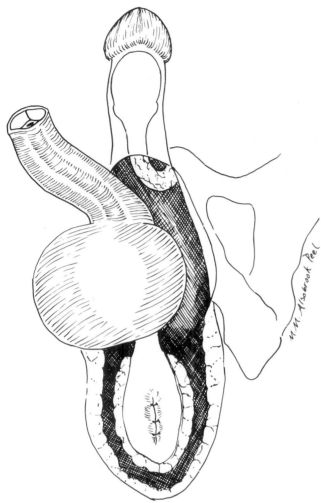

Figure 51–14. The extent of the perineal dissection for tumors involving the perineum and scrotum is depicted. Note that the scrotum, perineum, urethra, and corporeal bodies have all been dissected en bloc and are attached to the rectum, prostate, and bladder. Note also that the ischial rami have been skeletonized and that the levator muscles are included with the specimen. One testicle has been translocated into the penile skin tube with its tunica albuginea sutured to the glans of the penis, allowing for the preservation of a relatively normal appearance of the male external genitalia.

a myocutaneous gracilis flap or rectus muscle flap is employed to close it.[6] This dissection lends itself to intraoperative radiotherapy. The entire pelvis is open, allowing for unimpeded placement of the radiotherapy cone to any portion of the pelvis.

By keeping the small bowel out of the pelvis, postoperative complications are minimized. If the omentum is available, it is placed in the pelvis. Alternatively, it may be sutured to the sacral promontory to serve as a sling. When the omentum is not available or is of insufficient length, a polyglycolic acid mesh is sutured to the sacral promontory posteriorly and to the pubis anteriorly.[7, 8] This maneuver is effective only for the immediate postoperative period, as the mesh loses its strength in 2 to 4 weeks. The mesh is used if postoperative irradiation is to be given in

order to keep the small bowel out of the pelvis during the period of irradiation. Filling the pelvis with omentum or a rectus muscle flap is more effective in the long term and significantly reduces complications in the postoperative period.

Urinary intestinal diversion may be accomplished using a segment of left colon, thus eliminating an intestinal anastomosis, or using another segment of bowel. The techniques of diversion are discussed elsewhere in this text. For invasive cancers of the anus, perineum, and distal urethra, a groin dissection may be indicated in addition to the pelvic exenteration. This may be performed after completion of the exenterative procedure and urinary reconstruction. The procedure is a radical groin dissection and does not differ from that which is classically described.

POSTOPERATIVE MANAGEMENT AND COMPLICATIONS

Broad-spectrum antibiotics and fluids are continued in the postoperative period: the former until oral alimentation is resumed and the latter until the fifth

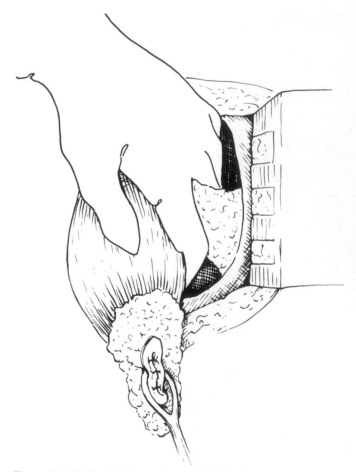

Figure 51–15. The inferior portion of the posterior lateral rectal pedicles is ligated and incised. These pedicles are the last attachments of the specimen to the pelvis.

postoperative day when the pelvic drain is removed. It is my practice to continue the oral prophylactic antibiotic for 1 month postoperatively. Oral alimentation is begun on the fifth postoperative day or after flatus, if no intestinal anastomosis was performed, or after a bowel movement, if an intestinal anastomosis was performed, whichever is longer.

There is an approximately 20 percent complication rate with this procedure. Wound problems, which include infections and dehiscence, and urinary complications, which include urine leak and ureteral obstruction, account for one third of the total. Gastrointestinal and pelvic complications account for one half of the total and include bowel leak, bowel obstruction, and abscess. These complications can be reduced considerably if the intestine is excluded from the pelvis by a sling, a tissue transfer technique as described, or both. The remainder of the complications include sepsis, thrombophlebitis, pulmonary emboli, and respiratory and cardiac difficulties. Perineal sinuses, bowel obstruction, and recurrent pelvic abscesses may occur over the long term.

Editorial Comment
Fray F. Marshall

The indications for total pelvic exenteration are infrequent. As pointed out by Dr. McDougal, however, tumors such as squamous cell carcinoma of the urethra, sarcoma of the prostate, and adenocarcinoma of the rectum may be palliated or at times cured by total exenteration. Urologists have the needed familiarity with the male pelvis for this procedure. The addition of excision of the rectum does not add greatly to the operation, as one might imagine, if the standard dissection for radical cystoprostatectomy has already been performed.

REFERENCES

1. Williams LF, Huddleston CB, Sawyers JL, et al. Is total pelvic exenteration reasonable primary treatment for rectal carcinoma? Ann Surg 207:670, 1988.
2. Kraybill WG, Lopez MJ, Bricker EM. Total pelvic exenteration as a therapeutic option in advanced malignant disease of the pelvis. Surg Gynecol Obstet 166:259, 1988.
3. Obson CA, Deckers PJ, Williams L, Mozden PJ. New look at pelvic exenteration. Urology 7:355, 1976.
4. Pearlman SW, Donahue RE, Stiegmann GV, et al. Pelvic and sacropelvic exenteration for locally advanced or recurrent anorectal cancer. Arch Surg 122:537, 1987.
5. McDougal WS, Koch MO. Phallic reconstruction during exenterative surgery for invasive urethral carcinoma. J Urol 141:1201, 1989.
6. Palmer JA, Vernon CP, Cummings BJ, Moffat FL. Gracilis myocutaneous flap for reconstructing perineal defects resulting from radiation and radical surgery. Can J Surg 26:510, 1983.
7. Clarke-Pearson DL, Soper JT, Creasman WT. Absorbable synthetic mesh (polyglactin 910) for the formation of a pelvic "lid" after radical pelvic resection. Am J Obstet Gynecol 158:158, 1988.
8. Buchsbaum HJ, Christopherson W, Lifshitz S, Bernstein S. Vicryl mesh in pelvic floor reconstruction. Arch Surg 120:1389, 1985.

Chapter 52

Vesical Fistulas

Michael J. Naslund

Vesicovaginal Fistula

A vesicovaginal fistula can be both distressing and disabling to the patient. Urinary incontinence, chronic infection, pelvic pain, and altered mental status are all common sequelae. Fortunately, almost all vesicovaginal fistulas can be closed with a proper surgical approach and meticulous attention to detail by the physician. In the United States, most vesicovaginal fistulas occur after hysterectomy or other gynecological surgery.[1] Other causes include cervical or bladder cancer, radiation therapy, and trauma during childbirth.[2] The presentation is usually straightforward with continuous leakage of urine per vagina. Also present are varying degrees of vulvar and perineal irritation, foul odor, and deposition of phosphate crystals on the introitus due to alkaline urine.

PREOPERATIVE MANAGEMENT

The diagnosis of a vesicovaginal fistula is usually obvious. Included in the differential diagnosis are ureterovaginal fistula, severe stress or urgency incontinence, and severe vaginitis. A complete urological evaluation should be performed, including urinalysis and culture, intravenous pyelogram, cystoscopy, and vaginoscopy. During cystoscopy, a diligent search should be made for multiple fistulas. The location of the ureteral orifices relative to the fistulas should be assessed. A retrograde pyelogram should be considered if a ureteral fistula is a possibility. A ureterovesico vaginal fistula may be present if a vesicovaginal fistula is located near a ureteral orifice.[3] When malignancy is a potential etiology, a deep biopsy should be performed.

If the source of the urinary leakage is unclear, a dye test can be performed. The vagina is packed with dry white gauze, and methylene blue is instilled into the bladder, care being taken to ensure that dye does not leak back out of the urethra. After approximately 20 to 30 minutes, the pack is removed. Blue dye on the pack suggests a vesicovaginal fistula. If the pack is wet with urine but not blue, this suggests a vesicoureteral fistula.

Urinary tract infection or vaginitis should be cleared with antibiotics before surgery. In some instances preoperative catheter drainage can lead to spontaneous closure of a small, simple fistula and can help clear the vaginitis and pruritus associated with larger fistulas.[4]

The timing of the repair can be a controversial decision, because patients and referring physicians often exert considerable pressure for early intervention. In general it is best to wait 3 to 4 months after onset of the fistula before considering reconstruction so that the fistula's size stabilizes and the inflammatory response subsides.[5]

If a fistula is recognized shortly after a surgical procedure, prompt repair can be considered when the patient's condition is satisfactory.[6] Some have advocated the administration of steroids in this setting.[7] In fistulas that occur after radiation therapy, surgical repair should be deferred 4 to 6 months or longer to allow time for maximal tissue healing. If recurrent carcinoma is present, one may choose not to attempt surgical reconstruction.

SURGICAL OPTIONS

There are several principles of fistula repair in the urinary tract. A tension-free, watertight, multilayered closure without overlapping suture lines is critical. All necrotic tissue should be excised and dead space should be avoided. A successful repair is much more certain if healthy vascularized tissue from another source can be interposed between the bladder and

426

vaginal suture lines. Adequate drainage of the bladder and wound is important postoperatively.

As mentioned previously, catheter drainage occasionally allows a small, simple vesicovaginal fistula to close spontaneously. Fulguration of small fistulas has also been successful.[4] Surgical reconstruction is usually the best treatment option. Such reconstruction can be done through a vaginal, transabdominal, or combined approach.

OPERATIVE TECHNIQUES

Vaginal Approach

The vaginal approach to a vesicovaginal fistula is the quickest and simplest procedure for reconstruction. Other advantages are low morbidity, less postoperative discomfort for the patient, and absence of an abdominal scar. One disadvantage is that exposure is often compromised for large or high-lying fistulas, making it difficult to completely excise all scar tissue and obtain a tension-free closure. Another disadvantage is the inability to bring omentum into the area for coverage of the repair.

Most surgeons prefer that the patient be in the lithotomy position for the vaginal approach. However, the jackknife position allows better visualization of the field so that a more complete and meticulous repair can be performed. To place a patient in the jackknife position, the hips are elevated on pillows and the legs are spread to the edge of the table and padded. The buttocks and inner thighs are retracted with tape to aid in the exposure. A narrow Deaver retractor can be used to retract the posterior vaginal wall and improve exposure. Often, a Foley catheter placed on traction gives added exposure of the anterior vaginal wall.[8] When the standard lithotomy position is used, a weighted vaginal retractor is placed in the vagina to retract the posterior vaginal wall. Traction on the cervix, on a Foley catheter placed through the fistula tract, or on both can also aid in exposure.

Turner-Warwick advocated a simultaneous abdominoperineal approach for repair of complicated vesicovaginal fistula. He suggested that any patient undergoing a vesicovaginal fistula repair should be positioned so that an abdominal approach can be used if the vaginal approach is inadequate.[9] In this position, the legs are placed in "skis" and elevated and abducted slightly. Both abdomen and vagina are prepared, and the operator sits between the patient's legs.

Whatever position is selected for the vaginal approach, the principles of fistula repair remain the same. Initially, the fistula and surrounding scar tissue are widely excised from both vaginal and bladder tissue (Fig. 52-1). Care must be taken not to injure the ureteral orifices when excising bladder tissue. If necessary, ureteral stents can be placed at the time of surgery. It is important to dissect the bladder and vaginal mucosa sufficiently to obtain a tension-free closure. A multilayered closure should be performed using absorbable sutures in both bladder and vagina with knots tied inside the lumen of each structure. Overlapping suture lines between bladder and vagina should be avoided, if possible.

Fistula repair is much more likely to be successful if normal vascularized tissue can be interposed between the vaginal and bladder suture lines. With the vaginal approach, one can consider using labial fibrofatty tissue as described first by Martius.[10] An incision is made lateral to the labia, and the underlying fat pad is dissected free of surrounding tissue. A tunnel is then created between the fat pad and the fistula repair, and the fat pad is sutured in place with absorbable sutures (Fig. 52-2). Other options for tissue interposition include a peritoneal flap,[11] a seromuscular intestinal graft,[12] the rectus abdominis muscle,[13] the bulbocavernosus muscle, and the gracilis muscle.[14]

Transabdominal Approach

The transabdominal approach is the choice of many urologists because of their familiarity with the anatomy of the site. The benefits of this approach

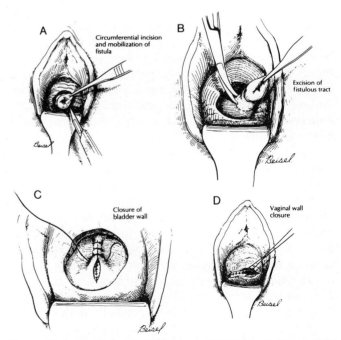

Figure 52-1. Vaginal repair of vesicovaginal fistula. *A,* The fistula is incised circumferentially and freed from the vaginal mucosa. *B,* The fistulous tract is excised from the bladder. *C,* The bladder wall is closed in multiple layers. *D,* The vaginal wall is closed in multiple layers with avoidance of overlying suture lines.

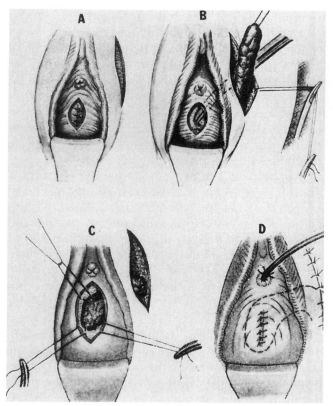

Figure 52–2. Martius technique of tissue interposition. *A,* An incision lateral to the labia majora is used to expose the underlying fat pad that is freed from surrounding tissues. *B,* A subcutaneous tunnel is created. *C,* The fat pad is pulled over the fistula site and sutured into place with absorbable sutures. *D,* Closure. (From Turner-Warwick R. Repair of urinary vaginal fistulae. In Operative Surgery, 4th ed. Butterworth, 1986. With permission of Butterworth & Co., Ltd.)

are excellent surgical exposure, easy visualization of ureters to avoid injury, and ability to interpose an omental or a peritoneal flap for coverage of the fistula repair. The vagina should be prepared into the operative field. A finger in the vagina aids in dissection around the fistula tract. In addition, a prepared vagina reserves the option of a combined abdominoperineal approach.

A midline vertical incision should be employed so that access to the transverse colon and stomach is obtainable in case the omentum must be mobilized from these structures. The peritoneum is dissected off the bladder, which is then opened vertically. The incision is extended posteriorly to bisect the bladder down to the fistula site. One can then separate the bladder from the vagina and excise fistula and scar tissue completely from each structure (Fig. 52–3). In difficult dissections, a Foley catheter placed into the fistula tract from the vagina can help delineate the proper plane of dissection. Bladder and vagina should then be closed separately in multiple layers with absorbable suture, ensuring that the knots face into the lumen of each structure.

At this point a decision needs to be made regarding

interposition of a peritoneal or omental flap. These procedures are not difficult to perform and there is no reason not to do one or the other. Parietal peritoneum from the lateral aspect of the pelvis can be mobilized and placed over the repair. It is important to use small, absorbable sutures to hold the peritoneum on the vagina. The peritoneum may be impossible to mobilize adequately in cases with severe scarring from infection or previous surgery.

The omentum is the best tissue for interposition for several reasons. The excellent blood supply keeps the omentum soft and supple and improves local tissue healing. If omentum is exposed to the interior of the bladder, it will become epithelialized with transitional epithelium; thus, in a large fistula, omentum can replace bladder or vaginal tissue. If re-exploration is necessary, the dissection of tissue planes is facilitated by the previous placement of well-vascularized omentum.

Omentum can almost always be mobilized adequately to extend into the pelvis via a retroperitoneal course lateral to the mobilized ascending colon (Fig. 52–4). If the omentum is too short to reach the pelvis, it can be mobilized from the greater curvature of the stomach by dividing the short gastric branches as described by Turner-Warwick.[9] All the short gastric arteries should be divided and ligated to prevent an arterial tear and subsequent omental hematoma (Fig. 52–4). A thick portion of omentum should be used to cover the fistula repair site. Omentum must extend well beyond the margins of the repairs; the omentum must be sutured to the vaginal wall with multiple absorbable sutures.

Drainage

Adequate drainage of the bladder and wound is critical to a successful fistula repair regardless of the surgical approach. It is advisable to employ both suprapubic and transurethral catheters to drain the bladder until postoperative bleeding has stopped. The urethral catheter can then be removed. This arrangement decreases the risk of potentially disruptive overdistention of the bladder. The pelvis is generally drained with a closed suction drain.

POSTOPERATIVE MANAGEMENT AND COMPLICATIONS

The patient is maintained on broad-spectrum antibiotics until all catheters and drains have been removed. She is allowed to ambulate the day after surgery and is instructed to avoid strenuous activity for 4 to 6 weeks. The suprapubic tube is left in place for at least 14 days, longer with large or complicated fistulas. Before removal, the patient is given a voiding

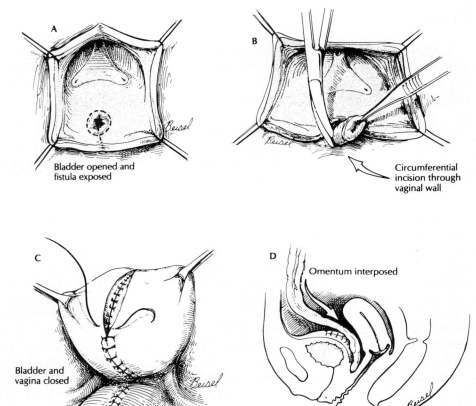

Figure 52–3. Transabdominal repair of vesicovaginal fistula. *A,* The bladder is opened and the incision is extended posteriorly to the fistula site. *B,* The fistulous tract is freed from the bladder and vaginal mucosa and excised. Bladder and vagina are completely separated. *C,* Bladder and vagina are closed in multiple layers with absorbable suture. *D,* Interposition of omentum between bladder and vagina. The omentum must be sutured in place on the vagina.

trial. She is advised to abstain from sexual intercourse for at least 6 weeks.

The complication of most concern is a recurrent urinary leak. Initial management should be reinstitution of catheter drainage for 2 to 3 weeks in the hope that further healing may occur. The primary reasons for a failed repair are excessive tension on the suture line, inadequate debridement of scar tissue before closure, postoperative bladder distention, abscess formation at the site of closure, and poor tissue healing due to radiation-induced damage or recurrent carcinoma. When considering reconstruction after a previously failed repair, one should give careful thought to the original approach and determine what additional techniques can be applied to obtain successful fistula closure.

Figure 52–4. Mobilization of omentum. *A,* The omentum is mobilized from the transverse colon. *B,* The short gastric branches are individually ligated to mobilize the omentum from the stomach. It is usually best to base the omental blood supply on the right gastroepiploic artery. *C,* All the short gastric branches should be divided to avoid a tear in the vessels *(inset).* The omentum is brought to the pelvis via a retroperitoneal course lateral to the mobilized ascending colon. An appendectomy is optional. (From Walsh PC, Gittes RF, Perlmutter AD, Stamey TA. Campbell's Urology, 5th ed. Philadelphia, WB Saunders, 1986.)

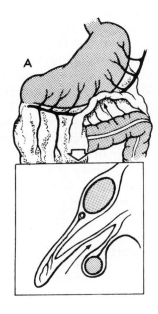
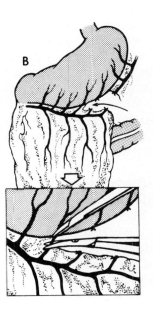
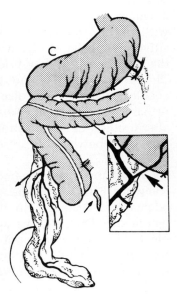

Summary

Vesicovaginal fistulas can be repaired with a vaginal, transabdominal, or combined approach. Wide excision of scar tissue and tension-free closure are critical principles of any fistula reconstruction. One should attempt to interpose normal, well-vascularized tissue between the bladder and vaginal suture lines. With a properly chosen surgical procedure and meticulous attention to detail, a urological surgeon should have a high success rate in closing vesicovaginal fistulas.

Vesicoenteric Fistula

A fistula between the bladder and bowel is usually caused by underlying bowel disease. The most common etiologies are diverticulitis, colon carcinoma, and Crohn disease.[15] Less common causes include penetrating trauma, bladder or cervical carcinoma, and appendicitis with a resultant appendicovesical fistula.[16] A vesicoenteric fistula is more common in males; the location of the uterus between the bladder and rectum offers females a degree of protection from formation of fistulas.[17]

The most common clinical presentation for a vesicoenteric fistula is a recurrent urinary tract infection, often with mixed fecal flora. Suprapubic pain and pneumaturia are also frequently present.[18] Pneumaturia can go unnoticed; however, its presence can be confirmed by instructing the patient to void while sitting in a filled bathtub and to watch for air bubbles.

With larger fistulas, fecaluria or the presence of food particles in the urine may be noted.

PREOPERATIVE MANAGEMENT

The diagnosis of a vesicoenteric fistula is often delayed. It is not unusual for a patient to have been treated with antibiotics for several months before this diagnosis. A pelvic computed tomographic (CT) scan without intravenous contrast material is the most sensitive diagnostic study, with the presence of air in the bladder as the key finding suggesting a fistula.[19] The presence of air is not pathognomonic for a vesicoenteric fistula; it can also be found in patients with urinary tract infections from air-forming organisms or after urethral catheterization. A paravesical mass and thickened bowel wall are other positive findings on CT.[19]

Cystoscopy is also a reliable diagnostic test for vesicoenteric fistula.[17, 18] The characteristic findings are edema and erythema in the bladder wall near the fistula site. The fistulous opening is usually not visible, but at times it is possible to pass a small catheter through the fistula and inject contrast material directly into the bowel. Common locations for a fistula in the bladder are the left dome or posterior wall in a patient with diverticular disease or Crohn colitis, and the right dome or posterior wall in a patient with Crohn ileitis or appendicovesicular fistula. An appendicovesical fistula can also be diagnosed with a CT scan.[20] The area of the fistula should be biopsied to rule out the presence of malignancy.

Other diagnostic tests include cystograms and barium enemas.[18] A barium enema can also be used to evaluate the status of the bowel. It has been suggested that a radiograph of a urine specimen taken after a barium enema with negative findings can demonstrate dye in the urine and confirm a subtle vesicoenteric fistula.[21]

SURGICAL TREATMENT

Spontaneous closure of a vesicoenteric fistula is rare, making surgical correction almost always necessary. In an otherwise healthy patient with no abcess or severe inflammatory process, a single-stage repair is usually adequate. In complicated cases and in infections that cannot be controlled with antibiotics, a staged repair with initial diversion of the urinary and fecal streams should be considered. The patient should undergo a cleansing bowel preparation and receive oral neomycin and erythromycin the day before surgery.

Surgical treatment involves resection of the diseased bowel segment and any involved bladder tissue. The bladder is then closed primarily. Treatment of bowel disease is usually best handled by a general surgeon and is not discussed in detail here. It is advisable to cover the bladder closure with omentum, as this will decrease the chance of recurrent fistula. A discussion on the use of omentum can be found earlier in this chapter. The pelvis is usually drained with a closed suction drainage system or a large Penrose drain. A Foley catheter is left indwelling for approximately 10 days. A cystogram is taken before catheter removal to rule out extravasation.

Summary

A vesicoenteric fistula is usually caused by underlying bowel disease. The urologist is often involved in the diagnostic evaluation. The usual presentation is recurrent urinary tract infections and pneumaturia. A pelvic CT scan and cystoscopy are the most useful diagnostic tests. Therapy centers on surgical repair of the bowel disease and closure of the bladder. Post-operative bladder drainage is important until healing is complete.

Editorial Comment
Fray F. Marshall

The principles of management of urinary fistula are discussed in detail in this chapter. In a complicated fistula, it is wiser to have the capability of both an abdominal and a perineal approach. Omentum can provide a significant vascularized pedicle of tissue that can be interposed. In general, it is probably not a good idea to rely on omentum exclusively to form part of the wall of the bladder. It is better to use it as an ancillary rather than a primary component of repair.

A ureterovaginal fistula can occur with a vesicovaginal fistula so that the upper urinary tract always needs investigation as well. Sometimes a significant component of stress incontinence may need correction at the same time. In patients who have had significant radiation and are not interested in sexual activity, colpocleisis (collapse of the upper vagina) can be utilized.[1]

1. Marshall VF. Vesicovaginal fistulas on one urological service. J Urol 121:25, 1979.

REFERENCES

1. Tancer NL. Observations on prevention and management of vesicovaginal fistula after total hysterectomy. Surg Gynecol Obstet 175:501, 1992.
2. Gerber GS, Schoenberg HW. Female urinary tract fistulas. J Urol 149:229, 1993.
3. Fichtner J, Voges G, Steindach F, Hohenfellner R. Ureterovesicovaginal fistulas. Surg Gynecol Obstet 176:571, 1993.
4. Nanninga JB, O'Conor VJ. The management of vesicovagina fistula: Suprapubic repair of vesicovaginal fistula. In Carlton CE Jr, ed. Controversies in Urology. Chicago, Year Book, 1989.
5. Wein AJ. Vesicovaginal fistula. In Resnick MI, Kursh E, ed. Current Therapy in Genitourinary Surgery. Philadelphia, BC Decker, 1987.
6. Belandy JP, Badenoch DF, Fowler CG, et al. Early repair of iatrogenic injury to the ureter or bladder after gynecological surgery. J Urol 146:761, 1991.
7. Collins CG, Pent D, Jones FB. Results of early repair of vesicovaginal fistula with preliminary cortisone treatment. Am J Obstet Gynecol 80:1005, 1960.
8. Scott FB. The management of vesicovaginal fistula: The case for vaginal repair of vesicovaginal fistula. In Carlton, CE. Jr, ed. Controversies in Urology. Chicago, Year Book, 1989.
9. Turner-Warwick R. The use of the omental pedicle graft in urinary tract reconstruction. J Urol 116:341, 1976.
10. Martius H. The repair of vesicovaginal fistulae with interposition pedicle graft of labial tissue. Zentralbl Gynakol 52:480, 1928.
11. Raz S, Dregg KJ, Nitti, VW, Sussman E. Transvaginal repair of vesicovaginal fistula using a peritoneal flap. J Urol 150:56, 1993.
12. Mraz JP, Sutroy M. An alternative in surgical treatment of post-irradiation vesicovaginal and rectovaginal fistulas: The seromuscular intestinal graft (patch). J Urol 151:357, 1994.
13. Menchaca A, Akhyat N, Gleicher N, et al. The rectus abdominis muscle flap in a combined abdominovaginal repair of difficult vesicovaginal fistulae: A report of three cases. J Reprod Med 35:565, 1990.
14. Patil U, Waterhouse K, Laungani G. Management of 18 difficult vesicovaginal and urethrovaginal fistulas with modified Ingelman-Sundberg and Martius operations. J Urol 123:653, 1980.
15. Moss RL, Rayn JA Jr. Management of enterovesical fistulas. Am J Surg 159:514, 1990.
16. Haas GP, Shumaker BP, Haas PA. Appendicovesical fistula. Urology 24:604, 1984.
17. Ral PN, Knox R, Barnard RJ, Schofield PF. Management of colovesical fistula. Br J Surg 74:362, 1987.
18. Kirsh GN, Hampel N, Shuck JN, Resnick MI. Diagnosis and management of vesicoenteric fistulas. Surg Gynecol Obstet 173:91, 1991.
19. Sarr MG, Fishman EK, Goldman SM, et al. Enterovesical fistula. Surg Gynecol Obstet 164:41, 1987.
20. Fraley EE, Reinberg Y, Holt T, Sneiders A. Computerized tomography in the diagnosis of appendicovesical fistula. J Urol 149:830, 1993.
21. Amendola MA, Agha FP, Dent TL, et al. Detection of occult colovesical fistula by the Bourne test. AJR 142:715, 1984.

Part V
URINARY DIVERSION

Chapter 53

Ureterosigmoidostomy

Terry D. Allen

The goal of any form of urinary diversion is to deliver the urine to the outside with a minimum of interference to life style and with a maximum of protection to the urinary tract. While no form of urinary diversion has achieved this goal to everyone's satisfaction, a close approximation to it has come from procedures that utilize one of nature's two natural sphincters: the external urethral sphincter as in the case of the intestinal neobladder, and the anal sphincter as in the case of ureterosigmoidostomy. Of the two, ureterosigmoidostomy is the older and thus has the longer track record for study—a fact that has exposed some of its weaknesses as well as its strengths. A clear understanding of the mechanisms responsible for some of the problems associated with the procedure is thus important if the operation is to take its rightful place among the options available today for urinary diversion.

PATHOPHYSIOLOGY

The entry of the ureters into a grossly infected area such as the colon would seem to represent a natural prescription for pyelonephritis, but this has not been the case in my experience. Tunneled implantation of the ureter through the wall of the colon produces a durable antireflux valve mechanism in most cases and, provided that the ureter is unobstructed and intracolonic pressure remains low, pyelonephritis in a ureterosigmoidostomy patient is not as common as generally thought. An obstructed anastomosis is a technical problem that can be overcome by attention to detail, but the obstruction caused by elevated intracolonic pressure is a more insidious threat. Normally, pressure within the colon receives little in the way of special attention; in urodynamic studies, intracolonic pressure is often considered equal to intra-abdominal

pressure for calculation purposes. This may be true for the colon in its natural state, but when it is filled with fluid, the colon behaves quite differently. Fisch and colleagues[1] have recorded intracolonic pressures in ureterosigmoid patients as high as 72 cm water, indicating that everything we have learned about compliance as it affects bladder function can be applied equally well to the colon in the ureterosigmoidostomy patient. For this reason, the importance of frequent evacuation of the bowel should be stressed to these patients, or consideration given to some form of detubularization of the colon to reduce intracolonic pressure.[1]

Since the monumental report by Ferris and Odel,[2] it has been appreciated that urine in contact with bowel mucosa has a potential to produce derangements in serum electrolytes. The extent of the problem varies with the intestinal segment involved, the surface area exposed, and the length of the exposure. The mechanism of derangement has been studied extensively by a number of investigators,[3–5] and it is now evident that the primary offender is the reabsorption of ammonia leading to a net gain in ammonium and chloride along with a net loss of sodium and bicarbonate. There is also a net loss of water and potassium. The result is a tendency to hyperchloremic acidosis and hypokalemia. In ureterosigmoidostomy patients with normal renal function and regular bowel evacuation, the abnormality may not appear critical. However, even minor derangements in electrolytes may lead to demineralization of bone, and it is best to consider administration of sodium bicarbonate or other alkali in doses sufficient to maintain serum bicarbonate at normal levels an integral part of the management of these patients.

Perhaps the greatest cause for concern in ureterosigmoidostomy patients is their tendency to develop colon cancer.[6] To some extent the attention that ureterosigmoidostomy has received in this regard is a consequence of its long history; newer information suggests that intestinal cancer may be a risk in any situation where bowel is chronically exposed to infected urine.[7] The exact mechanism of this complication is not entirely clear. The presence of nitrosamine, a potent carcinogen, in the urinary fecal flux has been suggested as a cause,[8] but the use of vitamin C to reduce nitrosamine levels has not been accompanied by a corresponding decline in the development of tumors in experimental animals.[9] Gittes found that a segment of ileum interposed between the urinary tract and the colon markedly reduced the incidence of colon cancer in rats, but the reason for this remains obscure.[10] Finally, it should be noted that the recorded incidence of colon cancer in ureterosigmoidostomy patients is not vastly different from the lifetime risk of the disease in the population at large, suggesting that the principal effect of ureterosigmoidostomy might be to accelerate the appearance of colon cancer in susceptible individuals. In any event, it does not seem justified to deny the option of ureterosigmoidostomy to appropriate candidates, although the decision to proceed with the operation carries with it the need for lifetime surveillance.

INDICATIONS AND CONTRAINDICATIONS

Ureterosigmoidostomy may be considered in any patient with adequate renal function and an intact anal sphincter whose bladder must be sacrificed for any reason. Patients with intractable urinary incontinence not amenable to surgical correction by conventional reconstructive procedures may also be candidates for the operation. Ureterosigmoidostomy is a particularly attractive option in children with anomalies such as bladder exstrophy, because it eliminates wetness while obviating the need for external appliances, catheters, and artificial sphincters. These devices are often poorly accepted by the young, especially as they approach adolescence when peer pressure makes any deviation from the norm almost intolerable.

Ureterosigmoidostomy is contraindicated in any patient with an incompetent anal sphincter, whether as a consequence of neurological disease, anorectal malformations, or anorectal surgery. It should also be considered with caution in anyone with an irradiated lower bowel because of the irritative bowel effect that may result, or anyone with reduced renal function because of the greater difficulty in controlling fluid and electrolyte balance. In general, it is best to avoid the operation altogether in any patient whose renal function is less than half normal. Dilated ureters pose a problem since they do not provide a very reliable antireflux mechanism, but this can be overcome by an interposed ileal segment with an intussuscepted valve[11] or by tapered implantation of the dilated ureters under the protection of a temporary diverting colostomy.

PREOPERATIVE MANAGEMENT

Preoperative assessment of the patient includes tests of renal function as well as studies to delineate the anatomy of the upper urinary tracts. A barium enema is generally not given as a routine unless disease of the colon is suspected. If there is a question regarding anal continence, anal manometrics may be undertaken, or a mixture of oatmeal and water approximating the texture of the expected urinary-fecal flux may be instilled into the rectum as a test before final commitment to the procedure is made.

The patient is placed on a clear liquid diet and the bowel is cleansed mechanically the day before the operation with laxatives and enemas or a gastrointestinal lavage solution such as GoLYTELY. The bowel is then sterilized by administration of appropriate antibiotics such as neomycin and erythromycin base or metronidazole orally, or by a wide-spectrum cephalosporin such as cefazolin parenterally.

OPERATIVE TECHNIQUE

The operation is performed with the patient in a supine position. If it is thought that ureteral stents will be needed, it is advisable to insert a rectal tube ahead of time so that it can be grasped from above and the stents affixed to it for later retrieval from below. The abdomen is generally opened through a lower midline incision to expose the lower ureters and the sigmoid and rectosigmoid portions of the colon. The peritoneum overlying each ureter is incised at the pelvic brim, and the ureters are identified and tagged by passing a tape or vessel loop around them. They are then transected at an appropriate level.

If the Leadbetter type of ureteral reimplantation is chosen (Fig. 53–1), the rectosigmoid is sutured to the medial margin of the previously incised peritoneum to fix it in position. The adjacent ureter is then laid on the bowel to identify an appropriate point for making a tunnel, and the wall of the ureter is sutured to the colon just proximal to the proposed tunnel. The tunnel is created in the tenia by incising it for a distance of about 5 cm, carrying the incision through the muscular wall of the colon but not through the mucosa itself. Care must be taken to cut all tissue and vascular bands over the mucosa and to dissect laterally between the mucosa and overlying muscle so that the mucosa bulges freely into the wound. Otherwise the resulting tunnel might be too tight,

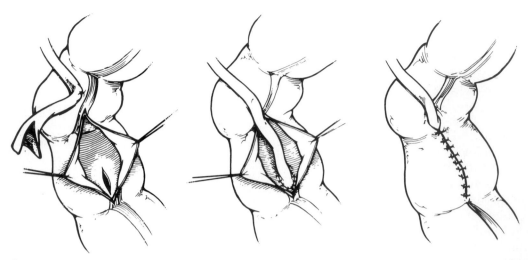

Figure 53–1. Leadbetter technique for ureterosigmoidostomy. The ureter is fixed to the wall of the colon adjacent to the tenia, and the tenia is incised distally for a distance of about 5 cm. The incision is carried down to the mucosa, and a small opening is made in the mucosa in the distal part of the trough. The end of the ureter is spatulated and sutured to the mucosal opening using fine catgut sutures, after which the wall of the colon is closed over the ureter, leaving it in a submucosal position.

and ischemia and secondary fibrosis of the terminal ureter might result.

A small opening is then made in the mucosa in the distal end of the trough. The spatulated ureter is sutured to the mucosal opening with fine absorbable sutures to achieve a meticulous mucosa-to-mucosa anastomosis. The ureter is then pushed down into the trough so that the muscular wall of the colon can be closed to leave the ureter in a submucosal position.

The right ureter is usually implanted into the descending rectosigmoid. However, when the bowel is sutured to the right pelvic wall to facilitate this anastomosis, the relationship of the rectosigmoid to the left ureter is such that a similar anastomosis between

the two is not generally practical. Instead, the left ureteral implantation is commonly made into the transverse sigmoid segment. The basic principle is the same, however: creating a tunnel in a readily accessible tenia.

As an alternative technique, the ureters may also be implanted through the open bowel (Fig. 53–2). With this technique the bowel is opened opposite the site of the implantation, and the ureter is brought through the bowel wall at an appropriate point to avoid any kinking. A tunnel is created distally by injecting saline submucosally along the line of the proposed tunnel, then dissecting beneath the bleb with tenotomy scissors to create a channel about 4 to 5 cm in length. The ureter is passed through the

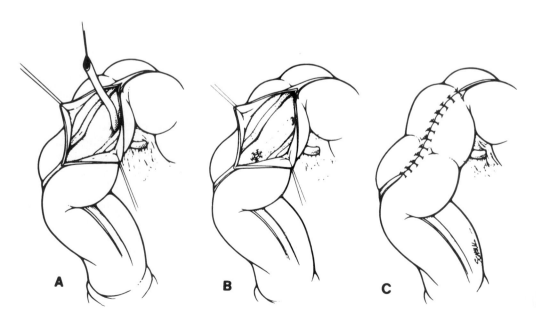

A   **B**   **C**

Figure 53–2. Open technique for ureterosigmoidostomy. The colon is opened opposite the site selected for implantation, and the ureter is brought through the wall of the colon. Distal to this point a tunnel is created by first lifting the mucosa off the underlying muscle by the submucosal injection of sterile saline and then passing narrow dissecting scissors submucosally along the line of injection for a distance of 4 to 5 cm. The ureter is then passed into the tunnel so created and sutured into position, after which the wall of the colon is closed.

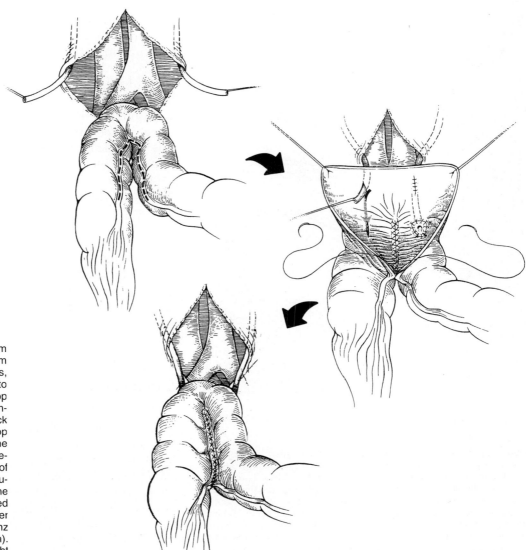

Figure 53–3. The sigma-rectum pouch. The posterior peritoneum is incised to expose the ureters, and the rectosigmoid is sutured to the sacral promontory. The loop of rectosigmoid so created is incised along a tenia, and the back walls of the two limbs of the loop are sutured together to create the back wall of the pouch. The ureters are pulled through the wall of the colon and implanted submucosally. The anterior wall of the pouch is then closed. (Adapted from Fisch M, Wommack R, Miller SC, Hohenfellner R. The Mainz pouch II (sigma rectum pouch). J Urol 149:258, 1993. Copyright Williams & Wilkins, 1993.)

tunnel so that it lies loosely in a submucosal position. A mucosa-to-mucosa anastomosis is accomplished within the lumen of the bowel, and the wall of the ureter is affixed to the wall of the colon externally. The colon is then closed.

Variations

For certain patients, variations in the basic operation may be appropriate. Hanley recommended a rectosigmoid bladder with a proximal colostomy either as a primary procedure or as a rescue operation for patients for whom the standard ureterosigmoidostomy proved unsatisfactory.[12] With proper colostomy care, it is possible to enjoy the benefits of a continent urinary reservoir without the annoyance of an external appliance.

Fisch and colleagues introduced the sigma-rectum pouch, created by detubularizing a segment of recto-

sigmoid into which the ureters are implanted (Fig. 53–3).[1] These investigators showed that detubularization of this portion of the colon decreased the intracolonic pressure substantially, thus reducing the risk of high-pressure reflux into the upper urinary tracts, while simultaneously lessening the chance of urinary incontinence.

An obstructed ureterosigmoidostomy with secondary hydroureteronephrosis may be salvaged by inserting an interposed ileal segment with an intussuscepted valve between the dilated ureters and the colon (Fig. 53–4), thus preserving the basic concepts of the ureterosigmoidostomy with respect to continence.[11] The same operation permits ureterosigmoidostomy to be performed in patients with dilated ureters. The key to the success of the interposed ileal segment is a durable valve created by intussuscepting a portion of the ileal segment and suturing one wall firmly to the ileum overlying it. To date, reflux has not been demonstrated proximal to a valve so constructed.

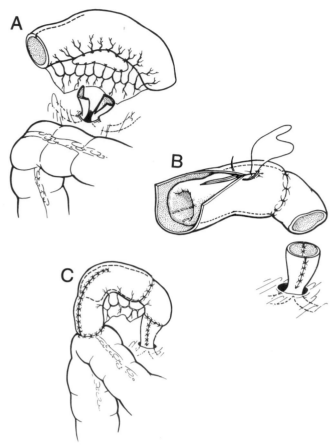

Figure 53–4. Ileal interposition procedure. A segment of ileum approximately 22 cm in length is disconnected from the fecal stream *(A)*. Its mesentery is divided in its midportion for a distance of about 6 cm and the ileum is intussuscepted upon itself to create a nipple valve. The nipple is stapled at the 4 and 8 o'clock positions, but at 12 o'clock the nipple is incised and sutured to the overlying ileal wall *(B)*. Proximally the ureters are attached to the ileum, while distally the ileum is anastomosed to the rectosigmoid colon *(C)*. (From Allen TD. Salvaging the obstructed ureterosigmoidostomy using an ileal interposition technique. J Urol 150:1195, 1993. Copyright Williams & Wilkins, 1993.)

POSTOPERATIVE MANAGEMENT AND COMPLICATIONS

Postoperatively, a rectal tube with or without ureteral stents should be left in place for several days to decompress the bowel and urinary tract while the anastomoses are healing. Most patients require alkali in some form, but the ideal maintenance dose may not be evident immediately. Serum electrolyte determinations should be made at appropriate intervals as titration of the alkali is carried out until stability is achieved. Patients should be instructed to evacuate their bowels at frequent intervals, not only to reduce urinary contact time and reabsorption of urine, but also to keep intracolonic pressure low and thus minimize the likelihood of incontinence.

The most common major complication of uretero-

sigmoidostomy is the development of hydroureteronephrosis, either as a consequence of a mechanical obstruction at the site of the ureterointestinal anastomosis, or because of high intracolonic pressures. Most of the other complications, such as pyelonephritis, renal scarring, urinary calculi, and loss of renal function, are generally the consequence of an underlying ureterointestinal obstruction. In some cases, this complication may force the selection of another form of urinary diversion, but often it can be overcome by using some of the techniques previously described without having to abandon ureterosigmoidostomy altogether.

Colon cancer remains a serious threat in these patients, but with careful surveillance it should be possible to detect this complication in sufficient time to deal with it effectively. For this reason, periodic guaiac examination of stools and annual colonoscopy should be implemented about 6 years after the procedure.

Summary

Despite its shortcomings, ureterosigmoidostomy has proven a durable option in urinary diversion, with survivors showing normal urinary tracts and stable renal function as long as 50 to 60 years after the operation. It is simple to perform, offers satisfactory continence with minimal interference in life style, and is associated with a complication rate not significantly different from that of other forms of urinary diversion. At a time when quality of life is being stressed as it is today, the advantages of ureterosigmoidostomy are provoking renewed interest in the procedure.

Editorial Comment
Fray F. Marshall

Ureterosigmoidostomy remains an option for continent urinary diversion. When it works well, it works exceedingly well. If there are problems, the urologist has to contend with both the urinary and alimentary tracts. I have one admonition—don't ever dilate the anus of a patient with exstrophy after ureterosigmoidostomy. Continence may change dramatically.

Ureterosigmoidostomy remains an option in some patients, but in view of many of the potential complications discussed in this chapter, it is usually best to obtain a radiographical study of the colon. A colon conduit can sometimes be created initially and later placed in continuity with the intestinal tract in a staged fashion, possibly with detubularization. Because of the long-term complications of infection, acidosis, and neoplasia, children may be less attractive candidates for this surgery.

REFERENCES

1. Fisch M, Wommack R, Müller SC, Hohenfellner R. The Mainz pouch II (sigma rectum pouch). J Urol 149:258, 1993.

2. Ferris DO, Odel HM. Electrolyte pattern of the blood after bilateral ureterosigmoidostomy. JAMA 142:634, 1950.

3. Boyce WH, Vest SA. The role of ammonia reabsorption in acid base imbalance following ureterosigmoidostomy. J Urol 67:169, 1952.

4. Stamey TA. The pathogenesis and implications of the electrolyte imbalance in ureterosigmoidostomy. Surg Gynecol Obstet 103:736, 1956.

5. Koch MO, Gurevitch E, Hill DE, McDougal WS. Urinary solute transport by intestinal segments: A comparative study of ileum and colon in rats. J Urol 143:1275, 1990.

6. Leadbetter GW Jr, Zickerman P, Pierce E. Ureterosigmoidostomy and carcinoma of the colon. J Urol 92:37, 1964.

7. Filmer B, Spencer JR. Malignancies in bladder augmentation and intestinal conduits. J Urol 143:671, 1990.

8. Stewart M, Hill MJ, Pugh RCB, Williams P. The role of N-nitrosamine in carcinogenesis at the ureterocolic anastamosis. Br J Urol 53:115, 1981.

9. Stribling MD, Cohen MS, Fagan JD, et al. The effect of ascorbic acid on urinary nitrosamines and tumor development in a rat animal model for ureterosigmoidostomy. Presented before the American Urological Association, Dallas, Texas, May 1989.

10. Gittes RF. Carcinogenesis in ureterosigoidostomy. Urol Clin North Am 13:201, 1986.

11. Allen TD. Salvaging the obstructed ureterosigmoidostomy using an ileal interposition technique. J Urol 150:1195, 1993.

12. Hanley HG. The rectal bladder. Br J Urol 39:693, 1967.

Chapter 54

Ileal Conduit Urinary Diversion

Ellen Shapiro

INDICATIONS

Although many new techniques for bladder replacement and continent urinary diversion are now being performed, the ileal conduit urinary diversion as described by Bricker[1] remains the standard for urinary diversion among urologists throughout the world. The ileal loop has proved to be a procedure with low morbidity and few complications. A patient with an ileal loop can maintain a favorable quality of life and preserve renal function.

The indications for ileal loop urinary diversion have evolved, especially in the younger patient with a neurogenic bladder or urological malignancy. The advent of clean intermittent catheterization in the early 1970s changed the present indications for urinary diversion. The urological disorders that continue to require ileal loop urinary diversion are (1) malignancy, (2) congenital anomalies, (3) neurogenic vesical dysfunction, and (4) trauma (Table 54–1).[2]

PREOPERATIVE MANAGEMENT

Once a decision has been made that a patient requires an ileal loop urinary diversion, a thorough preoperative evaluation is mandatory to ensure a successful intra- and postoperative course. This evaluation is especially important in the elderly. The surgeon must have complete knowledge of the patient's pertinent medical history, including medications, operations, and illnesses. This knowledge will ensure the proper postoperative administration of appropriate medications, such as antihypertensives, antiarrhythmics, insulin, and glucocorticoids, especially while the patient is not permitted oral intake. It is also important to determine whether the patient has had previous abdominal surgery or radiation therapy that may preclude the use of an ileal segment. The structural and functional integrity of the gastrointestinal system must be evaluated, especially in patients

with histories of inflammatory bowel disease, including regional enteritis, ulcerative colitis, and diverticulitis. These bowel disorders may further complicate the planned bowel surgery and limit the intestinal segments that can be used for urinary diversion.

If the patient has renal insufficiency, the use of jejunum is absolutely contraindicated because this segment is associated with a high incidence of metabolic abnormalities, which constitute the jejunal conduit syndrome.[3] This syndrome is characterized by nausea, vomiting, anorexia, and muscle weakness. The laboratory findings are azotemia, hyponatremia, hypochloremia, and hyperkalemic metabolic acidosis.

The preoperative planning for patients who are undergoing major abdominal surgery should include

---

TABLE 54–1. Indications for Ileal Loop Urinary Diversion

Malignancy requiring radical cystectomy or radical cystoprostatectomy
  Bladder (except for carcinoma confined to dome in absence of carcinoma in situ)
  Prostate (transitional cell carcinoma or local recurrence of adenocarcinoma following definitive radiation therapy)
  Urethra
  Urachal
  Advanced gynecological malignancy
  Advanced rectal malignancy
Congenital malformation
  Exstrophy (including noncandidates for primary functional closure and multiple failed attempts at continence)
  Posterior urethral valves with severe vesical dysfunction and renal insufficiency in preparation for renal transplantation
  Bilateral ureteral ectopia
Neurogenic vesical dysfunction
  Congenital
    Myelodysplasia
  Acquired
    Spinal cord injury
    Multiple sclerosis
Trauma
  Pelvic injury
  Radiation therapy (chronic cystitis, contracted bladder capacity, persistent hematuria)
  Persistent vesicovaginal fistula

a complete physical and laboratory evaluation with a complete blood count, serum chemistry findings, urinalysis, and urine culture. In the elderly or in patients with histories of pulmonary disease, pulmonary function tests, including arterial blood gas values, are indicated.

The patient's nutritional status should be assessed and appropriate supplementation given preoperatively. Although urinary diversion alone is not associated with appreciable blood loss, blood should be available for the patient, especially when ileal loop diversion is combined with radical pelvic surgery. Depending on the patient's preference, either autologous or directed donor blood products should be banked if the patient is unwilling to accept blood from the volunteer supply.

In addition to the aforementioned preoperative planning, it is imperative that the patient meet with the enterostomal therapist. It is also helpful for patients to speak with individuals who have successfully adapted to urinary diversions. During these preoperative meetings, a stomal site should be selected and marked.[4] The preferred stomal site is located in the right lower quadrant on a line joining the umbilicus and the anterosuperior iliac spine. The stomal site is located just medial to the lateral border of the rectus abdominis muscle. One must avoid placing the stoma near previous surgical scars or any distortions of the abdominal wall. A flat ring of metal or plastic is employed that simulates the urinary appliance faceplate. This ring is positioned and checked with the patient in various positions to assure that a large skin crease does not appear unexpectedly, leading to an improper fit of the appliance. The center of the stoma is marked with a small-gauge needle scratch over the site. Alternative quadrants for stomal sites should be evaluated in case a right lower quadrant stoma is not surgically feasible.

The patient is placed on a mechanical bowel preparation 2 days before surgery, and oral antibiotics for bowel sterilization are given (Table 54–2).[5, 6] A more vigorous bowel preparation is usually indicated in patients with neurogenic bowel dysfunction. Broad-spectrum parenteral antibiotics are not mandatory. Intravenous antibiotics can be administered preoperatively and continued for 24 hours postoperatively. On the evening of surgery, the patient is instructed on the use of incentive spirometry. The importance of early ambulation for the prevention of pulmonary emboli is reiterated.

Some surgeons may use perioperative minidoses of heparin or an intraoperative lower extremity compression device to help prevent the development of venous stasis during lengthy radical pelvic surgery. Electrolytes are evaluated to make sure no excessive losses during the bowel preparation have occurred. Patients are given intravenous hydration overnight.

OPERATIVE TECHNIQUE

The patient is placed in the supine position. After the patient has been intubated, a nasogastric tube is passed and checked to ensure that it irrigates freely. The patient's position is modified depending on whether the urinary diversion is being performed in combination with radical pelvic surgery. A midline vertical incision is made extending from the pubis just lateral to the midline and the umbilicus on the side away from the anticipated stoma site.[2, 7] The ureters are identified through incisions in the posterior peritoneum as they cross the bifurcation of the iliac vessels (Fig. 54–1). The ureters are mobilized, taking care to protect their blood supply, and transected 3 to 4 cm above their entry into the bladder. The distal ureteral margins are excised and submitted to pathology for frozen-section analysis to rule out malignancy or dysplasia when the diversion is performed for invasive bladder cancer. Ligating the ureters with chromic catgut suture results in ureteral dilation, which may aid in the ureteroileal anastomosis.

The ileocecal valve is identified. A routine appendectomy is performed in most patients. The distal ileum is tagged with a silk suture 12 cm from the ileocecal valve to ensure an isoperistaltic orientation of the segment. Approximately 20 cm of ileum are selected for the segment. The distal mesentery is divided in an avascular region between the ileocolic artery and the terminal branch of the superior mesenteric artery. The proximal mesentery is divided, leaving the first arcade of blood vessels intact. If excessive mesenteric fat is present and digital palpation of the vessels is difficult, the overhead light may be positioned opposite the surgeon to better illuminate the vascular arcades in the terminal ileum. The mesentery at the distal end of the segment is divided for approximately 8 cm so that the distal end of the segment can be mobilized through the abdominal wall without tension. The proximal mesentery is di-

---

TABLE 54–2. Protocol for Intestinal Antisepsis

Nichols-Condon Method
    Clear fluid diet 2 days before surgery
    Mechanical preparation using castor oil or magnesium sulfate in addition to enemas until clear
    Oral neomycin and erythromycin base administered on 2nd day; 1 gm of each antibiotic is given at 1, 2, and 11 PM. The operation is scheduled for 7:30 AM the next day.

Whole Gut Irrigation
    Patient ingests 1 L of chilled polyethylene-glycol-electrolyte lavage solution (GoLYTELY) per hour for a maximum of 5 hours or until rectal effluent is completely clear

A

B

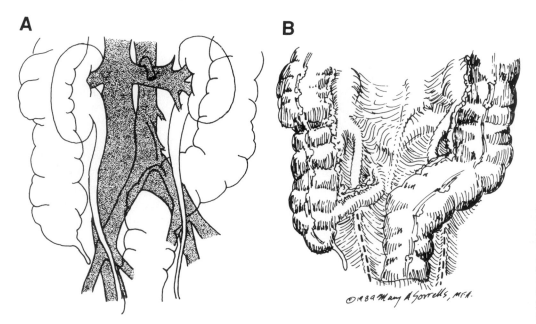

Figure 54–1. *A,* The ureters are identified crossing the iliac bifurcation. *B,* The left ureter is mobilized through an incision (*dotted lines*) in the posterior peritoneum lateral to the sigmoid colon. The right ureter is mobilized through a similar incision in the posterior peritoneum just above the pelvic rim.

vided, but only for a distance of approximately 4 cm to ensure adequate blood supply to the segment (Fig. 54–2).

Noncrushing bowel clamps are placed and the bowel is divided. The ileal conduit segment is positioned beneath the open ends of the ileum ("water under the bridge"). The proximal ("butt") end of the

ileal segment is closed with a Parker-Kerr running inverting 3-0 chromic catgut suture in two layers. A third layer of interrupted 3-0 chromic inverting serosal sutures may be used to reinforce the suture line. The clamp on the stoma end is removed and the segment is irrigated with warm saline (Fig. 54–3).

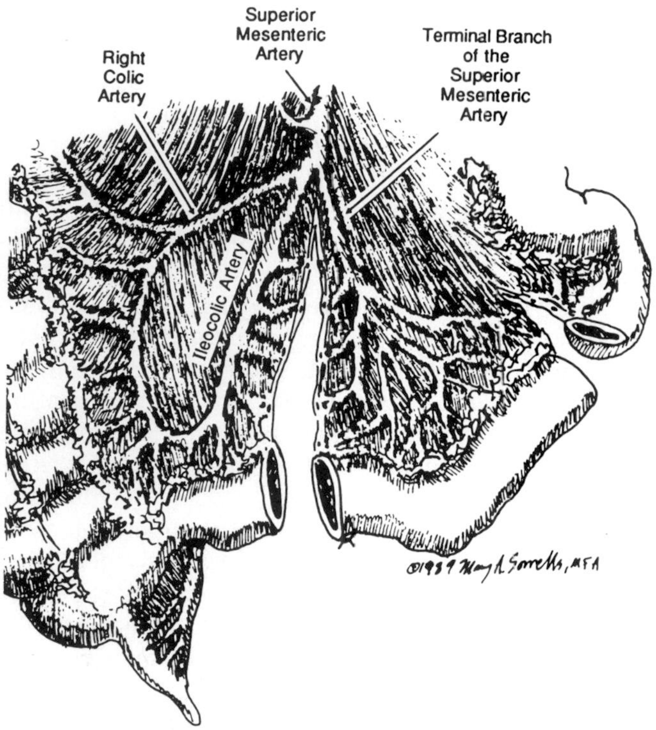

A standard two-layer bowel anastomosis is performed using a running transmural 3-0 chromic catgut suture line. The ends of the bowel are inverted and the anterior wall anastomosis is performed using the Connell stitch. The suture line is reinforced by interrupted 3-0 silk seromuscular sutures. Alternatively, a stapled anastomosis may be performed. The defect in the mesentery is approximated with multiple interrupted 4-0 silk suture to avoid internal herniation of the bowel (Fig. 54–3).

The left ureter is tagged with a chromic catgut suture and then passed behind the sigmoid mesentery in the avascular space just anterior to the sacral promontory and distal aorta, exiting through the incision on the right posterior peritoneum. The left posterior peritoneum is incised superiorly to permit the ureter to follow a smooth course without angulation (Fig. 54–4). A blunt curved clamp is placed through the distal open end of the ileal segment, and a small left ileotomy is made 2 cm from the butt end of the loop along its antimesenteric border (Fig. 54–5*A*). A 5 Fr. feeding tube is passed through the ileotomy. The ureter is spatulated medially and a holding suture is placed to secure the ureter to the ileum (Fig. 54–5*B*). A meticulous mucosa-to-mucosa watertight ureteroileal anastomosis is performed using interrupted 4-0 polyglycolic acid sutures. The sutures are tied on the outside of the urinary tract (Fig. 54–5*C*). A grooved director may facilitate visualization of the full-wall thickness of the ureter so that there is no mucosal

Right Colic Artery

Superior Mesenteric Artery

Terminal Branch of the Superior Mesenteric Artery

Ileocolic Artery

Figure 54–2. A routine appendectomy is performed. Approximately 20 cm of ileum is selected for the segment. The distal mesentery is divided between the ileocecal artery and the terminal branch of the superior mesenteric artery. The proximal mesentery is divided, leaving the first arcade of blood vessels intact.

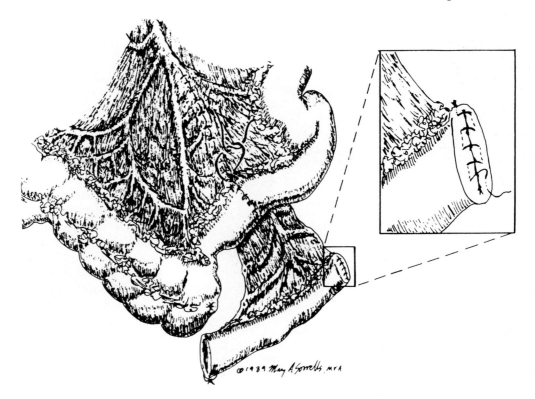

Figure 54–3. The bowel is divided and the ileal conduit segment positioned beneath the open ends of the ileum. The proximal end of the segment is closed with a two-layer running inverted Parker-Kerr suture. The inset shows the first layer of this closure. A third layer of interrupted inverting serosal sutures is placed. A standard two-layer bowel anastomosis is performed. The defect in the mesentery is closed.

exclusion. When half of the ureteroileal sutures are placed, the stent is passed up the ureter and irrigated. The right ileotomy is made and the ureteroileal anastomosis proceeds in a similar fashion. The loop is gently inflated with saline to ensure a watertight closure. The stents are sutured at the skin level at the end of the operation. They are trimmed at a right angle or obliquely to aid in their identification (right

or left). The use of stents remains the individual surgeon's preference, but they are absolutely indicated in patients who have received radiation therapy or who are undergoing ureteroileal revision.

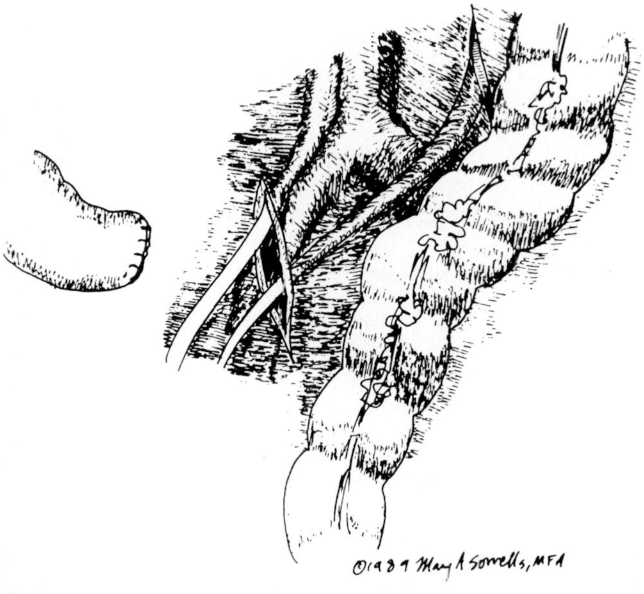

The right rectus fascia is placed on medial traction with a Kocher clamp. Stoma formation proceeds by grasping all layers of the abdominal wall with an Allis clamp. A button of skin is excised approximately the size of a quarter. Care is taken not to excise excessive subcutaneous tissue, to avoid retraction of the stoma (Fig. 54–6A). A cruciate incision is made in the anterior rectus fascia, and four 2-0 polyglycolic acid holding sutures are placed in the four quadrants of the rectus fascia (Fig. 54–6B). The rectus muscle is bluntly split and the posterior fascia and peritoneum are incised to permit passage of two fingers. A Babcock clamp is then passed through the stoma site, and the loop and stents are grasped and brought out several centimeters above the skin without tension (Fig. 54–6C). The ileal segment is inspected to ensure that the mesentery has not been twisted. The seromuscular layer of the ileum is fixed to the anterior rectus fascia using the previously placed 2-0 polyglycolic acid sutures. The stoma is created by forming a nipple employing the blunt end of a right-angled clamp to evert the mucosal edge (Fig. 54–6D). The mucosa is then sutured to the dermis with multiple interrupted 4-0 chromic catgut sutures. Before abdominal wall closure, closed suction drains are placed in the pelvis away from the ileal loop to avoid continuous suction near the ureteroileal anastomoses. Also, it is the preference of some surgeons to place a

Figure 54–4. The left ureter is passed behind the sigmoid mesentery in the avascular space just anterior to the sacral promontory and distal aorta. The left posterior peritoneum is incised superiorly to permit the ureter to follow a smooth course without angulation.

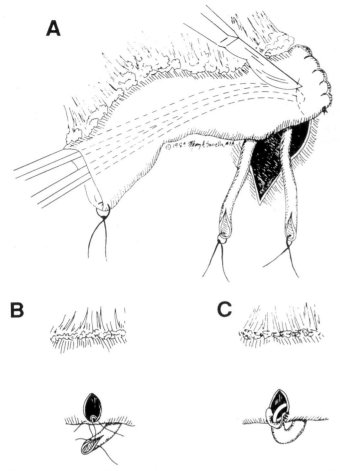

Figure 54–5. *A,* A blunt curved clamp is placed through the distal open end of the ileal segment, and a small left ureterotomy is made 2 cm from the butt end of the loop along its antimesenteric border. A 5 Fr. feeding tube is passed through the ileotomy. *B,* The ureter is spatulated medially. A holding suture is placed to secure the ureter to the ileum. A mucosa-to-mucosa watertight anastomosis is performed. *C,* When half of the ureteroileal sutures are placed, the stent is passed up the ureter. The loop is gently inflated with saline after the right ureteral anastomosis is completed.

formal gastrostomy instead of a nasogastric tube if extensive pelvic surgery has been performed.

Alternative Stoma Technique

An alternative to the end stomal loop is the Turn-bull-Hewitt end loop stoma (Fig. 54–7).[8] The bowel segment should be 8 to 10 cm longer than the segment for an end stoma. The rectus fascia is not sutured to the bowel; the distal segment is sutured closed. A loop of bowel is elevated through the stomal opening by placing gentle traction on an umbilical tape placed around the distal portion of the loop (Fig. 54–7*A*). Once the loop is elevated above the skin level, a glass rod is substituted for the tape and sutured to the skin. A transverse incision in the ileal segment is made through approximately three fourths of the ileal circumference (Fig. 54–7*B*). Everting 3-0

chromic catgut sutures are placed from the bowel to the dermis to mature the stoma (Fig. 54–7*C* and *D*). The rod is removed after about 1 week. A Turnbull-Hewitt end loop stoma permits a generous nipple to be fashioned without tension on the mesentery. This technique is advantageous in obese patients.

POSTOPERATIVE MANAGEMENT

Early ambulation and rigorous pulmonary toilet are essential elements of postoperative care. The nasogastric tube remains in place until bowel sounds are re-established, the abdomen is flat, and flatus is passed. The diet is subsequently advanced slowly over several days. Stent removal occurs after the patient is eating (about 1 week postoperatively). An intravenous pyelogram (IVP) is performed approximately 10 days postoperatively. The pelvic drains are removed if no extravasation is seen on the IVP and the drainage has been negligible.

Before discharge, the patient and family should be proficient and comfortable with the care of the stoma. The use of long-term antibiotics in a patient with an ileal loop diversion remains controversial. The urinary loop should be catheterized every 3 months to check the urine residual in the loop and ensure that the urine is not colonized with a urea-splitting

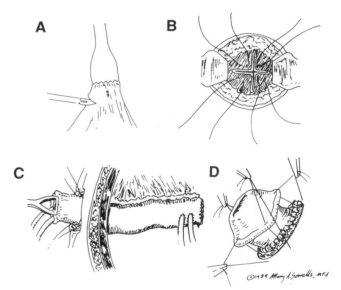

Figure 54–6. *A,* The right rectus fascia is placed on medial traction with a Kocher clamp. A "button" of skin approximately the size of a quarter is excised. *B,* A cruciate incision is made in the anterior rectus fascia, and four holding sutures are placed in the four quadrants of the rectus fascia. The rectus muscle is bluntly split, and the posterior fascia and peritoneum are widely incised. *C,* A Babcock clamp is passed through the stoma site, and the loop and stents are brought out several centimeters above the skin without tension. The seromuscular layer of the ileum is fixed to the anterior rectus fascia. *D,* The stoma is created by forming a nipple, using the blunt end of a right-angled clamp to evert the mucosal edge. The mucosa is sutured to the dermis.

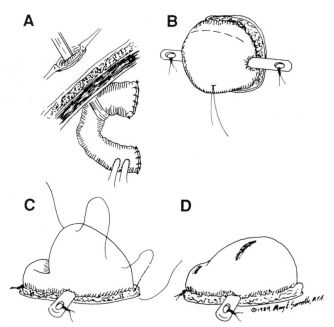

Figure 54–7. The bowel segment for a Turnbull-Hewitt end loop stoma is 8 to 10 cm longer than the segment for an end stoma. The distal segment is sutured closed. The loop of bowel is elevated through the stomal opening by placing gentle traction on an umbilical tape placed around the distal portion of the loop *(A)*. A glass rod is substituted for the tape and sutured to the skin *(B)*. A transverse incision in the ileal segment is made, encompassing about three fourths of the ileal circumference. Everting sutures are placed from the bowel to the dermis to mature the stoma *(C and D)*.

organism, which may lead to nephrolithiasis. If the loop has not been performed for invasive carcinoma of the bladder, an annual IVP can be alternated with an ultrasound examination (or a renal scan) and a plain film of the abdomen. If the patient has a history of bladder cancer, an IVP or loopogram may be performed that will satisfactorily evaluate recurrent upper urinary tract disease, stones, or obstruction. Electrolyte, blood urea nitrogen, and creatinine determinations should also be included in the yearly evaluation.

EARLY POSTOPERATIVE COMPLICATIONS

Wound Complications

Wound infection and dehiscence occurs more frequently (20 percent) when ileal loop diversion is combined with radical cancer surgery.[9] Malnutrition, diabetes, previous radiation therapy, and extreme obesity predispose patients to wound complications. In these circumstances, the surgeon should consider abdominal wall closure with monofilament and interrupted retention sutures. Wound infections usually require antibiotic therapy and local conservative care,

whereas dishiscence and possible evisceration necessitate emergent reclosure of the fascia.

Intestinal Complications

Intestinal complications are not uncommon and are usually manifested by a prolonged ileus (more than 6 days). Early postoperative bowel obstruction occurs infrequently (5 percent), whereas the incidence of late intestinal obstruction may be as high as 20 percent.[2, 9] Although some patients may ultimately require surgical exploration for intestinal obstruction secondary to adhesions and internal hernias, initial management with long gastrointestinal (Cantor) tube decompression may be a reasonable option, providing the patient's clinical status permits conservative treatment.

Ileal Loop Conduit Complications

The most common and deleterious complication of ileal diversion is a ureteroileal anastomotic urinary leak, which is usually detected within the first postoperative week.[10, 11] An increase in drainage from the pelvic drains and a concomitant decrease in urinary output from the conduit suggest urinary extravasation. The diagnosis is made radiographically with either an IVP or a loopogram. Intravenous administration of indigo carmine may be detected in the pelvic drains. Also, comparing glucose and creatinine levels in the serum and pelvic drain output is an additional method for establishing the presence of urinary extravasation. If stomal stenosis due to postoperative edema appears to be the cause (large loop residual), a 14 Fr. red rubber catheter is placed and sewn to the skin until drainage from the loop improves and stomal stenosis resolves. Failure of this conservative method to improve urinary extravasation may be due to leakage at the ureteroileal anastomosis. If urinary leakage does not improve after several days of external drainage, further drainage with percutaneous nephrostomy and antegrade stenting of the ureteral anastomosis may aid in the closure of a urinary fistula. Urinary diversion and hyperalimentation are instituted for at least 3 weeks. If these conservative measures fail to correct the urinary leakage, surgical revision will be required.

Late ureteroileal obstruction occurs in 5 to 10 percent of patients and its onset may be insidious, especially when it is unilateral.[2, 9, 10, 12] Causes of ureteral stricture include devascularization of the distal ureter due to excessive disruption of the ureteral adventitia, perianastomotic urinary leakage, and previous radiation therapy. Recurrent carcinoma and calculi can also cause late obstruction. The standard treatment for ureterointestinal anastomotic strictures is open surgical revision with excision of the strictured area and a stented reanastomosis of the ureter to the conduit. Endoscopic incision and balloon dilation have been shown to represent an acceptable first-line alternative to open surgery (89 vs. 71 percent success rate).[13] At this time, no large long-term series are available that compare open surgery and endourological techniques for repair of ureteroileal anastomotic strictures.[14] In select patients, ureteroileal anastomotic strictures can be managed with permanent indwelling stents, which develop a complete epithelial covering. This feature may avoid the potential problems of stone formation and urosepsis.

LATE COMPLICATIONS

Many excellent reviews are available on the long-term complications of ileal loop urinary diversion.[2, 9, 10, 12, 15, 17] The most common problems are discussed here briefly.

Stomal Complications

The incidence of stomal stenosis over 10 years may be as high as 50 percent in some early series.[15] Stomal revision may require the interposition of a skin flap into a vertical incision in the bowel.[16]

Prolapse of the bowel segment can occur if excessive length is left in the stoma.[2] Also, prolapse as well as parastomal and peristomal hernia may be due to inadequate fixation of the ileal segment to the anterior abdominal wall. If the loop does not drain properly because of prolapse or if a parastomal hernia leads to intestinal obstruction, revision of the loop with reduction of the hernia is indicated along with adequate fixation of the bowel to the abdominal wall with closure of the defect.[18] In 1992 the long-term complications of end versus loop ileal conduit stomas were reviewed.[19] Overall, stomal revisions were performed in only 5.5 percent of 458 patients. Although there was no difference in the incidence of complications between these two groups, prolapse occurred exclusively in the loop conduit group while stenosis occurred more frequently in the end stoma group. The study showed that in properly constructed end or loop ileal conduit stomas, functional results and complication rates were comparable. Long-term follow-up may demonstrate both obstructing and nonobstructing narrowings along the course of the ileal loop.[20] The pathogenesis may be due to a chronic inflammatory reaction or possible microvascular ischemia. These areas may respond to balloon dilation, or formal loop replacement may be required.

Renal Calculi

Renal calculi develop in 5 to 10 percent of patients with urinary diversions.[9, 12] Excessive conduit length or urinary stasis enhances the exchange of chloride for bicarbonate.[21] Chronic bicarbonate loss leads to calcium loss from bone and subsequent hypercalciuria. The combination of hypercalciuria, alkaline urine, and urea-splitting organisms promotes stone formation and growth. Prevention of calculus formation can be achieved by ensuring that the conduit drains well and that infections with urea-splitting organisms are treated promptly to avoid struvite stones. In patients who form struvite stones, urease-inhibiting agents may be useful, especially after the patient is rendered free of stones.

Renal Function and Pyelonephritis

Many reports suggest that renal deterioration occurs in patients with urinary diversion that is primarily due to obstruction (excessive residual urine) and infection.[12, 15-17] Although pyelonephritis occurs in 5 to 15 percent of patients, bacteriuria is present in 80 percent of patients with ileal loop urinary diversion. The incidence of pyelonephritis is not altered by preventive antibiotics. Therapy should be directed toward correcting any anatomical problems causing obstruction, urinary stasis, or both. Recurrent pyelonephritis may be avoided with long-term preventive antibiotic therapy or conversion of the ileal loop to a nonrefluxing colon conduit.

Editorial Comment
Fray F. Marshall

Many older cystectomy patients with medical problems are candidates for ileal conduit urinary diversion rather than the more complicated continent urinary diversion. The technique of construction of an ileal conduit has been well summarized. I sometimes use permanent suture as the final layer in the butt end of the ileal conduit. I do not think these sutures come into contact with the urine or cause any problems. A 5-0 or 6-0 monofilament absorbable suture can also be utilized for the ureteroileal anastomosis. I have generally excised a small seromuscular segment of ileum at the site of the ureteroileal anastomosis and then incised the mucosa. The suture is then placed into the mucosa, seromuscular layer, and the ureter as a single-layer anastomosis.

Ureteroileal strictures that develop late are not often successfully managed with balloon dilation, although it is frequently attempted. Ureteroileal strictures are recognized postoperative complications of an ileal conduit. If the strictures are short, endoscopic manipulations are often successful; if they are longer, operative intervention is often required. Chronic indwelling stents may suffice over the short term, but for the longer term in an otherwise healthy patient, avoidance of foreign hardware would seem reasonable.

REFERENCES

1. Bricker EM. Bladder substitution after pelvic evisceration. Surg Clin North Am 30:1511, 1950.
2. Hampel N, Bodner DR, Persky L. Ileal and jejunal conduit urinary diversion. Urol Clin North Am 13:207, 1986.
3. Kosko JW, Kursh ED, Resnick MI. Metabolic complications of urologic intestinal substitutes. Urol Clin North Am 13:2:193, 1986.
4. Noble MJ, Mebust WK. Creation of the urinary stoma. AUA Update Series, Vol 5, Lesson 13, 1986.
5. Nichols RL, Broido P, Condon RE, et al. Effect of preoperative neomycin-erythromycin intestinal preparation on the incidence of infectious complications following colon surgery. Ann Surg 178:453, 1973.
6. Fleites RA, Marshall JB, Eckhauser MI, et al: The efficacy of polyethylene glycol–electrolyte lavage solution versus traditional mechanical bowel preparation for elective colonic surgery: A randomized, prospective, blinded clinical trial. Surgery 98:708, 1985.
7. Richie JP, Skinner DG. Ureterointestinal diversion. In Walsh PC, Perlmutter AD, Gittes RF, Stamey TA, eds. Campbell's Urology, 6th ed. Philadelphia, WB Saunders, 1992.
8. Bloom DA, Lieskovsky G, Rainwater G, Skinner DG. The Turnbull loop stoma. J Urol 129:715, 1983.
9. Sullivan JW, Grabstald H, Whitmore WF. Complications of ureteroileal conduit with radical cystectomy: Review of 336 cases. J Urol 124:797, 1980.
10. Richie JP. Complications of urinary diversion. In Marshall FF, ed. Urologic Complications. Chicago, Year Book, 1986.
11. Libertino JA, Eyre RC. Plan for management of complications after ileal conduit diversion. AUA Update Series, Vol 3, Lesson 7, 1984.
12. Pitts WR, Muecke EC. A 20-year experience with ileal conduits: The fate of the kidneys. J Urol 120:154, 1979.
13. Kramolowsky EV, Clayman RV, Weyman PJ. Management of ureterointestinal anastomotic strictures: Comparison of open surgical and endourological repair. J Urol 139:1195, 1988.
14. Sanders R, Bissada NK, Bielsky S. Ureteroenteric anastomotic strictures: Treatment with Palmaz permanent indwelling stents. J Urol 150:469, 1993.
15. Middleton PW, Hendren WH. Ileal conduit in children at the Massachusetts General Hospital from 1955–1970. J Urol 115:591, 1976.
16. Smith ED. Follow-up study on 150 ileal conduits in children. J Pediatr Surg 7:1, 1972.
17. Schwartz GE, Jeffs RD. Ileal conduit urinary diversion in children: Computer analysis of long-term follow-up from 2 to 16 years. J Urol 114:285, 1975.
18. Marshall FF, Leadbetter WF, Dretler SP. Ileal conduit parastomal hernias. J Urol 114:40, 1975.
19. Chechile G, Klein EA, Bauer L, et al. Functional equivalence of end and loop ileal conduit stomas. J Urol 147:582, 1992.
20. Mitchell ME, Yoder IC, Pfister RC, et al. Ileal loop stenosis: A late complication of urinary diversion. J Urol 118:957, 1977.
21. Dretler SP. The pathogenesis of urinary tract calculi occurring after ileal conduit diversion: I. Clinical study II. Conduit III. Prevention. J Urol 109:204, 1973.

Chapter 55

Colon Conduit

Alex F. Althausen

INDICATIONS

Until the early 1970s an ileal loop conduit was the most popular form of urinary diversion in patients after anterior pelvic exenteration and other problems that required permanent supravesical diversion. Long-term follow-up, however, showed that there was loss of renal function, stomal stenosis, and pyelonephritis in a significant number of these patients.[1] This led to the use of a nonrefluxing colon conduit as an alternative to the ileal loop, which was refluxing.[2-4]

Although the indications for permanent noncontinent diversion have changed, there is still a population that benefits from this treatment. In general, this group includes patients who require evisceration for pelvic malignancies and those with severe malformations or neurological dysfunction of the lower urinary tract. Patients with failed ileal loops or a history of irradiated small bowel, and those who are unable to self-catheterize continent diversions, are also candidates for this surgery. The institutionalized patient with a cutaneous urinary diversion has special needs that most patients with loops do not have. A colon conduit has fewer long-term problems than its ileal counterpart and, without catherization, requires less urological nursing care.

PREOPERATIVE MANAGEMENT

Preoperatively, all patients should undergo a full medical and urological evaluation. This includes an intravenous urogram to determine urological anatomy and a barium enema to make sure that the large bowel is suitable for surgery. A medical history should exclude inflammatory large bowel disease. There should also be no familial predisposition to colonic cancer or polyposis. Metabolic and renal functions need to be assessed to be sure that they are adequate to handle the chemical abnormalities created by this form of diversion. The patient and family need to have preoperative teaching by the physician as well as the nursing service to define the benefits of the proposed surgery and the daily care involved once the patient leaves the hospital. This will help alleviate the "stigma" of the external stoma.

Three days before admission the patient is placed on a full liquid diet and daily mild cathartics such as magnesium citrate. One day before admission the diet is changed to clear liquids, and several liters of Go-LYTELY are imbibed. Nonintestinally absorbed oral antibiotics, e.g., neomycin, are also given to help sterilize the bowel. The patient should have enemas administered the night before surgery: it may be a disaster if the colon is not well prepared. An electrolyte-balanced solution is given intravenously to prevent dehydration during this intensive bowel preparation. If the urine is infected, antibiotics should be given pre- and intraoperatively.

The nurse clinician marks the stoma and has the patient wear the appliance while moving about in various positions to avoid the risk of future urinary leakage. On the day of surgery, pneumatic antiembolism boots are fitted and put into function when the patient is on the operating room table.

OPERATIVE TECHNIQUE

The details of the operation herein described are attributed to W. Hardy Hendren's modifications of previous ileal and colon conduit surgery. When strict attention is paid to the surgery, optimal results are obtained.

A thorough knowledge of colonic anatomy and its segmental blood supply is mandatory. The vasculature is shown in Figure 55–1. The ileocolic, right, and middle colic arteries supply the right and transverse colon. The left colic, sigmoidal, and superior hemorrhoidal vessels feed the descending and sigmoid colon. The middle and inferior rectal arteries, as terminal branches of the anterior division of the hypogastric artery, are sacrificed during radical cystectomy. Therefore, care is required in selecting the distal margin of the sigmoid

446

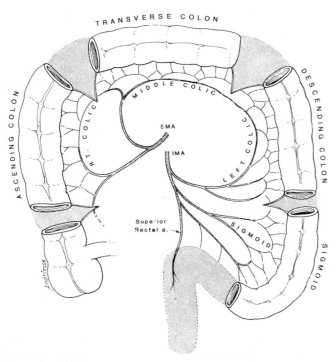

Figure 55–1. Anatomy of the colon. SMA, superior mesenteric artery; IMA, inferior mesenteric artery.

loop segment in order to preserve the blood supply of the rectum. This step necessitates identification and preservation of the superior rectal artery (the most inferior branch of the sigmoid vessels).

Through a midline abdominal incision the ureters are isolated and transected just below the pelvic brim, or above it if there has been previous irradiation. The ureters are then intubated with an 8 Fr. red rubber catheter. When the ureters are mobilized, as much length as possible should be preserved. It is also important to leave all the attached periureteral adventitia in place to minimize devascularization.

A suitable segment of colon is then selected with its blood supply, usually the proximal sigmoid. However, other segments may be chosen if the ureteral length is insufficient or if that section of bowel is in an irradiated field. The isolated colon has a tendency to shorten or go into "spasm." Therefore, it is advised that a longer segment be used, which may be trimmed later at the time of stoma formation.

When the conduit is isolated, the splenic, hepatic, or both colonic flexures need to be mobilized to assure that the end-to-end anastomosis of the remaining large bowel is without tension. A two layer interrupted 3-0 silk suture anastomosis is preferred to reestablish bowel continuity.

The conduit is fashioned for isoperistalsis. The proximal (base) end is closed with two running, inverting layers of 3-0 chromic catgut suture in the technique described as the Parker-Kerr stitch. The third layer is of interrupted 3-0 silk (Lembert) sutures.

Nonabsorbable or metal autosutures are not used because mucosal migration can cause calculus formation within the loop. The mesentery of the conduit should be mobile enough to allow for a clockwise, 180-degree rotation, as it is fixed to the retroperitoneum near the aortic bifurcation (Fig. 55–2). Rotation of the mesentery is not necessary if the conduit is based in the gutter, lateral to the ascending or descending colon. Mesenteric rotation is also not needed if the conduit is affixed higher in the midline above the aortic bifurcation.

Once the base of the loop is attached to the retroperitoneum, attention is focused on the creation of antirefluxing ureteral tunnels. The ratio of tunnel length to ureteral diameter should be about 4 or 5 to 1. The tunnel is created by infiltrating the seromuscular layer of the tenia with saline by way of a 25-gauge needle attached to a small syringe. The underlying mucosa should not be violated. The dissection is performed with a No. 15 surgical blade attached to a long, thin knife handle. Blunt dissection may be carried out employing the flat end of the knife handle or peanut gauze. In elevating this flap, the medial aspect of the seromuscular layer needs to be carefully mobilized lest the blood supply be disturbed. The end of the ureter is cut straight across, not spatulated. The ureter is then anastomosed end to side to the colonic mucosa at the distal end of the tunnel. The sutures are of 5-0 chromic catgut, interrupted, with knots on the inside

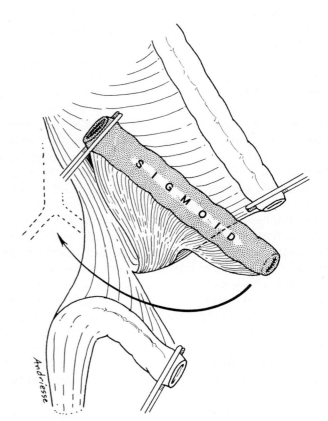

Figure 55–2. Rotation of the sigmoid conduit.

when possible. Meticulous technique must be used in handling the ureter so that a watertight anastomosis can be assured. The ureters are stented with a soft plastic feeding tube, 5 or 8 Fr., if previous obstruction was present or ureteral tapering was performed. The stents are left in place until the tenth postoperative day. With normal ureters, stents are not used.

The raised flap of the tenia is then reapproximated over the ureter with colored, 5-0 interrupted nonabsorbable sutures. This allows the surgeon to identify the ureteral tunnels if further surgery becomes necessary at another time. It is important to avoid angulation of the ureter as it enters the distal tunnel. If any doubt exists, a small transverse releasing incision can be made in the seromuscular flap.

The technique for constructing a nonrefluxing colon conduit is shown in Figure 55–3.

When a nonrefluxing colon conduit is not possible owing to greatly foreshortened ureters or when reflux is not a consideration in planning a urinary diversion, the ureters may be anastomosed to the colon in the standard ileal loop fashion (Fig. 55–4). In the 1960s Mogg and Syme paid little attention to antirefluxing anastomoses when they directed their efforts toward the isolated sigmoid conduit.[5]

The colon loop stoma is placed at the predetermined location. When this placement is not possible, it should be put below the beltline in either lower abdominal quadrant, but not as low as McBurney's point. In a patient with a previous stoma, it is best to place the new one at the old site unless urinary leakage or some other problem occurs. In a new case, a 3- to 4-cm circular incision is made into the skin and subcutaneous tissue. This skin plus tissue is then excised, and the anterior rectus fascia is cut into the shape of a Maltese cross. The rectus muscle is split along its fibers and the peritoneum is entered below it. Two fingers are then placed into the new stoma site and the fascia is further incised if an obstructing "shelf" exists. The conduit is pulled through the opening and secured to the fascial layers with 2-0 interrupted chromic catgut sutures placed in four quadrants. The colored sutures that were used to close the tenia are identified to make sure there is no chance that the ureteral anastomosis is caught above the posterior fascia. The colon loop is sutured again in four quadrants to subcutaneous tissue in such a way that an everting nipple is formed. The stoma is then matured to the skin with multiple 4-0 interrupted, chromic catgut sutures. It is usually placed 3 cm above the skin line, because about a 30 percent stomal shrinkage occurs 6 weeks after surgery. A stoma that is flush with the skin may cause surrounding dermatitis if the skin is constantly bathed with urine.

Figure 55–5 shows the technique of stoma construction.

STAGED URETEROCOLOCOLOSTOMY URINARY DIVERSION

Occasionally a patient who has undergone an antirefluxing colon conduit becomes a candidate for rediversion of the urine into the colon. This procedure is possible when the patient is young and has good anal sphincter tone. The staged ureterocolocolostomy has been successful in cases of bladder exstrophy and should be considered as an alternative in some adults in whom a primary ureterosigmoidostomy might normally be the procedure of choice.[6]

Obstruction and active upper tract infection have been contraindications to ureterosigmoidostomy. The incidence of pyelonephritis and hydronephrosis is decreased by isolating the ureterocolic anastomosis from the fecal stream. The construction of an antirefluxing colon conduit accomplishes these goals. Before the colocolostomy, the conduit is evaluated for the absence of reflux. The intravenous urogram should show no obstruction. Sterile urine and optimal renal function are necessary. Preoperative fecal continence and good anal sphincter tone are predictors of postcolocolostomy continence. However, an oatmeal retention enema is very helpful in stimulating the admixture of urine and stool.

The large bowel preparation is that used for the colon conduit. The loop is taken down and the distal 5 cm discarded once the distal limits of the ureteral tunnels have been identified. The conduit is then approximated to the rectosigmoid with a two-layer end-to-side anastomosis. A rectal tube is left in place for 7 to 10 days. The patient should wait at least 6 months before undergoing a colocolostomy. This is usually how long it takes to clear an active infection and to stabilize the upper tracts and renal function. Hypochloremic acidosis has not been a factor postoperatively. However, patients with marginal renal function need to avoid a high ash diet to decrease chloride intake and to evacuate the rectum every 2 to 4 hours. Carcinoma of the ureterocolic anastomosis has not yet been reported because the ureteral stumps are out of the fecal stream.

POSTOPERATIVE MANAGEMENT AND COMPLICATIONS

The colon conduit is usually not drained. However, if the surgery is associated with pelvic exenteration, ureteral tapering, or extensive dissection in an irradiated field, a half-inch Penrose drain is put at the base of the loop and brought out through a separate stab incision in the quadrant opposite from the stoma site. A suction drain may promote a urinary fistula. The Penrose drain is removed after the drainage has stopped and provided that the intravenous pyelo-

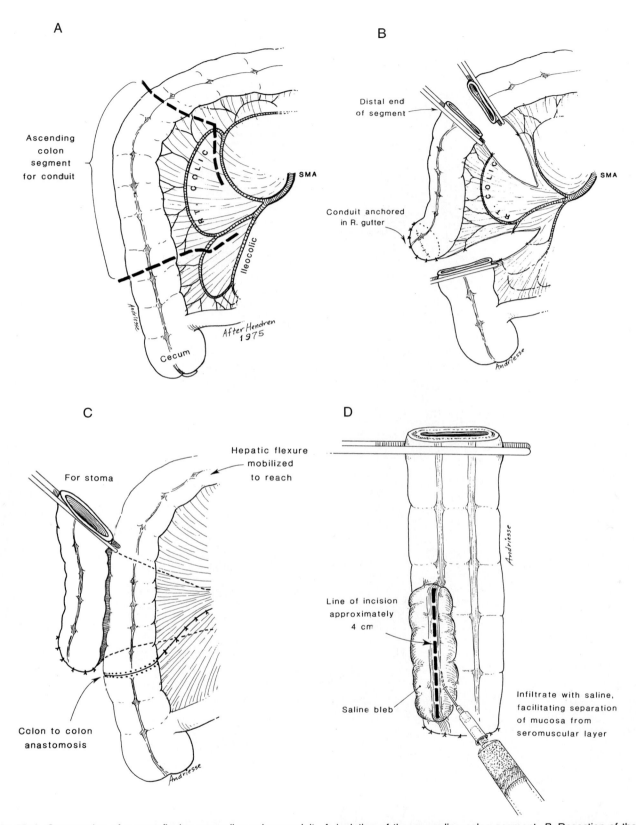

Figure 55–3. Construction of a nonrefluxing ascending colon conduit. *A*, Isolation of the ascending colon segment. *B*, Resection of the loop and fixation of the conduit base to the retroperitoneal gutter. *C*, Colonic reconstitution. *D*, Antirefluxing tunnel. *E*, Preparation of the tunnel flap. *F* and *G*, Ureterocolonic anastomosis. *H*, Completed antirefluxing conduit.

Illustration continued on following page

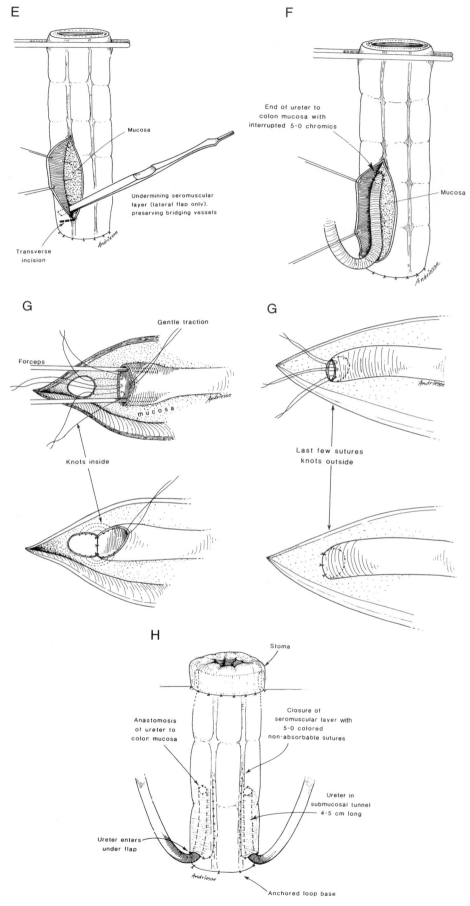

E

Mucosa

Undermining seromuscular
layer (lateral flap only),
preserving bridging vessels

Transverse
incision

Andriesse

F

End of ureter to
colon mucosa with
interrupted 5-0 chromics

Mucosa

Andriesse

G

Gentle traction

Forceps

mucosa

Knots inside

Andriesse

G

Last few sutures
knots outside

Andriesse

H

Stoma

Anastomosis
of ureter to
colon mucosa

Closure of
seromuscular layer with
5-0 colored
non-absorbable sutures

Ureter in
submucosal tunnel
4-5 cm long

Ureter enters
under flap

Anchored loop base

Andriesse

Figure 55–3 *Continued*

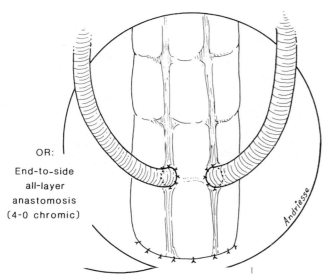

Figure 55–4. Refluxing of the uretercolonic anastomosis.

gram, 1 week postoperatively, shows no ureteral leakage. If the continuity of the intestinal anastomosis is suspect, the drain remains until the bowels begin to function normally. If ureteral stents are employed, they remain in place for at least 1 week. Stentograms should show intact anastomoses before the catheters are removed.

Non-nephrotoxic antibiotics are provided for the first 10 to 14 days and then prophylactically, with one fourth the normal dose, on a daily basis for the next 2 months. Sodium bicarbonate is given orally if hypochloremic acidosis becomes a problem in a patient with suboptimal renal function.

Althausen and colleagues reported an 8-year experience with 70 nonrefluxing colon conduit urinary diversions.[2] The mean follow-up was 3 years after diversion; 30 of these cases were in adults. Most patients (42) had preexisting urinary diversions, 36 of which were ileal loops. All the patients previously diverted showed deterioration of the upper tracts, persistent bacilluria while on medication, recurrent clinical pyelonephritis, and worsening of renal function.

The short-term follow-up revealed only five patients (7 percent) with clinical pyelonephritis. Pyelonephritis in ileal loop patients is reported to be as high as 22 percent. Of the 34 patients with consistently positive urine culture findings preoperatively, 7.8 percent remained positive. No patient with sterile urine before colon conduit surgery became infected.

The incidence of stomal stenoses in ileal loops has approached 55 percent. No children in the series of Althausen and colleagues had this problem; it was seen in only two adults, in whom vascular compromise was noted intraoperatively. Because of its bulk and vascular supply, the stoma develops less encrustation and less chance of fibrosis.

Chronic vesicorenal reflux may cause deterioration

of renal function.[7] Long-term experience with ileal loop urinary diversion has revealed deterioration of previously normal upper tracts as high as 68 percent. It is assumed that reflux and chronic bacilluria contribute to this problem. These patients have not been followed long enough to determine upper tract preservation. However, in this series only seven ureters persistently refluxed on loopograms.

Hyperchloremic acidosis occurred in one child and renal calculi in two adults. There were six ureterocolic anastomoses that became stenotic, two of which were tapered ureters. The other four were obstructed as a result of angulation at the proximal end of the tunnel where the ureter entered the colon.

No deaths were reported in these patients. Colon surgery is usually more hazardous than small bowel surgery. However, the surgical complication rate in this series compares favorably with that of ileal loops. Antirefluxing colon conduits have reduced the incidence of stomal stenosis, pyelonephritis, and probable renal damage. Meticulous attention to detail makes this a safe procedure in the patient who needs supravesical urinary diversion.

Editorial Comment
Fray F. Marshall

A place still exists for colon conduit urinary diversion. If any major complication, infection, radiation, or fistula has occurred in the pelvis and a urinary diversion is required, a colon conduit is frequently one of the better choices. An extensive dissection can be avoided in the pelvis and a very difficult operation can become less difficult.

In another situation, when a total exenteration is per-

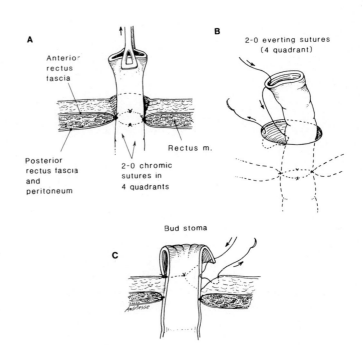

Figure 55–5. *A* to *C,* Construction of a stoma.

formed and the bowel is already divided, it makes good sense to use the distal portion of the colon as a form of urinary diversion so that another anastomosis is avoided.

REFERENCES

1. Middleton AW Jr, Hendren WH. Ileal conduits in children at the Massachusetts General Hospital from 1955 to 1970. J Urol 115:591, 1976.

2. Althausen AF, Hagen-Cook K, Hendren WH. Nonrefluxing colon conduit: Experience with 70 cases. J Urol 120:35, 1978.
3. Hagen-Cook K, Althausen AF. Early observations on 31 adults with nonrefluxing colon conduits. J Urol 121:13, 1979.
4. Hendren WH. Nonrefluxing colon conduit for temporary or permanent urinary diversion in children. J Pediatr Surg 10:381, 1975.
5. Mogg RA, Syme RR. The results of urinary diversion using the colon conduit. Br J Urol 41:434, 1969.
6. Nieh PT, Althausen AF, Dretler SP. Staged ureterocolostomy urinary diversion. J Urol 120:402, 1978.
7. Richie JP, Skinner DG. Urinary diversion: The physiological rational for nonrefluxing colon conduits. Br J Urol 47:269, 1975.

Chapter 56

Mitrofanoff Principle in Continent Reconstruction of the Lower Urinary Tract

Howard M. Snyder III and John W. Duckett

The last 25 years and especially the last 10 years have seen a burgeoning of techniques for the continent reconstruction of the lower urinary tract.[1, 2] Success is currently a result of much improved understanding of the physiology required for continent reconstruction. It is not the purpose of this chapter to review the techniques for the construction of an adequate low-pressure reservoir. A detubularized intestinal segment may be used successfully to either augment or totally replace an inadequate or absent bladder. The greatest challenge in continent reconstruction lies in the selection of a method for construction of a continence mechanism. Clean intermittent catheterization, as introduced by Lapides and coworkers,[3] has permitted attention to be focused on the creation of a continence mechanism that does not require spontaneous voiding and has been the real secret to the success of current continent reconstruction.

A brief review of the physiology of the types of continence mechanisms that have been used permits a better understanding of the development of the Mitrofanoff principle. A continence mechanism dependent purely on *hydraulic resistance* is typified by the Young-Dees-Leadbetter type of detrusor tubularization.[4–6] The resistance to leakage is provided by lengthening and narrowing, which cause an increased resistance to flow based on a simple hydraulic principle:

$$\text{Resistance} \propto \frac{\text{Length}}{\text{Diameter} \times \text{Tension in wall}}$$

The disadvantage of a hydraulic resistance lies in the fact that it does not increase with rising pressure within the bladder or urinary reservoir. Accordingly, once the threshold resistance to flow is overcome within the hydraulic channel, leakage will occur. While this effect can be a disadvantage, it may also be an advantage in that it provides a "pop-off" mechanism, which may avoid excessively high pressure within the reservoir that could be potentially dangerous and cause reservoir rupture. One of the most popular and successful current operations employing a hydraulic resistance is the Indiana continent urinary reservoir (Fig. 56–1).[7] The simplicity of a tapered ileal segment in continuity with the cecum as a detubularized reservoir provides an uncomplicated

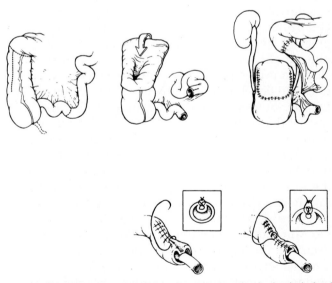

Figure 56–1. Indiana continent urinary reservoir. A detubularized (Heineke-Mikulicz reconfiguration) of the ascending and right transverse colon with continence dependent on hydraulic resistance from plicated terminal ileum. (From Rowland RG, Mitchell ME, Bihrle R, et al. J Urol 137:1136, 1987.)

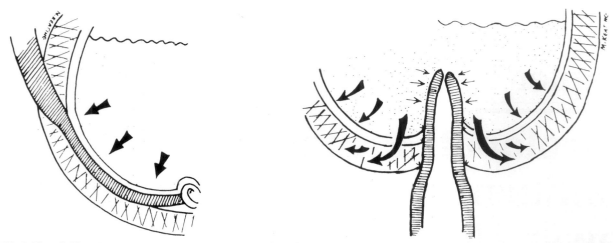

Figure 56–2. Flap *(left)* and nipple *(right)* valves. A nipple valve produces continence by intrareservoir pressure, which compresses the nipple. Unfortunately, this same pressure has a laterally distractive force at the base of the nipple, causing gradual effacement of the nipple and thus loss of continence. A flap valve results in continence by having the catheterizable tube supported in a *fixed* position on the inner wall of the reservoir, which is similar to a reimplanted ureter.

and rapidly constructed mechanism, which may lend itself particularly well to adults who are undergoing total cystectomy for cancer.

Nipple valves as continence mechanisms depend on pressure from within the reservoir to compress the nipple, thus preventing leakage (Fig. 56–2). The drawback of nipple valves is that these same compressive forces within the reservoir also generate laterally distractive forces at the base of the nipple that tend to lead to eventual flattening and eversion of the nipple, with loss of the continence mechanism.

One of the earliest repairs dependent on a nipple valve was the Gilchrist-Merrick procedure (Fig. 56–3).[8] Subsequently, multiple efforts were made to stabilize the nipple valve by further intussusception of the ileal segment into the cecum[9] or by formation of a wrap of the cecum around the terminal ileum.[10] Unfortunately, all efforts at nipple stabilization were plagued by loss of an effective valve in 30 to 50 percent of cases.[11, 12]

These problems led King and associates[11] and Hendren[13] to develop independently the technique of fixing the intussuscepted ileal nipple against the inner wall of the cecum (Fig. 56–4). This stabilization technique finally produced a high rate of preservation of a nonrefluxing valve mechanism. However, this modification of the nipple valve in essence changed the physiology of the continence mechanism from a nipple valve into a flap valve (see Fig. 56–2).

A *flap valve* mechanism for continence underlies the Mitrofanoff principle. An effective flap valve reflects the physiological principle one is achieving in a successful ureteral reimplantation into a normal bladder. A small-diameter supple tube (the ureter) is placed on the inner wall of the bladder with a relatively high length-to-diameter ratio. Filling of the bladder compresses the ureter and effectively pre-

vents reflux. The same flap valve can be employed in the creation of a continence mechanism to prevent leakage from a catheterizable tube. A flap valve is highly effective in avoiding reflux or leakage.[14] As pressure in the bladder or continent urinary reservoir rises, greater compression of the flap valve mechanism occurs, resulting in greater resistance to leakage.

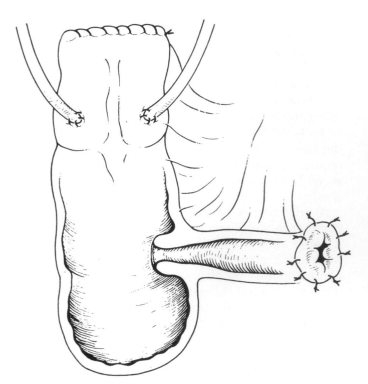

Figure 56–3. Gilchrist-Merrick operation. The ureters were anastomosed to the cecum, and the proximal ileum was brought to the skin as a continent catheterizable stoma. No effort was made to reinforce the natural nipple valve at the ileocecal valve, and the reservoir was not detubularized. (From Ashken MH. Urinary reservoirs. In Ashken MH, ed. Urinary Diversion. New York, Springer-Verlag, 1982, p 116.)

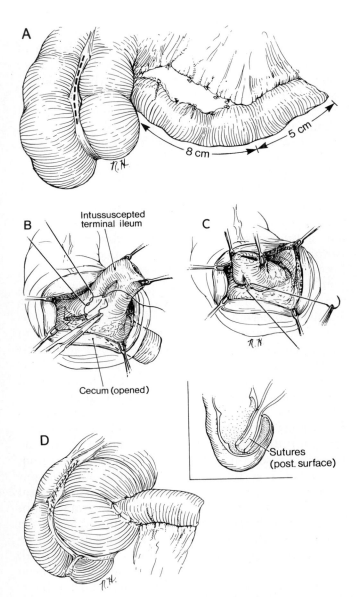

Figure 56–4. Conversion of an ileocecal nipple valve into a stable flap valve. Ileocecal intussusception with fixation of the nipple to the side wall of the cecum converts it into a stable flap valve. (From King LR, Robertson CN, Bertram RA. World J Urol 3:195, 1985.)

The fixed nature of a flap valve prevents loss of continence with increased filling and pressure.

Although a flap valve is a highly effective continence mechanism, it does carry one important drawback. The patient is completely dependent on intermittent catheterization of the reservoir. If this is not carried out in a timely fashion, sufficiently high pressures may be generated within the reservoir to lead to rupture. Thus, flap valve mechanisms for continent reconstructions lead to very successful outcomes but require meticulous patient compliance for safety.

THE MITROFANOFF PRINCIPLE

The development of the Mitrofanoff principle for continent lower urinary tract reconstruction followed the recognition by Mitrofanoff[15] that either the appendix or the ureter, when implanted on the inner wall of the bladder or urinary reservoir, creates a highly effective flap valve continence mechanism (Fig. 56–5). The Mitrofanoff principle involves using a small-diameter supple tube implanted on the inner wall of a reservoir to create a continent catheterizable channel dependent on a flap valve mechanism. The importance of a well-supported, small-diameter, supple tube in providing a successful flap valve mechanism was stressed. The ureter or appendix was ideal. The small-diameter tube was not only effective in helping to create an adequate length-to-diameter ratio but also facilitated catheterization, as the smaller lumen avoided problems with kinking and curling of the catheter. The classic approach of Mitrofanoff with either the appendix or ureter has been employed extensively at The Children's Hospital of Philadelphia.[16, 17] The technique has also been very successfully applied in many different medical centers.[18, 19] In our personal experience with more than 75 cases, the only failure has been with a boy early in our

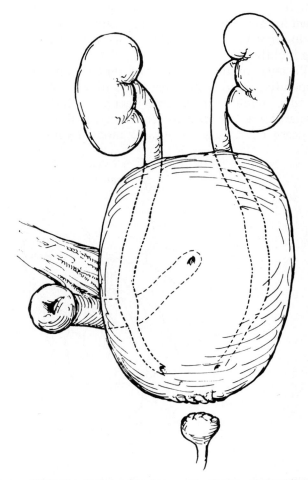

Figure 56–5. Appendicovesicostomy with closure of the bladder neck—Mitrofanoff. The submucosal course of the appendix creates a stable flap valve and thus a continent catheterization channel. The small diameter of the appendix facilitates catheterization. (From Duckett JW, Snyder HM. World J Urol 3:191, 1985.)

experience who developed necrosis of the appendix after overdissection.

APPENDICOVESICOSTOMY: TECHNICAL POINTS

Although one is naturally concerned that the appendix might not be a suitable catheterizable channel, making it important to have an alternative technique in mind whenever one does an appendicovesicostomy, we have yet to find an appendix that was not suitable. It is important to recognize that the appendicular artery represents the terminal branch of the superior mesenteric artery (Fig. 56–6). Accordingly, mobilization of the root of the mesentery, as one would carry out in starting a retroperitoneal node dissection, permits the cecum and appendix to be moved to almost any desired location within the abdomen. This maneuver permits the stoma of an appendicovesicostomy to be placed where it would be maximally convenient for the patient to catheterize. Placement within the umbilicus is cosmetically very satisfactory and has the advantage of obviating the need for much length of an appendix to bridge a thick abdominal wall, as the skin is fixed to the fascia at the umbilicus.

Because of the mobility of the cecum with the appendix, there is no great need to separate the appendix widely from the cecum, which avoids jeopardizing the appendiceal artery. If the appendix appears short, the intramural blood supply of the

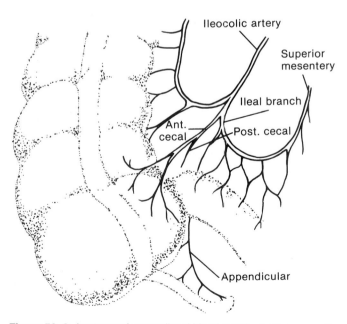

Figure 56–6. Anatomy of appendiceal blood supply. As the appendicular artery is at the terminal end of the superior mesenteric artery, the appendix and cecum can be moved widely by mobilizing the root of the mesentery. The appendix need not be widely separated from the cecum, and thus the appendicular artery is protected.

cecum permits a cuff of cecum to be taken with the appendix for tubularization to extend the length of the appendix. This maneuver is what we should have done in the early case mentioned in which overdissection led us to lose an appendix. With the exception of this case, however, we have not found cecal tubularization necessary. A fecalith does not preclude the utilization of an appendix; it can usually simply be milked out of the appendix.

The technical construction of the appendicovesicostomy is straightforward. The site for a stoma should be determined by considering convenience to the patient or by using a cosmetically favored site, such as the umbilicus or just above the pubic hair line to permit concealment. A small U-shaped skin flap is formed to interdigitate with the small cecal cuff taken with the appendix. The fascial opening below the skin stoma is fashioned generously, usually being made adequate to permit passage of an index finger. This is important to avoid constriction of the blood supply to the appendix and to avoid any kinking or angulation of the appendix as it traverses the fascia.

The bladder or intestinal reservoir is fixed with extramucosal nonabsorbable sutures immediately adjacent to the site of the stoma. This is important to avoid angulation that could make subsequent catheterization difficult. A submucosal tunnel within the intestinal reservoir or bladder can be fashioned from the outside, as in the technique of a Lich-Gregoir ureteral reimplant.[20] Alternatively, the submucosal course for the appendix can be created from within the reservoir by simple submucosal tunneling. If the mucosa is difficult to raise, a mucosal trough into which the appendix may be fixed can be created. Once the proposed course for the appendix has been constructed, it is placed into position and the interdigitating incision made in the small cecal cuff.

The anastomosis to the skin is carried out first with carefully placed interrupted sutures of polyglycolic or polyglactin acid. The advantage of completing the skin stoma first is that subsequently by traction on the appendix, the skin stoma will be displaced below the level of the skin, creating a more cosmetically attractive stoma. The appendix is gently drawn into its position supported on the inner wall of the reservoir, and its tip is amputated. The submucosal tunnel must be generous to avoid constriction of the appendiceal blood supply. If a mucosal trough technique is to be used, the appendix is fixed to the back wall of the trough to preserve good fixation. The appendix is kept on gentle traction as the distal end is anchored to the detrusor or intestinal reservoir with polyglycolic or polyglactin acid sutures. The object is to keep the appendix straight for ease in subsequent catheterization. The intrareservoir end of the appendix is matured with interrupted chromic sutures, taking care to avoid leaving any form of a lip at the junction of the appendix with the bladder or reservoir, which might catch a catheter.

It is important to practice catheterization of the appendix with the type of tube to be subsequently used for emptying. If any difficulty with catheterization is encountered, this is the time for correction to avoid problems later. If an existing bladder is to be utilized and augmented, we usually construct the appendicovesicostomy first and, as a last step, carry out the intestinal augmentation.

A word must be added about possible closure of the bladder neck. We do not favor surgically closing the bladder outlet unless all else fails to make the bladder outlet competent. Maintaining a patent urethra gives simple access to the bladder for cystoscopy and may provide a pressure pop-off mechanism, if the bladder is not emptied on time by intermittent catheterization. We would choose a fascial sling or Young-Dees-Leadbetter type of tubularization to increase the hydraulic resistance to urethral leakage before considering bladder neck closure. If bladder neck closure is needed, the best way to achieve it is by direct surgical division of the urethra at the bladder neck. This maneuver is done simply, even in previously operated on patients, by opening the bladder and identifying the proper plane for surgery, keeping a finger at the bladder neck as division of the urethra is carried out. Separation of the bladder from the urethra permits a secure layered closure. We and others have had difficulty with the technique advocated by Schneider and colleagues,[21] probably because it is actually quite difficult to completely remove the mucosa from the bladder neck before closure by serial pursestring sutures.

Postoperative adequate drainage is important. Often the patient undergoing such a reconstruction has spina bifida with a ventriculoperitoneal shunt. In such a situation, intraperitoneal postoperative drains should be of the closed type (Jackson-Pratt) and should be removed as early as possible (48 hours). In this situation, effective diversion of the urine helps to avoid problems. We routinely employ ureteral intubation with small feeding tubes. When there is no ventriculoperitoneal shunt and the ureters have not required reimplantation, ureteral stents may be omitted. A large-diameter (20 to 22 Fr.) Malecot suprapubic tube is placed, bringing it out through the bladder if possible, because leakage from the site of the suprapubic tube resolves most quickly if a bladder exit is selected. A small polyethylene feeding tube is left intubating the appendix until clean intermittent catheterization is begun.

POSTOPERATIVE CARE

Postoperative care involves leaving ureteral stents, if they have been used, in place for 5 to 7 days.

A longer period is appropriate if extensive ureteral remodeling has been carried out. Patients are generally discharged with the suprapubic tubes still in position and draining. In patients undergoing intestinal bladder augmentation or replacement, daily mechanical irrigation of the suprapubic tube to remove mucus is carried out. We have found the mechanical irrigation to be more important in removing mucus than the addition of acetylcysteine (Mucomyst) or normal saline, both of which do help render mucus less viscid and thus more easily removed. Three weeks after surgery the patient returns for a cystogram as an outpatient. If this evaluation shows no evidence of extravasation, the patient begins progressive clamping of the suprapubic tube and intermittent catheterization until comfortable with the tube clamped all night and until ease of catheterization has been established. These usually require only a few days. The suprapubic tube is removed also on an outpatient basis.

In the aftercare of an appendicovesicostomy, we emphasize to the patient the importance of generous use of a water-soluble lubricant with catheterization and gentle technique to avoid trauma to the appendix. Although this problem has not been our experience, it is possible for the mucosa of the appendix to be lacerated, leading to inflammation and stricture or obliteration of the appendiceal lumen. We usually start with a 10 or 12 Fr. polyethylene plastic catheter. At times, a coudé-tipped catheter may be useful. Many patients also find that aspiration with a syringe speeds the emptying of the reservoir.

We also emphasize the essential nature of meticulous compliance with frequent and complete reservoir evacuation to avoid the potential for high pressure in the reservoir, which could potentially damage the upper urinary tract or lead to reservoir rupture. Most patients catheterize between 4 and 6 times a day.

Suppressive antibiotics are usually given initially but are discontinued once it has been established that no reflux is occurring into the upper urinary tract. Virtually all patients with continent reconstructions involving intestine and intermittent catheterization experience at least transient asymptomatic bacteriuria. Brief courses of antibiotics are provided if a symptomatic reservoir infection occurs. The treatment is similar to that for uncomplicated cystitis.

Follow-up continues indefinitely with an ultrasound examination every 12 months, in the recognition that stone formation in such reservoirs is not rare. For reservoir stones, we have been successful in about half the cases in achieving complete dissolution through hemirenacidin (Renacidin). We discharge no patients who have had continent reconstructions, emphasizing to them that the ultimate long-term consequences of these reconstructions remain to be defined.

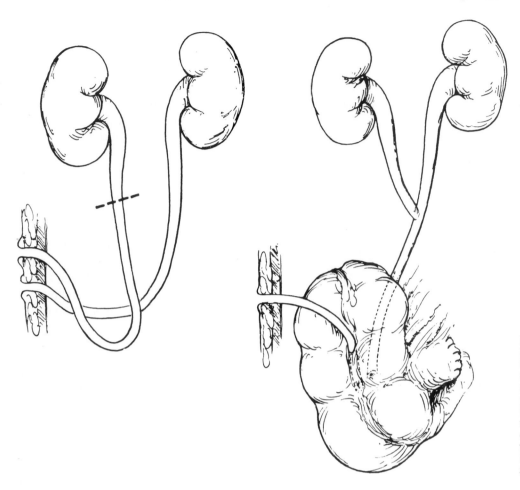

Figure 56–7. Continent catheterizable ureterostomy—Mitrofanoff. When there are two end-cutaneous ureterostomies, one distal ureter can be supported by its stomal blood supply, permitting the construction of a submucosal catheterizable continent flap valve attachment to an intestinal reservoir. A high transureteroureterostomy completes the repair. (From Duckett JW, Snyder HM. World J Urol 3:191, 1985.)

CATHETERIZABLE SKIN URETEROSTOMY

The ureter has been successfully utilized following the Mitrofanoff principle in two clinical situations. If the bladder has been removed and an end-cutaneous ureterostomy created, the distal ureter will obtain a supportive blood supply through its cutaneous anastomosis. Ashcraft and Dennis[22] showed experimentally in the dog that this effect may take place over as short a period as 6 weeks. The skin's blood supply to the distal ureter permits division of the ureter and preservation of the distal ureter as a continent catheterizable channel implanted with a submucosal tunnel into a continent reservoir (Fig. 56–7). A high transureteroureterostomy to the opposite ureter, which has its distal end implanted submucosally in the continent reservoir, completes the reconstruction. Gentle handling of the ureter is stressed to avoid injuring its intrinsic blood supply. The ureter from the upper tracts implanted into the reservoir and its joining transureteroureterostomy are usually diverted with internal ureteral stents until contrast studies show good healing, no extravasation, and free drainage.

The other clinical scenario in which the distal ureter is employed for a continent catheterizable channel arises when the ureter remains in contact with the bladder or a bladder remnant (Fig. 56–8). Here, the distal blood supply is from the trigone and must be carefully preserved. Accordingly, if the antireflux mechanism must be augmented, techniques that do not disturb the anastomosis of the ureter with the trigone are utilized. The submucosal tunnel may be extended by the use of the Lich-Gregoir technique,[20] the Hutch reimplant,[23] or the Gil-Vernet technique.[24]

As with the appendicovesicostomy, the catheterizable ureterostomy is left intubated after surgery until it is time to begin intermittent emptying by this route. Usually, a 6 or 8 Fr. feeding tube is left indwelling and catheterization begun with an 8 Fr. catheter. It is generally possible to use a 10 or 12 Fr. catheter for intermittent catheterization of the ureter within a few months after surgery. The technical points during catheterization and during follow-up are the same as those emphasized for an appendicovesicostomy.

ALTERNATIVE RECONSTRUCTIONS UTILIZING THE MITROFANOFF PRINCIPLE

Although the appendicovesicostomy followed by the catheterizable ureterostomy has been most com-

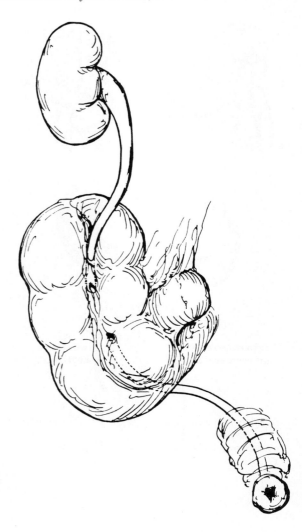

Figure 56–8. Continent catheterizable ureterostomy—Mitrofanoff. In a cloacal exstrophy variant, a solitary ureter was divided to provide two flap valve attachments to an intestinal reservoir. The distal segment maintained its blood supply from the small bladder remnant. (From Duckett JW, Snyder HM. World J Urol 3:191, 1985.)

monly used to apply the Mitrofanoff principle, the application of this principle is really limited only by the imagination of the reconstructive urological surgeon. A few examples will serve to illustrate this important point.

An appendicocecostomy (Penn pouch) utilizing the appendix with the cecal end brought to the skin has been successful at The Children's Hospital of Philadelphia (Fig. 56–9). An appendicocecostomy has also been used to bring the distal end to the skin and to implant the appendix into the cecum using a Lich-Gregoir technique (Fig. 56–10).[25, 26] It does not appear to matter whether the appendix is placed in an isoperistaltic or antiperistaltic submucosal course.

At The Children's Hospital of Philadelphia, we have tapered an existing ileal conduit and placed it as a catheterizable channel with a flap valve mechanism supported on the inner wall of an intestinal reservoir, as has Lobe.[27]

Hanna[28] intussuscepted a segment of the ileum and fixed it against the wall of the ileum to create what he calls a hemi-Kock pouch (Fig. 56–11). This pouch has been employed to create a continent catheteriz-

able stoma at the umbilicus and to bridge a gap between the upper urinary tract and bladder when the ureters are too short. Both Kock and Skinner and their colleagues[29, 30] have changed the physiology of the Kock continent catheterizable nipple into a flap valve mechanism by opening the mucosa on one side of the nipple, as well as the opposing side of the reservoir, fixing the nipple down to change it into a flap valve (Fig. 56–12).

The Kropp procedure[31] uses a small-caliber detrusor tube that maintains its blood supply from the bladder neck as a catheterizable continence mechanism implanted with a flap valve submucosal tunnel in the bladder (Fig. 56–13). Although some difficulties with catheterization have occurred, the continence mechanism has been highly successful.

Lobe and co-workers[32] took a small exstrophic bladder and totally tubularized this bladder into a small-caliber catheterizable tube, implanting it on the inner wall of an intestinal reservoir (Fig. 56–14). This successful reconstruction also follows the Mitrofanoff principle.

In a most innovating approach, Woodhouse[33] used

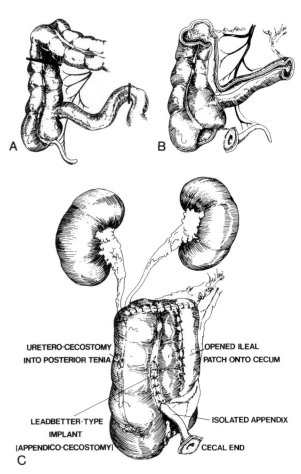

URETERO·CECOSTOMY
INTO POSTERIOR TENIA

OPENED ILEAL
PATCH ONTO CECUM

LEADBETTER·TYPE
IMPLANT
(APPENDICO·CECOSTOMY)

ISOLATED APPENDIX

CECAL END

Figure 56–9. Penn pouch—continent appendicocecostomy. *A,* The ileocecal segment and appendix are isolated, preserving bowel blood supply. *B,* The appendix is separated a short distance from the cecum, preserving the appendicular artery. The opened ileocecal segment is closed together to achieve detubularization and a low-pressure reservoir. *C,* The ureters and appendix are each implanted submucosally into the reservoir with creation of flap valves. The cecal end of the appendix becomes the skin stoma for a continent catheterizable channel. (From Duckett JW, Snyder HM. The Mitrofanoff principle in continent urinary reservoirs. Semin Urol 5:55, 1987.)

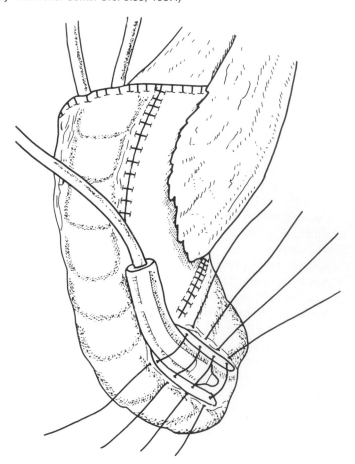

Figure 56–10. Mainz modification of the Penn pouch. The distal appendix is brought to the skin to serve as a catheterizable stoma. A Lich-Gregoire type of reimplant of the proximal appendix into the cecum creates a continent flap valve.

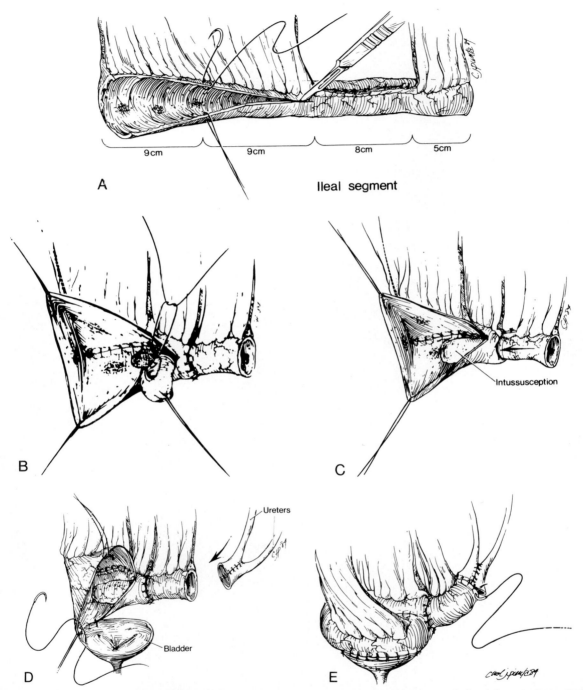

Ileal segment

Figure 56–11. Hemi-Kock pouch. A detubularized ileal pouch with an ileocecal intussuscepted segment is fixed down to the wall of the pouch to create a flap valve. This maneuver can be used to create a continent catheterizable channel or to create a nonrefluxing attachment of short ureters to an augmented bladder. (From Robertson C, King L. Urol Clin North Am 13:337, 1986.)

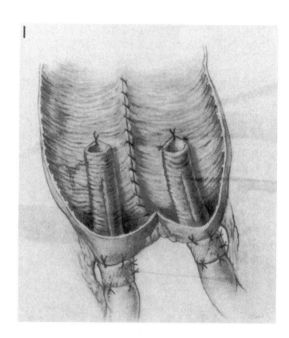

Figure 56–12. Skinner's modified Kock pouch. The nipple valves are fixed down to the inner wall of the reservoir, changing their physiology to that of a stable flap valve. (From Skinner DG, Lieskovsky G, Skinner EC, Boyd SD. Urinary diversion. Curr Probl Surg 24:399, 1987.)

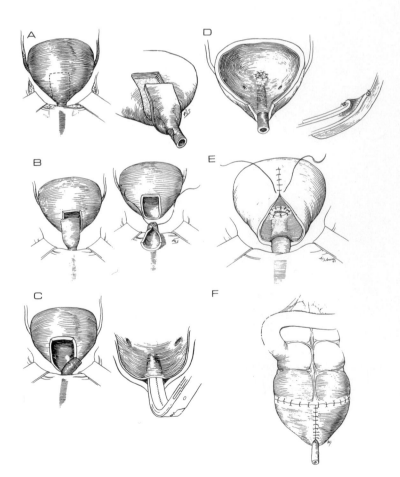

Figure 56–13. Kropp procedure. A detrusor tube based on the blood supply through the bladder neck is created. The anterior is shown; a posterior tube is also possible. The tube is tunneled submucosally in the bladder to create a flap valve mechanism for continent catheterization. (From Kropp KA, Angwafo FF. Urethral lengthening and reimplantation for neurogenic incontinence in children. J Urol 135:534, 1986.)

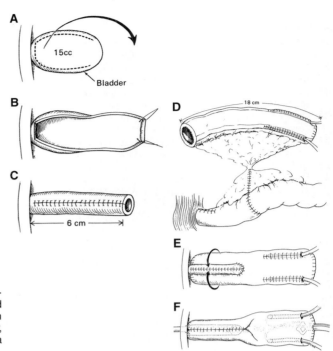

Figure 56–14. Lobe catheterizable bladder tube. *A* to *C,* The small exstrophic bladder is opened and tubularized. *D* to *F,* A detrusor tube is fixed to the wall of the colonic urinary reservoir by the technique of Nissen fundoplication, creating a stable flap valve. (From Lobe TE, Smey P, Anderson GF. A neo-urethral enteroplication for urinary continence in a case of cloacal exstrophy. J Pediatr Surg 20:616, 1985.)

a fallopian tube in a postpubertal woman to successfully create a continent catheterizable channel, utilizing the Mitrofanoff principle of a small-caliber catheterizable tube implanted with a flap valve continence mechanism into a bladder or intestinal reservoir.

These techniques illustrate the underlying, successful physiological elements inherent in the Mitrofanoff principle of continent lower urinary tract reconstruction. They lead us to continue to advocate this approach as a highly satisfactory solution to what has often been a difficult problem.

Editorial Comment

Fray F. Marshall

The Mitrofanoff principle is effective for achieving continence. As the authors point out, however, it can be so effective that bladder rupture may occur if catheterization is not performed. The patient's compliance is most important. The cutaneous "ostomy" can be placed in many different positions, including the umbilicus, which can provide for an excellent cosmetic result. When the ureter is divided and utilized for Mitrofanoff urinary diversion, the blood supply needs to be carefully maintained.

The continence of the Indiana or ileocecal pouch depends primarily on the ileocecal valve, not on the imbrication of the efferent ileal segment. It is probably easier and safer to imbricate the appendix in situ, leaving the blood supply intact, rather than dividing the appendix and reimplanting it. Tapered ileum can be reimplanted into bladder or bowel with a Mitrofanoff technique to provide for continence.

REFERENCES

1. King L, Stone AR, Webster GD, eds. Bladder Reconstruction and Continent Urinary Diversion. Chicago, Year Book, 1987.
2. Snyder HM. Principles of pediatric urinary tract reconstruction—a synthesis. In Gillenwater JY, Grayhack JT, Howards SS, Duckett JW, eds. Adult and Pediatric Urology, vol 2. Chicago, Year Book, 1987, p 1726.
3. Lapides J, Diokno AC, Silber SJ, et al. Clean intermittent self-catheterization in the treatment of urinary tract disease. J Urol 107:458, 1972.
4. Young HH. An operation for the cure of incontinence of urine. Surg Gynecol Obstet 28:84, 1919.
5. Dees JE. Congenital epispadias with incontinence. J Urol 62:513, 1949.
6. Leadbetter GW Jr Surgical correction of total urinary incontinence. J Urol 91:261, 1964.
7. Rowland RG, Bihrle R, Mitchell ME. The Indiana continent urinary reservoir. J Urol 137:1136, 1987.
8. Gilchrist RK, Merrick JW, Hamlin HH, et al. Construction of substitute bladder and urethra. Surg Gynecol Obstet 90:752, 1950.
9. Hendren WH. Reoperative uretera reimplantation: Management of the difficult case. J Pediatr Surg 15:770, 1980.
10. Zinman L, Libertino JA. Right colocystoplasty for bladder replacement. Urol Clin North Am 13:321, 1986.
11. King LR, Robertson CN, Bertram RA. A new technique for the prevention of reflux in those undergoing bladder substitution or undiversion using bowel segments. World J Urol 3:194
12. Mitchell ME, Rink RC. Urinary diversion and undiversion. Urol Clin North Am 12:111, 1985.
13. Hendren WH. Urinary undiversion and augmentation cystoplasty. In King LR, Belman AB, eds. Clinical Pediatric Urology, 2nd ed. Philadelphia, WB Saunders, 1985.
14. Malone PR, D'Cruz VT, Worth PHL, Woodhouse CRJ. Why are continent diversions continent? (abstract no. 536). Dallas, TX, AUA 84th Annual Meeting, May 1989.
15. Mitrofanoff P. Cystostomie continente trans-appendiculaire dans le traitement des vessies neurologiques. Chir Pediatr 21:297, 1980.
16. Duckett JW, Snyder HM. Continent urinary diversion: Variations on the Mitrofanoff principle. J Urol 135:58, 1986.
17. Duckett JW, Snyder HM. Use of the Mitrofanoff principle in urinary reconstruction. World J Urol 3:191, 1986.
18. Mollard P, Jourda R, Valla JS, et al. Colocystoplastie d'agrandissement et de substitution pour vessie neurologique congénitale de l'enfant. Chir Pediatr 24:54, 1983.
19. Monfort G, Guys JM, Lacombe GM. Appendicovesicostomy:

An alternative urinary diversion in the child. Eur Urol 10:361, 1984.

20. Gregoir W. Le traitement chirurgical du reflux vesico-ureteral congenital. Acta Chir Belg 63:431, 1964.

21. Schneider KM, Reid RE, Fruchtman B, et al. Continent vesicostomy: Surgical technique. Urology 6:741, 1975.

22. Ashcraft KW, Dennis PA. The reimplanted ureter as a catheterizing stoma. J Pediatr Surg 21:1042, 1986.

23. Hutch JA. Vesicoureteral reflux in the paraplegic: Cause and correction. J Urol 68:457, 1952.

24. Gil-Vernet JM. A new technique for surgical correction of vesicoureteral reflux. J Urol 131:456, 1984.

25. Gittes RF. Personal communication, 1989.

26. Fisch M, Riedmiller H, Hohenfellner R. Abstract 110, New Trends in Urology. Nijmegen, The Netherlands, Sept. 1989.

27. Lobe TE. Conversion of an ileal conduit into a neourethral entero-plication for urinary continence: Tips in its proper construction. J Pediatr Surg 21:1040, 1986.

28. Hanna MK. Personal communication, 1986.

29. Kock NG, Norlen L, Philipson BM, et al. The continent ileal reservoir (Kock pouch) for urinary diversion. World J Urol 3:146, 1985.

30. Skinner DG, Lieskovsky G, Skinner FC, Boyd SD. Urinary diversion. Curr Probl Surg 24:449, 1987.

31. Kropp KA, Angwafo FF. Urethral lengthening and reimplantation for neurogenic incontinence in children. J Urol 135:533, 1986.

32. Lobe TE, Smey P, Anderson GF. A neourethral enteroplication for urinary continence in a case of cloacal exstrophy. J Pediatr Surg 20:616, 1985.

33. Woodhouse CRJ, Malone PR, Cumming J, et al. The Mitrofanoff principle for continent urinary diversion. Br J Urol 63:53, 1989.

Chapter 57

Kock Pouch Urinary Diversion

Stuart D. Boyd, Eila Skinner, Gary Lieskovsky, and Donald G. Skinner

The aim of any urinary diversion after cystectomy should be to protect the kidneys from significant damage over patients' life span and to enable them to live as normal an existence as possible. There is no question that acceptance of the urinary diversion is a major issue in patients' quality of life. For years the standard urinary diversion in the United States was the ileal conduit, which required the patient to wear an external ostomy bag. In 1982, Kock introduced to the United States the concept of the "ideal" continent bladder substitute via a urinary reservoir that utilized antireflux and continence valves with detubularized ileum.[1] The problem with Kock's ileal reservoir, however, was that it was seemingly complicated to construct and the reoperation rate was extremely high.

Since 1982, our Department of Urology at the University of Southern California has been committed to refining this concept of continent urinary diversion. We have used the ileal reservoir as described by Kock and made a series of technical modifications in the continence and antireflux mechanisms aimed at reducing the incidence of late complications and the need for reoperation. From 1982 to 1994, over 1000 patients underwent various forms of continent urinary diversion and neobladders at our institution. In 711 patients, Kock ileal reservoirs were connected to the skin for continent cutaneous urinary diversion. Since the mid-1980s, on the basis of earlier work by Camey and LeDuc, clinical investigation of orthotopic lower urinary tract reconstruction utilizing neobladders modified from the Kock pouch has been instituted.[2] The neobladder obviates the need for a stoma and usually the need for intermittent catheterization. It has become an attractive alternative in men and more recently women who are undergoing radical cystectomy when the malignancy does not extend into the urethra. From 1986 to 1994, 361 patients (350 men, 11 women) had ileal neobladders anastomosed to the urethra after cystectomy at our institution. In addition, 15 patients had an ileoanal reservoir

diversion to allow voiding through the anus when the urethra is not present. In total, 768 male patients between 15 and 87 years of age and 319 female patients between 13 and 87 years of age underwent some form of Kock pouch diversion. The procedures were most often performed because of primary bladder malignancies but were also used to relieve the symptoms and complications of neurogenic and nonfunctioning bladders, and to convert to a continent diversion from some preexisting form of urinary diversion, usually an ileal conduit.

It is our opinion that some form of continent diversion should now represent the procedure of choice in most cystectomy patients. We believe our data underscore the fact that continent diversion can be accomplished with minimal complications, an excellent functional result, and high patient satisfaction. This concept now appears to be internationally accepted. At the Fourth International Consensus Conference on Bladder Cancer in Antwerp, Belgium, on March 16, 1993, the consensus opinion was that in the properly selected bladder cancer patient, urinary reconstruction to the urethra was the procedure of choice in most centers worldwide. Currently, approximately 90 percent of male patients and 80 percent of female patients requiring cystectomy at the University of Southern California undergo orthotopic lower urinary tract reconstruction. The remaining patients are routinely provided with a continent cutaneous diversion. Rarely is a ileal conduit utilized, mainly in the patient with an uncertain life expectancy or with various physical restrictions.

In summary, experience with these operations has established the following:

1. Continent diversions—whether to the skin, urethra, or rectum—can replace conduit diversions in most instances.

2. Continent diversions are not too difficult to perform or maintain.

3. Detubularized segments of bowel when refash-

465

ioned into reservoirs have improved compliance and have larger capacities than tubular segments.

4. Patients demand to be informed about these types of diversions and about the associated quality of life issues.

PATIENT SELECTION

Any patient who is a candidate for a conduit diversion is potentially suitable for a cutaneous Kock diversion as long as adequate small bowel is available. An in-depth psychological survey of continent Kock and conduit diversion patients conducted in 1987 revealed that there are definite advantages to continent diversions in terms of quality of life issues such as sexuality and interpersonal relations.[3] To benefit from continent diversion, however, the patient should have the intelligence, maturity, and manual dexterity to care for the diversion along with the life expectancy necessary to resume an active life style. Surgical indications for Kock diversion should include primary bladder cancers, radiation failures in cases of prostate or bladder cancer, neurogenic bladders, congenital abnormalities, refractory interstitial cystitis, and dissatisfaction or complication with another form of diversion.

Given the option, most patients would choose not to have a stoma. As noted above, bladder substitution with anastomosis of the reservoir to the urethra is an increasingly popular choice for males and more recently females with bladder cancer. As discussed in more detail below, however, bladder substitutes are typically not feasible in patients without a viable urethra; in men with tumor involving the anterior urethra, with prostatic stromal invasion by tumor, or with carcinoma in situ at the distal prostatic urethral margin; or in women with tumor at the bladder neck.

An alternative for internal diversion is the ileoanal reservoir,[4] which can be used in both men and women and is designed to eliminate the problems associated with ureteral implantation into the intact sigmoid. Experience with the ileoanal reservoir indicates that low pressures and high urinary volumes can be achieved without the urgency, frequency, and nocturnal fecaluria associated with the ureterosigmoidostomy. The antireflux nipple valve can effectively prevent ascending pyelonephritis. This is more complicated surgery, however, often requiring a temporary colostomy, and is not routinely recommended except in younger patients and especially those with a previous ureterosigmoidostomy that requires revision.

PREOPERATIVE EVALUATION

Preoperative bowel preparation is similar to that prescribed for ileal conduit patients.[5] A diet of clear liquids is begun 24 hours before surgery, and oral laxatives such as castor oil (Neoloid) or magnesium citrate are started the morning of the preoperative day. Later that day, oral neomycin and erythromycin base are given in measured doses. If the colon is to be opened, tap water and neomycin enemas are administered. The enterostomal therapist is invaluable in helping to predetermine stoma sites. If an ileal conduit diversion is being converted to a Kock diversion, it is important to examine the ureteral anastomoses radiographically before surgery. If free reflux up the ureters is seen on a loopogram and there is no evidence of ureteral anastomotic obstruction on intravenous pyelography, the base of the old conduit with its implanted ureters may be preserved at surgery to be anastomosed end to end with an appropriately shortened afferent limb of the Kock pouch.

OPERATIVE TECHNIQUE

Cutaneous Kock Diversion

The patient is placed in the hyperextended supine position on the operating table to provide optimal exposure of the pelvis and abdomen. A midline abdominal incision is used, curving to the left of the umbilicus and extending to the epigastrium. We tend to extend the incision up fairly high, as we also routinely use a gastrostomy tube at the end of the procedure. When a cystectomy is required, that portion of the procedure is completed first. If a previous conduit diversion is being converted to a Kock pouch, the small bowel and conduit are first well delineated. The viability of the ureteroileal anastomoses should have already been determined preoperatively, and the lower portion of the conduit with its implanted ureters should be saved if appropriate.

The diversion is begun by measuring out the amount of ileum to be used (Fig. 57–1). In patients without previous diversion, the distal ileal division (efferent end) should be about 20 cm from the cecum in a freely mobile area. This allows a long mesenteric division in the avascular plane between the terminal branch of the superior mesenteric artery and the ileal colic artery. Its division can be made back to the base of the mesentery and affords excellent mobility to the pouch and the efferent limb. In patients with existing ileal conduits, the previous small bowel anastomosis should be identified and excised. The previous mesenteric division should be opened, and the efferent end is begun at this point.

The individual segments of the reservoir are marked with silk sutures: 17 cm for the efferent (distal) limb, 22 cm for each of the two arms of the reservoir, and 17 cm for the afferent (proximal) limb.

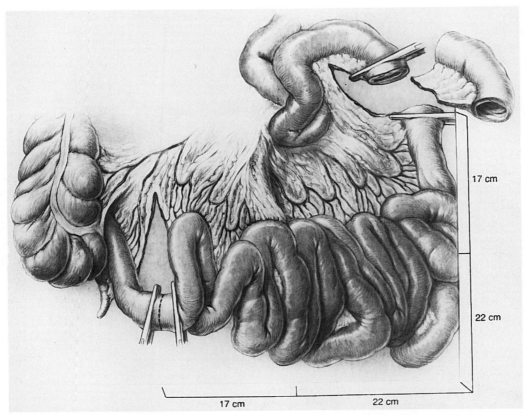

Figure 57–1. The ileum is measured out and resected as demonstrated. The removal of a 5-cm segment of ileum proximal to the afferent end provides improved mobility to the pouch and to the small bowel anastomosis.

About 5 cm of ileum proximal to the afferent end is routinely discarded along with a shallow mesenteric division. This provides improved mobility to the pouch and to the small bowel anastomosis, and because the proximal mesentery division can be quite short, an excellent blood supply to the pouch is ensured. A standard sutured or stapled small bowel anastomosis is performed, depending on the surgeon's preference. The mesenteric trap above the small bowel anastomosis is closed with running absorbable suture. The end of the afferent limb is closed with two-layer running 3-0 polyglycolic acid (PGA) suture. If stapling is used, this end is oversewn with 3-0 PGA suture so that the staple line is definitely excluded from the urine.

The two 22-cm ileal segments for the reservoir are laid out in a U shape directed caudally (Fig. 57–2). These segments may be further apposed with a running 3-0 PGA suture placed in the serosa just above the mesentery on each side; this helps keep the limbs aligned but is not mandatory. The reservoir segments are opened with the cautery knife just lateral to the apposed mesentery (Fig. 57–3). This incision is extended 2 or 3 cm up the afferent and efferent limbs along their antimesenteric border so that when the nipple valves are constructed, they are well separated. The back wall of the reservoir is closed with two-layer running 3-0 PGA suture (Fig. 57–4).

Next, the nipple valves for antireflux and incontinence are constructed. They are created from the afferent and efferent limbs by intussuscepting the bowel. The mesentery beneath the portion of the limbs to be intussuscepted is first divided for about 8 cm along the serosal border of the bowel (Fig. 57–5). This is best accomplished with the cautery knife opening the windows of Deaver and coagulating the individual vessels with forceps. The stripping of the mesentery is important: it allows the ileum to be easily intussuscepted and helps prevent late slippage or "extussusseption" of the valve.

An additional opening in the mesentery is made one vascular arcade beyond the 8-cm opening. A 1-cm strip of PGA mesh is passed through this additional opening to serve as an anchoring collar for the base of the nipple valve. This is most important for the efferent valve. We originally used Marlex for this purpose but discovered that Marlex tended to erode into the pouch over time and was subsequently a source of infection and stone formation.

The nipple valves are intussuscepted by passing two Allis forcep clamps halfway up the open limb to the anchoring collar, grasping the mucosa, and inverting the ileum into the pouch (Fig. 57–6). A valve at least 5 cm long can be created and still leave a lip of pouch at the opening for the reservoir closure. Staples are used to secure the valves. We previously

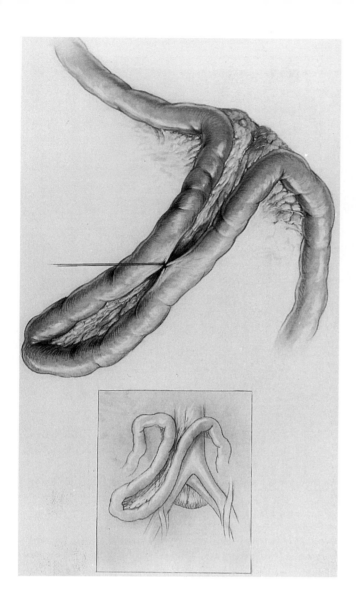

Figure 57–2. The 22-cm limbs of the reservoir are aligned and directed caudally in a U shape.

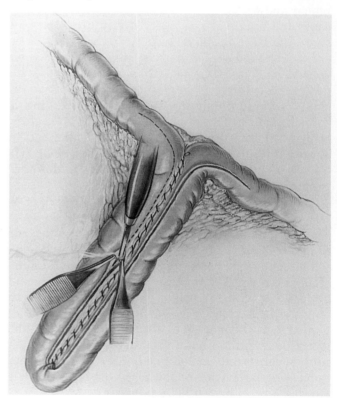

Figure 57–3. The reservoir segments are opened just next to the apposed mesentery. The incisions are extended for 2 to 3 cm up into the afferent and efferent limbs so that the subsequent nipple valves will be well separated.

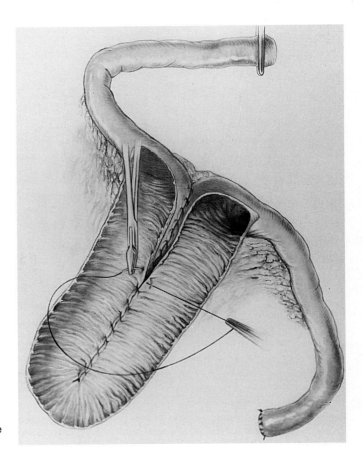

Figure 57–4. The back wall of the reservoir is closed with absorbable 3-0 polyglycolic acid (PGA) suture.

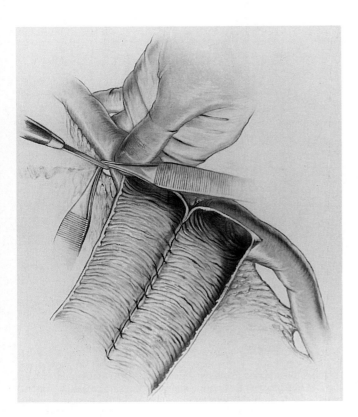

Figure 57–5. The mesentery beneath the portion of the limbs to be intussuscepted is divided for approximately 8 cm along the serosal border of the bowel approximately 1 cm beyond the opening of the limb.

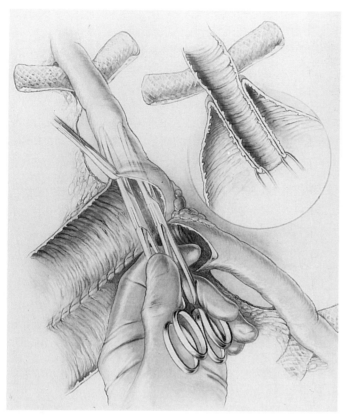

Figure 57–6. A 1-cm strip of PGA mesh is additionally passed through an opening in the mesentery, 1 cm distal to the 8-cm opening as noted in Figure 5.

used a standard TA-55 stapler with 4.8-mm staples to apply three rows of parallel staples. The TA-55 stapler uses a pin, however, and this creates a pinhole that needs to be separately closed with sutures at the base of each staple line. This pinhole has been noted to be an occasional site of a valve fistula. We now use a custom gastrointestinal appliance (GIA) stapler that places a double row of staples without a knife and does not create a pinhole. Two double rows of 3.5-mm staples are used (Fig. 57–7).

Regardless of the stapler used, the full 5.5 cm of the stapler should be used to create a nipple longer than 5 cm. The staple line should be arranged in the anterior half of the valve, leaving the posterior side of the valve free so that another row of staples can subsequently fix the nipple to the back wall of the pouch. The tip of the valve may appear dusky. There may even be some eventual sloughing of the tip, but the overall length of the valve should always be much longer than the needed functional length of 2.5 cm. The staples at the base of the valve are the most important for preventing "extususseption," and these staples tend to get buried in the mucosa. Staples at the tip of the nipples do not contribute to the maintenance of the valve, and could remain exposed and become a site of stone formation. The distal six

staples are therefore removed from the corresponding end of the staple cartridge before stapling.

The fixation of the nipple valve to the back wall of the pouch is important and can easily be accomplished with the stapler, either a TA-55 or GIA. The anvil of the stapler is slipped between the two leaves of the valve, and the valve is stapled to the back wall of the reservoir just next to the mesentery posteriorly (Fig. 57–8). This requires only two layers of tissue in the stapler, one wall of the nipple valve and the wall of the pouch. A standard full-length staple cartridge is used. Additional 3-0 PGA sutures are used to further secure the tip of the valve to the pouch wall (Fig. 57–9). This complete and secure fixation of the nipple valve to the pouch not only prevents long-term valve problems but also increases the efficiency of the antireflux and continence mechanisms as the reservoir fills and stretches.

The PGA mesh collar is anchored to the base of the valves and the ileal limb with solidly placed sutures

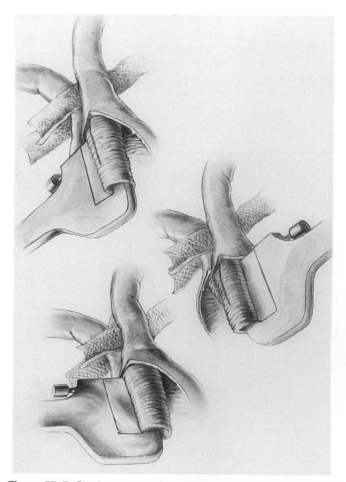

Figure 57–7. Staplers are used to create valves that are at least 5 cm long. We currently no longer utilize staplers with an aligned pin but use a custom gastrointestinal appliance (GIA) stapler that places a double row of staples without a knife and does not create a pinhole. Two double rows of 3.5-mm staples are used. The custom staplers have the distal six staples removed so that the staples do not end up in the tips of the valves.

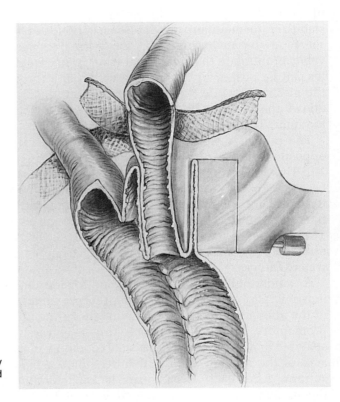

Figure 57–8. The nipple valve is fixed to the back wall of the reservoir by sliding the anvil of the stapler between the two leaves of the valve and outside the reservoir just next to the mesentery posteriorly.

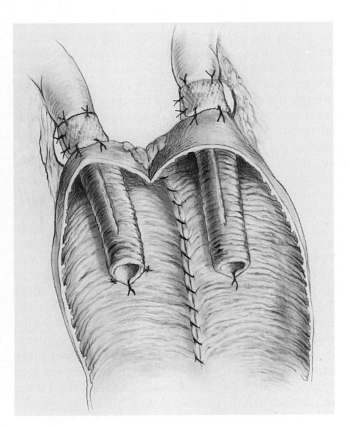

Figure 57–9. The nipple valves are additionally sutured to the back wall of the reservoir with 3-0 PGA suture. The PGA mesh collars are sutured to the base of the nipple valves and to the ileal limbs.

of 3-0 PGA (Fig. 57–9). This collar acts as a further stabilizer to maintain the intussusception and also serves as the anchoring point for fixing the efferent valve and limb to the abdominal wall. A 30 Fr. catheter can be passed up the nipple valves and through the mesh site while the mesh is being sutured. This allows the mesh to be affixed snugly without being too tight. The redundant mesh can be excised.

The pouch is closed by folding the ileum in the opposite direction to which it was opened (Fig. 57–10). This method of opening and closing is important because it causes the motor activities of the different ileal segments of the pouch to counteract themselves, thus creating an extremely low-pressure reservoir. The closure is accomplished with a two-layer running 3-0 PGA suture, meticulously placed to ensure watertightness.

A standard bilateral ureteroileal end-to-side anastomosis is performed after securing the proximal end of the afferent limb to the tissue overlying the sacral promontory (Fig. 57–11). Each ureter is carefully spatuled and anastomosed to a small opening on each side of the afferent limb with interrupted 4-0 PGA sutures. After each anastomosis is half completed, the ureters are routinely stented with 8 Fr. infant feeding tubes perforated with extra holes and passed up the afferent limb and valve. A small opening can be left in the pouch at the time of closure so that these ureteral stents can be secured to the end of the drainage catheter. These stents are removed when the drainage catheter is removed in approximately 3 weeks.

The stoma site is located and a 1.5-cm plug of skin removed. The diameter of the stoma should be smaller than that of a standard ileal stoma. The location for the stoma site can usually be chosen preoper-

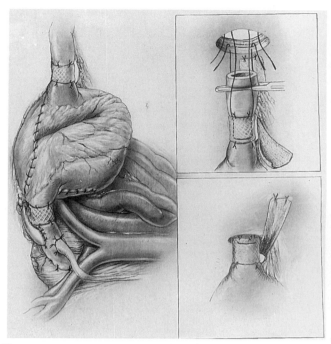

Figure 57–11. The distal end of the afferent limb is secured over the sacral promontory and standard bilateral ureteroileal end-to-side anastomoses are performed. The efferent limb is brought through the stoma site and secured with horizontal mattress sutures of No. 1 PGA to the rectus fascia. An additional 1-cm strip of Marlex mesh is used to secure the mesentery superiorly and prevent herniation.

atively by the enterostomal therapist, but the exact site should be selected after the pouch is created so that the efferent limb can reach this skin as perpendicular to the pouch as possible. This is especially important in an obese patient. The subcutaneous fat is opened directly beneath the stoma, and the anterior rectus fascia is exposed. A vertical incision is made through the rectus fascia, and the muscle and peritoneum are split just widely enough to accommodate the tips of two fingers. Two horizontal mattress sutures of No. 1 PGA are passed through each side of the anterior rectus fascial opening and positioned correspondingly through both sides of the efferent anchoring collar and the base of the valve (Fig. 57–11). Before these sutures are tied, an additional 1-cm strip of Marlex mesh is anchored with a No. 1 nylon suture to the posterior rectus fascia just cephalad and lateral to the abdominal wall opening for the stoma. This Marlex strut is brought through the window of Deaver in the mesentery adjacent to the PGA mesh (Fig. 57–11). An Allis clamp is used to bring the efferent limb carefully through the stomal opening while making certain not to cross the mattress sutures (these should be color coded to avoid confusion). The mattress sutures are securely tied, thus fixing the base of the efferent valve to the rectus fascia. When these sutures are properly placed and tied, the efferent limb should exit the pouch without angulation. An additional suture may be placed into the mesh and

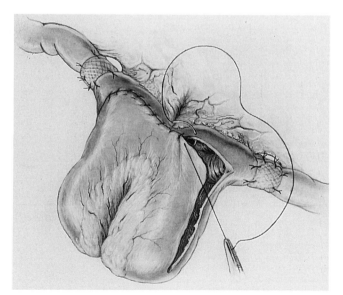

Figure 57–10. The reservoir is closed by folding the ileum in the opposite direction to which it was opened.

the fascial wall if further support is indicated. The Marlex strut is additionally secured to the abdominal wall medial to the mesentery with another 1-0 nylon suture (Fig. 57–11). The Marlex secures the mesentery side of the limb without risk of erosion, and prevents parastomal hernias and concomitant catheterization difficulties. All redundant efferent limb above the skin line is excised. A flush or slightly recessed stoma is completed by suturing the ileum circumferentially to the skin with interrupted 3-0 PGA.

A 30 Fr. Medina catheter should easily pass down the efferent limb and through the nipple valve and be positioned centrally in the pouch. Catheter placement should be performed before the abdominal wall is closed. Alternatively the catheter may be placed through a separate cystotomy incision and passed directly through the abdominal wall into the pouch. This avoids a catheter wearing against the valve during the healing period. The ureteral stents may be fixed to the tip of the catheter at this time and any remaining opening in the pouch closed. The catheter is irrigated to check the watertightness of the suture lines, and secured to the skin with two No. 1 nylon sutures. A 1-inch Penrose abdominal drain is placed through a separate stab incision and positioned down near the base of the pouch. The abdomen is closed.

Bladder Substitutes

The Kock neobladder utilizes the same construction technique as the cutaneous urinary diversion except that an efferent limb and a continence valve are not needed (Fig. 57–12). The urethra in males is prepared at the time of cystoprostatectomy just as would be done after a radical prostatectomy. However, the preparation of the urethra in females deserves specific mention. In the final stages of the female cystectomy, attention to surgical detail is critical to avoid damage to the vesicourethral junction, proximal urethra, and corresponding innervation that could jeopardize the continence mechanism. The posterior bladder wall is dissected off the anterior vaginal wall down to the bladder neck. If there is concern about adequate surgical margins at the posterior or base of the bladder, the anterior vaginal wall may be removed en bloc with the cystectomy specimen, thus requiring subsequent vaginal reconstruction. Nonetheless, minimal dissection should be performed anterior to the proximal urethra. In addition, the pubourethral suspensory ligaments, which also contribute to the continence mechanism, should be left intact. After the bladder is completely dissected and remains attached only to the urethra and bladder neck, a curved clamp should be placed across the bladder neck. Under tension, the urethra is transected

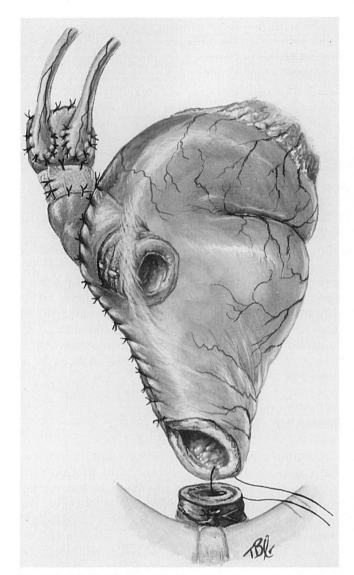

Figure 57–12. The Kock neobladder utilizes the same general configuration as the cutaneous reservoir but does not require the efferent limb or continence valve. A fingertip-sized opening is left in the down corner of the neobladder opposite the antireflux valve for anastomosis to the urethra.

just distal to the clamp. As the proximal urethra is transected, eight interrupted 2-0 PGA sutures are placed circumferentially in the urethra. These sutures are carefully set aside until the end of the diversion for reanastomosis to the Kock ileal reservoir.

Since the efferent limb and valve are not needed in the bladder substitute, the initial amount of ileum resected to construct the pouch is shortened by 17 cm. The proximal end of the ileal resection is initiated at the same point, about 20 cm from the cecum. The reservoir segments are aligned and opened, the back wall of the reservoir is sutured, and the antireflux valve is created and secured in the same fashion as previously described. The efferent end of the proximal reservoir segment is left open to be incorporated into the reservoir closure. The reservoir is folded and closed with two-layer running 3-0 PGA suture in the same fashion as the cutaneous reservoir except that the corner of the closure on the side opposite from the afferent limb is left open just enough to accommodate a fingertip (Fig. 57–12). This opening should be similar in size to the opening left in the bladder after a radical prostatectomy. The ureters are anastomosed to the afferent limb using the same end-to-side technique. The ureteral stents are similarly placed and fixed to the catheter used to drain the reservoir. The reservoir is anastomosed to the membranous urethra using eight 2-0 PGA sutures that have been preplaced circumferentially in the urethra at the time of the cystectomy. A 24 Fr. hematuria catheter with extra large drainage holes is passed per urethram into the reservoir after the posterior sutures are placed. The ureteral stents are sutured to the catheter tip with 4-0 nylon sutures before advancing the catheter all the way through the reservoir opening. The anterior sutures are placed in the reservoir opening, and all the sutures are tied, proceeding anterior to posterior. The ureteral stents are removed when the catheter is removed in 3 weeks.

Ileal Anal Reservoir

An alternative urinary diversion option for men and women requiring cystectomy and urethrectomy is some form of continent diversion to the rectum. The ureterosigmoidostomy fell out of favor in the past because of the late development of adenocarcinoma at the ureterocolonic anastomosis site and because of the high probability of renal damage due to infection, reflux, and stricture. This operation was also complicated by nocturnal incontinence, urgency, frequency, and hyperchloremic acidosis. To overcome these problems, we have investigated the use of the Kock neobladder anastomosed side to side to the rectum (Fig. 57–13). With this technique, the hemi-Kock reservoir is created like the Kock bladder substitute except that the folded reservoir is left open for about 12 cm on one side. The rectum is opened for a distance of about 12 cm up toward the sigmoid colon. A sigmoid nipple valve is created just proximal to the sigmoid opening by dividing the epiploica and the fat of the mesentery for 8 cm and intussuscepting a 4- to 5-cm valve, which is stabilized with staplers in the same manner as the Kock pouch valves.

The reason for this colon valve is to prevent reflux of urine back up the sigmoid, thus helping to avoid subsequent hyperchloremic acidosis. The hemi-Kock reservoir is anastomosed to the colon opening. The presence of the Kock neobladder permits a large-capacity reservoir of urine with the ureters above the antireflux valve and out of the fecal stream. The patient has the potential, therefore, of holding larger

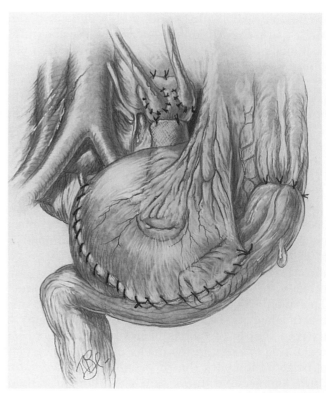

Figure 57–13. The Kock neobladder to the rectum is an alternative method for internal diversion to the rectum. The ureters are protected from the fecal stream. A valve may also be created in the colon to prevent urine reflux into the sigmoid.

volumes of urine under low pressures and, it is hoped, bypasses the risks of rectal incontinence, frequency, and hyperchloremic acidosis. Also, because the ureters are away from the rectum and feces, the risk of adenocarcinoma and renal damage should be low. Unfortunately, this is a much more complicated version of the continent diversion, and we have so far offered this option to only 15 patients. A diverting loop colostomy is usually performed proximally to temporarily divert the stool. The reservoir is drained through a rectal tube, and a catheter is brought through the skin and into the pouch by way of a defunctionalized proximal sigmoid. The ureteral catheters can also be brought through the reservoir and out the skin for independent drainage.

This procedure appears to work best in younger patients with good anal sphincter tone and a high degree of motivation. It is an excellent option for patients who have previously had an ureterosigmoidostomy and need revisional surgery because of complications. We still consider this form of diversion investigational, and it will most likely be offered only in unusual circumstances.

POSTOPERATIVE MANAGEMENT

The key to postoperative care lies in making certain that the reservoir is draining well. The drainage catheter should be irrigated every 4 hours with 50 ml of normal saline to keep it clear of mucus. Patients are instructed how to do this themselves, usually within the first 5 to 7 days. The catheters are routinely maintained for 3 weeks. Patients can typically be discharged to home health care within 7 to 10 days of the operation. They return at 3 weeks to have the catheter removed after radiological confirmation of complete healing. Patients who have the continent cutaneous diversion usually stay overnight during this return visit to become comfortable with their catheterization system.

Cutaneous diversion patients begin catheterizing with 20 Fr. coudé-tip reusable catheters every 2 or 3 hours. The catheterization interval is usually increased by 1 hour each week until the goal of catheterizing every 6 hours is reached. A small absorbency pad should be worn over the stoma to prevent mucous spotting of clothing.

Internal diversion patients need to perform Kegel-type perineal exercises after the catheter is removed. It usually takes bladder substitute patients several weeks before daytime continence is achieved. Continence is indeed uniformly excellent during the day but becomes more complex at night. About 60 percent of these patients become dry at night, and most of the remaining 40 percent can achieve acceptable nocturnal continence by planned awakening one to three times a night to void.

RESULTS AND COMPLICATIONS

Patient satisfaction with these procedures should be extremely high, but preoperative counseling is important to prioritize expectations. If patients undergoing construction of a continent reservoir are led to believe that this reservoir equals their natural bladder with the same level of care, they may consider the end result less than satisfactory.

Our experience, through much trial and error, demonstrates that the physical and psychological cost to the patient of a Kock intestinal reservoir diversion is comparable with that of a standard ileal conduit urinary diversion. Both types of diversion when combined with cystectomies carry operative mortality rates of 1 percent. Continent diversion requires approximately 1 to 2 hours' further operative time. The early complication rate for both types of diversions is 16 percent. These include infections, prolonged urinary leak, prolonged hospital stay, and bowel difficulties. Both types of surgery involve an average hospital stay of 8.5 days. The late complications of both operations are also surprisingly similar in number, although they tend to be of different types. The ureteroileal stenosis rate for both intestinal reservoirs and ileal conduits is 3 percent, as would be expected

since the anastomoses are identical. The ileal conduit has a 5 percent rate of stomal stenosis, while cutaneous continent diversions have essentially none because of the constant catheterization. Surprisingly, the rate of urethral anastomotic strictures in orthotopic diversions is also close to zero. Approximately 1 percent of continent cutaneous diversions develop difficult catheterization. The ileal conduit carries a 10 percent rate of pyelonephritis, while the ileal reservoirs have only a 1 percent rate because of the antireflux valve. Continent cutaneous diversions do carry a 7 percent rate of reoperation for urinary leakage at the skin, which is not an issue in the ileal conduit. These reoperations typically involve reconstruction of the continence valve. The antireflux valve runs only a 1 to 2 percent risk of stenosis, and this can usually be treated endoscopically. Intestinal reservoirs do have a higher incidence of stone disease (5 to 10 percent), but again these can typically be handled endoscopically.

As noted previously, many patients with bladder substitutes find that they need to void at least one to three times a night to stay dry. During sleep the resting pressure in the urethra tends to be low and does not benefit from the biofeedback of bladder filling. Therefore, as the reservoir fills at night, the sphincter mechanism cannot compensate by increasing its intrinsic tone, and leakage will ensue if patients do not anticipate and periodically empty the bladder. Complete reservoir emptying that uses increased abdominal pressure is extremely important in maintaining continence. Approximately 5 percent of patients may seek an artificial urinary sphincter at nighttime to control incontinence.

Factors that tend to favor continent diversion over conduit diversion gravitate toward quality of life issues. The patient acceptance rate with continent diversion is extremely high and there is a marked increase in self-confidence and self-image.[3] It is now well documented that patients with continent diversions develop better interpersonal and sexual relations after surgery than do patients with ileal conduits and urostomy bags. This improved outlook and potential normalization of life style should encourage patients with high-grade invasive bladder cancer and their physicians to adapt an earlier and more aggressive therapy by cystectomy when the potential for cure is highest.

DISCUSSION

The reintroduction of continent urinary diversion in the early 1980s was a major step forward for patients requiring cutaneous diversion. Realistically, however, most patients given the choice, would still opt to urinate per urethram if possible. The Kock ileal reservoir with its low internal pressures blends itself very nicely with both cutaneous diversion and orthotopic reconstruction to the urethra. It was originally thought that only men were good candidates for an orthotopic diversion after cystectomy, but this option is now considered just as appropriate in women.[6] Until recently, orthotopic urinary reconstruction was not technically feasible in women facing radical cystectomy because traditionally total urethrectomy was performed in all female patients and the continence mechanisms were poorly understood. Recent neuroanatomical studies of the female pelvis and urethra, however, have provided a better understanding of the female continence mechanism, and extensive pathological review of female cystectomy specimens suggests that the female urethra can be safely preserved in most women undergoing radical cystectomy.[7]

Performed correctly, orthotopic urinary reconstruction to the urethra is a viable option that provides female patients with complete continence and the ability to void per urethram without residuals. The bladder neck and proximal portion of the urethra are composed of smooth muscle and are innervated by the pelvic plexus running along the lateral aspect of the uterus, vagina, and bladder. A gradual transition with intermingling of this smooth muscle with striated muscle has been identified in the middle to lower third of the urethra.[8] This striated muscle, the so-called rhabdosphincter muscle with its major portion on the ventral aspect of the urethra, is innervated from branches of the pudendal nerve that run along the pelvic floor. Preservation of this musculature of the lower half of the urethra together with its nerve supply is crucial for urinary continence in females. It appears that maintaining the rhabdosphincter with this nerve supply should suffice to provide continence in female cystectomy patients undergoing orthotopic reconstruction to the urethra. Furthermore, cystectomy with removal of the uterus and cervix effectively denervates the bladder neck and proximal urethral sphincter mechanisms. These same anatomical studies support complete removal of the bladder neck with transection of the specimen at the urethrovesico junction, as continence is maintained only by the rhabdosphincter of the lower urethra.

Our own pathological examination of female cystectomy patients has further helped us understand the role of urethrectomy in female bladder cancers. A recent study of 67 female cystourethrectomy specimens revealed an overall risk of atypia, carcinoma in situ, or overt cancer within the urethra in 13 percent of patients.[7] Of the 67 pathological specimens, 6 percent also had anterior vaginal wall involvement. Interestingly, if no atypia or tumor was histologically seen to be present at the bladder neck, the woman was found to have no urethral or vaginal wall abnor-

mality. We believe that women without tumor at the bladder neck can be considered appropriate candidates for orthotopic urinary reconstruction to the urethra with preservation of the anterior vaginal wall. Careful preoperative evaluation with bladder neck biopsy and intraoperative frozen sections of the urethral margin of the cystectomy specimen are mandatory to exclude any abnormality at the anastomotic site that would preclude the proposed orthotopic reconstruction. With proper selection and informed consent, we consider that up to 80 percent of women undergoing cystectomy for transitional cell carcinoma of the bladder may be appropriate neobladder candidates.

Patient age or body habitus has not been a factor in selection for orthotopic reconstruction. In fact, the obese patient may be an ideal candidate for a neobladder. The need to negotiate a thick abdominal wall for a conduit or intermittent catheterization is eliminated. Although some investigators have reported difficulty in making an orthotopic reservoir reach the urethra, we have never found this to be the case when adequate mesenteric mobilization is utilized.[2]

Summary

Our extensive operative experience with the various forms of Kock continent ileal reservoir in more than 1000 patients since 1982 has clearly demonstrated the reliability and durability of this diversion system. Reflux can be reliably prevented and the upper urinary tracts protected. Patients can void or catheterize with confidence. Orthotopic diversions should now be available to a majority of patients, both male and female. Patients should be able to live a more normal life style with a positive self-image. We believe that our modifications of the ileal reservoir diversions have decreased the need for reoperation. These forms of continent urinary diversion have emerged as optimal operations, and continent urinary diversion in general has become the standard of care for most cystectomy patients. Ileal conduits should be reserved for poor-risk candidates with a short life expectancy or for those patients not motivated for continent diversion. Patients must still be aware, however, that complications can occur. An appropriate understanding of the continent diversion technique and its potential problems continues to be an essential prerequisite for the operation. Minor refinements of the Kock urinary diversion will continue to be made, but we believe that continent diversion, most often in the form of orthotopic reconstruction, can safely and wisely be offered to most patients.

Editorial Comment

Fray F. Marshall

These authors have demonstrated the success of continent urinary diversion. They have also demonstrated the feasibility of continent, orthotopic diversion in the female. Others have utilized less technically complex continent diversions without antireflux "nipples," but these authors have been among the leaders of continent diversion.

REFERENCES

1. Kock NG, Nilson AE, Nilsson LO, et al: Urinary diversion via a continent ileal reservoir: Clinical results in 12 patients. J Urol 128:469, 1982.

2. Camey M, Le Duc A: L'enterocystoplastie avec cystoprostatectomie totale pour cancer de la vessie. Ann Urol 13:114, 1979.
3. Boyd SD, Feinberg SM, Skinner DG, et al: Quality of life survey of urinary diversion patients: Comparison of ileal conduits versus continent Kock ileal reservoirs. J Urol 138:1386, 1987.
4. Kock NG, Ghoneim MA, Lycke G, Mahran MR: Urinary diversion to the augmented and valved rectum: Preliminary results with a novel surgical procedure. J Urol 140:1375, 1988.
5. Skinner DG: Technique of radical cystectomy. Urol Clin North Am 8:353, 1981.
6. Stein JP, Stenzl A, Esrig D, et al: Lower urinary tract reconstruction following cystectomy in women using the Kock ileal reservoir with bilateral ureteroileal urethrostomy: Initial clinical experience. J Urol 152:1404, 1994.
7. Stein JP, Cote RC, Freeman JA, et al: Lower urinary tract reconstruction in women following cystectomy for pelvic malignancy: A pathological review of female cystectomy specimens. J Urol 151:304A, 1994.
8. Colleselli K, Stenzl A, Posel S, et al: Hemi-Kock to the female urethra: Anatomical approach to the continence mechanism to the female urethra. J Urol 151:500A, 1994.

Chapter 58

The Ileal Neobladder

Richard E. Hautmann

Vesical reconstruction has undergone a tremendous evolution since the late 1980s. All segments of bowel have been used and numerous modifications of the original techniques have been described. While most authors claim that each type of reservoir offers the same advantages and disadvantages to the patient, it is clear that this statement is absolutely incorrect. The critical issue is continence. All reservoirs offer reasonable daytime continence, but nocturnal continence is critical. Depending on the definitions used, enuresis is common in most types of reservoirs, while some avoid this problem almost completely.

Cystectomy is usually connected with the problem of urinary diversion. In the past, urinary diversion with urostomy and an external device was a disfiguring operation. Nowadays, ideal diversion may include a stable upper urinary tract, continence, low reoperation rate, normal body image, and normal micturition. Therefore, the frequency of ileal and colon conduits has decreased to less than 50 percent in urological centers. These conduits are replaced by pouches with continent urostomy or by orthotopic bladder substitutes. The ileal conduit was the gold standard for supravesical diversion. Today, for male patients, bladder replacement by bowel segments with anastomosis to the urethra is the new standard. Total vesical replacement and voiding function of the bladder is expected after a radical curative cystectomy. The goal is to maintain quality of life or even enhance it by withdrawing the tumor symptomatology. The idea of imitating the storage function of the urinary bladder by bowel segments is more than 100 years old. In 1888, Tizzoni and Foggi replaced a bladder by an isoperistaltic segment of the ileum.[1] This method was taken up again in 1951 by Couvelaire and in 1979 by Camey and Le Duc.[2, 3] In 1982, after experimental investigations, Kock constructed a continent reservoir with a catheterizable stoma from a detubularized ileal segment in men.[4] This reservoir was modified by others to reduce complication and reoperation rates. Pouches were made from ileal and ileocecal segments, colon, sigmoid, and stomach. Basic theoretical application of urinary reservoirs was worked out by Hinman in 1988.[5] The correlation between bowel length and volume of the reservoir and compliance by viscoelastic qualities of the bowel wall was addressed.

INDICATIONS FOR AND CONTRAINDICATIONS TO CONTINENT URINARY DIVERSION

In general, all cystectomy patients are potential candidates for orthotopic bladder replacement. A contraindication is a noncompliant patient with a mental or physical disability. Poor renal function with elevated serum creatinine levels greater than 2.5 mg/dl is another contraindication because of the high absorbance capacity of the reservoir. However, in patients with preoperatively elevated creatinine due to renal obstruction, hydronephrosis should be relieved by percutaneous nephrostomy in an attempt to achieve recovery of renal function. A chronic inflammatory bowel disorder such as Crohn disease or ulcerative colitis is also a contraindication.

Contraindications to anastomosis of the reservoir to the urethra (Table 58-1) include transitional cell carcinoma of the prostate, tumor invasion into the prostatic stroma, and a multifocal tumor of the urethra. All these conditions require an urethrectomy at the time of cystectomy.

Relative contraindications are irradiation of the pelvis with more than 6000 rad, old age, lesion of the rectum during cystectomy, bladder cancer in the bladder neck, dysplasia or tumor in situ (Tis) in the prostatic urethra, and multifocal Tis/G3. To exclude these tumors, a urethrocystoscopy with biopsy of suspicious areas should be performed preoperatively. Patients with recurrent urethral strictures may not benefit from intestinal urethral anastomosis, and in

TABLE 58–1. Contraindications to Anastomosis of the Reservoir to the Urethra

Absolute	Mental or physical disability
	Incompliant patient
	Elevated serum creatinine (≥2.5 mg/dl) after relief of renal obstruction
	Chronic inflammatory bowel disease (Crohn disease, ulcerative colitis)
	Transitional cell carcinoma of prostate (stromal invasion) or urethra
	Direct tumor invasion into prostate
Relative	Pelvic irradiation with more than 6000 rad
	Old age (over 70 years)
	Tumor in bladder neck
	Carcinoma in situ of prostatic urethra
	Multifocal carcinoma in situ/G3
	Recurrent urethral strictures

these individuals a diversion to the skin might be better. In a case of irradiation or rectal lesion, a continent reservoir might be possible after creation of a temporary colostomy. A differentiation between physiological and chronological age is necessary. There should not be a limit for continent urinary diversion just because the patient is of a certain age, although the continence rate in men under 70 is higher. Continent reservoirs with a stoma as well as conduits are not ideally suitable for obese men owing to problems with catheterization or the external device. In these patients, an orthotopic bladder replacement may be an ideal solution.

CONSEQUENCES OF BOWEL RESECTION

In reservoirs using an ileocecal segment the ileocecal valve is lost. Consequences may include malabsorption of vitamin B_{12} and bile acids with subsequent diarrhea, steatorrhea, secondary hyperoxaluria, and intestinal osteopathy. Furthermore, bacterial contamination of the small bowel may occur. If a sole ileal segment is used, these side effects are minimal. In a case of bladder substitution by stomach, hemorrhagic cystitis, dysuria, and oxaluria were observed. Oxaluria is increased, as the stomach seems to be the critical site for intestinal oxalate absorption. In general, however, when ileum, ileocecum, sigmoid, or stomach is used, there is no definite evidence for the clear superiority of any bowel segment for bladder substitution.

SURGICAL OPTIONS

Complete detubularization of the bowel segment to create the ileal bladder and folding of the bowel to a spheric reservoir increase its radius nearly four times

compared with the original ileal segment, and its capacity by the square of four times the radius (Fig. 58–1A). The viscoelastic properties of the small bowel wall provide good compliance of the ileal bladder. Complete dissection of the longitudinal and circular intestinal musculature minimizes the incidence of bladder contractions, resulting in the highest capacity of all bladder substitutes described (Fig. 58–1B) and day and night continence in more than 90 percent of patients, without the need for artificial sphincters.

The surgical stress of the operation for the patient is comparable with that of an ileal conduit. As the function of the ileal bladder was never affected by tumor progression in our series,[10] the indications for bladder substitution include palliative cystoprostatectomy, high tumor burden, and previous chemotherapy. Solitary kidneys and serum creatinine concentrations of up to 2 mg/dl are not exclusion criteria for the ileal bladder.

An important criterion of the appropriateness of bladder replacement or external urinary diversion is the psychological and compliance status of the patient. The postoperative training period for bladder emptying, the attainment of control over continence, and the need for regular follow-up require a high degree of patient collaboration.

PREOPERATIVE MANAGEMENT

Patients selected for radical cystoprostatectomy and ileal bladder should undergo a tumor biopsy of the prostatic urethra (findings should be negative). Decompression of the dilated upper tracts by a percutaneous nephrostomy for 3 to 4 weeks may be useful for better tunneling of the distal ureters but is not mandatory. Before bladder augmentation, the diagnostic work-up includes intravenous pyelography, voiding cystourethrography, retrograde urethrography, urethrocystoscopy, and an extensive urodynamic evaluation. The day before surgery a central venous catheter is placed, and the patient is hydrated the night before the operation. Although the operation is carried out using general anesthesia, all patients receive an indwelling (epidural) catheter for better postoperative pain control. Twelve hours before surgery the bowel is flushed via a nasogastric tube with 3 to 5 L of a solution containing 1.4 g/L NaCl, 0.7 g/L KCl, 1.7 g/L $NaHCO_3$, 12.8 g/L $Na_2SO_4 \cdot 10\ H_2O$, 59.0 g/L PEG 4000. Intravenous broad-spectrum antibiotics are started the day before surgery and continued until the second postoperative day.

OPERATIVE TECHNIQUE

The patient is placed in the supine position to extend the distance between pubis and umbilicus. A

Intestinal Segments   Geometric Capacity   Reservoir Volumes from 60 cm Ileum

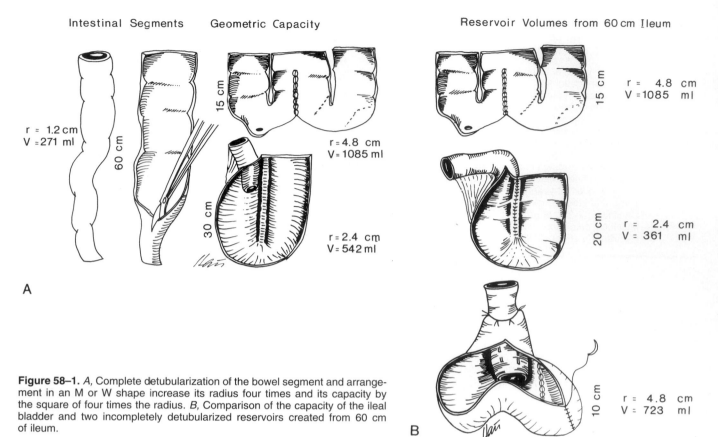

A

Figure 58–1. *A,* Complete detubularization of the bowel segment and arrangement in an M or W shape increase its radius four times and its capacity by the square of four times the radius. *B,* Comparison of the capacity of the ileal bladder and two incompletely detubularized reservoirs created from 60 cm of ileum.

B

midline abdominal incision is made extending from the pubis to approximately 5 cm proximally, above the umbilicus. Pelvic lymphadenectomy is carried out using the modified technique of Whitmore. Lymph nodes are not sent routinely for frozen-section analysis because the operation would be continued even in the presence of lymph nodes with microscopically positive findings. A standard cystoprostatectomy is then carried out as described in Chapter 50, and 1-cm sections of the distal ureters are sent for frozen-section analysis to make sure there is no tumor invasion. If the results are positive, the procedure is repeated until the distal ureters are found to be microscopically free of tumor.

To preserve continence, good exposure of the apex of the prostate and the proximal urethra is necessary (Fig. 58–2). The prostate is dissected from the urethra right at the apex, leaving a urethral stump 1.5 to 2 cm

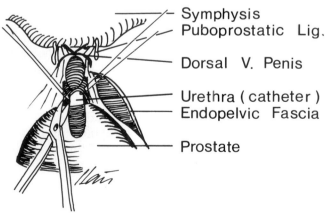

Symphysis
Puboprostatic Lig.

Dorsal V. Penis

Urethra (catheter)
Endopelvic Fascia

Prostate

Figure 58–2. Exposure of the prostatourethral junction before transection of the urethra. A long and intact urethral stump must be obtained to preserve continence.

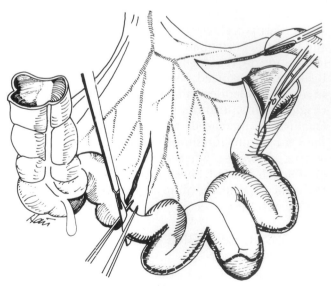

Figure 58–3. Selection of the ileal segment with an appropriate vascular supply and antimesenteric incision of ileum.

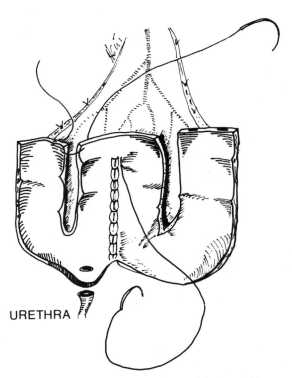

URETHRA

Figure 58–4. A W-shaped reconfiguration of the intestinal segment after detubularization and asymmetric incision of the ileal wall at the site of the anastomosis to the urethra, forming a U-shaped flap.

in length. After the urethra is dissected, six 2-0 double-armed Vicryl sutures are used for the anastomosis with the ileal neobladder, incorporating urethral mucosa and musculature, and are secured with mosquito clamps. Thus, retraction of the urethra into the pelvic floor is avoided. If the patient desires preservation of potency and no tumor extension is found, the nerve-sparing technique described by Walsh is performed.[6]

After cystoprostatectomy has been completed, a segment of small bowel, approximately 60 to 80 cm long and 15 cm proximal to the ileocecal valve, is selected (Fig. 58–3). The distal division of the mesentery along the avascular region between the ileocolic artery and the terminal branches of the superior mesenteric artery should extend to the base of the mesentery to provide maximal mobility and sufficient length to reach the urethral remnant. The proximal incision of the mesentery is made as short as possible to provide appropriate vascular supply to the ileal segment. The ileum is then divided between bowel clamps. A standard bowel anastomosis is performed using a two-layer interrupted technique with 4-0 Vicryl, and the mesenteric trap is closed.

The isolated bowel segment is thoroughly rinsed with saline or an iodine solution. The ileal section reaching down to the urethra is most easily identified and marked with a traction suture at the antimesenteric border. The bowel segment is then arranged in an M or W shape and secured by stay sutures or Allis clamps, positioning the traction suture in the bottom position

of the M or W, directed caudally toward the urethra. The entire ileal segment is opened strictly along the antimesenteric border except for a 5-cm section around the traction suture. At that point the incision of the ileum is made close to the anterior mesenteric border to create a U-shaped flap that facilitates anastomosis of the ileal bladder to the urethra (Fig. 58–3).

A flat plate of ileum is formed by connecting the antimesenteric borders of the M or W with 3-0 Vicryl running sutures (Fig. 58–4). No staples are used. The U-shaped flap serves as a new bladder neck. In the center of that flap, an incision of approximately the diameter of the little finger is made, and a 22 Fr. Foley catheter is placed through it. The six double-armed sutures, previously placed through the urethral stump for anastomosis with the ileal bladder, are now brought through the ileal wall at a distance of approximately 1 cm from the catheter (Fig. 58–5). With gentle traction on the catheter, the ileal plate is easily directed down to the urethra, and the sutures are tied from "inside" the ileal bladder, thus completing the ileourethral anastomosis (Fig. 58–6).

At this point, the ureters are implanted into the ileal bladder (Figs. 58–7 and 58–8). They are pulled through small separate incisions "inside" the ileal bladder at a convenient site in the natural course of the ureter. Care should be taken that the implantation is done as caudally as possible to prevent kinking of the ureters when the ileal neobladder is filled. Trac-

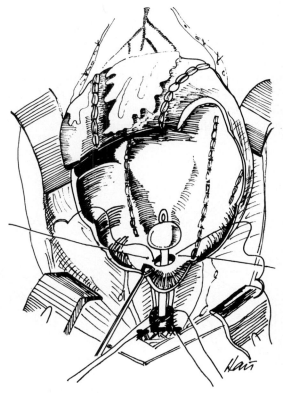

Figure 58–5. Anastomosis of the ileal plate to the urethral stump with six mattress sutures.

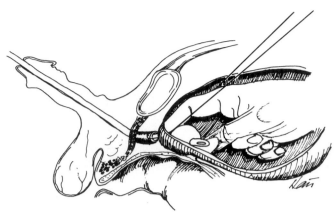

Figure 58–6. Lateral aspect of the ileourethral anastomosis. The sutures are tied from "inside" the ileal bladder.

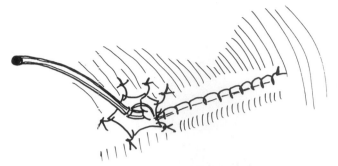

Figure 58–8. Completed ileoureteral anastomosis.

tion on the anastomosis or extensive mobilization of the ureters should be avoided.

The mucosa of the ileal wall is incised to create a mucosal sulcus approximately 3 cm in length and 1 cm in width. The entire thickness of the mucosa as far as the submucosa is removed. This maneuver is best achieved by folding the wall of the ileal neobladder 5 cm distal to the ureteral entry (Fig. 58–7A). In this way an adequate mucosal chip can be removed. The ureters are then spatulated and anchored to the muscular wall of the ileal bladder by three deep 4-0 Vicryl sutures. The mucosal edges of the sulcus are closed over the ureter with interrupted 4-0 catgut sutures (Fig. 58–7B). Thus the ureter is covered completely by ileal mucosa (Fig. 58–8). The ureter is fixed outside the seromuscular layer of the ileal neobladder as it enters the reservoir by one interrupted 3-0 Vicryl suture. This implantation technique, with the ureters lying in the mucosal sulcus on the muscular wall of the ileum neobladder, perfectly prevents reflux (Figs. 58–9 and 58–10). The 7 Fr. pigtail ureteral catheters employed for stenting the anastomosis are brought out of the skin through separate incisions.

The technique of ileal neobladder construction has been described in detail previously and has remained standardized since 1986.[7-10] A continued reanalysis of our results led to one noteworthy technical modification that has significantly decreased the incidence of ureteral complications and the need for reoperation. Initially, the ureters were implanted into the medial portions of the W (Fig. 58–10A). With increasing volume of the neobladder, this can cause ureteral kinking and occasional obstruction. Since 1989 we have preferred to implant the ureters in the lateral segments of the W (Fig. 58–10B). We continue to be pleased with the simple Le Duc technique of antireflux implantation.

A 12 Fr. cystostomy tube is placed, and the anterior wall of the ileal bladder is closed to a reservoir with 3-0 Vicryl running sutures starting at the lowest point. Two 20 Fr. silicone drains are placed into the small pelvis.

We have encountered no patient in whom the ileal neobladder would not reach the urethra. However, this part of the operation can be somewhat difficult in 10 percent of cases. Helpful methods include (1) loosening the retractor, which causes the abdominal wall to relax; (2) straightening the operative table and removing the sacral cushion, or bringing the patient

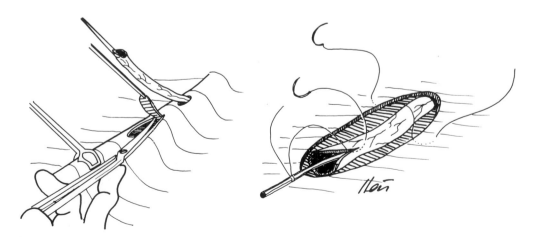

A   B

Figure 58–7. *A* and *B*, Ureteral implantation into the ileal plate.

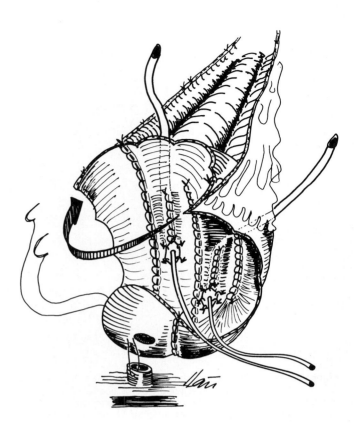

Figure 58–9. The ideal ureteral implantation is shown for the left ureter: implantation into the medial section of the W. The ureter is traveling underneath the mesentery and is implanted at the bottom of the ileal neobladder. With short ureters on the right side it may be necessary to cross the mesentery cranially. This step must not be taken with the left ureter!

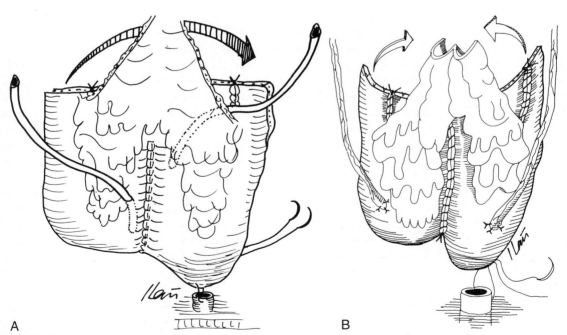

A   B

Figure 58–10. *A,* Our initial technique of ureteroileal anastomosis: ureters have been implanted into the medial portions of the W. Thus, the right ureter travels above and the left ureter below the mesentery of the ileal neobladder. With increasing volume of the neobladder, this can cause ureteral kinking and obstruction. *B,* Posterior view of the current method of ureteroileal anastomosis. Note that both ureters are now implanted in the lateral segments of the W.

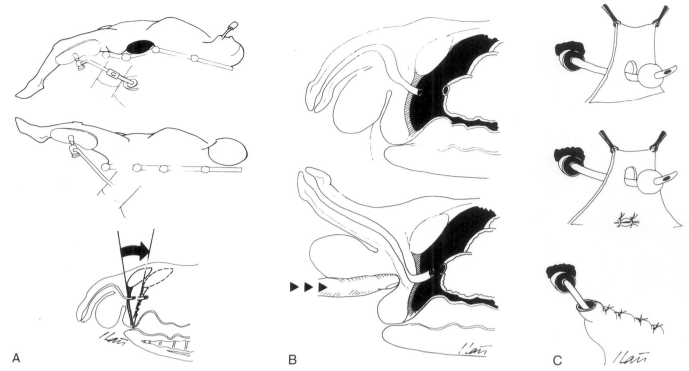

A B C

Figure 58–11. Methods to get the ileal neobladder to the pelvic floor. *A*, Changing the extended position of the patient to slightly supine and removal of the sacral cushion rotate the pelvic floor upward. *B*, Pushing up the perineum with a sponge stick or finger approximates the urethral remnant and neobladder. *C*, Moving the neobladder outlet closer to the tip of the U-shaped flap of ileal plate. If this still does not allow tension-free anastomosis, one should tubularize the U-shaped flap and perform direct (end-to-end) anastomosis.

with the legs abducted and knees and hips slightly flexed to a supine position, which causes the pelvic floor to rotate upward 2 to 3 cm (Fig. 58–11*A*); (3) when using a spreader bar table, pushing up the perineum with a sponge stick to gain another 2 to 3 cm (Fig. 58–11*B*); (4) freeing the descending colon and cecum as in retroperitoneal lymph node dissection; and (5) closing the neobladder outlet in the U-shaped flap (the intended site of the anastomosis of the neobladder to the urethral remnant) and moving it closer to the tip of the flap. If this maneuver fails, direct end-to-end anastomosis should be performed (Fig. 58–11*C*). Any incision into the mesentery of the neobladder should be avoided. The neobladder/mesentery should not be pulled roughly down to the pelvic floor.

If the ileal bladder is used for bladder augmentation, the surgical technique is similar to that of total bladder replacement, except that subtotal bladder resection is performed. The ileal bladder is anastomosed to the bladder remnant. In most cases, reimplantation of the ureters into the ileal bladder is advisable.

POSTOPERATIVE MANAGEMENT AND COMPLICATIONS

As soon as the patient does not need pain control via the indwelling epidural catheter, early mobiliza-

tion is important to prevent thromboembolic and pulmonary complications. All patients are kept on low-dose heparin for 3 weeks. Bowel stimulation is started on the second postoperative day.

Excessive mucus production of the ileal bladder may rarely cause a problem in the postoperative course by obstructing the urethral catheter and cystostomy. Therefore, the ileal bladder is rinsed via the cystostomy with 50 to 100 ml of saline twice a day, starting on the fifth postoperative day. Routinely, the ureteral stents are removed on the fourteenth postoperative day. As soon as the urine is in contact with the ileal bladder mucosa, reabsorption of urine electrolytes may occur. Therefore, the base excess is checked at weekly intervals for the first 4 weeks, and monthly thereafter. Approximately 50 percent of all patients need temporary alkalinizing therapy.

The urethral catheter is removed on the 21st postoperative day, after a cystogram has demonstrated complete healing of the ileourethral anastomosis. When, rarely, there is still leakage from the anastomosis, it is treated by prolonged catheter drainage until the leak has closed spontaneously.

After removal of the catheter, bladder emptying is usually achieved by abdominal straining. The cystostomy is removed as soon as the patient is able to empty the ileal bladder without significant residual urine. Most patients achieve full continence within 2 to 4 weeks, after spontaneous micturition has been initiated, but a few take up to 6 months to gain complete control over bladder emptying and continence. A special training program has been developed to aid competent sphincteric control. Late complications most often encountered, although rare, include acute urinary retention due to mucus obstruction and strictures of the ileourethral anastomosis. The problem of bladder outlet obstruction by excessive mucus production can be easily solved by catheterization and flushing of the ileal bladder. The patient should be advised to increase daily fluid intake to 3 L. Strictures of the ileourethral anastomosis are managed by careful transurethral urethrotomy.

If a patient develops urethral recurrence of bladder carcinoma, the ileal neobladder may be diverted to a reservoir with a wet stoma.

Complications of the procedure are divided into those related directly to the urinary reservoir construction and those not directly related to the ileal neobladder. Of our patients, 7.5 percent suffered general early complications unrelated to the neobladder that must be expected after any major operation, including thrombosis (2.5 percent), embolism (2 percent), wound infection (2.5 percent), and pneumonia (0.5 percent).[10] Specific early complications directly related to the reservoir construction and requiring surgery included prolonged ileus (4 percent), abscess drainage (2 percent), and insufficiency of the ileal anastomosis (0.5 percent). Thus, the early reoperation rate was 6.5 percent. Percutaneous transient nephrostomy and lymphocele drainage was established in six respectively 3 percent. It is noteworthy that 20 percent of our patients had prolonged decreased gastrointestinal function, which was treated conservatively.[10] Of the patients with leakage at the ileourethral anastomosis, 9 percent had prolonged catheter drainage until the leakage closed spontaneously.

Up to April 1992, 25 percent of the patients had died: 18 percent of metastatic bladder cancer and 7 percent of unrelated medical problems. Four patients (2 percent) suffered a urethral recurrence and 17 percent a pelvic recurrence.

Late Complications

Late complications requiring rehospitalization or reoperation have been acceptable. Reoperation was necessary for ileus (2 percent), abscess drainage (1 percent), a colon-reservoir fistula (1.5 percent), nephrectomy for hydronephrosis (1 percent), ureteral reimplantation for stenosis (3.6 percent), and transurethral incision of the urethroileal stricture (5 percent). Transurethral incision of preexisting urethral strictures was necessary in 2 percent of the patients. Mild temporary metabolic acidosis occurred in 47 percent (surveillance or sporadic oral medication), while 3 percent had severe metabolic disturbances requiring rehospitalization.

Upper Urinary Tract

A complete sonographic follow-up was available in 393 renoureteral units. In 286 units there was no upper tract dilation preoperatively and during the entire postoperative follow-up. A decrease in preoperative upper tract dilation was noted in 32 units and an increase in 73. In two units the degree of obstruction remained unchanged. Vesicoureteral reflux was found in 14 units. Compared with our first 100 patients, the urodynamic characteristics and the data on micturition remained unchanged.[10]

Continence

Information regarding continence was obtained by questionnaires mailed to the referring urologist or home physician. These were answered by the patients, frequently with immediate relatives present. The continence definition that we have used is strict. Complete nighttime and daytime continence was assumed if the patient was dry without the regular need for a condom catheter, alarm clock awakenings, and sanitary pads. However, if sanitary pads showed occasional spotting only and were worn for safety reasons, as reported by some patients, this was not defined as incontinence.

To assess the influence of the length of the postoperative period on the development of continence, patients were stratified according to length of follow-up. Continence rates were separately calculated for patients with a minimum follow-up of 6 months and 1, 2, 3, and 4 years, respectively. Continence was achieved by 6 months in 67 percent, 1 year in 72 percent, 2 years in 78 percent, 3 years in 85 percent, and 4 years in 90 percent of the various patient cohorts. Seven percent of patients reported nighttime incontinence at 6 months. The values at 1 to 4 years are 7, 5, 5 and 0 percent, respectively. Thus, no correlation between nighttime incontinence and the length of the postoperative period could be established.

Stress incontinence was defined according to the guidelines of the International Continence Society.[10] Grade 1 was observed by 6 months in 19 percent of patients, by 1 year in 17 percent, by 2 years in 12 percent, by 3 years in 4 percent, and by 4 years in 0 percent. Four patients reported severe stress incontinence (grade 2). This figure decreased to two patients after 2 years, and finally only one patient complained of stress 2 incontinence. Only two patients never had any form of continence (stress 3). No statistical tests were used for comparison of the five subgroups, since figures in some groups were too small. However, the data clearly suggest that daytime continence rates depend on the length of the postoperative period. Accordingly, long-term follow-up is necessary to assess the definitive outcome of the continence figures in continent urinary diversion. Stress incontinence may still improve even after 2 years.

Patients void two to ten times (average 5.1) during the day and zero to four times (zero times in 16 percent, once in 33 percent, twice in 34 percent, three times in 12 percent and four times in 5 percent) during the night (average 1.6). Almost all patients had some sensations of bladder fullness.

Of our patients, 3.6 percent required intermittent catheterization because of inability to void or to maintain a postvoid residual urine of less than 100 ml at 6 months. After more than 4 years, one of 20 patients was still unable to empty the bladder.[10]

The impact of patient age on the return of urinary control was examined for patients with a minimum postoperative follow-up of 2 years. The 2-year period was chosen because the cohort size at 3 or 4 years was considered inadequate. When patients were sorted by decades, urinary continence returned in 80 percent of those under 70 years old, while only 56 percent of those over 70 were continent. These data indicate that, for the older age group, achieving control of the external urethral sphincter is much more of a problem than for younger patients.

In discussing the complication rates shown in this study, it must be kept in mind that our study group is an unselected patient population.[10] Since 1986, all patients undergoing radical cystectomy with curative intent for the management of invasive bladder cancer received this form of diversion. Our early complication rate of 14 percent compares favorably with the experience of others.[11] However, unlike others and in contrast to our previous follow-up on our first 100 patients, we have now encountered some late complications requiring rehospitalization or reoperation.[9, 10] Overall, only 29.3 percent of our patients are without any complications, while 32 percent suffer significant complications, including neobladder-unrelated general early complications (7.5 percent), neobladder-related early complications (6.5 percent), and late reoperation (16 percent). The remainder of our patients experienced minor but not negligible problems, including prolonged decreased gastrointestinal function (20 percent) and leakage of the urethrointestinal anastomosis (9 percent), both treated conservatively. Further complications required transient nephrostomy (6 percent), lymphocele drainage (3 percent), and formal drainage of urinoma (2 percent).

Summary

Despite the fact that some price must be paid for excellent continence, natural voiding, and undisturbed body image, the ileal neobladder continues to be our procedure of choice for male patients after cystectomy provided that there is no evidence of prostatic or urethral involvement. Our results should stimulate earlier patient and physician acceptance of cystectomy. Our experience has yielded extraordinary results in terms of patient acceptance.

In conclusion, an orthotopic bladder replacement is the treatment of choice for male patients after cystectomy. Owing to high postoperative quality of life, it also produces higher acceptance for an early cystectomy by both patient and urologist. In female patients there is a concern about the radicality of the cystectomy if the urethra is left in situ. Furthermore, approximately 50 percent of female patients have to perform intermittent self-catheterization after bladder augmentation.

Editorial Comment
Fray F. Marshall

The ileal neobladder can provide continent micturition with a urethral anastomosis in the cystectomy patient. Although we have used the ileocolic neobladder in most of our reconstructions, the use of both large bowel and small bowel destroys the ileocecal valve, and the ileal neobladder does not. If large bowel disease is present, the ileal neobladder is an excellent alternative. We have tended to use the ileocolic bladder because the cecum often reaches the urethra somewhat more easily than the ileum, but in general at least one loop of ileum will reach the urethra.

The fact that the urethral sutures are tied inside the neobladder suggests that some difficulty may occur in some patients in getting the small bowel to reach the urethra. The urethral anastomosis does not seem to have been a major problem.

This operation is also performed without the use of nipples. This allows entire use of the ileal segment for bladder reconstruction.

In our experience a 12 Fr. cystostomy tube might be somewhat small if a mucus plug is present. We have generally selected larger cystostomy tubes. Many patients subsequently needed alkali replacement.

Dr. Hautmann and his group have now achieved significant long-term experience with this operation. The reoperation rates have remained quite low and the continence rates quite high. Overall, it has been a very successful operation.

REFERENCES

1. Tizzoni G, Foggi A. Die Wiederherstellung der Harnblase. Zentralbl Chir 15:15, 1888.
2. Couvelaire R. Le réservoir ileale de substitution après la cystectomie totale chez l'homme. J Urol (Paris) 57:408, 1951.
3. Camey M, Le Duc A. L'entero-cystoplastie après cystoprostatectomie totale pour cancer de la vessie. Ann Urol (Paris) 13:114, 1979.
4. Kock NG, Nilson AE, Nilsen LO, et al. Urinary diversion via a continent ileal reservoir: clinical results in 12 patients. J Urol 128:469, 1982.
5. Hinman F Jr. Selection of intestinal segments for bladder substitution: Physical and physiological characteristics. J Urol 139:519, 1988.
6. Walsh PC. Radical retropubic prostatectomy. In Walsh PC, Retik AB, Stamey TA, Vaughan ED Jr, eds. Campbell's Urology, 6th ed. Philadelphia, WB Saunders, 1992, p 2865.

7. Hautmann RE, Egghart G, Frohneberg D, Miller K. Die Ileum-Neoblase. Urologe A 26:67, 1987.
8. Hautmann RE, Egghart G, Frohneberg D, Miller K. The ileal neobladder. J Urol 139:39, 1988.
9. Wenderoth UK, Bachor R, Egghart G, et al. The ileal neobladder: Experience and results of more than 100 consecutive cases. J Urol 143:492, 1990.
10. Hautmann RE, Miller K, Steiner U, Wenderoth U. The ileal neobladder: 6 years of experience with more than 200 patients. J Urol 150:40, 1993.
11. Skinner DG, Boyd SD, Lieskovsky G, et al. Lower urinary tract reconstruction following cystectomy: Experience and results in 126 patients using the Kock ileal reservoir with bilateral ureteroileal urethrostomy. J Urol 146:756, 1991.

Chapter 59

Cutaneous Continent Ileocecal Reservoir

Randall G. Rowland

The first attempt at creating a continent urinary reservoir was a ureterosigmoidostomy performed in 1852 by Simon. Since that time, many other forms of urinary diversion have been reported. The first cutaneous ileocecal reservoir was reported by Verhoogen in 1908. In 1950 Gilchrist and associates described the first modern attempt at a continent reservoir constructed with an ileocecal segment. Although this reservoir applied many of the principles used today, it was not widely adopted, principally because of the lack of acceptance of intermittent catheterization at that time. The reservoir consists of a series of modifications of the Gilchrist procedure.

The most frequent indications for performance of a cutaneous continent ileocecal reservoir are extirpative procedures for pelvic malignancies, treatment of neurogenic bladders of either traumatic or congenital causation, and treatment of other congenital anomalies such as exstrophy. In adults the most common indication for a continent reservoir is a pelvic malignancy. In children the most frequent indication for a reservoir is a congenital anomaly.

Because a continent urinary reservoir is more complex to create and manage than a noncontinent urinary diversion, most surgeons believe that it is appropriate for patients to have a life expectancy of at least 1 year if they are going to be candidates for a continent reservoir. Patients must have a moderate degree of manual dexterity to allow intermittent catheterization of the reservoir. Most important, patients must have a high degree of motivation and a desire to be free of a urinary drainage appliance. This motivation is necessary to ensure their success in dealing with a continent reservoir, since this requires more work than a urinary conduit.

PREOPERATIVE MANAGEMENT

Before performing a continent urinary reservoir utilizing an ileocecal segment, a barium enema is ad-

ministered to evaluate the colon. This test may be excluded in younger patients who otherwise have normal bowel function and no history of bowel disease. The finding of extensive numbers of diverticuli, particularly on the right side of the colon, are a strong contraindication to the procedure. Previous bowel surgery in which lengthy segments of bowel were removed or in which the ileocecal segment was resected is a contraindication to creating a modified Gilchrist continent reservoir.

The patient usually has a 48-hour mechanical and 24-hour oral antibiotic bowel preparation. If possible, it is desirable to admit patients the day before surgery to assess the completeness of the bowel preparation and add enemas if needed. Patients should also be monitored for dehydration, and intravenous fluids given if needed.

OPERATIVE TECHNIQUES

The choice of incision is determined by the additional procedures indicated for the patient at the time of creation of the continent reservoir. If there are no compelling reasons for a different incision, the one choice is a midline incision extending from the symphysis pubis to approximately halfway between the umbilicus and the xiphoid process. This allows access to the pelvis for mobilization of the ureters as well as mobilization of the cecum and ascending colon up to the level of the transverse colon if needed.

Under normal circumstances, an ileocecal segment is isolated as shown in Figure 59–1. Approximately 8 to 10 cm of terminal ileum are resected along with 25 to 30 cm of cecum and ascending colon. The colon is reconfigured by splitting it along its antimesenteric border from the open, cephalad end caudally to approximately 1 to 2 cm from the very caudal tip of the

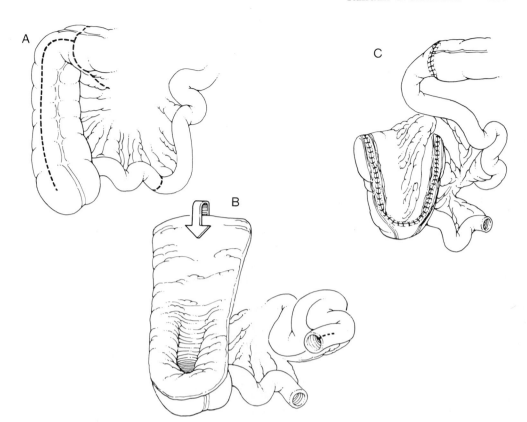

Figure 59–1. *A,* Dashed lines show the margins of resection used to create an ileocecal segment reservoir. The incision along the antimesenteric border is used to detubularize the colonic segment. *B,* Arrow indicates the direction in which the detubularized colon will be folded to create the reservoir. The dashed line on the distal segment of the ileum that will remain in the fecal stream indicates the area to be spatulated to compensate for the size discrepancy between the ileum and colon. *C,* The reservoir has been closed transversely in a Heineke-Mikulicz type of reconfiguration. The end-to-end ileocolostomy has been completed. Alternatively, an end-to-side stapled anastomosis can be performed.

cecum. If an appendectomy has not been previously performed, this is an ideal time to do so. After the efferent limb continence mechanism has been completed, the colon is folded over and closed transversely using one layer of synthetic braided absorbable 3-0 suture. Alternate sutures are locked to prevent shortening of the suture lines. Before total closure of the reservoir, a 22 or 24 Fr. Malecot catheter is placed through a separate stab wound in the anterolateral surface of the caudadmost portion of the cecum in a manner that will allow the cecostomy tube to be brought out directly through the anterior abdominal wall at the termination of the procedure.

Under normal circumstances the reservoir and efferent limb have a vascular supply based on the ileocolic and right colic arteries. In the case of a short cecum and ascending colon that would require taking a considerable portion of the transverse colon to achieve a colonic segment 25 to 30 cm in length, it is possible to take a shorter segment of cecum and ascending colon (15 to 20 cm) along with an additional 15- to 20-cm segment of ileum just proximal to the efferent limb segment. This additional segment of ileum can be split along its antimesenteric border and used as a patch on the reservoir. In this case the patch would be placed over the open, cephalad end and extended down the lateral margin of the colon to the level of the cecal cap. This procedure is illustrated in Figure 59–2.

The ileocolostomy can be performed by either a

hand-sewn end-to-end anastomosis with spatulation of a terminal ileum to compensate for the discrepancy in the size of the two bowel segments, or an end-to-side stapled anastomosis (see Fig. 59–1*C*).

The ureterocolic anastomoses can be carried out in one of two ways. Originally a tunneled Leadbetter type of implantation was performed along the tenia of the colon.[1] Figure 59–3 illustrates this method of anastomosis. Care must be taken to lead the left ureter under the colon mesentery so that there will not be a tendency to kink the ureter under the inferior mesenteric artery.

The Le Duc type of implantation (Fig. 59–4) is another satisfactory alternative for ureteral implantation.[2] If this type is chosen, it must be performed before final closure of the reservoir. Care must also be taken that the placement of the ureters is in the caudal half of the reservoir so that when the Heineke-Mikulicz reconfiguration is performed, the ureters will not be kinked by the folding of the reservoir.

Regardless of which style of ureteral implantation is chosen, 5 or 8 Fr. pediatric feeding tubes are used as ureteral stents, brought through the wall of the reservoir via separate stab wounds. A 3-0 chromic catgut suture is employed to secure the stent to the exterior wall of the reservoir.

The continence mechanism and efferent limb are created by stapling and plicating the terminal ileum segment. The original description of this technique included manual plication of the terminal ileum with

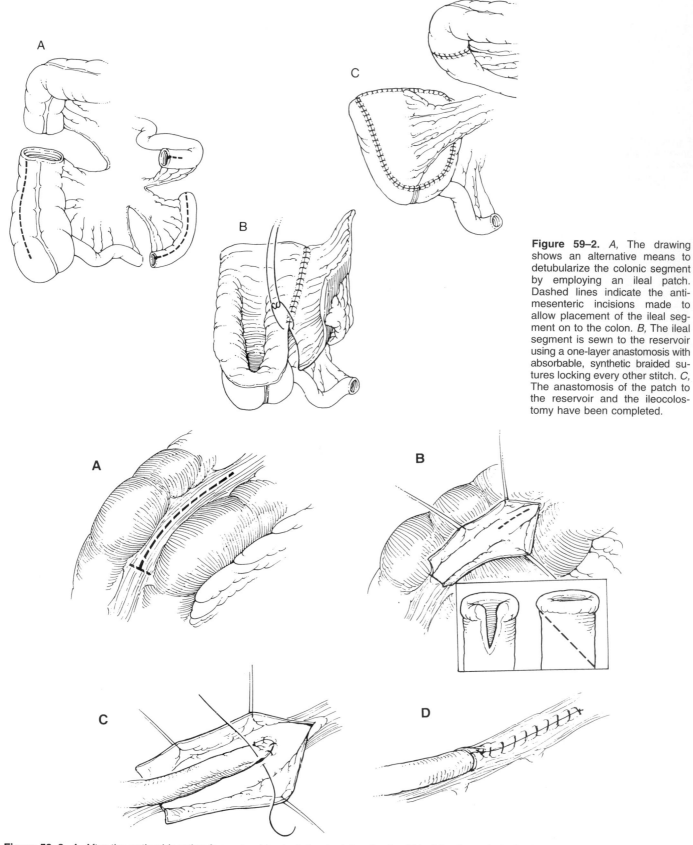

Figure 59–2. *A,* The drawing shows an alternative means to detubularize the colonic segment by employing an ileal patch. Dashed lines indicate the anti-mesenteric incisions made to allow placement of the ileal segment on to the colon. *B,* The ileal segment is sewn to the reservoir using a one-layer anastomosis with absorbable, synthetic braided sutures locking every other stitch. *C,* The anastomosis of the patch to the reservoir and the ileocolostomy have been completed.

Figure 59–3. *A,* After the optimal location for ureteral implantation is determined, a T incision is made in the tenia of the colon for a length of three to four times the diameter of the ureter. The cross-bar of the T creates a space for the ureteral hiatus. *B,* The edges of the tenia have been elevated to create a tunnel. A mucosal incision is made for formation of the ureteral orifice. The ureter is either spatulated or cut obliquely to increase the size of the ureteromucosal anastomosis. *C,* Interrupted 5-0 monofilament absorbable sutures are used to complete the anastomosis of the ureter to the colonic mucosa. *D,* The tenia is closed over the ureter with nonabsorbable 5-0 sutures. Each stitch is locked to prevent shortening of the tunnel.

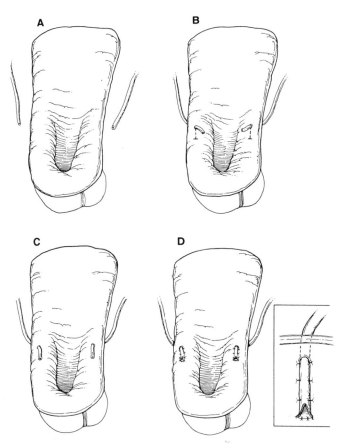

Figure 59–4. *A,* A Le Duc type of ureteral implantation is an acceptable alternative to tunneled implantation. The sites of implantation must be selected caudal to the halfway point of the segment to avoid kinking the ureter when the reservoir is folded over and closed. *B,* Inverted T incisions are made in the mucosa caudally from the point of penetration of the ureter through the colonic wall. *C,* The ureters are spatulated as shown by the dashed lines. *D,* Absorbable monofilament sutures are used to anastomose the ureter to the mucosa *(inset).*

3-0 silk Lembert sutures.[1, 3] Owing to difficulties with continence and catheterization of the efferent limb, the technique has been modified to take advantage of a stapling technique described by Bejany and Politano.[4]

Figure 59–5 shows the techniques involved in stapling the efferent limb and plicating the ileocecal valve area. The most important factor seems to be narrowing of the efferent limb in a uniform manner to promote ease of catheterization, and plication adjacent to the ileocecal valve to promote continence. Figure 59–5*E* and *F* shows a slight modification of Bejany's procedure. Placement of Lembert sutures at the ileocecal valve is substituted for placement of pursestring sutures. I believe that these sutures offer the same positive results in terms of continence as the pursestring sutures described by Bejany and Politano,[4] but they do not require dissecting the mesentery away from the terminal ileum to allow passage of the pursestring sutures.

Overall, one of the great advantages of creating the stapled and plicated efferent limb is that it allows intraoperative testing of the patient's continence as well as testing to make certain that the efferent limb will catheterize easily.

After the reservoir has been completed, it is placed in the orthotopic position in the right lower quadrant, and the stoma is led to either the right or left lower quadrants (Fig. 59–6). Alternatively, the reservoir can sometimes be placed in the pelvis and the efferent limb can lead to the anterior vaginal wall in females or to the urethral stump in males.

In most adults the orthotopic position is chosen because the most frequent indication for the continent reservoir has been the presence of a pelvic malignancy. Pelvic placement of a reservoir with perineal or urethral anastomosis of the efferent limb is more common in children being treated for congenital anomalies or neurogenic bladders. After the stoma and reservoir sites have been chosen, the cecostomy tube and ureteral stents are led out through a common anterior abdominal wall stab wound. The tubes are secured separately to the skin to allow for their removal at different time intervals. A closed drainage system such as a Jackson-Pratt drain is placed in the lower abdomen through a separate stab wound, which is usually located in the quadrant opposite the stoma site. The ureteral stents and cecostomy tube are attached to separate gravity drainage systems.

POSTOPERATIVE MANAGEMENT AND COMPLICATIONS

Most patients remain in the hospital for 7 to 10 days after surgery. During this immediate postoperative period they are taught to irrigate the cecostomy tube with 30 to 60 ml of saline approximately four times a day. This irrigation prevents obstruction of the cecostomy tube by mucous plugs. At the end of 1 week, radiographs are made after injection of contrast material into the stents. If free flow of contrast is seen around the stents into the reservoir and no gross leakage is noted, the ureteral stents are removed before discharging the patient from the hospital with the closed pelvic drain and cecostomy tube in place. Over the next 2 weeks, patients are instructed to irrigate the cecostomy tube three to four times a day at home to prevent obstruction with mucus.

Normally 3 weeks after surgery, patients are seen on an outpatient basis. A radiograph is made of the continent reservoir by filling the pouch through the cecostomy tube by gravity. If no reflux or leakage is noted, an intravenous pyelogram (IVP) is performed to verify that the upper tracts are functioning without evidence of significant hydronephrosis. After the integrity of the reservoir and upper tracts is confirmed, patients are started on intermittent catheterization

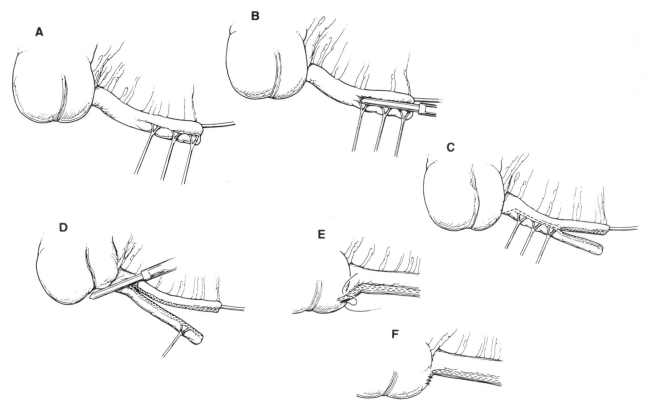

Figure 59–5. *A,* The efferent limb is narrowed by stapling techniques. Babcock clamps are used to grasp the antimesenteric surface of the bowel and a 12 Fr. catheter is placed through the ileum. *B,* A GIA stapler is used to create a smooth efferent limb by excising the redundant antimesenteric portion of the ileal segment. *C,* Additional cartridges of staples are used to divide the redundant bowel along the line indicated by the dashed line. *D,* The last staple cartridge is angled to prevent the staple line from extending into the cecum. *E,* The funnel-shaped segment of ileum created by the angling of the last staple cartridge is plicated to narrow the ileocecal junction to a straight tube of the same diameter as the remainder of the ileal segment. This procedure creates the continence mechanism. *F,* This shows the tubular effect achieved at the ileocecal junction by placing the plication sutures, five or six of which are usually required.

and the cecostomy tube is temporarily plugged. After they are able to catheterize successfully on two or three occasions, the cecostomy tube and pelvic drain are removed. They are observed on an outpatient basis for an additional 24 to 36 hours to ensure that

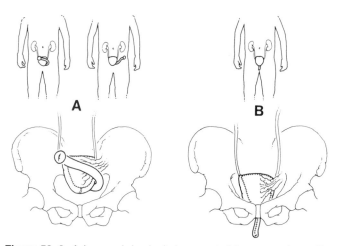

Figure 59–6. *A,* Lower abdominal placement of the reservoir creation of either a right or left lower quadrant stoma. *B,* Pelvic placement of the reservoir permits anastomosis of the efferent limb to the stump of the urethra (males) or perineum (females).

they are catheterizing well and that no problems with leakage or difficulty in catheterization are encountered. Initially, they are instructed to catheterize every 2 to 3 hours during the day and every 3 to 4 hours at night. Once patients have experienced at least a week without any evidence of incontinence, increasing intervals between catheterization are observed. It takes approximately 6 to 8 weeks to achieve a catheterization interval of 4 to 5 hours during the daytime and 4 to 6 hours at nighttime. During the postoperative period, both the blood urea nitrogen and creatinine values as well as the electrolyte values should be followed. A very slight hyperchloremic acidosis may be noted, but this rarely requires treatment.

In the early experience with the described continent urinary reservoir, efferent limb problems were the most common complications. Gradual modifications of the techniques involved in creation of the continence mechanism have dramatically reduced the complications encountered. Since stapling of the efferent limb has been adopted, difficulties with catheterization and incontinence have been virtually eliminated. Occasionally a parastomal hernia is encountered. In the early postoperative period, if hydronephrosis or leakage is present, the ureteral stents are left in place for an additional period until the problem has resolved. Long-term follow-up is required for any signs of development of ureterocolonic junction obstruction. This, of course, would be manifested by the development of hydronephrosis. When this obstruction occurs, both urodynamics of the reservoir and visualization of the upper tracts by radiological techniques are needed. If significant hydronephrosis occurs and no problem with increased pressure within the reservoir is noted, revision of the uretero-colonic anastomosis is needed. IVPs every 6 months in the first postoperative year are recommended. After this an IVP once a year or every other year should be sufficient monitoring for the development of hydronephrosis.

RESULTS

More than 97 percent of patients who have undergone the cutaneous continent ileocecal reservoir procedures have satisfactory daytime and nighttime continence. The average interval between catheterizations is greater than 4 hours during the daytime and approximately 6 hours at nighttime. At least 80 percent of all patients sleep the entire night without awakening to catheterize. During the daytime the average volume of catheterization is between 400 and 500 ml; nighttime or maximal volume is 700 to 1000 ml.

The complication and reoperation rates do not seem to be significantly different from those of standard urinary conduits. Careful long-term follow-up of these patients is required to further delineate these facts.

A technique has been developed for detubularizing and closing the reservoir with absorbable staples. I reported this technique in 1993[6] and am still gaining early experience with it. The results will be the subject of a future report.

Editorial Comment
Fray F. Marshall

The cutaneous ileocolic bladder involves a simpler operation than the Kock pouch. Resection and stapling of the efferent limb works well. The primary continent mechanism resides on the plicated ileocecal valve, not on the stapling of the efferent limb. The ureterocolic anastomosis is often more easily performed from the inside. We have tried to cover the ureter with colonic mucosa rather than perform a Le Duc reimplant. This operation works well and is an excellent choice for continent urinary diversion.

REFERENCES

1. Rowland RG, Mitchell ME, Bihrle R. The cecoileal continent urinary reservoir. World J Urol 3:185, 1985.
2. Camey M, Le Duc A. L'enterocystoplastie avec cystoprostatectomie totale pour cancer de la vessie. Ann Urol 13:114, 1979.
3. Rowland RG, Mitchell ME, Bihrle R, et al. The Indiana continent urinary reservoir. J Urol 137:1136, 1987.
4. Bejany DE, Politano VA. Stapled and nonstapled tapered distal ileum for construction of continent colonic urinary reservoir. J Urol 140:491, 1988.
5. Rowland RG, Kropp BP. Evolution of the Indiana continent urinary reservoir. J Urol 152:2247, 1994.
6. Rowland RG. Technique of the stapled Indiana pouch. Abstract presented at the North Central Section, American Urological Association. Meeting, Milwaukee, October 2, 1993.

Chapter 60

Total Bladder Substitution: Ileocolic Neobladder

Fray F. Marshall

Urinary diversion has evolved from ureterosigmoidostomy to the ileal conduit to various forms of continent urinary diversion. Most diversions have utilized a cutaneous anastomosis. In order to allow micturition, a urethral anastomosis to a bowel reservoir has become the preferred method of male urinary reconstruction in the appropriate patient. Although the bowel has been used for partial bladder substitution in patients with trauma, congenital anomaly, and neurogenic dysfunction, total reconstruction in the adult can now follow cystectomy for carcinoma. A description is given of total bladder reconstruction to the urethra after cystectomy for carcinoma.[1]

PREOPERATIVE MANAGEMENT

Careful evaluation of patients before consideration of continent urinary reservoir is important. This operation is longer, is more technically demanding, and has a higher theoretical complication rate than an ileal conduit. Advanced age, bowel disease, previous abdominal surgery, abdominal infections, prior radiation, other major medical problems, poor motivation, and poor nutrition can all constitute possible contraindications to this extensive surgery. In addition, it is very important to verify that in situ carcinoma is not present in the prostatic urethra. All patients undergo a biopsy of the prostatic urethra before cystectomy. If any atypia or in situ carcinoma is noted, the urethral anastomosis is not used. In one patient previous urethral biopsy findings were negative, but at the time of operation in situ carcinoma was found at the margin of the urethra. The form of diversion was changed at the time of operation. Preoperatively, all patients must realize that an ileal conduit or a continent cutaneous urinary diversion rather than a urethral anastomosis may be necessary.

Investigation includes a computed tomographic scan of the abdomen and chest. The usual blood studies are obtained, including liver function tests. A barium enema is given to make sure no colonic abnormalities are present.

The patient is placed on clear liquids 3 days before the operation. He is admitted 2 days before surgery and given an extensive bowel preparation, employing polyethylene glycol electrolyte (GoLYTELY). This preparation has worked well and appears to be better tolerated than many others. When the GoLYTELY is stopped the bowel movements stop, and the patient is not kept up all night before the operation. A standard oral antibiotic combination, usually neomycin and erythromycin, is given. Parenteral antibiotics are provided as well. In the past, ampicillin and gentamycin have been the chosen parenteral antibiotics.

OPERATIVE TECHNIQUE

A standard nerve-sparing radical cystoprostatectomy with associated lymph node dissection is performed (Fig. 60–1).[2] No prostatic apical tissue is left: this tissue can provide a source of transitional cell carcinoma or adenocarcinoma of the prostate. We have seen previously unrecognized adenocarcinoma of the prostate in cystoprostatectomy specimens in as many as 30 percent of patients. The apical dissection is critical to the success of the operation, not only for preservation of the neurovascular bundle and potency but also for an accurate cecal urethral anastomosis.

In the presence of grossly positive lymph nodes, we have not always proceeded with this form of urinary diversion. We have had patients with microscopical nodal disease who have received chemotherapy after creation of ileocolic neobladders.

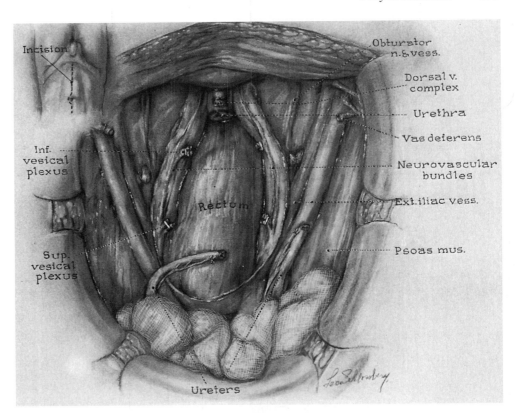

Figure 60–1. A nerve-sparing cysto-prostatectomy has been performed through a midline incision. The dorsal vein complex is ligated and the urethra is defined. All prostate has been removed. (From Marshall FF. J Urol 139:1266, 1988. Copyright by Williams & Wilkins.)

An appendectomy is performed and the right colon is mobilized extensively around the hepatic flexure so that essentially the entire right colon is available for the neobladder. An additional 30 cm of ileum is defined as well. Usually the cecum will descend to the urethra. All of this bowel is now available for a neobladder rather than a "wasting" bowel with a nipple formation.

A standard ileocolic anastomosis is then performed to reconstitute the bowel. Initially we utilized a sutured anastomosis, but we are now using the TLC50 and the RL60 staplers.* A generous side-to-side anastomosis is created, and the stapler reduces operative time. The bowel is then divided on its antimesenteric border.

The large bowel bleeds more than the small bowel, and electrocautery is applied to divide the large bowel. Scissors can be used to divide the small bowel (Fig. 60–2). The bowel is then placed in an S-shaped configuration, and after division stay sutures are placed. The posterior walls are sewn together from the inside with running 3-0 absorbable polyglycolic acid (PGA) sutures (Fig. 60–3). The entire bowel is not divided initially so that less bleeding occurs, and it is divided on its antimesenteric border as the suturing proceeds. After the posterior suture lines have been completed, the most dependent portion of cecum is identified and an 8-mm seromuscular portion excised. The mucosa is then incised and everted

with 4-0 chromic catgut sutures (Fig. 60–4). This eversion of mucosa provides for a better cecal urethral anastomosis, which will reduce the incidence of stricture. Either five or six 2-0 PGA sutures are used for a cecal urethral anastomosis, similar to a radical prostatectomy. We also fix the cecum to the posterior aspect of the symphysis, as in a Marshall-Marchetti or "pinup" operation.[3]

The left ureter is brought retroperitoneally under the mesocolon to the right side. It is easier to reimplant a ureter in a colonic than in a small bowel segment. Frozen sections are obtained to verify no carcinoma in situ in the ureter or urethra. Reimplantation of the left ureter may be the most difficult part of this operation. Although we have performed this reimplant from the outside, it is often easier to perform it from the inside, creating a submucosal tunnel (Fig. 60–5). A tacking suture is placed where the ureter enters the colon to hold the ureter in place (Fig. 60–6). A psoas hitch is performed to anchor the colonic wall to the psoas muscle and prevent migration of the neobladder at the site of the ureteral reimplant on filling.

The bladder is then closed and a 24 or 26 Fr. Malecot catheter brought through the colonic segment through a separate stab wound and out to the right abdomen. Next, 5 or 8 Fr. feeding tubes are placed as stents in the ureters and brought alongside this Malecot suprapubic tube. A 22 Fr. Foley catheter is left through the cecal urethral anastomosis. The colon is also fixed to the anterior abdominal wall at the site

---

*Ethicon, Johnson and Johnson Co, Somerville, New Jersey.

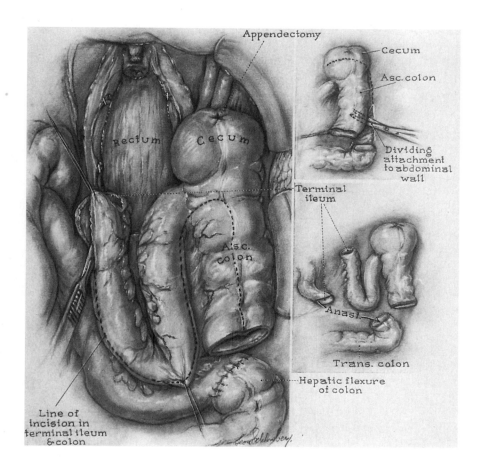

Figure 60–2. To construct the neobladder, 15 cm of ascending colon and 30 cm of ileum are utilized. Extensive mobilization of the right colon allows the descent of the cecum to the urethra. The ileocolic anastomosis is performed using the stapler to reduce operative time. The bowel is divided on its antimesenteric border through the ileocecal valve. (From Marshall FF. J Urol 139:1266, 1988. Copyright by Williams & Wilkins.)

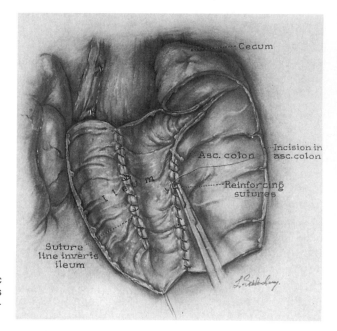

Figure 60–3. The posterior walls of the bowel are run with 3-0 polyglycolic acid absorbable sutures. Every 2.0 cm an interrupted reinforcing suture is placed. (From Marshall FF. J Urol 139:1266, 1988. Copyright by Williams & Wilkins.)

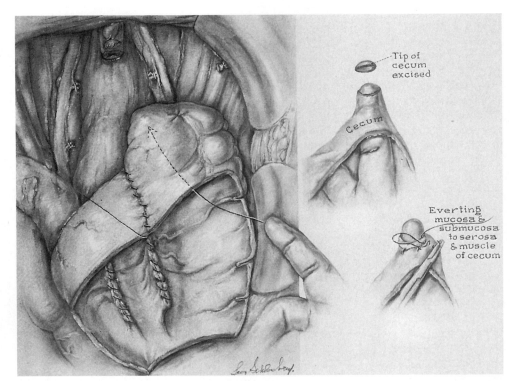

Tip of
cecum
excised

Cecum

Everting
mucosa &
submucosa
to serosa
& muscle
of cecum

Figure 60–4. The most inferior portion of the cecum is identified and an 8.0-mm seromuscular segment excised. The mucosa is incised and everted with 4-0 chromic sutures. (From Marshall FF. J Urol 139:1266, 1988. Copyright by Williams & Wilkins.)

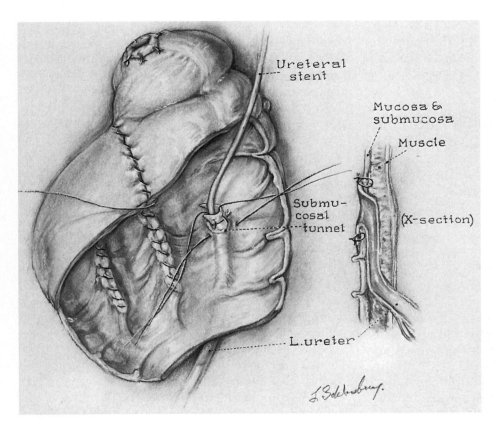

Ureteral
stent

Mucosa &
submucosa

Muscle

Submu-
cosal
tunnel

(X-section)

L.ureter

Figure 60–5. A submucosal tunnel is made through the colonic segment of the neobladder. Ureteral reimplants are performed with interrupted 5-0 absorbable sutures. An 8 Fr. feeding tube is generally left as a stent. (From Marshall FF. J Urol 139:1266, 1988. Copyright by Williams & Wilkins.)

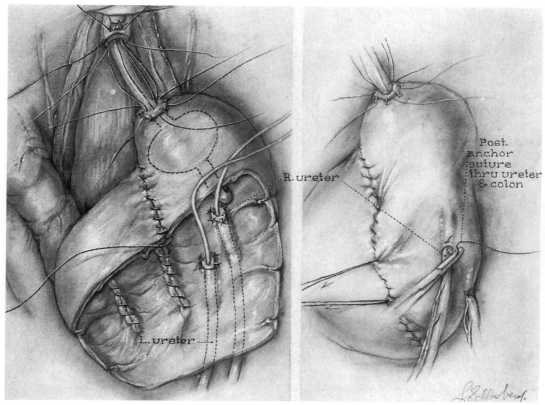

Figure 60–6. For the urethral cecal anastomosis, five or six 2-0 absorbable sutures are used. At the site of entrance of the ureter into the colon a small tacking suture is placed to anchor the ureter in this position. (From Marshall FF. J Urol 139:1266, 1988. Copyright by Williams & Wilkins.)

of the suprapubic cystostomy. Hemovac drains are placed. The bladder is then filled to make sure no leaks are obvious (Fig. 60–7).

POSTOPERATIVE MANAGEMENT AND COMPLICATIONS

Ureteral stents are usually removed after approximately 10 days and an intravenous pyelogram is obtained. The patient is sent home for 4 to 5 weeks with the suprapubic tube and urethral catheter in place. When the patient returns to the hospital, the urethral catheter is removed, the suprapubic tube is clamped, and a cystogram and cystometrogram are obtained. Often it takes a day or two for the patient to learn to void. He recognizes that "bowel gas sensation" really represents distention of the neobladder. The patient is still urged to void on a regular basis, even if he does not have obvious sensation. Usually after 1 to 2 days he learns the Valsalva maneuver, relaxes the perineal musculature, and voids with a reasonable stream to completion. The postvoid residuals are almost always under 50 ml after a few days. The suprapubic tube is then removed, and the patient is asked to return in a few months, or sooner if any problems exist. Sometimes

neobladders can enlarge, and usually they do enlarge over the course of the first 6 months. Patients are followed every 6 months with serum and radiological tests.

We have now performed many ileocolic bladder procedures and remain pleased with the results. In this highly selected patient population, relatively few complications have occurred, especially given the difficulty of the operation. Some patients have died of recurrent tumor. Most neobladders function well until death. Most patients have had excellent levels of continence, without wearing any pads and voiding almost to completion. Most patients have no eneuresis. Some patients have accidents if they do not get up at night to void or if they consume large quantities of fluids. Patients have been urged to void at least once a night, but some have not followed even that recommendation. Continence has been poorer in patients over the age of 70 years.

Once the urinary tract has become sterile, infections are infrequent. This form of closed continent urinary diversion will probably have fewer problems with infection than conduits or other forms of diversion with connection to the skin.

In a female or in a male patient with in situ carcinoma of the urethra, we have performed a cutaneous cecal reservoir as described by Rowland and col-

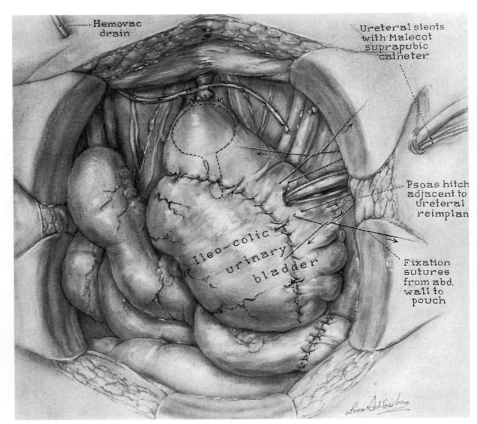

Figure 60–7. The neobladder is closed and the suprapubic Malecot catheter placed. The ureteral stents are brought out alongside the suprapubic tube. Absorbable sutures are placed in the colon adjacent to the ureteral reimplants to fix the neobladder at the site of the reimplantation (psoas hitch). The bladder is verified for any leaks and a Hemovac drain placed. (From Marshall FF. J Urol 139:1266, 1988. Copyright by Williams & Wilkins.)

leagues.[4] This reservoir has functioned very well. If difficulties are evident with specific bowel segments, a small bowel bladder can be constructed.[5] We have performed this operation with excellent results. The sigmoid colon can also be utilized.[6]

Vitamin B_{12} deficiency can develop in as many as 25 percent of patients.[7] Megaloblastic anemia may not be present because serum folate levels are normal. Neurological symptoms can theoretically develop and may be irreversible.

Although the ileocolic neobladder procedure is a long and demanding operation, continent micturition and sexual function can be maintained. Patients can enjoy a surprisingly normal existence.

REFERENCES

1. Marshall FF. Creation of an ileocolic bladder after cystectomy. J Urol 139:1264, 1988.
2. Walsh PC, Mostwin JL. Radical prostatectomy and cystoprostatectomy with preservation of potency: Results using a new nerve-sparing technique. Br J Urol 56:694, 1984.
3. Marshall VF, Marchetti AA, Krantz KE. The correction of stress incontinence by simple vesicourethral suspension. Surg Gynecol Obstet 88:509, 1949.
4. Rowland RG, Mitchell ME, Bihrle R. The cecoileal continent urinary reservoir. World J Urol 3:185, 1985.
5. Hautmann RE, Egghart G, Frohneberg D, Miller K. The ileal neobladder. J Urol 139:39, 1988.
6. Reddy PK. Detubularized sigmoid reservoir for bladder replacement after cystoprostatectomy: Preliminary report of new configuration. Urology 29:625, 1987.
7. Steiner, MS, Morton RA, Marshall FF. Vitamin B_{12} deficiency in patients with ileocolic neobladders. J Urol 149:255, 1993.

Chapter 61

Gastrocystoplasty and Bladder Replacement with Stomach

Michael C. Carr and Michael E. Mitchell

The treatment of dysfunctional and neurogenic bladder has been facilitated by clean intermittent catheterization, which has allowed the use of various segments of bowel for lower urinary tract reconstruction. Ileum, cecum, or sigmoid colon, as isolated flaps or in various shapes, combinations, and quantities, has been used to create a large and compliant reservoir for urine. Thus, procedures such as the Mainz, Kock, Indiana, and LeBag are now in common use. Long-term applications of several of these procedures have been reported, but many of these applications are relatively new. To this list must be added the use of stomach for lower urinary tract reconstruction, which has been popularized in the past several years.[1-3]

Unfortunately, side effects and problems have been noted with the use of various intestinal segments for a urinary reservoir. The experience with ureterosigmoidostomy led to the recognition of electrolyte abnormalities. Hyperchloremic metabolic acidosis was noted in many patients with ureterosigmoidostomies secondary to active resorption of chloride from urine by the descending and sigmoid colon. The large surface area and long contact time exacerbated this phenomenon.

The same electrolyte shifts are also noted for continent reservoirs of both large and small bowel and for segments of intestine used to augment the bladder or replace the ureter.[4] In patients with normal renal function, it is uncommon to note specific and significant electrolyte abnormalities, because homeostatic mechanisms usually correct for potential acidosis or hyperchloremia.[5] In young patients, however, the consequences of taxing buffer stores that are primarily dependent on the bone minerals are uncertain and worrisome. Patients with acute or chronic renal failure often manifest electrolyte changes if bowel is placed in the lower urinary tract; therefore, allow-

ances for increased acidosis and hyperchloremia must be made. With the active resorption of chloride, ammonia is also noted to be reabsorbed from the urine by passive diffusion or active transport, or both. In healthy patients, this is of no significance. In patients with diminished hepatic function, however, the net ammonia resorption may lead to coma. In addition, medications excreted unchanged in the urine that are absorbed by the bowel may reach toxic levels in a patient whose intestine is in contact with the urine.

Since bowel mucosa does not apparently change metabolic function, the consequences of its use in the lower urinary tract, other than electrolyte resorption, can be seen. Mucus production continues when intestinal mucosa is in contact with urine. Although differing in character depending on the bowel segment, mucus increases the viscosity and can congeal into clumps capable of obstructing small catheters or even the urethra. Patients on clean intermittent catheterization who have significant mucus are at risk for retention and possibly bladder rupture.[6] Such patients should irrigate with syringe aspiration on a daily basis, and continue such irrigations until mucus is clearly proved not to be a problem. Changes in mucus quantity and character are often early indications of infection, and analysis of urine from patients with intestinocystoplasty will show a significant cellular spin sediment. In contrast, patients with a gastrocystoplasty or gastric reservoir often have clear urine without obvious mucus.

The consequences of resection of a significant length of bowel for lower urinary tract reconstruction may be significant in patients with limited intestinal reserve. Loss of the ileocecal valve has resulted in transient diarrhea in some patients, but this has not been a significant or chronic problem in our experience. Patients with insufficient or radiated bowel are ideal candidates for stomach utilization, because this tissue is usually not missed as a resorptive surface and usually not in the field of radiation. Other long-term changes in bowel used in the urinary tract, which may be of great significance, are still unde-fined. Changes in the fibroelastic character of the segment may be of major importance. Tumors have been noted to develop in augmented bladder.[7] The potential for tumor to develop in intestine chroni-cally in contact with urine without fecal contamina-tion, however, is not known. The development of adenocarcinoma in patients with ureterosigmoidos-tomy is very disturbing but may represent a com-pletely different situation in which urine and feces are combined. It is hoped that the lower incidence of malignancy after cystoplasty is not just a function of shorter follow-up. Long-term rat studies in our laboratory and others have not demonstrated obvious potential for tumors to develop.

Spontaneous perforation of an augmented bladder and continent reservoir has also been noted. The risk of this serious, and sometimes lethal, complication is particularly associated with patients who have poor sensation (neurogenic bladder) and high outflow re-sistance, and with those who are not compliant with catheterizations. Spontaneous rupture of an aug-mented bladder has been observed in all bowel seg-ments but seems to be more likely in a patient with sigmoid augmentation.[8]

The effectiveness and efficacy of gastrocystoplasty was noted in several dog models.[9, 10] It became clear that stomach could be used to augment the bladder in the canine. Net excretion of chloride ions oc-curred, which supports a main buffer system of the urine (ammonium chloride). This permits the act of secretion of acid without the use of titratable acids that ultimately and potentially leads to the depletion of the buffer systems (Fig. 61–1). Ammonia resorption does not occur either, as has been observed when large and small bowel segments are used in the uri-nary tract. In a partial renal failure model, gastrocys-toplasty actually protected the dogs with chronic re-nal failure from the acidosis of chronic ammonium chloride loss. Theoretically, a patient with chronic acidosis and renal insufficiency could be protected, in part, by gastrocystoplasty, whereas large and small bowel in the same capacity would only serve to in-crease the acidotic state. This has proved to be the case clinically. The presence of acid in the urine may also contribute to the decrease in infections that likewise has been noted. This has been borne out by long-term study in rats. However, this study also noted changes in the augmented segments with meta-plasia, but no malignant degeneration.[11]

The use of stomach has proved invaluable in recon-structive procedures for patients with major complex problems. We have applied it to patients in whom no

Small or Large Bowel Wall

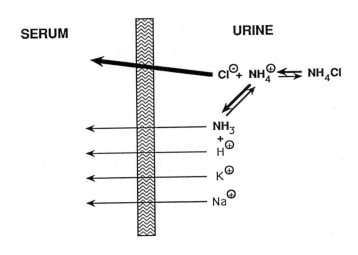

Stomach

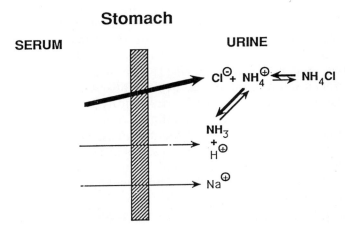

Figure 61–1. Large or small bowel actively resorbs chloride ion, which results in shifting of the equilibrium from ammonium chloride to ammonia and hydrogen ion. Ammonia is passively resorbed in the mechanism. The stomach actively excretes chloride into the urine, driving the equilibrium constant to ammonium chloride. Ammonia is thus locked in the urine. Hydronium ion, potassium, and sodium probably passively follow the chloride to preserve electrical neutrality.

other type of bowel was available for urinary recon-struction, including those with previous radiation and those with no large or reduced small bowel (the cloacal exstrophy group). Stomach has also been se-lected for patients with metabolic acidosis in whom the addition of large or small bowel would cause a worsening because of chloride and ammonia resorp-tion, and for patients with chronic and recurrent in-fections.

Urolithiasis has been noted increasingly in patients after augmentation cystoplasty.[12] Predisposing risk factors include the use of metallic staples, chronic intermittent catheterization with chronic bacilluria, chronic hyperchloremic metabolic acidosis, and mu-cus production from intestinal patches. No stones have been observed in several large series of gastrocystoplasty patients. Whether this relates to added buffering, a reduction in urease-producing urinary tract infections, or other processes not yet identified is unknown. Theoretically, it would be possible for stones to form in acid urine (e.g., uric acid, cysteine).

However, the more widespread application of gastrocystoplasties has led to the identification of some complications. Foremost among these is the so-called hematuria-dysuria syndrome, which is unique to the use of stomach in the urinary tract and has been seen in approximately 36 percent of children.[13] The symptoms are usually intermittent and self-limiting, and improve with time. The spectrum of severity is seen, ranging from intermittent dysuria and tea-colored urine to the rare occurrence of ulcer formation and bladder perforation. Most patients are controlled by intermittent use of H_2 blockers, sodium bicarbonate bladder irrigation, or oral bicarbonate therapy. A few children have required short-term use of oral omeprazole. The symptoms are more pronounced in adults, and in those children with sensate urethras in whom voiding is attempted or in whom there is wetness. The cause is believed to be related to hydrochloric acid production by the gastric segment and reduced buffering effect by urine. However, symptoms have been seen even with urine acidity in the normal range. There is a risk of peptic ulcer development in the gastric portion of a defunctionalized gastrocystoplasty. Patients with anuric states (e.g., renal failure or urinary diversion) should be treated with basic bladder irrigations, such as phosphate buffered saline or bicarbonate, to prevent this.

Patients with gastrocystoplasties who lose large amounts of hydrochloric acid, sodium, and potassium in the urine may become severely dehydrated and alkalotic. This usually occurs only when patients have significant salt losses from the bowel or kidney such as with severe diarrhea or emesis, salt-losing nephropathy, or (rarely) hypergastrinemia. The ensuing hyponatremic, hypochloremic alkalosis requires intravenous saline volume replacement and is usually easily corrected. It may be that excessive salt loss related to increased serum gastrin relates to reduced acid production in the stomach secondary to gastric resection. This can sometimes be reversed by carbonic acid (soda pop) with meals.

These newly recognized complications of gastrocystoplasty have led to efforts to eliminate gastric mucosa. A urothelium-lined bladder with gastrointestinal tract muscle augmentation of the detrusor muscle was attempted as early as 1955. Other demucosalized intestinal segments have been used in several other studies.[14, 15] Detrusorrhaphy or autoaugmentation results in a bladder lined with urothelium. The detrusor, however, is replaced with fibrous tissue or whatever happens to adhere, and this may result in inadequate bladder volume.[16] Dewan and Byard described an animal model combining the use of a demucosalized stomach muscle with bladder detrusorectomy.[17] The demucosalized augmentation with gastric flap (DAWG) uses a full-thickness urothelial graft in conjunction with a raw inner surface of incorporated stomach muscle/submucosa. This technique has now been applied to nine patients in a clinical setting.

OPERATIVE TECHNIQUE

Wedge (Mitchell) Gastrocystoplasty

Patient selection for gastrocystoplasty is no different from that for any bladder reconstruction procedure. Initially, the selection was limited to patients with a deficiency of bowel or with metabolic acidosis. The procedure is well suited, however, to patients who use small catheters or who would generally tolerate mucus and highly viscous urine poorly, and to those with chronic urinary infection problems.

Rigorous bowel preparation is generally not required. Most patients are placed on a liquid diet 48 hours before surgery and receive a bottle of magnesium citrate 24 hours before the procedure. Mechanical and antibiotic bowel preparations have been used in patients anticipating major reconstruction or who have had multiple previous abdominal procedures. Recently, because of restrictions on the length of hospital stays, patients have been admitted the day of surgery. When possible, all patients undergo preoperative video urodynamics and either an intravenous pyelogram or a nuclear scan. Every effort is made to sterilize the urine before the procedure. In children we have not thought it necessary to obtain an upper gastrointestinal series, but in adults this may be prudent.

The surgical procedure of wedge gastrocystoplasty is similar initially to that of antral resection. A long midline incision is made from the symphysis pubis to the xyphoid process. A self-retaining ring retractor is very useful in this procedure, which demands proper exposure deep in the pelvis and high in the epigastria.

In the case of gastrocystoplasty the bladder is initially explored through only the lower portion of the incision and opened in sagittal plane in the midline from the bladder neck (anteriorly) to the trigone (posteriorly) (Fig. 61–2). The upper portion of the incision and the peritoneum usually need to be opened only after the bladder preparation is complete. At this point, ureteral reimplantation is performed if necessary. It is also a good time to develop a plane around the bladder neck should this be necessary (as for implantation of an artificial sphincter or for a sling procedure). Pediatric feeding tubes are left in the

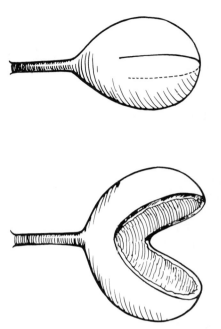

Figure 61–2. Bladder preparation should be performed before gastric resection. The bladder incision extends from the bladder neck anteriorly to just above the trigonal posteriorly. Ureteral reimplants and bladder neck surgery are usually done before gastric resection also. Pediatric feeding tubes are left in the ureters until after the augmentation is completed.

ureters to facilitate identification and prevent injury during the augmentation. The bladder is packed off with a moist sponge and the upper abdomen explored.

The stomach is brought well into the surgical field. It is helpful to use large Babcock clamps for this maneuver, taking care that they do not compromise or injure the gastroepiploic artery (GEA). The GEA is then carefully evaluated. Common observations at this point will be that the GEA along the left inferior margin of the greater curvature either is very thin or will apparently dive into the stomach wall. For this reason, it is usually preferable to base the wedge gastric flap on the *right* GEA. The greater omentum is then incised parallel to the GEA several centimeters inferior to this vessel (Fig. 61–3). The electrocautery and bipolar electrode can be used to do this very effectively. Larger vessels, however, may need to be ligated (Fig. 61–3). Although some of the omental vessels are quite significant, and it may seem preferable to base the wedge flap on these vessels, we have not done so to date, as it would necessitate bringing the blood supply of the flap anterior to the abdominal contents. The gastric wedge is next selected with the apex of the wedge close to, but not including, the lesser curvature of the stomach. The length along the greater curvature is usually about 9 to 15 cm, but this depends on the patient's age and size, and the anticipated final bladder volume. The position of the wedge will depend on the anticipated blood supply.

If the more constant right GEA pedicle is used, the wedge is usually taken closer to the cardia of the stomach. The rule of thumb is that the largest possible wedge should be taken and it should have the longest blood supply. Usually about one third to one half of the stomach is removed. The short arteries from the gastroepiploic pedicle to the stomach flap are kept intact. The others along the anticipated pedicle are carefully ligated in place and divided (Fig. 61–3). Great care must be taken during this portion of the procedure to make sure that the GEA is protected and not injured. It is sometimes helpful to gently apply papaverine solution on the artery along its entire length to prevent spasm.

The GEA at the distal end of the wedge is next divided. The 90-mm GIA stapler is used to resect the wedge. The staples in place prevent blood loss from the flap and stomach during repair of the stomach (Fig. 61–4). The wedge flap is wrapped in a moist sponge and placed in the pelvis, with a moist sponge over the pedicle to protect it during the gastric repair. The repair of the stomach resection is made in two layers: an outer layer of interrupted 3-0 silk sutures

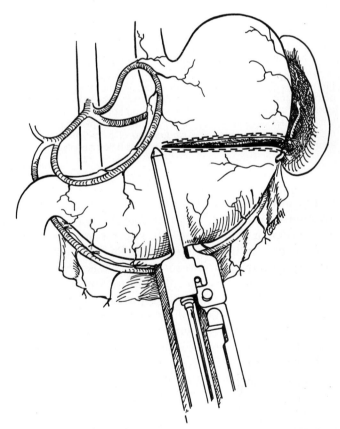

Figure 61–3. The omentum is incised several centimeters caudal and parallel to the gastroepiploic artery (GEA). Ligation and division of the short vessels between the GEA create the vascular pedicle. The triangular wedge is made as large as possible and usually measures 9 to 15 cm in length along the greater curvature. If the pedicle is based on the right GEA, the left GEA is divided as illustrated. The GIA stapler is then used to resect the segment as shown.

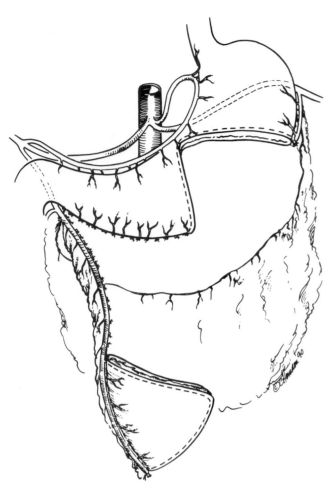

Figure 61-4. The flap has been removed and staples are left in place to prevent bleeding and leakage from the segment. A two-layer closure of the stomach is performed: an outer layer of interrupted 3-0 silk and an inner layer of 3-0 Monocryl. The staples may be left in the posterior suture line. The wedge flap is placed in moist saline sponges to prevent injury to the wedge and blood supply.

in the muscularis and serosa, and an inner layer of through-and-through running 3-0 Monocryl suture. The posterior interrupted silk sutures are placed before the gastric lumen is opened. The staples may be left in the posterior suture lines. A nasogastric tube is then positioned across the suture line and left in place until bowel motility is appreciated; this usually occurs on the fourth or fifth postoperative day. The wedge-shaped gastric flap is then brought with its blood supply through the mesentery of the transverse colon and through the root of the small bowel mesentery (Fig. 61-5). It therefore courses in a retroperitoneal position. One should make sure that there is no twisting of this pedicle in the process of placing the flap on the bladder. The wedge-shaped flap should reach well down into the pelvis without tension on the blood supply. If a further length of pedicle is required, this is secured by dissecting proximally at the gastroduodenal angle.

The wedge flap is next opened to form a parallelo-

gram-shaped flap. All the staples are removed. The posterior apex is then sutured into the area of the posterior bladder wall close to the trigone (Fig. 61-6). Running, locking through-and-through 3-0 Monocryl sutures are then used to sew the back wall in place. A second layer of 3-0 Vicryl sutures through the muscularis and serosa then ensure a watertight anastomosis. A Malecot catheter is usually placed before the anterior segment of the augmentation is sutured in place. The size of this catheter depends on the age of the patient, but it is usually preferable to have a larger than 14 Fr. tube. This tube is usually brought out through native bladder if possible, but it may exit through the flap. The ureteral catheters are left in place during the posterior anastomosis and may then be removed if reimplantation or tapering has not been performed. The anterior portion of the augmentation is then completed and the bladder tested to make sure that the suture lines are watertight. Any leaks must be repaired at this point.

We tend not to drain gastrocystoplasty patients. The omentum, which is still intact, is placed over the anterior portion of the bowel after the windows in the retroperitoneum have been closed with running chromic suture. With the omentum tucked over the bowel and behind the augmented bladder, the blad-

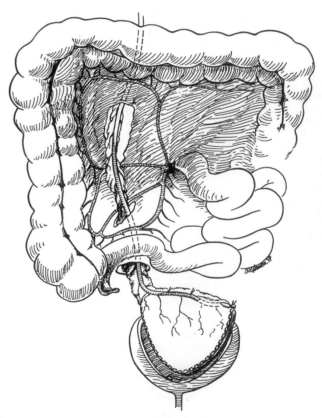

Figure 61-5. After closure of the stomach the flap is carefully brought through the base of the mesentery of the transverse colon and small bowel, and is positioned in the pelvis with its blood supply on the right side.

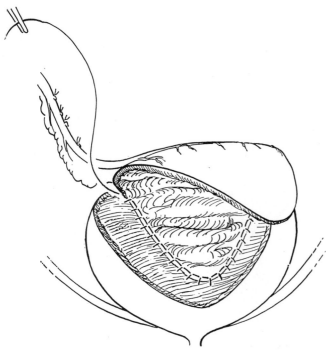

Figure 61–6. The staples are removed and the posterior aspect of the flap is sutured to the back wall of the bladder. A two-layer closure is used, beginning at the apex of the gastric wedge and the posterior aspect of the open bladder. The first layer is a running, locking 3-0 Monocryl suture; the second is a simple running 3-0 Vicryl suture.

der resides in a position close to the original. A careful check should be made that there is no tension on the pedicle of the flap.

Total Bladder Replacement with Wedge Flap

Total bladder replacement by stomach is possible with the wedge flap. After removal of the staples, the apex of the wedge is simply sutured to the urethra (Fig. 61–7). This may be feasible in a patient with an intact urethra (bladder replacement). Several options are available for patients requiring construction of a catheterizable reservoir. A distal ureter may be used as a catheterizable channel. The ureter can be tunneled in between mucosa and muscularis of the reservoir wall to provide continence. The appendix has been used in a similar manner (Fig. 61–8). A bladder tube, using a strip of the gastric flap, has been constructed successfully and is nippled into the reservoir to provide continence. This has resulted in a channel that is catheterizable and dry (Fig. 61–9). Our preference, however, is to use a tunnel technique for dryness with construction of a gastric reservoir. In bladder replacement it is usually most convenient to open the wedge completely and suture the posterior tip (which is usually the anterior apex of the wedge) onto the urethra. Subsequently, with the gastric seg-

ment open, ureteral reimplantation is easily performed in much the same way that a tunneled reimplant would be performed in the bladder. A plane between the mucosa and muscularis of the gastric flap is usually easily defined with sharp dissection. The anterior portion of the apex is then sewn to the anterior portion of the urethra, and the lateral aspects of the wedge are closed in a two-layer fashion with running 3-0 Monocryl and Vicryl. A suprapubic tube (a Malecot catheter) may be brought through the gastric tissue, but if this is done, it is advisable to suture the wall of the gastric reservoir to the anterior abdominal wall as for a gastrostomy. This prevents intraperitoneal leakage when the tube is subsequently removed. A catheterizable stoma should be constructed flush with adjacent tissue and in such a manner that catheterization can be performed without difficulty. A small V-flap of skin and spatulation of the catheterizable channel works well. *If catheterization is difficult in the operating room, it will be impossible out of the operating room.*

Demucosalized Gastric Flap Procedure

Augmentation of a bladder after detrusorrhaphy with demucosalized gastric flap (the DAWG procedure) is similar to gastrocystoplasty. The bladder is approached initially. It is helpful to have a Foley catheter in the bladder connected to a reservoir of irrigation saline that can be raised or lowered to fill or empty the bladder as desired. The bladder is filled to a pressure of approximately 20 cm of water and the detrusor incised in the midline sagittal plane. Great care is taken to preserve the transitional epithelium in finding the plane between the transitional epithelium and muscularis. It is easiest to use blunt and sharp dissection with the bladder full for this purpose (Fig. 61–10). If no holes are made in the epithelium, this usually proceeds very easily. Once a hole is made and the bladder is decompressed, it becomes very difficult to dissect the plane between the transitional epithelium and the bladder muscularis. We usually remove muscularis from two thirds to three quarters of the anterior and lateral wall of the bladder. The bladder is emptied by lowering the reservoir, and gently packed with moist sponges.

A gastric flap is obtained. Before it is brought into the pelvis, however, it is demucosalized. This is done very easily by removing the staples and placing four quadrant sutures for traction so that the flap is opened as a parallelogram. A vascular loop is gently placed around the pedicle with enough traction to temporarily interrupt blood supply to the pedicle. It takes approximately 10 to 15 minutes to sharply dissect the mucosa from the muscularis. Potts tenotomy scissors are used for this purpose (Fig. 61–11). The

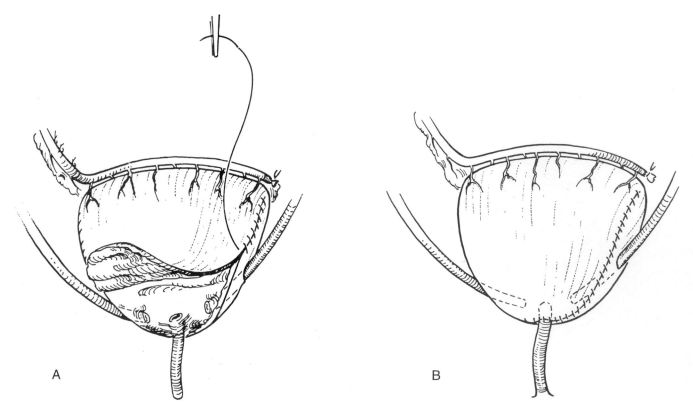

Figure 61–7. *A,* Total bladder replacement is feasible with a wedge gastric flap. The urethra may be sutured to the apex of the flap, which can be tubularized to provide a nice bladder neck. The ureters are reimplanted into the posterior gastric wall in a submucosal position. The urethra may be tunneled into the stomach if no external sphincter mechanism is present. *B,* Bladder closure is accomplished anteriorly. The triangular configuration later stretches to become spherical.

proper plane is easily found and tends to have a somewhat foamy appearance. Once the mucosa is removed, the pedicle vascular loop is loosened and bleeders are electrocauterized with the bipolar cautery. Most of the bleeding will be in the midline where the perforators follow the gastroepiploic pedicle. The demucosalized flap is brought into the pelvis as with any augmentation. The demucosalized flap is then laid directly on top of the outside of the bladder epithelium, raw surface to raw surface. Either a Penrose or suction drain is then placed between the transitional epithelium and flap and brought out through the abdominal wall (Fig. 61–12). This will be removed in approximately 48 hours. The demucosalized gastric flap is sutured in place using a running, locking 3-0 Vicryl suture as a single-layer closure. In an effort to keep the contact between the transitional epithelium and the demucosalized gastric flap, the bladder is kept partially filled at approximately 20 cm water pressure using a vented drainage system. This system is maintained for about 5 to 7 days. Subsequently, the patient is placed on either intermittent catheterization or intermittent clamping of a suprapubic tube. If a suprapubic tube is used, it is brought through the intact bladder wall rather than through the healing transitional epithelium and demucosalized gastric flap.

POSTOPERATIVE CARE

Management of the gastrocystoplasty patient is similar to that of any patient with intestinal augmentation. Mucus is generally not a problem and often irrigation of the bladder is not routinely performed. All patients are maintained on intravenous antibiotics initially and converted to chronic suppression for at least 2 months after surgery. H_2 blockade, usually consisting of ranitidine (1 mg/kg every 8 hours), is continued for 1 to 2 months postoperatively. If the patient then develops dysuria or perineal pain, the ranitidine is reinstituted until the symptoms resolve or the hematuria improves. Removal of the suprapubic tube is dependent on the ability of the patient to empty the bladder. A trial period of at least 1 week of continuous clamping is usually wise while the patient begins to void, otherwise intermittent catheterization is reinstituted. Finally, patients with anuria or dilute urine may rarely require irrigation with phosphate buffer if low pH and irritation is observed. Infection is less common with the gastrocystoplasty patient, but asymptomatic infection is usually not treated unless the organism is thought to be significant in terms of potential stone formation or the potential for pyelonephritis. Serum electrolytes should be followed periodically.

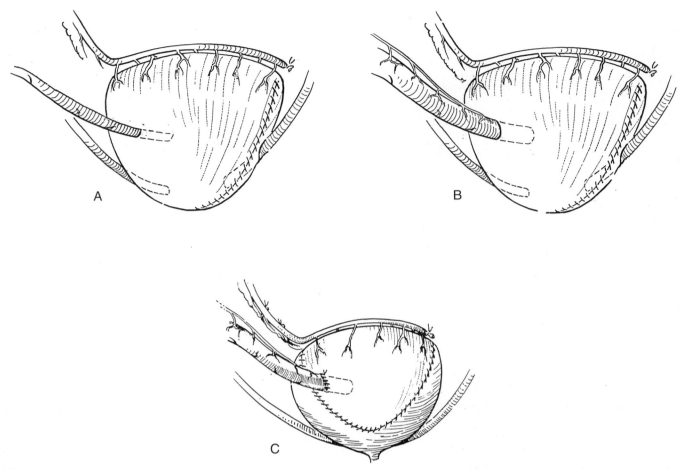

Figure 61–8. *A,* A distal ureter can be tunneled in between the mucosa and muscularis of the gastric reservoir, combined with a transuretero-ureterostomy or nephrectomy. *B,* The appendix may be tunneled into the reservoir to create a catheterizable stoma (Mitrofanoff procedure). *C,* In instances of gastric augmentation the appendix may be tunneled into the bladder or gastric segment. The latter is better because the appendix can be tunneled after the augmentation is completed.

For patients who have undergone the DAWG procedure, we have employed a system of humping the bladder drainage tube over the bed to increase the intravesical pressure. This is done to allow for coaptation of the seromuscular flap to the underlying epithelium during the healing phase, and is maintained for 5 to 7 days. The remainder of the postoperative care is the same as for patients who have undergone a gastrocystoplasty. Ranitidine has not been needed in these patients, since the gastric mucosa has been removed and an acidic environment is not present.

Our initial experience in 80 patients with stomach augmentation or replacement in bladder has been very encouraging. With an average follow-up of 4 years, all but three patients have shown either stable or improved renal function. All but seven patients are dry and urodynamics have demonstrated a marked improvement in compliance. Gastrin levels have not been elevated in our group and no patient has experienced duodenal or gastric ulceration. Early complications included gastric bleeding in one patient that did not require transfusion, a perivesical extravasation in one patient, and an obstruction of a ureter reim-

planted into the stomach in one patient. Delayed complications have included bowel obstruction in seven patients, spontaneous bladder perforation in three, and hematuria and/or dysuria in 28. Seventy-seven percent of patients on clean intermittent catheterization have had at least one positive urine culture. Our experience now extends to more than 80 patients with varied diagnoses, including neurogenic bladder, bladder exstrophy, exstrophy of the cloaca and urethral valves, and ectopic ureter. We have performed augmentation and bladder replacement in adults and children, although most of our experience is with younger patients. Stomach can be used to totally replace the bladder, but older male patients can experience urethral irritation. The advantages are little mucus, reduced infection, and the ability to easily tunnel ureters or a conduit as a catheterizable stoma, which make this a very appealing technique. We feel that in many clinical situations it has clear advantages over other tissues, particularly large and small bowel.

Our follow-up of patients who have undergone the DAWG procedure is limited. All have tolerated the

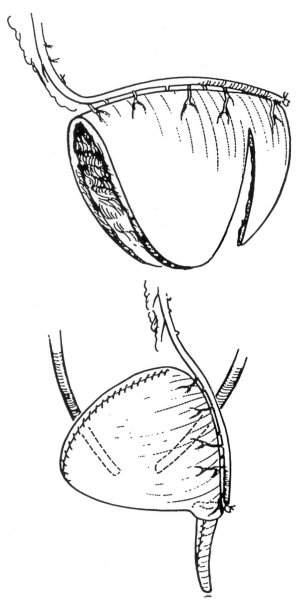

Figure 61–9. A gastric tube may be used when an appendix or distal ureter is not available. A proximal nipple can be constructed as shown to create a dry, catheterizable channel. The tunnel technique, in general, has proved more reliable than the nipple principle for dryness.

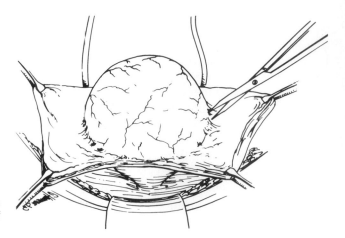

Figure 61–10. A combination of sharp and blunt dissection is used to perform the detrusorrhaphy. Distending the bladder with a reservoir of saline irrigation aids in the dissection.

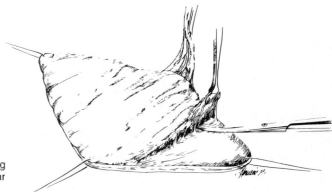

Figure 61–11. The gastric mucosa is sharply dissected from the underlying seromuscular layer. A vascular loop gently placed around the vascular pedicle minimizes the bleeding.

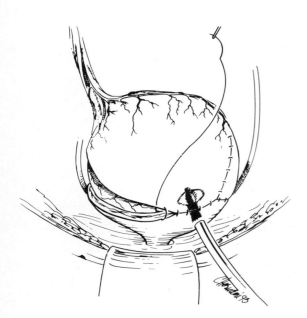

Figure 61–12. The seromuscular gastric flap is positioned over the bladder epithelium, and a Penrose or suction drain is placed between the transitional epithelium and flap. A single-layer closure using a running, locking 3-0 Vicryl suture completes the anastomosis.

procedure well. Postoperative urodynamics are necessary to demonstrate improvement in bladder capacity and compliance. For patients who have no problem with recurrent urinary tract infections or who have underlying renal insufficiency, the DAWG procedure may be an excellent alternative that avoids some of the complications of the traditional gastrocystoplasty.

Editorial Comment
Fray F. Marshall

The stomach has many favorable qualities in urinary tract reconstruction, including minimal mucus production, ease of ureteral reimplantation, and net secretion of acid. When other bowel is not available or damaged, stomach may be the primary choice for reconstruction. On the other hand, the hematuria-dysuria syndrome may be a significant problem, possibly more in adults. The demucosalized augmentation with gastric flaps (DAWG) procedure is innovative, but longer-term follow-up of these initial cases will be needed to justify its widespread use. For example, does scarring affect the later result? Stomach remains an option in urinary reconstruction, and the urologist should be aware of its possibilities.

REFERENCES

1. Sinaiko ES. Artificial bladder in man from segment of stomach. Surg Forum 8:685, 1957.
2. Leong CH. Use of the stomach for bladder replacement and urinary diversion. Ann R Coll Surg Engl 60:283, 1978.
3. Adams MC, Mitchell ME, Rink RC. Gastrocystoplasty: An alternative solution to the problem of urologic reconstruction in the severely compromised patient. J Urol 140:1152, 1988.
4. Koch MO, McDougal WS. The pathophysiology of hyperchloremic metabolic acidosis after urinary diversion through intestinal segments. Surgery 98:561, 1985.
5. Mitchell ME, Piser JA. Intestinocystoplasty and total bladder replacement in children and young adults: Follow-up in 129 cases. J Urol 138:579, 1987.
6. Elder JS, Snyder HM, Hulbert WC, Duckett JW. Perforation of the augmented bladder in patients undergoing clean intermittent catheterization. J Urol 140:1159, 1988.
7. Filmer RB, Spencer JR. Malignancies in bladder augmentations and intestinal conduits. J Urol 143:671, 1990.
8. Bauer SB, Hendren WH, Kozakewich H, et al. Perforation of the augmented bladder. J Urol 148:699, 1992.
9. Leong CH, Ong GB. Gastrocystoplasty in dogs. Aust N Z J Surg 41:272, 1972.
10. Kennedy HA, Adams MC, Mitchell ME, et al. Chronic renal failure and bladder augmentation: Stomach versus sigmoid colon in the canine model. J Urol 140:1138, 1988.
11. Klee L, Hoover DM, Mitchell ME, et al. Long-term effects of gastrocystoplasty in rats. J Urol 144:1294, 1990.
12. Blyth B, Ewalt DH, Duckett JW, Snyder HM. Lithogenic properties of enterocystoplasty. J Urol 148:575, 1992.
13. Nguyen DH, Bain MA, Salmonson KL, et al. The syndrome of dysuria and hematuria in pediatric urinary reconstruction with stomach. J Urol 150:707, 1993.
14. Oesch I. Neurourothelium in bladder augmentation: An experimental rat model. Eur Urol 14:328, 1988.
15. Salle JL, Fraga JC, Lucib A, et al. Seromuscular enterocystoplasty in dogs. J Urol 144:454, 1990.
16. Cartwright PC, Snow BW. Bladder autoaugmentation: Partial detrusor excision to augment the bladder without use of bowel. J Urol 142:1050, 1989.
17. Dewan PA, Byard RW. Autoaugmentation gastrocystoplasty in a sheep model. Br J Urol 72:56, 1993.

Chapter 62

Rectal Neobladders and Mainz Pouch II

Robert Wammack, Margit Fisch, and Rudolf Hohenfellner

EVOLUTION OF THE RECTAL NEOBLADDER

Even today the construction of a safe and simple continence mechanism remains difficult, and so it is not surprising that the pioneers of urinary diversion initially attempted to use a natural sphincter, i.e., the anal sphincter, to achieve urinary continence.

Early experience with ureterosigmoidostomy[1, 2] produced a high rate of infectious complications. Maydl first implanted the entire bladder trigone into the rectum in 1892[3] and his series of 173 patients demonstrated an operative mortality of 31 percent; 12.5 percent developed peritonitis and 24.4 percent had ascending infections.[4] It was believed that reflux of infected bowel contents and urine into the upper urinary tract was chiefly responsible for pyelonephritis and progressive renal function deterioration.

It was believed that the problem could be solved by separating the urinary and fecal streams. Mauclaire first published details of such a technique in 1895.[5, 6] Bowel continuity was disrupted at the level of the rectum, the ureters were implanted into the rectum stump, and a terminal sigmoid colostomy was created (Fig. 62–1). Apart from the colostomy, however, this technique has distinctive disadvantages. Ghoneim, who had used a modification of this procedure for more than 20 years in Egypt, described renal function loss in 30 percent of patients and nocturnal incontinence in up to 40 percent.[7] To maintain urinary and fecal continence and avoid a colostomy, Gersuny mobilized and pulled down the proximal sigmoid through the perineum anterior to the rectum (Fig. 62–2).[8] By this means the anal sphincter is used in an effort to achieve both bowel and urinary control. Heitz-Boyer and Hovelaque also created a rectal bladder, pulling the sigmoid through the pelvic floor

posterior to the rectum and passing it directly beneath the anal mucosa (Fig. 62–3).[9]

Reporting on a series of eight patients who had undergone the Gersuny procedure, Ghoneim and

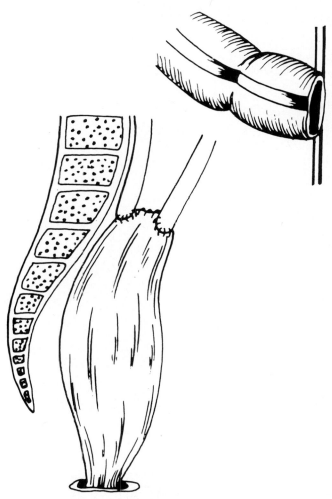

Figure 62–1. Mauclaire rectal bladder with total fecal exclusion and terminal colostomy.

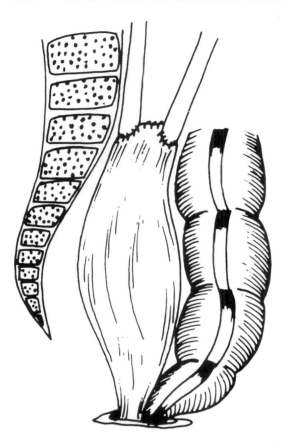

Figure 62–2. Gersuny operation: rectal bladder with perineal colostomy. The sigmoid is anterior to the rectum.

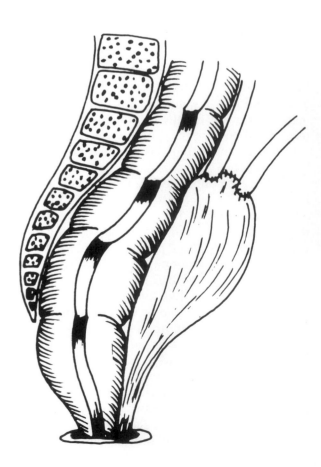

Figure 62–3. Heitz-Boyer and Hovelacque procedure: rectal bladder with perineal colostomy. The sigmoid is posterior to the rectum.

Shoukry concluded that even though all patients achieved good urinary continence, feces could pass suddenly without warning. In effect, the patients had an incontinent perineal colostomy.[10] Larger series reporting a satisfactory outcome were never published.

Aside from these procedures producing total fecal exclusion, several modifications have been published considering the possibility of partial fecal exclusion. The aim was to divide the urinary and fecal contents after ureterosigmoidostomy. Borelius suggested a side-to-side anastomosis between sigmoid and rectum (Fig. 62–4).[11] The ureters were anastomosed at the dome of the loop. Modelski in 1962[12] used a procedure devised by Descomps in 1909,[13] anastomosing the sigmoid terminolaterally to the anterior surface of the rectum, which had been previously transected. The ureters were implanted into the dome of the isolated rectum stump (Fig. 62–5). These principles have been revived recently. Kamidono implanted the ureters into a sigmoid pouch and performed an end-to-side sigmoidorectostomy.[14] Functionally, however, none of these procedures produced any clear advantage over conventional methods of ureterosigmoidostomy, as stored-up urine could freely reflux to the colon.

In summary, the isolated rectal bladder with a ter-

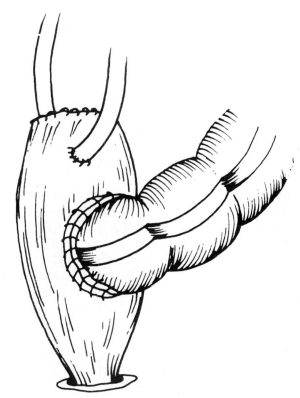

Figure 62–5. Descomps operation: rectal bladder with partial fecal exclusion.

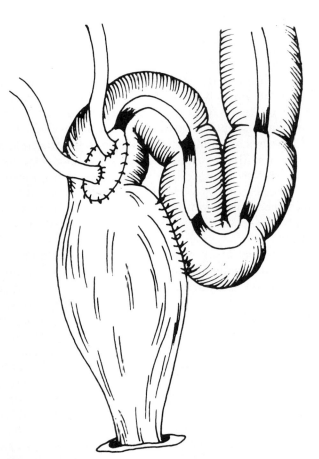

Figure 62–4. Borelius procedure: rectal bladder with partial fecal exclusion.

minal colostomy produced the most beneficial clinical results of the procedures reviewed thus far. Ghoneim, using a modification of the Mauclaire procedure,[5, 6] identified a high rate of incontinence (40 percent of patients),[15] recurrent pyelonephritis, and renal function impairment despite the separation of the urinary and fecal streams (30 percent of patients).[7] Furthermore, the terminal colostomy was problematic.

AUGMENTED AND VALVED RECTAL BLADDER

In 1969 Kock,[15a] in an attempt to construct a continent fecal reservoir, showed that a closed loop bowel segment, large or small, was capable of generating significant contractions. The pressure in the intact sigmoid colon can reach up to 200 cm H_2O during defecation, and the pressure waves that reach the distal colon with mass movements are 60 to 80 cm H_2O. These high-pressure conditions within the sigmoid colon and rectum produced by physiological bowel contractions were regarded as major causes of recurrent pyelonephritis and of nocturnal incontinence.

Curiously, back in 1907 Kocher proposed a most beneficial modification of the Maydl procedure (implantation of the trigone into the sigmoid colon) (Fig.

62–6) by means of distal sigmoid-to-sigmoid side-to-side anastomosis, and did so without advanced knowledge of bowel motility and pressure conditions (Fig. 62–7).[16] However, in 1907 the time for detubularization had not yet come and this idea was forgotten.

Ghoneim decided to augment the rectosigmoid with a segment of ileum in order to improve compliance, thus creating the so-called augmented rectal bladder.[17] Oral administration of alkalinizing drugs can be problematic in a noncompliant patient with limited possibilities of follow-up. The development of acidosis had to be prevented by other means. Urine could reflux into the descending and transverse colon, and the large absorbent surface increases the chances of biochemical disturbances. For this reason, an intussuscepted nipple valve was placed at the rectosigmoid junction to prevent urine from ascending into higher bowel segments (Fig. 62–8). Initially the ureters were implanted in the vicinity of the valve (Fig. 62–8C); later on the lower sigmoid colon was the preferred site of ureterointestinal implantation (Fig. 62–8D). A temporary colostomy was placed for protection closed after 6 to 8 weeks.

Operative Technique

The anterior wall of the rectum is incised longitudinally from the rectosigmoid junction to a level 3 to 5 cm distal to the peritoneal reflection. The incision is approximately 10 cm in length. The mesentery of the distal 10 cm of the sigmoid colon is mobilized and

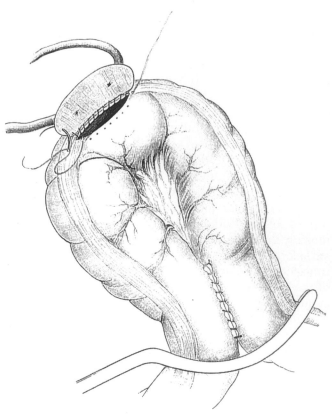

Figure 62–7. Kocher's modification of the Maydl procedure (implantation of the trigone into the sigmoid colon) by means of distal sigmoid-to-sigmoid side-to-side anastomosis.

defattened, and the appendices epiploicae are removed. Through the opened lumen of the rectum, the sigmoid is grasped by a pair of Babcock clamps and pulled down to form a 5-cm intussusception valve. The intussusception position is maintained by three or four rows of metallic staples applied at the base of the valve with an automatic stapling device. One row of the staples is placed on either side of the mesentery, and the other two in the opposite quadrants. An additional row is applied to anchor the valve to the wall of the rectum, providing additional stability and support.

The ureters are now anastomosed to the thus isolated pouch using an antireflux system. A buttonhole is cut at the summit of the nipple valve. A straight clamp is introduced between the two layers of the intussusception and parallel to the staple rows. The ureters are then pulled down through these tunnels. A stented mucosa-to-mucosa anastomosis is carried out between the ureter and the sigmoid using interrupted sutures of absorbable 4-0 material. This method was used initially,[18] but an alternative technique is readily available. A standard submucosal tunnel, following the procedure originally described by Goodwin and colleagues,[19] can also be adopted. For rectal augmentation, a 20-cm segment of the distal ileum is isolated. Its antimesenteric border is

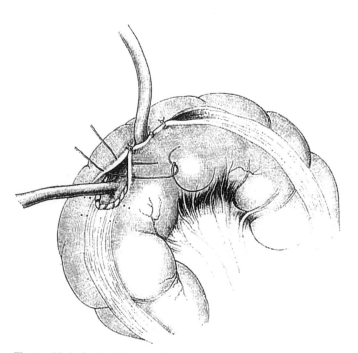

Figure 62–6. Implantation of the entire trigone into the rectum as described by Maydl.

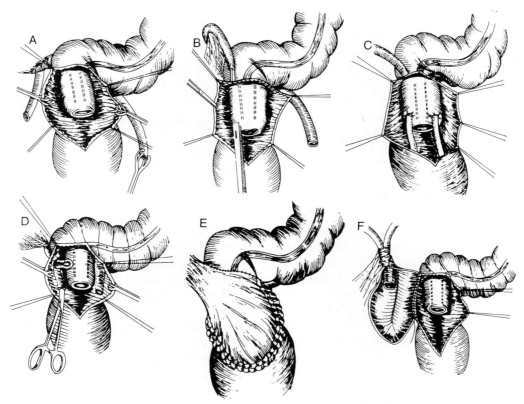

Figure 62–8. Surgical technique for the augmented and valved rectal bladder. *A,* Intussusception nipple valve. *B,* The ureter is pulled between the two layers of the intussusception. *C,* A stented mucosa-to-mucosa anastomosis is completed. *D,* Alternatively the ureters are implanted using a submucosal tunnel as described by Goodwin. *E,* The rectum is augmented with an ileal patch to improve compliance. *F,* When grossly dilated ureters are implanted, a second valve from ileum is used for reflux prevention.

opened and folded into a U shape, and the two adjacent borders are sutured together. This intestinal plate is then patched on the anterior wall of the open rectum.

If the ureters are grossly dilated, the above two methods are not suitable for reimplantation. Under such circumstances, Ghoneim creates a second antireflux valve from the ileum in connection with the patch used for augmentation. The ureters are then anastomosed to the afferent limb of this valve. For this procedure, the isolated segment of ileum should be 30 to 35 cm in length to provide adequate material for construction of the patch as well as the nipple valve.

Finally, a temporary transverse colostomy is made, which is closed after 6 to 8 weeks. The rectal pouch is drained by a tube for 3 weeks. Ureteric stents are removed after 10 days.[20]

Clinical Data

Filling proctometry revealed an adequate capacity of 500 to 800 ml and was achieved at a low pressure without segmental contractions. The pressure maximum did not exceed 30 cm of water.[21] Ghoneim, reporting a series of 109 patients, found all patients to be continent during the daytime with an emptying frequency of two to five times. All but six patients were dry at night with a voiding frequency of 0 to 2 times. There was no postoperative mortality. During the observation period (6 to 36 months), 32 died from recurrences and/or metastasis and two from cardiopulmonary problems. Follow-up intravenous pyelography revealed decompression or stability of the upper urinary tract in 88 percent of renal units. In the remainder, back pressure changes were seen because of stricture formation or reflux.[20]

SIGMA-RECTUM POUCH (MAINZ POUCH II)

This technique (augmented and valved rectal bladder, see Fig. 62–8), however, has several distinctive disadvantages. A bowel anastomosis has to be performed in order to use the ileal patch, staplers have to be implemented to secure the bowel invagination, and a second operative intervention is necessary to close the colostomy. All these additional steps are fraught with complications and turn the simple technique of ureterosigmoidostomy into an elaborate and complex procedure.

Applying Hinman's principles, we have developed

a novel modification of the classical technique of ureterosigmoidostomy, the sigma-rectum pouch (Mainz pouch II).[22] The idea was to lower the pressure within the rectosigmoid not by an elaborate augmentation but by simple detubularization, leaving the bowel in continuity. Detubularization of the intestinal tract eliminates mass contractions and high pressure peaks. In addition, the theoretical volume of the reservoir is increased.[23, 24]

Indications and Contraindications

Patients with a serum creatinine level below 1.5 mg/dl and a competent anal sphincter are good candidates for a sigma-rectum pouch. Those with severe diabetes or Parkinson's disease may have trouble with continence postoperatively. In such patients another form of urinary diversion might be preferable. Interestingly, there are also unfavorable rectodynamic evaluations in these patients. Moreover, pathologic conditions of the anal canal or rectum (e.g., hemorrhoids, old anal fissures) or the sigmoid (e.g., diverticulitis) are contraindications to the sigma-rectum pouch.

Women especially prefer the sigma-rectum pouch for continent urinary diversion because it is stomaless and they can continue to void in a sitting position. Previous radiotherapy or planned irradiation are contraindications. In patients with grossly advanced cancer, a sigma-rectum pouch should equally be avoided, so that in the dire case of pelvic recurrence the urinary reservoir is not located within the pelvic cavity.

Patient Preparation

Radiography by means of water-soluble opaque material is performed several days preoperatively to rule out diverticulosis or intestinal polyps. The risk of postoperative incontinence is psychologically a very serious complication that must be well assessed preoperatively. First, patients are given a 300-ml water enema, which they should be able to hold for 3 to 4 hours. Second, all patients scheduled for a sigma-rectum pouch receive a rectodynamic evaluation, including an anal sphincter profile.[25] Mechanical bowel preparation is performed in the usual manner, and all patients receive prophylactic antibiotic treatment during the peri- and postoperative periods. Immediately before surgery a multiperforate rectal tube is advanced through the anus far enough to be reached during surgery.

Operative Technique

In the vicinity of the junction between the sigmoid colon and rectum (Fig. 62–9), the intestine is opened

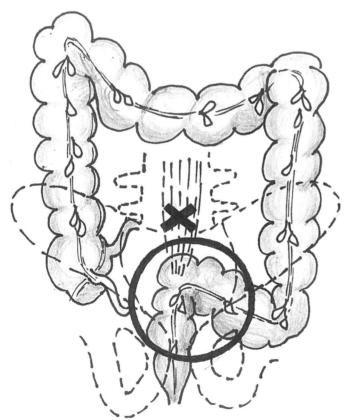

Figure 62–9. The area of the rectosigmoid junction is outlined. The *x* marks the later point of pouch fixation to the promontory.

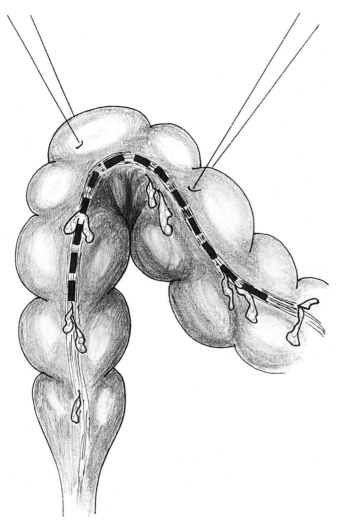

Figure 62–10. Leaving the bowel in continuity, the intestine is opened at its antimesenteric border over a length of 12 cm both distal and proximal to the rectosigmoid junction.

are placed parallel right and left to the medial running suture. The mucosa and the seromuscular layer are excised to create a wide buttonhole in between the two cranial stay sutures as an entrance of the ureter into the pouch. It is extremely important that the size of the buttonhole is twice as large as the diameter of the ureters. Subsequent obstruction by circular shrinkage of the intestinal wall can thereby easily be avoided. Starting from this incision, a submucosal tunnel over a length of 3.5 to 4 cm is dissected and the mucosa is incised at its distant end. The ureter is pulled through and the implantation is completed by single-stitch mucosa-to-mucosa sutures (Fig. 62–13). To secure the ureteral implantation, 6 or 8 Fr. ureteral stents are placed adjacent to the rectal tube. When dilated ureters are found, the open-end technique for ureteral implantation may be an alternative (Fig. 62–14). It is especially important to confirm that such ureters produce urine just before the ureterointestinal stitches are placed. Ureters with a thick wall and gross dilation easily kink and are strangulated by minute conditions. If no urine production is detectable, the ureter's path must be

at the taenia libera over a total length of 20 to 24 cm distal and proximal of this point (Fig. 62–10). As the length of the sigmoid varies greatly from individual to individual, the intestine is opened at a point that is most easily elevated by gently pulling on two stay sutures placed at the rectosigmoid junction.

By placing two stay sutures at the summit of the rectosigmoid, the split intestine receives the shape of an upsidedown U. A pouch plate is created by side-to-side anastomosis of the posterior wall, represented by the medial margins of the U by two-layer running sutures, using 4-0 polyglyconate for the seromuscular layer and 4-0 chromic catgut for the mucosa (Fig. 62–11). We believe that polyglyconate sutures should be avoided in children, as granulomatous tissue reactions have been observed in several instances.

The anastomosis presents a "pig-ear" at the proximal end. Subsequently, the left ureter is pulled through retroperitoneally to the right (Fig. 62–12). For ureteral implantation, four mucosal stay sutures

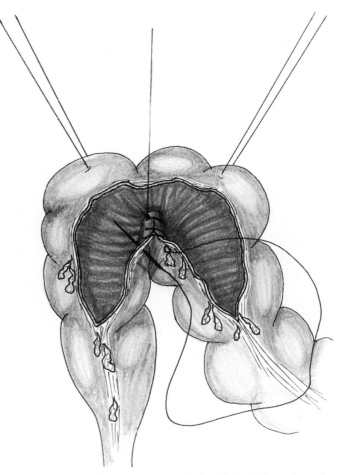

Figure 62–11. A pouch plate is created via side-to-side anastomosis of the posterior wall by means of two running sutures, 4-0 polyglyconate for the seromuscular and 4-0 chromic catgut for the mucosal layer.

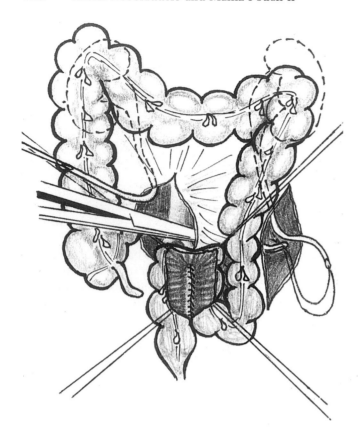

Figure 62–12. The left ureter is pulled through to the right side retroperitoneally.

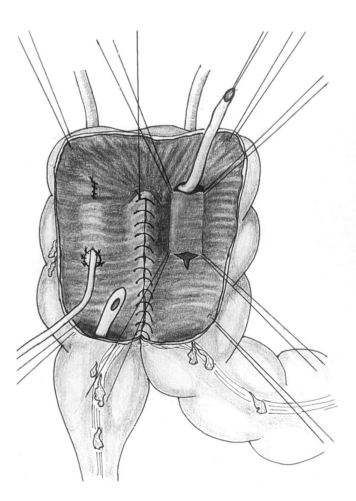

Figure 62–13. The ureters are implanted via a 3.5- to 4-cm long submucosal tunnel using the Goodwin-Hohenfellner technique.

third to fifth postoperative day, and the ureteral splints are removed around the eighth postoperative day.

Clinical Data

Between November 1990 and July 1993 73 patients (21 women and 43 men) received a sigma-rectum pouch at our institution. The mean age at the time of operation was 43.5 years, the youngest patient being 10 months old and the oldest 72 years. Twelve patients were children.

In 50 patients the indication for operative intervention was infiltrating bladder cancer. Nine patients had bladder exstrophy and five had incontinent epispadias. Five of the nine patients with bladder exstrophy had undergone no previous operations. These children had their bladder plate removed and in the same session received a Mainz pouch II. The other patients experienced repeated failed attempts at bladder closure and bladder neck reconstruction.

Four women had gynecological cancer (two carci-

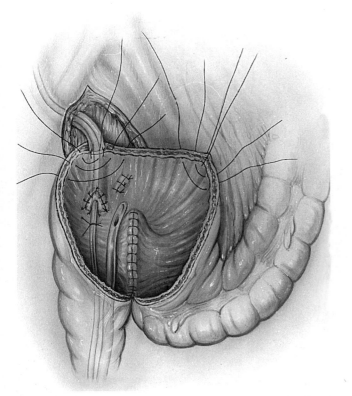

Figure 62–14. In case of dilated ureters, the open-end technique may be used for ureteral implantation. The figure depicts a case of ureteral reimplantation, the previous implantation site having been totally excised.

closely inspected. Novel techniques for implanting ureters damaged by irradiation or bilharziosis have been described by Abol-Enein and Ghoneim and may prove to be most beneficial during long-term follow-up.[26] The authors use two serous-lined extramural tunnels for this purpose. Figure 62–15 depicts the procedure as the ureters are being implanted into an ileal pouch; however, the identical technique can be used during construction of a sigma-rectum pouch.

The proximal end of the medial running suture presenting in the "pig ear" is evaginated dorsally and fixed to the anterior longitudinal cord of the promontory by two Bassini sutures (Fig. 62–16). If it is not possible to do this in a tension-free manner, the pouch may alternatively be fixed to the psoas muscle. Thus, dislocation of the pouch and consecutive kinking of the ureters are avoided. For closure of the anterior pouch wall, two-layer single-stitch sutures are used (5-0 polyglyconate for the seromuscular layer and 4-0 chromic catgut for the mucosal layer) (Fig. 62–17).

A gastrostomy (via a 12 Fr. Foley catheter) is usually placed intraoperatively. The patient receives intravenous hyperalimentation for about 5 days, and the gastrostomy is clamped around the third postoperative day and removed between the seventh and ninth day. The bowel tube is left in place until the

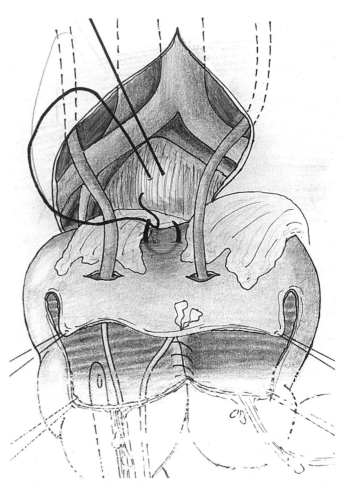

Figure 62–15. Pouch fixation to the anterior longitudinal cord in the area of the promontory without the risk of compromising the blood supply. Alternatively, the pouch may be fixed to the psoas muscle.

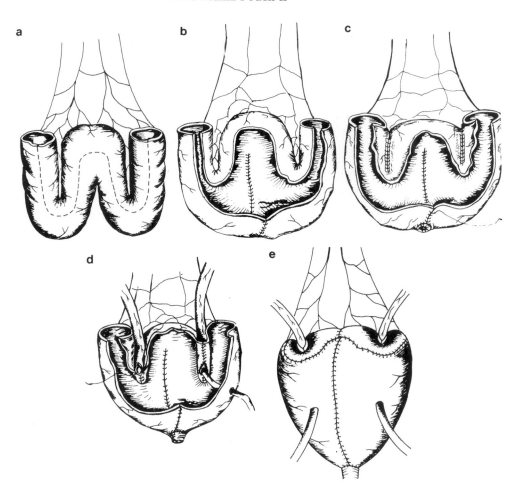

Figure 62–16. Technique of ureteral implantation in case of grossly dilated ureters as described by Abol-Enein and Ghoneim.[26] In this case a W-shaped ileal pouch is configured, producing two serous-lined intestinal troughs (a to c). The same technique can be used during construction of a sigma-rectum pouch. The ureters are laid in the troughs and anastomosed to the intestinal mucosa, and the tunnel is closed over the implanted ureter (d to e).

nomas of the cervix, 1 carcinoma of the vagina, and one leiomyosarcoma of the uterus) and underwent anterior exenteration and urinary diversion. One child had rhabdomyosarcoma. Three patients after severe pelvic trauma and urinary sphincter damage with total incontinence, and one woman with urogenital sinus, also received a sigma-rectum pouch.

Early Complications

There was no mortality related to the procedure. Four early complications (5.5 percent) were encountered.

An ileus required operative intervention on the seventh postoperative day, and a dislocated ureteral splint necessitated insertion of a nephrostomy tube on the second postoperative day in another patient. One patient with deep venous thrombosis had a pulmonary embolism without serious consequences. This same patient developed a suture dehiscence on the fourteenth postoperative day, which was surgically corrected. Another 66-year-old patient developed pneumonia, which subsided under antibiotic therapy.

Late Complications

Of the 73 patients, 69 were followed for a mean of 22 months (1 month to 33 months). Four patients with infiltrating bladder cancer died of their disease during follow-up. A total of eight late complications (10.9 percent) were observed that necessitated treatment.

Five patients (6.8 percent) developed stenosis at the ureteral implantation site. Three patients had antegrade balloon dilation, and two of these had to be surgically reimplanted later. Two patients had primary ureteral neoimplantation. All patients now have normal upper urinary tracts upon follow-up. It seems that when unilateral upper urinary tract dilation secondary to ureterocolic stricture becomes evident early after the operation, balloon dilation may be an effective form of treatment. Obstruction occurred 2 months postoperatively in the one patient in whom dilation was sufficient treatment. However, when scarring and fibrosis have taken place, dilation does not render satisfying results in the long term. This experience is shared by authors using balloon dilation to treat strictures in other forms of urinary diversion. When ureteral neoimplantation during open

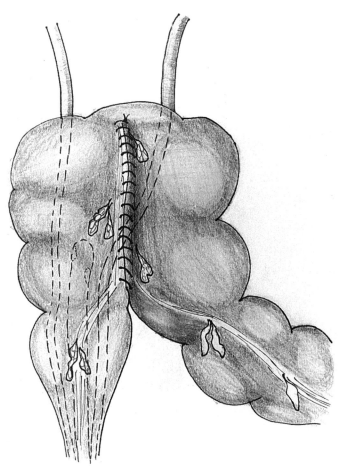

Figure 62–17. Closure of the anterior pouch wall using single-stitch sutures, 4-0 polyglyconate for the seromuscular and 4-0 chromic catgut for the mucosal layer.

surgery is inevitable, great care should be taken to avoid obstruction. Obstruction of these compromised ureters is much more dangerous than reflux.

Moreover, a 63-year-old patient under chemotherapy was readmitted 5 months after construction of the sigma-rectum pouch with slight anal bleeding. We performed rectoscopy using regional anesthesia and were able to coagulate the bleeding site. A common resectoscope was used for this purpose as in transurethral resection. The postoperative period was uneventful.

A large renal calculus occurred in a 51-year-old patient 5 months postoperatively.

The most serious late complication we have encountered was peritonitis 2 months after urinary diversion in a 51-year-old patient. Laparotomy was performed in another hospital and a rupture of the anterior pouch wall due to loosening of the anterior suture was found to be the cause. Primarily, a colostomy was performed. Two months later we closed the colostomy and resutured the anterior pouch wall. Since that time, we recommend the use of two-layer single-stitch sutures to complete the anterior and pos-

terior walls, as opposed to using a single, all-layer running suture as previously done.

Pressure Conditions

For scientific purposes, a modified technique of anorectal manometry, termed rectodynamics, was performed around the seventeenth postoperative day; after 3, 6, and 12 months; and annually thereafter. Rectodynamics represents a transfer of standard urodynamic techniques to the lower bowel.[25] A microtip catheter is inserted into the pouch. Under radiological guidance, one microtip is placed in the area of the sphincter; the other should float freely within the pouch (Fig. 62–18). Simultaneously, an electromyograph of the pelvic floor is registered along with the pouch, abdominal, sphincter, and differential pressure. Subsequently, an anal sphincter profile and a stress profile obtained during straining and coughing are documented.

The mean baseline pressure within the rectum during the preoperative examination was 23 cm H_2O. No significant correlation between baseline rectum pressure and filling volume was found. The same was true for all postoperative measurements. The basal pressures within the sigma-rectum pouch determined at different filling volumes on the seventeenth postoperative day, as well as 3 and 6 months postoperatively, were not statistically different from preoperative values.

During the rectodynamic evaluation, bowel contractions occurred (Fig. 62–19). The preoperative examination revealed a correlation between the filling volume and both the mean and maximal contraction pressures. The maximal contraction pressure was 72 cm H_2O during the preoperative investigation.

In the direct postoperative period, no bowel contractions were observed up to a filling volume of

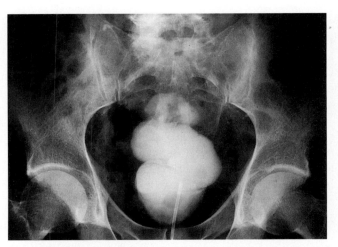

Figure 62–18. Contrast media–filled sigma-rectum pouch with a microtip catheter in place for rectodynamic evaluation.

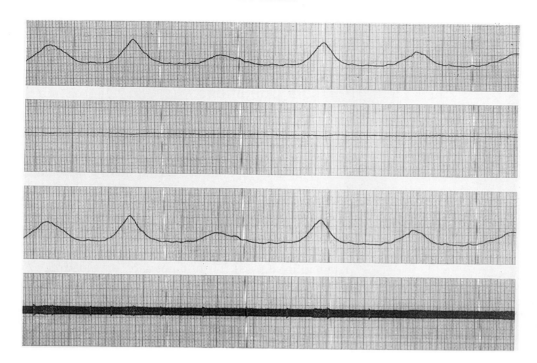

Figure 62–19. Preoperative rectodynamic measurement shows physiological bowel contractions in the area of the rectosigmoid junction. Normal pelvic floor EMG.

400 ml. Infrequent contractions up to 36 cm H_2O occurred thereafter. Three and 6 months postoperatively a correlation between bowel contractions and filling volume could no longer be found. The contraction pressures at rest were not significantly different from those during filling, even after administration of 500 ml of contrast media. The mean maximal closure pressure as determined during the preoperative examination was 77 cm H_2O (range 36 to 140 cm H_2O). Figure 62–20 shows the registration of such an anal sphincter profile. Reflux from the sigma-rectum pouch into the ureter was not seen in any case as determined by fluoroscopy and plain x-ray films during the rectodynamic evaluations.

Metabolics

The potentially life-threatening complication of hyperchloremic metabolic acidosis has received much attention in the literature. Prevention is of paramount importance. We recommend meticulous monitoring of the acid-base status and oral administration of alkalinizing drugs when the base excess drops below −2.5. Monitoring the serum electrolytes is not sufficient, as changes occur at a time when the acid-base metabolism has already decompensated. Not substituting early is like depriving a diabetic patient of insulin. Prevention rather than treatment is indicated. Oral sodium-potassium-hydrogen citrate has proved most beneficial for oral administration.

Of the 69 patients in long-term follow-up, 46 take alkalinizing drugs. As mentioned above, this high number is due to early preventive administration.

Secondary Malignancies

The development of secondary malignancies is a well-known risk after ureterointestinal anastomosis. From the first report of urinary diversion in 1852,[27] almost 80 years passed until Hammer in 1929 reported an associated malignant tumor.[28] The significance of this association was widely disregarded as late as 1975.[29] Filmer and Spencer reviewed several series with long-term follow-up and found carcinoma in the area of the ureterocolic anastomosis in 5 to 13 percent of patients.[30] In general, however, these patients represent a group who either have been lost to follow-up and present with symptoms of obstruction, or have not received proper surveillance. Surveillance programs found 16 to 41 percent of patients having at least one polyp, but none had invasive carcinoma.[31–33] Before surveillance programs, most patients developing premalignant colon polyps and subsequent colon cancer were simply going undetected. Colonic polyps are known to have malignant potential if left untreated. However, when treated, the risk of developing adenocarcinoma is alleviated.[33] A reliable tool in early detection of secondary malignancies is regular pouchoscopy, which we perform annually. For this purpose a microcontact cystoscope with an outer radius of 12 mm, designed by the Storz Company, is valuable. The use of this instrument permits a direct examination of the ureterocolic anastomosis using different magnifications. Malignancies can be detected at an early stage. Pouchoscopy should be performed by the urologist. There are many reports of gastroenterologists having biopsied the ure-

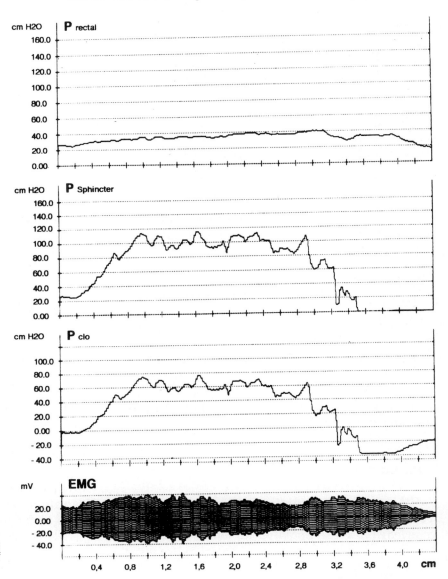

Figure 62–20. Anal pressure profile demonstrating a maximal closure pressure of nearly 120 cm of water.

teral implantation site in the belief that this was a polyp.

Continence

Four patients in our series reported minimal soiling of undergarments, but none of these required pads. One patient demonstrated second-degree stress incontinence; all others are totally continent. The 68-year-old woman with disturbing incontinence was able to hold a tap water enema for several hours, but produced a maximal closure pressure of only 45 cm H_2O during the sphincter profile testing portion of the rectodynamic investigation. We believe that the rectodynamic evaluation is also superbly suited to predicting postoperative continence whenever the anal sphincter is used as a continence mechanism during urinary diversion (Figs. 62–21 and 62–22).[25] As demonstrated in our series, clinical tests such as

holding a tap water enema for several hours are not sufficient.

The mean voiding frequency is five times during the day (range 2 to 8) and once at night (range 0 to 4). Nocturnal incontinence as well as urgency and frequency do not seem to be so much of a problem in Mainz pouch II patients as in patients having a rectal bladder or ureterosigmoidostomy. Imipramine hydrochloride was helpful for one patient who initially had to get up four times at night and now awakens only once at night to void.

Interestingly, almost all of patients who undergo postoperative M-VAC chemotherapy are incontinent during this treatment, even though they were perfectly continent beforehand. Imipramine hydrochloride is equally helpful in such instances, and complete continence is regained after chemotherapy. Some kind of toxic neuropathy involving the anal sphincter may explain this observation. This thesis is supported by the fact that when rectodynamics are

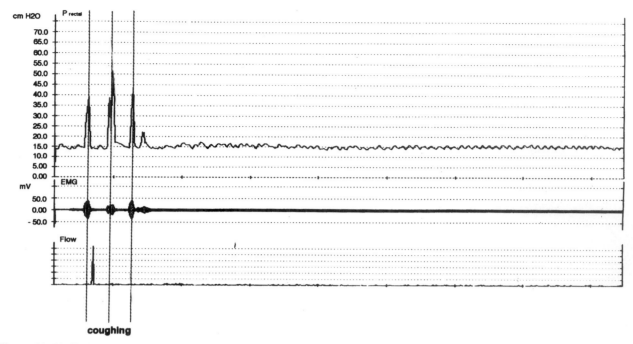

Figure 62–21. Preoperative rectodynamic measurement identifies anal sphincter incompetence. Incontinence is caused by coughing.

performed under chemotherapy, the sphincter profile is significantly reduced.

Summary

Although the implantation of the ureters into the rectosigmoid is associated with complications, the knowledge of these potential difficulties with over a

century of application permits many to be anticipated and treated before they become a serious medical problem. In properly selected patients desiring a continent urinary diversion, and with close monitoring (which has to be performed after any form of urinary diversion), anal sphincter controlled bladder substitutes represent a viable alternative to other surgical techniques.

After 25 years of experience of classical ureterosig-

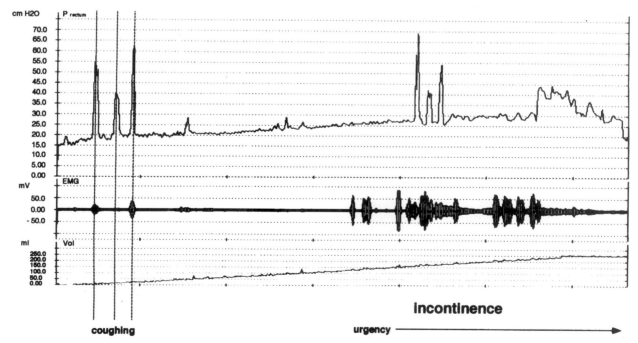

Figure 62–22. Preoperative rectodynamic measurement shows urgency and subsequent incontinence after the onset of high-pressure bowel contractions. Subconscious pelvic floor contractions as seen on the electromyogram cannot prevent leakage.

moidostomy in over 300 cases, we believe that the sigma-rectum pouch has many advantages over other forms of continent urinary diversion. A reservoir capacity, and safe and stable pouch fixation in the area of the promontory guaranteeing a straight ureteral path as well as low pressure even at high filling volumes, make this pouch a most attractive alternative to many forms of continent urinary diversion. The surgical technique termed the Mainz pouch II may serve to avoid or minimize the traditional shortcomings of classical ureterosigmoidostomy and may lead to a renaissance of ureterosigmoidostomy.

Editorial Comment
Fray F. Marshall

A detubulized rectal bladder appears to function well. Many of the problems similar to those involved in ureterosigmoidostomy, including acidosis, infection, and neoplasm, remain, but they have been addressed and reduced by these authors. If a perforation occurs, a colostomy is usually necessary. With these more favorable results, this operation might be considered more often.

REFERENCES

1. Smith T. An account of an unsuccessful attempt to treat extroversion of the bladder by a new operation. St Barth Hosp Rep 15:29, 1879.
2. Morestin G. Greffe de l'uretère dans le rectum. Ann Mal Org GU 11:224, 1893.
3. Maydl K. Über die Radikaltherapie der Ectopia Vesicae Urinariae. Wien Med Wochenschr 44:1113, 1169, 1256, 1894.
4. Hinman F, Weyrauch HM Jr. A critical study of the different principles of surgery which have been used in uretero-intestinal implantation. Trans Am Assoc Genitourin Surg 29:15, 1936.
5. Mauclaire P. De quelques essais de chirurgie expérimentale applicables au traitement: a) de l'extrophie de la vessie, b) des abouchements anormaux de rectum, c) les anus contre nature complexes. Proc Verb Ass Franc Chir IX Congr Paris 9:546, 1895.
6. Mauclaire P. De quelques essais de chirurgie expérimentale applicables au traitement de l'extrophie de la vessie et des anus contre natures complexes. Ann Mal Org Genurin 13:1080, 1895.
7. Ghoneim MA, Ashamallah AK. Further experience with the rectosigmoid bladder. Br J Urol 46:511, 1974.
8. Foges R. Wien Klin Wochenschr 11:990, 1898.
9. Heitz-Boyer M, Hovelaque A. Création d'une nouvelle vessie et d'une nouvelle urètre. J d'Urol 1:237, 1912.
10. Ghoneim MA, Shoukry I. The rectal bladder with perineal colostomy for urinary diversion. Urology 4:511, 1974.
11. Borelius J. Eine neue Modification der Maydl'schlen Operationsmethode bei angeborener Blasenektopie. Zentralbl Chir 30:780, 1903.
12. Modelski W. The transplantation of the ureters into the partially excluded rectum. J Urol 87:122, 1962.
13. Descomps P. Abouchement uréral dans le rectum exclu. Uretérostomie haute terminale après sigmoido-rectostomie basse termino-latérale. Arch Gen Chir 4:892, 1909.
14. Kamidono S, Oda Y, Hamami G, et al. Urinary diversion: Anastomosis of the ureters into a sigmoid pouch and end-to-side sigmoidorectostomy. J Urol 133:391, 1985.
15. Ghoneim MA, Shebab-El-Din AB, Ashamallah AK, et al. Evolution of the rectal bladder as a method for urinary diversion. J Urol 126:737, 1981.
15a. Kock NG. Intra-abdominal "reservoir" in patients with permanent ileostomy. Preliminary observations on a procedure resulting in fecal "continence" in five ileostomy patients. Arch Surg 99:223, 1969.
16. Kocher Th. Chirurgische Operationslehre. Verlag Gustav Fischer, Jena, 1907, p 1017.
17. Ghoneim MA, Shoukry I. The rectal bladder with perineal colostomy for urinary diversion. Urology 4:511, 1974.
18. Kock NG, Ghoneim MA, Lycke KG, et al. Urinary diversion to the augmented and valved rectum: Preliminary results with a novel surgical procedure. J Urol 140:1375, 1988.
19. Goodwin WE, Harris AP, Kaufman JJ, et al. Open, transcolonic ureterointestinal anastomosis: A new approach. Surg Gynecol Obstet 97:295, 1953.
20. Ghoneim MA. The modified rectal bladder: A bladder substitute controlled by the anal sphincter. Scand J Urol Nephrol Suppl 142:89, 1992.
21. Ghoneim MA, Ashamallah AK, Mahran MR, et al. Further experience with the modified rectal bladder (the augmented and valved rectum) for urine diversion. J Urol 147:1252, 1992.
22. Fisch M, Wammack R, Müller SC, Hoheufellnes R. The Mainz pouch II (sigma rectum pouch). J Urol 149:258, 1993.
23. Hinman F Jr. Selection of intestinal segments for bladder substitution: Physical and physiological characteristics. J Urol 139:519, 1988.
24. Koff SA. Guidelines to determine the size and shape of intestinal segments used for reconstruction. J Urol 140:1150, 1988.
25. Wammack R, Fisch M, Müller SC, et al. The rectodynamic evaluation. Assessment of anal continence in urology. Scand J Urol Nephrol 142 (Suppl):158, 1992.
26. Abol-Enein H, Ghoneim MA. A novel uretero-ileal reimplantation technique: The serous lined extramural tunnel. A preliminary report. J Urol 151:1193, 1994.
27. Simon J. Ectropia vesica (absence of the anterior walls of the bladder and pubic abdominal parieties); operation for directing the orifices of the ureters into the rectum; temporary success; subsequent death; autopsy. Lancet 2:568, 1852.
28. Hammer E. Cancer du colon sigmoide dix ans après implantation des uretères d'une vessie exstrophiée. J d'Urol 28:260, 1929.
29. Spence HM, Hoffmann WW, Pate VA. Exstrophy of the bladder. Long-term results in a series of 37 cases treated by ureterosigmoidostomy. J Urol 114:133, 1975.
30. Filmer B, Spencer JR. Malignancies in bladder augmentations and intestinal conduits. J Urol 143:671, 1990.
31. Starling JR, Uehling DT, Gilchrist KW. Value of colonoscopy after ureterosigmoidostomy. Surgery 96:784, 1984.
32. Berg NO, Fredlund P, Mansson W. Surveillance colonoscopy and biopsy in patients with ureterosigmoidostomy. Endoscopy 19:60, 1987.
33. Rainwater LM, Segura JW. Ureterosigmoidostomy. Probl Urol 5:299, 1991.

Chapter 63

Sigmoid Neobladder

Gang (Kevin) Zhang, Pratap K. Reddy, and Ali Cuneyid Iseri

Total bladder replacement with a bowel segment has become widely accepted as one of the best forms of urinary tract reconstruction after radical cystectomy for locally invasive bladder cancer. A variety of bowel segments and configurations to form a neobladder have been described, each having its advantages and disadvantages. In experienced hands, most forms of neobladder work well with quite acceptable functional characteristics. Since the mid-1980s the sigmoid colon has been used for neobladder reconstruction at our institution.[1] The sigmoid neobladder described in this chapter has many advantages. Unlike terminal ileum and right colon, the sigmoid colon is not associated with problems of malabsorption, including deficiencies of vitamin B_{12}, folic acid, and bile salts, and diarrhea.[2] In most patients, it is easy to reach the urethra for anastomosis. Restoration of bowel continuity is simple because the bowel anastomosis is lateral to the isolated segment and the small bowel can easily be packed away. Most important, because of the central location and the anatomy of the sigmoid, the ureters can readily be aligned to the neobladder with a reliable antireflux anastomosis. Like most other neobladders, a sigmoid neobladder is a low-pressure reservoir with good capacity and a nearly spherical shape. The continence rate is excellent. However, a few conditions may limit its use, such as a malignancy or severe diverticulitis. In some obese patients the sigmoid mesentery may be too short to reach the urethra for a tension-free anastomosis. Therefore, it is imperative for surgeons performing this type of operation to be familiar with a variety of techniques of neobladder creation to suit the anatomy of an individual patient.

PATIENT SELECTION

Currently, the sigmoid neobladder is created only in male patients undergoing radical cystectomy for invasive bladder cancer. Although neobladder recon-

struction requires a little more time than an ileal conduit, it does not necessarily increase morbidity.[3] Therefore, in general, any patient who is considered a suitable candidate for radical cystectomy should also be a candidate for a sigmoid neobladder. The most important factor in considering a neobladder is the patient's motivation to deal with the postoperative changes of voiding function and the possibility of performing intermittent self-catheterization. Obesity is not a limiting factor. On the contrary, these patients may benefit more from neobladder reconstruction because of the avoidance of stoma-related problems commonly seen in the obese. As mentioned, the only caution in some obese patients is that the sigmoid mesentery may not be long enough to reach the urethra. Patients with compromised renal function may not be suitable candidates for neobladder, and we do not advise the neobladder for patients with serum creatinine levels of more than 2.0 mg/dl.

Before the surgery, detailed discussions should be held to inform the patient and family about the perioperative course and functions of the neobladder, so that they can be well prepared to cope with the changes and do not have any unrealistic expectations. The patient should be informed that it may take 1 to 3 months to gain total daytime continence and that there is a possibility of enuresis after that. Both patient and family should also be cautioned that there is no long-term information about neobladder function and the possibility of the development of malignancy.

PREOPERATIVE EVALUATION

In addition to routine evaluation for radical cystectomy, there should be evaluation of the colon and prostatic urethra in these patients. A barium enema or colonoscopy should be performed. The presence of a malignancy precludes the use of sigmoid for a neobladder. The finding of diverticula in the sigmoid is not a contraindication to the use of sigmoid, but if extensive diverticulitis is present, the inflammatory changes in the sigmoid and mesentery may hinder its use. Patients who are considered candidates for any type of neobladder must undergo biopsies of the prostatic urethra. A finding of carcinoma in situ or invasion of transitional cell carcinoma to the prostatic urethra is a clear contraindication to a neobladder. However, the mere presence of multifocal tumors in the bladder or tumors close to the bladder neck without direct involvement of the prostatic urethra is not necessarily a contraindication. Nonetheless, it is advisable to have intraoperative frozen sections of the prostatic urethra and surgical margin at the prostatic apex. Finally, all patients should have a stoma site marked by a stoma therapist in case unexpected intraoperative events preclude the construction of a neobladder. The preoperative bowel preparation is the same as for radical cystectomy.

SURGICAL TECHNIQUES

The patient is placed in a modified dorsal lithotomy position using stirrups and thigh-high intermittent compression stockings as for radical retropubic prostatectomy.[4] Radical cystectomy and bilateral pelvic lymphadenectomy are performed in the standard fashion. The dorsal vein complex and the prostatic apex should be handled the same way as in radical prostatectomy to preserve the continent mechanism. One should avoid extensive blunt dissection at the posterior aspect of the membranous urethra. The prostate is transected at its apex, leaving no residual prostatic tissue. Frozen sections of the urethral margin are obtained. Before the sigmoid is finally chosen for the neobladder, one should assess the length of the sigmoid and its mesentery to determine whether it can easily reach the urethral stump. If the lowest point of sigmoid can be pulled down to reach the pubic symphysis, a tension-free sigmoidourethral anastomosis can be anticipated. To ensure a neobladder with adequate capacity and low pressure, 30 to 35 cm of sigmoid and descending colon is required. The sigmoid colon is first mobilized by incising the white line. With sharp and blunt dissection, the sigmoid and descending colon are isolated on a broad mesenteric pedicle based on the sigmoid arterial branches of the inferior mesenteric artery (Fig. 63–1). The division of the sigmoid mesentery should be short so that the sigmoid arterial branches are not disturbed. The divided segment of sigmoid and descending colon is packed medially and the colonic continuity is resumed by end-to-end anastomosis using a single layer of interrupted 3-0 polyglactin (Vicryl) suture. A stapling device can also be used if the surgeon prefers. In some patients the splenic flexure

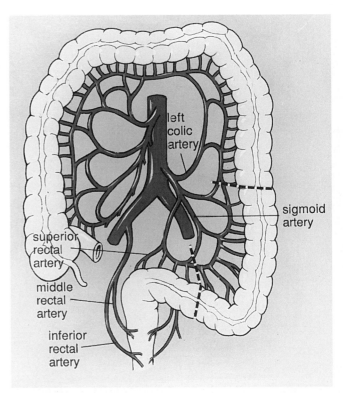

Figure 63–1. The sigmoid and descending colon is isolated on a broad mesenteric pedicle based on the sigmoid arterial branches of the inferior mesenteric artery. (From Reddy PK. Total bladder replacement. J Urol 145:51, 1991.)

may have to be taken down to ensure a tension-free colonic anastomosis.

To shorten the bowel anastomosis time for re-establishing bowel continuity, we have recently begun to use the biofragmentable bowel anastomosis ring (BAR). This is composed of two identical segments made of polyglycolic acid and 12 percent barium sulfate. The ring is fragmented in 15 to 23 days by absorption of water from the intestinal contents, leaving a satisfactory lumen. BAR rings of various diameters are available and their safety and efficacy have been well tested. We now routinely use the BAR ring, have encountered no complications, and consider it a useful tool for colon anastomosis (Fig. 63–2).

Neobladder Construction

The isolated sigmoid segment is cleansed with generous antibiotic irrigation until the return fluid is clear. The segment is then folded in a U shape and the most dependent part of this segment is marked as the site of urethral anastomosis. The colonic segment is completely detubularized by incising the medial tenia close to the mesenteric border (Fig. 63–3). To do so, we prefer to use an electrocautery with a cutting mode. Once the segment is completely opened up, a final inspection of the segment is made to con-

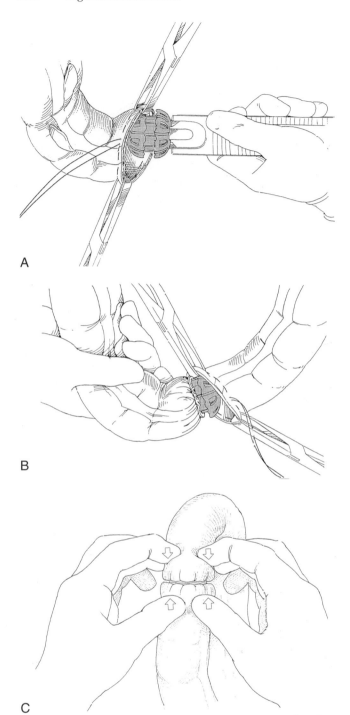

A

B

C

Figure 63–2. The techniques of using the biofragmentable bowel anastomosis ring. *A*, A pursestring suture with 4-0 Vicryl is placed 0.5 cm from the transection edge. The ring is inserted to the lumen of the distal colon with inserter. *B*, The pursestring suture is tied snugly over the edge of the half-ring, and the other half-ring is inserted to the proximal colon, which has a pursestring suture placed. *C*, After the other pursestring suture in the proximal colon is tied, the two halves of the ring are snapped together and the anastomosis is completed.

firm there are no unexpected pathologic conditions. The neobladder is formed by aligning the posterior walls of this sigmoid patch first. A few interrupted 2-0 Vicryl sutures are placed for the alignment, and then the entire posterior walls are closed with a single running 3-0 Vicryl suture (Fig. 63–4). If one chooses to perform ureterocolonic anastomosis within the pouch at this time, the ureteral anastomosis should be performed before the anterior wall of the pouch is closed. In the same fashion, the anterior wall of the sigmoid pouch is also closed with a single running

3-0 Vicryl suture. The formation of a neobladder is almost completed, with its opening only at the superior aspect of this pouch (Fig. 63–5). A 24 Fr. Malecot catheter is placed in the pouch and secured with a 3-0 chromic catgut suture. The superior aspect of the neobladder is left open until the anastomosis to the urethra is completed.

To further reduce operative time, we have recently started to use the Auto Suture Poly GIA 75-060 disposable surgical stapler. This device contains absorbable copolymer staples arranged in two, double-stag-

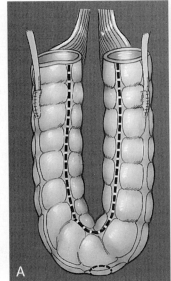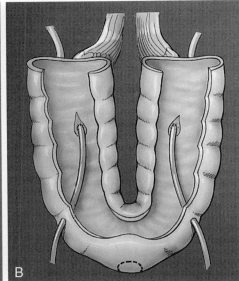

Figure 63–3. *A* and *B*, The colonic segment is completely detubularized by incising the medial tenia. (From Reddy PK. Total bladder replacement. J Urol 145:51, 1991.)

gered rows 75 mm in length. After the sigmoid segment is isolated and irrigated with antibiotic solution, the stapler is placed in the lumen and fired in the same manner as a standard GIA stapler (Figs. 63–5 and 63–6). Because of the length of the sigmoid segment, the completion of detubularization and pouch formation usually requires two firings. The advantage of this device is that it allows simultaneous detubularization and pouch construction, thus reducing operative time. In addition, the absorbable staples will not cause stone formation. With the stapler technique, the ureteral reimplantation should be performed through the exterior approach before detubularization and pouch formation.

The antireflux sigmoidoureteral anastomosis can be performed either from outside by the seromuscular technique as described by Leadbetter-Politano, or from within by the submucosal tunnel technique. With the first method, the ureterocolonic anastomosis should be completed before the colonic segment is detubularized. The ureters are brought anteriorly along the lateral tenia. To facilitate the anastomosis, the colonic segment is filled with normal saline to distend the wall. A 4- to 5-cm seromuscular incision is made along the lateral tenia; the ureter is anastomosed to the mucosal opening with interrupted 5-0 Vicryl sutures; and an 8 Fr. feeding tube is used as a stent, which is brought out anteriorly through the bowel wall. The stent should be secured with a 4-0 chromic catgut.

With the alternative method, the ureteral anastomo-

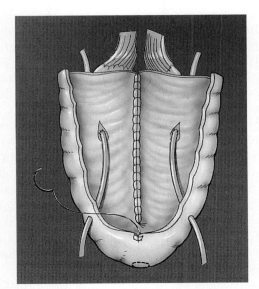

Figure 63–4. The posterior walls are closed with a running 3-0 Vicryl suture. (From Reddy PK. Total bladder replacement. J Urol 145:51, 1991.)

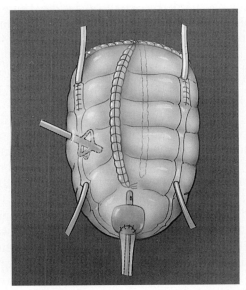

Figure 63–5. Completion of sigmoid neobladder.

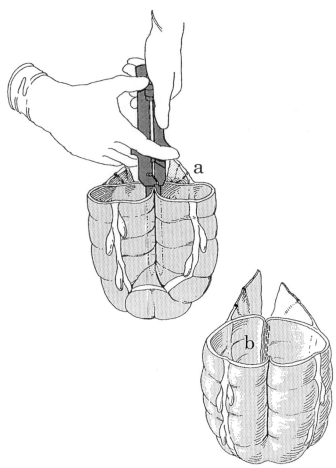

Figure 63–6. The detubularization and pouch formation of the colon are completed by firing the stapler with absorbable staples.

sis should be performed before the anterior wall of the colonic pouch is closed. Using a technique similar to the one described by Leadbetter-Politano, a 4- to 5-cm submucosal tunnel is created by a pair of fine scissors. Injection of normal saline into the submucosa may facilitate the creation of the tunnel. The ureter is then brought in through the submucosal tunnel and anastomosed directly to the full thickness of the colonic mucosa with interrupted 5-0 Vicryl sutures. Care must be taken at this point to avoid any kink of the ureter at its entrance to the colon pouch. Similarly, the ureteral anastomosis is stented with an 8 Fr. feeding tube, which is also brought out through a punch wound in the anterior wall of the pouch.

The neobladder is completed by its anastomosis to the urethral stump and closure of the superior part of the pouch. First, a small opening about 28 to 30 Fr. in size is made at the most dependent part of the sigmoid pouch as previously marked. This opening is stomatized by sewing the mucosa to the seromuscular edge with interrupted 4-0 Vicryl sutures. A watertight colonourethral anastomosis is completed with interrupted 2-0 Vicryl sutures over a 20 Fr. Foley catheter as in a radical prostatectomy. We usually place six

stitches for this anastomosis. After the proper positions of the Foley and Malecot catheters in the pouch are confirmed, the superior portion of the pouch is finally closed with running 3-0 Vicryl sutures, and the sigmoid neobladder reconstruction is completed. The ureteral stents and Malecot catheter are brought out through the anterior abdominal wall. Two Penrose drains are placed on either side of the neobladder and brought out through the abdominal wall as well. The abdominal incision is closed in a standard fashion.

POSTOPERATIVE MANAGEMENT

The ureteral stents, Foley catheter, and Malecot catheter are all connected to drainage. The Foley and Malecot catheters are irrigated gently with normal saline to flush out mucus, starting 24 hours after the surgery. The ureteral stents may be irrigated as needed. The amount of drainage from the Penrose drains varies and is usually peritoneal fluid. If there is an excessive amount, the urea nitrogen and creatinine in the fluid should be checked for the possibility of a urine leak. The Penrose drains can be removed once the drainage is minimal, which usually occurs on the third or fourth postoperative day. After patients have resumed normal bowel function and tolerated regular diet well, they can be discharged with the ureteral stents and catheters. They are instructed to irrigate the catheters at home. The ureteral stents are removed on the twelfth or thirteenth postoperative day. The Foley catheter is removed on the fourteenth postoperative day if there is no extravasation seen on a cystogram. The suprapubic tube is open to drainage until the 21st postoperative day. When the trial of voiding is successful, the Malecot catheter should be clamped. It is opened only to check residual urine each time after patients void. They are told to keep a diary to record the amount of voided urine and residual urine. If they void well with minimal residual urine, the Malecot catheter can be removed; this usually takes place in the third week after the surgery.

Patients are instructed to perform perineal exercise and use absorbent pads until complete continence is achieved. In the meantime, the use of a condom catheter to manage incontinence is ill advised, as patients may heavily depend on the condom catheter and jeopardize the perineal exercise. A baseline intravenous urogram, renal ultrasonogram, or renal scan should be obtained to make sure there is no obstruction of the upper tract after the Malecot catheter is removed.

These patients are followed every 3 months for the first year and every 4 to 6 months thereafter. At each follow-up visit, in addition to routine evaluation of

TABLE 63–1. Urodynamic Data

Follow-up	Maximal Capacity in ml (range)	Pressure of Capacity in cm H$_2$O (range)	Residual Urine in ml (range)
3 mo	450 (230–720)	40 (20–70)	26 (0–110)
1 yr	600 (380–780)	16 (10–25)	40 (4–80)
3 yr	620 (440–810)	15 (10–20)	45 (10–105)

the bladder cancer, they should be tested for residual urine, urine culture and cytology, and serum electrolytes. Voiding cystogram may be performed once a year to rule out reflux. Cystometrography is performed to determine the capacity and pressure of the neobladder. These patients should undergo a yearly intravenous pyelogram or renal ultrasonogram to evaluate the upper tracts. Flexible cystoscopy should be performed annually to rule out any development of neoplasms.

RESULTS

The results of a totally detubularized sigmoid neobladder in our first 27 patients have been reported in detail.[5] The daytime continence rate was 100 percent. The average interval between voidings was 4.5 hours (range 3 to 6 hours) during the daytime. In most patients, continence was obtained within 2 months; in a few, it took as long as 3 months. The nighttime continence rate was 67 percent and could well be managed by either absorbent pads or a condom catheter. Two patients with nighttime incontinence underwent artificial urinary sphincter implantation, which resulted in complete nighttime continence. The artificial urinary sphincter was deactivated during the daytime. At 6-month follow-up, the mean maximal capacity of the sigmoid neobladder was 580 ml (range 360 to 800 ml), the pressure at maximal capacity was 19 cm H$_2$O (range 12 to 30 ml), and the average residual urine was 35 ml (5 to 75 ml). The urodynamic data are summarized in Table 63–1. All patients resumed near-normal voiding function. They could sense a feeling of fullness or slight discomfort when the neobladder was full, and usually voided to completion. The mucus in the urine did not pose any problem. The perioperative and long-term complications are low. There was no renal function deteriora-

tion or serum electrolyte derangement in any patient except one. This individual, who had renal insufficiency with a serum creatinine level of 2.0 ml/dl before the neobladder reconstruction, developed progressive renal failure that eventually required dialysis. There was no perioperative mortality. So far, we have performed more than 60 totally detubularized sigmoid neobladders. The overall outcome continues to keep up with the excellent results in the first 27 patients, while the short- and long-term complications remain low.

Summary

In summary, the neobladder is perhaps the best form of urinary tract reconstruction after radical cystectomy. Sigmoid provides an excellent bowel segment for a neobladder. The procedure is technically simple, has no adverse metabolic sequelae, and provides a capacious reservoir with good continence and near-normal voiding function. The sigmoid colon's relatively thick wall allows a reliable antireflux ureteral anastomosis. In experienced hands, both short- and long-term morbidity is low. Thus, it significantly improves the quality of life in patients after radical cystectomy.

Editorial Comment
Fray F. Marshall

The sigmoid neobladder has many attractive features, including potential ease of construction and ureteral reimplantation, and less derangement of bowel function. Negative features include the presence of diverticuli, a potentially short mesentery, and possibly a smaller-volume neobladder.

REFERENCES

1. Reddy PK, Lange PH. Bladder replacement with sigmoid colon after radical cystoprostatectomy. Urology 29:368, 1987.
2. Koch MD, McDougal WS, Reddy PK, Lange PH. Metabolic alterations following continent urinary diversion through colonic segments. J Urol 145:270, 1991.
3. Reddy PK, Fraley EE, Lange PH. A comparative analysis of continent stomal reservoirs and neobladders to standard ileal conduit. J Urol 141:350A, 1989.
4. Lange PH, Reddy PK. Technical nuances and surgical results of radical retropubic prostatectomy in 150 patients. J Urol 138:348, 1987.
5. Reddy PK, Lange PH, Fraley EE. Total bladder replacement using detubularized sigmoid colon: Technique and results. J Urol 145:51, 1991.

Part VI

SURGERY OF THE PROSTATE

Chapter 64

Suprapubic Prostatectomy

Ray E. Stutzman

Suprapubic prostatectomy or transvesical prostatectomy consists of enucleation of hyperplastic adenomatous growth of the prostate performed through an extraperitoneal incision of the anterior bladder wall. This procedure does not involve total removal of the prostate because a tissue plane exists between the adenoma and the compressed, true prostate that is left intact when the procedure is properly performed.

Eugene Fuller of New York is credited with performing the first complete suprapubic removal of a prostatic adenoma in 1894.[3] This was a blind procedure with digital enucleation of the gland. Suprapubic and perineal drainage tubes were placed to wash out clots and control bleeding.[4]

Peter Freyer of London popularized the operation and subsequently published his results in over 1600 cases with a mortality rate of just over 5 percent.[1] The entire operation was usually a 15-minute procedure. A 2- to 3-inch midline suprapubic incision was made and the bladder was opened without opening the lateral tissue spaces or entering the space of Retzius. Digital enucleation of the prostate was then performed. One or two fingers were placed in the rectum for counterpressure while the suprapubic enucleation was accomplished. The prostatic fossa was left alone, as Freyer believed that the capsule and surrounding tissues at the bladder neck would contract enough to control bleeding, somewhat after the fashion of a uterus immediately after childbirth. He left an indwelling urethral catheter and a large suprapubic tube to evacuate clots.[2] The low mortality and morbidity rates were remarkable considering that no blood transfusions or antibiotics were available at that time. This blind enucleation remained popular for over 50 years.

The low transvesical suprapubic prostatectomy with visualization of the bladder neck and prostatic fossa and placement of hemostatic sutures has sup-

planted the blind procedure.[5, 7] This operation is presented here in more detail.

INDICATIONS

The indications for prostatectomy include acute urinary retention; recurrent or persistent urinary tract infections; significant or intractable symptoms from bladder outlet obstruction; recurrent gross hematuria caused by prostatic enlargement; pathophysiological changes of the kidneys, ureters, or bladder secondary to prostatic obstruction; bladder calculi secondary to obstruction; and decreased urine flow rate with or without high intravesical pressures. Over 90 percent of prostatectomies for benign prostatic hyperplasia are performed by transurethral resection. When the obstructive tissue is estimated to weigh more than 50 gm, serious consideration should be given to an open (suprapubic or retropubic) procedure. Ultrasonography is of value in determining the size of the prostate. Cystoscopic examination with measurement of the prostatic length is also of value and may aid in identification of other possible lesions in the bladder prior to planned enucleation. If sizable diverticula of the bladder justify removal, suprapubic enucleation of the prostate and diverticulectomy may be performed. Any large bladder calculi that are not amenable to easy fragmentation may also be removed during the open procedure. The possibility of ankylosis of the hip, preventing proper positioning for transurethral resection, must also be considered. The association of an inguinal hernia with an enlarged prostate may lead to an open procedure, as the hernia may be repaired via the same lower abdominal incision.[10]

Contraindications to a transvesical prostatectomy include a small fibrous gland, carcinoma of the prostate, and earlier prostatectomy in which most of the prostate has previously been resected or removed and the planes are obliterated.

PREOPERATIVE MANAGEMENT

The average age of patients is approximately 70 years. Many have histories of cardiovascular disease, chronic obstructive pulmonary disease, diabetes, or hypertension. A thorough evaluation of the patient is essential, as this is an elective procedure and bladder outlet symptoms could be managed by intermittent catheterization, indwelling Foley catheter, or suprapubic cystostomy. None of these are good alternatives if the patient is a reasonable surgical risk. It is preferable to evaluate the upper urinary tract with an intravenous urogram and a postvoid film if renal function is normal. A kidney-ureter-bladder (KUB) and renal sonogram may suffice. If the patient has documented urinary tract infection, this should be treated before elective surgery and may necessitate indwelling catheter drainage.

Informed consent is necessary, including discussion of the risks and complications of surgery.

Most patients can be evaluated as outpatients and admitted to the hospital on the day of surgery. This practice is cost effective and reduces the length of hospitalization.

SURGICAL TREATMENT

Suprapubic prostatectomy should accomplish the following:

1. Surgical access to the bladder neck and prostate with minimal disturbance to the tissue planes via a lower abdominal incision and low urinary bladder incision.

2. Transvesical enucleation of all adenomatous tissue within the surgical capsule leaving the remaining vascular, true prostate intact.

3. Accessibility to the vesical neck and proximal prostatic fossa, providing direct control and ligation of bleeding vessels near the bladder neck.

4. Accessibility of the bladder for cystolithotomy or diverticulectomy, if indicated.

5. Primary closure of the bladder with urethral and suprapubic catheter drainage.

The exposure of the prostatic fossa is comparable with that in retropubic prostatectomy; dissection of the retropubic space with a capsular incision is not necessary.

Spinal or epidural anesthesia is preferred in all prostatectomy procedures. If regional anesthesia is contraindicated, a general anesthetic with adequate relaxation may be utilized.

Blood transfusion is required in approximately 15 percent of patients undergoing suprapubic prostatectomy. It is prudent to have 2 or 3 units of blood available when contemplating an open prostatectomy. The safest transfusion is autologous blood. Individual units can be drawn a week apart while the patient is on oral iron medication.

OPERATIVE TECHNIQUE

The patient is placed in the supine position with the umbilicus positioned over the kidney rest. The table is slightly hyperextended, and the patient should then lie in a mild Trendelenburg position. The suprapubic area is shaved. A catheter is introduced into the urinary bladder, the bladder is irrigated and filled with 200 to 250 ml of water or saline, and the catheter is then removed. The abdomen and genitalia are prepared from nipple line to midthigh.

A vertical midline suprapubic incision is made through the skin and linea alba, the incision extending from below the umbilicus to the symphysis (Fig. 64–1). The rectus muscles are retracted laterally and the prevesical space is developed, sweeping the peritoneum superiorly. It is not necessary or desirable to expose the retropubic or lateral vesical spaces. For more adequate exposure, a self-retaining retractor is used.

Two sutures are placed in the anterior bladder wall below the peritoneal reflection. A vertical cystotomy

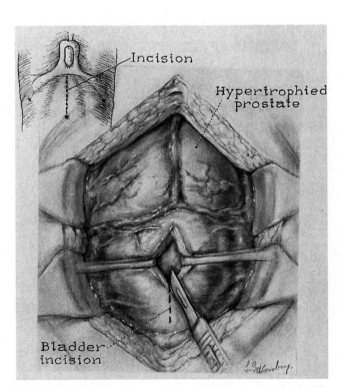

Figure 64–1. Suprapubic prostatectomy. Midline suprapubic incision. Vertical bladder incision exposing the bladder neck.

is then made and the incision opened down to within 1 cm of the bladder neck (Fig. 64–1). The bladder is inspected and the bladder neck and prostate can be visualized. A medium-sized Deaver retractor is placed into the open bladder retracting superiorly. A narrow Deaver is then placed over the bladder neck just distal to the trigone. This curved end of the Deaver retractor provides an excellent semilunar line for incising the mucosa around the posterior bladder neck just distal to the trigone (Fig. 64–2). By this method the ureteral orifices are well visualized and are not compromised. Metzenbaum scissors are then introduced at the 6 o'clock position, and by gentle dissection the plane between the adenoma and the capsule of the prostate is developed (Fig. 64–3).

The remainder of the procedure is done by digital dissection, freeing the posterior lobes down to the apex of the prostate and then circumferentially sweeping anteriorly (Fig. 64–4). The urethra is firmly attached at the apex; it is preferable to use scissors to sharply incise the urethra, keeping close to the prostatic adenoma in order not to cause injury to the sphincter and subsequent incontinence. With large glands it is often preferable to remove one lobe at a time. If a large intravesical protrusion of the middle lobe is found, this may be removed separately.

After removal of the adenoma, the prostatic fossa is inspected and a digital sweep made to ascertain the presence of any remaining nodular adenomatous

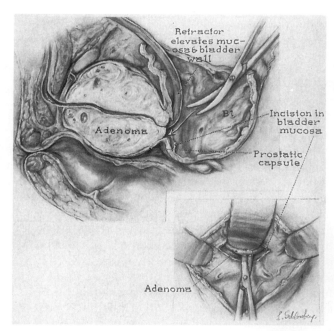

Figure 64–3. Suprapubic prostatectomy. A plane is established between the adenoma and capsule of the prostate by sharp dissection.

tissue. Usually, minimal bleeding occurs; however, bleeding frequently occurs in the 5 o'clock and 7 o'clock positions. The prostatic arteries enter the capsule and prostate at this level near the bladder neck. Suture ligature of these vessels is performed even without active bleeding (Fig. 64–5). Figure-of-eight sutures of 2-0 chromic catgut on a 5/8 circle needle will provide good hemostasis.

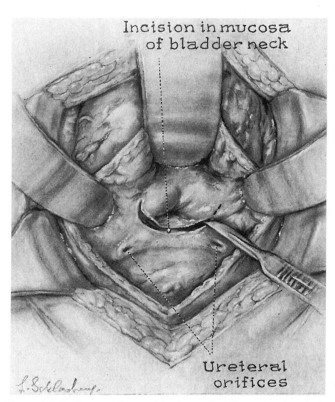

Figure 64–2. Suprapubic prostatectomy. Curvilinear incision in the mucosa of the posterior bladder neck.

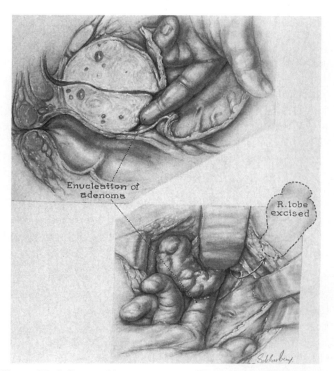

Figure 64–4. Suprapubic prostatectomy. Digital enucleation of an adenoma.

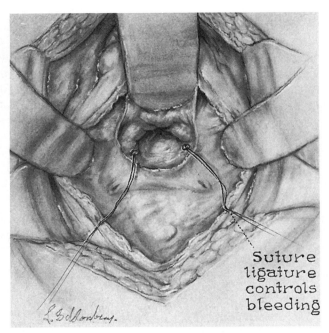

Figure 64–5. Suprapubic prostatectomy. Sutures are placed at 5 and 7 o'clock to control bleeding from major arterial vessels.

A 22 Fr. 30-ml bag, three-way Foley catheter is passed per urethra. A 26 or 28 Fr. Malecot suprapubic tube is passed through a separate stab wound in the anterior bladder wall and brought out through a stab wound in the lower abdominal wall (Fig. 64–6). A watertight single-layer interrupted closure of the bladder with either 2-0 chromic catgut or Vicryl suture is made, just missing the mucosa, but with full thickness of the muscularis and serosa. The balloon of the Foley catheter is inflated to 45 ml on no traction. A 4-0 chromic catgut pursestring suture is placed in the bladder wall around the suprapubic tube. This step prevents any leakage and helps to gently hold the suprapubic tube in position during wound closure. A Penrose drain is placed down to the cystotomy site and brought out through a separate stab wound. The bladder is irrigated until clear and checked for any significant leakage.

The wound is irrigated and the linea alba closed with a running no. 2 nylon or no. 1 polydioxanone suture.[9] The skin is approximated with skin staples. The drain and suprapubic tube are sutured to the skin with nylon sutures and a dressing is applied.

POSTOPERATIVE MANAGEMENT AND COMPLICATIONS

Excessive blood loss is the most common immediate complication encountered; approximately 15 percent of patients require blood transfusions. If excessive bleeding from the prostatic fossa is noted intraoperatively, two techniques are effective. Mala-

ment[6] described the placement of a no. 1 or 2 nylon pursestring suture around the vesical neck; the suture was then brought out through the skin and tied snugly. This maneuver effectively closes the bladder neck and tamponades the prostatic fossa, with control of bleeding. Approximately 24 to 48 hours after placement the suture is cut on one side and removed. O'Connor[8] described plication of the posterior capsule using 0 chromic catgut suture on a 5/8 circle needle. This plication narrows the fossa and results in effective hemostasis. Point fulguration of bleeders in the fossa may also provide hemostasis.

Antibiotics are not indicated for elective prostatectomy in patients who have had no urinary tract infections and have sterile urine. In cases of long-term indwelling catheters or preoperative infections, appropriate intraoperative antibiotics, usually a cephalosporin and an aminoglycoside, are indicated.

Mortality for open prostatectomy should be less than 1 percent. Myocardial infarction, pneumonia, and pulmonary embolus are the most common causes. Early ambulation, leg movement in bed, and breathing exercises decrease morbidity.

The patient is usually limited to intravenous fluids the day of surgery, but the following day can usually

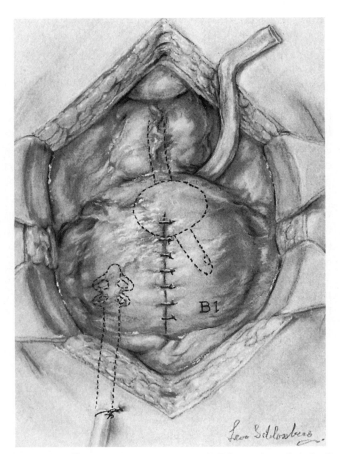

Figure 64–6. Suprapubic prostatectomy. A Foley catheter is indwelling per urethra. A Malecot suprapubic catheter and a prevesical Penrose drain are shown.

tolerate oral nutrition and often have a full diet. A stool softener or mild laxative is given to decrease straining with bowel movements and fecal impaction. Continuous bladder irrigation via the three-way Foley catheter is maintained for 12 to 24 hours. The Foley catheter is usually removed after 3 days, although the suprapubic catheter can be removed first. If the Foley catheter is removed first, the suprapubic tube is clamped at 5 days to give the patient a trial at voiding. It is removed the following day if voiding is satisfactory with little residual. The drain is removed a few hours after the suprapubic tube if no drainage occurs. The skin staples are removed on the seventh postoperative day and Steri-Strips are applied to the skin. On discharge from the hospital, the patient is encouraged to gradually increase his activity. He should be able to resume full activity 4 to 6 weeks postoperatively with outpatient visits at 3 and 6 weeks.

Delayed bleeding, as occasionally seen after transurethral resection of the prostate, is uncommon after suprapubic prostatectomy.

Wound infections occur in less than 5 percent of patients and are usually limited to the skin and subcutaneous tissue. Urinary fistulas have been reported. Rectal injury is very rare. Incontinence of urine is an uncommon complication that usually results from perforation and partial avulsion of the prostatic capsule, avulsion of the urethra at the apex of the prostate, or both. With careful enucleation of the adenoma, the capsule will not be perforated. With sharp excision of the urethra at the apex rather than avulsion, incontinence should not occur. Detrusor instability may cause stress and/or urge incontinence in some patients. Urethral stricture and bladder neck contracture occur most commonly as complications of transurethral resection and are uncommon after suprapubic prostatectomy. Erectile dysfunction after prostatectomy is reported but should not develop unless the capsule has been violated. Retrograde ejaculation is common. Postoperative epididymo-orchitis is uncommon but may occur early or late. This complication is usually seen in a patient who has had a long-term indwelling catheter or urinary tract infection.

Summary

Enucleation of the prostatic adenoma by a low suprapubic or transvesical approach is an excellent procedure applicable in approximately 10 percent of patients who present with significant bladder outlet obstructions. The operative mortality and morbidity are minimal.

Editorial Comment
Fray F. Marshall

Sometimes the bladder neck mucosa can be brought down into the proximal portion of the prostatic fossa with the hemostatic sutures at 4 and 8 o'clock. An attempt to surgically close the bladder neck around a catheter may theoretically create the possibility of bladder neck contracture. In the presence of significant bleeding, it may be helpful.

I have tended to prefer the retropubic prostatectomy rather than the suprapubic prostatectomy unless there is an intravesical gland, a bladder calculus, a bladder diverticulum, or some other specific reason to perform the operation suprapubically. However, the suprapubic operation has enjoyed great popularity over the years.

REFERENCES

1. Freyer PJ. A new method of performing prostatectomy. Lancet 1:774, 1900.
2. Freyer PJ. One thousand cases of total enucleation of the prostate for radical cure of enlargement of that organ. Br Med J 2:868, 1912.
3. Fuller E. Six successful and successive cases of prostatectomy. J Cutan Genitourin Dis 13:229, 1895.
4. Fuller E. The question of priority in the adoption of the method of total enucleation, suprapubically, of the hypertrophied prostate. Ann Surg 41:520, 1905.
5. Harvard BM. Low transvesical suprapubic prostatectomy with primary closure. In Campbell MF, ed. Urology, 1st ed. Philadelphia, WB Saunders, 1954.
6. Malament M. Maximal hemostasis in suprapubic prostatectomy. Surg Gynecol Obstet 120:1307, 1965.
7. Nanninga JE, O'Connor VJ Jr. Suprapubic and retropubic prostatectomy. In Walsh PC, Perlmutter AD, Gittes RF, Stamey TA, eds. Campbell's Urology, 5th ed. Philadelphia, WB Saunders, 1986.
8. O'Connor VJ Jr. An aid for hemostasis in open prostatectomy: Capsular plication. J Urol 127:448, 1982.
9. Poole GV Jr. Mechanical factors in abdominal wound closure: The prevention of fascial dehiscence. Surgery 97:631, 1985.
10. Schlegel PN, Walsh PC. Simultaneous preperitoneal hernia repair during radical pelvic surgery. J Urol 137:1180, 1987.

Chapter 65

Nerve-Sparing Radical Retropubic Prostatectomy

John F. McCarthy and William J. Catalona

The use of radical prostatectomy has produced excellent cure rates in appropriately selected patients whose prostate cancer is organ confined. In the past, many patients shied away from the classical radical prostatectomy, fearing the potential complications of sexual impotency and urinary incontinence. In the early 1980s, Walsh developed a modified approach to the performance of radical retropubic prostatectomy based on detailed knowledge of the surgical anatomy.[1] With an appreciation of this anatomy, preservation of both urinary continence and erections can be achieved in most patients.[2] We present our technique in this chapter.

INDICATIONS

The ideal candidates for nerve-sparing radical prostatectomy are men whose tumor is confined to the prostate and whose life expectancy is 10 years or more. In most instances, cancer that has extended to either local or distant sites will not be cured by radical prostatectomy.

PREOPERATIVE EVALUATION

Preoperative evaluation of a patient with prostate cancer should include measurement of serum prostate-specific antigen (PSA) and acid phosphatase concentrations as well as a radionuclide bone scan. Transrectal prostatic ultrasonography has become an integral part of the biopsy process and can be helpful in determining the local extent of the carcinoma. Optional imaging studies include abdominal and pelvic computed tomographic scanning or magnetic resonance imaging, which are best reserved for patients with poorly differentiated tumors and those with high serum PSA concentrations (more than 20 ng/ml).

Preoperatively, we have the patient donate 1 or 2 units of autologous blood to decrease the chance of receiving nonautologous transfusions. Alternatively, we treat the patient with erythropoietin in anticipation of performing intraoperative hemodilution. The day before surgery, the patient should have a light dinner. The evening before surgery, we have the patient insert a bisacodyl rectal suppository. A sodium biphosphate enema is given to mechanically cleanse the rectum after the suppository has induced a bowel movement. A first-generation cephalosporin is administered on call to the operating room.

In the operating room, thigh-high elastic hose are placed on the patient. He is positioned with his legs on spreader bars, and the operating table is flexed (Fig. 65–1). This allows an assistant to use a sponge forceps to displace the perineum in a cranial direction, which enhances the exposure of the urethral stump for the surgeon and facilitates the performance of the vesicourethral anastomosis (Fig. 65–2). A 22 Fr. Foley catheter is inserted after the patient has been prepared and draped, and the sterile drainage bag remains on the surgical field for the duration of the operation.

SURGICAL TECHNIQUE

We begin the operation with a midline lower abdominal incision. The linea alba is incised and the prevesical space entered. With care to avoid disrupting the lymphatic tissue lateral to the external iliac vein and to avoid compression of the vein itself, a Balfour retractor is placed. A modified pelvic lymphadenectomy is performed, removing only the lymph nodes medial to the external iliac vein. Care

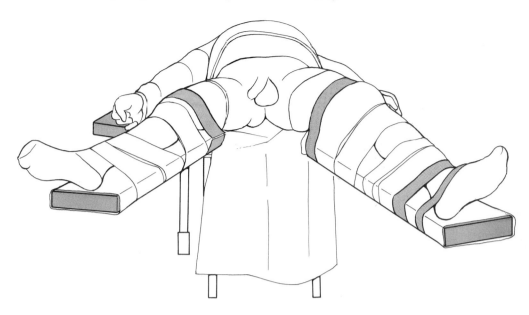

Figure 65–1. The patient is positioned with his legs on spreader bars and with the break in the table situated in line with the anterosuperior iliac spine. By breaking the table, the distance between the umbilicus and the symphysis pubis is maximized, improving visualization of the pelvic structures.

is taken during the lymphadenectomy to preserve any accessory arterial branches to the corpora cavernosa that arise from the distal external iliac or obturator arteries. The excised lymph node packet is sent for frozen-section examination, unless the patient has decided to have the prostate gland removed even if there are pelvic lymph node metastases. If the frozen-section examination reveals metastatic cancer, it is unlikely that the patient will be cured by radical prostatectomy, and the operation is terminated.

After completing the lymphadenectomy, the adipose and areolar tissue is swept gently from the anterior surface of the prostate and the endopelvic fascia to expose the puboprostatic ligaments. Care is taken to avoid injury to the perforating branches of Santorini's plexus that pierce the endopelvic fascia between the puboprostatic ligaments and pass cephalad on the anterior surface of the bladder.

The endopelvic fascia is pierced with the scissors in the groove between the levator ani muscles and the lateral border of the prostate. Inside the endopelvic fascia, the lateral surface of the prostate is covered by a smooth, glistening membrane overlying the lat-

eral portion of Santorini's plexus. Strands of the levator ani muscles are gently dissected off the prostate to the level of the urogenital diaphragm. Often, venous tributaries pass from the levator ani muscles to the prostate just lateral to the puboprostatic ligaments (Fig. 65–3). These vessels are ligated laterally, then clamped medially with a delicate snub-nose right-angled clamp. After the vein is transected sharply, its medial portion is ligated. When the endopelvic fascia has been opened from the base to the apex of the prostate, the superficial branch of Santorini's plexus is gently retracted medially, and the puboprostatic ligaments are placed on stretch and divided close to the pubic symphysis. Care is taken not to divide the puboprostatic ligaments too medially or too far under the pubic symphysis to avoid injuring the dorsal venous complex.

After the puboprostatic ligaments are divided, the lateral surfaces of the urethra are palpated. The groove between the anterior surface of the urethra and the dorsal venous complex is developed with a pinching motion of the left index finger and thumb. An extra-large right-angled clamp is then passed in

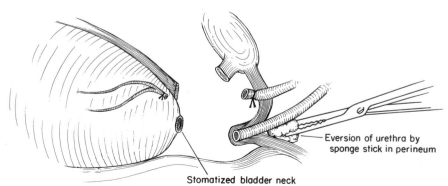

Stomatized bladder neck

Eversion of urethra by sponge stick in perineum

Figure 65–2. An assistant standing between the patient's legs uses a sponge forceps to displace the perineum in the cephalad direction. This everts the urethral stump and facilitates the performance of the vesicourethral anastomosis.

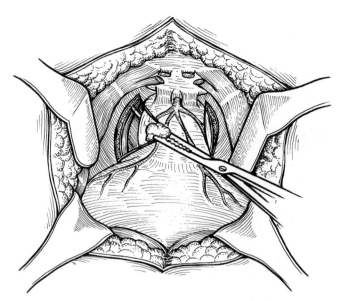

Figure 65–3. The endopelvic fascia is opened. Using a sponge forceps, the prostate may be retracted medially to free any strands of the levator ani muscle fibers that remain attached to the prostate. Often, small crossing veins are encountered that require ligation.

the avascular plane anterior to the urethra. A No. 1 polyglycolic acid ligature is grasped and passed around the dorsal venous complex. The plane between the urethra and the dorsal venous complex is then developed gently, first with a right-angled clamp and then with a pedicle clamp (Fig. 65–4). This facilitates tight ligation of the dorsal venous complex. A 2-0 chromic catgut suture ligature is placed in the anterior surface of the prostate to reduce back-bleeding from Santorini's plexus.

The right-angled clamp is then passed behind the dorsal venous complex and its jaws are spread. Under direct vision, the dorsal venous complex is transected with a scalpel. Back-bleeding from the dorsal venous complex is controlled with a running 2-0 polyglycolic acid hemostatic suture. It is important to obtain good hemostasis so that the apical dissection of the prostate may be performed in a relatively bloodless field. If the dorsal venous complex ligature slips off, the complex is oversewn using a 2-0 chromic catgut su-

ture on a 5/8 circle needle. The goal in oversewing the complex is to pass the suture just through the lateral borders of the complex itself in its anterior, middle, and posterior aspects. Wide, imprecisely placed sutures may damage the neurovascular bundles.

The anterior surface of the urethra is palpated between the neurovascular bundles. The circumurethral sphincter muscle and the anterior wall of the urethra are incised with a scalpel without dissecting around the lateral or posterior surfaces of the urethra. The incision should not be carried too far laterally, where it may injure the neurovascular bundles. The urethral catheter is exposed and carefully hooked with a delicate right-angled clamp. Gentle traction on the clamp in a cephalad direction exposes the posterior wall of the urethra. The catheter is divided and placed on cephalad traction, the posterior urethral wall is sharply transected, and the fibromuscular bands tethering the apex of the prostate are incised using sharp dissection.

The lateral pelvic fascia is incised from the apex of the prostate to the base. A delicate right-angled clamp may be used to elevate the lateral pelvic fascia from the underlying veins on the surface of the prostate. Small perforating vessels are secured with hemoclips, ties, or ligatures to ensure adequate control. The posterolateral groove between the prostate and the neurovascular bundles is developed using sharp and blunt dissection (Fig. 65–5), allowing the prostate to assume a more anterior position in the pelvis. The dissection is carried distally, following the curve of the prostate until the rectourethral muscle is encountered. The rectourethral muscle and the inferior extension of Denonvilliers' fascia are isolated posterior to the prostate and medial to the neurovascular bundles. The rectourethral muscle is then incised, along with the remaining fibrovascular attachments to the apex of the prostate, exposing the prerectal fat (Fig. 65–6).

The lateral aspect of the prostate is then dissected from the neurovascular bundles, which allows the latter to retract laterally. The plane between the pros-

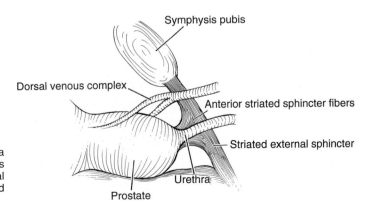

Figure 65–4. The dorsal venous complex lies anterior to the urethra and the circumurethral sphincter mechanism. A right-angled clamp is passed in the avascular space between the urethra and the dorsal venous complex to develop a plane for passage of a ligature around the complex.

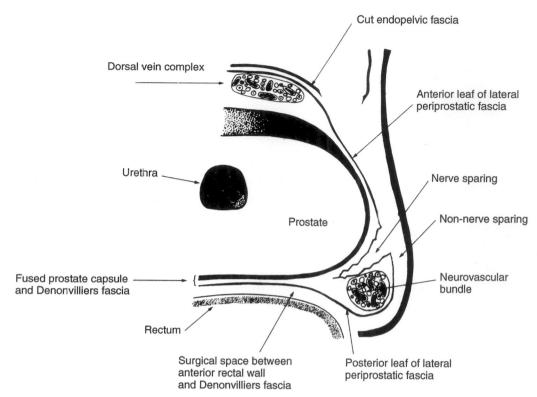

Figure 65–5. In performing nerve-sparing radical prostatectomy, the neurovascular bundles are sharply dissected from the prostate and allowed to retract laterally and posteriorly.

tate and the rectum is developed by passing an index finger between the prostate and the rectum in the midline. In a case of extensive fibrosis, the dissection is performed sharply. The dissection is carried cephalad until the portion of Denonvilliers' fascia covering the ampullary portions of the vasa deferentia and the seminal vesicles is exposed. Denonvilliers' fascia is incised with the cautery. The scissors are then used to develop the proper plane beneath Denonvilliers' fascia and the underlying seminal vesicles. Denonvilliers' fascia is incised laterally toward the neurovascular bundles to expose the proper plane of dissection for the prostatic vascular pedicles.

The prostatic pedicles are divided by inserting the right-angled clamp medial to them, with the tip of the clamp directed almost parallel to the lateral surface of the prostate (Fig. 65–7). The prostatic pedicle is ligated laterally, taking care to place the tie medial to the neurovascular bundle. The pedicle is divided close to the prostate. This dissection is performed on both sides to a point just cephalad to the seminal vesicles. Care is taken when dissecting near the seminal vesicles to avoid injuring the neurovascular bundles that are situated just lateral to the seminal vesicles. The seminal vesicles are freed from the bladder base using sharp and blunt dissection, and a pedicle clamp is used to further develop this plane. Two hemostatic sutures of 3-0 chromic catgut are placed in the lateral bladder pedicles, one just lateral to the

prostate and another just medial to the neurovascular bundles. It is important to avoid including the seminal vesicles in these sutures. The lateral bladder neck fibers are partially incised with the cautery, but are not incised through their entire thickness.

The anterior bladder neck is transected in the natural groove between the bladder and the prostate. We use a scalpel for this to avoid cautery injury to the tissues that will be included in the vesicourethral anastomosis. The bladder neck opening is enlarged with scissors, and the catheter is pulled through and used as a tractor on the prostate. The posterior bladder neck is incised with the cautery. The muscular attachments between the bladder and prostate are isolated with a right-angled clamp, clipped with hemoclips, and divided.

The seminal vesicles are dissected first along their lateral edges, carrying the plane of dissection medially. Many small perforating arteries enter the lateral and terminal portions of the seminal vesicles. These are secured with small hemoclips. The ampullae are freed using sharp and blunt dissection, and then clipped and transected. After the seminal vesicles have been dissected to their tips and the hemoclips placed, the surgical specimen is removed. At this point, the pelvis is carefully inspected for hemostasis. Most small bleeders on the neurovascular bundles stop bleeding spontaneously, but some may require 4-0 chromic catgut suture ligatures. It is important

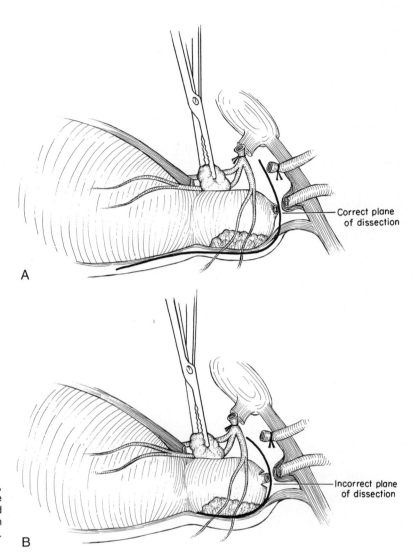

Correct plane
of dissection

A

Incorrect plane
of dissection

B

Figure 65–6. *A* and *B*, After in situ division of the urethra, the rectourethral muscle is transected in order to enter the correct plane between the anterior rectal wall and Denonvilliers' fascia. Failure to enter the correct plane can lead to dissection in a plane within the prostatic capsule. This can produce cancerous surgical margins.

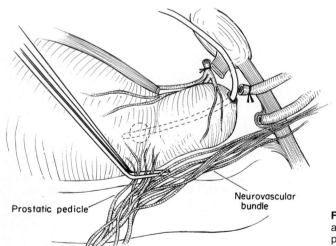

Prostatic pedicle

Neurovascular bundle

Figure 65–7. The prostatic pedicles are ligated with 2-0 silk ligatures and then transected. Passing the right-angled clamp too close to the prostate can result in a cancerous surgical margin; passing it too far laterally can injure the neurovascular bundles.

not to use the cautery for hemostasis on the neurovascular bundles, to avoid cautery injury to the cavernosal nerves.

Reconstruction of the bladder neck begins by everting the anterior bladder neck mucosa with a right-angled clamp. The mucosa and underlying detrusor muscle are grasped with a delicate Allis clamp. Three everting sutures of 3-0 chromic catgut that encompass mucosa and underlying muscle are anchored in the groove formed by the cut edge of the bladder neck muscle. Tying these sutures everts the mucosa. The bladder neck is closed in a tennis racket fashion, with the handle of the racket directed posteriorly. Bladder neck closure is accomplished through a single-layer closure of interrupted 2-0 chromic catgut sutures. Each suture must include both muscle and mucosa, and care should be taken to avoid compromising the ureteral orifices. The bladder neck is closed to a size of approximately 22 to 24 Fr. (Fig. 65–8).

An 18 Fr. catheter with a 30-ml balloon is passed through the urethra. The assistant provides pressure on the perineum with a sponge forceps to better expose the urethral stump for the surgeon. Doubly armed 2-0 chromic catgut sutures are used for the vesicourethral anastomosis. A 5/8 circle needle is used to place the anterior sutures at the 10 and 2 o'clock positions. The suture is passed from inside the urethra to the outside, avoiding placing it into the neurovascular bundles. The tip of the catheter is grasped and brought out of the wound to expose the posterior lip of the urethral stump. The posterior sutures are similarly placed at the 5 and 7 o'clock positions. The other ends of the sutures are placed in the corresponding positions on the bladder neck. These sutures encompass mucosa and muscle and exit at the edge of the mucosa. The catheter tip is placed in the bladder, and the bladder neck is guided gently toward the urethral stump. The anastomotic sutures are tied carefully under direct vision. The bladder is then irrigated free of clots, suction drains are placed in the pelvis, and the incision is closed.

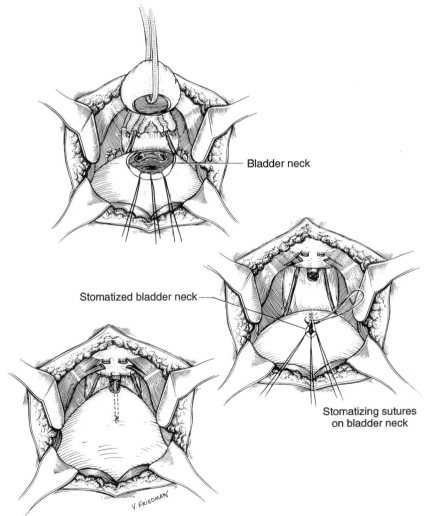

Bladder neck

Stomatized bladder neck

Stomatizing sutures on bladder neck

V. FRIEDMAN

Figure 65–8. After the seminal vesicles have been dissected out, the prostate gland is removed. The bladder neck is stomatized using 3-0 chromic catgut sutures. The handle of the tennis racket closure is performed with a single layer of interrupted 2-0 chromic catgut sutures that include both muscle and mucosa. After placement of the anastomotic sutures, the reconstructed bladder neck is brought to the urethral stump over a catheter and the sutures are tied.

POSTOPERATIVE CARE AND MONITORING

We routinely manage postoperative pain with intramuscular ketorolac. The initial dose of 60 mg is given intraoperatively, with 30-mg injections every 6 hours thereafter for 24 hours. Care is needed when prescribing this medication for older patients, patients with renal insufficiency, or those with a history of peptic ulcer disease. With this regimen, we have achieved excellent pain relief without significant complications. By avoiding the use of narcotic pain relievers, postoperative sedation is greatly reduced and return of bowel function occurs more quickly.

Patients begin a mechanical soft diet on the morning of the first postoperative day and are advanced to a regular diet on the morning of the second day. The suction drains are removed when their output is less than 50 ml per shift, usually by the second or third postoperative day. The Foley catheter is removed 2 weeks after surgery, at which time the first postoperative serum PSA measurement is made. Oral antibiotics are begun the day before catheter removal and are continued for 2 weeks thereafter.

The serum PSA concentration should fall to an undetectable range within 2 to 3 weeks after surgery, although in patients with higher preoperative PSA levels it takes longer. Patients whose serum PSA concentrations remain at a detectable level postoperatively usually have distant metastases or a large residual tumor burden. Adjuvant external beam radiation therapy usually fails to provide durable responses in most such patients.

We customarily follow patients whose surgical margins are positive with semiannual digital rectal examinations and serum PSA testing. If the PSA concentration begins to rise after being initially undetectable and if restaging shows no distant metastases, we recommend external beam radiation (6000 rad) to the pelvis. The results to date are encouraging.[3] In patients with extensively positive surgical margins, we usually recommend adjuvant external beam radiation therapy beginning about 3 months after the prostatectomy.

COMPLICATIONS

With contemporary surgical techniques, radical retropubic prostatectomy is well tolerated, with perioperative mortality rates well below 1 percent and total postoperative complication rates (excluding erectile dysfunction and temporary urinary incontinence) around 5 percent.[4] Complications associated with the operation can be divided into those that occur intraoperatively and those that occur postoperatively.

Intraoperative

The most common intraoperative problem encountered with radical retropubic prostatectomy is acute blood loss. Careful attention to anatomical detail is of the utmost importance in reducing blood loss. With an average blood loss of 1200 to 1500 ml and the almost routine need for blood transfusion, we request that our patients donate 1 or 2 units of autologous blood before surgery. This autologous blood, along with the performance of intraoperative hemodilution and autotransfusion, obviates the need for nonautologous blood transfusions in more than 90 percent of patients. We have also had promising results with preoperative administration of erythropoietin combined with intraoperative hemodilution and autologous transfusions.

Other intraoperative complications are related to inadvertent injury to adjacent structures. Rectal injury is a rare complication that occurs in less than 1 percent of cases.[4] Careful transection of the rectourethral muscle under direct vision decreases the risk of rectal injury. Small rectal injuries identified intraoperatively can be repaired primarily. Large rectal defects or injuries in irradiated patients should be managed with a temporary diverting colostomy.

Ureteral injury, which can occur during either pelvic lymphadenectomy or radical prostatectomy, is also a rare complication. The most important aspect of management is intraoperative recognition. Efflux of urine from each ureteral orifice should be noted during the operation, and no urine should be seen to accumulate outside the bladder. If a ureteral injury is identified, ureteroneocystostomy should be performed.

Postoperative

Deep venous thrombosis and pulmonary embolism are serious complications of radical prostatectomy. We have seen a deep venous thrombosis rate of 0.8 percent and a pulmonary embolus rate of 2.3 percent.[4] A high index of suspicion should be maintained to detect either of these complications. Any unexplained fever, shortness of breath, tachycardia, tachypnea, or minimal lower extremity edema or tenderness should be completely evaluated. We anticoagulate patients with full-dose intravenous heparin if we suspect pulmonary embolism, and then stop the heparin if the definitive evaluation is negative.

Additional complications in the early postoperative period include wound hematoma (0.7 percent), atrial fibrillation (0.6 percent), myocardial infarction (0.4 percent), and lymphocoele (0.4 percent).[4]

The most common late complications of nervesparing prostatectomy include bladder neck contracture, impotence, and urinary incontinence. In our series, 5 percent of patients developed bladder neck contracture, although in our last 310 cases the contracture rate fell to 0.6 percent. The reduction in contractures has probably occurred because we now fashion the bladder neck to 22 to 24 Fr. rather than 18 Fr. and are careful to achieve mucosa-to-mucosa approximation. Bladder neck contracture can be managed initially with dilation, and if this fails, with cold knife incision.

The most feared and disabling complication after prostatectomy is urinary incontinence. Using our technique of avoiding dissection around the urethra during the apical dissection to prevent injury to the circumurethral sphincter mechanism, we have achieved immediate postoperative continence in more than 50 percent of patients. In the remaining patients, urinary control usually returns in three phases: phase I, patients are dry when lying down at night; phase II, they are dry when ambulating; and phase III, they are dry when rising from a seated position. We have achieved continence (no protective measures to keep clothing dry) in 94 percent of patients.[5] There appears to be no significant correlation between continence and age of the patient, pathological stage, previous transurethral resection, and the performance of nerve-sparing surgery.

The delineation of the neurovascular anatomy by Walsh has significantly decreased the incidence of postoperative impotence.[1] After bilateral nerve-sparing surgery, return of erections occurs more often in young men and in those with organ-confined cancer. Men under 60 years of age who undergo a bilateral nerve-sparing procedure and have pathologically organ-confined disease are most likely to regain potency (78 percent). Overall, in our patient population, erections returned in 63 percent of patients treated with a bilateral nerve-sparing procedure and 41 percent of those receiving a unilateral nerve-sparing procedure.[5] Generally, potency returns slowly over a period of 3 to 6 months, with some patients continuing to improve for up to 18 months or longer.

Summary

Radical retropubic prostatectomy is the preferred treatment for men with localized prostate cancer whose life expectancy is 10 years or more, because of its unsurpassed ability to control the primary tumor. With current understanding of the sphincteric and neurovascular anatomy, excellent cancer control can be achieved with a low incidence of postoperative incontinence and impotence.

Editorial Comment
Fray F. Marshall

Dr. Catalona's extensive experience demonstrates very nicely the technique of radical retropubic prostatectomy. Control of the dorsal vein complex remains paramount in the dissection. Careful dissection of the urethra and sphincter may allow early return of continence. Previously the urethra was often extensively mobilized, and this mobilization may be detrimental to early continence. Ketorolac administration with avoidance of opiates may also allow earlier return of bowel function and earlier discharge from the hospital.

With these refinements in technique, the blood loss has been reduced and continence has improved. Compared with a perineal prostatectomy, blood loss may still be somewhat higher, but potency rates are not often reported with perineal prostatectomy. In addition, lymph nodes are not inspected with a perineal approach, although the incidence of positive lymph nodes in a favorable patient may be quite low.

REFERENCES

1. Walsh PC, Lepor H, Eggleston JC. Radical prostatectomy with preservation of sexual function: Anatomical and pathological considerations. Prostate 4:473, 1983.
2. Walsh PC. Radical prostatectomy with preservation of sexual function: Evolution of a surgical procedure. AUA Update Series Vol 5, lesson 5, 1986.
3. McCarthy JF, Catalona WJ, Hudson MA. Effect of radiation therapy on detectable serum prostate specific antigen levels following radical prostatectomy: Early versus delayed treatment. J Urol 151:1575, 1994.
4. Keetch DW, Andriole GL, Catalona WJ. Complications of radical retropubic prostatectomy. AUA Update Series Vol 13, lesson 6, 1994.
5. Catalona WJ, Basler JW. Return of erections and urinary continence following nerve sparing radical retropubic prostatectomy. J Urol 150:905, 1993.

Chapter 66

Radical Perineal Prostatectomy

David F. Paulson

Radical perineal prostatectomy is one of the two commonly accepted methods for surgical extirpation of the prostate. The operative procedure, once thought to be the ideal method for control of prostatic carcinoma, fell into disuse in the late 1960s and early 1970s, partly because of the belief that radical surgery was not a reasonable method for control of apparent organ-confined prostatic malignancy and partly because of an increasing tendency of surgical training programs to provide only retropubic experience. Recently, it has become more acceptable to consider perineal prostatectomy as an equivalent method for surgical control of prostatic malignancy.[1-3]

PATIENT SELECTION

If one adheres to the philosophy that surgical treatment of prostatic malignancy is appropriate only for patients with disease clinically confined to the prostate, preoperative staging maneuvers should be those designed to ensure, to the best of one's ability, that the disease is confined to the prostate.[4, 5] Patients are subjected to preoperative isotopic bone scanning to check that metastatic disease does not exist and also to provide a baseline against which future studies may be compared. Further, patients must have a serum acid phosphatase level on colorimetric or enzymatic assay that is within the normal range, as experience has indicated that patients whose levels are abnormally elevated have an 85 percent probability of showing clinical failure at a distant site 4 years after the date of operative intervention.[6] Lastly, all reasonable efforts must be made to determine that the patient has no metastatic lymph node extension. This can be accomplished by staging pelvic lymphadenectomy through a lower abdominal incision or by laparoscopic surgery during anesthesia prior to that needed for the perineal prostatectomy, or this surgical staging may be accomplished under the same anesthetic. Recent data (unpublished personal observa-

tions) have demonstrated that, in patients with non-palpable disease, whose prebiopsy prostate-specific antigen (PSA) reading is less than 20 ng/ml, and whose Gleason sum is less than 7, the probability of lymph node extension is so small that preoperative lymphadenectomy may be discarded and they may be subjected to radical perineal prostatectomy without physical assessment of the regional lymph nodes.

PREOPERATIVE PREPARATION

The patient is given an osmotic mechanical bowel preparation the day before surgery, with nonabsorbable oral antibiotics the evening before the procedure. On the morning of surgery a neomycin enema is given 2 to 3 hours before the scheduled operative procedure. Broad-spectrum antibiotics are given parenterally on call.

CONTRAINDICATIONS

Patients who have significant competing risks of death that are estimated to arise 10 years from the projected date of surgery are not considered candidates for radical prostatectomy. Those who have undergone an open transcapsular or transvesical prostatectomy are not thought to be candidates for perineal prostatectomy owing to fixation of the prostatic capsule and/or bladder within the pelvis, which may prevent an adequate urethrovesical anastomosis from being established. Patients who are massively obese may not be able to tolerate the exaggerated lithotomy position, as the intra-abdominal contents may drive the diaphragm into the chest and prevent adequate respiration even at increased ventilatory pressures. Previous pelvic radiation, other pelvic surgery, and abdominoperineal resection are not contraindications to surgery except when the previous therapy has compromised the bladder neck.[7]

545

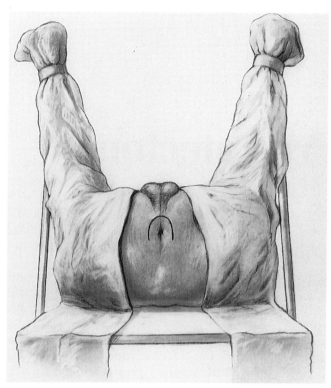

Figure 66–1. In the exaggerated lithotomy position, the weight of the patient is borne across the upper back, and positioning is maintained by towels or pillows placed beneath the sacrum or small of the back. (From Skinner DG, Lieskovsky G. Diagnosis and Management of Genitourinary Cancer. Philadelphia, WB Saunders, 1988.)

OPERATIVE PROCEDURE

Patient Positioning

The procedure may be accomplished on a standard operating table using any available form of leg support (Fig. 66–1). My preference is to use candy-cane stirrups, wrapping the feet to ensure that the straps do not place excessive pressure on bony prominences. There is no need to wrap the legs or to place them in alternating pressure stockings. For proper positioning, the patient is placed far from the head of the table, the small of the back being brought to the edge of the table with the buttocks extending approximately 8 to 12 inches over the end of the table. There is no necessity to use shoulder braces to stabilize the patient by producing counterpressure on the upper body and shoulders. With the patient properly positioned, his weight is borne across the upper back while sandbags or folded towels placed beneath the sacrum and the small of the back maintain elevation of the pelvis. The legs and feet are rotated toward the head, and when the patient has been properly positioned, the perineum is parallel to the floor. The ischial tuberosities can be palpated and should lie in a line parallel or just posterior to the anus (Fig. 66–2).

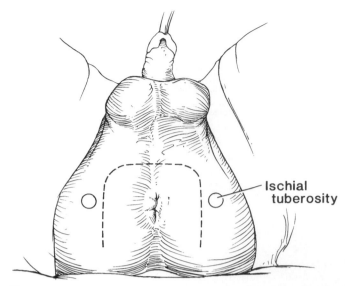

Figure 66–2. The incision is a generous inverted U and is carried posteriorly to the anus.

Exposure of the Prostate

A skin incision is made 1.5 cm anterior to the anal verge, extended posterolaterally on either side of the anus medial to the ischial tuberosities (Fig. 66–2), and continued behind the anus on either side. The ischiorectal space is now opened. To create this space, a defect is created in the superficial perineal fascia on either side of the central tendon using the cutting cautery. The surgical space in the ischiorectal fossa is developed by placing a finger into this defect perpendicular to the floor (Fig. 66–3). The finger is then curved toward the operating surgeon, and the

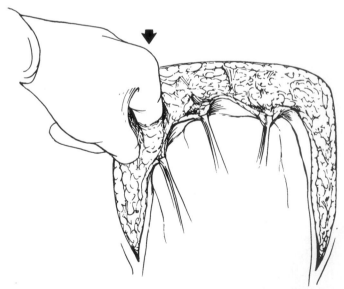

Figure 66–3. The anus is excluded from the field by the use of drapes and Allis clamps. The fibrofatty tissue to either side of the midline is incised with cautery to permit access to the ischial rectal fossa.

overlying fibrofatty tissue is incised with the cutting cautery. The surgeon may then place a finger on either side of the rectum and identify its position relative to the central tendon. The next maneuver is designed to sever the central tendon and allow the anus and rectum to be displaced posteriorly. The surgeon passes a finger anterior to the rectum and beneath the central tendon. The central tendon is a fibromuscular tissue that inserts posteriorly on the tip of the coccyx, flows around the rectum, and inserts on the perineal body. This fibromuscular tissue must be divided so that the anus and rectum can be displaced posteriorly. Once the surgeon has passed a finger anterior to the rectum and beneath the central tendon, the central tendon is divided in its entirety with cautery, a line of incision being made as close as possible to the skin margin (Fig. 66–4). The surgeon may wish to mark the muscular extension of the central tendon either with surgical clips or with a black silk suture so that it can be identified during final reconstruction of the perineum.

After division of the central tendon, the anus will drop posteriorly and, with upper traction on the perineal body, the rectourethralis may be identified as well as the glistening surface of the anterior rectal fascia (Fig. 66–5). With the Metzenbaum scissors held in such a way that their curve approximates the curve of the rectum, and by gently spreading the scissors on either side of the midline, with blunt dissection, the anterior surface of the rectum can be exposed and mobilized on either side of the rectourethralis to and beyond the level of the prostatic apex (Fig. 66–5).

The next maneuver is designed to place the rectourethralis on tension. To accomplish this, an examining finger is placed in the rectum to place downward pressure on the rectum while an assistant elevates the perineal body in the opposite direction. A finger may now be placed on either side of the rectourethralis to further open this space by blunt dissection. Next, using Metzenbaum scissors, the rectourethralis is incised in the midline only. As this tissue is divided with Metzenbaum scissors, it will be seen to be white and largely avascular. The series of cuts should be made to the level of the prostate, at which point the rectum will be seen to be displaced posteriorly and the prostate will be visualized anteriorly. The tissue that appears to either side of the midline is that portion of the levator sling that supports the prostate and pelvis. Although this may be divided, it is preferable to leave this tissue intact so that this muscular sling may be brought together in the midline to support the urethrovesical anastomosis at the completion of the operative procedure.

The next maneuver is designed to fully expose the prostate laterally and posteriorly. This can be easily

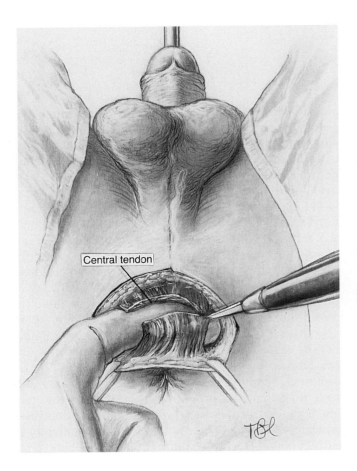

Figure 66–4. The central tendon is isolated by placing a finger anterior to the rectum and is divided at the skin margin. (From Skinner DG, Lieskovsky G. Diagnosis and Management of Genitourinary Cancer. Philadelphia, WB Saunders, 1988.)

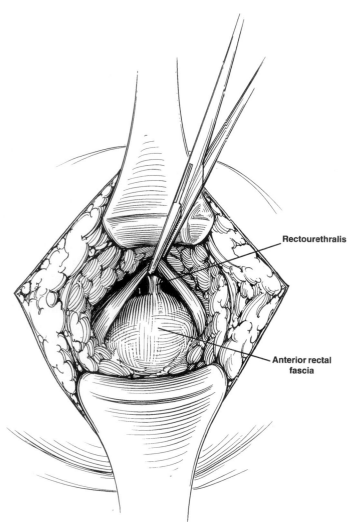

Rectourethralis

Anterior rectal fascia

Figure 66–5. The muscular fibers overlying the anterior rectal fascia are elevated and, with the anterior rectal fascia as a guide, a plane is established on either side of the rectourethralis to the base of the prostate.

accomplished by using a bronchial or Kitner dissector, placing the instrument medial to the levator sling and lateral to the margin of the prostate. With inward and downward pressure, the prostate and neurovascular fascia can be separated from the levator sling to the level of the reflection of the endopelvic fascia onto the bladder. This is largely an avascular plane. Once this area has been developed on both the right and left side of the prostate, exposure is maintained by the use of baby Deaver retractors. Fixed retractors may be used, but I prefer hand-held retractors to facilitate exposure.

Attention is now turned to developing a plane between the rectum posteriorly and the prostate anteriorly. After the prostate has been exposed in the manner described above, the posterior aspect of the prostate will be covered with musculature that is seemingly continuous with the anterior rectal surface. By downward pressure on the rectum, the margin between rectum and prostate can be identified, and these fibers may be divided with Metzenbaum or Strully scissors. Once these muscular fibers have

been divided, digital dissection will establish a plane between the prostate and seminal vesicles anteriorly and the rectal surface posteriorly.

Note that the Lowsley retractor has not been mentioned at any time during the maneuvers described above. The Lowsley prostatic retractor is placed on the urethra, and the bladder and blades are opened. The Lowsley may or may not be necessary and may be replaced by a curved sound. This retractor is not used at any time except to stabilize the prostate while it is being liberated from the levator sling on either side, or when it is being elevated to permit identification of the plane between rectum and prostate posteriorly. Anterior or downward pressure on the handle of the Lowsley retractor will cause the prostate to move into the operative field and will decrease markedly the amount of exposure between the bony pelvis and the prostatic surface. The movement is similar to pulling a cork from the inside of a wine bottle into the neck of the bottle and then attempting to dissect between the cork and the bottle neck.

Exposure of the Prostatic Apex, Urethra, and Neurovascular Fascia

The prostate has been exposed laterally and posteriorly. It is now time to expose the apex of the prostate, identify the urethra, determine whether the neurovascular fascia will be sacrificed unilaterally or bilaterally, and then divide the urethra from the apex of the prostate. To accomplish this, the surgeon should palpate the prostate laterally to ascertain whether there is palpable disease on the side of the negative biopsy. If there is any suggestion of such disease, it is my current opinion that the neurovascular fascia should be sacrificed on this side. It is also my belief that the neurovascular fascia should always be sacrificed on the side of the positive biopsy.

With the prostate exposed and still covered posteriorly with fibromuscular tissue, the surgeon may palpate the Lowsley retractor in the urethra at the apex of the prostate. With scissors, the fibers overlying the apex of the prostate and the urethra are incised only in the midline. With blunt dissection utilizing a bronchial or Kitner dissector, the prostatic apex is displaced posteriorly and the urethra exposed in the midline. This dissector may then be pushed on either side of the urethra, medial to the neurovascular tissues that flow off the prostate and that parallel the urethra, to separate them from the urethra. Once this plane has been accomplished, if the surgeon intends to sacrifice the neurovascular fascia at the apex, the tissue may be divided. If the surgeon proposes to preserve the tissue, the neurovascular fascia is dissected with sharp dissection off the prostatic substance from the apex to the base of the prostate (Fig. 66–6).

In either instance the surgeon may, with digital dissection to the right and left of the urethra, separate prostatic substance from beneath the dorsal venous complex and liberate prostatic substance from the detrusor musculature. It may be necessary to excise some of the investing fascia on either side in order to further expose the apex of the prostate. Once the apex of the prostate and the urethra have been fully mobilized, a right-angled clamp is placed around the urethra, the Lowsley retractor is removed, and the urethra is divided at the apex, the patient side margin being tagged with 2-0 suture to permit its easy identification during reconstruction.

After division of the urethra, a Young prostatic tractor (or a straight Lowsley retractor) is passed through the urethra into the bladder, and the blades are extended. The extended blades permit the sur-

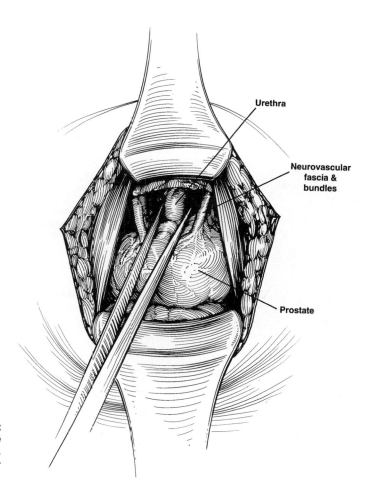

Urethra

Neurovascular fascia & bundles

Prostate

Figure 66–6. The urethra may be exposed in the midline at the apex of the prostate and the neurovascular fascia separated from the urethra. This fascial layer, which is adherent to prostatic substance, may be preserved or sacrificed in accordance with the extent of disease.

geon to identify the bladder wall and also to manipulate the operative specimen. Allis clamps or a tenaculum may be placed on the apex of the prostate to draw the prostate into the operative field and to permit identification of the plane between prostate and detrusor fibers. With blunt dissection, the plane between prostate and detrusor can be developed to the right and left of the bladder neck.

The bladder neck is then sharply divided between 10 and 2 o'clock using curved Metzenbaum scissors, a large curved clamp is passed through the prostatic urethra from apex to bladder neck, and a Foley catheter of any size is grasped and brought out through the apex of the prostate, the catheter being held as a loop and used for manipulation of the specimen. With traction on the Foley catheter and the tenaculum, the prostate is further mobilized on either side of the bladder neck and cut away from the bladder laterally. There is no need to use surgical clips at this level; any bleeding points encountered can be successfully controlled after division with electrocautery. Once the prostate is maximally mobilized but still adherent to the posterior bladder neck, the curved Metzenbaum scissors are passed behind the bladder neck and the posterior bladder neck is sharply divided. This now allows the bladder to retract into the pelvis.

With traction on the prostate to bring it further into the operative field, the surgeon should incise with scissors the fibromuscular tissue overlying the vas

deferens and seminal vesicles in the midline. This is an avascular structure and these tissues may be divided with impunity. Once the vasa deferentia have been identified in the midline, the surgeon can begin to mobilize the lateral vascular pedicles to the prostate. This is accomplished by using a right-angled clamp and passing it lateral to the seminal vesicles but medial to the vascular pedicle to the prostate (Fig. 66–7). Once this space has been identified, the vascular pedicles may be controlled with surgical clips, or they can be sharply divided and controlled by electrocoagulation. In fact, using the seminal vesicles as an anatomical marker, the seminal vesicles can be entirely encircled at the base of the prostate, investing tissue sharply divided to fully mobilize the prostate. If, for technical reasons, the surgeon should decide not to so mobilize the prostatic specimen, the specimen may be elevated anteriorly by direct upward traction on the tenaculum, and the fibrous tissue (Denonvilliers' fascia) overlying the seminal vesicles and vas deferens in the midline can be incised transversely. With this accomplished, using either a tonsillar or a right-angled clamp, a plane can be established between the seminal vesicles medially and fibrovascular tissue posterolaterally, this tissue being controlled either with surgical clips before division or by electrocautery after division. Once the fibrovascular tissue and vascular pedicles have been controlled on both the right and left sides, the specimen

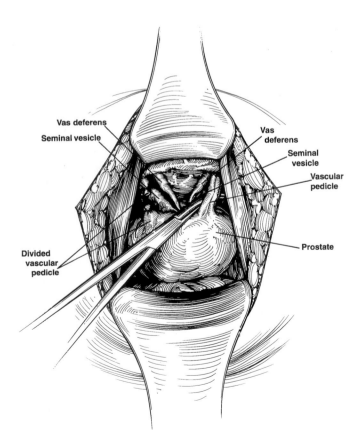

Figure 66–7. The seminal vesicles bilaterally are the landmarks the surgeon uses to identify the plane for control of the vascular pedicles of the prostate. A right-angled clamp may be passed lateral to the seminal vesicles and medial to the vascular pedicle. This tissue is divided sharply and vascular control established either mechanically or with electrocautery.

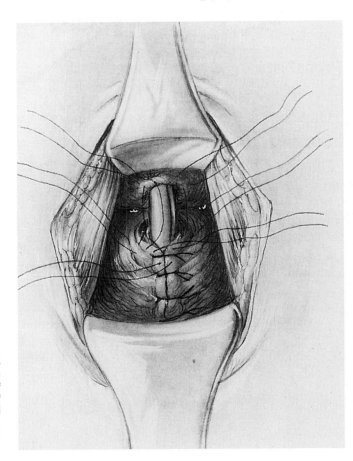

Figure 66–8. The anastomosis between the urethra and bladder neck, closed previously from 6 o'clock to 12 o'clock with interrupted 0 absorbable suture, is accomplished by four-quadrant sutures of 00 absorbable sutures. The direct anastomosis is supported by Dees' modification of the vest sutures in which 0 absorbable sutures, at each quadrant of the vesical neck closure, are brought through the perineal body and secured anterior to anterior, posterior to posterior. (From Skinner DG, Lieskovsky G. Diagnosis and Management of Genitourinary Cancer. Philadelphia, WB Saunders, 1988.)

is held in place only by the seminal vesicles and vas deferens.

The specimen is then displaced posteriorly and each vas deferens is isolated in the midline, controlled with surgical clips, and divided. The specimen may then be elevated in the operative field and, with alternating sharp and blunt dissection, the seminal vesicles may be exposed either in their entirety or for a distance of 2 to 3 cm. If the surgeon elects not to remove the seminal vesicles in their entirety, they can be controlled at a distance of 2 to 3 cm from the prostate itself with surgical clips before division, and the specimen then removed.

Control of Surgical Margins

The posterior bladder neck is grasped at 6 o'clock and bladder neck margins are taken, going from 6 through 8 to 12 o'clock and from 6 through 4 to 12 o'clock. A traction suture is placed at 6 o'clock and tension is maintained on the posterior bladder neck by the weight of a Kelly clamp on this traction suture.

Attention is then turned to covering the raw detrusor anteriorly with bladder mucosa. This is accomplished by using 4-0 absorbable suture and bringing the bladder mucosa up onto the raw surface of the detrusor between 9 through 12 to 3 o'clock. That

portion of the detrusor that extends from 3 through 6 to 9 o'clock need not be covered with mucosa, as this portion will be closed in the racket handle.

After the anterior bladder neck has been covered with vesical mucosa, 0-strength absorbable sutures are placed outside-inside, inside-outside, approximately 0.5 cm from the 12 o'clock midline. These will be brought through the perineal body later and tied beneath the skin to support the direct urethrovesical anastomosis.

Urethrovesical Reconstruction

An 18 Fr. Foley catheter is now passed through the urethra. The previously placed 2-0 suture is used to identify the urethra as it penetrates the transverse perineal diaphragm, and 2-0 absorbable sutures are placed in the urethra at 2, 4, 8, and 10 o'clock. The two sutures being placed at 4 and 8 o'clock into the urethra are driven into the mucosa-covered bladder neck approximately 0.5 cm from the 12 o'clock midline, so that a mucosa-to-mucosa approximation will occur. The Foley catheter is placed into the bladder and the balloon inflated (Fig. 66–8). The bladder neck is closed from 6 to 12 o'clock with interrupted 0 absorbable sutures, the closure being made tight around the 18 Fr. Foley catheter. At this point the

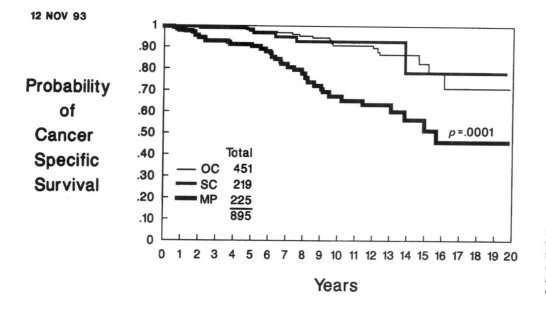

Probability of Cancer Specific Survival

p =.0001

	Total
OC	451
SC	219
MP	225
	895

Years

Figure 66–9. Kaplan-Meier projections of cancer-specific survival for patients with organ-confined (OC), specimen-confined (SC), and margin-positive (MP) disease.

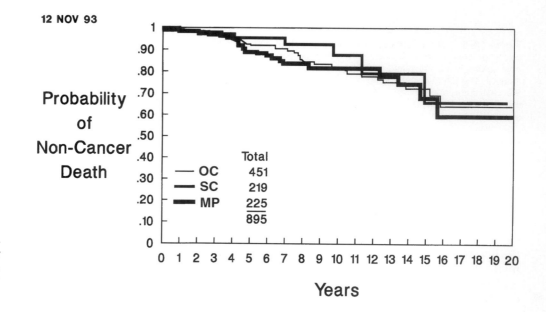

Probability of Non-Cancer Death

	Total
OC	451
SC	219
MP	225
	895

Years

Figure 66–10. Kaplan-Meier projections of noncancer deaths for patients with organ-confined, specimen-confined, and margin-positive disease.

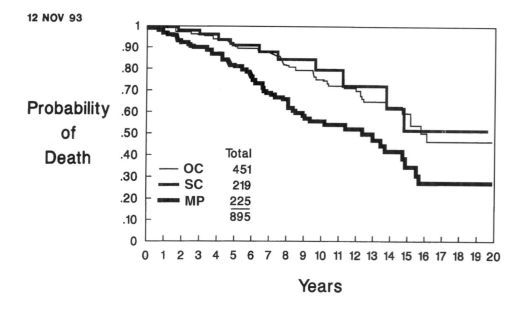

Probability of Death

	Total
OC	451
SC	219
MP	225
	895

Years

Figure 66–11. Kaplan-Meier projections of overall deaths for patients with organ-confined, specimen-confined, and margin-positive disease.

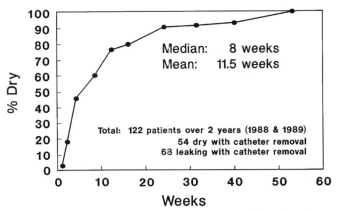

Figure 66–12. Time to continence for 121 patients operated on before the mucosa-to-mucosa anastomosis.

two urethral sutures that have been placed at 10 and 2 o'clock are brought into the reconstructed bladder neck approximately 0.5 cm to either side of the racket handle closure.

The four 2-0 absorbable sutures are then snugly tied. Once the direct urethrovesical anastomosis has been secured, the four 2-0 absorbable sutures previously placed in the bladder neck anteriorly and the last two used in the racket handle posteriorly are brought through the transverse perineal body on the right and left side of the urethra using a No. 8 surgeon's needle, and are tied securely beneath the skin.

The fibers previously identified as being a portion of the levator sling that supports the prostate are brought together in the midline with interrupted 2-0 absorbable sutures, and the wound is drained with a Penrose drain. The central tendon is reconstructed using interrupted absorbable 2-0 sutures, and the skin margins are then closed with vertical mattress sutures of 2-0 absorbable material.

POSTOPERATIVE CARE

The patient is mobilized within 6 to 8 hours after surgery and oral intake is initiated within 8 hours

TABLE 66–1. Potency Rates Among 121 Consecutive Patients Undergoing Radical Perineal Prostatectomy

73/122 (60%) patients potent preoperatively
22/74 (77%) patients considered candidates for potency preservation
17/22 (77%) patients potent within 1 year after surgery

TABLE 66–2. Operative Parameters Among 121 Patients Undergoing Radical Retropubic Prostatectomy (RRP) or Radical Perineal Prostatectomy (RPP)

	RPP (n = 122)	RRP (n = 51)	p Value
Age (yr)	66.2	66.9	.74
Preoperative hematocrit (%)	43.0	42.0	.85
Estimated blood loss (ml)	565	2000	<.001
Transfusions (units)	0	3	<.001
Operative time (min)	203	225	.001
Anesthesia time (min)	268	290	.192

after surgery. He is placed on oral antibiotics plus a stool softener. Discharge is routinely on the morning of the third or fourth postoperative day. The catheter is left in place for 18 days and then removed by either the operating or referring surgeon.

RESULTS

Cancer-specific survival is seen to be a function of the extent of disease in the histopathological specimen and can be segregated into organ-confined, specimen-confined, or margin-positive malignancy (Figs. 66–9 to 66–11). The time to continence for perineal prostatectomy is identified in Figure 66–12.[8, 9] Note that 50 percent of the patients surveyed in this review were continent the moment the catheter was removed. Potency rates are as given in Table 66–1.[10–12]

The most remarkable difference is in blood loss, as noted in Table 66–2. Note also that the relative costs of radical perineal prostatectomy versus radical retropubic prostatectomy give a significant advantage to the former (Table 66–3). Patients are discharged on the fourth or fifth postoperative day and catheters are routinely removed 2 weeks after discharge. The occasional patient with perineal urine leakage is maintained on catheter drainage until the leakage ceases, the catheter being removed after 5 days of dryness. Patients are followed at 6-month intervals

TABLE 66–3. Relative Cost of Radical Retropubic Prostatectomy (RRP) Versus Radical Perineal Prostatectomy (RPP)

	RRP 1	RRP 2	RRP 3	RPP
Bed care	$3241	$2902	$3932	$2542
OR costs	2503	2556	2832	1813
Anesthesia	785	750	840	628
Recovery room	441	326	358	334
Transfusion	520	505	402	71
Average total cost	$11,418	$10,609	$12,565	$8824
Average length of stay (days)	7.5	6.6	8.9	6.0

with PSA determinations during the first 5 years and at yearly intervals thereafter.

Editorial Comment
Fray F. Marshall

Perineal prostatectomy is being performed more commonly. It has the advantages of decreased blood loss and perhaps less patient discomfort. It carries the disadvantages of no pelvic lymphadenectomy and lower potency rates. With smaller incisions and improved analgesia, we are frequently discharging patients 4 days postoperatively after a radical retropubic prostatectomy. Perineal prostatectomy may be a reasonable alternative in impotent patients with a low incidence of positive nodes.

REFERENCES

1. Anscher MS, Prosnitz LR. Postoperative radiotherapy for patients with carcinoma of the prostate undergoing radical prostatectomy with positive surgical margins, seminal vesicle involvement and/or penetration through the capsule. J Urol 138:1407, 1987.
2. Paulson DF, Moul JW, Walther PJ. Radical prostatectomy for clinical stage T1-2N0M0 prostatic adenocarcinoma: Long term results. J Urol 144:1180, 1990.
3. Paulson DF, Moul JW, Walther PJ, Robertson JE. Postoperative radiotherapy of the prostate for patients undergoing radical prostatectomy with positive margins, seminal vesicle involvement and/or penetration through the capsule. J Urol 143:1178, 1990.
4. Paulson DF. The prognostic role of lymphadenectomy in adenocarcinoma of the prostate. Urol Clin North Am 7:615, 1980.
5. Paulson DF. Localized prostatic carcinoma: The case for radical surgery. In Fitzpatrick J, Krane R, eds: The Prostate. New York, Churchill Livingstone, 1989, p 327.
6. Whitesel JA, Donohue RE, Mani JH, et al. Acid phosphatase: Its influence on the management of carcinoma of the prostate. J Urol 131:70, 1984.
7. Paulson DF, Frazier HA. Radical prostatectomy. In Krane RJ, Siroky MB, Fitzpatrick JM, eds: Clinical Urology. Philadelphia, JB Lippincott, 1994, p 1020.
8. Kaplan EL, Meier P. Nonparametric estimation from incomplete observations. J Am Stat Ass 53:457, 1958.
9. Cox DR. Regression models and life tables. J Roy Stat Soc B 34:187, 1972.
10. Catalona WJ, Dresner SM. Nerve-sparing radical prostatectomy: Extraprostatic tumor extension and preservation of erectile function. J Urol 134:1149, 1985.
11. Eggleston JC, Walsh PC. Radical prostatectomy with preservation of sexual function: Pathological findings in the first 100 cases. J Urol 134:1146, 1985.
12. Walsh PC, Lepor H, Eggleston JC. Radical prostatectomy with preservation of sexual function: Anatomical and pathological considerations. Prostate 4:473, 1983.

Chapter 67

Prostatectomy: New Technologies Including Laser, Microwave, Ultrasound Surgery, and Stents

Leonard G. Gomella

The treatment of obstructive symptoms due to benign prostatic hypertrophy (BPH) is an area of rapid change. For over 50 years, urologists have utilized the electrosurgical transurethral prostatectomy (TURP) in most of these patients. Currently, urologists are investigating a wide array of "minimally invasive therapies" as alternative treatments for BPH.

The impetus for these new technologies has come from several areas. Several scientific publications have recently questioned the safety of TURP. Studies suggesting increased mortality in the first 90 days after TURP have been widely publicized.[1] An American Urological Association (AUA) Cooperative Group Study found an 18 percent morbidity rate immediately after TURP, which included a 6.4 percent transfusion rate, a 2 percent incidence of transurethral resection (TUR) syndrome (e.g., confusion, nausea, seizures), and up to a 2 percent occurrence of significant cardiac events.[2] Delayed sequelae of TURP may include strictures, bladder neck contractures, stress urinary incontinence, occasional impotence, and an almost uniform incidence of retrograde ejaculation.[3]

Advances in medical technology, such as the impact of extracorporeal shock wave devices on the management of stone disease, led to additional investigations into the treatment of bladder outlet obstruction.[1] Balloon dilation of the prostate has generally been disappointing and is infrequently used. Newer technologies such as lasers, microwave hyperthermia, ultrasound ablation, and stents, as well as pharmacological manipulations are challenging the "gold standard" TURP in the management of BPH.

Newer prostatectomy techniques offer the potential of a less morbid and costly procedure. At the present time, laser prostatectomy is undergoing widespread application and testing in the United States and abroad. Although some of the new technologies such as microwave hyperthermia, ultrasound ablation, and stents are approved in other countries, these are mainly limited to investigational use in the United States. Laser prostatectomy will be the focus of this chapter, with a brief overview of some of the other technologies.

The Food and Drug Administration (FDA) has approved most of the laser fibers noted in this chapter for "destruction of soft tissues in the urinary tract" and one manufacturer's fiber for destruction of "prostate tissue." In spite of multiple studies indicating the efficacy and safety of this technology, to date no laser fiber has been *specifically* approved by the FDA for the treatment of BPH.

Laser prostatectomy can often be performed on an outpatient basis, is not associated with significant blood loss or TUR syndrome, and allows the potential for normal ejaculation by preservation of the bladder neck.

INDICATIONS

The indications for prostatectomy using newer technologies are generally similar to transurethral resection of the prostate. Patients with persistent and progressive symptoms of bladder outlet obstruction, e.g., decreased force of stream, hesitancy, intermittency, and nocturia due to BPH, are potential candidates. Although one or more troubling symptoms is the usual indication for prostatectomy, the complications associated with an enlarged prostate, e.g., bladder calculi, renal insufficiency, retention, and recurrent infection, are also indications. At present, laser prostatectomy may have limitations with larger glands (larger than 80 to 100 gm), depending on the technique used. Although anticoagulation with warfarin (Coumadin) is a problem for patients treated with electrosurgical TURP, treatment with noncontact laser prostatectomy has been successful.[4]

PREOPERATIVE EVALUATION

The diagnosis of symptomatic BPH that requires intervention must be clearly established. At a minimum this should include a careful history and physical examination, assessment of voiding dysfunction such as the AUA symptom score, routine laboratory and urine studies, and serum prostate-specific antigen (PSA). Objective measurement of urinary flow rates, postvoid residual urine, and pressure flow studies are potentially valuable but may not be mandatory for all patients.[5] Since no tissue is obtained during procedures such as routine laser prostatectomy, transrectal ultrasound-directed biopsy should be performed if there is any suspicion of prostate cancer, such as an abnormal digital rectal examination or elevated PSA. Cystoscopy is also helpful to define the lobar anatomy or to rule out any other pathological condition that may be causing symptoms. It also provides guidance regarding the laser technique to be used and an estimate of the amount of tissue to be removed, since patients with very large glands (larger than 80 to 100 gm) are not considered ideal candidates for procedures such as laser prostatectomy by many experienced clinicians. Clearance to undergo a procedure, provided by a medical specialist, is often necessary in this traditionally older patient population.

Patients should be counseled preoperatively about all the alternative therapies for symptomatic BPH (e.g., watchful waiting, drugs, surgical techniques) and about the potential risks and benefits for an individual patient. In particular, laser surgery is often viewed by patients so favorably that their expectations about the procedure and recovery may be too high. Depending on the technique used, symptoms may require weeks or months to resolve, and there may be a potential need for a variable period of catheterization. Lastly, although the short-term follow-up data are promising, laser prostatectomy is a relatively new procedure with few long-term follow-up data.

LASER PROSTATECTOMY: OPERATIVE TECHNIQUES

Basic Principles

An understanding of basic laser tissue interactions is essential to the performance of laser prostatectomy.

In addition, the subtle differences between the various laser fibers must be well understood by the operating surgeon to ensure a successful outcome.

A variety of surgical lasers are commercially available, including the carbon dioxide, holmium, argon, diode, Nd:YAG, and KTP lasers. The neodymium:yttrium-aluminum-garnet (Nd:YAG) laser is currently the primary laser energy source of choice to treat BPH. The emission from the Nd:YAG laser can be passed through a flexible fiber and is not well absorbed by fluids such as blood or irrigation solutions, making it ideal for laser prostatectomy. Nd:YAG laser energy is absorbed by tissues, resulting in a zone of protein denaturation and coagulation necrosis when the tissue is heated above 60°C (Fig. 67–1). At temperatures above 100°C, the tissue vaporizes, meaning that tissue liquids and some solids are turned into vapors of water and hydrocarbons. Potassium titany L phosphate (KTP) is primarily an incising/vaporizing wavelength.

"Laser prostatectomy" is a very broad concept that actually refers to two distinct approaches. One approach is noncontact coagulation, also referred to as the "free beam technique," "right-angle fiber technique," or "visual laser ablation of the prostate" (V-LAP). The Nd:YAG laser energy is used to photocoagulate the prostate tissue in order to induce coagulation necrosis. The laser penetrates a variable depth into the tissue, depending on the power and duration of the exposure, typically 10 to 12 mm into the prostate. This results in thermal coagulation necrosis and delayed sloughing of the prostate for a variable period, usually several weeks to months after the procedure. Noncontact laser prostatectomy does not remove any significant amounts of tissue at the time of the procedure, and no specimen is obtained as part of the standard electrosurgical prostatectomy.

In the other laser approach, the tissue is primarily removed at the time of the procedure by vaporization. This is accomplished by either contact laser vaporization or noncontact high-power density vaporization (HPDV) (cavitation). Here there is immediate loss of tissue with minimal penetration (2 mm) beyond the point of vaporization, meaning that there is minimal sloughing of tissue postoperatively. This can be accomplished by either specifically designed contact laser probes or noncontact probes that can be placed in approximation with the tissue and can function in a high-power density mode.

Laser Fibers

According to the design and application of the laser fiber, the prostate tissue is treated by immediate removal through vaporization, delayed sloughing, or a combination of the techniques. A representative

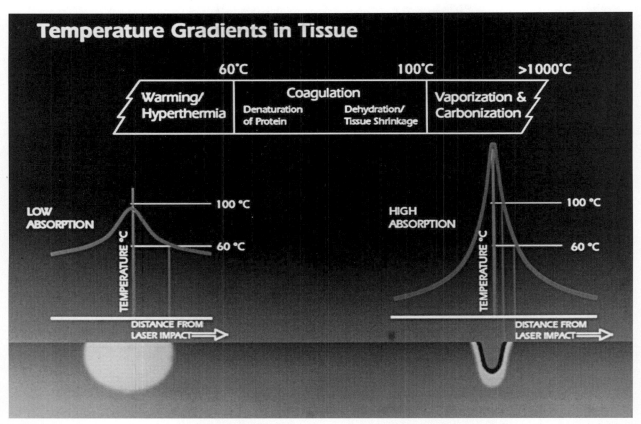

Figure 67–1. Illustrative example of tissue gradients in tissue. Heating prostate tissue with a laser to 60° to 100°C induces coagulation necrosis that is the hallmark of the "noncontact" prostatectomy. Contact lasers and laser tips that rely on high-power density vaporization heat the tissues well above 100°C. (Courtesy of Dr. Terry Fuller.)

sampling of laser fibers is shown in Table 67–1 and Figures 67–2 and 67–3. As can be seen from Table 67–1, most commercially available fibers rely on non-contact coagulation of the tissue as the primary means of tissue destruction.

The laser energy leaves the noncontact laser fiber and is dispersed in a lateral direction at varying angles of incidence by either a reflective (mirror) or refractive (prism) technology (Fig. 67–4). It is important to note that certain fibers (e.g., Prolase I, Ultraline, ADD/Stat) can act both in a vaporization fashion when held in approximation with tissue and in a noncontact fashion when not touching tissue. True contact lasers (e.g., SLT Contact System) rely on the interface between the synthetic sapphire tip and have essentially no effect when not touching tissue. This is an important differentiating factor in performing laser prostatectomy. The surgeon must understand that "contact" with tissue is not necessarily the same as pure contact laser vaporization. Lastly, many fibers (e.g., Urolase, SideFire) must be intentionally held off the tissue, since prolonged tissue contact with the open-face reflective mirror and prostate tissue may cause the reflector to burn out. Hooded noncontact laser fibers (in which the reflective mechanism is shielded by a protective transparent dome) are less likely to be damaged by tissue contact and in many cases are designed specifically to be used in approximation with the tissue.

All fiber assemblies must be connected to a compatible laser system. In most cases the laser generator and fiber connect by an SMA (standard military adaptor) connector. Some fibers, however, rely on proprietary connectors (Table 67–1). All Nd:YAG laser devices rely on a He:Ne (helium neon) red aiming beam to determine the site of laser impact, since the Nd:YAG wavelength is invisible. KTP laser energy is visible as a green light. Except for the TULIP II system (see later), which relies primarily on an integrated ultrasound probe to direct the procedure, all other fibers are designed to be used through a cystoscope system, since the procedure is controlled under vision either directly through the cystoscope or on a video system.

Laser safety practices (e.g., protective eyewear, laser safety sterile drapes, laser control nurse) are established at each hospital on the basis of national guidelines and must be followed for all laser procedures.

Anesthetic Considerations

Laser prostatectomy can be performed using any suitable technique. However, one of its potential ad-

TABLE 67–1. Overview of Laser Fiber Delivery Systems Used in Laser Prostatectomy

Laser Fiber	Manufacturer/ Distributor	Primary Tissue Effect**	Distal Tip Type	Distal Tip Diameter	Lateral Beam Angle (degrees)	Beam Divergence (degrees)	Laser Connector	Notes
ADD	Laserscope (San Jose, CA)	NCC	Refractive (total internal reflection) Hooded dome with metal cannula	1.1 mm	70	15–20	Proprietary Laserscope (KTP/YAG); SMA-905 for YAG	Dual wavelength; can switch between Nd:YAG for coagulation and KTP for incision and vaporization
ADD/Stat	Laserscope (San Jose, CA)	HPDV and NCC	Refractive (total internal reflection) Hooded quartz dome	1.8 mm	70	15–20	Proprietary Laserscope (KTP/YAG); SMA-905 for YAG	Dual wavelength; can switch between ND:YAG for coagulation and KTP for incision and vaporization; tolerates prolonged tissue contact
Contact Laser System	SLT (Surgical Laser Technologies) (Oaks, PA)	Vaporization	Synthetic sapphire	MTRL-10 5 mm MTRL-6 3.5 mm MTRL-3 2.2 mm (large round) MD-6 3.5 mm (chisel)	NA	NA	Proprietary SLT Contact Connector	Resusable probes; disposable low-cost fibers; SREF 15 Semirigid endoscopic fiber recommended; pure contact probes have effect only when in contact with tissue
Diffuser Tip	Indigo (Palo Alto, CA)	Interstitial coagulation	Fused silica	Introducer sleeve 1.8 mm/diffuser 1.2 mm	NA	NA	Proprietary Indigo diode laser	Interstitial technology; not yet FDA approved in US; available in 1- and 2-cm distal tip designs; 360° radial diffusion into tissues
Laser Peripherals DBLF-60S	Laser Peripherals (Minnetonka, MN)	HPDV and NCC	Refractive (Prism) Hooded quartz dome	1.7 mm	78	12–15	SMA-905	
Prismlase	Planet Medical (Oceanside, CA)	HPDV and NCC	Refractive (Prism) Hooded quartz dome	1.8 mm	80	14	SMA-905	
Prolase I	Endocare (Cytocare) (Aliso Viejo, CA)	HPDV and NCC	Refractive	2.0 mm	90	15	SMA-905	

Product	Company (City)	Mode	Optics	Fiber/Probe size	Angle	Power	Connector	Comments
Prolase II	Endocare (Cytocare) (Aliso Viejo, CA)	NCC	Refractive	2.0 mm	45	35	SMA-905	
Rotalase XT	Xintec (Oakland, CA)	NCC	Reflective (gold mirror) Open	2.0 mm	90	30	EZ, Sharplan, SM-905	
SFB	SLT (Oaks, PA)	NCC	Reflective (Gold mirror) Open	3.3 mm	90	30	Proprietary SLT Contact Connector	Reusable probe; disposable low-cost fibers; SREF 15 semirigid endoscopic fiber recommended
SideFiber 1800	CeramOptec (San Jose, CA)	HPDV and NCC	Refractive (Prism) Hooded quartz dome	1.8 mm	80	14	SMA-905	
SideFire	Myriadlase (Forest Hill, TX)	NCC	Reflective (Gold mirror) Open	2.1 mm	105	15	SMA-905	
Side Focus II	Domier (Kennesaw, GA)	HPDV and NCC	Refractive (Prism) Hooded quartz dome	1.8 mm	80	22	SMA-905	
TULIP II	Intrasonics (Burlington, MA)	NCC	Refractive (Prism) Enclosed inside ultrasound balloon	Probe 20F Balloon expanded size 48 Fr.	90	NA	SMA-905	Replaces TULIP I; integrated ultrasound visualization system; greatly improved ultrasound visualization over original design; not FDA approved in US
UltraGold	Surgitek (Racine, WI) Cabot Medical (Langhorne, PA)	NCC	Reflective (gold mirror)	2.1	90	30	SMA-905 or Modified Sharplan 905	
Ultraline	Circon-ACMI (Stamford, CT) LaserSonics (Milpitas, CA)	HPDV	Refractive (Prism) Hooded	2.0	80	20	SMA-905	
Urolase	Bard (Covington, GA)	NCC	Reflective (gold mirror)	2.5	90	30	SMA-905, Proprietary SLT Connector	

HPDV, high-power density vaporization; NCC, noncontact coagulation; NA, not applicable.

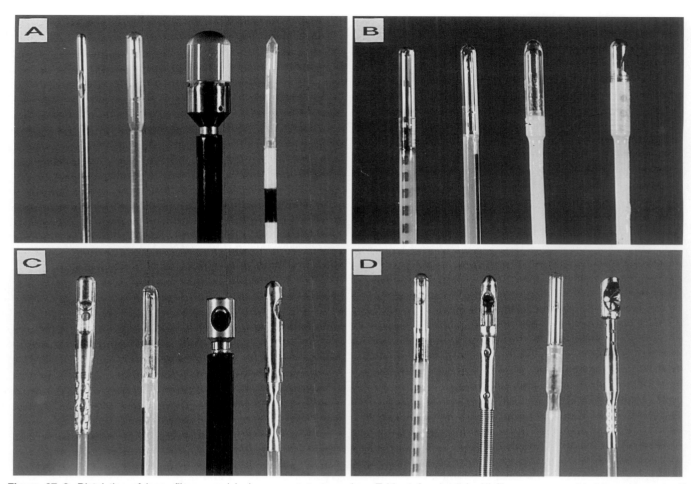

Figure 67–2. Distal tips of laser fibers used in laser prostatectomy (see Table 1 for details). All fibers were provided by and used with permission of the manufacturer. *A,* ADD, ADD/Stat, MTRL-10 (Contact Laser), Interstitial Diffuser tip. *B,* Laser Peripherals DBLF-60S, Prismlase, Prolase I, Prolase II. *C,* Rotalase XT, SFB, SideFiber 1800, SideFire. *D,* Side Focus II, UltraGold, Ultraline, Urolase.

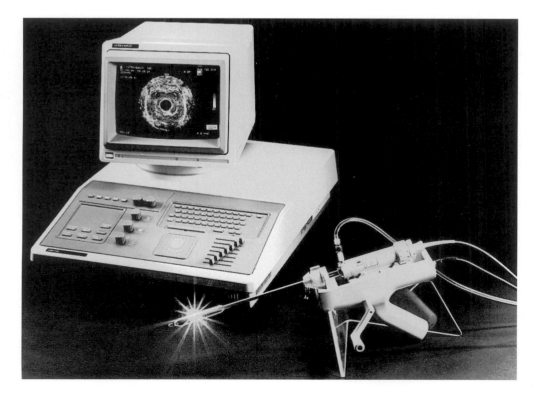

Figure 67–3. The TULIP II includes an integrated 360-degree ultrasound device that allows visualization of the procedure and is connected to a separate Nd: YAG laser generator. (Courtesy of Intrasonics.)

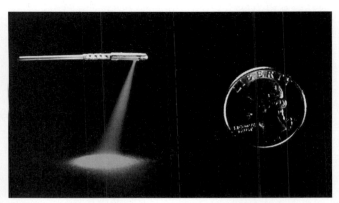

Figure 67–4. The lateral beam angle varies by manufacturer of noncontact lasers. This is an example of a 105-degree angle of the SideFire fiber. (Courtesy of Myriadlase.)

vantages is that it is a less invasive procedure than electrosurgical TURP and there is the potential for limiting the amount and duration of anesthesia. Laser prostatectomy is relatively quick and can often be performed with a minimal hospital stay or on an outpatient basis. Most clinicians currently prefer to use a short-acting regional or a general anesthetic. Patients may experience some discomfort during the procedure from instrumentation, bladder distention, or the heating of the prostate tissue. Noncontact techniques also require prolonged exposure to a given site on the prostate, and patient movement may make this difficult. Leach and associates have advocated the use of local anesthesia to perform the noncontact technique.[6] A periprostatic block is performed transperineally and light intravenous sedation with midazolam (Versed) is administered. The ultimate choice of anesthetic technique should be agreed on by surgeon, anesthesiologist, and patient. Preoperative antibiotics (oral quinolone or intravenous aminoglycoside) are standard for transurethral surgery and given according to the surgeon's preference.

Noncontact Coagulation

Noncontact coagulation is the laser prostatectomy approach that has been most extensively studied in the peer-reviewed literature. The first clinical experience with the current generation of lateral-firing laser fibers using the noncontact technique was reported by Costello and associates.[7] Although slight variations have been reported, the technique promoted by Kabalin with the Urolase fiber is widely used and is presented here.[8] Any free beam laser fiber can be substituted, but the surgeon must be aware of the incident lateral beam angle of the device (Table 67–1). This ensures that the laser energy is directed to the appropriate site.

A standard 22 Fr. cystoscope or a newer continuous

flow "laser" cystoscope can be used. The length of the prostatic urethra from bladder neck to verumontanum is determined. Since the effective diameter of the tissue ablation by the noncontact technique is up to 2 cm, four-quadrant photocoagulation is planned every 2 cm along the prostatic urethra. As demonstrated in Figure 67–5, prostatic urethral lengths of less than 2.5 cm require only one four-quadrant treatment. If the length is between 2.5 and 4 cm, an additional treatment cycle may be needed.

There is virtually no fluid absorption during the laser procedure, and room temperature sterile water or saline is often used. A constant flow of irrigating solution is needed to ensure cooling of the laser tip and help prevent tissue adherence. On rare occasions a temporary suprapubic tube (Stamey type) may be necessary to ensure continuous flow. The laser fiber is checked for power output using a laser power meter to verify the integrity of the fiber, and the fiber is loaded through the bridge and passed into the bladder. Noncontact fibers have an adjustable "torque" control handle that allows the tip to be oriented accurately. There have been several reports of laser settings ranging from 20 to 60 watts (W) over varying time periods. On the basis of dosimetry studies, the current recommendations from several investigators are that the energy be applied at 40 W for 90 seconds in continuous time mode. Acceptable results have also been reported for 60 W and 60 seconds,[9] but there is a concern that the higher wattage may yield more superficial vaporization and less efficient deep coagulation necrosis.[10] The fiber should not be moved, nor should the time interval be interrupted: these may lead to inadequate tissue penetration. A stop watch is used to time each treatment.

The typical prostate is treated around the clock in the 2, 4, 8, and 10 o'clock positions with 7200 joules

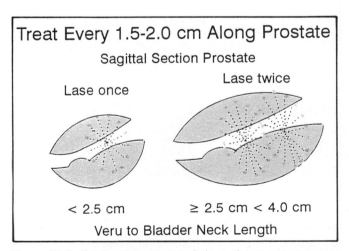

Figure 67–5. For the noncontact technique, the verumontanum to bladder neck length is determined. For prostatic urethral length of less than 2.5 cm, one treatment is given around the clock as shown in Figure 67–6. Longer prostatic urethral lengths may require additional treatments. (Courtesy of Dr. John Kabalin.)

(J) (40 W × 90 sec = 7200 W/sec) in each quadrant (Fig. 67–6). Larger prostates, with increased volume of lateral lobe tissue, may benefit from the sextant technique (Fig. 67–6) in which the prostate is also treated with 7200 J at the 3 and 9 o'clock positions to ensure overlapping of the zones of coagulation necrosis.

If the prostatic urethral length is less than 2.5 cm ,the around-the-clock treatment is performed in the midprostatic urethra, approximately 1 cm from the bladder neck. When the prostatic urethra is between 2.5 and 4.0 cm in length, a second treatment is given approximately 2 cm distal to the first, making sure that it is not beyond the verumontanum.

The laser energy is directed into the substance of the prostate as shown in Figure 67–7. The He:Ne red aiming beam indicates the point of impact on the urethra. The opening of the tip of the laser should be held off the tissue during the laser application to prevent tissue sticking to and burning out the reflective mirror of the open-face fibers (Fig. 67–8). If tissue becomes adherent, the laser should be gently cleaned

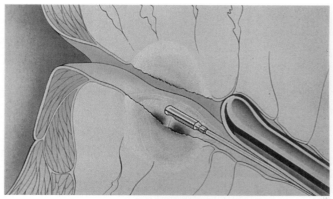

Figure 67–7. Example of a noncontact prostatectomy indicating the concentric zone of coagulation necrosis that is induced. Note that this type of open-face reflective fiber must be held off the tissue. (Courtesy of Myriadlase.)

with a moist, sterile gauze pad. (*Note*: It is a good practice to allow the bladder to empty between each 90-second "lasing" and clean the tip. The hooded laser fibers tend to be more resistant to tissue adherence but also benefit from gentle cleaning.) As the treatment progresses, there is blanching and occa-

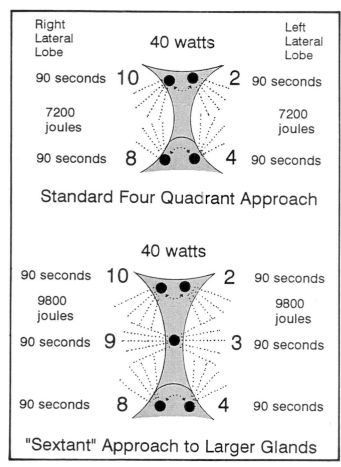

Figure 67–6. The standard noncontact approach is to treat with 40 watts for 90 seconds around the clock at the 2, 4, 8, and 10 o'clock positions. Note that the laser is directed into the substance of the gland. Larger prostates may require additional treatments using the sextant approach to ensure that there will be overlapping areas of coagulation necrosis. (Courtesy of Dr. John Kabalin.)

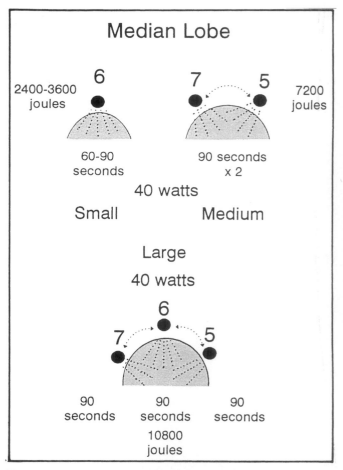

Figure 67–8. The median lobe can be treated before or after the lateral lobes are coagulated using the noncontact technique. (Courtesy of Dr. John Kabalin.)

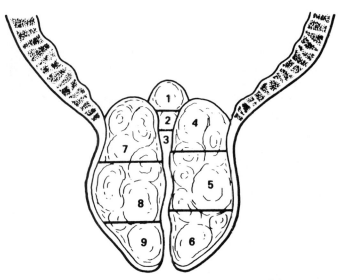

Figure 67–9. Sequence of contact laser vaporization of the prostate. Since the contact laser relies on a pushing technique, the tissue at the bladder neck is vaporized first, and one then works outward to the apical tissue.

sionally some superficial vaporization of the tissue. Sometimes there is an audible "pop" caused by rapid vaporization of submucosal tissues and subsequent rupture of the intact overlying mucosa ("popcorn effect"). Recall that with this noncontact technique the goal is to induce a deep tissue effect that can be obtained only by a continuous laser application for the specified period. These superficial effects are unrelated to the deep tissue changes and cannot be used to guide the duration of the laser application.

If there is obstructing median lobe tissue, it can be treated either before or after the lateral lobes. Smaller lobes can be given 40 W for 90 seconds at the 6 o'clock position, and additional treatments given as needed for larger lobes (Fig. 67–9).

Occasionally minimal bleeding is encountered, often due to cystoscope trauma in the urethra. Activating the laser and using a back-and-forth "painting" technique usually coagulates the superficial bleeding vessels.

Postoperatively a 16 Fr. Foley catheter is left in place on a leg bag for 3 to 10 days. Irrigation is not necessary and oral antibiotics are continued until the catheter is removed. The duration of catheterization is determined by the size of the prostate and the amount of energy applied (larger prostate: more energy, longer catheterization). With a preoperative history of retention or mild bladder dysfunction, the catheter may be left for up to 4 weeks. There is transient initial swelling associated with the coagulation necrosis that necessitates the catheterization. Dissolution of the treated prostate tissue takes several weeks, so patients will note a gradual improvement in symptoms and in flow rate with time. They may note passage of minute particulate matter or of whit-ish, cloudy urine as the prostate tissue passes. It appears that complete resolution of symptoms with the noncontact technique is around 2 to 4 months. Irritative voiding symptoms can be troubling for some patients but tend to resolve with time. Anti-inflammatory agents have had mixed results in eliminating the irritative symptoms in these patients.

TULIP Procedure

Although technically a non-contact prostatectomy, the transurethral laser-induced prostatectomy (TULIP) device is unique since it combines a laser and ultrasound monitoring system.[11] The original TULIP system has now been replaced by TULIP II, with improvements that include full 360-degree higher-resolution ultrasound visualization and the option to directly visualize the urethra endoscopically (see Fig. 67–3). The laser connects to any standard SMA-905 Nd:YAG laser. The device is available in several European countries and is investigational in the United States.

After cystoscopic examination, a small-caliber suprapubic tube is placed. The bladder is left full, and the TULIP is lubricated and passed into the urethra. There is a marker that is palpated rectally to ensure proper orientation. The distal balloon is pressurized to 2 atmospheres and the ultrasound examination is conducted to identify the depth of tissue, the bladder neck, and the external sphincter. The polymer balloon is transparent to the Nd:YAG laser energy. Using a laser energy of 35 W, passes are from the bladder neck to the apex, moving the control handle of the laser at a rate of approximately 1 mm/sec. The delivery handle has an orientation system that allows the laser to be directed at 12 positions around the clock face. Typically, five to seven passes are needed from the 3 o'clock to the 9 o'clock position for the average prostate. Foley catheter drainage is normally maintained for less than 1 day and the suprapubic tube removed approximately 1 week later. As with most laser prostatectomy techniques, there can be transient irritative voiding symptoms.

Contact Laser Vaporization

Pure contact vaporization of the prostate is generally recommended for patients with a resectable gland size of less than 30 gm, making it suitable for most patients who are candidates for transurethral prostatectomy.[2, 3, 12] It has the advantage of providing an open fossa at the end of the procedure. Larger glands can now be treated with a so-called hybrid approach combining preliminary noncontact coagulation with vaporization of a channel (see below). Contact laser ablation of the prostate (CLAP) is usually performed with regional anesthesia. The contact laser tips are reusable and the fiber is disposable. The fluid-cooled semirigid fiber (SREF 15) is connected to the Nd:YAG contact laser (SLT) and passed through a standard 23 Fr. cystoscope. This fiber improves the ability of the tip of the probe to maintain approximation with the tissue. The synthetic sapphire contact tip of choice (MTRL-10 is recommended because of the larger vaporizing surface) is connected to the fiber and passed through the cystoscope sheath. The tips can be reused, typically four to five times. The contact tip works best when a small amount of char builds up in the contact surface. The probe should be inspected for excessive pitting before use and the fiber calibrated before it is passed into the cystoscope.

The primary effect from the contact laser is at the tip. The laser is set on 40 to 50 W continuous mode and the tip is applied to the luminal surface of the gland. At that point the tip is in contact with the tissue and there is immediate vaporization equal to the size of the contact tip. There is minimal depth of penetration beyond the point of vaporization, with rapid dissipation of the energy. The sequence of vaporization is noted in Figure 67–9. Since this is a "pushing" technique, tissue at the bladder neck (or median lobe if present) is vaporized initially, with subsequent tissue removal moving more distally. There is a 1- to 2-second delay before the tissue begins to vaporize and the fiber can be passed through the tissue. A contact laser tip must remain in approximation with and pressure must be applied to the tissue for there to be an acceptable effect. The vaporization of tissue continues until the prostatic urethral lumen is judged to be adequate, as with standard electrosurgical TURP. There is no TUR syndrome associated with the contact laser prostatectomy, and since tissue is resected, there can be minimal bleeding.[13] The CLAP procedure can be more time consuming than the noncontact technique, but the immediate removal of tissue using probes specifically designed to vaporize tissue is appealing.

Urethral catheter drainage is maintained for approximately 48 to 72 hours, usually on an outpatient basis since continuous bladder irrigation is not required. Improvement in the urinary stream is usually prompt because most tissue removal occurs at the time of the procedure. However, there may be transient irritative voiding symptoms lasting 2 to 3 days. Some investigators have reported immediate removal of the catheter with good outcome, but patients may experience transient edema or discomfort that may interfere with early catheter removal.

Noncontact Vaporization

Several investigators, including Childs and Fournier and Narayan, have modified the noncontact technique to perform HPDV (cavitation), allowing the noncontact laser to vaporize and remove tissue.[14, 15] This procedure has been called TUEP (transurethral evaporation of the prostate).[16] This relies primarily on the hooded laser fibers (e.g., Prolase I, Ultraline, ADD/Stat) that can be held in approximation with the tissue without damaging the reflective mechanism in the tip.

One approach is the drag-and-twist technique of fiber movement.[15] A hooded fiber such as the Ultraline is used through a standard or continuous flow cystoscope. Furrows are created in the prostate, starting just distal to the bladder neck and extending to the verumontanum at the 1, 4, 8, and 11 o'clock positions. They are created by activating the laser set at 60 W while touching the tissue for 5 to 7 seconds to initiate the vaporization. The fiber is then rotated in a 30- to 45-degree arc while being withdrawn slowly at a rate of 1 to 1.5 cm/min (Fig. 67–10A). Both the cystoscope sheath and the fiber are moved. The motion back and forth over a wide area is necessary to ensure adequate vaporization and prevent formation of a deep narrow crater that could perforate the prostate.

The furrows, when created properly, resemble the tissue removed with a resectoscope loop (Fig. 67–10B). Vaporization of the furrows can be repeated as necessary to increase the depth. A series of parallel furrows are then created between the 1 to 5 o'clock and 8 to 11 o'clock positions to vaporize the remaining tissue and create a fossa that resembles a prostate resected by electrocautery but in a much more hemostatic fashion (Fig. 67–10C).

There can be "etching" (creation of a small frosted spot) of the protective cap where the laser exits the

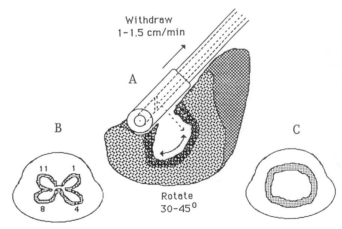

Figure 67–10. Technique for high-power density vaporization using a hooded fiber such as the Ultraline. *A*, The fiber is rotated in a 30- to 45-degree arc and withdrawn at a rate of 1 to 1.5 cm/sec. *B*, This is repeated to create a series of furrows at 1, 4, 8, and 11 o'clock in the prostatic urethra from the bladder neck to the veru. *C*, The intervening tissue is vaporized, resulting in a fossa that resembles a transurethral prostatic resection (TURP) defect. (Courtesy of Drs. P. Narayan and G. Fournier.)

fiber after approximately 30,000 J of energy have been expended. This may cause a slight decrease in the vaporizing capacity of the fiber, and some investigators recommend increasing the laser output to 80 W after 50,000 J have been used to compensate for this etching effect.[15] Fiber failure may occur at very high levels (approximately 150,00 J) owing to reflector failure when the etched area perforates.

The catheter is removed immediately or after several days, depending on the amount of tissue resected. Improvement in voiding is usually prompt.

Hybrid Laser Prostatectomy Techniques

Several investigators are attempting to address the initial swelling and irritative voiding symptoms associated with the noncontact technique by allowing at least a partial removal of the obstructing tissue at the time of the procedure.

Sacknoff has proposed combining initial noncontact laser ablation with a standard electrosurgical TURP (Turpette).[17] Another potential improvement in laser prostatectomy is the CHRP (coagulation and hemostatic resection of the prostate) approach: noncontact coagulation followed by contact laser vaporization of a channel utilizing interchangeable tips.[13] The bladder neck is incised using the contact tip at the end of the procedure. These newer approaches allow the immediate creation of a voiding channel with virtually no blood loss and continued improvement from the effects of deep coagulation necrosis.

Complications

In most preliminary series the immediate complication rates appear to be far less than those seen with electrosurgical TURP.[7, 13, 16, 18] There is no TUR syndrome and there are no reports in the literature of significant perioperative morbidity. Rare complications include bladder neck contractures, urethral strictures, and urinary tract infections. Repeat procedures have been reported in the early experience with most of these techniques. Most troubling is the irritative voiding experienced by some patients, which may respond to anti-inflammatory agents or urinary tract agents such as Urised. Patients with larger prostates treated by noncontact techniques occasionally require prolonged intermittent catheterization. As the number of patients reported in the literature increases, the overall perspective of complications will become more clear.

Results

The results of the Nd:YAG, noncontact,[6, 8, 11, 18] noncontact HPDV,[14-16] contact,[12, 19, 20] and hybrid laser

prostatectomy[17] techniques are reported in the literature. All techniques are showing promise in the treatment of symptomatic BPH. As the various fibers and alternative techniques are investigated by clinicians, the advantages and limitations of each are being appreciated.

The noncontact technique is relatively quick to perform and is not associated with intraoperative bleeding. However, some patients may be troubled by prolonged periods of irritative voiding symptoms or retention as the obstructing tissue is sloughed.[8, 14, 15] Vaporization has the advantage of immediately removing tissue, but larger gland sizes (above 20 to 30 gm of resected tissue) may necessitate prolonged operating time.[21] The improvements and modifications in the laser prostatectomy procedures will continue to occur at a rapid rate. With increased awareness of the importance of hemostatic vaporization, increasing contact laser tip sizes and improving the durability of the HPDV fibers will be a priority of manufacturers of laser fibers.

MICROWAVE THERAPY

Microwave therapy of the prostate is approved in many countries but is still considered investigational in the United States. This technology refers to two distinct tissue applications: hyperthermia and thermotherapy.[1] Hyperthermia involves heating the prostate to a target range of 42° to 44°C over several treatment sessions. Thermotherapy, usually administered only transurethrally, heats the prostate at a single session up to 55°C. The mechanism of action on the tissues is not clearly defined and may include alterations in alpha receptors and hence bladder neck–prostate tone, periurethral necrosis, and small vessel necrosis. Histological studies have demonstrated larger areas of induced necrosis with the thermotherapy approach.[22, 23]

The devices rely primarily on microwave thermal heating of the tissues administered through either a transurethral or rectal delivery system. The site of the energy generator typically includes some type of cooling jacket to prevent destructive heating of tissues immediately around the probe.

There is a lack of accepted uniform treatment protocols with respect to route (rectal or urethral), time duration, number of treatments, and target temperature. The use of this new modality awaits confirmation in ongoing trials; most studies suggest that microwave therapy is palliative rather than curative.[22]

ULTRASOUND ABLATION

High-frequency focused ultrasound (HIFU) acoustic ablation of the prostate is one of the newest technologies being investigated for BPH. HIFU relies on delivering ultrasound energy and resultant tissue destruction (target tissue heated to 70° to 90°C) at a distant point without injury to the tissue in the path of the ultrasound beam.[24]

The Sonablate device (investigational in the United States) consists of a combination ultrasound imaging/therapy probe that is placed in the rectum. The target therapy zone (periurethral tissue between the bladder neck) is visualized with a urethral catheter, which is removed before the therapy. The beam is focused and treatment begun at the bladder neck, progressing to the verumontanum in seven different sectors 2 degrees apart. Catheter drainage is maintained for 1 to 4 days. General anesthesia has been used in most patients; studies of intravenous sedation are under way.

A potential advantage of this technology is that the urethra is not manipulated and postprocedure discomfort is reduced. Short-term data are encouraging, and prospective trials comparing the therapy with sham and TURP will define the role of this promising modality.

PROSTATIC STENTS

Stents are being investigated for several applications in the urinary tract, including refractory strictures, sphincterotomy, and BPH. They are investigational in the United States but approved for a variety of uses in Europe. Stents are widely used in Europe, primarily in a palliative role in patients who are not considered surgical candidates for TUR, but many stents have a role in a wide group of symptomatic BPH patients.[1, 23] Several manufactures are developing prostatic urethral stents, including the Uro-Lume Wallstent (American Medical Systems), Intra-Prostatic Stent (Advanced Surgical Intervention), and Prostacath (Pharma-Plast).

As an illustrative example of stent technology, the UroLume Wallstent is a prosthetic, nonmagnetic alloy that is woven into a mesh.[24] The design is flexible and self-expanding with no elastic recoil. When deployed in the prostatic urethra via a special cystoscopic device, it has the capability of expanding to 42°F or 1.4 cm in internal diameter (Fig. 67–11). Various lengths are available to fit from bladder neck

to urethra, and when deployed the stent holds the prostatic urethra in an open position. A regional or general anesthetic is preferred. After 3 to 6 months the stent often becomes covered by the prostatic urethral epithelium. Although these stents are well tolerated, they may require removal because of irritative voiding symptoms.

Summary

We are in the earliest stages of these new, minimally invasive surgical interventions for bladder outlet obstruction. Electrosurgical TURP became refined over many years of clinical observations and manufacturing advances. Although the resectoscope continues to be a standard and trusted surgical device, its dominant position in the definitive treatment of symptomatic BPH is being seriously challenged.

Editorial Comment
Fray F. Marshall

New technology is starting to partially replace transurethral resection of the prostate. The laser has the advantage of ease of use, no bleeding, and absence of TUR syndrome. On the other hand, it has the deficiencies of no specimen and often a delayed recovery. Transurethral resection of the necrotic tissue may avoid bleeding, removes this tissue, and shortens recovery time. Vaporization of a small prostate gland may be performed without resection of any tissue. The place of high-intensity focused ultrasound and microwave therapy remains to be determined. Urethral stents may be helpful over the short term but in the longer term may become problematic in management.

REFERENCES

1. Watson GM. Minimally invasive therapies of the prostate. Minim Invas Ther 1:231, 1992.
2. Mebust WK, Holtgrewe HL, Cockett ATK, et al. Transurethral prostatectomy: Immediate and postoperative complications: A Cooperative Study of 13 participating institutions evaluating 3,885 patients. J Urol 141:243, 1989.
3. Holtgrewe HL, Mebust WK, Dowd JV, et al. Transurethral prostatectomy: Practical aspects of the dominant operation in American urology. J Urol 141:248, 1992.
4. Bolton DM, Costello AJ. Management of benign prostatic hyperplasia by transurethral ablation in patients treated with warfarin anticoagulation. J Urol 151:79, 1994.
5. McConnell JD, Barry MJ, Bruskewitz RC. Benign prostatic hyperplasia: Diagnosis and treatment. Agency for Health Care Policy and Research. Clin Pract Guides 8:1, 1994.
6. Leach GE, Sirls L, Ganabathi K, et al. Outpatient visual laser-assisted prostatectomy under local anesthesia. Urology 43:149, 1994.
7. Costello AJ, Browscher WG, Bolton DM, et al. Laser ablation of the prostate in patients with benign prostatic hypertrophy. Br J Urol 69:603, 1992.
8. Kabalin JN. Laser prostatectomy performed with a right angle firing neodymium:YAG laser fiber at 40 watts power setting. J Urol 150:95, 1993.
9. Shanberg AM, Lee IS, Tansey LA, et al. Depth of penetration of

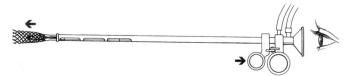

Figure 67–11. The UroLume Wallstent is deployed in the prostatic urethra using a specially designed endoscope. (Courtesy of Della-Corte Publishing.)

the neodymium:yttrium-aluminum-garnet laser in the human prostate at various dosimetry. Urology 43:809, 1994.

10. Kabalin JN, Gill HS. Dosimetry studies utilizing the urolase right angle firing neodymium:YAG laser fiber. Lasers Surg Med 14:145, 1994.

11. McCullough DL, Roth RA, Babayan RK, et al. Transurethral ultrasound guided laser induced prostatectomy: National human cooperative study results. J Urol 150:1607, 1993.

12. Gomella LG, Lotfi MA, Milam D, et al. Contact laser vaporization of the prostate for benign prostatic hypertrophy. SPIE proceedings. Lasers Urol 2129:92, 1994.

13. Gomella LG, Lotfi MA, Reagan GR. Laboratory parameters following contact laser ablation of the prostate for benign prostatic hypertrophy. Techniques in Urology (in press).

14. Childs SJ. High power density prostate cavitation. Lasers Surg Med Suppl 6:313A, 1994.

15. Fournier GR, Narayan P. Factors affecting size and configuration of neodymium:YAG (Nd:YAG) laser elsions in the prostate. Lasers Surg Med 14:314, 1994.

16. Narayan P, Fournier G, Indudhara R, et al. Transurethral evaporation of prostate (TUEP) with ND:Yag laser using a contact free beam technique: Results in 61 patients with benign prostatic hyperplasia. Urology 43:813, 1994.

17. Sacknoff EJ. Laser prostatectomy with a Turpette: Evolution of a new technique. Lasers Surg Med Suppl 6:312A, 1994.

18. Childs S, Coles RS, Dixon C, et al. Prospective randomized study comparing transurethral resection of the prostate with visual laser ablation of the prostate. J Urol 149:467A, 1993.

19. Daughtry JD, Rodin BA. Transurethral laser resection of the prostate. Lasers Surg Med 10:269, 1992.

20. Sadoughi MS. Transurethral contact Nd:YAG laser ablation of the prostate. J Urol 149:465A, 1993.

21. Smith JA. Benign prostatic hypertrophy. In Smith JA, ed. Lasers in Urologic Surgery. St. Louis, Mosby-Year Book, 1994, p 83.

22. Matzkin H. Hyperthermia as a treatment modality in benign prostatic hyperplasia. Urology 43:17, 1994.

23. Monda JM, Osterling JE. Medical and minimally invasive treatments for benign prostatic hyperplasia. Curr Probl Urol 2:100, 1992.

24. Bhirle R, Foster RS, Sanghvi NT, et al. High intensity focused ultrasound for the treatment of benign prostatic hyperplasia: Early United States clinical experience. J Urol 151:1271, 1994.

25. Milroy E, Chapple CR. The UroLume stent in the management of benign prostatic hyperplasia. J Urol 150:1630, 1993.

Chapter 68

Needle Biopsy of the Prostate

William H. Cooner and W. Holt Sanders

The diagnosis of prostate cancer depends on microscopical examination of material obtained by tissue sampling, regardless of whether the disease is suspected by digital palpation, abnormal serum markers, or sonographic visualization. A variety of approaches to prostatic biopsy have been used, including open surgical biopsy as well as needle biopsy performed transperineally or transrectally. Material can be aspirated for cytological examination, or tissue cores can be obtained. Digital guidance is often used to direct prostate biopsy, but visual guidance under sonographic control has become a widely practiced procedure during the past few years.

TECHNICAL FACTORS

Fine Needle Aspiration versus Core Biopsy

Larger areas of the prostate can be sampled by aspiration than by core biopsy, even if multiple cores are obtained. Some physicians with access to highly skilled cytological expertise are confident of the accuracy of cytological interpretation. Others prefer to have core confirmation of the presence of cancer, especially before instituting therapy, the nature of which may be influenced by the location from which the core was obtained, the degree of tumor differentiation, and the extent of cancer within the core.

Digital versus Sonographic Needle Guidance

Some investigators report higher yields when biopsy is done under sonographic control than when it is performed under digital guidance,[1, 2] whereas others report little difference between the two methods.[3, 4] Comparative evaluation among these studies is impossible because of important technical differences

in the sonographic equipment used in the different studies and the issue of whether the biopsies were performed transperineally or transrectally. Today, biopsy is most commonly performed transrectally under either method of guidance.

It is clear that large, palpable cancers can be sampled accurately under either digital or sonographic guidance. However, if biopsy of an area about which there is a high degree of tactile suspicion yields negative tissue, repeat biopsy sonographically often yields cancer.[2, 5] Most palpable cancers are visible by sonography, and small cancers can be biopsied under visual control with greater confidence that the abnormal area has been sampled than is possible by digital guidance. This is because peripheral zone cancers tend to remain relatively thin during their early development as a result of confinement between the surgical capsule and the true capsule of the gland (Fig. 68–1).[6] Since it is not possible to appreciate by palpation the depth of needle penetration into the

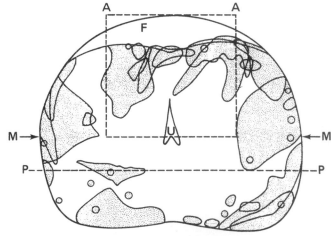

Figure 68–1. Transaxial plane through the prostate reveals the locations of small carcinomas found in cystoprostatectomy specimens removed for bladder cancer. These incidental tumors tend to be very thin. (From McNeal JE, et al. Stage A versus stage B adenocarcinoma of the prostate: Morphological comparison and biological significance. J Urol 139:61, 1988. Copyright Williams & Wilkins, 1988.)

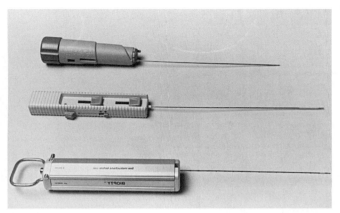

Figure 68–2. *From top to bottom*, the Monopty, the ASAP, and the Biopty automatic biopsy instruments.

Several automatic instruments are produced today (Fig. 68–2). They all operate well and obtain satisfactory cores. Factors that influence choice are cost (the reusable instruments cost more initially but are less expensive in the long run, since only the needle need be changed for each patient), ease of use (some require that the needle be disassembled from the instrument for core removal between biopsies, a somewhat time-consuming procedure), and the personal preference of the operator.

Biopsy Needle Configuration

Almost all spring-firing biopsy instruments thrust forward 23 mm as they are activated. The needle notch in which tissue will be acquired begins 5 mm from the distal end of the tip, so it is necessary to make sure that the area to be sampled lies within that distance proximal to the tip of the needle (Fig. 68–3).[7] Therefore, the operator must know the distance between the dots on the biopsy line of the particular sonographic instrument being used in order to be sure that the desired area will be encompassed by the needle notch.

SONOGRAPHIC INSTRUMENT CONFIGURATION. Prostatic needle biopsy can be done under ultrasonic guidance either transperineally or transrectally. Any of the three types of scanners (rotary, linear array, sector) can be used for biopsy (Fig. 68–4). It is essential that the examiner understand the specific attributes of the instrument, since each is markedly different in its application.

Rotary scanners display the prostate only in transverse views by emitting sound at a right angle circumferentially around the end of the probe. They can be used for transperineal biopsy only. Biopsy needles are inserted in a slot of a needle guide that corresponds to an appropriate biopsy dot on a line generated by the sonogram instrument. The needle approaches the scan plane at a right angle and does not appear on the sonogram monitor until the instant it penetrates the scan plane. Thus, the needle is seen only as a point, and while it continues to be seen at that point as the needle is advanced, the location of the needletip is not visible once the scan plane is

gland, visual guidance is helpful in ensuring that the needle does not actually penetrate the lesion and sample tissue too deeply within the prostate.

Sonographically suspicious areas that are not palpable can be biopsied, of course, only under visual guidance.

When a palpable lesion is not seen by ultrasound examination, sonographic control is still helpful in taking multiple cores through the area in which the abnormality was felt. Coordination by a single examiner between the location of a tactile abnormality and its geographical location visually is a great help. Since neither tactile nor visual biopsy guidance is perfect, both should be considered when a palpable lesion cannot be seen by sonography.

Biopsy Instruments

The spring-operated automatic biopsy instruments available today acquire tissue cores within a fraction of a second after discharge, and they avoid the almost inevitable needle notch displacement encountered with manipulation of the slower manual needles. This rapid action of the automatic instruments also avoids tissue crushing at the core edges, with the result that cores are superior to those obtained with manual needles. This is true even though the automatic needles are of smaller caliber (usually 18 gauge) than most manual needles (usually 14 gauge).

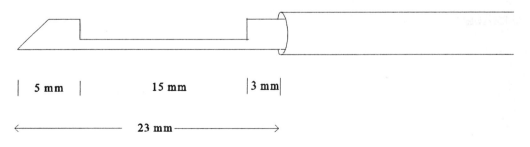

Figure 68–3. Needle architecture. Note that the tip of the needle extends 5 mm beyond the notch in which the tissue will be harvested.

| 5 mm | 15 mm | |3 mm| |

← 23 mm →

METHODS OF TRANSDUCER SWEEP

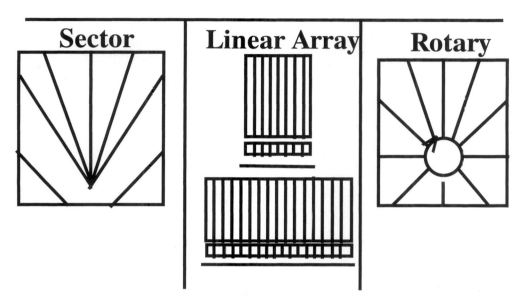

Figure 68–4. A sector scanner, a linear array scanner, and a rotary scanner.

traversed. As a consequence, needle location is indicated only in the X axis (laterolaterally) and Y axis (anteroposteriorly) of the patient. No Z axis (cephalocaudad) location is seen.

Linear array scanners emit their sound, somewhat like the teeth of a comb, in a line parallel to the long axis of the scanner. They display the gland in longitudinal views only. This type of scanner lends itself well to transperineal biopsy, but transrectal biopsy can present problems. In transperineal biopsy the needle is passed through an appropriate slot in a guide affixed to the instrument corresponding to a line generated on the monitor. In this instance the monitor displays Z-axis needle excursion as the needle advances progressively through the scan plane. When a linear array scanner is used for transrectal biopsy, the biopsy channel must pass through the center of the scanner at an angle that will allow it to be seen on the monitor. Biopsy of lesions near the apex of the prostate is quite satisfactory, but use of local anesthesia into the anal verge is important in order to obtund the pain occasioned by insertion of a needle through it. Biopsy of lesions more cephalad in the prostate, or in the seminal vesicles, may be impossible transrectally because of inability to advance the scanner far enough into the rectum to reach the desired area. Should that occur, it is necessary to convert the biopsy to the transperineal route.

Sector scanners sweep their sound back and forth across the prostate from a common point, similar to the sweep of a windshield wiper. Scanners of this type provide both transverse and longitudinal views of the gland and accommodate either transperineal or transrectal biopsy. Thus, they are the most versatile scanners available for this purpose.

Sector scanners change the view from transverse to longitudinal by one of two distinctly different means, each of which has a marked effect on biopsy technique. Scanners that emit sound directly at their distal end from transducers that are fixed within the probe housing must be rotated through 90 degrees to change the scan plane. The biopsy guide is affixed to the outside of the scanner, and the guideline is visible as a series of dots generated on the monitor. The advancing needle is displayed throughout its excursion in either transverse or longitudinal planes, since the needle guide is affixed to the scanner housing.

In other sector scanners the scanning transducer can be rotated from a transverse to a longitudinal plane within the scanner housing by turning a lever on the probe. Biopsy in the transverse plane shows the needle only as a point, exactly as in the case of a rotary probe (Fig. 68–5A). Thus, Z-axis location is not displayed. However, when the transducer is rotated to the longitudinal position, the Z axis is visible, since the advancing needle traverses the center of the scan plane. These instruments have an axis that is common to both planes of view, and it is helpful to be able to switch back and forth between planes for assurance that an area to be sampled is located accurately in all three planes (Fig. 68–5).

ACCURACY OF SONOGRAPHICALLY GUIDED BIOPSY. Almost all biopsy needles in use today, whether spring-advanced or manual, have beveled tips. This promotes spreading of the needle notch so

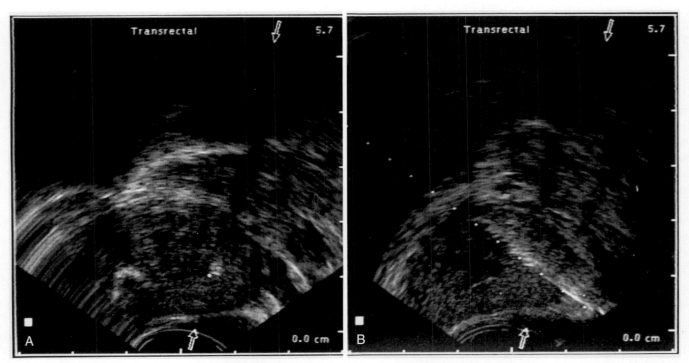

Figure 68–5. A single biopsy needle trajectory is seen in both the transaxial and longitudinal planes centered on the rotational axis between the arrows at the top and bottom of the screen. *A,* Biopsy in the transverse plane of the sector scanner shows the needle as a point only. *B,* Biopsy in the longitudinal plane shows the entire trajectory of the needle.

that the acquired tissue core is as wide as possible. As a result of the bevel, however, needles tend to deflect from the guideline slightly as they strike the posterior surface of the prostate and advance into it. This deflection can be minimized by making sure that the point of the needle, rather than the flat side of the bevel, strikes the back of the prostate first. All currently available spring-firing biopsy instruments are arranged so that the point of the needle will strike the prostate first if the widest part of the handle is oriented toward the feet of the patient (the dictum of "fat feet") (Fig. 68–6).

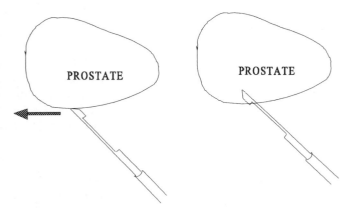

Figure 68–6. The dictum of "fat feet": The point of the needle will strike the prostate first if the wide portion of the biopsy instrument is oriented toward the feet of the patient.

LESION-DIRECTED VERSUS SYSTEMATIC WIDE-AREA BIOPSY. Hodge and associates reported an enhanced yield of cancer obtained by combining sonographic biopsy of visible, palpable cancers with systematic six-sextant biopsies.[8] The efficacy of wide-area biopsy compared with directed biopsy of either tactilely or visually suspicious lesions has been further clarified.[9] As a result of these studies, systematic area biopsies have become an integral part of a proposed algorithm for prostate cancer detection.[10]

BIOPSY TISSUE HANDLING. It is important that the physician who performs the biopsies work out with the pathologist tissue handling techniques that are satisfactory to both, so that as much information as possible can be obtained from the submitted material.

ASPIRATION FOR CYTOLOGY. Fine needle aspiration can be done either transperineally or transrectally under either digital or sonographic control. There are several completely acceptable methods for preparing cytological specimens, but many pathologists have a strong preference for one method over another. It is critical, therefore, to discuss with the local pathologist how tissue should be affixed to slides. One technique is to eject the aspirate onto a microscope slide and to spread the material as thinly as possible with the edge of a second slide. Immediate spraying with a fixative cements the tissue to the slide. A common mistake is to be too stingy with the fixative; it is important to flood the slide with fixative solution.

CORE SAMPLES. In addition to specifying the location of tactilely or visibly suspicious lesions, sextant biopsy sites are precisely documented. Cores are rolled out onto glove paper, a procedure that avoids tissue destruction caused by its being raked off with a needle or hemostat. The distal end of each core is marked with vital dye or India ink (Fig. 68–7), after which the paper bearing each core is cut out and dropped into fixative in an appropriately identified bottle. Rolling the core out on paper ensures that it will be relatively straight when fixed, aiding in tissue processing and interpretation. If there is a possibility that DNA ploidy determination will later be required from the biopsy specimen, the fixation fluid used should be one, e.g., 10 percent formalin, that does not preclude future studies on archival tissue.

If carcinoma is found in a core, the pathologist can determine not only its grade but the length of the tumor within the core, thus allowing an estimation of the minimal volume of the tumor. He or she can also specify the distance between the carcinoma and the inked end of the core, which, along with its microscopical appearance, helps determine the site of tumor origin (transition zone or outer gland).

PREOPERATIVE EVALUATION

PATIENT SELECTION. The natural history of prostate cancer is not clearly defined, and there is uncertainty about the prognosis and optimal therapy in individual patients. While exceptions certainly exist, it seems prudent to concentrate diagnostic efforts on patients who have a life expectancy of at least 10 years on the basis of actuarial data, performance status, and comorbidity.

HISTORY. In addition to obtaining general information about the patient's medical history, it is important to make specific inquiry into factors that directly affect evaluation of the prostate and the proposed prostatic biopsy.

The dates and results of previous digital rectal examination and the levels of prostatic serum markers, especially prostate-specific antigen (PSA), are helpful. Any history of previous prostatic surgery, including prostatic biopsy, should be obtained, along with details of tissue findings.

Other information should include coexisting conditions that may presage an increased biopsy complication rate, especially infection and bleeding. Recent episodes of lower urinary tract infection may indicate the need for intensification of antimicrobial prophylaxis. A history of prolonged or excessive bleeding from minor trauma suggests the need for formal coagulation studies. One should ask if the patient is taking any medications that have an anticoagulant effect. Although there are anecdotal reports of prostatic biopsy without complications in patients taking warfarin (Coumadin), biopsy under these circumstances is probably best avoided. It has not been determined whether other medications that inhibit platelet adhesion should be stopped before prostatic biopsy. The need to know whether carcinoma exists and the risk of biopsy should be balanced against the risk to the patient of stopping drugs that have an anticoagulant effect.

The physician should inquire about the existence of any internal prosthetic materials, such as heart valves or orthopedic devices, so that appropriate antimicrobial prophylaxis can be administered. A history of previous anal surgery that might affect probe insertion should be obtained.

Inquiry about the family history of both paternal and maternal relatives is pertinent in view of the increased risk of prostate cancer in patients who have family members with the disease.[11]

PHYSICAL EXAMINATION. This should include tactile evaluation of the size and consistency of the prostate, as well as assessment of any factors, such as a rectal mass, that might impede probe insertion. Anal spasm or scarring can usually be handled by digital anal dilation with appropriate topical or local anesthesia.

LABORATORY STUDIES. Urinalysis is needed to assess possible urinary tract infection before biopsy. The level of serum PSA provides vital adjunctive information. Formal coagulation parameters are not determined in the absence of any history of a bleeding tendency.

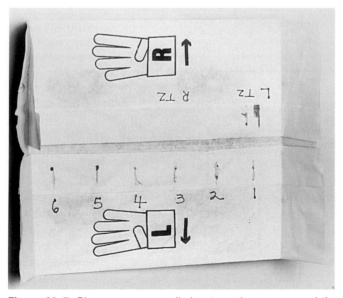

Figure 68–7. Biopsy cores are rolled out on glove paper, and the distal end is marked with India ink.

INFORMED CONSENT. As is the case with any invasive procedure, the patient must be told of the potential risks and benefits of prostatic biopsy.

BIOPSY TECHNIQUE

PATIENT PREPARATION. Administration of a Fleet enema before sonography and biopsy is helpful in eliminating rectal gas that often interferes with sonographic visualization of the prostate. It also seems wise to minimize driving fecal material into the prostate with the biopsy needle. While no studies document the need for prophylactic antimicrobials, they are commonly employed. One common regimen consists of a fluoroquinolone on the morning of biopsy and for 3 days afterward. Alternatively, an aminoglycoside can be given. Enhanced coverage is appropriate for patients with internal prostheses.

PATIENT POSITION. Sonographic examination and biopsy of the prostate can be performed with the patient in the prone jackknife, supine, or lateral decubitus position. For better patient comfort and ease of probe manipulation by right-handed examiners, the left lateral decubitus position is usually employed.

ANESTHESIA. With the availability of spring-loaded biopsy instruments that acquire tissue rapidly and almost painlessly, anesthesia is needed only if the biopsy is to be carried out transperineally. Even then, local anesthesia usually suffices. Sedation, analgesia, or anesthesia is rarely needed for transrectal biopsy. Local anesthesia into the anal verge is required if transrectal biopsy near the prostate apex is to be performed with a linear array scanner.

Digitally Guided Biopsy

Aspiration of prostatic material for cytological examination as well as core biopsy is possible under digital guidance and can be performed either transperineally or transrectally. Digital guidance is essentially limited to biopsy of areas of palpable abnormality, since wide-area biopsy of the gland by this technique provides little assurance that material is obtained accurately from all areas of the gland.

TRANSPERINEAL. After insertion of a well-lubricated finger into the rectum, the examiner passes the sampling needle through the perineum just anterior to the anus. When the needle point is felt through the rectal wall, it is directed into the area of suspicion. The finger is then backed away from the lesion, and the biopsy mechanism is activated to remove the desired tissue. If a spring-firing instrument with a safety feature is used, it is wise to keep the safety engaged until the instant of discharge.

Since aspiration needles of small gauge may bend as they are advanced transperineally, their direction into the prostate can be facilitated by first passing a 14-gauge Tru-Cut needle into the prostate, removing the inner element, and then using the outer element as a guide through which the aspiration needle can be passed.

TRANSRECTAL. Digital guidance is accomplished by pressing the needletip against the tip of the well-lubricated finger and inserting both into the rectum simultaneously. The fingertip then locates the area to be sampled, and the needle is advanced into the lesion and activated. When using a spring-firing instrument with a safety feature, it is advisable to keep the safety engaged until the finger is backed well away from the area to be sampled before firing. Even if the instrument is not equipped with a safety setting, the examiner must remember to back the finger away before firing in order to avoid inadvertent injury.

A small-caliber needle for cytological aspiration can be stabilized and directed by passing it through a hand-held needle guide, equipped with a disc-shaped stabilizer that fits in the palm, and designed specifically for aspiration of prostate tissue.

In an effort to reduce possible infection from transrectal biopsy, some operators prefer to use a double-glove technique in which it is necessary to direct the needle between the two gloves to the fingertip without penetrating the gloves. This is easy to accomplish by using scissors to shorten the plastic sheath in which the needle is packaged, passing the sheath between the gloves to the fingertip, inserting the needle through the sheath until it is felt at the fingertip, and then directing the needle into the lesion.

Sonographically Guided Biopsy

ASPIRATION. Carried out under sonographic guidance, aspiration is performed by inserting the needle until its tip is seen within the desired area. The needle is then passed in and out several times until aspirate appears at the transparent hub of the needle or within the aspiration syringe. If wide-area aspiration is performed, it is necessary to withdraw the needle from the aspiration channel, reposition the transducer to another location, and then repeat the process.

TRANSPERINEAL. Using a longitudinally oriented transducer, the operator inserts the biopsy needle through the needle guide of the sonogram probe until it appears on the screen at the proximal end of the biopsy line. The needle is advanced until its tip is 5 mm from the area to be sampled so that the 15-mm needle notch encompasses the area of interest. The biopsy instrument is then activated and the needle immediately withdrawn. If a transversely oriented transducer is used, it is advanced until it intersects the scan plane, appearing as a bright dot corresponding to the biopsy dot on the monitor. It should be pulled back approximately 5 mm from the point at which it is no longer seen so that tissue can be taken within the 15-mm range of the needle notch. The biopsy instrument is then activated, at which point the needle will again be seen at the biopsy point. It should then be removed promptly.

Transperineal Biopsy After Abdominoperineal Resection

Prostatic evaluation in men who have undergone rectal ablation presents a unique problem. Transperineal biopsy of the gland is possible by application of a sonographic biopsy probe directly on the perineum. While the image obtained is not as good as that through the rectum and usually does not allow clear visualization of individual lesions, it does permit localization of the gland sufficient for wide-area biopsy. An end-firing prostatic probe can be used, although limited tissue penetration due to the transducer's high sound frequency may impede visibility. If this happens, use of a surface probe of lower frequency is usually needed.

TRANSRECTAL. The operator inserts the biopsy needle through the needle guide of the sonogram probe until it appears on the screen at the proximal end of the biopsy line. The needle is advanced until its tip is 5 mm from the area to be sampled so that the 15-mm needle notch encompasses the area of interest. The biopsy instrument is then activated and the needle immediately withdrawn.

If an end-firing probe is used for biopsy in a longitudinal plane, the biopsy guideline is oriented over the desired gland area by levering the probe to the appropriate side. Biopsy can be accomplished in any desired plane with end-firing probes, since their rotation produces gland views in an infinite number of planes. If a side-firing probe is used for biopsy in a longitudinal plane, the biopsy guideline can be moved to the desired location by either levering the probe or rotating it. Leverage produces biopsy planes that are more nearly parallel to the lateral margins of the gland and enhance the acquisition of outer gland tissue.

SAFETY CONSIDERATIONS. When performing biopsy, one should attempt to avoid large vascular structures if possible. Such structures posterior to the

gland and at the apex are usually visible, and the probe can almost always be reoriented so that the desired area can be sampled without penetrating them. Anteriorly, vessels in the plexus of Santorini can usually be avoided by placing the tip of the biopsy needle at least 23 mm proximal to them before the biopsy instrument is activated. In performing biopsy of areas in the anterior aspect of the prostate, it is sometimes impossible to avoid passing the needle at least 5 mm through the anterior surface of the gland, particularly if an end-firing probe is used. Angulation of the probe will usually allow the area of interest to be approached from a direction that avoids impingement on large vessels.

It is important that the sonographic probe not be moved in the rectum once the needle strikes the rectal wall. Thus, it is vital that the needle remain confined within the biopsy channel until the area to be sampled is aligned properly on the biopsy guideline. The needle protrudes from the distal biopsy port before becoming visible on the monitor (Fig. 68–8). If the operator does not take this into account, damage may occur to the rectal wall or to vessels therein as the needletip is raked back and forth during lesion positioning on the guideline. This can be avoided if the needle is placed just into the proximal part of the needle guide, and the hands holding the probe and the biopsy instrument are locked together (the "rule of finger") (Fig. 68–9).[12]

Four maneuvers performed immediately after core acquisition further promote safety. First, the prostate should be viewed throughout its entirety for evidence of expanding hyperechoicism, characteristic of blood within the gland. Second, if an interface balloon is used around the transducer, it should be deflated. The probe should then be backed away from the posterior prostatic surface, thus allowing the tissue between it and the anterior rectal wall to expand and to be examined from one side of the prostate to the other. Expanding blood in that location is usually markedly hypoechoic, since it dissects through the

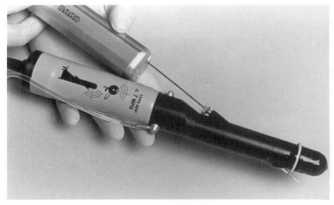

Figure 68–8. The needle protrudes from the distal biopsy port before becoming visible on the monitor.

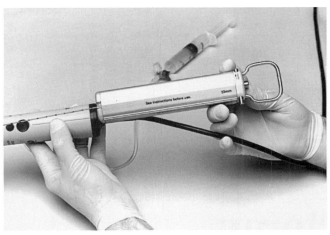

Figure 68–9. The "rule of finger." The fifth finger of the right hand is hooked around the wire from the probe. This prevents the biopsy needle from inadvertently projecting out of the ultrasound probe.

tissues without the advantage of tamponade, as is the case with intraprostatic bleeding confined by the capsule of the gland. Third, the probe should be slowly removed from the rectum and its sheath inspected for evidence of excessive blood. Fourth, digital palpation of the prostate and its surrounding tissue should be carried out for localized areas of hematoma or for general thickening of tissue between rectal wall and prostate. If any of these four maneuvers shows evidence of possible bleeding, pressure on the affected area for about 5 minutes is usually all that is required.

POSTOPERATIVE MANAGEMENT

PATIENT INSTRUCTIONS. The patient is given a prescription for a fluoroquinolone and instructed to continue this for 3 days after the biopsy. He is cautioned to report immediately to the physician any significant bleeding in the urine or stool, as well as any difficulty in voiding. He is also told that any developing fever should be reported immediately to the physician, who should consider this to be impending septicemia until proved otherwise. The patient must be seen without delay, appropriate urine and blood cultures obtained, and parenteral antimicrobial therapy started pending culture results. The need to monitor the patient's vital signs and to administer parenteral therapy indicates that this has to be done in an inpatient setting.

COMPLICATIONS. The most significant complications of prostatic biopsy are septicemia and bleeding. In over 4000 sonographically guided biopsies we have performed, fever occurred in 1.0 percent of patients who received no prophylactic antimicrobials, compared with less than 0.1 percent in those who received fluoroquinolone prophylaxis. The statistical significance of this difference cannot be determined because of small numbers and low incidence.

Many patients have transient hematuria after prostate biopsy, and hematospermia may be present for several weeks after biopsy of the seminal vesicles. However, these are rarely of sufficient magnitude to require treatment.

Another complication occasionally seen is rectal bleeding, sometimes severe enough to require anoscopic ligation. A small amount of blood with the first postbiopsy stool is common.

Editorial Comment
Fray F. Marshall

Needle biopsy of the prostate has changed significantly with the advent of transrectal ultrasound and spring-loaded biopsy guns. This chapter provides an excellent guide to needle biopsy of the prostate. We have been inclined to obtain small tissue cores rather than needle aspirates because of the occasional difficulty of cytological interpretation of aspirates only. In addition, no Gleason grade can be given with an aspirate. Many patients do not consider that aspirin is a medication, so we specifically tell patients not to take aspirin 2 weeks before the biopsy.

REFERENCES

1. Rifkin MD, Kurtz AB, Goldberg BB. Sonographically guided transperineal prostatic biopsy: Preliminary experience with a longitudinal linear-array transducer. AJR Am J Roentgenol 140:745, 1983.
2. Weaver RP, Noble MJ, Weigel JW. Correlation of ultrasound-guided and digitally directed transrectal biopsies of palpable prostatic abnormalities. J Urol 145:516, 1991.
3. Resnick MI. Transrectal ultrasound guided versus digitally directed prostatic biopsy: A comparative study. J Urol 139:754, 1988.
4. Ajzen SA, Goldenberg SL, Allen GJ, et al. Palpable prostatic nodules: Comparison of US and digital guidance for fine-needle aspiration biopsy. Radiology 171:521, 1989.
5. Hodge KK, McNeal JE, Stamey TA. Ultrasound guided transrectal core biopsies of the palpable abnormal prostate. J Urol 142:66, 1989.
6. McNeal JE, Price HM, Redwine EA, et al. Stage A versus stage B adenocarcinoma of the prostate: Morphological comparison and biological significance. J Urol 139:61, 1988.
7. Kaye KW. Prostate biopsy using automatic gun: Technique for determination of precise biopsy site. Urology 34:111, 1989.
8. Hodge KK, McNeal JE, Terris MK, et al. Random systematic versus directed ultrasound guided transrectal core biopsies of the prostate. J Urol 142:71, 1989.
9. Flanigan RC, Catalona WJ, Richie JP, et al. Success rate of digital rectal examination (DRE) and transrectal ultrasonography (TRUS) in localizing prostate cancer. J Urol 149:288A, 1993.
10. Oesterling JE, Cooner WH, Jacobsen SJ, et al. Influence of patient age on the serum PSA concentration: An important clinical observation. Urol Clin North Am 20:671, 1993.
11. Carter BS, Beaty TH, Steinberg GD, et al. Mendelian inheritance of familial prostate cancer. Proc Natl Acad Sci USA 89:3367, 1992.
12. Cooner WH: Reducing rectal injury from sonographically-guided transrectal needle biopsy of prostate. The "rule of finger." Urology 36:191, 1990.

Part VII

SURGERY OF THE SEMINAL VESICLES

Chapter 69

Seminal Vesiculectomy

David F. Paulson

Seminal vesiculectomy was one of the earliest urological procedures. The indications ranged from seminal vesicular tuberculosis to arthritis and rheumatoid disease. Today, surgery on the seminal vesicles is rarely indicated, as inflammatory disease is usually responsive to broad-spectrum antibiotics. However, in cases in which the disease process is unresponsive to pharmaceutical management, surgical removal of the seminal vesicles may be warranted.

The seminal vesicles arise as lobulated organs from outpouchings of the vas deferens. In the adult, they measure approximately 7 cm in length and distally they join the ampullae of the vas deferens to form the ejaculatory ducts. The latter lie within prostatic substance and open into the prostatic urethra on the colliculus seminalis on either side of the prostatic utricle. The seminal vesicles lie between the posterior wall of the bladder and the anterior surface of the rectum. This anatomical position permits several surgical approaches. The arterial supply of the seminal vesicles arises from branches of the medial and inferior vesical arteries.

PREOPERATIVE EVALUATION

Inflammatory disease within the seminal vesicles is characterized by hematospermia accompanied by severe pain at the time of ejaculation. The pain may persist for many hours after ejaculation and is characterized as low abdominal discomfort. It may be of sufficient intensity to discourage sexual activity. Rectal examination will identify tenderness and induration in one or both seminal vesicles and prompt the diagnosis of seminal vesiculitis. Seminal vesicle pa-

thology is best identified by contrast retrograde seminal vesiculograms or by ultrasound examination.

Few diseases of the seminal vesicles require surgery. However, in cases in which chronic symptomatic inflammation of the seminal vesicles can be documented or other disease of the seminal vesicles is suspected, surgical removal of the vesicles is appropriate.

OPERATIVE TECHNIQUE

The seminal vesicles can be approached transvesically or transabdominally, or through the perineum or sacrum (Fig. 69–1). The perineal approach is conducted in the manner of radical prostatectomy with posterior displacement of the rectum. The seminal vesicles are identified at the base of the prostate and followed proximally. They are then mobilized and removed in their entirety. An incision can also be made in the lower abdomen, with the bladder mobilized anteriorly. With an incision made in the cul-de-sac, the seminal vesicles are exposed by anterior displacement of the bladder. This surgical approach is difficult owing to the position of the seminal vesicles deep in the pelvis and the restricted operating field available between the anteriorly displaced bladder and the posteriorly displaced rectum.

The vesicles are approached most easily through the posterior wall of the bladder. The retropubic space is opened through either a transverse suprapubic or a midline lower abdominal incision. The bladder is opened through a vertical cystotomy. The ureteral orifices should be identified and catheterized. The seminal vesicles can then be exposed through either a posterior midline incision, splitting the trigone

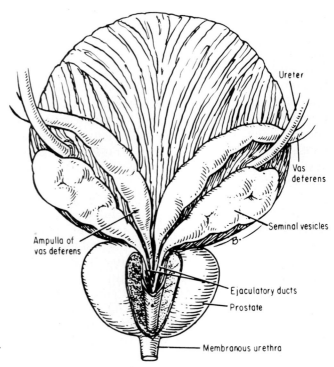

Figure 69–1. Anatomical relationships of the seminal vesicle, vas deferens, bladder, and prostate as viewed from behind.

and displacing the ureters laterally, or a transverse incision distal to the ureteral orifices and proximal to the bladder neck, allowing superior displacement of the posterior bladder neck to permit visualization of the seminal vesicles (Fig. 69–2).

I prefer a midline posterior vesical incision, splitting the trigone in the midline and displacing the ureteral orifices laterally. The incision should be carried sharply through the bladder musculature to gain access to the retrovesical structures. With alternating sharp and blunt dissection, the seminal vesicles and ampullae of the vas deferens can be identified. The investing fibers should be mobilized with blunt dis-

section and the vessels cauterized as they are encountered. Early identification of the ampullae of the vas deferens, with dissection carried proximally along these structures, will permit mobilization of a 3- to 5-cm segment of the vas deferens. The latter then should be divided and the proximal end controlled with an absorbable suture or nonabsorbable metallic clip. Subsequent traction on the portions of the ampullae that remain with the operative specimen will elevate the seminal vesicle into the operative field. The vesicle should be identified and additional attention directed to mobilization of its tip. Once the tip of the seminal vesicle is identified, it can be grasped

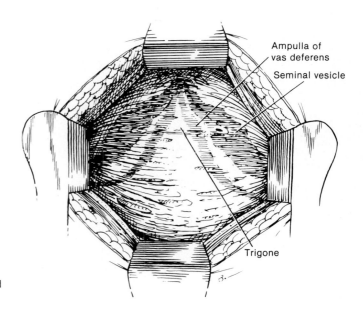

Figure 69–2. Anatomical relationships of the seminal vesicle as viewed through the posterior wall of the bladder from the head of the table.

in noncrushing forceps, such as a Babcock clamp, and mobilized with alternating sharp and blunt dissection. As the seminal vesicle and the associated ampullae of the vas deferens are mobilized, they will be seen to join to form the ejaculatory duct as they enter into the prostatic substance. At this point the ejaculatory duct can be cross-clamped, divided, and suture ligated with an absorbable suture material or controlled with a metallic clip. Transvesical seminal vesiculectomy does not carry with it any hazard of postoperative impotence.

After removal of the seminal vesicle, the retrovesical space should be drained. Careful digital exploration will permit the creation of a tunnel behind the trigone that emerges lateral to the bladder wall. A curved clamp can be passed through this tunnel, and a Penrose drain grasped and led into the retrovesical space. This drain is brought out through either the lateral aspect of the incision or a separate stab wound. The posterior vesicostomy incision should be closed in two layers with running 2-0 chromic catgut sutures, one suture being used to approximate the detrusor and the second being used for mucosal closure. The ureteral catheters inserted preoperatively should be brought out of the contralateral bladder wall, through the inferior abdominal wall via separate stab wounds, and left in place for 3 to 5 days. This precaution will prevent postoperative edema producing ureteral obstruction. The ureteral catheters should be removed on successive days so that postoperative anuria will not be encountered.

Editorial Comment
Fray F. Marshall

Relatively few indications exist for seminal vesiculectomy, especially since tuberculosis is not often encountered in the United States. The anterior approach to the seminal vesicle, with division of the bladder posteriorly and a vertical incision between the ureteral orifices, has been an excellent way to expose the seminal vesicle without injuring the neurovascular bundle and creating impotence.

Cysts of the seminal vesicle can become infected and require removal. Patients who had transurethral incisions of such cysts through the bladder developed recurrent seminal vesiculitis and epididymitis that required removal of the seminal vesicles. These patients did very well postoperatively.

REFERENCE

1. Paulson DF. The prostate. In Genitourinary Surgery. Philadelphia, Churchill Livingstone, 1984.

Part VIII

SURGERY OF THE URETHRA IN THE MALE

Chapter 70

Surgery of Anterior Urethral Strictures

Gerald H. Jordan

A urethral stricture is a scar in the spongy erectile tissue of the corpus spongiosum that underlies the urethral epithelium, and in some cases extends into the adjacent tissues. Contraction of this scar reduces the area of the urethral lumen; when severe, it causes profound changes in the dynamics of voiding.

With publication of his technique for urethral stricture excision in 1914, Hamilton Russell described the first truly "modern" approach to the treatment of urethral stricture disease.[1] After excising the area of the stricture, he reanastomosed the remaining urethra to the respective dorsal wall and left the ventral wall to granulate and heal by secondary intention. Unfortunately, his approach was limited by the lack of knowledge of the deep penile and superficial genital blood supplies and a poor understanding of tissue transfer techniques at that time. Today, using applied anatomic principles and modern tissue transfer techniques, urethral reconstruction (i.e., urethral scar revision) can yield excellent functional and cosmetic results.

SURGICAL ANATOMY

Neither the penis nor the scrotum has a subcuticular adipose layer. The dartos fascia is immediately beneath the skin of the penis, with the superficial lamina of Buck's fascia lying beneath the dartos fascia. Surrounding both the dorsal neurovascular structures and the corpus spongiosum in envelope fashion, Buck's fascia is closely applied to the tunica albuginea of the corpora cavernosa. The anterior ure-

thra is that portion of the urethra that, throughout its course, is invested by either the corpus spongiosum or the spongy erectile tissue of the glans penis. For purposes of discussion, the anterior urethra is divided into three sections: the bulbous urethra, the pendulous urethra, and the fossa navicularis (Fig. 70–1). The bulbous urethra, lying proximally, is the portion that is widest in caliber; more importantly, it is where the corpus spongiosum is invested by the

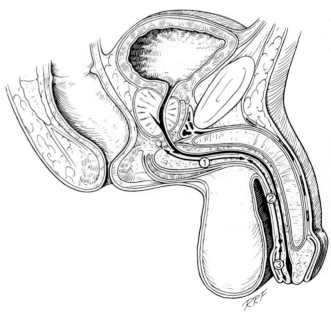

Figure 70–1. Sagittal section of the pelvis illustrating the portions of the anterior urethra: 1, bulbous urethra; 2, pendulous or penile urethra; 3, fossa navicularis.

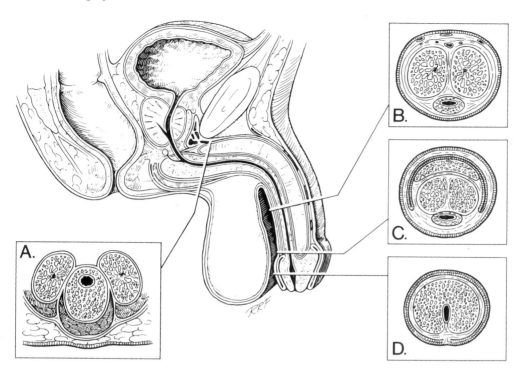

Figure 70–2. Sagittal section of the pelvis with corresponding sections of the base of the penis and urethra: A, bulbous urethra; B, midpendulous urethra; C, distal penile or pendulous urethra; D, fossa navicularis.

midline fusion of the ischial cavernosus musculature (Fig. 70–2). Here the urethra is eccentrically placed within the corpus spongiosum, closer to the dorsal penile structures. Moving distally, one finds the pendulous or penile urethra. More centrally placed within the corpus spongiosum, it is in an area that is relatively uninvested. Finally, in the area of the urethra where the corpus spongiosum has flared to become the spongy erectile tissue of the glans penis, is the fossa navicularis.

The corpus spongiosum is characterized by a dual blood supply. The deep internal pudendal artery gives off a prominent scrotal branch and then extends as the common penile artery (Fig. 70–3). The proximal branches of the common penile artery (arteries to the bulb and the circumflex cavernosal arteries)

represent the proximal arterial supply to the corpus spongiosum. The artery then bifurcates to become the profunda artery of the corpora cavernosa and the dorsal artery. The dorsal artery extends and arborizes into the spongy erectile tissue of the glans penis. The corpus spongiosum is therefore arterialized proximally via the circumflex cavernosals and arteries to the bulb and distally via the arborizations of the dorsal artery. The dual vascularity of the corpus spongiosum has significance for reconstructive surgery. If the blood supply of the corpus spongiosum is kept intact, it can be vigorously mobilized both proximally and distally. The venous drainage of the glans and corpora cavernosa provide the venous drainage of the corpus spongiosum.

Quartey described his microdissection and microinjection studies of the superficial penile vascular supply in 1983,[2] demonstrating that vasculature to be dependent on the superficial and deep external pudendal vessels, which are medial branches of the iliofemoral system. These branches are given off in Scarpa's fascia and extend to the penis (Fig. 70–4).

There is some controversy surrounding the true nature of this blood supply. It is my opinion that these vessels arborize to become a true fasciocutaneous blood supply. However, the fasciocutaneous system of vascularity should not be viewed as a blood supply based on the fascia itself. The fascia simply serves as the trellis for the vine; there is a superficial and deep plexus associated with the fascia and perforators associated with the fascial septa. Because the fascial plexuses are the true blood supply to the genital skin islands, these skin islands can be widely

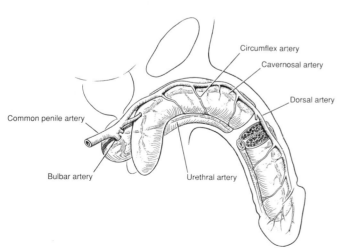

Figure 70–3. Deep arterial supply to the penis.

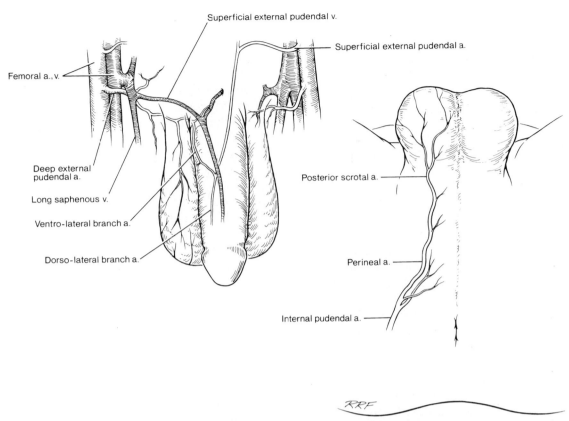

Figure 70–4. Superficial blood supply to the genital skin. *Left,* Distribution of the superficial external pudendal artery. *Right,* Distribution of the perineal artery and scrotal artery. (From Jordan GH, Schlossberg S. Using tissue transfer for urethral reconstruction. Contemp Urol 5:13, 1993. Copyright Medical Economics.)

mobilized and aggressively transposed, and to a point the fascial flap can be twisted. In short, the fascia is the flap and the skin is the passenger. At the point where the deep internal pudendal artery becomes the common penile artery, it has in essence bifurcated, the other branch being the perineal artery. The perineal artery extends anteriorly in the crease of the groin, giving off the labial scrotal arteries. These branches are believed to arborize to become a fascial blood supply associated with the tunica dartos of the scrotum. The blood supply of the perineal artery also appears to operate in concert with the superficial external pudendal blood supply. An understanding of this blood supply has allowed the entire genital skin to be viewed as a donor site (provided it is nonhirsute).

PREOPERATIVE EVALUATION

Patients who have urethral strictures often have obstructive voiding symptoms or urinary tract infections, including prostatitis and epididymitis. Some patients have urinary retention; on close inquiry, however, many of them will have tolerated voiding symptoms for some time before the obstruction. When a patient cannot void, an attempt is made to

pass a urethral catheter. If the catheter will not pass, the nature of the obstruction should be determined using a dynamic retrograde urethrogram, if possible. In many instances, acute dilation may not be the best course for the patient. When there is doubt, a suprapubic cystostomy catheter should be placed to treat the acute situation. This allows time for a treatment plan to be devised.

The treatment of strictures must vary according to the anatomy of the stricture. Therefore, the pathological anatomy (length, location, depth, and density of scarring) must be precisely defined for a plan of reconstruction to be formulated. Urethrograms should be dynamic studies accomplished while the contrast material is injected and while the patient is voiding.[3] Films in more than one projection may be necessary to visualize the stricture. In addition, pelvic radiography studies often show evidence of loss of elasticity in the urethra proximal and distal to the stricture, and this length of involvement should be considered in the treatment plan. Because the pressure generated by the bladder is transmitted to this portion of the urethra, voiding films should illustrate dilation proximal to the stenosis, if that area of the urethra is normal. A coning down or irregularity of this segment of the urethra is evidence of its involvement and indicates that the distal scar may have kept it dilated by hydrodynamic pressure/hydrodilation. Unless this segment is included in the repair, voiding pressure will be lowered after relief of the distal obstruction, causing it to contract and the obstruction to recur. Finally, during surgery, it is important to evaluate the urethra proximal and distal to the portion being operated on and to include all involved areas in the repair. In some cases, it may be beneficial to "defunctionalize" the urethra for a time (approximately 3 months) to allow the hydrodilated segments to "declare themselves."

The depth and density of the scar in the urethra (spongiofibrosis) are derived from the appearance of the urethral outline on contrast studies and fixation and induration noted at urethroscopy. Ultrasound studies also suggest that this modality may make evaluation more precise.[4-6] "High-frequency ultrasonography of the penis and urethra *may* demonstrate additional scarring along the urethra, particularly in the anterior urethra."[7] With definition of the stricture and application of an appropriate plan, urethral stricture disease can be treated with fewer procedures and better results than with the application and reapplication of simpler techniques until the surgeon is forced to move on to more complex therapy.

Dilation and internal urethrotomy are still useful for strictures that involve the epithelial and superficial segments of the urethra. However, the success of internal urethrotomy is clearly related to the depth and length of the stricture. Patients with short strictures that involve only the superficial spongy tissue seem to have reliable and good results from internal urethrotomy, whereas those having deep, multiple, or complex strictures predictably have poor results from internal urethrotomy. In the past, all patients were first treated using internal urethrotomy, and those failing to respond eventually received an open reconstruction. Using today's tissue transfer techniques, one-stage open surgical procedures have significantly more predictable results and, despite their complexity, are easier to perform than their multistage predecessors. Therefore, only patients with stricture disease known to respond well to a particular procedure should be offered that procedure. Patients with strictures that do not fit into a classification calling for a simple procedure must be treated at the outset with a more complex operation selected according to the anatomy of the stricture. Dedicated treatment by "conservative, repetitive procedures" that fail to cure the stricture can, at best, be regarded as management of the stricture. If such a course is elected, surgeons must be honest with themselves and their patients regarding the goals of such a course, including advising patients of the availability of complex reconstructive techniques that do offer the potential for cure.

OPERATIVE TECHNIQUES

Instrumented strictures or strictures that are in evolution may be unpredictable and yield unpredictable surgical results. In cases in which instrumentation has been necessary, at least 6 weeks but preferably 3 months should elapse before reconstruction to allow the urethra to stabilize. If the patient develops severe voiding symptoms, urinary tract infection, or retention during this waiting period, suprapubic diversion should be established. It is important to remember that urethral reconstruction is a scar revision in which the surgeon is trading a functionally poorly tolerated scar for a new, predictable, and functionally well tolerated scar.

Dilation

For strictures that consist of mucosal folds or superficial scars in the spongy tissue, dilation can be curative; however, it is most commonly used only as a management tool. I favor balloon dilation for acute dilation, and soft catheter dilation for chronic dilation.

If dilation is to be effective for management of a stricture, it must be carried out in such a way that further trauma is not caused to the urethra. The stricture should be gradually stretched, not disrupted. Tearing the strictured area will lead to further scarring, with an increase in the depth and density of the fibrosis. Intervals between instrumentation should be separated by 6 to 12 months. Recurrent obstructive symptoms, requiring shortening of the interval, are evidence of a change in the character of the stricture and call for a change in the treatment plan. Even without such symptoms, all patients undergoing dilation as a management tool should be periodically reevaluated using radiography and flexible cystoscopy.

Internal Urethrotomy

As a curative modality, internal urethrotomy should be limited to mucosal folds, strictures with an iris-like configuration, and strictures with only superficial spongiofibrosis. Strictures at the level of the suspensory ligament associated with urethral instrumentation, such as a transurethral resection (TUR), are commonly associated with deep fibrosis, and even though short often do not respond to internal urethrotomy. Likewise, straddle injury strictures, also usually associated with deep fibrosis, do not respond to internal urethrotomy.

For internal urethrotomy to be curative, the incision must extend through the depth of the spongiofibrosis, disrupting the stricture/scar so that the underlying soft elastic tissue can allow expansion of the urethral lumen. Internal urethrotomy sets into play the "forces" of healing by secondary intention. Success depends on the completion of re-epithelialization before wound contraction re-establishes the stricture. Diversion and stenting allow the urethra to regenerate and they increase the diameter of the stricture, but a scar always remains. Either temporary or permanently implanted stents have been proposed as a method to oppose wound contraction while allowing the progress of re-epithelialization to continue to completion. In some patients this concept appears to be a valid one. However, the long-term effects and success of implantable stents are not currently known, and they must be used with the utmost caution.

Internal urethrotomy may also be used in combination with dilation for patients who, because of their general condition, are not candidates for open reconstructive surgery. In these cases, an internal urethrotomy is performed; the incision should be deep enough to allow passage of a reasonably sized silicone catheter. The catheter is left in place for 10 to 14 days to allow for the onset of healing. When the catheter is removed, the patient is provided with a 20 or 22 Fr. catheter (Rusch Coudé-tipped catheter: Catalog no. 221800, Willy Rusch AG., P.O. Box 1633, D-7050 Waiblingen, Germany) and instructed to pass it through the area of stricture three or four times weekly. After 3 to 4 months, the interval is reduced. Satisfactory voiding should be achieved with self-dilation only once or twice a week by that time. When self-dilation is discontinued, the stricture typically recurs and requires a more definitive procedure.

Excision and Anastomosis

It is now certain that the most dependable technique of anterior urethral reconstruction is the complete excision of the area of fibrosis and primary reanastomosis of normal anterior urethra. Adhering to the following technical points will yield the best results: (1) totally excise the area of fibrosis; (2) widely spatulate the urethral reanastomosis to create a large ovoid anastomosis; and (3) ensure a tension-free anastomosis.

The success of this procedure relies on the fact that the corpus spongiosum can be vigorously mobilized. When the length of mobilization is limited, this procedure in general is limited. However, with vigorous mobilization, development of the intracrural space, and detachment of the bulbospongiosum from the perineal body (Fig. 70–5), significant lengths of stricture can be excised and and the urethra anastomosed. Care must be taken when detaching the bulbospongiosum from the perineal body to limit the dissection

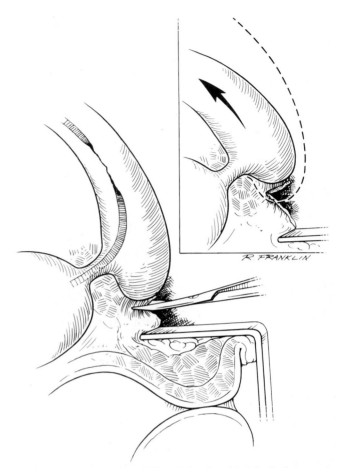

Figure 70–5. Mobilization of the bulb by detaching the bulbospongiosum from the perineal body. (From Schlossberg SM, Jordan GH. Mediguide to Urology: A Practical Approach to Treatment of Anterior Urethral Stricture. New York, Lawrence A. Della Corte, 1994.)

and not disrupt the proximal blood supply (arteries to the bulb). In general, strictures 1 to 2-cm long are easily excised with reanastomosis of the remaining urethra, and, in some cases, strictures as long as 3 to 4 cm can be totally excised and a primary anastomosis of the anterior urethra performed.

After excision of the stricture and mobilization of the urethra, spatulating incisions are performed (Fig. 70–6). Several polydioxanone sutures (PDS) are used to approximate the urethra dorsally, bringing together the adventitia of the spongiosum. The urethral epithelium is then reapproximated in a watertight fashion, using small absorbable monofilament suture. After the anastomosis is tested for water tightness, the remaining adventitia of the corpus spongiosum is closed with PDS, and the mobilized urethra is reattached to the corpora cavernosa or the triangular ligament with interrupted Vicryl sutures.

When the anastomosis is complete, the repair is stented with a soft silicone catheter and the urine diverted. The length of time and manner in which urinary diversion for urethral reconstruction are carried out have been controversial. Webster and co-

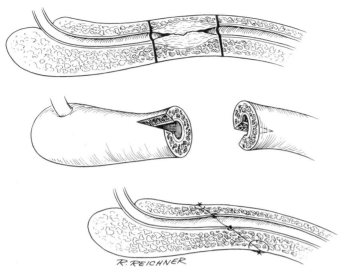

R. REICHNER

Figure 70–6. Technique of excision with spatulated anastomosis for stricture of the anterior urethra. (From Jordan GH. Urethral stricture and stricture disease. In Droller MJ, ed. Surgical Management of Urologic Disease: An Anatomic Approach. St. Louis, Mosby-Year Book, 1992.)

workers[3] employed fenestrated urethral catheters for diversion in their cases, calculating the mean length of time of diversion before disappearance of extravasation on a urethrogram following repair. For an end-to-end anastomosis the time necessary for healing was 10 days, for an "island flap" procedure the mean time was 16 days, and after full-thickness skin graft repair it averaged 21 days.

I prefer the use of suprapubic urinary diversion and thin-walled silicone tubes placed in the urethra as stents. I do not use fenestrated stents. In posterior repairs I pass a silicone Foley catheter through the urethra into the bladder as a stent and use a suprapubic tube for urinary diversion. For more distal repairs, I place thin-walled silicone tubes, extending a few centimeters proximal to the repair, and secured at the urethral meatus with 4–0 Prolene sutures sewn through the glans and loosely tied. I have chosen 14 Fr. tubing to stent urethroplasties in adult patients because silicone tubing larger than 14 Fr. has a thick and incompressible wall.

Grafts for Urethral Reconstruction

For the purpose of urethral reconstruction, four types of grafts have been used: full-thickness skin grafts, meshed split-thickness skin grafts, buccal mucosal grafts, and bladder epithelial grafts. Examining the microvasculature to the skin, the deep plexus (subdermal plexus) is distributed at the interface between the dermis and the subcutaneous skin. Consisting of rather large vessels that are sparsely distributed, it communicates with an intradermal plexus

via perforators. The intradermal plexus is roughly distributed at the juncture of the superficial adventitial dermis and the deeper reticular dermis, and consists of smaller vessels that are more numerous in their distribution. This distribution influences the take characteristics of a full-thickness compared with a split-thickness graft, because a split-thickness skin graft (exposing the intradermal plexus) has many more vessels exposed on its deep surface than a full-thickness skin graft (exposing the subdermal plexus) (Fig. 70–7).

Full-thickness skin grafts, which have been thought of as noncontracting, do contract by 10 to 15 percent, and grafts taken from areas of the body where the skin is thick are likely to contract more than full-thickness units that are thin. This contraction must be considered when the graft is designed. In addition, after a full-thickness graft is harvested, all of the underlying fibrovascular tissue must be removed from its dermal aspect without thinning the graft. Careful preparation of the dermal aspect of the graft optimizes apposition of the dermis to the vessels to the graft bed. Preputial skin is the full-thickness skin best suited for urethral reconstruction, and other areas should be avoided whenever possible.

Split-thickness skin grafts (STSG) can contract as much as 100 percent in unsupported tissue. For this reason, and because collagen deposited beneath the epidermal layer during the healing of split-thickness grafts causes them to remain brittle and lack compliance, split-thickness skin grafts are not considered satisfactory for use in single-stage urethral reconstruction. However, in the early 1980s, Schreiter and Noll[8] began their experience with the use of split-thickness skin grafts placed in staged fashion as a mesh graft. In this case, the STSG is placed open, supported at the first stage. The second stage is then a tubularization of the graft, after a period to allow for graft maturity and take and stability of contraction.

Problems with the use of skin grafts and situations in which nonhirsute genital skin is not sufficient for the repair have led to the investigation of other donor

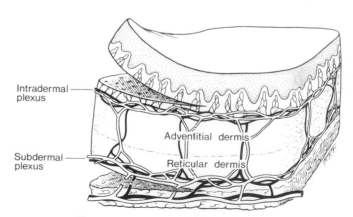

Figure 70–7. Microvasculature of the skin.

sites. The microvascularity of a bladder epithelial graft is similar to that of the skin, consisting of two plexuses—a deep laminar plexus and a superficial laminar plexus—that are distributed like the microvasculature of the skin. With maturation, it is truly hairless, and it maintains good compliance. Bladder epithelial grafts have been useful in some situations, but there are problems with the graft, particularly when it is brought distally to the meatus. Care must be taken to avoid letting the bladder epithelial graft dry out during the reconstructive surgery, because this tissue seems particularly prone to desiccation injury.

Although Humby first studied the use of buccal mucosal grafts in 1941,[9] they have not been widely used until recently. A buccal mucosal graft differs in its microvascularity from a skin graft in that the microvasculature of the lamina propria of the buccal mucosa has been shown to be fairly uniformly distributed, without a layered distribution as seen in the skin and bladder. This uniform microvasculature allows a buccal mucosa graft to be cut at various levels of the lamina without affecting the take characteristics of the graft. However, despite the level of graft harvest, the contraction characteristics appear to be similar to those of a full-thickness skin graft. From early experience, buccal mucosal grafts appear to be versatile, but the greatest experience with them has been for reconstruction in hypospadias or complicated hypospadias. Whereas it remains to be seen whether there is any advantage to the use of buccal epithelial grafts, they may have the same limitations as other grafts.

For good graft take, the tissues of the graft bed must be appropriate. Avascular scar tissue, fat, and exposed bone are not good graft beds. Rapid neovascularization of the graft is dependent on a well-vascularized graft bed as well as on adequate immobilization of the graft to reduce disruption of the delicate new vessels as they form. Graft failures result from mechanical factors that prevent tight apposition of the graft to its host bed, bleeding and hematoma beneath the graft, necrosis in the bed, or infection. Finally, contraction of a graft is a factor not only of its composition, but also of the bed on which it is placed, and because the tissues of the penis are not fixed, they offer little resistance to contracture. To resolve these problems, I do not use a graft when a flap would be more appropriate.

Flaps for Urethral Reconstruction

The term *flap* implies transfer of a composite of tissues with the blood supply intact or re-established in the recipient area by microvascular surgical anastomosis (free flap). In the case of flaps for reconstruction of the urethra, the term flap is, by definition, a composite of skin and the underlying tissues. Flaps do not take, they survive. If a flap survives, it does not contract. If a flap does not survive, the tissue is completely lost, because it will not take as a graft.

Two classifications of vascularity apply to skin flaps: a direct cuticular pattern and a musculocutaneous/fasciocutaneous pattern. In the cuticular pattern the segmental vessels communicate with prominent vessels that lie superficial to the fascia of the body wall and have distinct, predictable, cuticular vascular territories. A classical example of a flap with a direct cuticular blood supply is the groin flap. In a musculocutaneous/fasciocutaneous pattern, the blood supply is associated either with vessels to the underlying muscles, or with vessels that perforate through fascial septa. The fascial vessels are distributed on the fascia via superficial and deep plexuses that connect the perforators to the subdermal plexus of the overlying skin. In the case of skin islands elevated on muscle or fascia, the muscle/fascia represent the flap carrying the skin island or paddle, and the vasculature of the island is that of the muscle or fascia. In these systems the vasculature cannot be thought of as a single axial vessel, but as a supply based on a single axial vessel with wide arborization. A classical example of a musculocutaneous flap is a gracilis muscle flap with a skin island/paddle. The fasciocutaneous system has been demonstrated to be useful for urethral reconstruction in particular and for genitourinary reconstructive surgery in general.

Applications of genital skin islands, mobilized on either the dartos fascia of the penis or the tunica dartos of the scrotum, should not be considered as separate procedures per se, but as different applications of a single concept.[2] Placing hirsute skin in the urinary tract can usually be avoided today, and skin islands should therefore be taken from the areas of genital skin redundancy that is not hirsute. If the redundancy of the penis is dorsal, the skin island is commonly oriented transversely and mobilized on the dorsal dartos fascia, after the techniques described by Duckett[10] and Standoli.[11]

If the redundancy is of the penile skin in general, it is efficient to mobilize the island as a ventral longitudinal island. This island can either be ventrally mobilized on a lateral dartos flap for transposition and inversion into a penile urethral stricture, or vigorously mobilized on the entire ventral dartos fascia and transposed to the area of the perineum requiring proximal pendulous urethral stricture repair. If the redundancy is transversely oriented, a mechanically efficient flap can be mobilized. These islands are frequently oriented across the midline, because the extension of hirsute skin onto the ventrum of the penis often requires the use of transversely oriented islands. Similar to the ventral longitudinal island, they are mobilized on the entire ventral dartos fascia and are easily transposed to the area of the proximal bulbous urethra.

Longer skin islands can be mobilized by orienting the island both ventrally and transversely at the distal extent on the entire ventral fascial blood supply. Known as the "hockey-stick orientation," these islands are useful for reconstructing long segments of the bulbous urethra, with extension out into the proximal pendulous urethra.

An island oriented longitudinally is somewhat limited in length, and 11 to 12 cm is usually the most that can be obtained with this orientation. If there is any redundancy to the penile skin at all, however, the island can be oriented circumferentially ("circular skin island"). A circular skin island is mobilized on the entire penile dartos fascia. This is accomplished by first degloving the skin in the layer superficial to Buck's fascia, then elevating the dartos pedicle by developing the layer between the superficial dartos and the deep plexus of the penile skin. Whereas McAninch and colleagues prefer to divide these islands ventrally, leaving the dorsal pedicle intact,[4] I prefer to divide the pedicle dorsally, leaving the ventrum intact, when it is reliable. I have achieved more mechanical efficiency with transposition when the fascia is split dorsally, and there does not appear to be an advantage to leaving the fascia intact dorsally, because the vessels come onto the fascia in a ventral lateral orientation and begin to arborize almost immediately.

Scrotal skin islands should not be used in preference to penile skin islands, but, when necessary, can be used without hesitancy. Scrotal skin islands are elevated on the tunica dartos of the scrotum. The tunica dartos, unlike the dartos fascia of the penis, has a significant muscular component that can cause the surgeon to mobilize islands that are redundant. In some cases of extremely long stricture disease, scrotal islands can be combined with penile islands in a so-called double-island technique. Using double islands, reconstructions as long as 18 to 20 cm have been accomplished. The double-island technique requires redundancy of penile skin along with redundancy of nonhirsute scrotal skin. With careful consideration of the pedicle in the island design, so that areas of the fascial flap are not inadvertently devascularized, the island can be mobilized either on a unilateral/ipsilateral pedicle or on contralateral pedicles.

There are also situations in which there is limited nonhirsute skin to be mobilized as an island. As an alternative to the use of a split-thickness skin graft, I have investigated the use of epilated midline genital skin islands. The epilations require anesthesia, and because hair grows in crops, it may be necessary to perform multiple epilations. The interval between epilations should be 6 to 8 weeks, and urethral recon-

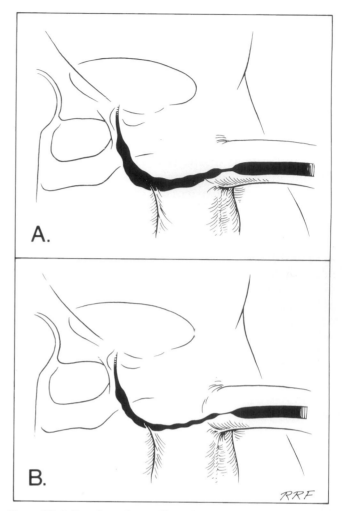

Figure 70–8. Drawings of x-ray films of a 16-year-old boy with severe proximal anterior urethral stricture disease. *A,* Appearance of the urethrogram at the time of discontinuing catheter dilation. *B,* Anterior urethra at the time of reconstruction. Note the totally obstructing segment at the penoscrotal junction with marked stenosis of the proximal urethra once the forces of hydrodilation have been removed.

struction cannot be accomplished until 10 to 12 weeks after the last epilation. Adhering to these tenets, however, one can be assured of placing true nonhirsute skin into the urethra. As with scrotal islands in general, the actual repair involves elevating the scrotal portion on the tunica dartos and meticulously tailoring that portion of the island to avoid redundancy and an iatrogenic diverticulum. I have reserved the application of this procedure to the difficult cases of panurethral stricture disease and have enjoyed gratifying success to date.

Experience with urethral reconstructive surgery has made it clear that onlay procedures yield a higher success rate than tubularized grafts and skin islands. There are situations in which tubularized segments cannot be avoided. However, by combining aggressive mobilization and excision of either the entire stricture or a portion of it, the length of these segments can often be limited.

The case of a teenager with complex bulbous urethral stricture disease who had developed a totally obstructing segment illustrates this principle (Fig. 70–8). A circular skin island was outlined on the penile skin, with careful tailoring of dimensions (Fig. 70–9). The skin island was elevated as described above. The vascular pedicle was divided dorsally and the island transposed to the perineum. A long area of completely obstructed urethra was excised. The vascular pedicle was divided dorsally and the island transposed to the perineum. A long area of completely obstructed urethra was excised. The proximal corpus spongiosum and urethra were then vigorously mobilized, with detachment of the midline fusion of the ischial cavernosus musculature, the corpus spongiosum from the triangle ligament, and the bulbospongiosum from the perineal body. This limited but did not completely avoid the length of the tubu-larized segment. The corpus spongiosum was then spatulated on its dorsal aspect, from the distal aspect to the area of the membranous urethra, and the skin island was laid into the urethrostomy defect with the distal island tubularized. The urethra and corpus spongiosum were returned to their normal path, and a widely ovoid anastomosis was created between the distal limits of the tubularized segment skin island and the normal distal anterior urethra.

Reconstruction of the Fossa Navicularis

Strictures of the fossa navicularis are a particular challenge to the surgeon. Although strictures of other portions of the anterior urethra require careful attention to attain a good functional result, repair of strictures of the fossa must also yield a good cosmetic

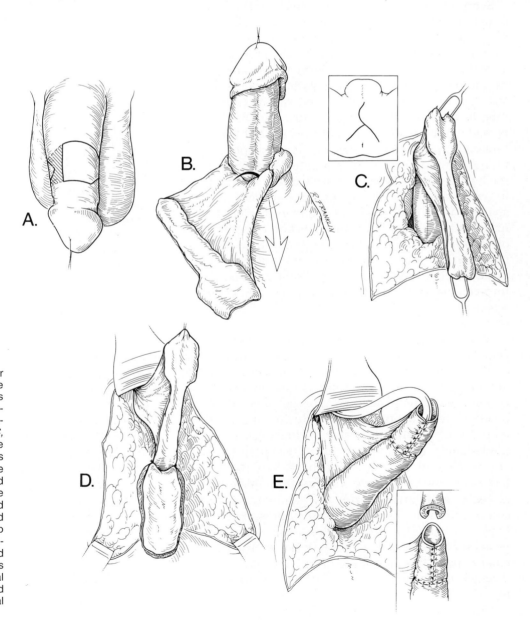

Figure 70–9. Technique of a circular island flap for reconstruction of the bulbous urethra. *A,* The island is marked circumferentially on the penile skin. *B,* The skin island is elevated on the penile dartos fascia. *C,* A lambda incision is created in the perineum, and the skin island is transposed to the perineum. *D,* The corpus spongiosum has been divided at the point of total obstruction. The proximal urethra has been spatulated on the dorsal wall, and the skin island is in the process of being inlaid into that segment. *E,* The skin island onlay is complete; note the tubularized section. The corpus spongiosum is then transposed back to its normal anatomical position with a spatulated anastomosis created to the proximal portion of the distal anterior urethra.

result. Graft repairs have been used with success in select cases of strictures of the fossa navicularis, but, in general, I prefer the use of fascial flap/skin island procedures.[12, 13] Both transversely and longitudinally oriented skin island procedures have been described. Although it is more mechanically efficient to transpose a transversely oriented island to the area of the meatus and fossa navicularis, there are cases in which the island must be oriented longitudinally and the island then advanced into the area of the fossa navicularis and meatus. Relatively large series with both modalities of elevation have been described, with excellent functional and cosmetic results.

PREOPERATIVE AND POSTOPERATIVE MANAGEMENT AND COMPLICATIONS

Every effort is made to undertake urethral reconstruction in the presence of sterile urine. When possible, orally administered antibiotics are used to sterilize the urine. When this is not feasible, the patient is admitted to the hospital for intravenous antibiotics, beginning approximately 12 to 24 hours before reconstruction. In cases in which an indwelling suprapubic tube is in place, sterilizing the urine preoperatively is made much easier if the cultures are not "chased." I maintain patients on a suppressive dose of antibiotics (Macrobid, Procter & Gamble Pharmaceuticals, Inc., 1327 Eaton Avenue, Norwich, NY 13815-1799) in combination with agents to suppress bladder spasms. With this treatment regimen, bacterial colonization will occur, but symptoms and complications of colonization are minimal. For graft repairs, intravenous antibiotics are continued through the fourth postoperative day (graft take). For flap procedures, intravenous antibiotics are continued for 48 hours, when the patient is switched back to a suppressive antibiotic regimen.

When the patient is operated on in the supine, frog-leg, or split-leg positions, Kendall stockings are applied before the administration of anesthesia and left in place until the patient is ambulatory. When patients are to be placed in an exaggerated lithotomy position, Ted stockings are used during the procedure in place of pneumatic Kendall stockings. However, immediately after the procedure, Kendall stockings are applied in all cases. We have had remarkably few occurrences of deep venous thrombosis in our patients, and attribute the low incidence of these complications to the vigorous use of pneumatic stockings. If a patient has any factors that would predispose him to deep venous thrombosis, we use subcuticular heparin, beginning preoperatively and extending through the period of diminished ambulation/bed rest.

The use of the exaggerated lithotomy position is attended by some positioning morbidity. Angermeier and Jordan examined a large series of our patients[14] and determined that 15.8 percent of patients placed in the exaggerated lithotomy position suffered some neuropraxic phenomena. Fortunately, these complications resolve spontaneously and quickly, and patients are not distressed by their occurrence if they have been warned preoperatively. We have not had any complications with compartment syndrome, and we attribute this to the careful positioning measures that we undertake while placing the patient in the exaggerated lithotomy position.

After the procedure the patient is taken to the postanesthesia care unit for recovery, and transferred to the routine surgical floor for his subsequent postoperative course. For single-stage graft techniques, I keep the patient at bed rest for 4 to 5 days. For a meshed split-thickness skin graft repair, the bolster is left in place for 5 to 7 days, and the patient is kept at bed rest throughout that course (in reality, it is difficult to ambulate with the bolster in place). For fascial flaps/skin island procedures, the patient is kept at bed rest for 2 to 3 days, depending on edema, and ambulated and discharged from the hospital shortly thereafter.

Most of our patients remain stented and diverted for 2 days. Although Webster's data suggest that diversion could be shortened, a 21-day healing period has worked well for our patients and we continue to use that interval. For single-stage graft repairs, diversion is usually continued for 28 postoperative days.

The obvious major complication encountered with urethral reconstruction is recurrence of the stricture. Graft and flap loss are fortunately extremely rare today. Also fortunate is the fact that perineal wound infections are quite rare. Flaps obviously tolerate wound infection much better than grafts. The treatment of wound infection is as for wound infections in any other part of the body: drainage, healing by secondary intention or delayed primary closure, and continued diversion. With the use of antibiotics, as described, and suction drains, we have not had a perineal wound infection at this center in over 5 years.

The anatomical approach to urethral reconstruction implies the aggressive application of open urethral reconstructive techniques. The aim of this chapter is not to teach any given procedure, but to provide the concepts and basis for all procedures useful for urethral reconstruction. Adhering to the concepts described, we have enjoyed approximately 90 to 95 percent success, even in the most challenging of cases.

REFERENCES

1. Russell RH. The treatment of urethral stricture disease by excision. Br J Surg 2:375, 1914.

2. Quartey JKM. One stage penile/preputial cutaneous island flap urethroplasty for urethral stricture: A preliminary report. J Urol 129:284, 1983.

3. Webster GD, Koefoot RB, Sihelnik SA. Urethroplasty management in 100 cases of urethral stricture: A rationale for procedure selection. J Urol 134:892, 1985.

4. McAninch JW, Laing FC, Jeffery B. Sonourethography in the evaluation of urethral strictures: A preliminary report. J Urol 139:294, 1988.

5. Gluck CD, Bundy AL, Fine C, et al. Sonographic urethrogram: Comparison to roentgenographic techniques in 22 patients. J Urol 1401:404, 1988.

6. Merkle W, Wagner W. Sonography of the distal male urethra—a new diagnostic procedure for urethral strictures: Results of a retrospective study. J Urol 140:1409, 1988.

7. Devine CJ, Jordan GH. Surgery of anterior urethral strictures. In Marshall FF, ed. Operative Urology. Philadelphia, WB Saunders, 1991, p 307.

8. Schreiter F, Noll F. Meshgraft urethroplasty using split-thickness skin graft or foreskin. J Urol 142:1223, 1989.

9. Humby G. A one stage operation for hypospadias. Br J Surg 29:84, 1941.

10. Duckett JW. The island flap technique for hypospadias repair. Urol Clin North Am 8:503, 1981.

11. Standoli L. One stage repair of hypospadias: Preputial island flap technique. Ann Plast Surg 9:81, 1989.

12. Jordan GH. Reconstruction of the fossa navicularis. J Urol 128:102, 1987.

13. DeSy WA. Aesthetic repair of meatal stricture. J Urol 132:678, 1984.

14. Angermeier KW, Jordan GH. Complications of the exaggerated lithotomy position: A review of 177 cases. J Urol 151:866, 1994.

Chapter 71

Reconstruction of the Membranous Urethral Stricture

George D. Webster

The male urethra may be conveniently divided into four parts that are both anatomically and functionally distinct: the prostatic, membranous, bulbar, and pendulous portions. The management of stricture disease is in large part dictated by the anatomical division affected. Strictures of the membranous urethra, which is also known as the sphincter active or the posterior urethra, are most commonly associated with pelvic fractures. These are usually caused by distraction injuries that tear the urethra partially or completely. Complete tears result in discontinuity of the urethra, which is more correctly termed a distraction defect than a stricture. In fact, approximately 10 percent of pelvic fractures result in membranous urethral disruption; approximately 90 percent of such injuries are caused by motor vehicle accidents and the remainder by falls and crush injuries.[1, 2] In the past, the initial management of these injuries, along with the repair of the urethral distraction defect that often resulted, usually involved multiple procedures and considerable morbidity. Currently, techniques for the repair of urethral distraction defects have evolved so that most may be managed by a one-stage repair usually performed through the perineum alone, provided that proper management was instituted at the time of the initial injury.

EXTENT OF URETHRAL INJURY AFTER PELVIC FRACTURE

In general, injuries to the membranous urethra after pelvic fracture may be categorized as urethral elongation injuries, partial urethral disruptions, or complete urethral disruptions. When the pelvic ring is disrupted, the prostate, being firmly attached to the pubis by the puboprostatic ligaments, is often dislocated from its normal anatomical position, stressing the fascial attachments to the pelvic floor and the urethra. If the degree of distraction is not severe, the membranous urethra may remain in continuity, although the expanding pelvic hematoma may float the vesicoprostatic unit cephalad, elongating and compressing the posterior urethra (Fig. 71–1). This stretching of the membranous urethra may result in intramural fibrosis and therefore functional impairment of the distal intrinsic sphincter mechanism. It usually does not result in a urethral stricture and, assuming that the bladder neck is uninjured, this impairment of the distal sphincter mechanism may be clinically inapparent until a later date when a transurethral resection of the prostate (TURP) ablates the bladder neck mechanism! In approximately one third of all ure-

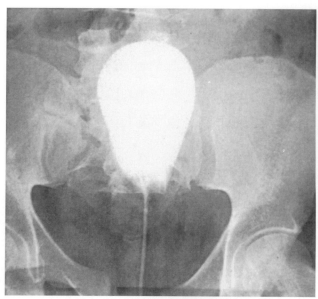

Figure 71–1. Distraction injury of the posterior urethra in pelvic fracture. Elongation of the urethra without rupture has occurred, and the bladder has risen on the pelvic hematoma.

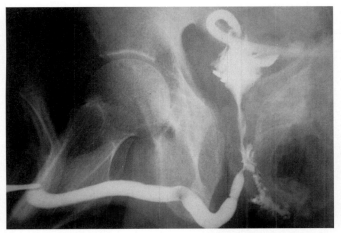

Figure 71–2. Partial urethral tear. Retrograde urethrogram showing urethral continuity but extravasation at the site of membranous urethral injury.

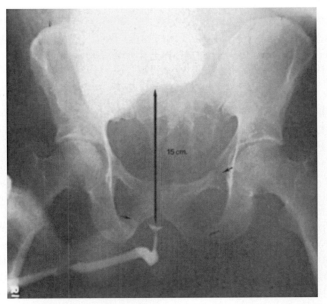

Figure 71–4. Combined urethrogram and cystogram in a patient who had massive urethral separation after pelvic fracture membranous urethral injury. This patient is an appropriate candidate for hematoma evacuation and realignment.

thral injuries after pelvic fracture the urethra is only partially torn, and the potential exists for this injury to heal without stricture or with only a short stricture that may be manageable by either dilation or direct vision internal urethrotomy (Fig. 71–2). It is critical that a partial urethral tear not be converted to a complete tear by attempts at urethral catheterization. In most cases, however, a complete urethral disruption results (Fig. 71–3). The pelvic hematoma that accompanies pelvic fracture usually displaces the prostate and bladder cephalad. However, provided that the displacement is not excessive, with the passage of time and reabsorption/reorganization of the hematoma the prostate will descend to a relatively anatomical position, and a short urethral distraction defect will be the result. In some cases the displacement of the bladder and prostate is massive so that it is futile to anticipate natural descent to an anatomical position (Fig. 71–4). Associated bladder neck and rectal

injury and compound pelvic fractures with massive perineal and integumentary disruption present more complex situations, so the initial management should be different and subsequent repair of the urethral distraction defect is often more complex.[3]

SPHINCTER ANATOMY AND ITS SURGICAL SIGNIFICANCE

The entire posterior urethra from bladder neck to bulbomembranous junction is sphincter active. Under normal circumstances, continence is maintained at the bladder neck, which is normally closed except during periods of detrusor contraction.[4] When this internal or proximal sphincter is compromised, continence may still be maintained by the distal mechanism, which commences at the verumontanum and extends from 3 to 4 cm distally to the bulbomembranous junction. In the past this external sphincter was thought to be part of a urogenital diaphragm external to the membranous urethra. It is now clear that this concept of a urogenital diaphragm is a myth,[5, 6] and that in reality continence at the external sphincter is due entirely to the 3- to 4-mm intramural muscle component rather than any external compressive force. In fact, the only muscle components external to the membranous urethra fuse posteriorly and are incapable of a sustained urethral compression, but are capable of brief volitional contraction to interrupt the urinary stream. When the distal sphincter is destroyed by urethral injury after pelvic fracture, continence becomes completely dependent on the bladder

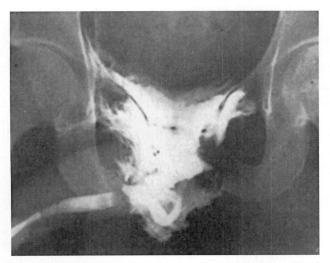

Figure 71–3. Total transection of the urethra. Urethrogram showing extravasation and no urethral continuity.

neck, so every effort must be made to preserve its function. If it is compromised by associated injury or subsequent scarring, its reconstruction may be necessary as a part of the urethroplasty.

MANAGEMENT OF MEMBRANOUS URETHRAL INJURY ASSOCIATED WITH PELVIC FRACTURE

Prostatomembranous urethral injury occurs in approximately 10 percent of patients sustaining pelvic fracture, most being the result of automobile or occupational injury. The magnitude of the initial trauma will determine the amount of prostatovesical displacement on which the degree of urethral injury will depend. In most pelvic fractures the urethra either is not injured or is simply contused and/or elongated with minimal residual sequelae. If urethral disruption does occur, it may be partial or complete, and retrograde urethrography will diagnose the extent. Patients with contusion/elongation injury require a temporary urethral Foley catheter, but those with a partial tear in whom retrograde urethrography will show continuity but some extravasation are best managed by suprapubic cystostomy alone until the urethra heals. Urethral catheterization is injudicious in this scenario, for it may convert a partial into a complete tear.

Management of the patient with total prostatomembranous urethral disruption is controversial. Once the diagnosis is made by retrograde urethrography, excretory urography should also be performed to evaluate the upper tracts and bladder; bladder rupture occurs simultaneously in up to 10 percent of cases. A few cases demand immediate surgical intervention.[7] These include the patient with an associated rectal injury in whom early exploration is needed to evacuate the contaminated hematoma and to perform a colostomy. Urethral realignment over a stenting catheter is appropriate in such cases. Patients in whom both the prostatomembranous urethra and the bladder neck are injured by the fracture should also undergo exploration so that the bladder neck can be debrided and repaired. This is to improve the chance of continence. In most cases, however, the situation is not complicated by these events, and a decision must be made regarding the timing and means of intervention. There are a number of options.

Immediate Urethral Realignment

Advocates of immediate urethral realignment stress the advantage of the immediacy of managing the problem, thereby avoiding the need for prolonged suprapubic catheterization while awaiting secondary repair. In this approach the injury is explored at the time of presentation, the pelvic hematoma being evacuated and the urethra realigned over a stenting catheter using one of a variety of techniques. Unfortunately, conditions are rarely ideal for cautious surgery soon after pelvic fracture, and early exploration often results in catastrophic new bleeding. A historical review by this author of 15 reported series encompassing 301 patients managed in this fashion showed that only 69 percent of them had stricture-free healing of the urethra in any event.[7] Forty of 201 (20 percent) were incontinent and 102 of 252 (40 percent) were impotent. This is in sharp contrast to the results of accumulated series of 236 patients managed by delayed intervention in whom only four (1.7 percent) were incontinent and 26 (11 percent) impotent.

Follis et al recently advocated immediate management, reporting on the outcome of 33 patients with complete prostatomembranous urethral disruptions, 20 of whom were managed by immediate realignment while 13 were managed by initial cystostomy alone and delayed urethroplasty.[8] Potency was totally preserved in 55 percent of the primary realignment group compared with 33 percent of the delayed repair group, and the authors suggest this as an advantage of early intervention. However, injury characteristics in the patients selected for these two forms of management can account for such differences. Patients with more severe injuries tend to be managed by delayed intervention. These authors comment on the morbidity of early intervention and suggest that critically unstable patients are not appropriate candidates for such management. However, the text of this study shows that two of the patients selected for early realignment did require massive blood transfusion, and both required arteriographic embolization of bleeding vessels. This is one of the major complications of such management, and it is not possible to predict preoperatively which patients might develop such life-threatening complications. These authors criticize delayed intervention in view of their own poor success rate with delayed posterior urethroplasty, noting that nine of the 13 required secondary procedures. This does not reflect the customary outcome of posterior urethroplasty as reported in the literature, however, where success rates higher than 90 percent can be achieved.[9] The one certain valid argument for immediate realignment is that fewer patients will develop a stricture requiring urethroplasty. Sixty-five percent of their 33 patients healed without stricture, whereas 100 percent of those managed with suprapubic tube alone with planned delayed elective urethroplasty developed strictures.

Herschorn et al also reported on immediate catheterization, with a concluding comment that careful urethral catheter realignment, either immediately or within 5 weeks of injury, is safe and obviates total urethral closure.[10] Their method of catheterization was retrograde or antegrade, using the linked catheter technique primarily; they comment that 54 percent of patients managed in this fashion subsequently developed a stricture during follow-up and required urethrotomy or dilation, and no patients developed incontinence. These authors also suggest that the rate of impotence was related to the extent of injury rather than to its management. This series is slightly different from the one discussed above in that of the 13 managed by catheterization, eight were catheterized immediately after the injury (two retrograde and six by surgical antegrade transvesical placement), and in five the catheter was placed within a mean of 3 weeks after injury. This "delayed" catheterization might avoid the risk of catastrophic hemorrhage, and this paper does not imply that delayed placement altered the outcome.

Delayed Primary Repair

Delayed primary repair requires that the patient with prostatomembranous urethral disruption from pelvic fracture be managed by suprapubic catheter placement at the time of injury, and that the disruption then be realigned endoscopically over a stenting catheter or repaired surgically at the next opportunity (usually within the first 10 days) when the patient's general condition has stabilized. The advantage of this technique is purported to be that it avoids the high risk of pelvic exploration during the immediate postinjury period.

Mundy reported 17 men with pelvic fracture urethral distraction defect in whom he performed abdominal exploration with pelvic hematoma evacuation and sutured anastomotic repair over a stenting catheter.[11] In 12 cases the site of injury was immediately subprostatic, but he noted that in five the rupture was as much bulbar as membranous urethral; however, in all cases he was able to place six anastomotic sutures. Follow-up was not long at the time of publication, but his personal communication states that thus far no patients have required subsequent urethroplasty and four have needed dilation or urethrotomy. Five of the 13 are potent and none are incontinent.

I have similar unreported experience with delayed primary repair, performed per perineum rather than abdominally. The advantage of the perineal approach is the simplicity of the anastomosis and the lesser operative morbidity as compared with the laparotomy approach. A disadvantage, however, is that many patients cannot be placed in the lithotomy position so soon after pelvic fracture injury.

Cohen et al reported five cases with complete posterior urethral disruption following pelvic fracture managed by endoscopic realignment 7 to 19 days after injury.[12] This was performed using a flexible endoscope passed through a suprapubic tract and a rigid or flexible cystoscope negotiated per urethra. Once a guidewire was negotiated across the injury, a catheter could be guided over the wire and left indwelling for 5 to 10 weeks. These patients performed intermittent self-catheterization for up to 6 months after catheter removal. There was a successful outcome in four; one patient was unable to perform the self-catheterization and ultimately required urethroplasty because of obliteration. Two patients were potent and none were incontinent. One criticism of these authors' technique relates to their use of Foley catheter traction, presumably to facilitate healing at the realigned injury.

SECONDARY REPAIR OF DISTRACTION DEFECT AFTER PELVIC FRACTURE URETHRAL INJURY

The delayed management of membranous urethral injuries falls broadly into two categories: (1) endoscopic procedures, including direct vision internal urethrotomy and urethral dilatation; and (2) open surgical procedures, including anastomotic and substitution urethroplasties. Procedure selection is dictated by the nature of the urethral defect (obliterative or nonobliterative); the length of the defect; the presence of complicating factors, such as urethral cavitation, fistulas, or bladder neck injury; and, to some degree, by the treatment philosophy of the surgeon.

Delayed Endoscopic Management of Posterior Urethral Strictures and Distraction Defects

The role of urethral dilation and direct vision internal urethrotomy has been well established for the treatment of nonobliterative membranous urethral strictures after partial urethral tears. Although these procedures are recommended as first-line therapy, it must be recognized in these cases that few strictures are cured, most requiring long-term dilation management and many needing eventual open urethroplasty. Unfortunately, these procedures may result in worsening of the associated periurethral fibrosis and spongiofibrosis, sometimes making subsequent surgical management more difficult.

More controversial is the use of visual urethrotomy in the management of obliterative membranous urethral defects, better known as "cut to the light" technique. Variations of this technique have been described by both Barry and Marshall and in many

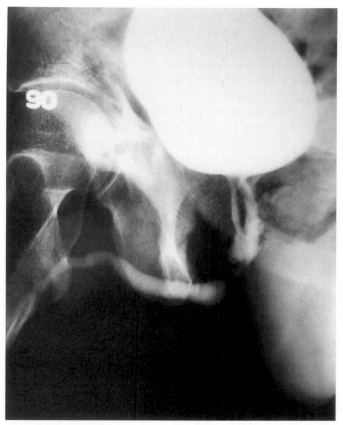

Figure 71–5. Endoscopic ("cut to the light") management of an established pelvic fracture urethral distraction defect has resulted in a false passage that has traversed the bladder neck, ultimately compromising future continence. (From Webster GD, MacDiarmid SA. Posterior urethral strictures. In Webster GD, Kirby R, King LR, Goldwasser B, eds. Reconstructive Urology. Boston, Blackwell Scientific, 1993, p 690.)

other small series.[13, 14] A 1993 report by Spirnak et al presented five patients with distraction defects less than 3 cm in length managed for an average of 4 months after injury.[15] Once urethrotomy had been accomplished through the obliterated segment, a stenting catheter was left in place for 3 to 7 days, and after removal the patient was placed on a 3-month regimen of urethral self-dilation. These authors noted three totally successful outcomes an average of 31 months after treatment, while two who failed to perform self-dilation required repeat urethrotomy. Of the latter two patients, one now has a successful outcome, but the other has required urethroplasty.

Although this procedure, if successful, may spare the patient an open urethroplasty, it may result in a number of complications. False passages may be created that bypass the sphincter (Fig. 71–5), and fistulas may be established between urethra and rectum. At best, if successful, the procedure re-establishes urethral continuity but the channel created lies in dense scar and generally requires long-term dilation, and often eventual surgical urethroplasty.

The role of this technique in the management of

pelvic fracture urethral distraction defects remains to be established by long-term follow-up of larger series of cases. Optimal techniques (radiographical vs. stylet directed vs. endoscopically guided) need to be established, as do patient inclusion criteria for the technique (length of defect) and appropriate timing (from time of injury). It is likely that until these questions are answered the procedure cannot universally replace the surgical management of these defects, and enthusiasm for this nonoperative approach must be tempered with caution.

Delayed Surgical Repair of Pelvic Fracture Urethral Distraction Defects

There is no panacea for the management of posterior urethral distraction defects, but it is these authors' belief that the optimal repair is by a one-stage anastomotic procedure, preferably performed through the perineum alone.[16, 17] This repair has proved remarkably versatile and has been successfully used for distraction defects as long as 7 cm. It is these authors' opinion that only extremely complex strictures will require an abdominoperineal approach or a substitution urethroplasty. In this author's current experience, fewer than 5 percent of cases will be classified as complex because of associated adverse local features affecting repair selection, and these features are noted in Table 71–1. Certainly, those reconstructive urologists dealing primarily with war injuries rather than automobile injuries will note a higher incidence of such complicated cases.

PROGRESSIVE PERINEAL APPROACH FOR REPAIR OF POSTERIOR URETHRAL DISTRACT DEFECTS. I prefer a delay of at least 3 months before embarking on repair. Longer delays have not proved advantageous, and the proposal that the length of the distraction defect reduces with time is not borne out by experience. Combined cystography/retrograde urethrography will have evaluated the complexity and length of the defect, the competence of the bladder neck, and the normality of the anterior urethra, and the antegrade and retrograde cystoscopy are performed to verify the radiographic findings and also

---

TABLE 71–1. Features Associated with Complex Posterior Urethral Strictures

Long urethral defect
Chronic periurethral cavity
Rectal, cutaneous, and periurethral bladder base fistula
Incontinence
Associated anterior urethral stricture
Factors limiting surgical access
History of previous failed repair

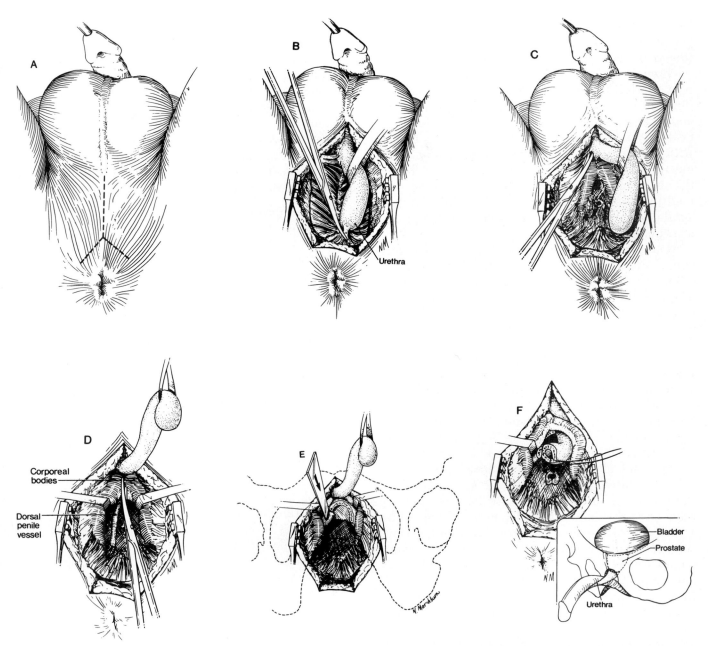

Figure 71–6. Perineal repair of pelvic fracture urethral distraction defects. *A,* A midline perineal incision is bifurcated posteriorly. *B,* After the bulbospongiosus muscle is dissected from the bulbar urethra, it is circumferentially mobilized proximally to the obliterative defect. Incision of the posterior urethral attachments (scissors) facilitates mobilization. *C,* Once transected posteriorly, the urethra is mobilized distally as far as the suspensory ligament of the penis, if necessary. *D,* The penile corporeal bodies are separated, right from left, from the crus distally for 5 to 7 cm. The dorsal penile vessels dorsal to the corpora lie beneath the inferior ramus of the pubis above. *E,* A channel is excised from the inferior ramus of the exposed pubis between the separated corporal bodies using a bone osteotome and/or bone rongeur. *F,* The corporeal body is circumferentially dissected, and the mobilized urethra is rerouted around it and through the resected bony defect. The mobilized bulbar urethra is spatulated dorsally for anastomosis to the posteriorly spatulated prostatomembranous urethra. *Inset,* The supracrurally rerouted urethra is shown traversing the resected inferior bony defect to facilitate bulboprostatic anastomosis. (From Webster GD, MacDiarmid SA. Management of posterior urethral injuries. In Hendry WF, Kirby RF, eds. Recent Advances in Urology. London, Churchill Livingstone, 1993.)

to rule out any bladder stones present as a result of the long-term catheterization.

The patient is placed in the lithotomy position and both abdomen and perineum are prepared in case combined retropubic access is required intraoperatively. Excellent exposure of the posterior urethra can be attained by a midline perineal incision bifurcated posteriorly and by division of the bulbospongiosus

muscle in the midline (Fig. 71–6*A*). The bulbar urethra is then circumferentially mobilized as far proximally as the obliterated segment, where it is transected, and distally to a few centimeters distal to the crura (Fig. 71–6*B*). The anterior urethra is in essence converted to a "urethral flap," depending on collateral retrograde blood supply from the corpora cavernosa and glans. Any previous anterior urethral surgery or strictures and significant hypospadias may jeopardize the blood supply to the flap, precluding this mobilization and dictating an alternative repair.

Through the suprapubic tract, a urethral sound is next carefully negotiated through the prostatic urethra until its tip can be palpated in the perineum, and a vertical incision is then made through the perineal scar onto its tip. Adequate exposure is obtained with a nasal speculum inserted retrogradely into the membranoprostatic urethra, allowing one to spatulate the membranous urethra at 6 o'clock as far proximally as the verumontanum. The bulbar urethra is similarly spatulated to ensure a 40 Fr. bulboprostatic anastomosis.

At this point, it will become apparent whether a simple tension-free anastomosis is possible or whether further lengthening procedures are required. These further maneuvers, which are carried out in a progressive stepwise fashion as the need for further lengthening is required, are as follows[17]:

1. *Further circumferential mobilization to the suspensory ligament.* Careful dissection is required to avoid dissection into the spongy tissue, which could jeopardize the blood supply of the "flap." Mobilization should not proceed beyond the suspensory ligament, to avoid penile chordee (Fig. 71–6C). Up to 3 cm of lengthening can be obtained by this maneuver owing to the elasticity of the healthy bulbar urethra.

2. *Separation of the proximal corporeal bodies.* If the urethra is allowed to course between the separated corporeal bodies rather than over them, at least 1 to 2 cm of apparent urethral lengthening can be achieved. The proximal 4 to 5 cm of the corporeal bodies can be separated by careful sharp dissection along a relatively avascular plane in the midline (Fig. 71–6D). Beyond this point the corporeal bodies are more intimately connected, making further separation too difficult.

3. *Inferior pubectomy.* The above two maneuvers achieve a tension-free anastomosis in approximately 50 percent of cases. A further 1 to 2 cm can be gained by redirecting the urethra through a bony channel excised from the inferior pubic bone using an osteotome and bone rongeur (Fig. 71–6E); this facilitates the anastomosis in an additional 28 percent of cases. In an attempt to preserve the laterally situated neurovascular bundle along the inferior surface of the pubis, bone excision must be limited to the midline.

4. *Rerouting the urethra around the corporeal body.* As a final maneuver, the urethra can be laterally rerouted around the corporeal body and through the tunnel created by the inferior pubectomy (Fig. 71–6F). A tunnel is created in the soft tissue around the corporeal body, taking care to stay away from the corporeal body, and thereby preventing damage to the neurovascular bundle close to its surface. This supracrural rerouting achieves at least a further centimeter of urethral lengthening and is required in about 23 percent of cases. It is difficult to predict preoperatively which patients will require these final two maneuvers, since urethrograms estimate only the length of the distraction defect in one radiographic plane and give little information about associated spongiofibrosis and urethral elasticity. Subsequent transurethral instrumentation or insertion of a penile prosthesis has not been adversely affected by the new course of the urethra.

The Anastomosis. A long nasal speculum is inserted retrogradely into the prostatic urethra, and under direct vision a mucosa-to-mucosa bulboprostatic anastomosis is performed using interrupted 3-0 polyglycolic acid sutures. The verumontanum is an important landmark and identification of the prostatic urethral mucosa is of utmost importance. With needles bent into a J shape (Fig. 71–7), each suture is inserted before being individually tied. The needles are advanced through the prostatic urethral edge from outside to inside, the point of the needle being retrieved within the prostatic urethra and advanced until clear, and then removed. Approximately eight sutures are inserted, starting at the 12 o'clock position and proceeding clockwise before being tied individually in the same order as they were inserted.

A 16 Fr. fenestrated silicone catheter is inserted after the anastomosis is complete along with a suprapubic cystostomy tube. A periurethral Jackson-Pratt drain is inserted for wound drainage and in most cases is removed on the third postoperative day.

Urethral stenting with an indwelling Foley catheter is required for approximately 2 to 3 weeks and is removed only after a retrograde urethrogram around the catheter has proved no extravasation. The suprapubic catheter is usually removed on the same day after a successful trial of voiding. I routinely repeat the retrograde urethrogram 3 and 12 months postoperatively.

Results. The author has recently updated his originally reported experience (74 cases) using this technique in 113 cases of pelvic fracture distraction defects. Patients' ages ranged from 9 to 69 years (mean 36 years) and the causes of injury were automobile related in 71 and occupational in 42. Defects ranged from 1.5 to 7 cm (only three cases were strictures) and a successful, stricture-free outcome was achieved in 110 cases. The maneuvers used to facilitate the tension-free anastomosis are shown in Table 71–2. Complications were uncommon and included temporary peroneal nerve dysfunction in four and persistent incontinence due to preexisting bladder neck dysfunction in two. These were managed successfully by artificial urinary sphincter implantation (cuff around bladder neck).

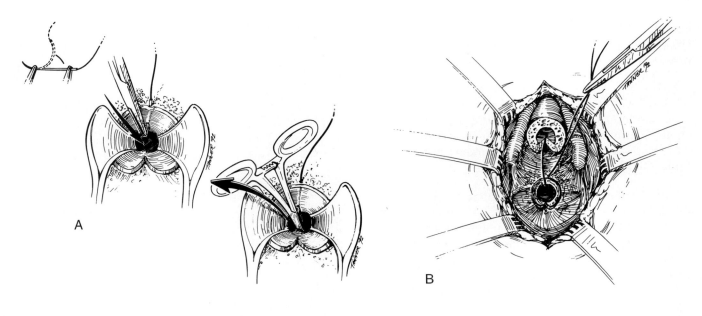

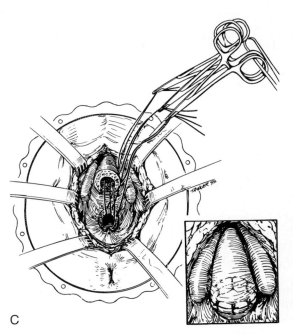

Figure 71–7. *A,* Bulboprostatic anastomosis is facilitated by use of a standard suture needle bent into a J shape. The needle is advanced through the prostatic urethral edge, and the needle tip is retrieved in the prostatic lumen. The needle is advanced through the bladder neck to clear the needle and then withdrawn. *B,* Suture placement is begun with the 12 o'clock suture in the prostatic urethra. *C,* Sequential sutures are then placed in a clockwise direction around the prostatic urethral opening but are not tied. Hemostats placed on the end of each suture are stacked sequentially on an Allis clamp. After approximately eight sutures have been placed, they are individually tied, starting with the 12 o'clock suture and proceeding clockwise. A catheter is inserted after suture placement and tying. (From Webster GD, MacDiarmid SA. Management of posterior urethral injuries. In Hendry WF, Kirby RF, eds. Recent Advances in Urology. London, Churchill Livingstone, 1993.)

Mark et al have recently looked at the potency status of this group of patients.[18] Of 92 patients in whom follow-up data could be obtained, it was noted that 57 patients (62 percent) remained potent in the long term with a median follow-up of 48 months and that, importantly, the operation did not render impotent any patient who was preoperatively potent. Self-injection with vasoactive agents was successful in 24 of 27 impotent patients (89 percent), suggesting a predominant neurological etiology. Of 30 patients in whom original postinjury radiographs could be examined, it was possible to correlate the pattern of bony injury with incidence of impotence, and it was found that bilateral pubic rami fractures correlated with impotence: 13 of 15 were impotent, whereas 11 of 15 with unilateral fractures or no fractures remained potent! Disruption of the cavernous nerves

TABLE 71–2. Maneuvers to Facilitate Anastomosis

Urethral mobilization	9 (8%)
Corporeal separation	46 (41%)
Inferior pubectomy	31 (28%)
Supracorporeal rerouting	26 (23%)
	113 (100%)

lateral to the prostatomembranous urethra behind the symphysis pubis is the most likely cause of impotence in this injury.

FACTORS MILITATING AGAINST PERINEAL ANASTOMOTIC REPAIR. As noted earlier, a number of uncommon complicating factors may render this repair inappropriate, but in our recent experience they account for fewer than 5 percent of cases (see Table 71–1).

Long Urethral Defect. This situation may be avoidable by early intervention after the initial pelvic fracture in patients with massive pelvic hematoma and resultant "pie-in-the-sky" bladder. The perineal approach, employing all the tension-relieving maneuvers, has been used to successfully repair 7-cm long defects, and in such cases good positioning and lighting are important. The tubed perineoscrotal flap procedure or a tubed full-circumference substitution urethroplasty has been suggested for such cases, but these give suboptimal results.

Chronic Periurethral Cavity. In some cases the pelvic hematoma liquefies and evacuates through the urethra, leaving cavities within the pelvic floor that become epithelialized and ultimately may be a source of chronic infection and stone formation. These epithelialized pelvic floor diverticula may become infected and discharge into the rectum, creating fistulas, or result in osteomyelitis. When identified, they suggest the need for an abdominoperineal repair so that the pelvis can be "cleaned out" and omentum brought into the pelvis to facilitate absorption and healing.

Rectal, Cutaneous, and Periurethral Bladder Base Fistulas. These may occur from the injury itself, from the above complication of pelvic floor abscess, or from inept urethral instrumentation, particularly at the time of "cut-to-the-light" endoscopic urethroplasty. They do not necessarily preclude an anastomotic repair.

Incontinence. As noted earlier, after pelvic fracture injury and particularly after the urethroplasty, continence resides in the bladder neck mechanism. Any previous bladder neck surgery or injury may be predictive of incontinence after repair. However, in my experience mild incompetence of the bladder neck does not necessarily translate into postoperative incontinence, and for this reason, I hesitate to perform bladder neck reconstruction at the time of the urethroplasty. Individualized management is needed in such cases; in some patients simultaneous or staged bladder neck reconstruction may suffice, and in others an artificial urinary sphincter has been implanted as a secondary procedure (Fig. 71–8).

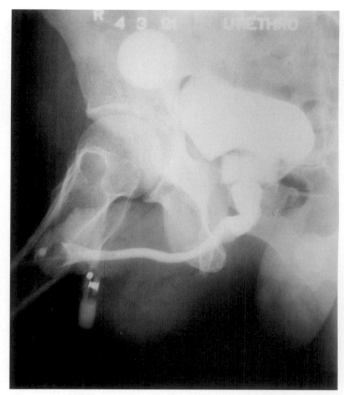

Figure 71–8. Patient with a bladder neck artificial urinary sphincter secondarily implanted to achieve continence after successful four-step perineal urethroplasty for pelvic fracture injury in the face of an incompetent bladder neck. (From Webster GD, MacDiarmid SA. Posterior urethral strictures. In Webster GD, Kirby R, King LR, Goldwasser B, eds. Reconstructive Urology. Boston, Blackwell Scientific, 1993, p 696.)

Associated Anterior Urethral Stricture. This may complicate the repair because of inability to achieve the lithotomy position to obtain exposure. Such a stricture does not necessarily preclude a perineal approach, but it may dictate that the urethra be circumferentially mobilized perineally and the anastomosis performed abdominally.

History of Failed Repair. Once an earlier repair has failed, the subsequent salvage procedure has a number of additional problems to contend with, not the least of which is the fixation of the bulbar urethra in the perineal scar. Surprisingly, however, anastomotic repairs as described above are still possible in most cases. If these are not possible, however, a one-stage substitution urethroplasty using a pedicled island of skin mobilized from the penis on its subcutaneous vascular pedicle, or a staged scrotourethral inlay-type procedure, may be necessary.

COMBINED ABDOMINOPERINEAL TRANSPUBIC APPROACH FOR MORE COMPLEX INJURIES. Some of the features mentioned above indicate a need for this repair, the chief of which are fistulous tracts, inability to achieve the lithotomy position, and pelvic floor cavities. Bladder neck incompetence, as noted above, is not in itself an indication for abdominoperineal repair, and I prefer to defer its management to a secondary procedure unless an abdominal approach is indicated for other reasons.

If required, a lower midline abdominal incision is made after the perineal dissection of the anterior urethra has been completed as previously described. The bulbar urethra transected at the level of the obliteration and the corporeal bodies separated and, if needed, a small wedge inferior pubectomy performed. The prevesical and retropubic spaces are carefully dissected down to the level of the apex of the prostate, staying close to the periosteum of the retropubis until communication with the perineal dissection is made. To avoid injury to the bladder neck, it is wise to open the bladder high on its anterior wall so that an intravesical finger can help direct the retropubic dissection. It is rarely necessary to excise the entire anterior wedge of pubis, as previously described by Waterhouse et al[19]; equally good access is achieved by partial removal of the posterior surface of the pubis using a Capener gouge.[20] The inferior wedge pubectomy will have been completed through the perineum and the intrapelvic dissection will communicate with the perineum at this location in front of the prostate. This wide anterior access facilitates the anastomosis to the spatulated prostatic urethra, and the retropubic bone removal improves access to the pelvic floor to deal with the complicating features, which, as previously discussed, are the indication for this approach. Most important is that the omental wrap be fashioned into a pedicle and placed around the anastomosis and bladder neck, filling the space resulting from bony excision.

SUBSTITUTION URETHROPLASTY. This approach was the preferred technique of many surgeons, particularly after Morehouse et al reported good outcomes in 1972.[21] Now, these repairs should be used only when there is associated anterior urethral stricture disease compromising the retrograde urethral blood flow, or in the rare situation when the distraction defect is too long (over 7 cm) for primary anastomosis. Substitution procedures may be performed in one or two stages. The one-stage repairs include pedicle skin island and free full-thickness skin graft repairs; two-stage procedures include a variety of scrotourethral inlay operations sometimes combined with full-thickness or meshed split-thickness skin graft inlay. The complexities of the individual situation will dictate which repair is most appropriate, but tubed full-thickness skin grafts generally do poorly in pelvic fracture cases because of the lack of a well-vascularized bed for the free graft, and one should always strive to complete the repair in one stage.

Summary

This discussion indicates that patients may be managed endoscopically or by open surgery, either immediately after injury, by delayed primary repair, or by secondary repair some months later. The appropriateness of each of these options is controversial. My opinion is that immediate exploration at the time of injury carries too great a morbidity to be justified and should be reserved for cases demanding pelvic exploration because of associated rectal injury or bladder injury involving the bladder neck. Gentle trial catheterization is justifiable, recognizing the fact that it is generally successful only if the tear is partial. In this event, stricture-free healing can be anticipated in a small number of cases, although most will require intermittent dilation or urethrotomy. Delayed primary repair would seem to embrace the advantages of early resolution of the problem while avoiding the morbidity of immediate surgery. The results reported in the literature indicate that early surgical repair by anastomosis carries a high success rate. Endoscopic delayed primary management has been reported only in small series, but the results have been acceptable, justifying continued interest. Secondary repair by perineal anastomotic urethroplasty 3 months or more after the injury (at which time a suprapubic tube is placed) is indicated for those who are inappropriate candidates for or who fail the above techniques. This is certainly the best approach for the patient who is hemodynamically unstable at the time of injury or who has other major visceral or integumentary injuries, for the patient whose early management was in a peripheral hospital setting, or in situations when the managing surgeon has little experience with urethral injury. This latter technique has improved the outcome very substantially in patients with pelvic fracture urethral distraction defect, and is probably still the optimal approach except in carefully selected patients in the hands of surgeons experienced in the management of urethral injuries.

Editorial Comment

Fray F. Marshall

This chapter provides an excellent comprehensive approach to traumatic urethral obliteration. As outlined, this step-by-step approach should allow for excellent management of these potentially difficult injuries. Although we have described the use of endoscopic reconstruction of urethral transections, not all patients are candidates for endoscopic reconstruction. In addition, multiple procedures are typically required for these endoscopic cases. This approach allows a single operation to fix the problem.

REFERENCES

1. Glass RE, Flynn JT, King JB, Blandy JP. Urethral injury and fractured pelvis. Br J Urol 50:578, 1978.
2. Cass AS, Godee CJ. Urethral injury due to external trauma. Urology 11:607, 1978.
3. Turner-Warwick R. Complex traumatic posterior urethral strictures. J Urol 118:564, 1977.

4. Turner-Warwick R. Clinical urodynamics. Urol Clin North Am 13:30, 1979.

5. Turner-Warwick R. Urethral stricture surgery. In Current Operative Surgery: Urology. London, Bailliere Tindall, 1988, p 160.

6. Chilton C. The distal urethral sphincter mechanism and the pelvic floor. In Mundy AR, Stephenson TP, Weir AJ, eds. Urodynamics: Principles, Practice and Application. Edinburgh, Churchill Livingstone, 1984, p 9.

7. Webster GD, Mathes G, Selli C. Prostatomembranous urethral injuries: A review of the literature and a rational approach to their management. J Urol 130:898, 1983.

8. Follis WH, Koch MO, McDougal WS. Immediate management of prostatomembranous urethral disruptions. J Urol 147:1259, 1992.

9. Webster GD, Ramon J. Repair of pelvic fracture posterior urethral defects using elaborated perineal approach: Experience with 74 cases. J Urol 145:744, 1991.

10. Herschorn S, Thijssen A, Radomski SB. The value of immediate or early catheterization of the traumatized posterior urethra. J Urol 148:70, 1992.

11. Mundy AR. The role of delayed primary repair in the acute management of pelvic fracture injuries of the urethra. Br J Urol 68:273, 1991.

12. Cohen JK, Berg G, Carl GH, Diamond DD. Primary endoscopic realignment following posterior urethral disruption. J Urol 146:1548, 1991.

13. Barry JM. Visual urethrotomy in the management of the obliterated membranous urethra. Urol Clin North Am 16:2, 1989.

14. Marshall FF. Endoscopic reconstruction of traumatic urethral transections. Urol Clin North Am 16:313, 1989.

15. Spirnak JP, Smith EM, Elder JS. Posterior urethral obliteration treated by endoscopic reconstitution, internal urethrotomy and temporary self-dilation. J Urol 149:766, 1993.

16. Webster GD, Sihelnik S. The management of strictures of the membranous urethra. J Urol 134:469, 1985.

17. Webster GD. Perineal repair of membranous urethral stricture. Urol Clin North Am 16:303, 1989.

18. Mark SD, Keane TE, Vandemark RM, Webster GD. Impotence following pelvic fracture urethral injury: Incidence, etiology and management. Br J Urol 75:62, 1995.

19. Waterhouse K, Abrahams JI, Gruber H, et al. The transpubic approach to the lower urinary tract. J Urol 109:486, 1973.

20. Turner-Warwick R. Complex traumatic posterior urethral strictures. J Urol 118:564, 1977.

21. Morehouse DD, Belitsky P, MacKinnon K. Rupture of the posterior urethra. J Urol 107:255, 1972.

Chapter 72

Urethral Fistula and Diverticula

Kenneth A. Kropp

It is convenient to discuss the surgical treatment of urethral diverticula and fistula together because the principles and techniques are similar. In this chapter principles are discussed in the text. Details of the surgical techniques are elaborated in the legend accompanying each figure.

Female Urethral Diverticulum

INDICATIONS

The chance of finding a urethral diverticulum in a woman is directly related to the urologist's awareness of and effort to diagnose this entity. The classic symptoms are the "three Ds": dysuria, dyspareunia, and dribbling. They are present, according to most published series, in 30 to 90 percent of these patients. An exception to these findings is a series of 37 patients reported by Leach and Bavendam.[1] In this series, the three most common symptoms were stress incontinence (51 percent), recurrent infections (40 percent), and urgency incontinence (35 percent). This change most likely reflects greater thoroughness in their evaluation of women with lower urinary tract complaints.

PREOPERATIVE EVALUATION

The physical examination usually reveals a bulging suburethral mass, which may produce a generous urethral discharge when the urethra is stripped. Radiographical confirmation is generally obtained from an intravenous pyelogram (IVP). One should request either a postvoid film to include the bladder neck-urethral area or a standing voiding cystourethrogram (VCUG) to evaluate urethral hypermobility and an incompetent bladder neck. If not demonstrated, a positive-pressure or double-balloon urethrogram is necessary. Transvaginal ultrasonography using a 7-mHz sagittal probe should also be helpful in confirming the size and extent of the diverticulum. At urethroscopy the location of the orifice of the diverticulum can usually be demonstrated by various techniques and provides essential information in planning surgical correction. Urodynamic and other tests can then be done if irritable bladder or incontinence symptoms are present.

Surgical correction begins with appropriate preoperative antibiotics based on urine and urethral discharge culture and sensitivity results. Although "excess" tissue is observed as a result of pressure expansion by the diverticulum, this tissue is abnormal because of associated inflammation. This tissue represents thinned out urethra and periurethral supporting structures and, to a lesser extent, thinned out anterior vaginal wall. The surgeon must be aware of this factor as the surgical plan is developed.

Leach has proposed a classification system for female urethral diverticula (Table 72–1).[2] The system is based on accurate assessment of the diverticulum by physical examination, VCUG, and cystourethroscopy. Adoption of this system should aid the surgeon in planning therapy and allowing valid comparisons of various therapies and postoperative complications between various reported series.

OPERATIVE TECHNIQUE

The two basic types of open surgical correction of female diverticula are vaginal marsupialization and excision. The marsupialization technique of Spence

TABLE 72–1. Classification of Diverticula Using the L/N/ S/C3 System

L	=	Location—i.e., distal, middle, proximal with or without extension beneath the bladder neck.
N	=	Number—whether single or multiple.
S	=	Size—expressed in centimeters (two dimensional).
C3	=	Configuration, Communication, Continence
		Configuration (C1)—single, multiloculated, or saddle shaped.
		Communication (C2)—communication site with the urethral lumen.
		Continence (C3)—is genuine stress incontinence present?

and Duckett[3] is shown in Figure 72–1. This technique is best suited for the more distal diverticulum and involves midline incision of the urethra, urethrovaginal septum, and vagina back to the opening of the diverticulum. The long-term results of this technique have been reviewed by Roehrborn.[4] Downs[5] reported on a technique of marsupialization of the diverticular patch by excision of the anterior vaginal wall (Fig. 72–2).

Excision techniques are generally more difficult but also more appealing because they remove the pathological entity and reconstruct the normal anatomy. Several surgical approaches are available for transvaginal excision. Figure 72–3 illustrates a technique of raising laterally based vaginal flaps following a midline incision through the anterior vaginal wall over the diverticulum. A second layer of pubocervical fascia is developed before beginning the dissection of the diverticular sac. After the communication of the diverticulum with the urethra has been identified and excised, the urethral defect is closed, followed by closure of the pubocervical fascia and laterally based vaginal flaps. The vaginal flaps can be trimmed asymmetrically to avoid overlapping suture lines.

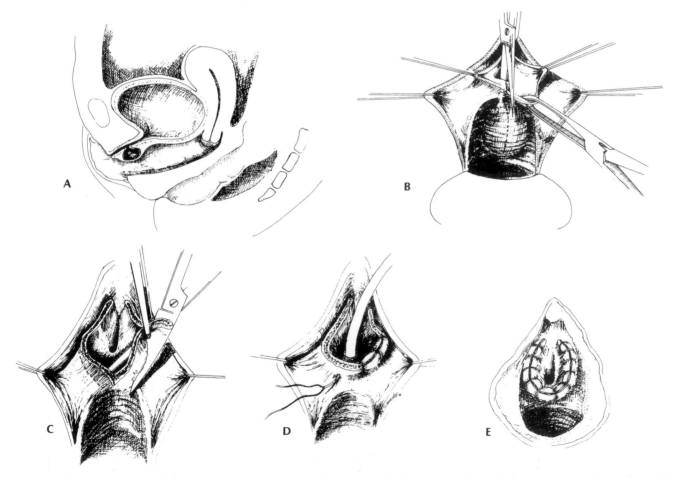

Figure 72–1. Marsupialization technique of Spence and Duckett: lithotomy position. Special requirements include traction sutures on the labia majora and minora opposite the urethral meatus, a weighted vaginal retractor, and a cystourethroscope for identification of the diverticular opening and placement of an identifying ureteral catheter. *A,* The urethral diverticulum is shown in coronal section. Note the communication with the urethra in the middle or distal urethra. *B,* Traction sutures are placed on either side of the urethral meatus. An incision is made from the urethral meatus back into the diverticulum, incising the urethra, the urethrovaginal septum, and the anterior vaginal wall. This incision can be made with the Bovie needle electrode, scalpel, or scissors as shown. *C,* The redundant vaginal mucosa and the floor and side walls of the diverticulum are excised. *D,* The vaginal mucosa is sutured to the urethral mucosa, creating a generous meatotomy. *E,* Closure is completed. (From Kropp KA. Urethral fistula and diverticula. In Glenn JF, ed. Urologic Surgery, 3rd ed. Philadelphia, JB Lippincott, 1983, p 729.)

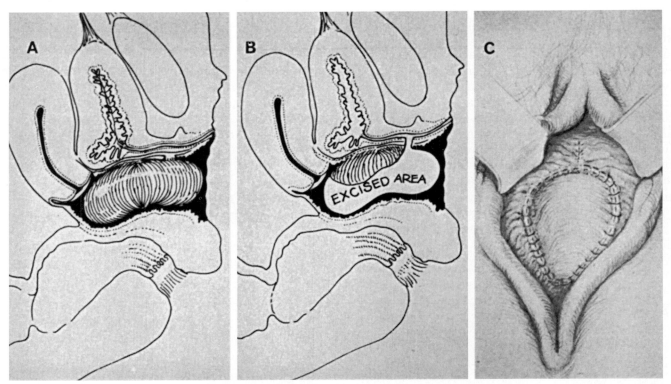

Figure 72–2. Marsupialization—saucerization technique of Downs: lithotomy position. Special requirements include traction sutures on the labia majora and minora opposite the urethral meatus and weighted posterior vaginal retractor; a coagulum for filling the diverticulum: and punch cystotomy. *A,* After a longitudinal vaginal incision over the diverticulum, the distal and lateral diverticular sac is dissected from the surrounding tissues. The opening into the urethra is identified and amputated. The urethra is closed. *B,* No attempt is made to separate the proximal diverticular sac from the bladder neck area. The dissected-free wall and a portion of the vaginal wall are excised. *C,* The vaginal mucosa is sutured proximally to the excised edges of the diverticular sac, and the distal vaginal mucosa is reapproximated. (From Downs R.A. Urethral diverticula in females. Urology 29:201, 1987.)

Figure 72–3. Excision of a female urethral diverticulum: lithotomy position. Special requirements include traction sutures on the labia majora and minora opposite the urethral meatus, a weighted posterior vaginal retractor, a coagulum for filling the diverticulum, a Foley catheter for tamponade of the bladder neck, a pursestring suture around the catheter at the meatus, and punch cystotomy. *A,* The diverticulum in coronal section. *B,* A midline vaginal incision has been made over the diverticulum. *C,* Laterally based vaginal and pubocervical fascial flaps are developed. The diverticulum is dissected completely to its entrance into the urethra and amputated. The urethral mucosa is closed. *D,* The periurethral fascia is reapproximated under the urethral repair. *E,* The excess vaginal mucosal flaps are trimmed equally and resutured. Alternatively, the excess vaginal mucosa can be removed on one side only, which avoids overlying suture lines. (From Kropp KA. Urethral fistula and diverticula. In Glenn JF, ed. Urologic Surgery, 3rd ed. Philadelphia, JB Lippincott, 1983, p 727.)

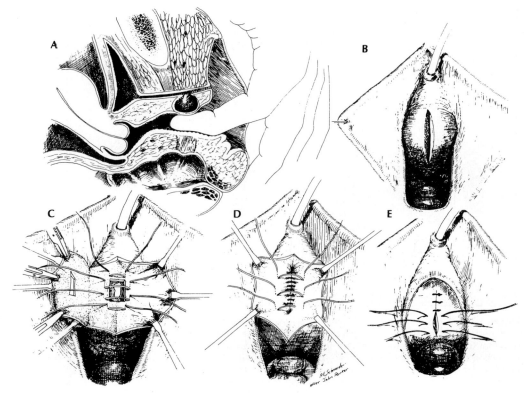

Figure 72–4 demonstrates another vaginal flap technique first described by Sholem and colleagues[6] and refined by Leach and colleagues.[7] In this technique, a proximally based U-shaped vaginal flap is developed fully to expose the extent of the diverticulum. Pubocervical fascial flaps are developed from the midpoint of the diverticulum proximally and distally. After the diverticular sac and urethral communication are excised, the urethral defect is closed longitudinally, the pubocervical fascia closed transversely, and the trimmed U-shaped vaginal flap resutured.

In the aforementioned excision techniques, it is helpful to fill the diverticulum with a coagulum to aid in completing the dissection before entering the diverticulum. Figure 72–5 shows a technique de-scribed by Moore[8] of deliberately entering the diverticulum initially by a transvaginal stab wound through which a Foley or Fogarty catheter is placed. The balloon is inflated in the expectation that it will completely fill the diverticulum and aid in the dissection.

Excision of a large, complex-shaped, proximal diverticulum can create a large defect with little adequate supporting tissue. In these instances a Martius bulbocavernosus fat pad graft[9] can be transferred into the area to further support the repair (Fig. 72–6).

POSTOPERATIVE MANAGEMENT AND COMPLICATIONS

In all of these described excisional techniques, a peridiverticular reaction (inflammation and fibrosis)

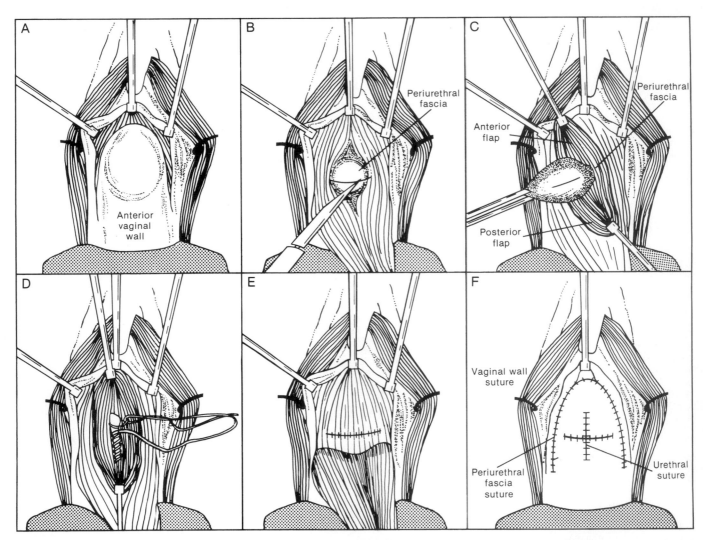

Figure 72–4. Excision of a female urethral diverticulum: lithotomy position. Special requirements include labial traction sutures, a weighted posterior vaginal retractor, a coagulum, a Foley catheter, and punch cystotomy. *A,* Inverted U-shaped incision with the apex of the U just proximal to the urethral meatus, and the limbs of the U carried proximally over the diverticulum. The vaginal flap is raised, keeping the dissection directly onto the vaginal flap. *B,* The pubocervical fascia is incised transversely and dissected off the diverticular sac. *C,* Complete mobilization of this fascia into proximal and distal flaps that completely exposes the diverticulum. *D,* The communication with the urethra is identified and amputated and the urethral defect closed with absorbable sutures. *E,* The proximal and distal flaps of pubocervical fascia are closed transversely. *F,* The vaginal flap is trimmed, if necessary, and resutured. (From Leach GE, Bavendam TG. Female urethral diverticula. Urology 30:407, 1987.)

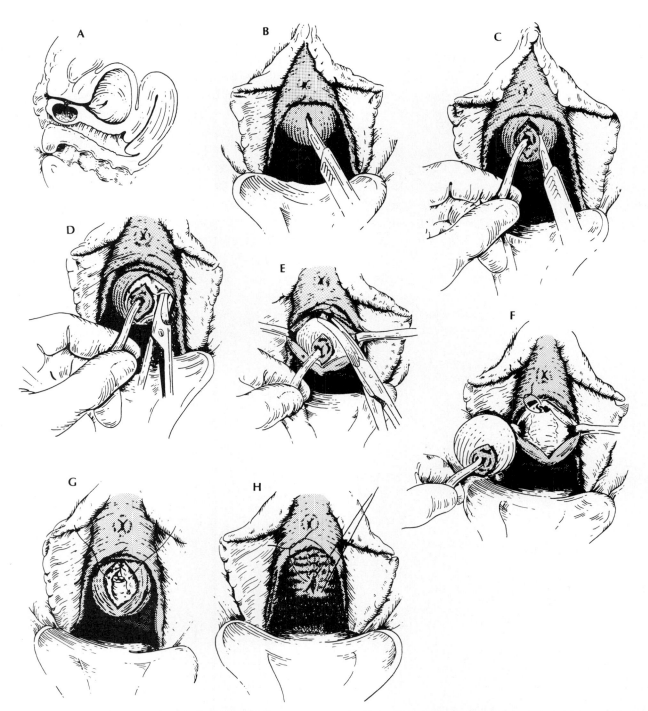

Figure 72–5. Excision of female urethral diverticulum (Moore technique): lithotomy position. Special requirements include labial traction sutures opposite the urethral meatus, a weighted posterior vaginal retractor, a 8 Fr. urethral Foley balloon catheter, suprapubic cystotomy, and a coagulum. *A,* Coronal section of the diverticulum. *B,* The anterior vaginal wall is exposed and a stab wound made into the diverticulum with either the needle-tip Bovie or scalpel as shown. Insert the 8 Fr. Foley catheter with the tip cut off and inflate the balloon to fill the diverticulum. *C,* Place a pursestring suture around the catheter. Incise the vaginal mucosa elliptically. Place a urethral catheter (not shown). *D,* Dissect against the wall of the diverticulum with curved scissors, moving the catheter from side to side to reach the neck of the diverticulum. *E,* Amputate the neck of the diverticulum transversely upon the urethra. *F,* Close the urethra transversely. *G,* Reapproximate the cervicovaginal fascia under the urethra. *H,* Close the vaginal mucosa. (From Kropp KA. The female urethra. In Glenn JF, ed. Urologic Surgery, 2nd ed. Hagerstown, Harper & Row, 1975, p 758.)

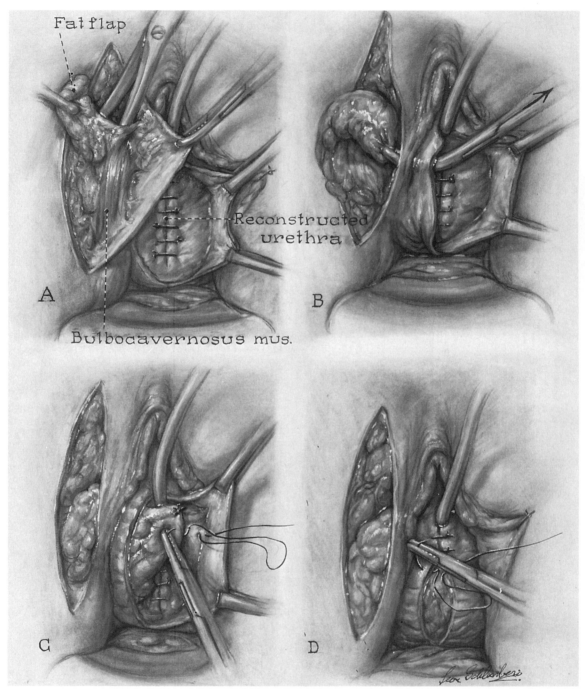

Figure 72–6. A Martius bulbocavernosus fat pad graft for urethrovaginal or vesicovaginal fistula repair. *A,* The lateral margin of the labia majora is opened by a vertical incision and the fat pad adjacent to the bulbocavernosus muscle is mobilized, leaving a broad pedicle attached at the inferior pole. *B* and *C,* The fat pad is drawn through a tunnel beneath the labia minora and vaginal mucosa and sutured with 3–0 delayed-absorbable sutures to the fascia of the urethra and bladder. *D,* The vaginal mucosa is mobilized widely to permit closure in the midline. The vulvar incision is closed with interrupted 3–0 delayed-absorbable sutures and drained if necessary. (From Thompson JD. Vesicovaginal fistula. In Thompson JD, Rock JA, eds. Te Linde's Operative Gynecology, 7th ed. Philadelphia, JB Lippincott, 1992, p 815.)

may make the operation more difficult than the surgeon may anticipate. Therefore, timing of the procedure is important and should not be attempted until acute inflammation and urinary infection have been controlled with appropriate antibiotics. Urinary diversion can be accomplished with a urethral Foley catheter, a suprapubic tube, or both. Patients should be given anticholinergics to prevent bladder spasms and premature urination across the repair. Antibiotic or povidone-iodine (Betadine)-soaked vaginal packing helps support the repairs and decreases edema and hematoma formation. All these measures help reduce the incidence of postoperative infection and fistula formation.

Urinary incontinence after diverticulectomy, although a rarely reported complication, is probably more common than recorded. Postoperative proximal urethral-bladder neck fistulas may account for some cases of incontinence. Minor degrees of preoperative stress incontinence may not be recorded by the surgeon and may become worse after surgical excision. The filled urethral diverticulum may actually prevent incontinence, such as periurethral polytetrafluoroethylene (Teflon) does when used for treating incontinence. Periurethral diverticular infection may destroy or weaken normal urethral supporting tissues.

We are indebted to the work of Reid and associates[10] and Leach and Bavendam[1] for pointing out the importance of thorough preoperative evaluation, including urodynamics, and the feasibility of simultaneous urethral suspension procedures at the time of diverticulectomy.

Urethrovaginal Fistula

INDICATIONS

Urethrovaginal fistula is an acquired lesion secondary to surgical or obstetrical trauma or periurethral abscess with fistula formation. Seldom are middle and distal urethral fistulas associated with complaints related to urination or infection. A proximal urethral-bladder neck fistula is a major problem because it is frequently associated with total incontinence. The repair of these bladder neck fistulas is discussed under repair of the bladder neck and vesicovaginal fistula.

OPERATIVE TECHNIQUE

Figure 72–7 demonstrates the repair of a small urethrovaginal fistula and includes excision of the fistulous tract and three-layer closure. An alternative to this technique, which avoids overlapping suture lines, is to develop an eccentric vaginal flap that is advanced into the defect.

Although large vesicovaginal fistulas are uncommon, their repair basically incorporates the principles of a second-stage urethroplasty. The large segment of ventral urethral wall that is missing can be closed with a Thiersch tube technique, utilizing vaginal mucosa. This type of repair needs to be reinforced with additional tissue, which can be one of the bulbocavernosus muscles freed from the labia majora and transferred medially. Usually vaginal wall tissue is sufficient and can be mobilized laterally to be comfortably sutured in the midline. The steps in this repair are shown in Figure 72–8. Wang and Hadley[11] recently demonstrated the use of rotated vascularized Martius, labial, and buttock flaps for the repair of complex radiation and artificial sphincter erosion fistulas. These are well illustrated in this article. The principles of urinary diversion and avoidance of premature voiding are the same as those outlined for urethral diverticular surgery.

Male Urethral Diverticulum

INDICATIONS

Urethral diverticula in men are frequently seen in association with distal urethral stricture disease. The diverticulum forms when a periurethral abscess drains back into the urethra rather than out to the skin. An exception is the diverticula seen in paraplegics and quadriplegics with indwelling urethral Foley catheters. Surgical correction can follow or can be done simultaneously with surgical correction of the distal stricture.

OPERATIVE TECHNIQUE

Urinary infection and peridiverticular inflammation should be controlled with antibiotics, urinary

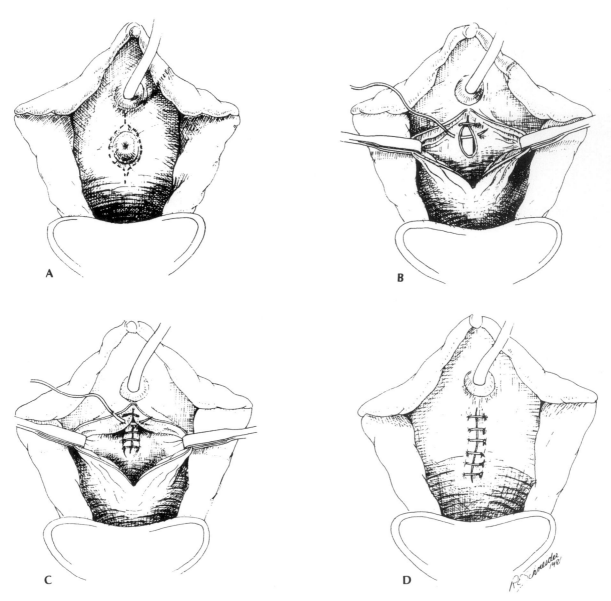

Figure 72–7. Repair of a urethrovaginal fistula: lithotomy position. Special requirements include labial traction sutures, a weighted posterior vaginal retractor, suprapubic punch cystotomy tubes, and a urethral Foley catheter. *A,* At the midline an elliptical incision is made around the fistula. *B,* The pubocervical fascia is developed laterally and the urethra closed. *C,* The pubocervical fascia is reapproximated in the midline. *D,* The vaginal mucosa is closed. (From Kropp KA. Urethral fistula and diverticula. In Glenn JF, ed. Urologic Surgery, 3rd ed. Philadelphia, JB Lippincott, 1983, p 734.)

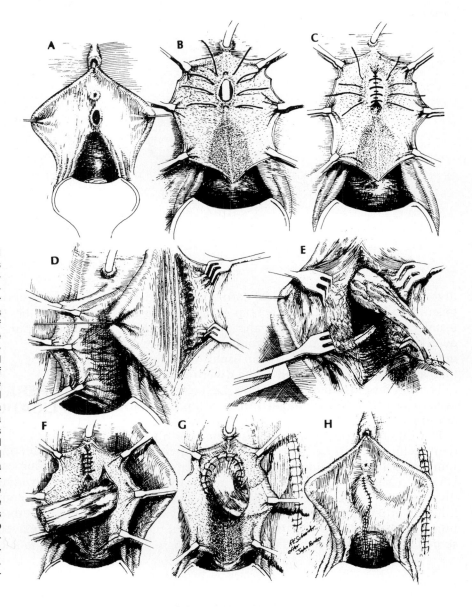

Figure 72–8. Repair of a large urethrovaginal fistula: lithotomy position. Special requirements include labial traction sutures, a weighted posterior vaginal retractor, suprapubic punch cystotomy, and a urethral Foley catheter. *A,* Anterior vaginal wall exposed. An elliptical incision is made around the fistulous tract, leaving a cuff of vaginal tissue. The incisions meet and are carried proximally to the bladder neck and distally to the urethral meatus. *B,* Vaginal mucosal flaps are developed laterally. *C,* The cuffs of vaginal mucosa around the fistulous tract are mobilized medially, turned inward, and closed in the midline over the catheter. *D,* The labia majora on one side are retracted medially and a vertical incision made. *E,* The bulbocavernosus muscle is dissected from above downward and transsected at its insertion into the perineal body. A tunnel is developed beneath the labia minora and majora, large enough to accommodate the freed bulbocavernosus muscle. *F,* The bulbocavernosus muscle is drawn through the tunnel. *G,* The bulbocavernosus muscle is tacked to the undersurface of the urethra to cover the urethral closure. *H,* The vaginal mucosa is reapproximated. (From Kropp KA. Urethral fistula and diverticula. In Glenn JF, ed. Urologic Surgery, 3rd ed. Philadelphia, JB Lippincott, 1983, p 735.)

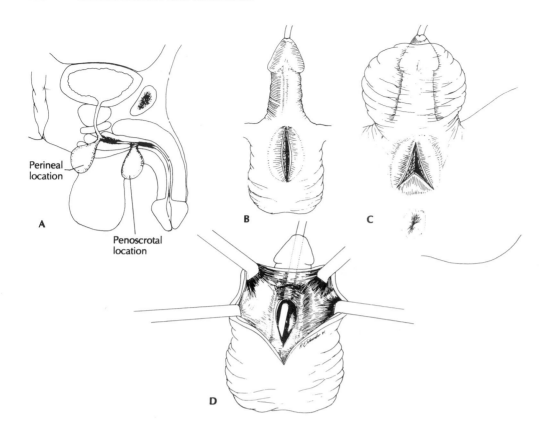

Figure 72–9. Excision of a male urethral diverticulum. Either the lithotomy or supine position is selected for the penoscrotal diverticulum, and lithotomy for the perineal diverticulum. Special requirements include suprapubic punch cystotomy, a urethral Foley catheter, a coagulum, and the Turner-Warwick retractor. *A,* Position of a penoscrotal and bulbous urethral diverticulum. *B,* Midline incision for the penoscrotal or perineal location or *C,* an inverted Y incision for the bulbous urethral diverticulum. *D,* The diverticulum has been excised, leaving a urethral defect. The urethral defect, if small, is closed longitudinally. A large urethral defect, as shown here, is either marsupialized for later staged closure or covered with a dartos-based vascularized graft of adjacent skin. (From Kropp KA. Urethral fistula and diverticula. In Glenn JF, ed. Urologic Surgery, 3rd ed. Philadelphia, JB Lippincott, 1983, p 726.)

diversion, or both before surgical correction is undertaken. Because of its mass effect, an excess of skin is usually available for coverage and tailoring so that overlying suture lines can be avoided. Conversely, a deficit of healthy urethral tissue usually occurs so that, at times, part of the wall of the diverticulum has to be used for closure of the urethra. Layers of dartos fascia can often be developed to cover the urethral closure.

The lithotomy position can be selected for all patients who undergo excision of a urethral diverticulum, regardless of its location. A midline or various U- and Y-shaped incisions can be made over the diverticulum. It is easier to dissect the coagulum-filled diverticulum intact than the unfilled diverticulum. Figures 72–9 and 72–10 show excision of penoscrotal and bulbous urethral diverticula.

The urethral repair is done over a urethral catheter, which can be used for diversion alone or with a suprapubic punch cystotomy.

POSTOPERATIVE MANAGEMENT AND COMPLICATIONS

Anticholinergics should be administered until voiding resumes, usually on the tenth to fourteenth postoperative days.

The most common complication is the development of a urethrocutaneous fistula. The repair of this fistula is delayed for 4 to 6 months to allow tissue induration to subside.

Urethrocutaneous Fistula

INDICATIONS

Urethrocutaneous fistulas occur in males with severe stricture disease. The fistula is usually secondary to an associated periurethral abscess that drains to the skin. More common are the fistulas that occur as complications of urethroplasty. Urethroplasties have

as the second stage a closure of a urethrocutaneous fistula. Once established, the fistula seldom closes spontaneously, even when distal obstruction is relieved. Repair of these fistulas can be done at the time of correction of the urethral stricture or it can be delayed. No attempt should be made to close a postoperative urethroplasty fistula until all tissue re-

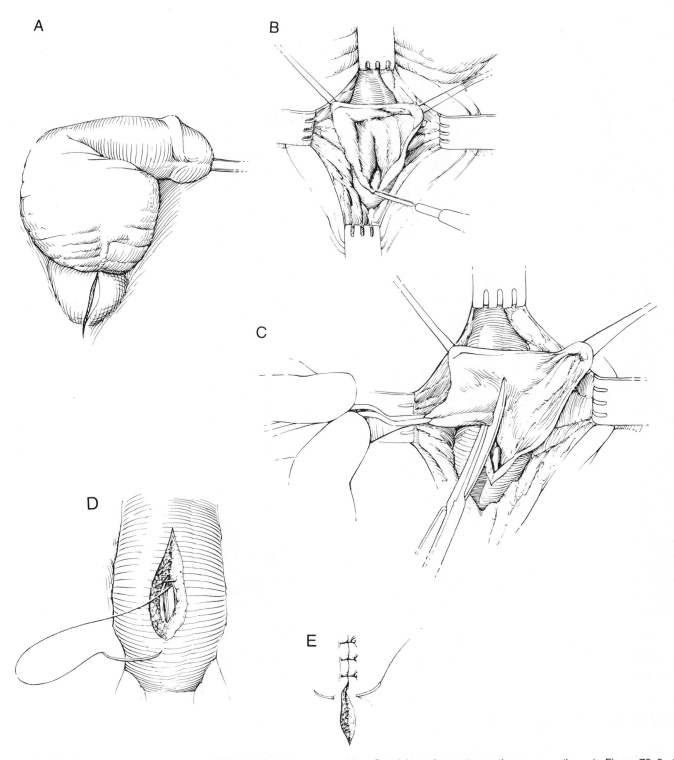

Figure 72–10. Excision of a bulbous urethral diverticulum: lithotomy position. Special requirements are the same as those in Figure 72–9. *A,* The midline incision is over the diverticulum. Develop flaps of skin and Colles fascia laterally, freeing the diverticulum from the surrounding bulbocavernosus muscle. *B,* Enter the diverticulum in the midline with the Bovie. Place stay sutures on the diverticular sac. *C,* Excise the walls of the diverticulum, leaving enough for urethral closure in case the opening into the urethra is large. *D,* Close the urethral defect. If possible, close the bulbocavernosus muscle over the urethral closure. *E,* Close Colles fascia and skin. (From Hinman F Jr. Atlas of Urologic Surgery. Philadelphia, WB Saunders, 1989.)

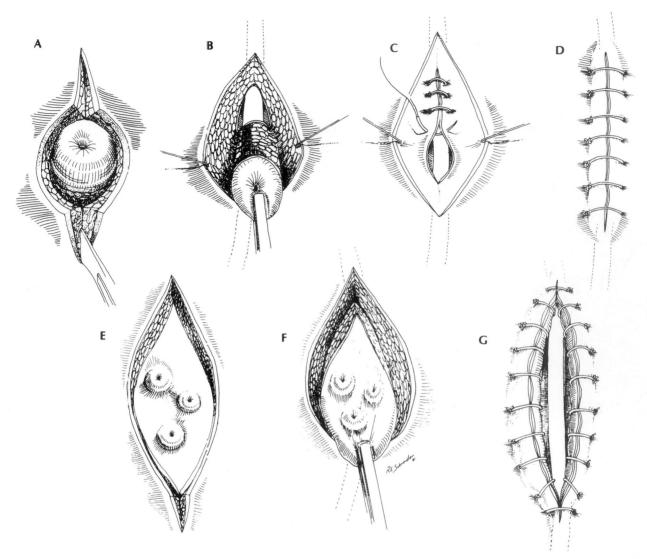

Figure 72–11. *A* to *D,* Repair of a simple urethrocutaneous fistula. *E* to *G,* Repair of more extensive or multiple fistulas. The position is dependent on the location. Special requirements include suprapubic punch cystotomy and methylene blue for staining the fistulous tract. *A,* An elliptical incision is made around the fistulous tract. *B,* The fistulous tract is dissected to its entrance into the urethra and excised. *C,* The urethra is closed over a catheter. *D,* The dartos and skin are closed in layers. *E,* An elliptical incision is made around all fistulous tracts. *F,* The fistulas and adjacent involved tissue are excised along with the urethral wall. *G,* The urethral mucosa is sutured to the skin as in a first-stage Johanson procedure. (From Kropp KA. Urethral fistula and diverticula. In Glenn JF, ed. Urologic Surgery, 3rd ed. Philadelphia, JB Lippincott, 1983, p 731.)

action has subsided, usually 4 to 6 months after the urethroplasty.

OPERATIVE TECHNIQUE

A variety of surgical techniques are available for closing fistulas. Common to most of the small fistulae are complete excision of the fistulous tract, including skin, intervening tissue, and urethra. The tissues are closed primarily, or the urethra is marsupialized (Fig. 72–11). Whenever possible, it is preferable to avoid overlying suture lines. This can be accomplished by either mobilizing skin flaps for rotation into the area of repair (Figs. 72–12 and 72–13) or using adjacent

scrotum to temporarily cover the repair after the method of Cecil (Fig. 72–14).

Some fistulas associated with large urethral defects can be closed by either mobilizing vascularized flaps of adjacent skin to cover the urethral defect (Fig. 72–15) or utilizing a full-thickness, tubed skin graft as shown in Figure 72–16. Many of these techniques are described elsewhere in this text.

POSTOPERATIVE MANAGEMENT

If the fistulous tract is small and overlying suture lines have been avoided, the patient may void immediately after the repair. However, in most cases an

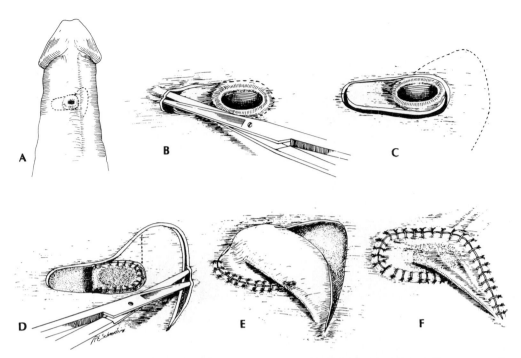

Figure 72–12. Wise's closure method utilizing a rotational flap: supine position. Special requirements are the same as those in Figure 72–11. *A,* The skin incisions are outlined with a marking pen. *B* and *C,* The skin flap for closure of the fistula is mobilized. *D,* The skin flap is turned over the fistula and sutured. The rotational flap for skin coverage is mobilized. *E* and *F,* The rotational flap is rotated to cover the fistula repair, and the skin closure is completed. (From Kropp KA. Urethral fistula and diverticula. In Glenn JF, ed. Urologic Surgery, 3rd ed. Philadelphia, JB Lippincott, 1983, p 737.)

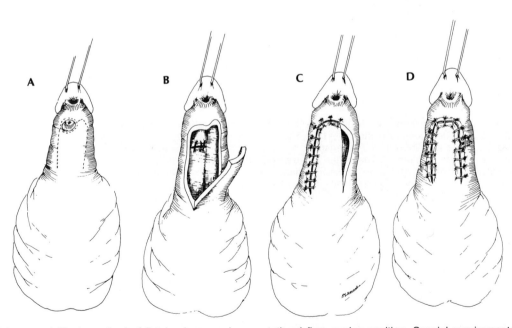

Figure 72–13. Belman and King's method of fistula closure using a rotational flap: supine position. Special requirements include those as described in Figure 72–11. *A,* A traction suture has been placed through the glans penis. The lines of incision are marked. *B,* The fistulous tract is excised and the urethra closed. The rotational flap is elevated. *C* and *D,* The flap is rotated to cover the urethral closure and the skin closed. (From Kropp KA. Urethral fistula and diverticula. In Glenn JF, ed. Urologic Surgery, 3rd ed. Philadelphia, JB Lippincott, 1983, p 736.)

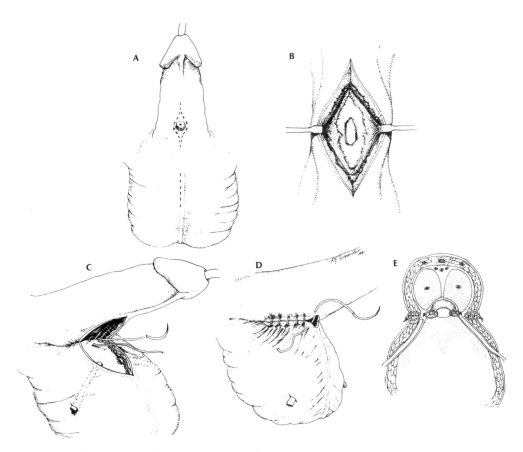

Figure 72–14. Repair of a urethrocutaneous fistula using a modified Cecil urethroplasty closure: supine or lithotomy position. Special requirements include those as described in Figure 72–11. *A,* The incisions are marked on the penis and scrotum. *B,* The fistulous tract and surrounding inflammatory tissue are excised. *C,* A corresponding longitudinal opposing scrotal incision is made. The edges of the urethra are sutured to the dartos layer of the scrotum. *D,* The edges of the penile incision are sutured to the edges of the scrotum. *E,* Drains are placed laterally through separate stab wounds and up to the urethral-dartos suture line. (From Kropp KA. Urethral fistula and diverticula. In Glenn JF, ed. Urologic Surgery, 3rd ed. Philadelphia, JB Lippincott, 1983, p 732.)

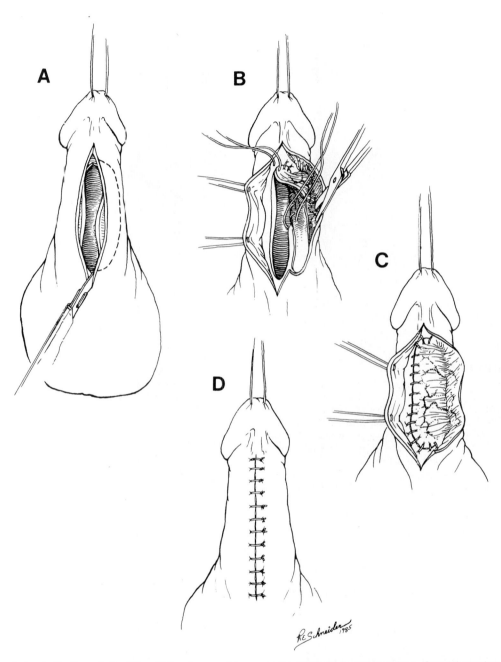

Figure 72–15. Vascularized skin flaps (after Orandi) for closure of large urethral defects: supine position. Special requirements are the same as those described in Figure 72–11. *A,* The fistulous tracts and adjacent inflammatory tissue are excised, creating a large urethral defect. An island of adjacent skin is outlined (*dotted lines*). *B,* A dartos-based vascular pedicle is developed and the skin island turned over and sutured to the urethral defect as a patch. *C,* Completed suture of the vascularized skin island. *D,* Penile skin closed over the repair. (From Kropp KA. Strictures of the male urethra. In Gillenwater JY, ed. Adult and Pediatric Urology. Chicago, Year Book, 1987.)

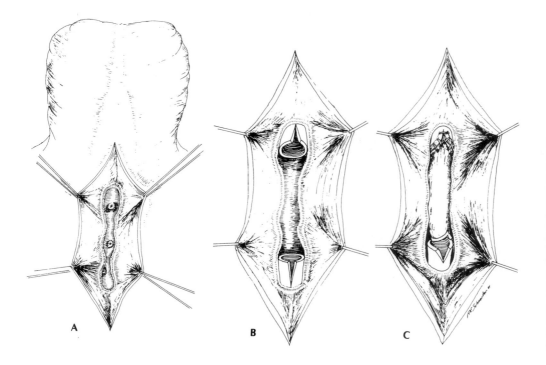

Figure 72–16. Repair of perineal urethrocutaneous fistulae: lithotomy position. Special requirements are the same as those described in Figure 72–11. *A,* Multiple perineal fistulae are isolated by an elliptical skin incision. *B,* The fistulas along with surrounding tissue and involved urethra are excised back into normal tissue. *C,* The urethra is replaced with a full-thickness tube skin graft. (After Devine CJ. J Urol 116:444, 1976.) (From Kropp KA. Urethral fistula and diverticula. In Glenn JF, ed. Urologic Surgery, 3rd ed. Philadelphia, JB Lippincott, 1983, p 733.)

indwelling Foley catheter or a suprapublic tube is used to divert the urine away until the repair has healed.

Editorial Comment

Fray F. Marshall

In females, urethral diverticula probably represent sequelae of previous infections. Marsupialization is a relatively safe way to manage this problem, although a female "hypospadiac" urethra can result. If a large urethral fistula involving the bladder neck is present in a female patient, a posteriorly based buttock flap can provide excellent vascularized tissue for reconstruction. In a male patient, a large urethral fistula or diverticulum really is managed as a urethroplasty as outlined in an excellent way by Dr. Kropp.

REFERENCES

1. Leach GE, Bavendam TG. Female urethral diverticula. Urology 30:407, 1987.
2. Leach GE, Sirls LT, Ganabathi K, Zimmern PE. LNSC3: A proposed classification system for female urethral diverticula. Neurourol Urodynam 12:523, 1993.
3. Spence HM, Duckett JW. Diverticulum of the female urethra: Clinical aspects and presentation of a simple operative technique for cure. J Urol 104:432, 1970.
4. Roehrborn CG. Long-term follow-up study of the marsupialization technique for urethral diverticula in women. Surg Gynecol Obstet 167:191, 1988.
5. Downs RA. Urethral diverticula in females. Urology 29:201, 1987.
6. Sholem SL, Wechsler M, Roberts M. Management of the urethral diverticulum in women: A modified operative technique. J Urol 112:485, 1974.
7. Leach GE, Schmidbauer CP, Hadley HR, et al. Surgical treatment of female urethral diverticulum. Semin Urol 4:33, 1986.
8. Moore TD. Diverticulum of the female urethra: Improved technique of surgical excision. J Urol 68:611, 1952.
9. Thompson JD. Vesicovaginal fistula. In Thompson JD, Rock JA, eds. Te Linde's Operative Gynecology, 7th ed. Philadelphia, JB Lippincott, 1992, p 815.
10. Reid RE, Gill B, Laor E, et al. Role of urodynamics in management of urethral diverticulum. Urology 28:342, 1986.
11. Wang Y, Hadley HR. The use of rotated vascularized pedicle flaps for complex transvaginal procedures. J Urol 149:590, 1993.

Chapter 73

Urethrectomy with Preservation of Potency

Charles B. Brendler and Patrick C. Walsh

Preservation of potency in a patient who is undergoing urethrectomy is more difficult than in a patient who is undergoing radical cystoprostatectomy alone. The reason is that the cavernous nerves travel posterolaterally in direct apposition to the urethra as they traverse the urogenital diaphragm.[1-4] Dissection of the nerves away from the urethra is more difficult in this region because of the surrounding muscle of the urogenital diaphragm and the decreased operative exposure. Nevertheless, it is possible to preserve potency in men who are undergoing urethrectomy using the modified technique described here.

OPERATIVE TECHNIQUE

The patient is initially positioned supine, with the table broken at the umbilicus and tilted to effect the Trendelenburg position until the legs are parallel to the floor (Fig. 73–1A). A radical cystoprostatectomy with preservation of the cavernous nerves is performed as described by Schlegel and Walsh.[5]

After ligation and division of the dorsal vein of the penis, a 0 silk suture is passed around the urethra and ligated to prevent spillage of urine around the urethral catheter (Fig. 73–2A). An umbilical tape is then passed around the urethra and gentle traction exerted cephalad. Using a Kutner dissector, the urethra is dissected from the urogenital diaphragm, removing only urethral mucosa and smooth muscle and leaving the striated muscle of the urogenital diaphragm behind (Fig. 73–2B). As the dissection continues, the neurovascular bundles lying immediately posterolateral to the membranous urethra are gently pushed away (Fig. 73–2C and D). This dissection continues until the membranous urethra has been liberated completely from the urogenital diaphragm. The urethra is then transected and the catheter drawn

cephalad into the wound (Fig. 73–2E). The remaining pedicles to the prostate and bladder are divided. The specimen is removed.

If a frozen-section analysis of the membranous urethra produces negative findings for carcinoma but a subsequent urethrectomy is planned, we prefer to delay the urethrectomy at least 2 weeks to avoid excessive mobilization of the cavernous nerves simultaneously from the pelvis and through the perineum.

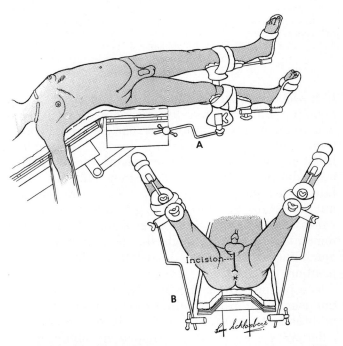

Figure 73–1. A, Patient position for radical cystoprostatectomy. The umbilicus is placed over the break of the table, and the table is fully flexed and tilted to effect the Trendelenburg position until the legs are parallel to the floor. B, Patient position for urethrectomy. The leg braces are elevated until the hips are flexed 60 degrees and the knees are fully extended. (From Brendler CB, Schlegel PN, Walsh PC. Urethrectomy with preservation of potency. J Urol 144:270, 1990. Copyright Williams & Wilkins.)

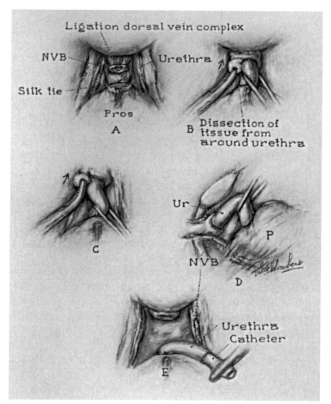

Figure 73–2. *A,* Urethra ligated with 0 silk suture to prevent spillage of urine around the catheter. *B,* Mobilization of the membranous urethra from the urogenital diaphragm with a Kutner dissector. *C,* Further mobilization of the membranous urethra. *D,* Lateral view showing the membranous urethra fully mobilized with neurovascular bundles (NVB) displaced posterolaterally. *E,* The urethra transsected and a catheter drawn cephalad into the wound. The neurovascular bundles are seen intact lateral to the urethra. (From Brendler CB, Schlegel PN, Walsh PC. Urethrectomy with preservation of potency. J Urol 144:270, 1990. Copyright Williams & Wilkins.)

If, however, a frozen-section analysis of the membranous urethra is positive for carcinoma, a simultaneous urethrectomy is performed. The patient is repositioned for the urethrectomy in the exaggerated lithotomy position simply by raising the leg braces until the hips are flexed 60 degrees and the knees fully extended (see Fig. 73–1*B*). The extra few minutes it takes to change the patient's position are worthwhile, because it facilitates dissection of the remaining urethra through the perineum. This is much more difficult to do using a low lithotomy position.

The perineal dissection of the urethra is done in the usual fashion with minor modifications. Either a midline or transverse perineal incision can be used. Alternatively, an inverted Y-shaped incision provides excellent exposure of the bulbar urethra (see Fig. 73–1*B*). Once the perineal skin and subcutaneous tissue have been incised, a Turner-Warwick ring retractor is positioned over the incision and provides excellent exposure. The bulbocavernosus muscle should be divided sharply in the midline posteriorly

to the level of the central perineal tendon to expose the bulbar urethra (Fig. 73–3). The anterior urethra is then dissected from the penis and brought into the perineum. The penis is reconstructed in the usual way.

Dissection of the bulbar urethra then begins. The relatively avascular tissues anterior to the bulbar urethra directly beneath the symphysis pubis are dissected first. This maneuver allows the urethra to be displaced anteriorly, facilitating exposure of the posterolateral bulbar urethral arteries and reducing the chance of inadvertent injury to these vessels (Fig. 73–4). The bulbar urethral arteries should be controlled with hemoclips (Fig. 73–5*A* and *B*) rather than fulgurated to avoid injuring the internal pudendal arteries from which the bulbar urethral arteries arise and that provide arterial supply to the corpora cavernosa (Fig. 73–5*C*). Having dissected the membranous urethra from above through the pelvis, the perineal dissection is usually completed without difficulty (Fig. 73–6).

Editorial Comment

Fray F. Marshall

Two of the primary maneuvers in preservation of potency during urethrectomy include initial extensive mobilization of the urethra in the retroperitoneum at the apex of the prostate. The neurovascular bundle is dissected off the urethra. Mobilization of the urethra to the level of the

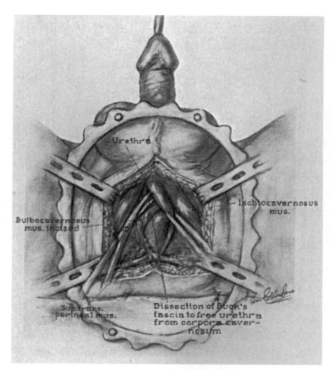

Figure 73–3. Turner-Warwick ring retractor positioned and the bulbocavernosus muscle incised to expose the bulbar urethra. (From Brendler CB, Schlegel PN, Walsh PC. Urethrectomy with preservation of potency. J Urol 144:270, 1990. Copyright Williams & Wilkins.)

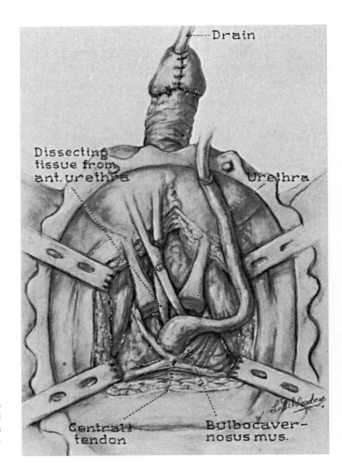

Figure 73–4. Initial dissection of tissue anterior to the bulbar urethra to facilitate subsequent exposure and control of posterolateral bulbar urethral arteries. (From Brendler CB, Schlegel PN, Walsh PC. Urethrectomy with preservation of potency. J Urol 144:270, 1990. Copyright Williams & Wilkins.)

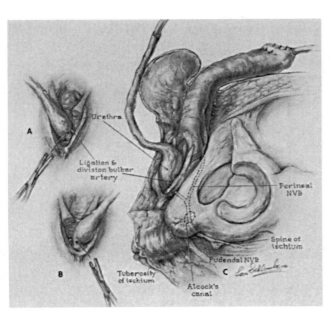

Figure 73–5. *A* and *B,* Ligation of bulbar urethral arteries with hemoclips. *C,* Lateral view showing the relationship between the internal pudendal and bulbar arteries. The bulbar arteries should not be fulgurated in order to prevent injury to the internal pudendal arteries from which they arise and that provide arterial supply to the corpora cavernosa. (From Brendler CB, Schlegel PN, Walsh PC. Urethrectomy with preservation of potency. J Urol 144:270, 1990. Copyright Williams & Wilkins.)

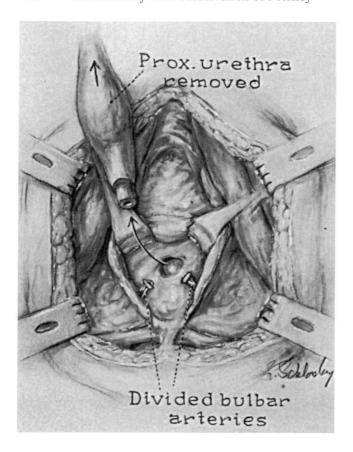

Prox. urethra
removed

Divided bulbar
arteries

Figure 73–6. Completed urethrectomy. Dissection of the bulbar urethra is completed without difficulty because the membranous urethra has previously been mobilized through the pelvis. (From Brendler CB, Schlegel PN, Walsh PC. Urethrectomy with preservation of potency. J Urol 144:270, 1990. Copyright Williams & Wilkins.)

urogenital diaphragm can be accomplished and the dissection from below is facilitated. During the perineal dissection the bulbar arteries often bleed and extensive fulguration in this area may be deleterious to the neurovascular bundle. Clips are potentially much less injurious.

One further note of caution needs to be given regarding the use of stirrups of any sort in patients undergoing a concomitant cystectomy and urethrectomy. In spite of all efforts to pad legs, I have seen peroneal nerve palsies as well as compartment syndromes in patients who have had lengthy operations. For that reason, I have more recently used the split-leg fluoroscopy table as an alternative. The exposure in the perineum is not quite as good but can still be quite adequate in a patient who has already had extensive mobilization of the urethra with the retroperitoneal dissection.

REFERENCES

1. Walsh PC, Donker PJ. Impotence following radical prostatectomy: Insight into etiology and prevention. J Urol 128:492, 1982.
2. Lue TF, Zeineh SJ, Schmidt RA, and Tanagho EM. Neuroanatomy of penile erection: Its relevance to iatrogenic impotence. J Urol 131:273, 1984.
3. Lepor H, Gregerman M, Crosby R, et al. Precise localization of the autonomic nerves from the pelvic plexus to the corpora cavernosa: A detailed anatomical study of the adult male pelvis. J Urol 133:207, 1985.
4. Brendler CB, Schlegel PN, Walsh PC. Urethrectomy with preservation of potency. J Urol 144:1990.
5. Schlegel PN, Walsh PC. Neuroanatomical approach to radical cystoprostatectomy with preservation of sexual function. J Urol 138:1402, 1987.

Chapter 74

Artificial Sphincter in the Treatment of Male Urinary Incontinence

Eduardo Kleer and David M. Barrett

PREOPERATIVE EVALUATION

The incontinent patient most likely to benefit from the implantation of an American Medical Systems 800 artificial genitourinary sphincter (AGUS) is one with normal detrusor contractility and compliance associated with sphincteric incompetence. Typically, this occurs with postprostatectomy incontinence. Patients with incontinence after trauma, radiation, or neurological disease are also likely to benefit from the implantation of an AGUS. Postprostatectomy incontinent patients obtain a 90 to 96 percent improved continence rate and a 90 percent satisfaction rate after AGUS implantation.[1, 2] The preoperative evaluation before implantation should consist of a history; physical examination; urinalysis; urine Gram stain, culture, and sensitivity; urodynamics; radiological imaging of the urinary tract; and urethrocystoscopy.

In patients with a history of postprostatectomy incontinence, it is important to determine the length of time since the surgery; the severity of the incontinence in terms of pads worn per day; whether it is improving, worsening, or stabilized; and the quality of the urinary stream. A minimal period of 6 months should be allowed between the time of prostatectomy and consideration of AGUS implantation, as postprostatectomy incontinence can improve dramatically during this time. In addition, it is important to ask if the patient has been on a regular program of pelvic strengthening exercises and has undergone a trial of pharmacological therapy. Pelvic strengthening exercises and the use of anticholinergic and/or alpha-sympathomimetic agents may sometimes allow patients with minimal to mild incontinence to achieve a level of socially acceptable incontinence without

surgery. A history of a dribbling flow of stream may indicate a bladder neck contracture, urethral stricture, or meatal stenosis resulting in overflow incontinence. Patients with postprostatectomy strictures should be questioned regarding the number, frequency, and time of the last dilation. A history of strictures is not a contraindication to AGUS implantation unless they are located at the site where the cuff needs to be implanted. However, repeated urethral instrumentation in the presence of an AGUS may predispose the patient to cuff erosion.

It is also important to obtain a thorough history regarding strictures and their treatment in patients with a history of incontinence after radiation or trauma. Patients with a history of post-traumatic urethral reconstruction are better served by placement of the cuff around the bladder neck, whereas those who have undergone previous bladder neck reconstruction benefit more from placement of the cuff around the bulbous urethra.

In patients with incontinence secondary to neurological disease such as myelodysplasia, it is important to verify that a trial of pharmacological treatment and intermittent catheterization has failed to enhance outlet resistance and/or increase bladder capacity to a point that results in socially acceptable incontinence. In patients with neurological disease, it is recommended that the sphincter cuff be implanted around the bladder neck rather than the urethra, as the result seems to be more physiological.[3] Many of these patients require intermittent catheterization to completely empty their bladders. Catheter-induced trauma is less likely to occur if the sphincter cuff is around the bladder neck rather than the bulbous urethra, where the tissue is thinner and less well vascularized.

621

On physical examination, many patients with chronic urinary incontinence have various degrees of dermatitis on the lower abdomen and pelvis. In these patients, it is best to insert a Foley catheter several days before implantation to promote healing and reduce the possibility of infection. It is also important to look at the location of previous abdominal scars, since it is preferable to implant the reservoir away from these scarred areas. Rectal examination should be performed to rule out recurrent cancer in postprostatectomy patients and to assess anal sphincter tone.

Urinalysis, culture, and sensitivities are performed to ensure urine sterility before AGUS implantation and thus minimize the likelihood of infection.

All patients with a history of neurological disease should undergo an intravenous pyelogram and a voiding cystourethrogram to exclude upper tract or bladder structural abnormalities that would require repair before or during sphincter implantation.[3] Grade 2 reflux or greater should be corrected before or during implantation. Retrograde urethrograms are indicated in patients with a history of recurrent strictures, pelvic trauma, or urethral reconstruction.

Urodynamics is the next step in the work-up of the possible candidate for AGUS implantation. Patients with detrusor instability and/or small-capacity, poorly compliant bladders are poor candidates for AGUS implantation, but pharmacological agents or bladder augmentation may render them suitable for the procedure. The bladder must be able to hold volumes greater than 400 ml and maintain an intravesical pressure of less than 40 cm of water.[4]

Urethrocystoscopy is also necessary before implantation of an AGUS to evaluate any false passages, strictures, contractures, diverticula, or foreign bodies. It is important to note the location of the urethral defect. For example, a stricture in the distal or mid-bulbous urethra may prevent implantation of the occlusive cuff at this level, and an alternative site should be chosen. In postradiation patients, cystoscopy is important to determine tissue viability before AGUS implantation and decrease the risk of subsequent urethral erosion.[3–5]

OPERATIVE TECHNIQUE

Patients are admitted to the hospital on the morning of the surgical procedure. Those undergoing bladder neck cuff placement should be told to have a limited lower bowel preparation the night before surgery. Parenteral broad-spectrum antibiotics should be administered on call to the operating room. Hair removal is carried out just before surgery. Patients undergoing the bladder neck cuff operation are positioned supine with their legs slightly abducted; those receiving the bulbous urethral cuff are placed in the lithotomy position. A rectal tube is placed in patients who will have bladder neck cuff placement. A full 10-minute iodophor skin scrub should be performed. Draping should allow access to the lower anterior abdominal wall and perineum. A 12 Fr. Foley catheter is subsequently inserted. An antibiotic solution should be available and used frequently for irrigation during the procedure.

Bladder Neck Cuff Placement

A lower abdominal midline incision is made and carried down into the retropubic space. The dissection should be extraperitoneal, as the peritoneal cavity does not need to be opened. Blunt dissection around the bladder neck is begun superior to the endopelvic fascia and inferior to a point where the ureters empty into the posterior aspect of the bladder. With the Foley catheter in place, the demarcation of the bladder neck and proximal portion of the urethra can be palpated. The plane is established between the posterior aspect of the bladder neck and the anterior surface of the rectum (Fig. 74–1). Palpation of the rectal tube may help identify the anterior surface of the rectum. Usually, a combination of blunt and sharp dissection allows complete circumferential dissection. The width of this plane should be approxi-

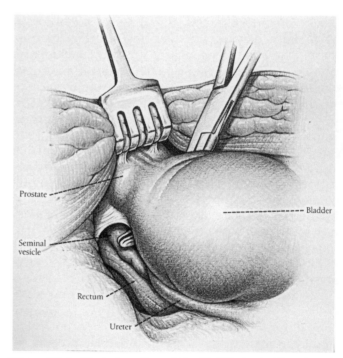

Figure 74–1. Blunt dissection of the bladder neck. The plane is established between the posterior aspect of the bladder neck and the anterior surface of the rectum. Dissection is begun superior to the endopelvic fascia but inferior to a point where the ureters empty into the posterior aspect of the bladder. (Drawing by William B. Westwood, courtesy of LTI Medica®. Copyright 1988 by Learning Technology, Inc.)

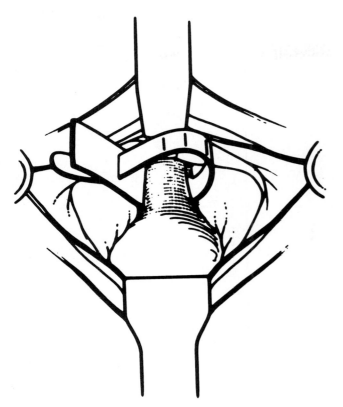

Figure 74–2. The bladder neck is circumferentially measured with the calibrated measuring strap and must be circumferentially dissected. The width of the plane should be approximately 2 cm to allow unrestricted placement of the cuff. (Courtesy of American Medical Systems, Inc., Minnetonka, Minnesota.)

mately 2 cm to allow unrestricted placement of the cuff. A tape is passed around the bladder neck, and the bladder is filled with antibiotic solution to reveal any small tears that may have been created during the dissection. If present, they may be closed with

3-0 or 4-0 absorbable sutures. However, if a rectal injury is identified, it should be closed primarily and the procedure abandoned for a later date. The bladder neck is circumferentially measured with the calibrated measuring strap (Fig. 74–2). The indwelling Foley catheter need not be removed before this measurement unless the size is greater than 12 Fr. In men, an 8- to 14-cm cuff may be necessary. The properly sized cuff is then passed underneath the bladder neck and snapped into place (Fig. 74–3). The tubing from the cuff is passed through the belly of one rectus muscle and through the anterior abdominal wall fascia on the side of the patient where the pump will be placed. This tubing should penetrate the rectus muscle and fascia and into the deep subcutaneous tissues from 3 to 4 inches above the pubic symphysis. A curved shod clamp is used on the end of the cuff tubing closed with only one click.

The pressure balloon reservoir is placed in the prevesical space. Its tubing penetrates the rectus muscle next to the tubing of the cuff. A straight shod clamp closed with only one click is left on the end of the reservoir tubing (Fig. 74–4). Before the balloon is filled, the prevesical space is drained and the anterior abdominal wall fascia closed with absorbable sutures. After completion of the closure, the balloon is filled with 22 ml of isosmotic contrast medium. A 61- to 70-cm water pressure reservoir is routinely used in most patients. With a Hegar dilator, a lateral hemiscrotal pocket is developed for the control assembly (Fig. 74–5). The pump is placed in an optimally dependent position with the activation/deactivation button laterally, easily palpable against the skin (Fig. 74–5). A curved shod clamp should be on the control tubing to the cuff and a straight shod clamp on the control tubing to the reservoir, each with only one

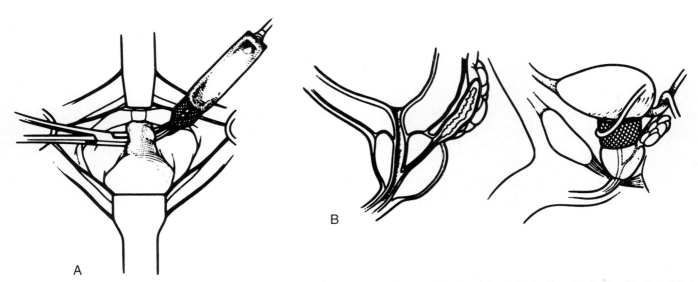

Figure 74–3. *A,* The properly sized cuff is passed underneath the bladder neck and strapped in place while gentle opposing traction is applied to the tab and tubing. Care should be taken that the tubing attached to the cuff is directed toward the side where the pump and reservoir will be inserted. *B,* Sagittal view of the cuff site. (Courtesy of American Medical Systems, Inc., Minnetonka, Minnesota.)

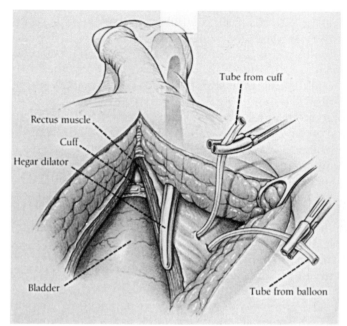

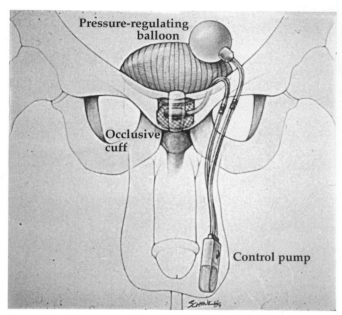

Figure 74–4. After the cuff and reservoir tubes are brought through the rectus muscle, a Hegar dilator is used to create a deep pocket through the subcutaneous tissues above Scarpa's fascia into the right hemiscrotum. The control assembly will be placed in this pocket. (Drawing by William B. Westwood, courtesy of LTI Medica®. Copyright 1988 by Learning Technology, Inc.)

Figure 74–6. The implantation of the artificial genitourinary sphincter (AGUS) with a bladder neck cuff has been completed.

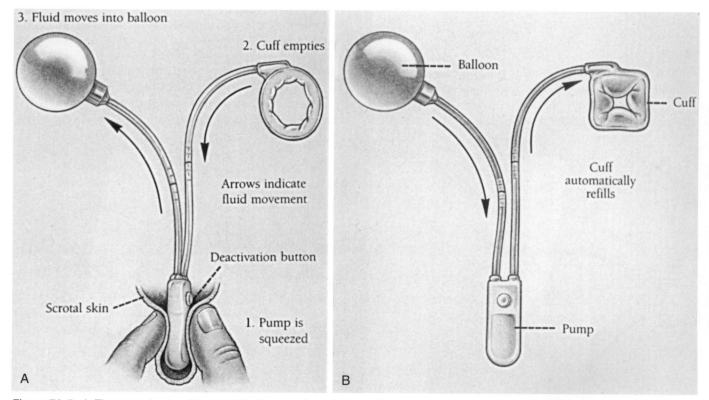

Figure 74–5. *A,* The pump is placed in an optimally dependent position with the activation/deactivation button laterally. This button must be easily palpable against the scrotal skin. To void, the patient squeezes the pump through the scrotal skin. *B,* When the patient stops squeezing the pump, the cuff will begin to refill automatically. (Drawing by William B. Westwood, courtesy of LTI Medica®. Copyright 1988 by Learning Technology, Inc.)

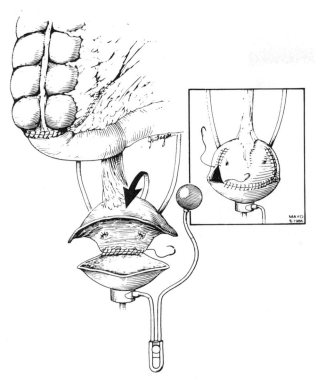

Figure 74–7. In performing bladder augmentation intestinocystoplasty concomitantly with AGUS implantation, the cuff should be placed around the bladder neck when possible. The cuff should not be impinging on any of the suture lines. (By permission of Mayo Foundation.)

click. Appropriate connections are made between the AGUS components using straight connectors tied in place with 2-0 Prolene sutures (Fig. 74–6). Connections may also be made with the quick-connect connectors. The incision is closed in layers with absorbable sutures. After the device has been tested and cycled, the cuff is left in an open deactivated position.

As discussed earlier, patients with detrusor instability and/or small-capacity, poorly compliant bladders may require concomitant bladder augmentation intestinocystoplasty at the time of AGUS implantation. The cuff should be placed around the bladder neck when possible, since many of these patients will require clean intermittent catheterization (Fig. 74–7).[6] The augmentation cystoplasty should be completed before insertion of the AGUS. Ample space should be allowed around the bladder neck area for the cuff to be placed without impinging on any of the suture lines.

Bulbous Urethral Cuff

A small perineal incision is made over the bulbous urethra (Fig. 74–8). With a Young retractor superiorly and a Gelpi retractor for lateral exposure, the bulbous urethra is dissected circumferentially (Fig. 74–9). If

possible, dissection should be carried out around the bulbocavernosus muscle and a plane established between it and the tunica albuginea of the corporeal bodies. This plane allows the cuff to be placed around the bulbocavernous muscle and not directly on the bulb of the urethra, to reduce the risk of erosion. The width of this dissection must be adequate to accommodate the 2-cm width of the cuff. Care is taken not to injure the urethra at the 12 o'clock position, the point at which dissection is most difficult and most urethral injuries occur. If the urethra is injured, it may be possible to close the defect primarily with 4-0 or 5-0 absorbable sutures; a different site on the urethra can then be selected for cuff placement. Routinely, a 4.5-cm cuff is passed tab first beneath the urethra (Fig. 74–10) and snapped into place while gentle opposing traction is applied to tab and tubing. Care should be taken to direct the tubing attached to the cuff toward the side where the pump and reservoir will be inserted. A curved shod clamp closed with only one click is placed around the cuff tubing for later identification.

Subsequently, a small transverse incision is made in the lower abdominal wall to the side where the pump and reservoir will be located. In general, this should be the side of hand dominance. After the anterior fascia is exposed, it is vertically incised for a short distance and a pocket bluntly developed be-

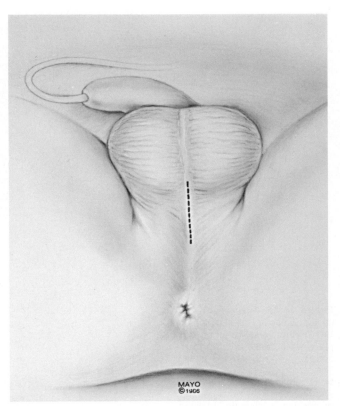

Figure 74–8. With a Foley catheter in place, a small perineal incision is made over the bulbous urethra. (By permission of Mayo Foundation.)

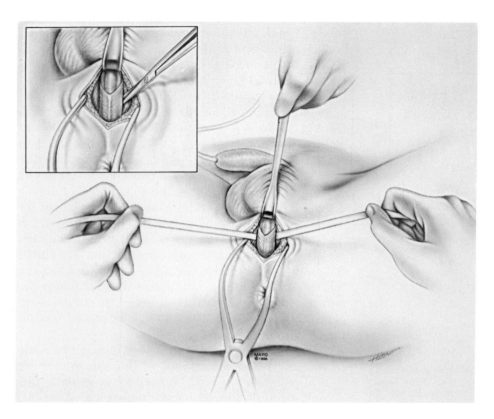

Figure 74–9. With a Young retractor superiorly and a Gelpi retractor for lateral exposure, the bulbous urethra has been circumferentially dissected. The width of this dissection must be sufficient to accommodate the 2-cm width of the cuff. *Inset,* Sharp dissection is used to enter a plane between the bulbocavernous muscle and the tunica albuginea of the corporeal bodies to gain circumferential access. (By permission of Mayo Foundation.)

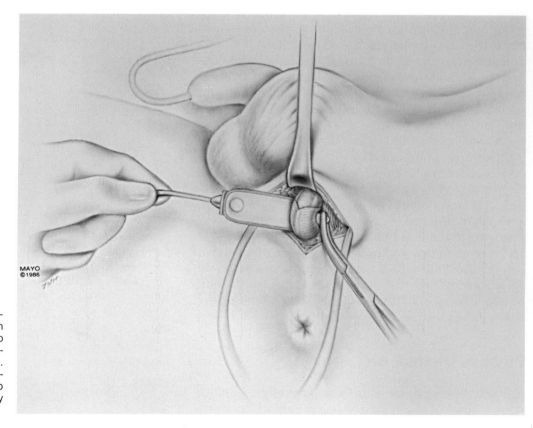

Figure 74–10. Routinely, a 4.5-cm cuff is passed tab first beneath the urethra and snapped into place while gentle opposing traction is applied to tab and tubing. The tubing should be directed toward the side where the pump and reservoir will be inserted. (By permission of Mayo Foundation.)

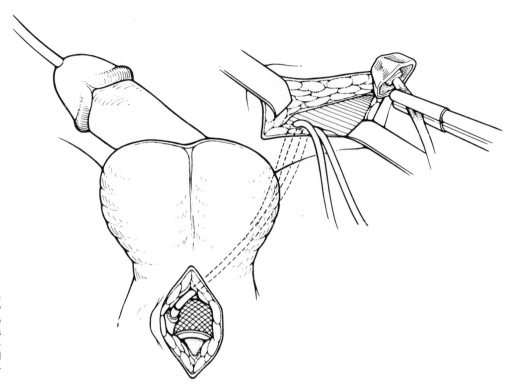

Figure 74–11. The deflated balloon reservoir is placed in a pocket below the belly of the rectus muscle. The cuff tubing has been guided to this area through the subcutaneous tissues. (Courtesy of American Medical Systems, Inc., Minnetonka, Minnesota.)

low the belly of the rectus muscle, extraperitoneally, to allow placement of the deflated balloon reservoir (Fig. 74–11). The reservoir tubing is brought through a separate stab incision in the anterior rectus fascia. The reservoir is subsequently filled with 22 ml of isosmotic contrast medium, and a straight shod clamp is placed around the tubing and closed with only one click to prevent fluid loss. A 61- to 70-cm water pressure reservoir is routinely used in most patients with uncomplicated bulbous urethral cuffs. In high-risk patients the 51- to 60-cm pressure reservoir is used to minimize tissue pressure ischemia. After ensuring that the inflated balloon is well accommodated within the rectus pocket, the fascial defect is closed with running absorbable sutures.

A long clamp is then passed from the plane superior to the rectus fascia, above Scarpa's fascia, to the area of the perineal incision (see Fig. 74–10). The cuff tubing is grasped and guided to the area of the lower quadrant incision. Next, a lateral subcutaneous hemiscrotal pouch is created with Hegar dilators, where the pump is placed in an optimally dependent position with the activation/deactivation button laterally (see Figs. 74–4 and 74–5). The activation/deactivation button must be easily palpable against the skin. Once a satisfactory position for the pump has been assured, a Babcock clamp is placed around it and the scrotal skin to prevent its proximal migration when the tubing is connected. The pump tubing that will be connected to the cuff tubing should have a curved shod clamp around it, while a straight shod clamp should be placed around the other tubing that will be connected to the reservoir tubing.

All the appropriate tubing connections are next made (Fig. 74–12). The cuff tubing is attached to the control assembly tubing with a right-angled connector to prevent kinking. The balloon and the control assembly tubing are attached with a straight connector. These connectors can be tied in place with 2-0 Prolene or may be assembled with the quick-connect tubing connections.

The incisions are closed in layers with absorbable sutures, and the AGUS is left in a cuff open deactivated position after the device has been tested and cycled. Pressure dressings are applied.

POSTOPERATIVE MANAGEMENT

The Foley catheter is removed the following day. The patient should have ice packs to the scrotum and/or perineum for the first 24 hours postoperatively to minimize edema and hematoma formation. Some patients experience a transient postoperative continence secondary to tissue edema around the cuff site. Once the incontinence recurs, they are advised to use diapers or condom drainage devices. The use of penile clamps is discouraged. In the rare instances in which the patient is unable to urinate, intermittent self-catheterization with a small-caliber catheter should be instituted.

The AGUS is activated 6 to 8 weeks postoperatively

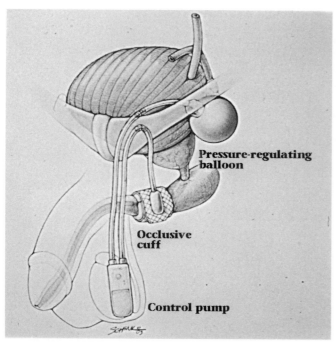

Figure 74–12. The implantation of the AGUS with a bulbar urethral cuff has been completed. (From Barrett DM, Furlow WL, Goldwasser B. The artificial urinary sphincter. In Yalla SV, McGuire EJ, Elbadawi A, Blaivas JG, eds. Neurourology and Urodynamics: Principles and Practice. New York, Macmillan, 1988, pp 474–488. Reproduced with permission of McGraw-Hill, Inc.)

by firm compression of the pump. The deactivation button will switch into the activated configuration, allowing fluid to circulate through the control assembly. Activation can be monitored by "inflate/deflate" radiographs that confirm filling of the cuff after activation. During this clinic visit, it is beneficial to reeducate the patient regarding the AGUS operation.

Patients who are dry at night in a recumbent position are instructed to deactivate the AGUS before falling asleep. This reduces the risk of ischemia to the underlying urethra or bladder neck. Patients who have diminished flow rates may require a second pumping to allow enough time to adequately empty the bladder before cuff recompression occurs. Patients unable to completely empty the bladder, such as those with neurogenic bladders or bladder augmentations, should use intermittent self-catheterization. The sphincter cuff must be deflated before the catheter is inserted into the bladder.

POSTOPERATIVE COMPLICATIONS

Hematoma formation is the most common minor complication of sphincter implantation. It has the potential to displace the pump into an unfavorable location for external manipulation. A large hematoma may need to be drained to prevent discomfort and enhance healing.

Cuff erosion is most common in the first 3 to 4 months after implantation. Its incidence has decreased dramatically, affecting only three of 144 patients in a recent series, since the introduction of the AMS 800 narrow-backed cuff design.[7] Cuff erosion prior to activation implies an unrecognized iatrogenic injury to the urethra or bladder neck. Cuff erosion may present as pain or swelling in the cuff or pump area, recurrent incontinence, urethral discharge, and/or urosepsis. Retrograde urethrography and urethroscopy confirm the diagnosis. Surgical removal of the cuff is mandatory. The remaining sphincter components should be removed if there is also purulent drainage. If the erosion is clean and uncomplicated, only the cuff needs to be removed and a stainless steel plug is used to temporarily occlude the tube leading to the pump. Copious irrigation of the surrounding area with antibiotic solution and drainage may prevent subsequent infection around the device components. For bulbar urethral erosions, a 12 or 14 Fr. silicone catheter is left indwelling. For bladder neck erosions, an 18 Fr. silicone catheter should be left indwelling for 2 to 4 weeks or until the retrograde urethrographic picture is normal.

Once complete healing occurs and there is no evidence of infection, a new cuff may be inserted. Bladder neck cuff replacement is facilitated if, at the time of cuff removal, the eroded opening is closed with absorbable sutures and a thin silicone strip placed around the bladder neck. This facilitates reoperation and cuff replacement in the plane maintained by the silicone strip. On the other hand, if infection cannot be ruled out at the time of cuff removal, the peritoneum should be opened and an omental wrap positioned around the bladder neck to facilitate redissection. The patient should be forewarned that, despite these precautionary measures, bladder neck cuff reimplantation may be impossible. In the case of a urethral cuff, another location around the bulbar urethra should be selected for reimplantation.

In cases of infected sphincter components, the entire device should be removed and the wound copiously irrigated and drained. Reimplantation may be considered at a later date.

Recurrent urinary incontinence after successful sphincter implantation requires a systematic approach to identify the problem.[8, 9] The control assembly should be checked to make sure it is in the activated state. If an "inflate/deflate" film is normal, cystoscopy should be performed to rule out an erosion. Mechanical malfunction may result from fluid leakage, tube kinks and disconnections, or control pump malfunction. The most common site of fluid leakage is the cuff. Another potential site of mechanical failure is occlusion of the control assembly secondary to debris. Urodynamics should be performed to evaluate for detrusor hyperreflexia. Incontinence after AGUS implantation may also result from suboptimal occlusive pressure secondary to urethral atrophy or suboptimal occlusive cuff pressure. Reduction in cuff size is an option for compensation of recurrent or persistent incontinence in a patient with an otherwise normally functioning sphincter. In patients with bladder neck cuffs, dissection of the implanted cuff is more difficult, and it is recommended that an attempt be made to raise the balloon pressure initially. Results may also sometimes be improved with pharmacological agents that decrease detrusor contractility or enhance outlet resistance.

Patients with neurological disorders such as myelomeningocele who have undergone AGUS implantation may be at risk for developing upper tract deterioration secondary to high voiding pressures; they thus require regular follow-up. This should consist of an excretory urogram or ultrasonographic assessment of the kidneys and urodynamic evaluation, beginning within the first 3 to 6 months postoperatively. Should hydronephrosis develop, treatment is based on decreasing detrusor pressure, which may be accomplished by increasing the frequency of intermittent catheterization, anticholinergics, and bladder augmentation if needed.

Editorial Comment

Fray F. Marshall

The most common indication for an artificial urinary sphincter in the male is usually seen after radical retropubic prostatectomy or after transurethral resection of the prostate. This operation can be most helpful in these circumstances and generally works quite effectively. Although mechanical failures occur, I have seen patients with sphincters functioning for more than 10 years. With erosion, it may be possible to reconstruct the urethra with an end-to-end anastomosis and, at a later date, replace the sphincter with a lower-pressure system. In patients with neurological disease, urodynamic evaluation is important; the urodynamic findings may change after implantation of a sphincter.

REFERENCES

1. Gundian JC, Barrett DM, Parulkar BG. Mayo Clinic experience with use of the AMS 800 artificial urinary sphincter for urinary incontinence following radical prostatectomy. J Urol 142:1459, 1989.
2. Gundian JC, Barrett DM, Parulkar BG. Mayo Clinic experience with use of the AMS 800 artificial urinary sphincter for urinary incontinence after transurethral resection of prostate or open prostatectomy. Urology 41:318, 1993.
3. Barrett DM, Goldwasser B. The artificial urinary sphincter: Current management philosophy. American Urological Association Updates, Vol 5, lesson 32, 1986.
4. Petrou SP, Barrett DM. The expanded role for the artificial sphincter. American Urological Association Updates, Vol 10, lesson 16, 1991.
5. Light JK. Implantation of the AMS 800 artificial urinary sphincter. Probl Urol 7:402, 1993.
6. Strawbridge LR, Kramer SA, Castilla OA, et al. Augmentation cystoplasty and the artificial genitourinary sphincter. J Urol 142:297, 1989.
7. Leo ME, Barrett DM. Success of the narrow-backed cuff design of the AMS 800 artificial urinary sphincter: Analysis of 144 patients. J Urol 150:1412, 1993.
8. Furlow WL, Barrett DM. Recurrent or persistent urinary incontinence in patients with the artificial urinary sphincter: Diagnostic considerations and management. J Urol 133:792, 1985.
9. Marks JL, Light JK. Management of urinary incontinence after prostatectomy with the artificial urinary sphincter. J Urol 142:302, 1989.

Part IX

SURGERY OF THE SCROTUM, TESTIS, AND PENIS

Chapter 75

Simple and Radical Orchiectomy

Brad A. Wolfson, Jacob Rajfer, and Andrew Freedman

The testis is both an exocrine and an endocrine organ. Its major functions are to produce spermatozoa and testosterone. The testis may require removal (orchiectomy) when affected by various diseases or trauma. The major indications for orchiectomy include epididymo-orchitis that has failed to respond to medical therapy or has progressed to abscess formation; testicular torsion, where detorsion has failed to relieve the ischemia leading to total infarction; and testicular cancer. Besides these intrinsic diseases of the testis, the testicles may require removal if surgical castration is contemplated for the management of metastatic prostate cancer.

The testes can be removed via the scrotal (simple orchiectomy) or inguinal (radical orchiectomy) approach. If suspicion of a testicular carcinoma exists, the inguinal route is utilized to gain initial control of the testicular vessels. For all other disease states that require orchiectomy, a simple transscrotal approach is used.

Simple Orchiectomy

OPERATIVE TECHNIQUE

A simple orchiectomy may be performed with the patient under general, regional, or local anesthesia.[1] A longitudinal incision in the midline scrotal raphe gives exposure to each testis and is relatively bloodless. The dartos muscle is sharply divided down to the tunica vaginalis, which is identified by its bluish hue. The tunica vaginalis is incised longitudinally, exposing the testis, the epididymis, and the spermatic cord. The testicular vessels and vas deferens are identified, clamped separately, and divided. These cord structures are ligated individually with a nonbraided suture. Strict hemostasis of the wound and skin edges is obtained, utilizing the cautery. Closure of the wound is done in two layers. The dartos is closed with a running 3–0 chromic suture, and the skin is approximated with interrupted vertical mattress 4–0 chromic sutures. A turban pressure dressing of gauze fluffs and a scrotal supporter are applied for 24 hours.

POSTOPERATIVE MANAGEMENT AND COMPLICATIONS

The most frequent complication is postoperative hemorrhage with the development of a scrotal hematoma. Hematomas can be quite substantial and cause severe pain with increased risk of infection. The incidence can be reduced with meticulous attention to intraoperative hemostasis and with a pressure dressing. Some surgeons advocate the placement of a scrotal drain for 24 hours postoperatively. If a hematoma occurs, it should be drained only if it becomes large, extremely tender, or infected.

630

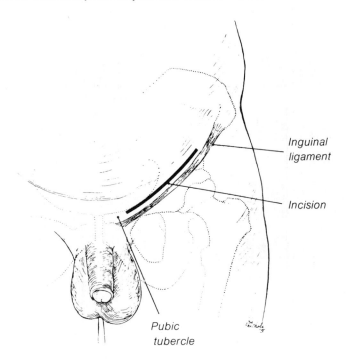

Figure 75–1. The line of incision runs parallel to the inguinal ligament and is approximately 8 cm long. (From Crawford ED, Borden TA. Genitourinary Cancer Surgery. Philadelphia, Lea & Febiger, 1982.)

Radical Orchiectomy

OPERATIVE TECHNIQUE

Radical orchiectomy has long been the standard initial therapy for testicular cancer. Despite this practice, up to 10 percent of testicular tumors are diagnosed after a nonclassic orchiectomy as the initial surgical management.[2] The patients so treated are at increased risk of local recurrence and may require aggressive local surgical salvage.[3]

Radical inguinal orchiectomy should be performed using general or spinal anesthesia. A transverse incision in the skinfold above the inguinal ligament yields good exposure and cosmetic effect (Fig. 75–1). Camper's and Scarpa's fasciae are divided to expose the external oblique fascia and the external inguinal ring. The external oblique fascia is incised in the direction of its fibers from the external inguinal ring to the level of the internal inguinal ring. The ilioinguinal nerve is identified and dissected from surrounding tissue. The spermatic cord is isolated and snugly encircled with a Penrose drain prior to manipulation of the testicle (Fig. 75–2). The testis is then delivered into the wound.

Attachments of the external spermatic fascia and the cremaster muscle to the scrotal wall are bluntly dissected until the gubernacular attachment to the lower pole of the testis is reached. This fibrous band is divided between hemostats. The testicular vessels and vas deferens are clamped individually at the level of the internal inguinal ring, and the spermatic cord is divided between hemostats and ligated (Fig. 75–3). The vessels should also be ligated with a nonabsorbable suture that is cut long to allow identification of the spermatic cord if retroperitoneal lymphadenectomy is performed. Strict hemostasis is obtained using cautery. The external oblique fascia is closed with a running 3–0 Dexon suture and the skin with a running 4–0 Dexon subcuticular suture. A pressure dressing of gauze fluffs and a scrotal supporter are applied.

POSTOPERATIVE MANAGEMENT AND COMPLICATIONS

As with simple orchiectomy, the most frequent complication is the development of a scrotal hematoma. Meticulous hemostasis and application of a pressure dressing for 24 hours can minimize this problem. The use of a scrotal drain should be discouraged.

Editorial Comment
Fray F. Marshall

The vertical incision in the midline raphe does work well for bilateral orchiectomy, but I have generally used a transverse incision on each side in the skin folds. Ordinarily,

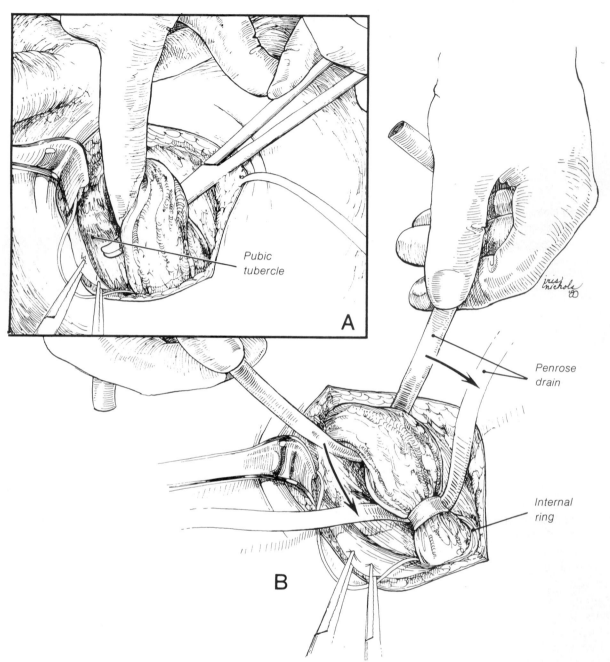

Figure 75–2. *A*, The Penrose drain is placed around the spermatic cord at the level of the pubic tubercle. *B*, After the cremasteric vessels have been divided, the Penrose drain is doubled around the spermatic cord and clamped securely, 1 inch from the internal ring. (From Crawford ED, Borden TA. Genitourinary Cancer Surgery. Philadelphia, Lea & Febiger, 1982.)

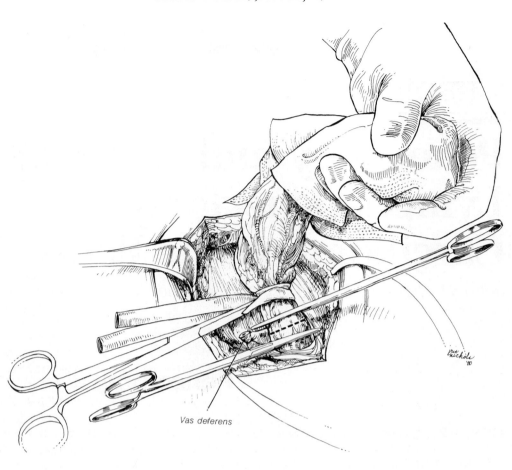

Figure 75–3. The vas deferens and spermatic vessels are individually ligated with nonabsorbable suture. Note that the testicle has been wrapped with a towel to prevent contamination. (From Crawford ED, Borden TA. Genitourinary Cancer Surgery. Philadelphia, Lea & Febiger, 1982.)

Vas deferens

hemostasis should be excellent. I have not left a drain because I am not sure what purpose it serves other than to drain blood.

An attempt should be made to fully open the inguinal canal with a radical orchiectomy and to divide the spermatic vessels and cord at the internal inguinal ring. I have opened several inguinal incisions during a retroperitoneal lymph node dissection to remove all of the spermatic cord because the cord was ligated well away from the internal inguinal ring.

REFERENCES

1. Kaye KW, Lange PH, Fraley EE. Spermatic cord block in urologic surgery. J Urol 128:720, 1982.
2. Giguere JK, Stablein DM, Spaulding JT, et al. The clinical significance of unconventional orchiectomy approaches in testicular cancer: A report from the testicular cancer intergroup study. J Urol 139:1225, 1988.
3. Thurner S, Hricak H, Carrol PR, et al. Imaging the testes: Comparison between MR imaging and US. Radiology 167:631, 1988.

Chapter 76

Penectomy and Inguinal Lymphadenectomy for Carcinoma of the Penis

John W. Colberg, Gerald L. Andriole, and William J. Catalona

Penectomy

GENERAL CONSIDERATIONS

Cancer of the penis accounts for only 0.3 to 0.6 percent of all malignancies in male patients.[1] The most common histological type is squamous cell carcinoma. For most patients, surgical excision is the most effective means of controlling the tumor and remains the treatment of choice. Histological confirmation of penile carcinoma by biopsy is usually the first step, followed by clinical staging, definitive resection of the primary tumor, and possible regional lymphadenectomy. There are several surgical approaches to resecting the primary tumor; the surgeon's choice depends on the size, location, and depth of invasion of the primary tumor.[2]

Patients with small superficial lesions on the prepuce are usually best managed with circumcision provided that adequate surgical margins are obtained. Small noninvasive lesions arising on the skin of the penile shaft may also be managed by wide local excision with primary skin closure. However, local recurrences have occurred in up to 50 percent of patients treated with circumcision alone; therefore, only the smallest lesions should be treated in this fashion, and patients must be closely monitored for local recurrence.

Carcinoma in situ, especially erythroplasia of Queyrat, is often managed successfully with topical 5-fluorouracil cream. Laser ablation, using a neodymium:yttrium-aluminum-garnet (Nd-YAG) or CO_2 laser, has also been employed in selected patients with small, superficial, or superficially invasive penile cancers. Deeply infiltrative penile cancers, however, cannot be adequately controlled with laser surgery.

Mohs micrographic surgery has also been employed for the treatment of selected patients with small, superficial penile cancers.[3] Adapted from the local excision of skin cancers, Mohs surgery is usually performed by a dermatologist who has special training in this technique. The Mohs technique involves excision of the penile lesion and microscopical examination of the underside of each layer by systematic inspection of serial sections. There are two standardized approaches: (1) the fixed-tissue technique, in which the tissues are fixed with zinc chloride paste before the excision of the successive layers; and (2) the fresh-tissue technique, in which the tissues are excised in the fresh, unfixed state and evaluated by frozen section. The entire course of treatment may last up to 7 days, usually on an outpatient basis. After the entire tumor has been excised, the surgical defect is allowed to heal by secondary intention. In appropriately selected patients, excellent control of the primary tumor has been achieved; however, local recurrences have been reported.

When penile lesions are not amenable to irradiation, local excision, laser ablation, or Mohs micrographic surgery, more extensive surgical therapy consisting of partial or total penectomy is indicated. The goal of partial penectomy is complete tumor excision with a 2-cm margin, while leaving an adequate residual penile stump, usually of 3 cm, for micturition in the standing position. If this is not possible or if the tumor involves the proximal penile shaft, total penectomy with creation of a perineal urethrostomy is indicated. For extensive, proximal primary tumors, total emasculation consisting of total penectomy, scrotectomy, and orchiectomy is recommended. More aggressive approaches have also included cystoprostatectomy, resection of the lower abdominal wall and pubic symphysis, and, in extreme cases, hemipelvectomy.

PREOPERATIVE EVALUATION

A biopsy of the penile lesion is usually necessary to confirm the diagnosis and to assess the grade and invasiveness of the tumor. Occasionally, a frozen section at the time of partial or total penectomy is adequate to confirm the diagnosis in cases that are clinically obvious.

The primary lesion and the patient's urine should be cultured before surgery. Appropriate broad-spectrum oral antibiotics are recommended for 3 to 5 days before surgery. Parenteral antibiotics are administered 1 hour preoperatively and continued for 24 to 48 hours after surgery. As part of informed consent, the patient should be advised of all possible intraoperative findings and surgical options, including the possibility that total penectomy may be necessary.

OPERATIVE TECHNIQUE

Partial Penectomy

The patient is positioned supine on the operating table (Fig. 76–1). If a total penectomy is a possibility, the dorsal lithotomy position or the use of spreader bars is advisable. A povidone-iodine scrub of the lower abdomen, pelvis, and genitalia is performed and the patient is appropriately draped.

The tumor-bearing distal penis is covered with a sterile glove or condom that is sutured in place to avoid gross contamination or spillage of tumor cells. A ½-inch Penrose drain is placed around the base of the penis to function as a tourniquet to diminish blood loss during the procedure. A sterile marking pen may be used to outline the margin of resection, which should be at least 2 cm proximal to the tumor. A circumferential incision is made in the skin and through the subcutaneous tissues of the penis. The superficial and deep dorsal veins and arteries should be individually ligated with 3-0 chromic catgut. Buck's fascia is then incised to expose the urethra and the corpora cavernosa. The corpora cavernosa are transected 2 cm proximal to the tumor. The corpus spongiosum is transected about 1 cm distal to the transected corpora cavernosa. The amputated specimen is sent for frozen section of the proximal margin.

The transected ends of the corpora cavernosa are closed with interrupted mattress sutures of 2-0 polyglycolic acid (Vicryl), being certain to include Buck's fascia, the tunica albuginea, and the intercavernosal septum. After the cavernosa are closed, the tourniquet is released and hemostasis is obtained.

The urethra is spatulated approximately 1 cm dorsally and sutured to the skin edges with interrupted 4-0 chromic catgut. The remainder of the penile skin is closed vertically with interrupted 4-0 chromic catgut sutures. Some surgeons prefer to pull the spatulated urethra through a 1-cm crescentic buttonhole in a dorsal skin flap, but the final cosmetic result is comparable with that achieved by other techniques of wound closure. Redundant penile skin may be excised. An 18 Fr. silicone catheter is left indwelling for urinary drainage, and a light compressive dressing is applied.

Total Penectomy

The patient is positioned in the dorsal lithotomy position (Fig. 76–2). A povidone-iodine scrub of the lower abdomen, pelvis, perineum, and genitalia is performed and the patient is appropriately draped. Special adhesive drapes are used to exclude the anus from the operative field. A sterile glove or condom is used to cover the tumor.

A vertical elliptical incision is made around the base of the penis at least 2 cm from the tumor margin. The incision is deepened through the fascial layers to expose the corpora cavernosa and corpus spongiosum. Dorsally the suspensory ligament of the penis is divided, and the deep dorsal penile vessels are sutured ligated at the level of the urogenital diaphragm.

Ventrally, Buck's fascia is incised and the plane between the corpus spongiosum and the corpora cavernosa is developed. The urethra is mobilized from the corpora cavernosa and divided. The corpora cavernosa are dissected proximally and are transected when a 2-cm proximal margin has been obtained. The transected ends of the corpora cavernosa are oversewn with hemostatic sutures of 2-0 Vicryl. It is not necessary to dissect the crura of the corpora off the pubic bone unless the cancer appears to infiltrate close to the margin. The specimen is sent for frozen section of the proximal margin.

The urethra is mobilized proximally up to the urogenital diaphragm. A 1-cm ellipse of skin and subcutaneous tissue is removed in the region of the central perineal body to create the perineal urethrostomy. The urethra is tunneled without angulation to this site, spatulated ventrally, and approximated to the skin edges using interrupted sutures of 3-0 chromic catgut.

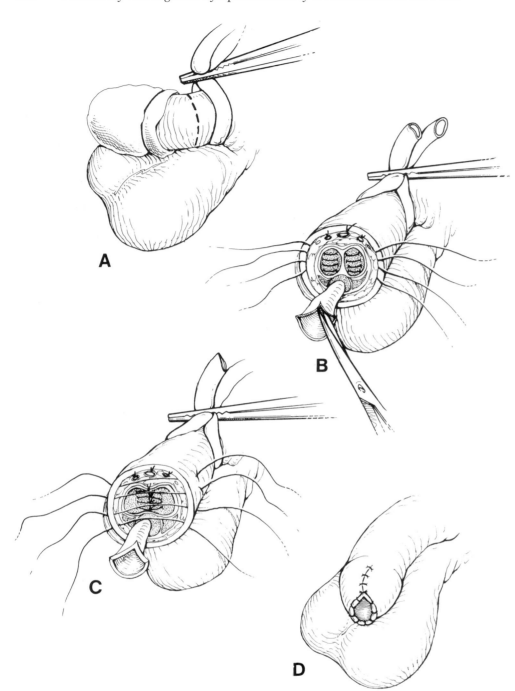

Figure 76–1. Technique of partial penectomy for invasive carcinoma of the penis. *A*, Isolate the tumor in a condom or sterile glove. Apply a ½-inch Penrose drain as a tourniquet. Incise the skin circumferentially 2 cm proximal to the tumor margin. *B*, Divide the corpora cavernosa and dissect the urethra in the corpus spongiosum distally for at least 1 cm. Spatulate the urethra on its dorsal surface. *C*, Close the ends of the corpora cavernosa with interrupted 2-0 polyglycolic acid (Vicryl) sutures. *D*, The urethra is sutured to the skin. The remainder of the penile skin is closed vertically.

The skin incision is closed transversely by transposing the scrotum anteriorly; this keeps the scrotum away from the perineal urethrostomy. A closed suction drain (Jackson-Pratt or Blake) or small ½-inch Penrose drain is left to drain the bed of the penile amputation. An 18 Fr. silicone catheter is passed through the urethrostomy and left indwelling.

POSTOPERATIVE MANAGEMENT AND COMPLICATIONS

Few postoperative complications are encountered following partial or total penectomy. Complications may usually be avoided by careful attention to the technical details of this operation. Early complications include wound infection and wound hematoma. These can be avoided by copiously irrigating the wound and obtaining meticulous hemostasis. Broad-spectrum antibiotics administered both preoperatively and postoperatively are also helpful in preventing wound infection. If wound infection or hematoma does occur, it is best treated by open drainage and secondary healing.

Urinary extravasation may occur under the skin flaps if a watertight urethrostomy is not achieved. Replacing the urethral catheter until healing is com-

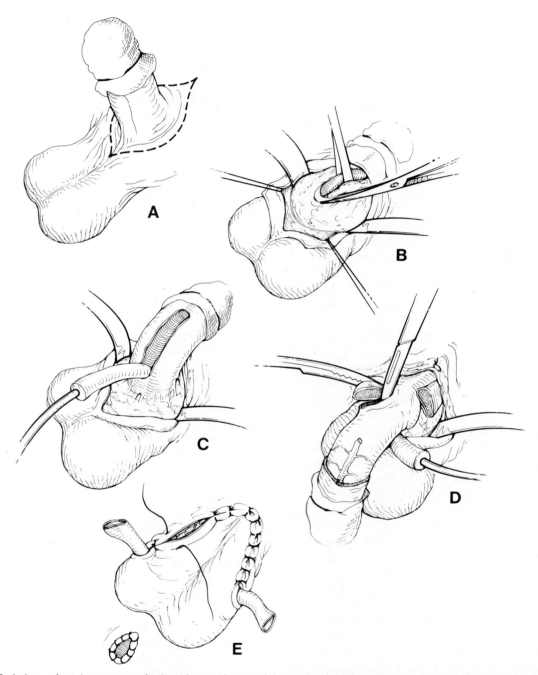

Figure 76–2. Technique of total penectomy for invasive carcinoma of the penis. *A*, Isolate the tumor in a condom or sterile glove. A vertical elliptical incision is made around the base of the penis at least 2 cm from the tumor margin. *B*, Buck's fascia ventrally is incised; the urethra is mobilized from the corpora cavernosa. *C*, The urethra is dissected proximally and transected. *D*, The corpora cavernosa are dissected proximally and are transected when a 2-cm proximal margin has been obtained. The transected ends of the corpora cavernosa are oversewn with hemostatic sutures of 2-0 polyglycolic acid. *E*, A 1-cm ellipse of skin and subcutaneous tissue is removed overlying the perineal body to create the perineal urethrostomy. The urethra is tunneled without angulation, spatulated ventrally, and sutured to the skin with interrupted 3-0 chromic sutures. The skin incision is closed transversely. Penrose or closed suction drains are left to drain the bed of the penile amputation.

plete usually is successful. It may be necessary to place extra sutures to achieve a watertight closure.

Late complications include stricture of the urethrostomy. This is best managed by dilation with metal sounds or meatotomy. If these fail, surgical revision is indicated. Strictures can be avoided by adequately spatulating the urethra, using tension-free sutures, and providing a well-vascularized urethral stump.

Early ambulation on postoperative day 1 is encouraged. Drains should be removed in 48 hours if there is scant drainage. The urethral catheter is removed in 3 to 5 days.

Inguinal Lymphadenectomy

INDICATIONS

The role and timing of inguinal lymphadenectomy in patients with carcinoma of the penis remain controversial.[4, 5] Noninvasive means of determining the true status of the lymph nodes are inaccurate. The traditional recommendation has been for surveillance on a 1- to 3-month basis if the inguinal lymph nodes are not enlarged or palpable following excision of the primary tumor and antibiotic administration. If the inguinal lymph nodes remain enlarged after a 4- to 6-week course of appropriate antibiotic therapy or if they become enlarged during surveillance, an ilioinguinal lymphadenectomy is indicated.

Surveillance management in patients with clinically negative lymph nodes has been recommended despite the acknowledged inaccuracy of clinical staging. For the 80 percent of patients who have pathologically uninvolved lymph nodes, this approach is advantageous because it spares them the morbidity of groin dissections. Conversely, for the 20 percent of patients who have occult microscopic metastases in clinically negative inguinal lymph nodes, withholding excision until they become grossly enlarged may squander an opportunity for cure. In most series, the majority of patients with positive lymph nodes who have been cured have had clinically nonpalpable metastases.[6] Many patients cannot be cured after nodal metastases have become clinically evident.

To identify patients in whom inguinal lymphadenectomy is necessary, Cabanas has recommended sentinel node biopsy.[7] However, several investigators have reported that removal of such a limited number of lymph nodes to determine the necessity of lymph node dissection is unreliable because there may be skip metastases.[8, 9] Some of these patients have developed incurable metastases despite careful follow-up after bilateral, negative findings on sentinel lymph node biopsy.

Because of the inaccuracy of clinical staging and the poor results of surveillance, increasing numbers of investigators have recommended standard inguinal lymphadenectomy for patients with clinically normal lymph nodes as well as those with clinically involved inguinal lymph nodes.[6] Recommendations for the standard ilioinguinal lymphadenectomy include[10]:

1. Persistent palpable lymphadenopathy after 4 weeks of adequate antibiotic therapy following resection of primary tumor.
2. Histologically or cytologically confirmed metastases.
3. Development of inguinal adenopathy in a patient with a history of penile carcinoma.
4. Large, proximal primary lesions.
5. Stage II cancer, either clinically evident or proved by imaging studies.
6. Palliation.

The morbidity of the standard inguinal lymphadenectomy may be considerable, with a 30 to 50 percent incidence of severe lymphedema and skin flap necrosis. This procedure may be unnecessarily radical for patients who have clinically negative nodes.

A modification of the standard inguinal lymphadenectomy has been developed as another option for patients with clinically negative findings on inguinal lymph node dissection.[11] The modified groin dissection differs from the standard one in that (1) the skin incision is shorter; (2) the extent of the node dissection is less, excluding the regions lateral to the femoral artery and caudal to the fossa ovalis; (3) the saphenous veins are preserved; (4) the transposition of the sartorius muscle is eliminated; and (5) the subcutaneous tissue superficial to Scarpa's fascia is preserved. This technique has been associated with less morbidity than the standard lymphadenectomy and is believed to be less likely to produce false-negative results than sentinel lymph node biopsies. If the nodes are found to contain metastases, a complete inguinal and pelvic lymphadenectomy is performed. With the advent of laparoscopic surgery, a laparoscopic pelvic lymph node dissection may be an option in selected patients.[12]

SURGICAL ANATOMY OF THE LYMPHATIC DRAINAGE OF THE PENIS

The lymphatic drainage of the penis involves three sequential groups of lymph nodes (Fig. 76–3). The

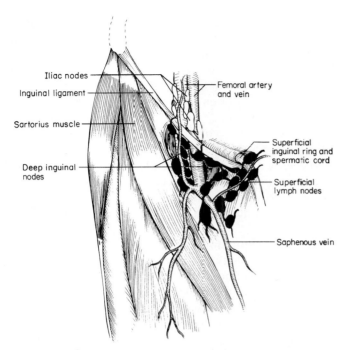

Figure 76–3. The pattern of lymphatic drainage of the penis involves three sequential groups of lymph nodes: the superficial inguinal lymph nodes that are superficial to the fascia lata, the deep inguinal lymph nodes that are deep to the fascia lata and surround femoral vessels, and the iliac lymph nodes that surround the external iliac artery and vein cephalad to the inguinal ligament.

ing follow-up, a unilateral standard groin dissection is recommended.

PREOPERATIVE MANAGEMENT

In preparation for inguinal dissection, the patient should receive a 4- to 6-week course of broad-spectrum oral antibiotic therapy following treatment of the penile lesion. This allows for reduction of any regional adenopathy and sterilization of any nodal infection and minimizes the potential for postoperative wound infections. The patient should be in optimal metabolic condition for this extensive procedure.

OPERATIVE TECHNIQUE

Modified Inguinal Lymphadenectomy

The limits of dissection of the modified inguinal lymphadenectomy in relation to the standard inguinal lymphadenectomy are shown in Figure 76–5. After general anesthesia (or continuous epidural anesthesia) has been induced, the patient is positioned with his legs on padded spreader bars. Sequential

first group are the superficial inguinal lymph nodes, situated at the anterior and medial aspects of the saphenofemoral junction, superficial to the fascia lata. The next group of lymph nodes are the deep inguinal lymph nodes, which are clustered around the femoral vessels deep to the fascia lata. The third group of lymph nodes are the iliac nodes in the pelvis, which receive afferent drainage under the inguinal ligament from the deep inguinal lymph nodes.

Anatomical studies have grouped the superficial inguinal lymph nodes into four quadrants and a central zone (Fig. 76–4).[13] These areas are defined in relation to horizontal and vertical lines that cross at the saphenofemoral junction. The lymphatics of the penis pass directly to the medial and central zones and occasionally to the superolateral zone. Lymphatic drainage from the penis usually does not go to the inferolateral zone unless there is massive adenopathy.

Clinical studies have demonstrated that in 80 percent of patients with lymph node metastases from carcinoma of the penis, only the nodes in the superomedial quadrant are involved. Bilateral modified groin dissection is therefore a reasonable alternative for sentinel lymph node biopsy for patients with invasive carcinoma of the penis with clinically negative findings on lymph node biopsy. In patients with clinically or histologically positive inguinal adenopathy, a standard bilateral lymphadenectomy is still recommended. When unilateral adenopathy develops dur-

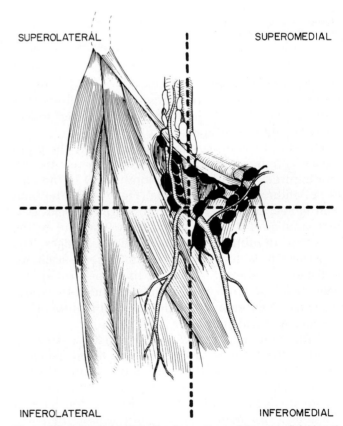

Figure 76–4. Anatomical studies have grouped the superficial lymph nodes into four quadrants defined in relation to the saphenofemoral junction. The lymphatics of the penis pass primarily to the central portions of the medial quadrants and the superolateral quadrant.

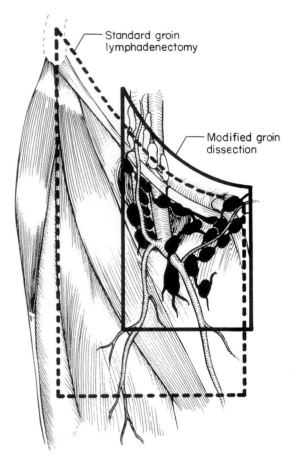

Figure 76–5. Limits of dissection of the modified and standard inguinal lymphadenectomy.

compression stockings are placed on the patient's lower extremities. A povidone-iodine scrub of the pelvis, genitalia, and lower abdomen is performed, and the patient is draped.

The skin incision is made 1.5 cm below the groin crease and is approximately 10 cm in length, extending from lateral to the femoral artery to the area of the adductor longus muscle (Fig. 76–6). The incision is deepened to the level of Scarpa's fascia. Dermal sutures of 3-0 silk are used to manipulate the skin flaps to minimize trauma to the skin edges. The superior flap is developed deep to Scarpa's fascia for a distance of about 8 cm. After the superior flap has been developed, the dissection is extended to expose the external oblique fascia, the external inguinal ring, and the spermatic cord.

A funiculus of adipose and lymphatic tissue can be identified coursing from the base of the penis to the superficial inguinal lymph nodes in the superomedial aspect of the incision. The funiculus is clamped, ligated, and divided close to the base of the penis. The main lymphatic drainage of the penis passes into the superficial nodes through the funiculus. The spermatic cord is reflected medially, and the superior portion of the rectangular bloc of lymphatic

tissue is mobilized inferiorly to the level of the inguinal ligament, dissecting it off the external oblique fascia and the spermatic cord.

The inferior flap is now developed for a distance of 6 cm below the incision in a plane deep to Scarpa's fascia. The saphenous vein is identified in the center of the surgical field, emerging from the package of tissue bearing the lymph nodes. The vein is isolated and dissected, and its numerous small tributaries are ligated and divided (Fig. 76–7). The plane of dissection is deepened to the level of the fascia lata. The inferior portion of the lymphatic package is dissected off the fascia lata up to the level of the saphenofemoral junction.

After the saphenous vein has been dissected to its junction with the femoral vein, the limit of the dissection is defined laterally by the femoral artery. The dissection of the lymphatic package progresses in a lateral-to-medial direction. The superficial lymph nodes are dissected off the saphenofemoral junction and surrounding tissues. The saphenous vein is carefully preserved. As the dissection proceeds, the numerous lymphatic channels encountered are isolated and individually ligated. The superficial nodes medial to the saphenofemoral junction are then dissected off the surface of the adductor longus muscle. The superficial dissection is completed by freeing the remaining attachments from the medial aspect of the inguinal ligament.

After the superficial lymph node package has been removed, the deep inguinal nodes clustered around the femoral vein are dissected superiorly to the level of the inguinal ligament, where they are ligated and

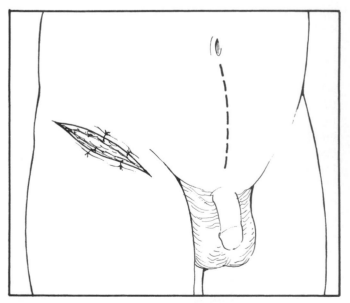

Figure 76–6. Modified inguinal lymphadenectomy. The skin incision is placed 1.5 cm below the groin crease, extending for 10 cm. A midline extraperitoneal incision is used if pelvic lymphadenectomy is performed.

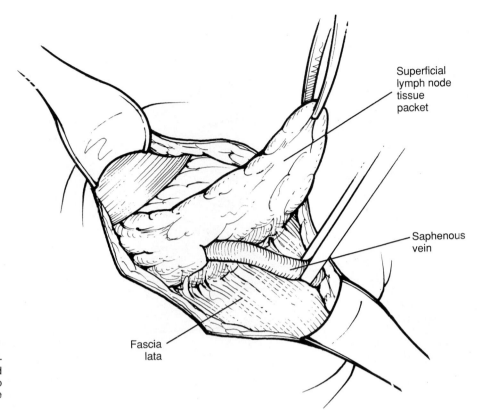

Superficial
lymph node
tissue
packet

Saphenous
vein

Fascia
lata

Figure 76–7. Modified inguinal lymphadenectomy. The saphenous vein is dissected and retracted but not divided. All tissue anterior to the vessel and between the vein fascia of the thigh is removed.

divided (Fig. 76–8). Lymphatic channels pass from the deep inguinal lymph nodes cephalad to the iliac nodes under the inguinal ligament. The most cephalad of the deep inguinal nodes is the node of Cloquet.

The deep inguinal lymph nodes are excised from the medial and lateral surfaces of the femoral vein and from the anterior surface of the femoral artery.

If the inguinal lymph nodes contain metastases on

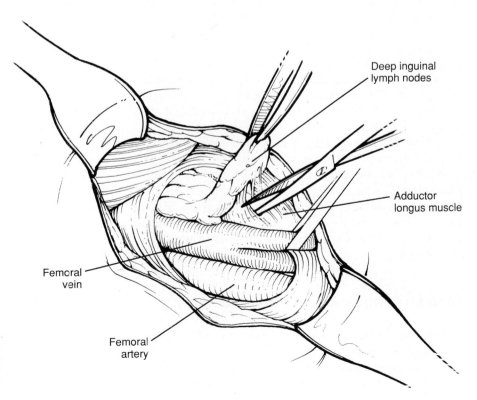

Deep inguinal
lymph nodes

Adductor
longus muscle

Femoral
vein

Femoral
artery

Figure 76–8. Modified inguinal lymphadenectomy. The lateral margin of the deep node dissection exposes the femoral artery. Only the deep inguinal nodes medial to the femoral artery and vein are removed.

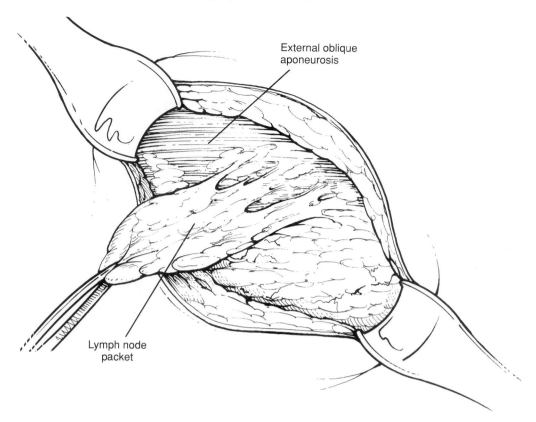

External oblique
aponeurosis

Lymph node
packet

Figure 76–9. Standard inguinal lymphadenectomy. The proximal skin flap is developed and the superficial fascia is dissected down to the external oblique aponeurosis.

examination of frozen or permanent sections, a bilateral pelvic lymph node dissection is performed through a midline extraperitoneal abdominal incision (see Fig. 76–6). The lymph node dissection is carried distally to skeletonize the external iliac artery and vein where they pass under the inguinal ligament. The pelvic lymphadenectomy performed in connection with penile cancer should extend more distally than that performed for prostate or bladder cancer. It is important not to leave unresected lymph nodes between the deep inguinal lymph node group and the iliac group. The inguinal ligament is approximated to Cooper's ligament to prevent the development of a femoral hernia.

The subcutaneous tissue is closed with 3-0 plain catgut sutures. The skin is approximated with staples or with a subcuticular suture of 4-0 Vicryl. The sartorius muscle is neither detached nor rotated to cover the femoral vessels with the modified groin dissection. Closed suction drains (Jackson-Pratt or Blake) are left under the flaps of the groin dissection and in the pelvis.

Standard Inguinal Lymphadenectomy

The boundaries of the standard complete inguinal lymphadenectomy are shown in Figure 76–5. This area is bounded superiorly by a line from the anterior superior iliac spine to the superior margin of the

external inguinal ring. It is bounded laterally by a line running inferiorly from the anterior superior iliac spine for a distance of 20 cm, medially by a line running inferiorly from the pubic tubercle for a distance of approximately 15 cm, and inferiorly by a line joining the medial and lateral boundaries. Various incisional approaches have been described. For cases that require bilateral dissection, a parallel incision 1.5 cm below the groin crease beginning inferior to the anterior superior iliac spine and extending below the pubic tubercle is recommended.

After the inguinal incision has been made, it is deepened to the level of Scarpa's fascia. The superior and inferior skin flaps are raised to the margins defined by the area of dissection. Meticulous attention is given to the development of these skin flaps. A common error is to make the skin flaps too thin. The flaps must include the thick layer of subcutaneous adipose tissue, leaving only a thin layer of Scarpa's fascia containing the superficial lymph nodes. All vessels and lymphatic channels are meticulously divided between fine catgut ligatures or electrocoagulated throughout the dissection to minimize lymph leakage. In cases in which large nodes are present and protrude to the skin, it may be impossible to leave sufficient subcutaneous tissue. In this situation it is advisable to excise the skin en bloc with the lymph nodes and to cover the defect with a myocutaneous flap.

Once the skin flaps have been created, the lymph

node dissection is begun superiorly. The plane of dissection is deepened to the fibers of the external oblique aponeurosis approximately 4 to 5 cm above the inguinal ligament (Fig. 76–9). The fascia lata is incised and reflected from the adductor longus and sartorius muscles, defining the medial and lateral extent of the dissection. The node-bearing tissues covering the sartorius muscle are stripped downward, defining the lateral border of the femoral triangle (Fig. 76–10). Medially, the node-bearing tissues are stripped from the adductor longus muscle. Inferiorly, the dissection is deepened to the fascia lata to come across the apex of the femoral triangle. The greater saphenous vein is encountered and divided between ligatures. More recently, authors have recommended preserving this vein after dissecting away all lymphatic tissue. The large package of node-bearing tissue is then dissected off the underlying tissues from the inferolateral to the superomedial margin. All fibrofatty and nodal tissues are dissected off the anterior and lateral aspects of the femoral vessels (Fig. 76–11). The profunda femoris branch is identi-

fied as it arises from the posterior aspect of the femoral artery, 3 cm distal to the inguinal ligament. This artery should be identified and preserved. Lateral to the femoral artery, the femoral nerve lies deep to the muscle fascia. It is not necessary to dissect the nerve because no significant nodal tissue exists in the region. The dissection proceeds superiorly and medially, freeing the entire package until its only attachments are deep to the inguinal ligament. These attachments are isolated and divided and the inguinal nodes are removed en bloc. Alternatively, if a pelvic lymph node dissection is performed simultaneously, both the pelvic and inguinal lymph nodes can be delivered en bloc. The specimens are carefully labeled so that the extent of regional disease may be accurately determined.

The sartorius muscle is divided at its origin to the anterior superior iliac spine and is rotated medially to cover the femoral vessels (Fig. 76–12). Its origin is sutured to the inguinal ligament superiorly, and its margins are sutured to the muscles of the thigh adjacent to the femoral vessels. This maneuver protects the femoral vessels from erosion should a wound infection or a major flap necrosis develop. The inguinal ligament is sutured to Cooper's ligament with interrupted 2-0 Vicryl sutures to close the femoral canal medial to the femoral vein to prevent postoperative hernia. Closed suction drains (Jackson-Pratt or Blake) are placed in the bed of the inguinal dissection and brought out inferiorly through the skin of the thigh. The subcutaneous tissue is closed with interrupted 3-0 plain catgut or Vicryl to eliminate dead spaces and prevent fluid collections. Excess or nonviable skin is excised and the skin edges are approximated with staples or a subcuticular suture of 4-0 Vicryl (Fig. 76–13).

POSTOPERATIVE MANAGEMENT AND COMPLICATIONS

The patient is maintained at bedrest for approximately 1 week to allow the groin flaps to adhere to the underlying tissue. For patients undergoing a modified lymph node dissection this may be shortened to 3 to 5 days. Sequential compression stockings are kept in place below the limits of the dissection. The closed suction drains are left in place until the 24-hour drainage output is less than 30 ml, usually by 5 to 7 days postoperatively. The urethral catheter is removed at 48 hours. Broad-spectrum antibiotic therapy is continued for 1 week postoperatively. Despite use of sequential compression stockings during the period of immobilization, thromboembolic complications may occur. Prophylactic minidose heparin may be indicated in selected patients. However, heparinization may cause prolonged lymphatic drainage

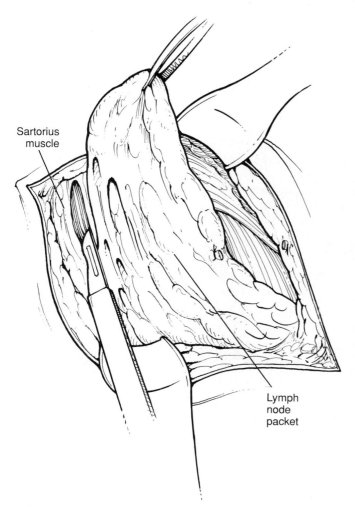

Sartorius muscle

Lymph node packet

Figure 76–10. Standard inguinal lymphadenectomy, showing the outer limit of dissection at the lateral margin of the femoral triangle.

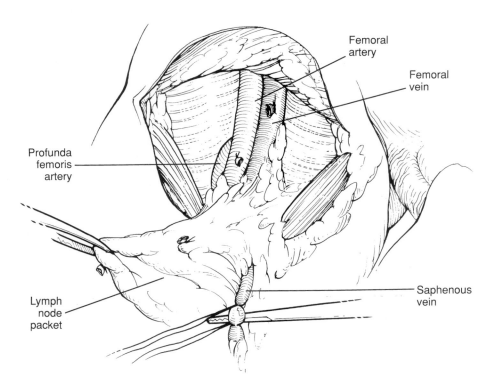

Figure 76–11. Standard inguinal lymphade-nectomy, showing the distal limit of dissection at the apex of the femoral triangle.

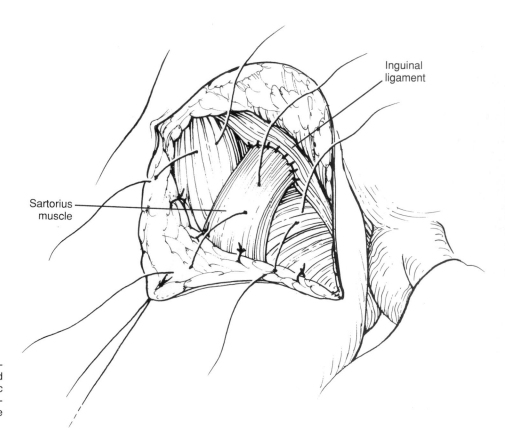

Figure 76–12. Standard inguinal lymphad-enectomy. The sartorius muscle is divided from its origin at the anterosuperior iliac spine and rotated medially, where it is sutured to the inguinal ligament over the femoral vessels.

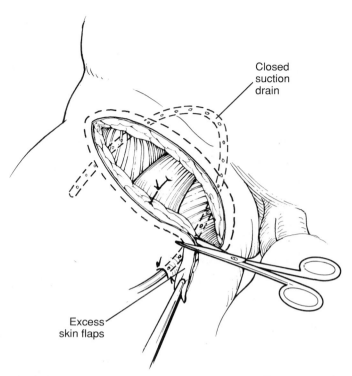

Figure 76–13. Standard inguinal lymphadenectomy. The excess skin is excised, and a large closed suction drain is placed in the wound and brought medially.

Closed suction drain

Excess skin flaps

or lymphocele formation under the skin flap. When wound healing appears well established, ambulation can be resumed. Fitted elastic stockings and elevation of the lower extremities reduce the incidence and severity of postoperative lymphedema.

Studies have reported a 30 to 50 percent incidence of significant morbidity and a mortality rate of up to 3 percent from a standard ilioinguinal lymph node dissection. The most common complications include wound infection, flap necrosis, lymphocele, lymphedema, thrombophlebitis, and hemorrhage from erosion into the femoral vessels. The significant morbidity associated with this dissection results from the wide excision of lymphatics, the devascularization of skin flaps, and the interruption of collateral lymphatics. Results from the modified groin dissection suggest that the morbidity may be substantially less.

Necrosis of the flaps may occur if the skin flaps are too thin, devascularizing the overlying skin, or when the tissue is traumatized during the dissection. Meticulous attention during the procedure may help prevent these complications. The management of skin flap necrosis depends upon the extent of necrosis involved. If the area of necrosis is small, debridement with secondary healing may be appropriate. If the necrosis is larger, split-thickness skin grafting or rotation of a myocutaneous flap may be indicated. Infection can precipitate skin flap necrosis. Infection is best treated by drainage and antibiotic therapy.

Hemorrhage from the femoral vessels is a uncom-

mon occurrence if transposition of the sartorius muscle has been performed. Lymphoceles should be initially managed by local aspiration. If the lymphocele reaccumulates, percutaneous drainage is indicated until this resolves. Chronic lymphedema of the lower extremities has been reported in as many as 40 percent of patients. It is best managed with waist-high compression stockings, elevation, and diuretic therapy. Patients should be examined every 3 months for 2 years, then semiannually for another 2 years.

Summary

Excision of the primary tumor and the regional lymph nodes is the mainstay of treatment for cancer of the penis. Patient selection and surgical technique are extremely important in controlling this disease while minimizing the morbidity and functional loss associated with surgery. Several options are available for the treatment of the primary tumor, depending upon its location, size, and depth of infiltration. Clinically negative inguinal lymph nodes may be managed by observation alone, by sentinel lymph node biopsy, or by modified inguinal lymphadenectomy. Standard inguinal lymphadenectomy is necessary to control histologically confirmed regional lymph node metastases. A pelvic lymph node dissection is performed if metastatic disease is detected in the inguinal lymph nodes.

Decisions regarding the treatment of penile carcinoma should be tempered by the fact that delays in diagnosis and therapy are common. Prompt recognition may result in the diagnosis and treatment of more favorable, early-stage cancers. Surgical excision is the only effective means of curing this disease. Neither adjunctive radiation therapy or chemotherapy is effective in salvaging patients who have not been cured by primary surgical therapy.

Editorial Comment
Fray F. Marshall

The efficacy of lymphadenectomy is questioned with the treatment of many genitourinary tumors. It can be therapeutic in penile cancer. The modified inguinal lymphadenectomy can be performed with lower morbidity. In higher risk patients with high-grade, invasive disease, the modified inguinal lymphadenectomy may be considered even with clinically negative lymph nodes. Important points in the operation include thicker subcutaneous flaps, preservation of the saphenous vein, less extensive resection, and closure of a potential femoral hernia site.

REFERENCES

1. Gloeckler-Ries LA, Hankey BF, Edwards, BK (eds). Cancer Statistics Review. National Cancer Institute, National Institutes of

Health Publication No. 90-2789, Bethesda, National Institutes of Health, 1990.

2. Horenbas S, van Tinteren H, Delemarre JFM et al. Squamous cell carcinoma of the penis. II. Treatment of the primary tumor. J Urol 147:1533, 1992.

3. Mohs FE, Snow SN, Larson PO. Mohs micrographic surgery for penile tumors. Urol Clin North Am 19:305, 1992.

4. Das S, Crawford ED. Carcinoma of the penis: Management of the regional lymphatic drainage. In Crawford ED, Das S, eds. Current Genitourinary Cancer Surgery. Philadelphia, Lea & Febiger, 1990, p 373.

5. Horenbas S, van Tinteren H, Delemarre JFM et al. Squamous cell carcinoma of the penis. III. Treatment of regional lymph nodes. J Urol 149:492, 1993.

6. McDougal SW, Kirchner FD Jr, Edwards RG et al. Treatment of carcinoma of the penis: The case for primary lymphadenectomy. J Urol 136:38, 1986.

7. Cabanas RC. An approach for the treatment of penile carcinoma. Cancer 39:456, 1977.

8. Perinetti EP, Crane DB, Catalona WJ. Unreliability of sentinel lymph node biopsy for staging penile carcinoma. J Urol 124:734, 1980.

9. Wespes E, Simon J, Schulman CC. Cabanas approach: Is sentinel node biopsy reliable for staging penile carcinoma? Urology 28:278, 1986.

10. Abi-Aad AS, deKernion JB. Controversies in ilioinguinal lymphadenectomy for cancer of the penis. Urol Clin North Am 19:319, 1992.

11. Catalona WJ. Modified inguinal lymphadenectomy for cancer of the penis with preservation of saphenous vein: Techniques and preliminary results. J Urol 140:306, 1988.

12. Rukstalis DB, Gerber GS, Vogelzang NJ, et al. Laparoscopic pelvic lymph node dissection: A review of 103 consecutive cases. J Urol 151:670, 1994.

13. Daseler EH, Anson BH, Reimann AF. Radical excision of the inguinal and iliac lymph glands: A study based upon 450 anatomical dissections and upon supportive clinical observations. Surg Gynecol Obstet 87:679, 1948.

Chapter 77

Surgery for Priapism

Jamil Rehman, Farhad Parivar, Serge Carrier, and Tom F. Lue

Priapism is a painful and persistent erection that is not associated with sexual excitement or desire and does not subside after sexual intercourse or masturbation. It involves the corpora cavernosa only. Low-flow (ischemic) priapism is a urological emergency similar to compartment syndrome. If untreated it can cause necrosis and fibrosis of cavernous tissue and lead to impotence. Electron microscopic studies show that after 24 hours of priapism there is necrosis of smooth muscle, destruction of endothelium with exposure of basement membrane, and thrombocyte adhesion.[1]

Priapism can be divided into two types: low flow (ischemic) and high flow (nonischemic). Adequate evaluation to identify the cause and type of priapism is essential before initiation of therapy because the treatment of the two types of priapism is considerably different.

PATIENT EVALUATION

The history should include questions regarding medications, illicit drug use, hematological history, family history of sickle cell disease or trait, concurrent medical problems, recent sexual activity, trauma, and previous surgery. The physical examination should be sufficiently detailed to uncover subtle neurological deficits, pelvic masses, and abnormalities of the perineum, prostate, and genitalia. In most cases the corpus spongiosum is not involved, but edema and induration of penile skin may occur.

Laboratory tests should include a complete blood count, urinalysis, and hemoglobin electrophoresis, if indicated. Coagulopathy screening or any other appropriate tests dictated by the history and physical findings are mandatory.

Penile blood gas estimation is an integral part of the evaluation of priapism. The aspiration of dark-appearing blood that is markedly hypoxic, acidotic, and hypercapnic is diagnostic of veno-occlusive is-

chemic priapism. In nonischemic priapism, blood gas determination will demonstrate normal oxygen and carbon dioxide levels consistent with arterial blood.

Cavernosal arterial blood flow can be quantitated using duplex or color Doppler ultrasonography. This is essential in the evaluation of nonischemic priapism.

TREATMENT

The therapeutic goals are (1) to avert the unwanted erection, (2) relieve pain, and (3) preserve potency. These goals can be achieved by surgical or nonsurgical means. In ischemic priapism the goal is to create a temporary venous drainage route from the corpus cavernosum to one of the following: the glans, the corpus spongiosum, the dorsal vein of the penis, or the saphenous vein. The ensuing high-flow state caused by vasodilator substances released by ischemic and necrotic tissue will thus produce an iatrogenic high-flow (nonischemic) priapism for several days. In nonischemic priapism the goal is to control the deregulated arterial flow by angiographic embolization or surgical ligation of the ruptured arterial branch.

Nonsurgical Treatment

Alpha-adrenergic agonist therapy is a very effective first-line medical therapy and can be used in virtually all cases of ischemic priapism of less than 36 hours' duration. After 36 hours, damaged smooth muscle will no longer respond to alpha agonists, and surgery is required to avert the condition. Our preferred therapeutic regimen is aspiration plus injection of 250 to 500 μg saline-diluted phenylephrine solution every 3 to 5 minutes until detumescence. This therapy is not recommended for nonischemic priapism: it is ineffective and may result in acute systemic hypertension secondary to release of phenylephrine into the systemic circulation through the wide-open venous channels.

Surgery for Ischemic Priapism

Distal Glans-Cavernosum Shunts

WINTER SHUNT. A Winter shunt[2] is the least invasive of shunting procedures. The dorsum of the glans penis is infiltrated with local anesthetic. An 18-gauge needle is inserted through the same needle site and advanced through the septum between the glans and one corpus cavernosum. The dark stagnant blood is aspirated and the corpus cavernosum flushed with saline. Once the blood return is bright red, the needle is removed and replaced with a Tru-Cut biopsy needle (Travenol) in a closed position. The outer sheath is held steady while the inner needle (obturator blade) is piercing the tunica albuginea and entering the corpora. The sheath is advanced over the needle (obturator), as would be done for prostate biopsy, coring out a segment of tunica albuginea, creating a fistula between the glans and corpus cavernosum. The procedure is repeated until four fistulas have been created, two on each side.

Detumescence may occur immediately or slowly over the next few hours. In infants, one biopsy-created fistula should be sufficient. For children up to the age of puberty, a single fistula in each corpus cavernosum should suffice. Brisk bleeding from the puncture site is not uncommon and should be controlled with a figure-of-eight 3-0 chromic catgut suture.

Winter recommends this procedure as the first step in management. If unsuccessful, the next step is a shunt between the corpus cavernosum and spongiosum. If that fails, the third step would be a saphenous vein-to-cavernosum shunt.

Comment.   The advantage of the Winter shunt is that it can be performed under local anesthesia in the emergency room or office. The disadvantage is that it is not effective in 50 percent of ischemic priapism cases because of the small size of the shunts. It is difficult to repair if the shunt persists.

GOULDING MODIFICATION. Goulding's modification[3] of the Winter shunt uses Kerrison rongeurs to create the shunt. A small stab incision is made in the dorsal glans penis to insert the instrument. A scalpel blade is pushed through the septum between the glans and corpus cavernosum to allow the rongeur to be placed in a position to remove a button of the septal tissue. The same procedure is quickly carried out on the other side; if there is a delay, the second corpus cavernosum softens and cannot be adequately palpated and punctured.

Comment.   An interesting idea but the procedure is not easy once the corpus cavernosum is decompressed. It also carries a higher risk of persistent fistula.

DATTA MODIFICATION. Datta's modification[4] of the Winter shunt uses a skin biopsy punch for creation of a bigger shunt than created by a biopsy needle. A small 2- to 4-mm incision is made in the glans sufficient to admit a skin biopsy punch. This instrument is briskly rotated and pressed to incise septal tissue. The loosened septal tissue is grasped with a hemostat and pulled out through the incision and excised.

Comment.   This has the advantage of producing a more effective shunt. The disadvantage is that it may destroy more erectile tissue in the glans and has a higher risk of persistent fistula.

KILINC MODIFICATION. Kilinc's modification[5] of the Winter shunt uses an indwelling trocar with multiple 3-mm side holes introduced through a stab incision in the glans. The obturator is advanced 1 cm into the tunica albuginea of the corpus cavernosum. The trocar is pushed forward by gentle rotation until it reaches the tip of the obturator. Upon removal of the obturator, the entrapped blood will drain. The corpus cavernosum is then irrigated with saline solution containing 10 percent heparin through a 25-gauge needle inserted through the trocar. A plug is placed in the open end of the trocar. The side holes act as a shunt. Glandular tissue around the trocar is sutured in a U-shaped manner to prevent bleeding from the cut edges. A similar process is repeated on the other side of the glans to hasten detumescence. The trocar is left in place for 2 to 24 hours. Intermittent compression is provided with a pediatric blood pressure cuff applied to the penis.

Comment.   The advantage of this modification is that it ensures an open shunt when the trocar is in place. The disadvantage is that the blood pressure cuff impedes venous drainage. Heparin solution may cause excessive bleeding from the wound. The trocar may cause more tissue damage than other methods.

EBBEHOJ SHUNT. In the Ebbehoj shunt,[6] a fistula is created under local anesthesia between the corpus cavernosum and the glans using a knife placed via the coronal sulcus. A No. 11 blade is inserted parallel to the dorsal surface of the penis into the corona glandis at its most protruding point. The tip of the knife is carried forward (deep and inward) in the substance of the glans. A small cut is made sideways and then the knife is rotated 90 degrees with the cutting edge toward the tunica albuginea. The tunica albuginea is penetrated at its tip and cut open for a length of 1 cm to create an effective shunt.

Comment.   The advantage of the Ebbehoj shunt is that it can create an effective and adequate-sized shunt. The disadvantage is that the terminal branch of the dorsal nerve and artery may be damaged when cutting in the coronal sulcus.

AL-GHORAB SHUNT. In an Al-Ghorab shunt,[7] local anesthesia is induced and a 2-cm transverse incision is made on the dorsum of the glans penis 0.5 to 1 cm distal to the coronal ridge. The glans is hinged back to expose the tips of the bulging corporeal bodies. The distal portion of the corpora cavernosa is identified immediately below the incision. A 5 × 5-mm segment of tunica albuginea is removed from each corpus cavernosum, including a portion of the septum, using sharp dissection. Grasping the core with a Kocher clamp facilitates this procedure. When detumescence has occurred, the skin is sutured back superficially so as not to obliterate the spongy vascular space of the glans penis.

Comment. The advantage of this procedure is that it creates a large shunt and should be more effective than Winter's shunt. The disadvantage is that the transverse cut on the glans may cut the terminal portion of the dorsal nerve branches, resulting in anesthesia or hypoesthesia of the glans. The chance of persistent fistula is high.

HASHMAT-WATERHOUSE SHUNT. In the Hashmat-Waterhouse shunt,[8] the patient is placed in the frog-leg position and regional or general anesthesia is induced. A 4-mm incision is made in the glans lateral to the external urethral meatus. A No. 11 blade is then introduced into the incision in the glans and plunged into the corporeal body. Dark, thick blood will gush out at this point. Both corpora are then milked until all dark blood has been squeezed out and replaced with fresh red blood. Irrigation of the corpus cavernosum is then performed with an irrigation fluid containing a 1-ml ampule of phenylephrine in 10 ml normal saline. The glans is then closed with a horizontal mattress suture of 3-0 chronic cat gut. No compression dressing is used.

Comment. The advantage of this shunt is that there is less chance of injury to the terminal branches of the dorsal artery and nerve. The disadvantage is that irrigation with phenylephrine solution in priapism of several days' duration and tissue damage may cause further ischemia of the tissues.

Proximal Shunts

QUACKELS SHUNT (CAVERNOSUM-SPONGIO-SUM). In a Quackels shunt,[9] the patient is placed under regional or general anesthesia and an 18 Fr. Foley catheter is placed in the bladder to facilitate intraoperative identification of the corpus spongiosum. The shunting technique can be unilateral or bilateral, depending on whether priapism subsides after the first shunt. With the patient in the lithotomy position, a vertical skin incision is made on the ventral aspect of the penis over the area of the bulbous urethra. The bulbocavernous muscle is reflected off

the urethra in the midline and preserved. The groove between the corpus cavernosum and the corpus spongiosum (which is easily compressible and flaccid) is exposed. A longitudinal incision is made in the tunica albuginea of the corpus cavernosum (which is turgid). The stagnant dark viscid blood is evacuated and the corpora irrigated with normal saline. Appearance of fresh arterial blood is the end point of irrigation. An equal-size incision is made in the corpus spongiosum opposite the cavernosal incision to create a fistula at the level of the urethral bulb (although the incision may be sufficient, it is better if a 1-cm long ellipse of tissue is removed from both sides). The shunt is completed by anastomosis of the anterior and posterior walls of each opposing incision with 5-0 continuous running polyglycolic acid suture. If detumescence is unsatisfactory, an identical procedure is performed on the contralateral side. The second shunt should be about 1 cm proximal or distal to the first to minimize tension on the spongiosal suture line.

Comment. The shunt should be called cavernosum-urethral bulb shunt to emphasize that it should be created in the perineum between bulb and crura. If placed in the pendulous urethra or penile base, it will not be effective and will carry a higher risk of urethral injury. The advantage is that it can be an effective treatment for priapism even in cases of severe distal penile edema or thrombosis. The disadvantage it that it is more difficult to repair if the fistula persists. It is more time consuming and needs to be performed in the operating room.

ODELOWO SHUNT (CAVERNOSUM-SPONGIO-SUM). The Odelowo shunt[10] is similar to Quackel's shunt except for interposition of saphenous vein between the two structures, allowing for a wider anastomosis. The cavernospongiosum groove is obliterated with a posterior row of 5-0 monofilament vascular sutures. A longitudinal incision is made in the spongiosum approximately halfway between the sutured cavernospongiosum groove in the midline. An appropriate length of previously prepared saphenous vein graft is laid open and trimmed to size. Anastomosis of the vein to the superficial lips of the spongiosum and cavernosum incision using 5-0 or 6-0 vascular suture is completed. A chordae-like deformity of the penis caused by unequal flaccidity or frank persistence of priapism on the contralateral side at this stage calls for anastomosis on that side. The saphenocavernosum anastomosis may be performed with 3-0 or 4-0 vascular sutures.

Comment. This procedure is time consuming and rarely necessary.

GRAYHACK SHUNT (CAVERNOSUM-SAPHENOUS VEIN.) A Grayhack shunt[11] is carried out under general anesthesia, with the patient in a supine and slight frog-leg position. The first incision is made over the saphenofemoral junction 3 to 4 cm below

TABLE 77–1. Surgical Procedures for Ischemic Priapism

Distal Shunt
- Ebbehoj   (1974)
- Winter   (1976)
- Goulding   (1980)
- Datta   (1986)
- Al-Ghorab   (1981)
- Hashmat et al. (1993)
- Kilinc   (1993)

Proximal Shunt
- Quackels   (1964)
- Odelowo   (1988)

Cavernosum-venous shunt
- Grayhack et al. (1964)
- Barry   (1976)

the inguinal ligament and extended distally in the line along the saphenous vein. The vein is mobilized for 8 to 10 cm distal from the fossa ovalis to bridge the gap between the saphenofemoral junction and the root of the penis. The tributaries are divided and ligated individually using nonabsorbable suture. The distal end of the mobilized vein is ligated and cut. The second incision, 1 inch long, is placed vertically over the lateral aspect of the penile shaft near the base of the penis. It is extended through all layers, including Buck's fascia, down to the tunica albuginea. Using blunt finger dissection, a tunnel is created between the two incisions. The distal cut end of the saphenous vein is passed through this subcutaneous tunnel without tension, torsion, or angulation. An ellipse of tunica albuginea, 1.5 × 0.5 cm, is excised from the corpora cavernosa. The distal end of the vein is spatulated to match the aperture made in the tunica albuginea, and the anastomosis is completed with continuous 5-0 suture. If detumescence does not ensue, the procedure is performed on the contralateral side.

Comment.   This procedure is effective but time consuming.

BARRY SHUNT (CAVERNOSUM-DORSAL VEIN). In a Barry shunt,[12] the corpus cavernosum is anastomosed to the superficial or deep dorsal vein of the penis. These veins are not involved in priapism. A 4-

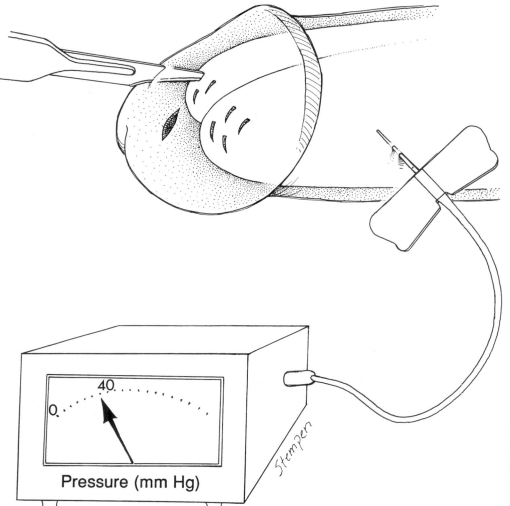

Figure 77–1. A glans-cavernosum shunt is made using a No. 11 blade. Stagnant blood is milked until the return becomes fresh red. Intracavernosal pressure is monitored. Maintenance of pressure of 40 mm Hg or less for 10 minutes or more is indicative of an adequate shunt.

Pressure (mm Hg)

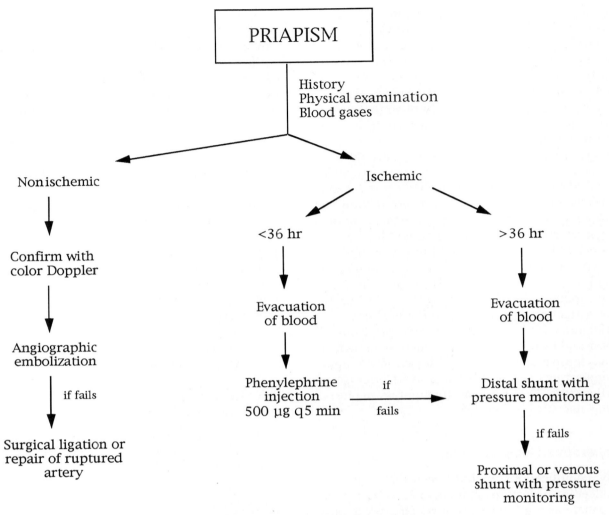

Figure 77–2. Algorithm for treatment of priapism.

cm skin incision is made at the base of the penis extending through the subcutaneous tissue and Buck's fascia. The superficial or deep dorsal vein is dissected from surrounding tissue, ligated distally, and divided. The proximal limb is spatulated on its ventral surface. An incision is made in the corpus cavernosum at the intended site of anastomosis. The spatulated vein is anastomosed to the corpus cavernosum.

Comment.   There are several advantages of a Barry shunt. It is effective treatment even in cases of distal penile edema or thrombosis. If the fistula persists, it can be repaired easily. It can be recommended for patients with recurrent priapism. A rubber band can be applied at the base of the penis to temporarily obstruct the persistent fistula if necessary.

The disadvantage is that it is more time consuming than a glans-cavernosum shunt. Pulmonary embolism has been reported after a venous shunt.

All the above shunts are listed in Table 77–1.

Preferred Methods

In ischemic priapism less than 24 to 36 hours in duration, we prefer aspiration and intracavernous

injection of diluted phenylephrine solution (250 to 500 μg) every 3 to 5 minutes until detumescence.

In ischemic priapism of more than 36 hours' duration, we prefer to perform a glans-cavernosum shunt with a No. 11 blade knife (Fig. 77–1) under regional or general anesthesia. The stagnant blood is milked out by hand, followed by irrigation with normal saline, not heparin solution, until the return is red. We believe monitoring of the intracavernous pressure[13] is very useful in determining how many shunts are needed to provide adequate drainage and prevent recurrence. If the intracavernous pressure can be maintained below 40 mm Hg for 10 minutes after the skin over the glans is closed, a successful shunting procedure is ensured.

The preferred treatment algorithm is summarized in Figure 77–2.

Postoperative Management

After the shunting procedure, the drainage of the corpora cavernosa is through the deep and superficial dorsal veins and the corpus spongiosum. A circular compressive dressing is to be condemned, because this may cut off all the draining pathways and result in further ischemia and even tissue necrosis. Occasional squeezing and milking of the corpora cavernosa by hand will help keep the shunt open and prevent recurrence. In case of recurrence, forceful milking may reopen the clotted shunt so that further surgery can be avoided. A pediatric cuff with an intermittent cycle is not necessary.

The penis will often appear to be partially erect even when an effective shunt has been created because of edema of the corporeal bodies and penile skin. When in doubt, blood gas determination can help differentiate induration due to edema (normal blood gases) from recurrence (abnormal blood gases).

Perioperative antibiotics should be given to all patients with ischemic priapism. Catheters should be removed as soon as possible and avoided in a cavernosum-spongiosum shunt. If treatment is successful, the patient may be discharged the next day.

In patients with intractable recurrent priapism, either oral alpha-adrenergic agents such as ephedrine or phenylpropanolamine or self-injection of alpha-adrenergic drugs can be useful to avert priapism at an earlier stage. Oral estrogen to suppress nocturnal erections may also be helpful.

Postoperative Complications

Early complications include recurrence of priapism, bleeding, infection, skin necrosis, cellulitis, abscess, gangrene, and urethral injury. The risk of postoperative infection must be anticipated and adequate perioperative antibiotics administered. Late complications include urethrocutaneous fistula, urethral stricture, and impotence, secondary to fibrosis of vascular spaces and failure of the venous shunt to close spontaneously. The most frequent complication of sickle cell priapism is recurrence.

Patients with prolonged or repetitive episodes of priapism are highly likely to suffer erectile dysfunction after resolution of the condition (secondary to fibrosis). In most studies, postoperative potency varies from 54 to 57 percent. Older hypertensive patients with priapism and those with repeated episodes from sickle cell disease have a poor prognosis for future potency. Traumatic priapism appears to have the best prognosis. Treatment of nonischemic priapism by selective pudendal artery embolization has the highest chance of success in preserving potency.

Pulmonary embolism has been reported after cavernosaphenous and cavernodorsal vein shunts. It is believed that this may directly relate to early shunt thrombosis. In other shunts, the spongiosum or glans act as a filter to prevent emboli from entering the venous circulation.

About 50 percent of patients develop some degree of erectile dysfunction regardless of the duration of the priapism or the method of management. Therefore, a carefully worded informed consent explaining the possibility of impotence should be obtained from the patient. This is an area of high medicolegal importance.

Surgery for Nonischemic Priapism

A history of perineal blunt trauma and a painless fluctuating erection strongly suggests a nonischemic priapism. Cavernous blood gas analysis will show arterial blood levels of P_{O_2} and P_{CO_2}. Color duplex ultrasound is helpful in identifying the high flow and the site of the ruptured artery, which confirms the nonischemic nature of the disease.

Angiographic embolization of the injured artery is the treatment of choice. If this is not successful, surgical exploration and ligation of the ruptured arterial branch will be necessary.

Editorial Comment
Fray F. Marshall

A logical approach to the management of priapism is given. Priapism is most commonly ischemic. The algorithm is well presented in the table.

REFERENCES

1. Spycher MA, Hauri D. The ultrastructure of erectile tissue in priapism. J Urol 135:142, 1986.
2. Winter CC. Cure of idiopathic priapism: New procedure for creating fistulas between glans penis and corpora cavernosa. Urology 8:399, 1976.
3. Goulding FJ. Modification of cavernoglandibular shunt for priapism. Urology 15:64, 1980.
4. Datta NS. A new technique for creation of a cavernoglandular shunt in the treatment of priapism. J Urol 136:602, 1986.
5. Kilinc M. A modified Winter procedure for priapism treatment with a new trochar. Eur Urol 24:118, 1993.
6. Ebbehoj J. A new operation for priapism. Scand J Plast Reconstr Surg 8:241, 1974.
7. Wendel EF, Grayhack JT. Corpora cavernosa–glans penis shunt for priapism. Surg Gynecol Obstet 153:586, 1981.
8. Hashmat AI, Rehman J. Priapism. In Hashmat AI, Das S, eds. The Penis. Philadelphia, Lea & Febiger, 1993, p 219.
9. Quackels R. Cure of patient suffering from priapism by cavernospongiosal anastomosis. Acta Urol Belg 32:5, 1964.
10. Odelowo EO. A new caverno-spongiosum shunt with saphenous vein patch graft for established priapism. Int Surg 73:130, 1988.
11. Grayhack JT, McCullough W, O'Connor VJ, et al. Venous bypass to control priapism. Invest Urol 1:509, 1964.
12. Barry JM. Priapism: Treatment with corpus cavernosum to dorsal vein of penis shunts. J Urol 116:754, 1976.
13. Lue TF, Hellstrom WJ, McAninch JW, et al. Priapism: A refined approach to diagnosis and treatment. J Urol 136:104, 1986.

Chapter 78

Surgical Treatment of Peyronie's Disease

Timothy M. Roddy and Robert J. Krane

Although initially described more than 250 years ago, Peyronie's disease remains a therapeutic dilemma for physicians today. The dilemma can be attributed to a persistent lack of knowledge about the disease's etiology as well as to the fact that the natural course of the disease, its effect on the tunica albuginea and erectile tissue, and the potential risks and benefits of medical and surgical therapy are unpredictable.

Peyronie's disease should be considered in the differential diagnosis of any process associated with a penile mass or penile curvature (Table 78–1). The hallmark of the disease is a fibrotic plaque on the corpus cavernosum that is usually readily palpable. The plaque can be located dorsally, laterally, or ventrally and can vary in size from millimeters to virtually the entire length of the penile shaft, with an average size of 2 cm. About 20 to 30 percent of patients have multiple plaques.

The clinical manifestations are usually evident only during erection. Painful erection is often the initial reason for seeking medical evaluation. Penile curvature with erection may also be evident, with curvature in the direction of the lesion. Another symptom, occurring in about half the patients, is diminished rigidity or diminished sustaining capability.

Painful erection can be successfully treated in most patients. Penile curvature and diminished rigidity are more difficult treatment problems.

The age range for presentation is usually in the fourth or fifth decade, although reports include patients from the teens and into the eighties.[1-3] The duration of symptoms at clinical presentation varies from days to years but generally averages 6 to 15 months.[2-4]

No single factor has been clearly identified as the cause of Peyronie's disease. Genetics, trauma, and atherosclerosis may likely be the major predisposing factors.

INDICATIONS AND CONTRAINDICATIONS FOR SURGERY

One further dilemma of Peyronie's disease is not only how to treat but whom to treat. The disease is often self-limited, although the natural course without treatment remains an unknown. The disease is not life-threatening, and in the patient for whom sexual function is not a consideration, no treatment seems justified in terms of morbidity and cost.

Most conservative therapies have excellent responses in terms of pain resolution (Table 78–2). Improvement in penile curvature, regression of plaque size, and recovery of sexual function are more variable and unpredictable. Conservative management for at least 6 months to 1 year is indicated for most patients before surgery is considered. The presence of calcified plaques or stable disease for more than 6 months may warrant earlier surgical intervention. Surgery is contraindicated in the presence of progres-

---

TABLE 78–1. Differential Diagnosis of a Penile Mass or Curvature

Congenital curvature of penis
Chordee with or without hypospadias
Thrombosis of dorsal artery of penis
Cavernosal thrombosis, hereditary hemoglobinopathy
Fibrosis secondary to local trauma
Leukemic infiltration of corpora cavernosum
Benign or malignant primary or secondary tumors
Ventral curvature secondary to urethral stricture disease
Late syphilitic lesions
Fibrosis secondary to severe urethritis with abscess
Penile infiltration with lymphogranuloma venereum

TABLE 78–2. Nonsurgical Therapy for Peyronie's Disease

Investigator	No. of Patients	Therapy	Results
Peyronie,[5] 1743	3	Water baths	100% cure
Helvie et al,[6] 1972	37	Orthovoltage	29 improved, 9 no change, 2 worse
Martin,[7] 1972	77	Orthovoltage	26 curves, 43 improved
Furlow et al,[8] 1975	90	Orthovoltage	No improvement in SX for treated group
Duggan,[9] 1964	87	High- vs. low-dose XRT	83% improved with high-dose; 71% improved with low-dose XRT
Carson et al,[10] 1985	40	Orthovoltage/external beam radiation	13 improved, 24 no change, 3 worse
Fricke and Olds,[11] 1939	31	Radium	16 with good/fair results
Soiland,[12] 1944	9	Radium/XRT	8 improved
Burford,[13] 1940	18	Radium	15 cured/improved
Burford and Burford,[14] 1957	96	Radium	74 cured/improved
	31	Radium/vitamin E	26 cured/improved
Scardino et al,[15] 1949	23	Vitamin E	100% pain free; 90% improved curve; 91% improved plaque
Zarafonetis et al,[16] 1959	21	Potaba	100% pain free; 82% improved curve; 75% plaque improvement
Persky et al,[17] 1967	13	DMSO	6 subjectively improved
Bodner et al,[18] 1954	17	Steroid injections	16 cured/improved
Williams et al,[19] 1980	42	Triamcinolone injection	14 cured/improved
DeSanctis et al,[20] 1967	38	Steroid injections + Vitamin E/Potaba/XRT	31 improved
Rothfeld et al,[21] 1967	12	Steroid iontophoresis	100% pain free; 66% improved curve
Whalen,[22] 1960	15	Histamine iontophoresis	12 improved
Miler and Ardizzone,[23] 1983	25	Ultrasound with topical steroids	19 with "some benefit"
Frank and Scott,[24] 1971	25	Ultrasound with topical steroids	92% subjective improvement
Gelbard et al,[25] 1983	9	Topical β-aminopropionitrile	3 with subjective improvement
Gelbard et al,[26] 1985	31	Bacterial collagenase injections	93% pain free; 67% with improved curve
Morales et al,[27] 1975	12	Parathormone injections	100% pain free; 67% improved curve
Oosterlinck and Renders,[28] 1975	10	Procarbazine	90% no change
Morgan and Pryor,[29] 1978	34	Procarbazine	91% no change or worse
Bystrom,[30] 1976	18	Procarbazine	56% good/excellent; 39% no change
Strachan and Pryor,[31] 1988	5	Systemic prostacyclin	80% not improved

SX = symptoms; XRT = external radiation therapy; DMSO = dimethyl sulfoxide.

sive disease. Any chance for spontaneous regression should be considered before surgical intervention.

PREOPERATIVE EVALUATION

Clinical examination remains the first means of assessing the extent of Peyronie's plaque. A patient's photographs can be used to corroborate his history and are important documentation to keep in the medical records. Most investigators would agree that it is difficult to determine exact localization, depth, and extent by palpation and in most cases the plaques will be underestimated.[32] Plain radiographs can be used to look for calcification within the plaques. Xeroradiography gives a better soft tissue resolution and is a more sensitive test, however.

High-resolution superficial sonography with a water bath allows a detailed objective assessment of the plaque. In addition, multiple areas of involvement can be defined.[33] The presence of calcification within the plaque is also well visualized with sonography. Sonography permits precise definition of the size and depth of the plaque, which are important considera-

tions in planning reconstructive surgery. The presence of calcification also defines the plaque as more likely longstanding and less likely to resolve with conservative medical therapy.[34] Sonography can also be used to follow plaque regression, either as a result of natural processes or as a response to medical therapy or surgery.

Simple cavernosography has limited utility in the diagnosis of Peyronie's disease and is not without risks. If necessary, the degree of curvature can be assessed by using saline to create an artificial erection. Saline artificial erections are most useful in the operating room at the time of reconstructive surgery. When performing cavernosography, careful consideration must be given to the osmolar concentration of the contrast agent. One case of cavernosal thrombosis and complete fibrosis of the erectile tissue was reported after cavernosography.[35]

In patients with symptoms of erectile insufficiency, dynamic infusion cavernosometry and cavernosography (DICC), using intracavernosal vasoactive drugs, helps delineate the cause of the erectile dysfunction. It also allows prompt visualization of the degree of curvature. Sonography is more accurate in assessing

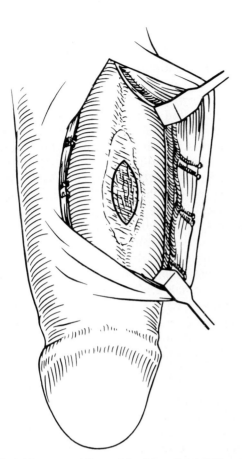

Figure 78–1. Exposure of Peyronie's plaque by elevation and protection of dorsal nerves and vessels. (From Glenn J. Urologic Surgery. Philadelphia, JB Lippincott, 1983.)

OPERATIVE TECHNIQUES AND RESULTS

In 1910 Horwitz[36] performed an operation for severe penile curvature and removed a portion of the tunica albuginea opposite the curvature without covering the defect. One month postoperatively his patient resumed normal intercourse.

Lowsley and Gentile[37] stated that Peyronie's disease was "incurable in the late stages" without surgery. They reported a 74 percent cure rate in their 23 patients who underwent plaque excision and free fat grafting. Lowsley originally described the procedure in 1943 and advocated early surgery because "tissues respond better."

Devine and Horton[38] sought a stronger replacement to cover the tunical defect. They believed that free fat grafts did not have the tensile strength to withstand corporal engorgement during erection. Their preliminary work employed grafts with autogenous dermis, artery, vein, and fascia. All the grafts except dermis became contracted and scarred. The dermal grafts were obtained from the abdominal wall and required special harvesting instruments. (Figures 78–1 to 78–3 illustrate the technique of plaque resection and dermal graft placement.)

Postoperatively, patients were treated with vitamin E for 1 year. All seven patients from the initial report were doing well, the longest follow-up being 3.5

the deep extent of the plaque and is the most objective means of assessing plaque dimensions at any stage of the disease.

Before reconstructive surgery the patient should clearly understand what the goals and risks of this therapy entail. An honest, straightforward discussion of the disease with the patient (and his partner) will allow the physician to ascertain whether the patient has realistic expectations for surgery. The primary goal of surgery is to straighten the penis, allowing resumption of normal intercourse. No surgical procedure can be advocated as capable of restoring normal rigidity if this is compromised preoperatively. Although reports have been made of improved rigidity in a limited number of patients in the literature, this recovery of function is unpredictable. If the patient has no interest in resuming an active sex life, most likely there is no indication for surgery. Surgery for the resolution of pain will cause more problems than it will solve. Painful erections can be managed conservatively with excellent results. No surgery should be undertaken until the disease progression has stopped and the penile deformity, sexual dysfunction, or both have stabilized.[10] It is essential that the physician have an objective assessment of erectile function preoperatively.

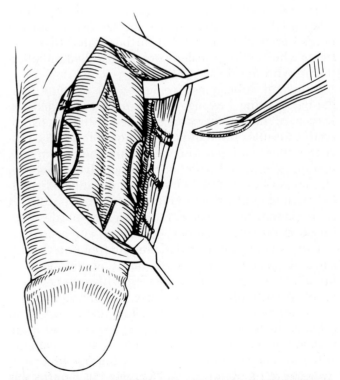

Figure 78–2. Removal of Peyronie's plaque and stellate incisions in the tunica albuginea. (From Glenn J. Urologic Surgery. Philadelphia, JB Lippincott, 1983.)

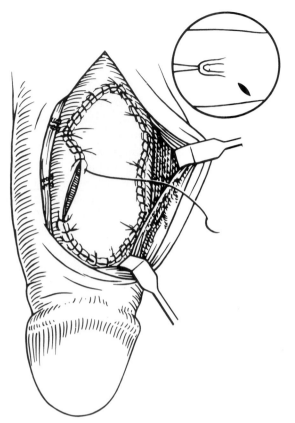

Figure 78–3. Graft secured in place with widely spaced 4-0 to 5-0 Prolene; edges are approximated with running sutures of 4-0 Vicryl. (From Glenn J. Urologic Surgery. Philadelphia, JB Lippincott, 1983.)

years. Devine[39] stated that "patients with Peyronie's disease who are impotent are not candidates for the dermal graft procedure." He further stated that "patients who had large lesions or who had had radiation therapy did not do as well."

Wild and colleagues[35] reviewed 50 patients after dermal grafting (average follow-up 17 months); 70 percent of the patients were satisfied with the postoperative results. Intercourse was possible for 53 percent of those patients who were potent before surgery. It is not mentioned whether postoperative impotence was a result of residual chordee or diminished rigidity. Dermal graft surgery is technically more difficult in a patient with prior radiation or intralesional injection therapy secondary to fibrosis and scarring.

The issue of postoperative erectile function is critical and must be assessed in terms of preoperative functional status. Is the difficulty with intercourse a problem with curvature, rigidity, sustaining capability, or all three? Melman and Holland[40] reported no success in their seven patients in terms of restoring potency using a dermal graft. Five of seven patients with normal rigidity but severe chordee preoperatively were impotent postoperatively (18 months follow-up). Hicks and associates[41] and Hall and Turner[42] reported that 80 percent of their patients had a return

of normal function with dermal grafts. Green and Martin[43] reported that 67 percent of their preoperatively impotent patients regained potency after dermal grafting.

Jones and co-workers[44] believed that 75 percent of patients who failed to resume intercourse after dermal grafting experienced this problem because of psychogenic factors. Performance anxiety was thought to be the major factor, and careful counseling involving the patient (and sometimes his partner) led to resolution of the problem. Preoperative mental preparation of the patient is just as important as the physical preparation so that he understands the procedure and has realistic expectations for postoperative recovery as well as surgical results. The need for special graft harvesting instruments and a second graft incision also made dermal grafting less desirable. Delayed graft contracture with recurrent chordee and the rare development of cysts and swellings in association with retained hair follicles and sebaceous cysts under the graft have been late complications of dermal grafts.

Nesbit[45] presented a surgical treatment for congenital penile curvature in 1965 that involved removing ellipses of tunica albuginea from the longer convex side of the corpus cavernosum (Fig. 78–4). Pryor and Fitzpatrick[46] were not satisfied with their postoperative potency results after dermal grafts (eight of eight patients) and performed Nesbit's operation in 23 patients with Peyronie's disease. All their patients had correction of penile curvature and 87 percent resumed satisfactory intercourse. Of 16 patients with diminished potency preoperatively, 13 returned to normal after surgery. Some degree of penile shortening occurs with the Nesbit procedure but had little effect on coital function.

Other series report similar excellent results (77 to 100 percent) for resumption of satisfactory intercourse using the Nesbit procedure.[30, 47, 48] Bailey and associates[49] reviewed 179 patients after the Nesbit procedure and found poor results in 14 percent at 3 months and 28 percent at 3 years. Devine and Horton[50] stated that the Nesbit procedure "is not applicable for the major bend we have seen in most of our patients."[50] Essed and Schroeder[51] proposed a slight variation in the Nesbit operation by not excising tunica albuginea but using "reeving" sutures on the convex side of the corpora to straighten the penis. They reported success in all five patients they treated, but larger clinical trials are needed. Lemberger and colleagues[52] further modified Nesbit's procedure by making a longitudinal incision in the corpora, without excising tunica, and closing the defect transversely. As a result, 94 percent had the curvature corrected, 94 percent resumed satisfactory intercourse, and 67 percent who were impotent preoperatively had potency restored.

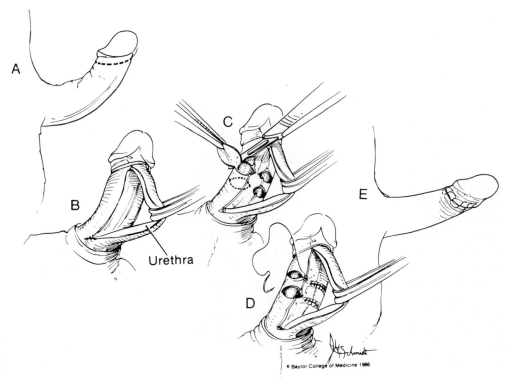

Figure 78–4. *A* to *E*, The Nesbit procedure for correction of dorsal chordee. (From Fishman IJ. Urol Clin North Am 16:73, 1989.)

In the search for simpler grafting materials, Das and Maggio[53] employed autogenous tunica vaginalis in dogs and found it very satisfactory. It was not difficult to procure without special instruments, well accepted at the graft site, pliable enough to accommodate the engorgement with erection, and firm enough to prevent ballooning with erection. At 6 months the graft could not be histologically differentiated from the tunica albuginea. Das and Amar[54] and Amin and colleagues[55] reported 100 percent success with autogenous tunica vaginalis grafts. Devine and Horton[50] stated that "tunica vaginalis, although acceptable for small lesions, is not strong enough for large grafts." The use of other graft materials, including lyophilized dura,[56] synthetic Dacron,[57, 58] and Dexon mesh,[59] has been reported, but the results are no better than those from other series. Synthetic grafts carry the risk of a foreign body reaction but require no second incisions for harvesting of autogenous graft material. All procedures need long-term follow-up to validate preliminary data, and no surgical therapy to date has clearly established itself as the best option.

Reconstructive surgery has potential complications that must be understood by the patient preoperatively. Any procedure carries the risk of failure or of making the patient worse. Postoperative glans anesthesia has been reported in some instances but is less likely when care is taken during the dissection around the dorsal neurovascular bundle. Bipolar cautery only should be utilized during reconstructive surgery to prevent thermal injury to adjacent tissue.

The use of penile prostheses in patients with Peyronie's disease has been controversial. These are used in patients who complain of preoperative erectile dysfunction. Bailey and associates[49] stated that "analysis of the results shows that patients presenting with severe impairment or complete failure of erection were likely to have an unsatisfactory outcome due to postoperative persistence of the erectile inadequacy." Ideally, surgical treatment of Peyronie's disease would result in a painless, straight, and natural erection that is sufficient for intercourse. If curvature, but otherwise normal rigidity, is the reason for sexual dysfunction, surgery to correct angulation is indicated. It may then be necessary to use a prosthesis if a potency problem occurs after surgery. When the primary complaint is impotence or flaccidity distal to the plaque, placement of a penile prosthesis (semirigid or inflatable) may be the best course of action.[49, 60–64] Penile implants can be placed to straighten the penis and restore potency. If further surgery is necessary after the prosthesis is placed, excising the plaques with grafting, plicating the corpus opposite the area of persistent curvature, or simply incising the plaques over the prosthesis with cautery should straighten the penis. Caution should be exercised if cauterizing over a polyurethane (Bioflex) prosthesis. No damage to a silicone prosthesis should occur when the cautery is used in this fashion.

In a case involving reoperation for a failed previous attempt to correct penile curvature, the loss of normal landmarks and tissue planes makes surgery very difficult. Fishman[65] recommends the use of a duplex Doppler ultrasound intraoperatively to identify the dorsal arteries as well as the use of magnifying loupes to improve visualization and avoid damage to the dorsal neurovascular bundle.

To date no reports have been published on the effectiveness of intracorporeal injection of vasoactive drugs as treatment for postreconstructive potency problems. This alternative therapy would allow correction of the angulation with surgery and pharmacological agents to supplement natural erections, if necessary postoperatively. Should the patient fail to respond to injection therapy, a prosthesis could be placed.

Any patient with Peyronie's disease debilitating enough to prevent intercourse must have his options carefully presented in relation to his needs. Is he interested in resuming his sex life? What is his present functional status in terms of penile curvature, rigidity, and sustaining capacity? Is the disease progressive or stable? On the basis of these findings, the best surgical alternative can be offered to suit his needs.

ERECTILE DYSFUNCTION

Ashworth[66] stated in 1960 that "the onset of Peyronie's disease heralds the end of effective sexual life." Impotence is the presenting complaint in 4 to 5 percent of patients with Peyronie's disease.[3] The normal physiology of erection has been provided in various reports.[67–69] The flaccid state of the penis is maintained by the pulsatile release of the adrenergic neurotransmitter norepinephrine, which keeps the smooth muscle of the corporeal lacunar spaces in a constricted state. The hemodynamic changes that initiate the erectile process are neurogenically mediated. They involve inhibition of the adrenergic (constrictive) tone in lacunar smooth muscle as well as direct relaxation of the lacunar and arteriolar smooth muscle of the helicine arterioles. Arteriolar smooth muscle relaxation leads to increased arterial inflow. This smooth muscle relaxation appears to be mediated by a nonadrenergic/noncholinergic neurotransmitter and an endothelial-derived vasoactive relaxation factor (nitric oxide).

Corporal veno-occlusion is an essential aspect of normal erection and occurs as a mechanical phenomenon in response to lacunar smooth muscle relaxation and erectile tissue expansion within the corpora. The corpora fill with blood and the peripheral, subtunical emissary venules become compressed against the tunica albuginea. This compression mechanically occludes the oblique emissary venous drainage from the corpora during erection. Corporeal

body pressure under these circumstances is then able to approach mean arterial pressure.

Corporeal veno-occlusive dysfunction (CVOD) has been termed *failure to store* erectile dysfunction.[70] If the expanding corporeal lacunar smooth muscle/ erectile tissue complex cannot effectively compress the emissary venules against the tunica albuginea, continued drainage during erection ensues ("venous leak"). This drainage is manifested as the inability to maintain corporeal body pressure, with resulting insufficient erectile rigidity, or the inability to sustain rigidity. Electron microscopical examination of the smooth muscle under the tunica albuginea in Peyronie's disease reveals it to be abnormal, which may contribute to venous leak.[71, 72]

Healthy tissue elasticity and compliance are essential to normal venous occlusion. Stecker and Devine[73] reported 17 patients with preoperative documentation, i.e., of erectile insufficiency nocturnal penile tumescence (NPT) monitoring, who underwent plaque excision with dermal grafting. Of these patients, 71 percent had subjective improvement of erectile function after surgery. No objective postoperative data of erectile function are given.

Paulson[74] stated that "removal of the plaque did improve penile blood flow" in these patients after dermal grafting. It is possible, however, that the graft restored normal veno-occlusive function in this area of the tunica, accounting for the improved erectile status.

Pryor[75] stated that Peyronie's disease caused impotence in one of four ways: (1) psychological (performance anxiety), (2) deformity preventing coitus, (3) flail penis, and (4) impaired erection. Those with psychological problems responded well to counseling. Those with deformity showed improvement after surgery to straighten the penis. Pryor described a subgroup of patients with "localized cavernous fibrosis" with absent tumescence in the area of fibrosis and an unstable penis with erection. He stated that "impaired distal erection in men with Peyronie's disease . . . is often due to impaired blood supply," implying that arterial insufficiency may be a contributing cause. Pryor concluded that venous leakage is not a "major factor in the erectile failure associated with Peyronie's disease."

Devine and Horton stated that "Peyronie's disease by itself does not cause impotence, but the psychologic effect of the distortion and pain can have a profound effect. . . . A venous leak is rarely found."[50]

Metz and associates[76] reported that "abnormal drainage from the cavernous body seems to indicate this condition as the underlying pathological mechanism leading to erectile impotence in patients with Peyronie's disease . . . it seems more likely that the fibrous tissue might interfere mechanically with the normal function of the drainage system in the area."

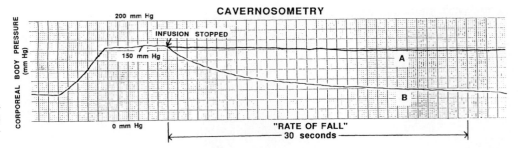

CAVERNOSOMETRY

Figure 78–5. Composite cavernosometrogram with normal curve (*A*) and corporal veno-occlusive dysfunction curve (*B*).

They measured ^{133}Xe washout after visual sexual stimulation and revealed insufficient corporal veno-occlusion in 11 of 15 impotent men. Cavernosography demonstrated CVOD in eight of 12 patients. Visual sexual stimulation is a variable, unpredictable means of promoting erection. Intracavernosal injection of vasoactive drugs provides a more controlled situation under which to perform DICC. CVOD is a dynamic phenomenon and is not visualized at surgery or in any excised plaque specimens. It can be suspected by history and confirmed with DICC under conditions that attempt to reproduce normal erections.

Figure 78–5 is a composite cavernosometrogram from a DICC. The corpora cavernosa have been infused with heparinized saline until a pressure of 150 mm Hg is reached, and at this pressure the infusion is stopped. The decrease in corporeal body pressure measured over a 30-second interval should not exceed 40 mm Hg. *Curve A* represents a normal rate of decay in corporeal body pressure from 150 mm Hg over a 30-second interval in a patient with a normal veno-occlusive mechanism. *Curve B* is consistent with CVOD in which the corporeal body pressure cannot be maintained because of abnormal veno-occlusion. Figures 78–6 and 78–7 represent cavernosograms that identify specific locations of abnormal venous drainage.

It is not currently agreed in the literature whether Peyronie's disease leads to veno-occlusive dysfunction based on a lack of elasticity in the tunica albuginea. The debate concerning CVOD as the primary mechanism causing erectile insufficiency associated with Peyronie's disease is not resolved. Overlap is seen in the patient population with Peyronie's disease with regard to other known vascular risk factors for CVOD (smoking, diabetes mellitus, elevated serum cholesterol level, atherosclerosis, hypertension, and obesity).

On the basis of the normal mechanism of erection, the pathophysiology of Peyronie's disease involving the tunica albuginea and, in some instances, the underlying erectile tissue, and the cavernosometric documentation of veno-occlusive dysfunction, it appears that the most reasonable explanation for erectile dysfunction in the setting of Peyronie's disease involves

CVOD. Any direct cause-and-effect relationship at this time has not been proved and must still be considered speculative. The fact that some patients have reported subjective improvement in erections after surgery that straightens the penis but leaves the plaque alone would argue for another unidentified factor being involved in some cases.

Summary

The diagnostic and therapeutic advances made in the management of Peyronie's disease have not resulted in a consistently reliable medical or surgical cure. The lack of an understanding of the basic pathophysiology of the disease process and the lack of an animal model for in vitro study have limited progress. In vitro investigation using cell culture techniques seems most promising at this time. Careful patient selection and longer follow-up periods in

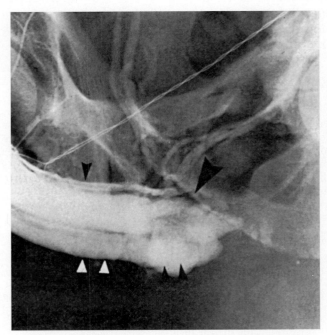

Figure 78–6. Cavernosogram with marked corporeal veno-occlusive dysfunction. Abnormal drainage patterns identified are the dorsal vein (*single small arrow*), corpus spongiosum (*double arrows*), and proximal cavernosal venous system (*large arrow*).

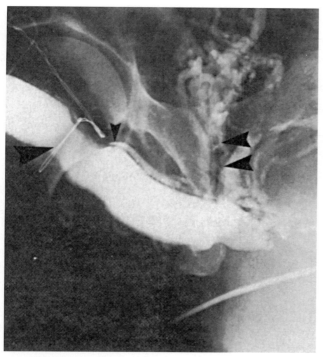

Figure 78–7. The circumferential corporeal filling defect (*large arrow*) is the Peyronie's plaque. The dorsal vein (*small arrow*) can be seen exiting the area of the plaque. Markedly abnormal proximal venous drainage can be seen in the internal pudendal system (*double arrows*).

large series will define what treatment regimen will best serve a clinical situation. Erectile dysfunction must be carefully evaluated and documented so that the treatment offered to the patient is based on his individual needs. An honest and open approach to the disease so that the patient understands his options will help offset some of the frustration in dealing with Peyronie's disease.

Editorial Comment
Fray F. Marshall

Peyronie's disease can occur in variable forms. The less severe form may require no treatment. In the more severe form with erectile dysfunction, straightening of the penis can be facilitated by placement of a penile prosthesis. As the authors state, surgery for pain alone causes more problems than it solves.

REFERENCES

1. Billig R, Baker R, Immergut M, Maxted W. Peyronie's disease. Urology 6:409, 1975.
2. Mira JG. Is it worthwhile to treat Peyronie's disease? Urology 16:1, 1980.
3. Williams JL, Thomas GG. The natural history of Peyronie's disease. J Urol 103:75, 1970.
4. Chilton CP, Castle WM, Westwood CA, Pryor JP. Factors associated in the aetiology of Peyronie's disease. Br J Urol 54:748, 1982.
5. Peyronie F, de la. Sur quelques obstacles qui s'opposent a l'ejaculation naturelle de la semence. Memoires de l'Académie de Chirurgie 1:318, 1743.
6. Helvie WW, Ochsner SF. Radiation therapy in Peyronie's disease. South Med J 65:1192, 1972.
7. Martin CL. Long time study of patients with Peyronie's disease treated with irradiation. AJR 114:492, 1972.
8. Furlow WL, Swenson HE Jr., Lee RE. Peyronie's disease: A study of its natural history and treatment with orthovoltage radiotherapy. J Urol 114:69, 1975.
9. Duggan HE. Effect of x-ray therapy on patients with Peyronie's disease. J Urol 91:572, 1964.
10. Carson CC III, Coughlin PWF. Radiation therapy for Peyronie's disease: Is there a place? J Urol 134:684, 1985.
11. Fricke RE, Olds JW. The radium treatment of Peyronie's disease. AJR 42:545, 1939.
12. Soiland A. Peyronie's disease or plastic induration of the penis. Radiology 42:183, 1944.
13. Burford EH. Fibrous cavernositis. J Urol 43:208, 1940.
14. Burford EH, Burford CE. Combined therapy for Peyronie's disease. J Urol 78:265, 1957.
15. Scardino PL, Scott WW, Ant M. The use of tocopherols in the treatment of Peyronie's disease. Ann NY Acad Sci 52:390, 1949.
16. Zarafonetis CJD, Horrax T. Treatment of Peyronie's disease with potassium para-aminobenzoate (Potaba). J Urol 81:770, 1959.
17. Persky L, Stewart BH. The use of dimethyl sulfoxide in the treatment of genitourinary disorders. Ann NY Acad Sci 141:551, 1967.
18. Bodner H, Howard AH, Kaplan JH. Peyronie's disease: Cortisone-hyaluronidase-hydrocortisone therapy. J Urol 72:400, 1954.
19. Williams G, Green NA. The non-surgical treatment of Peyronie's disease. Br J Urol 52:392, 1980.
20. DeSanctis PN, Furey GA. Steroid injection therapy for Peyronie's disease: A 10-year summary and review of 38 cases. J Urol 97:114, 1967.
21. Rothfeld SH, Murray W. The treatment of Peyronie's disease by iontophoresis of C^{21} esterified glucocorticoids. J Urol 97:874, 1967.
22. Whalen WH. A new concept in the treatment of Peyronie's disease. J Urol 83:851, 1960.
23. Miller HC, Ardizzone J. Peyronie's disease treated with ultrasound and hydrocortisone. Urology 21:584, 1983.
24. Frank IN, Scott WW. The ultrasonic treatment of Peyronie's disease. J Urol 106:883, 1971.
25. Gelbard M, Lindner A, Chvapil M, Kaufman J. Topical beta-aminopropionitrile in the treatment of Peyronie's disease. J Urol 129:746, 1983.
26. Gelbard MK, Lindner A, Kaufman JJ. The use of collagenase in the treatment of Peyronie's disease. J Urol 134:280, 1985.
27. Morales A, Bruce AW. The treatment of Peyronie's disease with parathyroid hormone. J Urol 114:901, 1975.
28. Oosterlinck W, Renders G. Treatment of Peyronie's disease with procarbazine. Br J Urol 47:219, 1975.
29. Morgan RJ, Pryor JP. Procarbazine (Natulan) in the treatment of Peyronie's disease. Br J Urol 50:111, 1978.
30. Bystrom J. Induratio penis plastica. Scand J Urol Nephrol 10:21, 1976.
31. Strachan JR, Pryor JP. Prostacyclin in the treatment of painful Peyronie's disease. Br J Urol 61:516, 1988.
32. Mohar N, Rukavina B, Uremovic V. Ultrasound diagnostics as a method of investigation of plastic induration of the penis. Dermatologica 159:115, 1979.
33. Fleischer AC, Rhamy RK. Sonographic evaluation of Peyronie's disease. Urology 17:290, 1981.
34. Altaffer LF III, Jordan GH. Sonographic demonstration of Peyronie's plaques. Urology 17:292, 1981.
35. Wild RM, Devine CJ Jr, Horton CE. Dermal graft repair of Peyronie's disease: Survey of 50 patients. J Urol 121:47, 1979.
36. Horwitz O. Plastic operation for the relief of an incurvation of the penis. Ann Surg 51:557, 1910.
37. Lowsley OS, Gentile A. An operation for the cure of certain cases of plastic induration (Peyronie's disease) of the penis. J Urol 57:552, 1947.

38. Devine CJ Jr., Horton CE. Surgical treatment of Peyronie's disease with a dermal graft. J Urol 111:44, 1974.

39. Devine CJ Jr. Evaluation of the dermal graft inlay technique for the surgical treatment of Peyronie's disease. (Editorial Comment.) J Urol 120:421, 1978.

40. Melman A, Holland TF. Evaluation of the dermal graft inlay technique for the surgical treatment of Peyronie's disease. J Urol 120:421, 1978.

41. Hicks CC, O'Brien DP III, Bostwick J III, Walton KN. Experience with the Horton-Devine graft in the treatment of Peyronie's disease. J Urol 119:504, 1978.

42. Hall WT, Turner RW. Experience with Devine-Horton dermal patch graft for Peyronie's disease. Urology 9:407, 1977.

43. Green R Jr., Martin DC. Treatment of Peyronie's disease by dermal grafting. Plast Reconstr Surg 64:208, 1979.

44. Jones WJ Jr., Horton CE, Stecker JF Jr., Devine CJ Jr. The treatment of psychogenic impotence after dermal graft repair for Peyronie's disease. J Urol 131:286, 1984.

45. Nesbit RM. Congenital curvature of the phallus: Report of three cases with description of corrective operation. J Urol 93:230, 1965.

46. Pryor JP, Fitzpatrick JM. A new approach to the correction of the penile deformity in Peyronie's disease. J Urol 122:622, 1979.

47. Frank JD, Mor SB, Pryor JP. The surgical correction of the erectile deformities of the penis of 100 men. Br J Urol 53:645, 1981.

48. Coughlin PWF, Carson CC III, Paulson DF. Surgical correction of Peyronie's disease: The Nesbit procedure. J Urol 131:282, 1984.

49. Bailey MJ, Yande S, Walmsley B, Pryor JP. Surgery for Peyronie's disease. A review of 200 patients. Br J Urol 57:746, 1985.

50. Devine CJ Jr, Horton CE. Peyronie's disease. Clin Plast Surg 15:405, 1988.

51. Essed E, Schroeder FH. New surgical treatment for Peyronie's disease. Urology 25:582, 1985.

52. Lemberger RJ, Bishop MC, Bates CP. Nesbit's operation for Peyronie's disease. Br J Urol 56:721, 1984.

53. Das S, Maggio AJ. Tunica vaginalis autografting for Peyronie's disease. An experimental study. Invest Urol 17:186, 1979.

54. Das S, Amar AD. Peyronie's disease: Excision of the plaque and grafting with tunica vaginalis. Urol Clin North Am 9:1, 1982.

55. Amin M, Broghamer WL Jr., Harty JI, Long R Jr. Autogenous tunica vaginalis graft for Peyronie's disease: An experimental study and its clinical application. J Urol 124:815, 1980.

56. Collins JP. Experience with lyophilized human dura for treatment of Peyronie's disease. Urology 31:379, 1988.

57. Lowe DH, Ho PC, Parson CL, et al. Surgical treatment of Peyronie's disease with Dacron graft. Urology 19:609, 1982.

58. Schiffman ZJ, Gursel EO, Laor E. Use of Dacron graft in Peyronie's disease. Urology 25:38, 1985.

59. Bazeed MA, Thuroff JW, Schmidt RA, et al. New surgical procedure for management of Peyronie's disease. Urology 21:501, 1983.

60. Raz S, DeKernion JB, Kaufman JJ. Surgical treatment of Peyronie's disease: A new approach. J Urol 177:598, 1977.

61. Carson CC, Hodge GB, Anderson EE. Penile prosthesis in Peyronie's disease. Br J Urol 55:417, 1983.

62. Subrini L. Surgical treatment of Peyronie's disease using penile implants: Survey of 69 patients. J Urol 132:47, 1984.

63. Gangai M, Rivera LR, Spence CR. Peyronie's plaque: Excision and graft versus incision and stent. J Urol 127:55, 1982.

64. Bruskewitz R, Raz S. Surgical considerations in the treatment of Peyronie's disease. Urology 15:134, 1980.

65. Fishman IJ. Corporeal reconstruction procedures for complicated penile implants. Urol Clin North Am 16:73, 1989.

66. Ashworth A. Peyronie's disease. Proc Roy Soc Med 53:652, 1960.

67. Broderick GA, Lue TF. Priapism and the physiology of erection. AUA Update Series Vol. 7, Lesson 29.

68. Lue TF, Tanagho EA. Physiology of erection and pharmacological management of impotence. J Urol 137:829, 1987.

69. Saenz de Tejada I, Goldstein I, Krane RJ. Local control of penile erection. Nerves, smooth muscle and endothelium. Urol Clin North Am 15:1, 1988.

70. Goldstein I. Nomenclature and classification. Presented at the Third Biennial World Meeting on Impotence. Boston, Massachusetts, October, 1988.

71. Smith BH. Peyronie's disease. Am J Clin Pathol 45:670, 1966.

72. Vande Berg JS, Devine CJ, Horton CE, et al. Peyronie's disease: An electron microscopic study. J Urol 126:333, 1981.

73. Stecker JF Jr., Devine CJ Jr. Evaluation of erectile dysfunction in patients with Peyronie's disease. J Urol 132:680, 1984.

74. Paulson DF. Evaluation of erectile dysfunction in patients with Peyronie's disease. (Editorial Comment.) J Urol 132:681, 1984.

75. Pryor JP. Peyronie's disease and impotence. Acta Urol Belg 56:317, 1988.

76. Metz P, Ebbehoj J, Uhrenholdt A, Wagner G. Peyronie's disease and erectile failure. J Urol 130:1103, 1983.

Chapter 79

Gangrene of the Male Genitalia

Franklin C. Lowe

The pathophysiology of gangrene of the male genitalia can result as a consequence of infectious, traumatic, or vasculogenic causes (Table 79–1). The major differentiation in approach and management of this entity depends on whether it is infectious gangrene or dry gangrene, usually vasculogenic in origin. Infectious gangrene of the penis, scrotum, and perineum is best known as Fournier gangrene. Classically, infectious gangrene can result from idiopathic, colorectal, or genitourinary processes. In addition, most traumatic (mechanical or postsurgical) causes lead to the development of progressive synergistic and necrotizing fasciitis. Therefore, most patients with genital gangrene need emergency intervention to prevent further tissue destruction and death. Mortality noted for this entity can approach 50 percent.[1] Patients with only dry gangrene can be treated promptly but usually do not require emergency intervention.

PREOPERATIVE MANAGEMENT

Diagnosis of Fournier gangrene can usually be made from clinical examination findings of fever; edematous genitalia with areas of eschar and frank necrosis; and cellulitic changes or crepitus, extending into the perineum and onto the abdominal wall. Once these are recognized, prompt evaluation and therapy are required. Initial evaluation includes a complete history including sexual practices and a complete physical examination including an appropriate rectal examination. Retrograde urethrography is usually performed to rule out lower urinary tract causes, in particular urethral strictures and urinary extravasation. In about 25 percent of patients Fournier gangrene is caused by pathological entities of the urinary tract.[2] An abdominal radiograph is obtained to rule out any intra-abdominal process as well as to evaluate the abdomen for the presence and extent of perifascial gas. Blood, urine, and pus specimens should be obtained for both Gram staining and culturing before the initiation of antibiotic therapy.

The current literature and our experience indicate that multiple aerobic and anaerobic organisms can be obtained in most cases of infectious gangrene.[3] The most commonly cultured organisms are gram-negative rods from the Enterobacteriaceae family and gram-positive streptococci and staphylococci. *Bacteroides fragilis* and streptococci are the most frequently found anaerobes. Therefore, appropriate antibiotic coverage should include gentamicin (4.5 mg/kg/day), metronidazole (500 mg q6h), and penicillin G (2 million units q4h). The rationale for this combination is that the aminoglycoside covers the gram-negative rods, metronidazole covers *Bacteroides* species and anaerobes, and penicillin G covers anaerobes, streptococci, enterococci, and *Clostridium* species. Other frequently used antibiotics, in a combination with one or more of the previously mentioned antibiotics, include ticarcillin with clavulanic acid (3.1 gm q6h), ampicillin (2 gm q4h), and clindamycin (600 mg q6h). Cephalosporins should not be given in place of the penicillin because enterococci and anaerobic streptococci coverage is inadequate. However, some of the third-generation cephalosporins (cefoxitin, ceftazidime) provide adequate gram-negative and *Bacteroides* coverage and can be used in place of gentamicin and metronidazole.

In addition to the initiation of antibiotic therapy, metabolic stabilization of the patient is usually required before early surgical intervention. Almost half of the patients with Fournier gangrene are diabetic, and treatment for hyperglycemia and acidosis is frequently needed.[4] Azotemia and dehydration are also commonly found in these often febrile and septic patients; therefore, aggressive fluid management usually with lactated Ringer's solution is necessary. Approximately 10 to 20 percent of patients are in septic shock at the time of initial examination and require immediate transfer to an intensive care unit for medical management with intravenous fluids, antibiotics,

TABLE 79–1. Causes of Gangrene of the Male Genitalia

Infectious (Fournier gangrene)
  Idiopathic
  Genitourinary
    Urethral stricture
  Colorectal
    Perirectal abscess
    Fissura in ano
Traumatic
  Thermal
  Chemical
  Mechanical
    Scratches
    Human bites
    Coitus
    Fellatio
    Anal intercourse
Vasculogenic
Arterial
  Tourniquet syndrome
    String
    Hair
    Condom catheter
    Rubber bands
    Rings
  Embolic
    Streptokinase therapy
    Abdominal aortic aneurysm
    Arterial heroin injection
  Progressive atherosclerosis
    Azotemia secondary to hyperparathyroidism
    Diabetes mellitus
Venous
  Venous thrombosis
    Compression dressings
    Vena cava thrombosis
    Priapism
Miscellaneous
  Warfarin therapy
  Kaposi sarcoma
  Wegener granulomatosis
  Idiopathic thrombocytopenic purpura
  Disseminated intravascular coagulation

and vasoactive medications. Once stabilized, emergent surgical intervention is also needed.

SURGICAL OPTIONS

The extent and cause of the disease process usually dictate the operative approach. If retrograde urethrography has demonstrated either urinary extravasation or significant urethral disease, proximal urinary diversion via either trocar or open suprapubic cystostomy is necessary. Extensive penile involvement or edema is another strong indication for urinary diversion. If perirectal disease is present, proctoscopy should be performed at the beginning of the surgical procedure. A diverting colostomy should be performed when significant rectal involvement is noted.

Classical teaching recommends prompt and aggressive surgical debridement and excision to drain infected tissues and limit the progression of tissue ne-

crosis. Excision was carried out until clearly viable tissue was encountered. This maneuver was frequently extensive. Scarpa's fascia of the abdominal wall is contiguous with the dartos of the penis and Colles' fascia of the perineum; therefore, extensive spread of the infectious gangrene process can occur along these planes.[2] However, the resulting large open wounds would then need extensive reconstructive surgery—including rotational flaps and skin grafts to achieve closure. Therefore, the current trend has been to leave marginal tissue to try to limit the need for extensive reconstructive surgery for wound closure. Secondary excision of demarcated areas provides the best chance for conserving skin. However, this approach usually requires repeat debridements every 48 to 72 hours until the infection is controlled and the devitalized tissues are excised.

Orchiectomy was also previously recommended in the management of this disease; however, the testes, with their own separate blood supply, are almost always viable. Orchiectomy is rarely necessary unless the spermatic cord itself is involved. However, completely denuded testes need to be either covered with skin grafts or buried in subcutaneous upper thigh pockets. Fortunately, sufficient scrotal tissue frequently remains to regenerate, expand, and provide adequate coverage.

Multiple incisions with drainage may obviate the need for more aggressive debridement and excision.[5] Multiple through-and-through Penrose drains can provide adequate drainage (Fig. 79–1). This technique is particularly useful when crepitus extends up the abdominal wall, without full-thickness skin and subcutaneous necrosis.

I excise only frankly necrotic tissue and place mul-

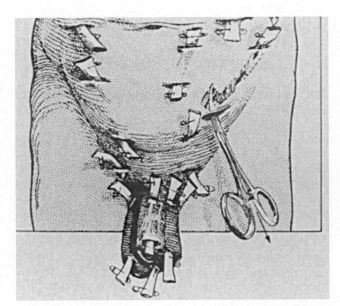

Figure 79–1. Radical drainage of the penis, scrotum, and abdominal wall with Penrose drains. (From Kearney GP, Carling PC. Fournier's gangrene: An approach to its management. J Urol 130:697, 1983.)

tiple drains. Careful exploration of the perineum, genitalia, and abdomen for loculations is mandatory at the time of initial surgical intervention. I usually place a trocar cystostomy unless the process has extended onto the abdominal wall; in that case, an open suprapubic cystostomy is performed.

OPERATIVE TECHNIQUE

Several examples follow to provide an outline for various surgical techniques.

Localized to the Scrotum

The patient should be placed in the dorsal lithotomy position with the lower abdomen, genitalia, and perineum prepared into the operative field. Usually, a Foley catheter is inserted and the bladder filled with 300 to 500 ml sterile normal saline. Once the bladder is easily palpable, a percutaneous trocar cystostomy tube is placed. Usually, a small skin incision is made approximately 2 fingerbreadths above the pubic symphysis. A 4-inch, 22-gauge spinal needle is used to determine the depth of the bladder below the skin and the angle required for insertion of the larger cystostomy tube into the bladder. Once inserted, the cystostomy is held in place with nylon sutures.

An incision is made around the frankly necrotic eschar areas of the scrotum. It is carried down through the layers of scrotal wall until viable tissue is encountered, usually the parietal layer of the tunica vaginalis or spermatic fascia. The necrotic area is excised; some of this material is sent for culture. Bovie cauterization of bleeding vessels is achieved. The wound is copiously irrigated with antibiotic (bacitracin and kanamycin) solution. A Kelly clamp

is inserted above the viable layers and tunneled until it reaches the edges of the edematous or questionable tissues—usually in the groin creases. A skin incision is made onto the tips of the Kelly clamp until exposed. Penrose drains are then brought through the tissue to the area of excision. Two or three drains are usually placed. Subsequently, the drains are sutured in place and brought out inferiorly through the scrotal defect. The subcutaneous tissues and dartos muscle are reapproximated if possible, using interrupted 2-0 chromic sutures. Several 2-0 Prolene retention sutures are placed through all layers for wound closure. The skin edges are left open. The wound is dressed with gauze fluffs and a scrotal supporter/T-binder.

If the loss of the scrotal skin is extensive, either split-thickness skin grafts or pedicle flaps might be needed for reconstruction. Before scrotal reconstruction, the infection must be controlled and the wounds cleaned and appropriately debrided.

Scrotal reconstruction can be undertaken with split-thickness grafts for both partial and total loss. The anterolateral aspect of the thigh is the donor site most frequently selected. The skin is harvested with an air-powered dermatome after the site has been cleaned, shaved, and coated with mineral oil. The donor site is covered with oxygen-permeable or oxygen-impermeable polyurethane film dressings. Previously, petrolatum or Congo red–impregnated gauze was commonly used to cover the donor sites.

The thickness of the graft can vary from 0.010 inch (thin) to 0.018 inch (thick). The thickness of the graft is usually determined by a combination of factors—the skin of the donor site and the size and location of the recipient site. Subsequently, the graft is meshed to improve chances for a complete "take" by allowing drainage through the pores and to permit coverage of

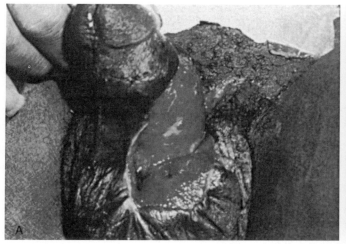 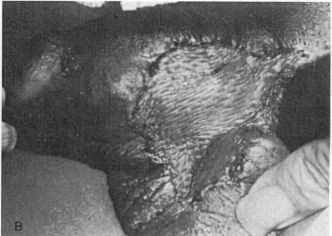

Figure 79–2. Partial scrotal and penile skin loss from infectious gangrene secondary to direct injection of heroin into the scrotum. *A,* The wound after three operative procedures and a week of hyperbaric oxygen therapy. *B,* The wound after successful split-thickness skin grafting with meshed, 0.016-inch-thick graft.

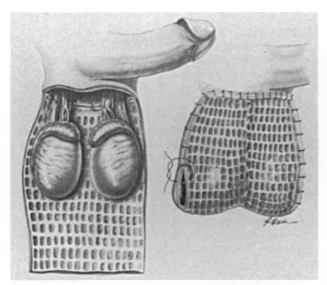

Figure 79–3. Technique for meshed, split-thickness skin grafting for total scrotal loss. (From Howards SS. Surgery of the scrotum and its contents. In Walsh PC, Gittes RF, Perlmutter AD, Stamey TA, eds. Campbell's Urology, 5th ed. Philadelphia, WB Saunders, 1986, p 2956.)

the denuded area (Fig. 79–2). When the grafts are placed into position they should be stretched as little as possible to minimize postoperative contractures. The skin grafts can be both sutured, using absorbable 4-0 chromic suture, and stapled, using small staples, into place, then dressed with Adaptic gauze and gauze dressings.

For total scrotal reconstruction, either meshed split-thickness skin grafts (Fig. 79–3) or rotational flaps based upon the arterial supply for the medial circumflex and obturator arteries can be used (Fig. 79–4). The reconstruction of the scrotum with flaps

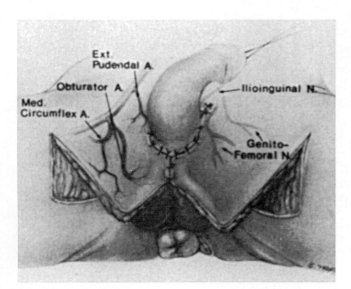

Figure 79–4. Arterial and neural supply of medial thigh rotational flaps used for scrotal reconstruction. (From McAninch JA. Management of genital skin loss. Urol Clin North Am 16:387, 1989.)

is a staged procedure that involves initial drainage and debridement of the scrotum, placement of the testicles into medial thigh pouches, and rotation and closure of the flaps with grafting of the thigh defects (Fig. 79–5).

Localized to the Penis

Patients with penile cellulitis/gangrene frequently have not been circumcised. Initially, placement of a percutaneous suprapubic cystostomy and a dorsal slit are performed to control infection and allow full demarcation of the eschar and necrotic tissues. Subsequent eschar excision is undertaken and as much tissue as possible is preserved (Fig. 79–6). The debrided areas are usually still heavily contaminated and edematous; therefore, reconstruction is not performed immediately. Meshed xenograft (pigskin) can be applied and stapled into position. This process involving debridement and xenografting frequently needs to be repeated. Once the wound is clean and granulating, reconstruction can be undertaken (Fig. 79–7). The inner foreskin can sometimes provide adequate coverage. Otherwise, skin grafting is needed.

A full-thickness graft can be taken from the groin area, with primary closure of the donor site, or from the inner forearm or upper arm. In the case of the upper arm, the donor area requires a split-thickness skin graft from the lateral thigh. Split-thickness grafts are usually taken from the anterolateral thigh.

Extensive Genital and Abdominal Wall Involvement

With clear extension of the process into the groin area and lower abdominal wall, an open suprapubic cystostomy tube is inserted. A Pfannenstiel skin incision is made because it can provide a "firewall" to prevent further extension onto the abdominal wall. The rectus fascia is opened vertically in the midline. Two 2-0 chromic stay sutures are placed into the bladder muscle. Bovie cautery is used to make a small 2- to 3-cm opening at the anterior surface of the bladder near the dome. Once the mucosa is opened, a 22 Fr. Malecot catheter, which has been previously loaded on a Kelly clamp, is inserted into the bladder. A 2-0 chromic pursestring suture is then used to close the defect around the cystostomy tube. The tube is secured to the bladder with another 2-0 chromic suture. The tube is brought out through the fascia, which is closed with interrupted nonabsorbable monofilament sutures.

Debridement of necrotic tissues is undertaken. Penrose drains are placed into all areas of crepitus and cellulitis. These drains can be removed sequentially,

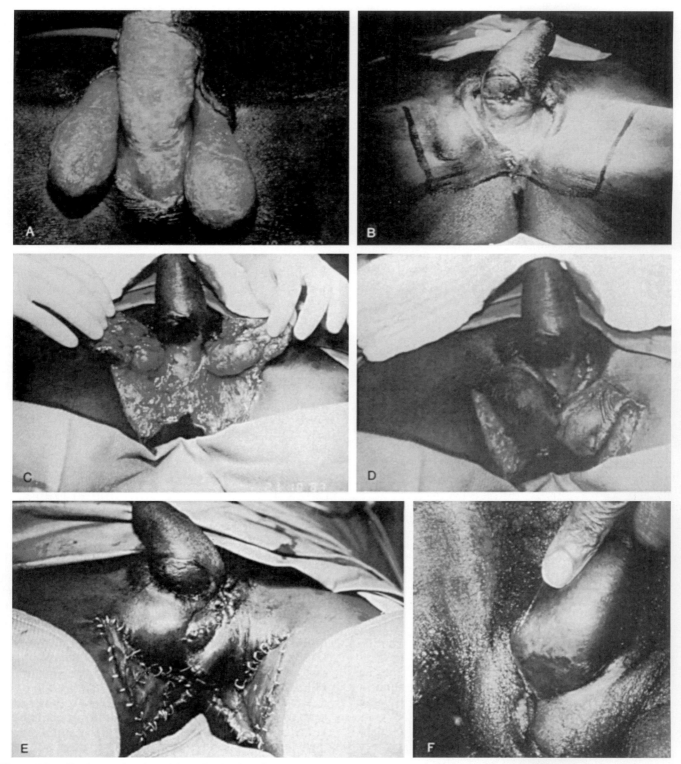

Figure 79–5. Total scrotal and partial penile skin loss from idiopathic Fournier gangrene of the scrotum. *A,* Testicles exposed. *B,* The testicles were placed in medial thigh pouches, and partial grafting of penis took place. *C,* Testicles attached to mobilized flaps. *D,* Flaps and testicles rotated medially. *E,* Nonmeshed, split-thickness grafts stapled into defects created by rotational flaps. *F,* Six weeks postoperatively. (Courtesy of Dr. Joel Studin.)

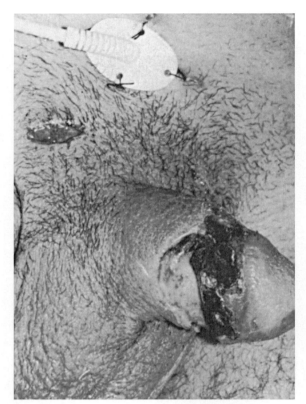

Figure 79–6. Infectious gangrene of the penis resulting from accidental teeth injury to the subcoronal area during fellatio. After placement of a percutaneous suprapubic cystostomy tube and debridement, Penrose drains are used to curtail the infection. Note the drain site from previous Penrose drains as well as residual necrotic eschar. The patient underwent further debridement and skin grafting.

once the infectious process has been controlled. After further bedside and whirlpool debridements, the wounds are reconstructed primarily or with skin grafts (Fig. 79–8).

Dry Gangrene

Dry gangrene usually does not require supravesical urinary diversion. When the process invades the glans penis (Fig. 79–9), standard partial penectomy can be performed. Following a circumcisional subcoronal incision, the penile skin is retracted proximally, exposing the corpora. Guillotine amputation, usually without a tourniquet, is undertaken with attempts at providing a slightly longer urethra. The urethra is spatulated on its dorsal surface. The corpora cavernosa are closed to the midline septum with interrupted 2-0 polyglycolic acid sutures. The urethra is sutured circumferentially to the penile skin with interrupted 4-0 chromic sutures. The remainder of the penile skin is closed over the corporeal bodies in two layers. A Foley catheter is inserted and left in place for several days.

When the scrotum is involved, these affected areas can frequently be simply excised (Fig. 79–10). The

scrotal skin edges are undermined until closure in two layers can be performed. Interrupted 2-0 or 3-0 chromic sutures are used for the dartos and subcutaneous layers; interrupted 4-0 chromic sutures are used for the skin.

POSTOPERATIVE MANAGEMENT AND COMPLICATIONS

The major complication for a patient with infectious gangrene is the continued progression of the infection, leading to further necrosis of the tissues as well as to septic shock and death. Mortality rates average 30 to 40 percent. Progression requires repeated operations with debridement and drainage. The attending physician should have a low threshold for reoperating on these patients to prevent further progression of the infection and worsening of the sepsis. When the infection is fulminant despite repeated interventions and antibiotics, hyperbaric oxygen therapy should be utilized.

Meticulous attention must be given to postoperative wound care. Frequent examinations, at least twice a day, need to be performed, particularly in the early postoperative period. About 48 hours after surgery, whirlpool therapy is usually initiated. Drains are usually removed after the patient's fever has subsided and the wounds are stabilized. It is not uncommon for a patient to undergo several operative debridements to prepare the sites for subsequent closure.

Antibiotic therapy is altered according to the pus and tissue culture and sensitivity findings. Appropriate therapy is usually continued for 7 days after the resolution of fever. Renal function must be closely monitored for a patient receiving aminoglycosides. Determinations of peak-and-trough antibiotic levels are frequently useful in selecting the proper dosage.

Nutritional support and vitamin therapy are important aspects of wound care. Either intravenous alimentation or enteral feedings are important in patients with markedly increased metabolic needs. Our patients usually receive vitamin supplements, including daily multivitamins, ascorbic acid, zinc sulfate, and ferrous sulfate.

Summary

Prompt recognition of gangrene of the male genitalia with appropriate surgical interventions and antibiotic therapy can usually prevent loss of the genitalia, progression of sepsis, and death. Delayed wound closure can be obtained through the utilization of existing remaining skin, skin grafts, or flaps. With the current trend toward minimizing debridements and

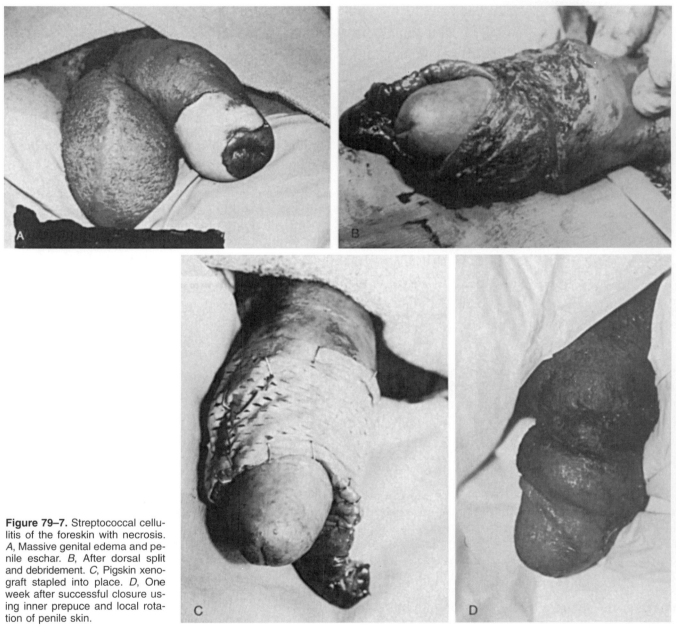

Figure 79–7. Streptococcal cellulitis of the foreskin with necrosis. *A,* Massive genital edema and penile eschar. *B,* After dorsal split and debridement. *C,* Pigskin xenograft stapled into place. *D,* One week after successful closure using inner prepuce and local rotation of penile skin.

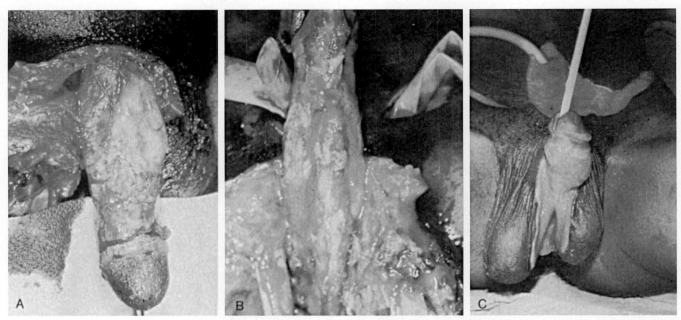

Figure 79–8. Fournier gangrene of the penis and scrotum with fascial necrosis extending onto the abdominal wall. *A*, The debrided penis still shows whitish eschar on the dorsum. *B*, Penrose drains from groins into each hemiscrotum. The ventral surface of the penis is shown after debridement. *C*, After control of infection. Note the large-bore suprapubic cystostomy tube, denuded penis, and scrotal/perineal defect. The abdominal wall, perineal, and scrotal areas were closed primarily. Split-thickness skin grafts were used to cover the penile shaft.

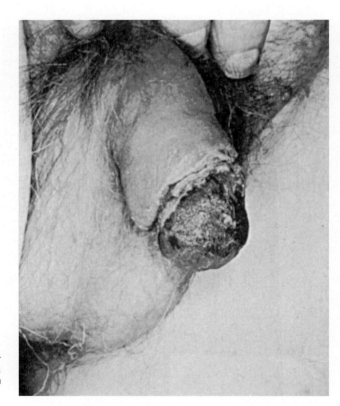

Figure 79–9. Dry gangrene of the glans penis due to metastatic calcification from secondary hyperparathyroidism. (From Lowe FC, Brendler CB. Penile gangrene: A complication of secondary hyperparathyroidism from chronic renal failure. J Urol 132:189, 1984.)

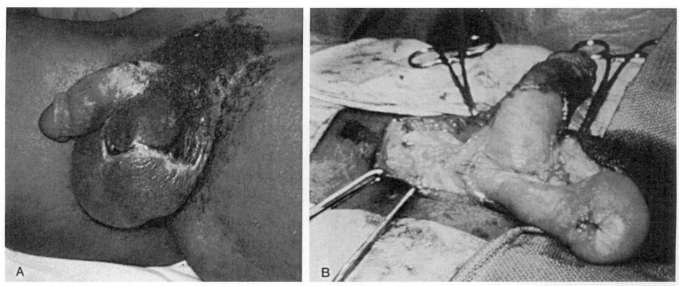

Figure 79–10. Dry gangrene of the scrotum secondary to injection of heroin into the femoral vessels. *A,* Scrotal eschar. (From Somers WJ, Lowe FC. Localized gangrene of the scrotum and penis: A complication of heroin injection into the femoral vessels. J Urol 136:11, 1986.) *B,* Intraoperative view after excision of eschar.

the increasing use of extensive Penrose drainage, it is hoped that fewer patients will require extensive wound closure.

Editorial Comment

Fray F. Marshall

Gangrene of the male genitalia carries a high mortality and requires aggressive treatment as outlined by Dr. Lowe in this chapter. Multiple debridements may be necessary as well as aggressive medical management of infection and associated disease, particularly diabetes.

REFERENCES

1. Spirak JP, Resnick MI, Hampel N, Persky L. Fournier's gangrene: Report of 20 patients. J Urol 131:289, 1984.
2. Lamm RC, Juler GL. Fournier's gangrene of the scrotum: A poorly defined syndrome or a misnomer? Arch Surg 118:38, 1983.
3. Jones RB, Hirschmann JV, Brown GS, Tremann JA. Fournier's syndrome: Necrotizing subcutaneous infection of the male genitalia. J Urol 122:279, 1979.
4. Cohen MS. Fournier's gangrene. AUA Update Series, vol. 5, no. 6, 1986.
5. Kearney GP, Carling PC. Fournier's gangrene: An approach to its management. J Urol 130:695, 1983.

Chapter 80

Vascular Surgery For the Treatment of Impotence

Jonathan P. Jarow and Anthony DeFranzo

Our understanding of erectile physiology increased considerably with the advent, approximately one decade ago, of intracorporeal pharmacological stimulation of erections. Intracorporeal administration of vasodilators has been used in the study of erectile physiology in animal models, in diagnostic testing of impotent patients, and as a form of therapy. It is now known that the creation and maintenance of an erection in man is based on a delicate hemodynamic balance between arterial blood flow into the corpora and restriction of venous outflow.[1] This process is critically dependent on normal compliance of the corporeal sinusoidal tissues and tunica albuginea. Despite all the tremendous advances we have seen over the past 10 years, most patients seen today cannot be cured of their impotence. Instead, we provide treatments that restore sexual function to a degree, but the patients remain dependent on these therapies for life. Examples include penile implants, vacuum erection devices, and pharmacological erection therapy. It is the exceptional patient in whom we can cure erectile dysfunction and restore normal sexual function without any further therapy.

The development and advancement of vascular surgery for the management of impotence has been based on the belief that a patient can be cured of impotence if a specific underlying vascular cause can be identified and surgically corrected. For example, a patient with impotence secondary to traumatic injury of the penile arterial blood supply could be cured by an arterial bypass procedure analogous to coronary bypass surgery. Conversely, a patient with difficulty in maintaining erections because of veno-occlusive dysfunction could be cured by venous ligation surgery. The logic behind this approach to patients with vasculogenic impotence makes sense in theory, but the clinical results have been disappointing in practice.[2] Part of the problem lies in our incomplete understanding of erectile physiology and the inadequacy of our diagnostic tests. Most patients with vasculogenic impotence have either primary or secondary damage to the sinusoidal tissues, which prevents a good response to therapy even if the vascular abnormality can be corrected. In addition, we have a very limited understanding of the neural control of erections and no accurate method to assess its function. Therefore, we can only guess whether a patient with supposed arteriogenic impotence after a pelvic fracture has concomitant neurogenic impotence. Potentially, there are some patients who are excellent candidates for these surgical procedures, but our current ability to identify them is limited.

Numerous surgical procedures to correct vasculogenic impotence have been reported. The discussion in this chapter is limited to the three main operations used to treat arterial occlusive disease, veno-occlusive dysfunction, and combined venous and arterial disease. Artery-to-artery bypass is used to correct arterial occlusive disease in a patient with an otherwise normal phallus. Venous ligation surgery is used in patients with normal arterial inflow and evidence of veno-occlusive dysfunction. Finally, arterialization of the penile veins may be used in patients with a combination of veno-occlusive dysfunction and arterial occlusive disease, or in patients with impotence caused by arterial disease and whose penile vascular anatomy prohibits a simple arterial bypass.

PREOPERATIVE EVALUATION

A complete description of the standard evaluation of impotent patients is not within the scope of this chapter. Therefore, comments are limited to features specifically relevant to patients being considered for vascular surgery. A history should be obtained and physical examination performed to determine risk factors for vasculogenic impotence and identify any contraindications for vascular surgery. A history of pelvic or perineal trauma may suggest an arterial lesion. Even minor trauma may produce significant lesions, especially if chronic in nature, such as those related to bicycle riding.[3] A history of penile fracture or primary impotence may be suggestive of veno-occlusive disease. Elderly patients or patients with systemic diseases such as atherosclerosis and diabetes mellitus are not good candidates for vascular surgery. Cigarette smoking is another contraindication to vascular surgery. The phallus should be carefully palpated for plaques, since venous incompetence is frequently associated with Peyronie's disease but not curable with venous ligation surgery.[4]

Pharmacological erection testing is used to screen impotent patients for vascular disease, since a complete response to pharmacological agents usually rules out significant vascular disease.[5] Conversely, an incomplete response to a pharmacological agent does not always signify significant vascular disease because there is sometimes an overriding psychogenic clinical effect in anxious patients. Using a high dose of triple drug mixture in combination with self-stimulation and repetitive testing helps to limit the false-positive rate but also increases the risk of priapism. Further diagnostic testing for surgically correctable vasculogenic impotence is indicated only in a patient who fails to respond to the drug appropriately, is a potential candidate for vascular surgery, and is interested in that form of therapy. Duplex Doppler ultrasonography is often utilized to assess the penile arteries, and dynamic infusion cavernosometry and cavernosography (DICC) to assess the penile veno-occlusive mechanism. Arteriographic definition of the penile arterial anatomy is mandatory before arterial bypass surgery is performed because impotent patients frequently have variant arterial anatomy. The criteria for normal for all these diagnostic studies are based on very limited clinical data and are poorly defined. The possibility of misdiagnosis is significant, especially in patients labeled venogenic.[6] Therefore, formal sleep laboratory testing may be indicated to completely rule out a significant psychogenic component in these patients. The final diagnosis of vasculogenic impotence should be based on multiple studies, since no single laboratory test or diagnostic study is completely reliable. Patients undergoing vascular surgery should be fully informed of the potential risks and alternative therapies because of the limited success and investigational nature of these procedures.

OPERATIVE PROCEDURES

Arterial Bypass

Patients with discrete proximal arterial lesions, good distal runoff, and no evidence of veno-occlusive disease are the best candidates for arterial bypass surgery. The choice of donor and recipient vessels is dependent on the patient's anatomy and the surgeon's preference. However, the most common procedure performed is an anastomosis between the inferior epigastric and the proximal dorsal artery. An alternative donor vessel to the inferior epigastric artery is a reversed saphenous vein graft attached to the superficial femoral artery. An alternative to the dorsal artery is the cavernous artery.[7] However, the location of the cavernosal artery within the corpora makes this approach more difficult than necessary. Preoperative arteriography is mandatory to establish the presence of a good donor vessel and to choose an appropriate recipient artery. Variant penile arterial anatomy is present in up to 80 percent of impotent men.[8] Common variants include both dorsal arteries originating from the same penile artery and distal cavernosal perforators from the dorsal artery. Patients with classic penile arterial anatomy are best served by an end-to-end anastomosis to the proximal dorsal artery on the side of the lesion to maximize blood flow into the corpora. The presence of distal cavernosal perforators may require an end-to-side anastomosis to an intact dorsal artery or an end-to-end anastomosis to the distal portion of the dorsal artery to maximize blood flow into the corpora. An intraoperative arteriogram may be necessary if the preoperative arteriogram does not adequately visualize the intrapenile arterial anatomy.

The procedure is performed with the patient in the supine position. A transverse or paramedian abdominal incision is performed to harvest the inferior epigastric artery (Fig. 80–1). It is important to handle the donor vessel gently and avoid cautery close to the main trunk. Small arteriole side branches are frequent and should be managed with bipolar cautery. One or two venae comitantes run with the artery with numerous crossing branches; these may be controlled with bipolar cautery. The artery is harvested to or just beyond the umbilicus from the underside of the rectus abdominis muscle. The inferior epigastric artery is usually still larger in diameter than the dorsal penile artery at this level. Systemic heparin (5000 U) is administered just before the artery is ligated superiorly. A topical vasodilator such as bupivacaine (Marcaine) is applied with a warm sponge and attention turned to the penile vascular anatomy. A separate incision at the base of the penis is used to expose the dorsal penile arteries. A short pubic tunnel is created beneath the fascia of the anterior rectus sheath between the two incisions. The inferior epigastric vessels are passed through the tunnel with care not to twist or kink the artery. A segment of the dorsal artery is carefully dissected and prepared for anastomosis by stripping away loose tissue attached to the adventitia. The operative microscope is then

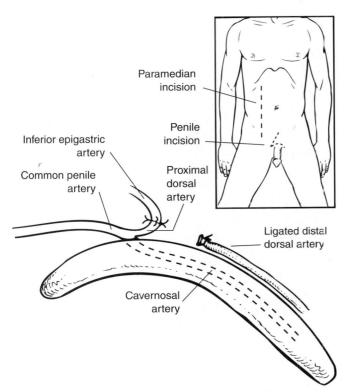

Paramedian incision

Penile incision

Inferior epigastric artery

Common penile artery

Proximal dorsal artery

Ligated distal dorsal artery

Cavernosal artery

Figure 80–1. Penile arterial bypass surgery is performed using a combined approach through the abdomen to harvest the inferior epigastric artery and through the base of the penis to gain access to the dorsal artery (*inset*). The inferior epigastric artery is brought down to the base of the penis through a subfascial tunnel and anastomosed to the proximal end of a dorsal artery in an end-to-end fashion.

used to prepare the arteriotomies and perform the anastomosis. Because of the large relative size of the inferior epigastric artery compared with the dorsal penile artery, an end-to-end anastomosis is technically easier. An end-to-side anastomosis may be necessary, depending on the pattern of penile arterial blood flow. The goal of the microsurgical revascularization is to direct blood flow into the corpora. An on-the-table intraoperative arteriogram of the penile arterial anatomy may be necessary in selecting the type and direction of the arterial anastomosis to maximize blood flow into the corpora.[9] The anastomosis is performed with interrupted 10-0 nylon suture on a tapered needle with care taken to exclude adventitia from the lumen and to avoid tension on the anastomosis. Low-molecular-weight dextran (40 percent) is administered intravenously in a 100-ml bolus immediately upon completion of the arterial anastomosis and then maintained at 20 ml/hr for 5 days. The patient is also started on one aspirin daily. No further heparin is administered because there is a high complication rate associated with the combined use of heparin and dextran. A drain is placed for the abdominal incision. The patient should avoid cigarette smoke and foods containing vasoconstrictors. Sexual activity should be avoided for 6 weeks.

Penile Vein Ligation

Penile vein ligation is performed on patients with veno-occlusive dysfunction and without evidence of either arterial or psychogenic impotence. Preoperative cavernosometry demonstrates the severity of venous leakage, and cavernosography determines the site of leakage. The normal venous drainage of the penis includes the superficial and deep dorsal veins, the cavernosal and crural veins, and occasionally the corpus spongiosum. All these venous systems can be approached through a single inguinoscrotal incision at the base of the penis.[10] Placing the patient in the lithotomy position enhances exposure for the proximal dissection beneath the symphysis pubis. The penis may then be degloved through this incision to expose both the dorsal veins and any communication to the corpus spongiosum (Fig. 80–2). The deep dorsal vein or veins (frequently there are more than one) are completely resected from the trifurcation located 2 to 3 cm proximal to the glans penis all the way to beneath the symphysis pubis. All circumflex and emissary veins are ligated as well. The cavernosal veins can be identified at the hilum of the penis after the suspensory ligaments are detached. Optical magnification with loupes and intraoperative Doppler ultrasonography are helpful in the hilar dissection to avoid inadvertent ligation of the arteries. Crural veins visualized on preoperative cavernosography may be ligated after further dissection along the lateral aspect of the corpora. It is critical to approximate the suspensory ligament in multiple layers upon completion of the venous dissection to prevent significant penile shortening.

This procedure may be performed on an outpatient basis under general or regional anesthesia. Sexual activity should be delayed for several weeks after the procedure. Complications include penile paresthesia, penile shortening, and hematoma formation. Patients who do not experience a return of adequate sexual function postoperatively may have been converted to responders to vasoactive injections. An alternative approach to open surgical penile vein ligation is percutaneous ablation of the penile veins.[11] Access to the penile veins for sclerotherapy may be obtained through the femoral vein, a deep dorsal vein cutdown, or both.

Arterialization of the Dorsal Vein

Arterialization of the deep dorsal vein to correct vasculogenic impotence was first described by Virag.[12] He subsequently modified his procedure several times and other investigators have also suggested modifications. The procedure has been employed with limited success in patients with isolated veno-

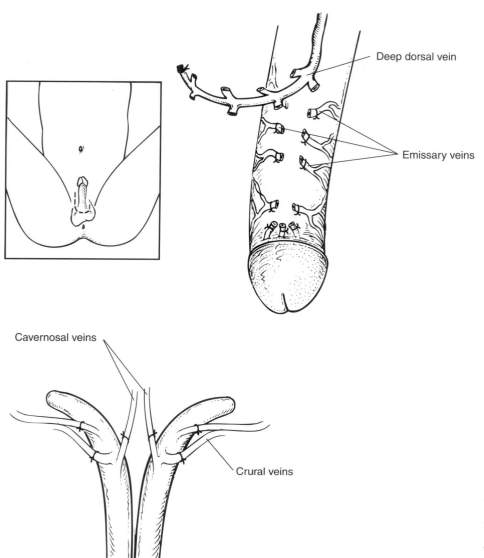

Figure 80–2. Penile vein ligation is performed through an inguinoscrotal incision (*inset*). The penis is degloved and the entire length of the deep dorsal vein or veins is resected while the emissary and circumflex veins are ligated. The cavernosal and crural veins may be ligated after the suspensory ligament of the penis is severed.

genic impotence, pure arteriogenic impotence, or combined disease. This procedure theoretically impedes venous outflow through the deep dorsal vein at the same time as it increases intracorporeal arterial blood flow. Thus, the balance between arterial inflow and venous outflow is significantly shifted to enhance penile engorgement. The patient is prepared in a manner similar to that for the straightforward arterial bypass operation. The inferior epigastric artery is harvested through a separate abdominal incision as described earlier. The deep dorsal vein is isolated at the base of the penis through a separate incision at the base. An isolated segment of the deep dorsal vein with its emissary veins intact should be prepared by ligating the deep dorsal vein both proximally near the hilum of the penis and distally before its trifurcation near the glans penis (Fig. 80–3). The inferior epigastric artery is brought down through a tunnel beneath the fascia of the anterior rectus sheath.

Again, it is important not to twist or kink this vessel. A venotomy is then created in the side of the deep dorsal vein. The deep dorsal vein has intact venous valves that prevent retrograde flow into the corpora except in patients with massive venous leakage. These venous valves must be ablated for this procedure to have any significant benefit over simple ligation of the deep dorsal vein. A Leather valvulotome or Fogarty balloon catheter may be used to mechanically disrupt the valves. Alternatively, the valves can be excised through a venotomy using microsurgical techniques. All these methods carry the risk of damage to the intima of the venous wall, resulting in eventual clotting of the anastomosis. In addition, disruption of the valves within the deep dorsal vein does not guarantee that blood flow will extend all the way into the corporeal sinuses. Therefore, the valves of the emissary veins must be ablated as well. The anastomosis between the inferior epigastric artery

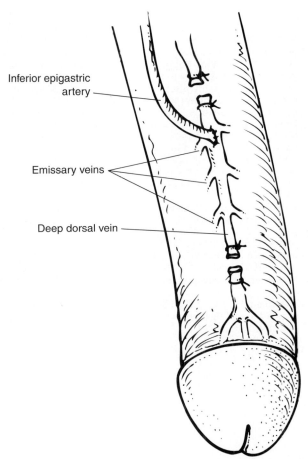

Figure 80–3. The deep dorsal vein of the penis may be arterialized via an end-to-side anastomosis from the inferior epigastric artery. It is important to ligate the dorsal vein distally to prevent hypervascularity of the glans penis and to disrupt the venous valves.

Inferior epigastric artery

Emissary veins

Deep dorsal vein

and the deep dorsal vein is performed in an end-to-end or end-to-side fashion with interrupted 10-0 nylon sutures.

The overall success rate of this procedure has been disappointing. Modifications of this procedure have been developed to improve the success rate. Virag described a modification in which a window is created in the corpora by excising an ellipse of tunica albuginea. The arterialized segment of the dorsal vein is then anastomosed to the corpora in a side-to-side fashion in an effort to increase the blood flow directed into the corpora. Hauri described an alternative technique whereby the dorsal artery is anastomosed side to side to the arterialized dorsal vein segment in an effort to increase blood flow and maintain the patency of the anastomosis.[13]

Postoperative management includes placement of a drain and systemic anticoagulation as described for the arterial bypass procedure. Postoperatively, the patient should avoid cigarette smoke and foods containing vasoconstrictors. Sexual activity should be delayed for at least 6 weeks to avoid disruption of the anastomosis. A major complication of this procedure is hypervascularity of the glans penis.[14] This is caused by excessive blood flow reaching the glans penis through arterialized collateral veins. Hypervascularity of the glans penis is usually seen in the early postoperative period but may appear late. Treatment consists of ligation of the collateral veins located between the arterialized segment of the deep dorsal vein and the glans penis. Intraoperative Doppler ultrasonography is helpful in identifying these arterialized collateral veins. The dorsal arteries should be spared to prevent ischemic damage to the glans. Alternatively, the inferior epigastric artery can be ligated proximal to the anastomosis if the original procedure was not effective in restoring potency.

Summary

The introduction of surgical procedures to cure vasculogenic impotence was greeted with a great deal of initial enthusiasm because of limitations in other therapies. Unfortunately, the published long-term results of these procedures fall far short of our initial expectations. Numerous surgical techniques have been developed and modified and none appear to significantly improve outcome. The reported success rate for arterial surgery ranges from as low as 50 percent to as high as 90 percent, depending on the population treated, the method employed, and the length of follow-up.[2] Long-term results of venous ligation surgery have been extremely disappointing: approximately 30 percent of the procedures are successful.[15] The current sentiment is that many or all of these procedures should be abandoned. The gaps in our understanding of erectile physiology and the flaws in our diagnostic evaluation may lead to a misdiagnosis and inappropriate application of these surgical therapies. We have learned which patients will not benefit from these procedures. These include any patient with end-organ disease of the penis, including elderly and diabetics, and patients with severe ischemic vascular disease. Many patients who are thought to have veno-occlusive dysfunction potentially suffer from psychogenic impotence. DICC is the least standardized test, and the lack of a gold standard method for the diagnosis of veno-occlusive dysfunction is a major handicap. The best candidates for vascular surgery are young, healthy patients with an identifiable segmental vascular pathological entity, such as patients with traumatic injuries or those with congenital abnormalities. However, these patients are rare and represent only a small fraction of those with impotence seen in a standard practice. Patients undergoing penile vascular surgery should be made aware of the potential risks, alternative therapies, and the investigational nature of these procedures.

Editorial Comment
Fray F. Marshall

I agree with Dr. Jarow's and Dr. DeFranzo's summary and assessment of vascular surgery for impotence.

REFERENCES

1. Carrier S, Brock G, Kour NW, et al. Pathophysiology of erectile dysfunction. Urology 42:468, 1993.
2. Sharlip ID. The role of vascular surgery in arteriogenic and combined arteriogenic and venogenic impotence. Semin Urol 8:129, 1990.
3. Levine FJ, Greenfield AJ, Goldstein I. Arteriographically determined occlusive disease within the hypogastric-cavernous bed in impotent patients following blunt perineal and pelvic trauma. J Urol 144:1147, 1990.
4. Lopez JA, Jarow JP. Penile vascular evaluation of men with Peyronie's disease. J Urol 149:53, 1993.
5. Pescatori ES, Hatzichristou DG, Namburi S, et al. A positive intracavernous injection test implies normal veno-occlusive but not necessarily normal arterial function: A hemodynamic study. J Urol 151:1209, 1994.
6. Montague DK, Lakin MM, Medendorp SV, et al. Infusion pharmacocavernosometry and nocturnal penile tumescence findings in men with erectile dysfunction. J Urol 145:768, 1991.
7. Konnak JW, Ohl DA. Microsurgical penile revascularization using the central corporeal penile artery. J Urol 142:305, 1989.
8. Jarow JP, Pugh VW, Routh WD, et al. Comparison of penile duplex ultrasonography to pudendal arteriography. Variant penile arterial anatomy affects interpretation of duplex ultrasonography. Invest Radiol 28:806, 1993.
9. Bare RL, DeFranzo A, Jarow JP. Intraoperative arteriography facilitates penile revascularization. J Urol 151:1019, 1994.
10. Miller EB, Schlossberg SM, Devine CJ Jr. New incision for penile surgery. J Urol 150:79, 1993.
11. Yu GW, Schwab FJ, Melograna FS, et al. Preoperative and postoperative dynamic cavernosography and cavernosometry: Objective assessment of venous ligation for impotence. J Urol 147:618, 1992.
12. Virag R, Zwang G, Dermange H, et al. Vasculogenic impotence: A review of 92 cases with 54 surgical operations. Vasc Surg 15:9, 1981.
13. Hauri D. A new operative technique in vasculogenic erectile impotence. World J Urol 4:237, 1986.
14. Jarow JP, DeFranzo AJ. Hypervascularity of the glans penis following arterialization of the dorsal vein. J Urol 147:706, 1992.
15. Freedman AL, Neto FC, Mehringer CM, et al. Long-term results of penile vein ligation for impotence from venous leakage. J Urol 149:1301, 1993.

Part X

OUTPATIENT SURGERY

Chapter 81

Vasectomy

Michael J. Naslund

A properly performed vasectomy is the most reliable form of male contraception. A vasectomy should be reserved for emotionally stable and motivated individuals who can fully comprehend the advantages and disadvantages of the procedure. Given the high rate of litigation associated with this procedure, it is critical to obtain informed consent before surgery. The decision to undergo a vasectomy must ultimately be made by the patient after proper counseling. If the patient is married, it is important that his spouse agree with the decision.

PREOPERATIVE MANAGEMENT

The surgeon should make every effort to ensure that the patient understands the risks and benefits of vasectomy. The patient should know the procedure is designed to be irreversible and thus permanent and that recanalization has been reported in only approximately 0.8 percent of cases.[1] Postoperative complications include pain, scrotal hematoma, sperm granuloma, and injury to the vascular supply of the testis. The patient should be made aware of the possibility that sperm autoantibodies may form after vasectomy.[2] He should be told of other options regarding contraception. In selected cases, he should be given the opportunity to bank sperm preoperatively in case he desires children in the future. The patient should also be informed of the possibility that vasectomy may increase the future risk of developing prostate cancer.[3, 4]

The patient is examined preoperatively to ensure that each vas deferens is palpable and that anatomical problems, such as large hernias and hydroceles, are not present that may preclude or complicate the vasectomy.

Surgical preparation is quite simple. The scrotum is shaved, usually by the patient himself, on the day of surgery. Antibiotics are generally not given.

OPERATIVE TECHNIQUE

Unless the patient has had previous scrotal surgery, vasectomy can almost always be done using local anesthesia. A suitable agent is 1 or 2 percent lidocaine. An incision can be made on each side of the scrotum or a single vertical incision along the median raphe. Before an incision is made, the vas deferens is separated as much as possible from surrounding tissue and held firmly between thumb and forefinger. Local anesthetic is then injected into the scrotal skin, the subcutaneous tissue, and the vas deferens itself. One should then wait 2 to 3 minutes for the local anesthetic to permeate the surrounding tissues before making a 1- to 2-cm scrotal incision (Fig. 81–1A). The vas deferens and surrounding tissue are grasped with a towel clip to prevent the vas from falling back into the scrotum (Fig. 81–1B). The fascia around the vas is then incised and a 2- to 3-cm segment of vas dissected free. The towel clip is repositioned around the isolated vas deferens (Fig. 81–1C). It is important that dissection of the vas deferens be made away from the epididymis to facilitate a future vasovasostomy, if desired.

Metal clips are placed on the vas 1.5 cm apart, and a 1-cm segment of vas is excised and sent for pathological examination (Fig. 81–1D). Needlepoint electrocautery or thermal cautery (a red-hot wire) is utilized to fulgurate the vasal lumen distal to the clips for added protection against recanalization. There is evidence that thermal cautery may be more effective at sealing the ends of the vas than electrocautery.[5] An alternative technique is to occlude the vasa with sutures instead of clips or to use only a

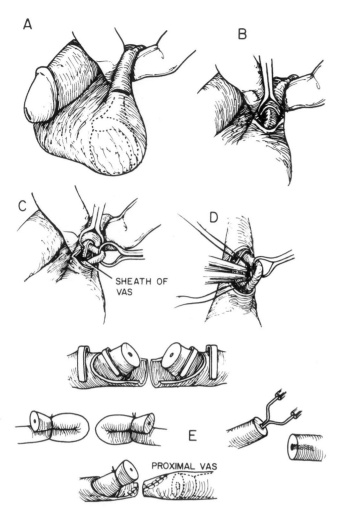

Figure 81-1. Technique of vasectomy. *A*, The vas deferens is palpated and held between the thumb and forefinger. After local anesthetic is injected, an incision is made over the vas deferens. *B*, The vas deferens and fascial sheath are grasped with a towel clip. *C*, The fascial sheath is incised and a 2- to 3-cm segment of vas is isolated with a towel clip. *D*, The vas deferens is clipped or tied and a 1-cm segment is excised. *E*, The distal vasal lumen is fulgurated with cautery. The proximal vas is buried in subcutaneous tissue. (From Gerlser WL. The scrotum. In Surgical Urology, 5th ed. Chicago, Year Book, 1985.)

needlepoint cautery in the vasal lumen. The proximal vas is then buried in subcutaneous tissue so that it lies in a different tissue plane from the distal vas, to decrease the chance of recanalization (Fig. 81-1*E*). Each end of the vas and the surrounding tissue should be inspected for bleeding before closure. A similar procedure is then performed on the other side.

Closure is done in two layers. First, a running 3-0 chromic suture is used to close the tunica vaginalis, and then interrupted chromic sutures are used to close the skin and dartos muscle layer. The skin sutures can be placed subcutaneously to decrease patient concern in the postoperative period. A compression dressing should be placed around the scrotum.

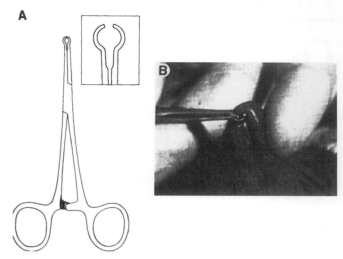

Figure 81-2. *A*, Extracutaneous vas deferens fixation ring clamp. *B*, The vas deferens in the ring clamp after the scrotal skin is first stretched with the clamp. (From Li S, Goldstein M, Zhu J, Huber D. The no-scalpel vasectomy. J Urol 145:341, 1991. Copyright Williams & Wilkins, 1991.)

The patient should be instructed to wear a scrotal support for 7 to 10 days.

An alternative technique, the "no-scalpel" vasectomy, has been described by Li et al.[6] The vas deferens is grasped with the fingers beneath the median raphe, and local anesthetic is administered as described above. An extracutaneous vas deferens fixation ring clamp is pressed onto the skin overlying the vas to stretch the scrotal skin before the clamp is locked around the vas (Fig. 81-2). One blade of a sharpened curved hemostat is used to pierce the scrotal skin and the vas in the midline (Fig. 81-3). The single blade is withdrawn, and both blades are then introduced through the puncture opening and spread to expose the vas wall, which is grasped by piercing the wall again with one blade of the clamp and then grasping the vas and rotating the clamp to deliver the vas from the puncture hole (Fig. 81-4). The ring clamp is then repositioned over the vas to facilitate exposure (Fig. 81-5). Vas deferens excision and occlusion can be performed using the techniques dis-

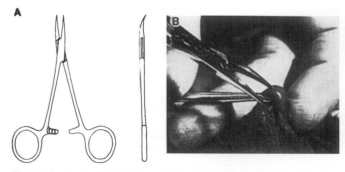

Figure 81-3. *A*, Sharpened curved hemostat. *B*, One blade of the hemostat is used to puncture the scrotal skin and vas deferens. (From Li S, Goldstein M, Zhu J, Huber D. The no-scalpel vasectomy. J Urol 145:341, 1991. Copyright Williams & Wilkins, 1991.)

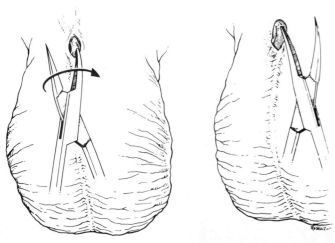

Figure 81–4. After the scrotum is spread to expose the vas wall, one blade again pierces the vas deferens. The clamp is then rotated to deliver the vas from the scrotum. (From Li S, Goldstein M, Zhu J, Huber D. The no-scalpel vasectomy. J Urol 145:341, 1991. Copyright Williams & Wilkins, 1991.)

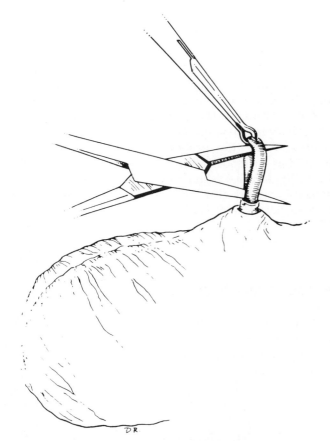

Figure 81–5. Fixation ring clamp repositioned on the vas deferens to facilitate excision and occlusion of the vas. (From Li S, Goldstein M, Zhu J, Huber D. The no-scalpel vasectomy. J Urol 145:341, 1991. Copyright Williams & Wilkins, 1991.)

cussed above. Sutures are usually not necessary for closure with this technique.

POSTOPERATIVE MANAGEMENT

The patient must be instructed to consider himself fertile until he returns for semen analysis in 6 to 8 weeks. It takes eight to ten ejaculations to clear sperm from the distal vas deferens. The patient must therefore continue contraception during that interval. No sperm should be seen on the postoperative semen analysis. If even one sperm is noted, the patient should be instructed to return in 2 to 3 weeks for another check.

Summary

Bilateral vasectomy is a simple and highly successful procedure for male contraception. Candidates for this procedure should be selected carefully, and informed consent must be obtained. Vasectomy can almost always be done utilizing local anesthesia and carries few significant postoperative complications.

Editorial Comment
Fray F. Marshall

Vasectomy is an effective form of contraception. Patients never expect any problems with "lesser procedures," such as vasectomy or circumcision. Complications need to be explained in detail, and the patient should understand that vasectomy is a permanent procedure. If the man has had no children and is young, other forms of contraception should be recommended in most instances.

REFERENCES

1. Esho JO, Ireland GW, Cass AS. Recanalization following vasectomy. Urology 3:211, 1974.
2. Alexander NJ, Fulgham DC, Plunkett ER, Whitkin SS. Antisperm antibodies and circulating immune complexes of vasectomized men, with and without coronary events. Am J Reprod Immunol Microbiol 12:38, 1986.
3. Giovannucci E, Ascherio A, Rimm EB, et al. A prospective cohort study of vasectomy and prostate cancer in U.S. men. JAMA 269:873, 1993.
4. Giovannucci E, Tosteson TD, Speizer FE, et al. A retrospective cohort study of vasectomy and prostate cancer in U.S. men. JAMA 269:878, 1993.
5. Schmidt SS, Minckler TM. The vas after vasectomy: Comparison of cauterization methods. Urology 40:468, 1992.
6. Li S, Goldstein N, Zhu J, Huber D. The no-scalpel vasectomy. J Urol 145:341, 1991.

Chapter 82

Varicocelectomy, Hydrocelectomy, Spermatocelectomy, and Testicular Biopsy

Jonathan P. Jarow

VARICOCELECTOMY

Indications

A varicocele is an abnormal dilation of the pampiniform plexus of the testis. Varicoceles can occur bilaterally but are more common unilaterally on the left side. Since the time of Aulus Cornelius Celsus (first century AD), they have been noted to be associated with ipsilateral testicular atrophy. Although numerous causes have been suggested, the exact pathogenesis of how these vascular lesions adversely affect the testes is unknown. The acute presentation of a large unilateral right varicocele suggests the presence of a retroperitoneal lesion and warrants further investigation with ultrasonography.

The prevalence of varicoceles in the general population has been estimated to range from 13 to 15 percent.[1] Varicoceles are usually asymptomatic. When large, however, they are often associated with pain or testicular atrophy, both of which are indications for repair. The management of varicoceles in the pediatric age group is controversial. The current consensus is to repair varicoceles in adolescents who have either ipsilateral testicular atrophy or testicular growth failure.[2] Prophylactic varicocelectomy in an adolescent with grossly normal testes has not been shown to have a positive effect upon either future testicular development or fertility.

The incidence of varicocele cases in adult male infertility clinics has been reported to range from 35 to 40 percent.[3, 4] The lesion has been associated with

abnormalities in testicular steroidogenesis[5] and spermatogenesis,[6] but the exact pathophysiology is unknown. Although the efficacy of varicocelectomy in an otherwise asymptomatic infertile man remains controversial,[7] the preponderance of evidence suggests that varicocelectomy in the male partner of an infertile marriage who demonstrates abnormalities on semen analysis that cannot be attributed to other known causes will result in improvement of the seminal variables in up to 70 percent and in a pregnancy rate of approximately 40 percent.[8]

Preoperative Management

A varicocele is diagnosed by palpation of the spermatic cord within the scrotum with the patient standing upright and both before and after a Valsalva maneuver. On the basis of this examination, the varicocele is graded by size as large (easily visible), moderate (palpable both before and during the Valsalva maneuver), or small (impulse felt only with the Valsalva maneuver). Various diagnostic tests have been advocated for the detection of varicoceles not easily palpable within the scrotum, including Doppler ultrasound examination of the spermatic veins[9]; internal spermatic vein venography[10]; and scrotal examination by ultrasound,[11] radioisotope scanning,[12] and thermography.[13] Varicoceles detected by these imaging studies in a patient without a palpable abnormality are considered subclinical. All of these tests are subject to false-positive and false-negative results and are rarely needed in clinical practice. In addition, the repair of a subclinical varicocele is of questionable value. However, these radiological imaging studies can be useful in treating an infertile patient who is suspected of having a potentially recurrent or persistent varicocele after surgical repair.

Treatment Options

Varicoceles are associated with reflux of blood through incompetent valves of the internal spermatic vein. These valves are normally located within several centimeters of the junction of the internal spermatic vein with the renal vein or the inferior vena cava.[14] On rare occasions, blood may reflux through the external spermatic venous system.[15] Therefore, the ideal site for varicocele ligation would be within the scrotum, where all incompetent channels of both venous systems could be ligated. However, because of the multiplicity of veins at this level and the potential damage to the testis if the gonadal artery is injured, Palomo[16] recommended a retroperitoneal approach. Using this approach, all the internal spermatic veins can be ligated in the retroperitoneum near the internal inguinal ring. This operation has been successful in most cases and has not been associated with testicular damage when the internal spermatic artery is also ligated. Unfortunately, this approach does not allow for the ligation of the external spermatic veins, which may sometimes play an important role in recurrence or persistence of a varicocele. An approach either within the inguinal canal (the Ivanissevich approach) or below the inguinal canal (subinguinal approach) allows for the identification and ligation of both the external and the internal spermatic veins.

The percutaneous approach is an alternative to surgery and has gained in popularity over the last decade. The procedure is performed on an outpatient basis, and access to the internal spermatic vein is gained via catheterization of the femoral vein after local anesthesia has been induced. A variety of materials have been used to occlude the internal spermatic vein, including sclerosing agents,[17] metal coils,[18] and balloons.[19] Initial reports revealed a relatively high failure rate, particularly when the procedure is performed for varicoceles on the right side. However, later reports by radiologists experienced in the use of this technique reveal a success rate comparable with that of open surgical procedures, with the advantage of a short convalescence period.[19] Unfortunately, this approach, like the Palomo approach, does not allow for the occlusion of the external spermatic veins. Therefore, either an inguinal or a subinguinal surgical approach is now recommended in the treatment of varicoceles in infertile men. The percutaneous approach has its greatest utility in patients with questionable persistent or recurrent varicoceles after surgical correction.

Operative Technique

Subinguinal Approach

The spermatic veins may be easily ligated under local anesthesia using the subinguinal approach. A transverse incision is made at the junction of the scrotum with the abdominal wall just lateral to the pubic tubercle. Blunt dissection is used to deliver the spermatic cord, which is then supported by a Penrose drain. The floor of the incision is inspected for any collateral veins, which should be ligated if observed. The testicle can be delivered through the incision to facilitate ligation of all collateral veins.[20] However, this maneuver is extremely uncomfortable to a patient under local anesthesia and has never been shown to yield results superior to those of the standard microsurgical subinguinal technique. Optical magnification with either the surgical microscope or loupes is mandatory to avoid injury to lymphatics and the gonadal artery. In addition, intraoperative Doppler ultrasonographic examination and topical administration of vasodilators will aid in the identification of the spermatic arteries.

The cremasteric muscle is divided in a transverse fashion to expose the testicular vessels and vas deferens below. The vas deferens should be separated from the other spermatic cord structures and left undissected. The arteries and lymphatic vessels are identified and preserved. All of the venous channels including the small vessels adherent to the artery should be ligated with either hemoclips, silk ligatures, or bipolar cautery, depending on the size and location of the vessel. The cremasteric muscle is then reapproximated using chromic suture upon completion of the dissection. The skin is closed with absorbable suture.

Inguinal Approach

The patient is placed on the operating room table in the reverse Trendelenburg position. An incision is made starting two fingerbreadths above and lateral to the ipsilateral pubic tubercle and extending laterally along the skin lines of the inferior abdominal wall. If the patient is markedly obese, it is important to retract the panniculus superiorly in an effort to reduce the depth of the incision. The incision should be carried down to the external oblique fascia using blunt dissection, and the fascia cleared to identify the external inguinal ring and the inguinal ligament. The external oblique fascia is then sharply incised

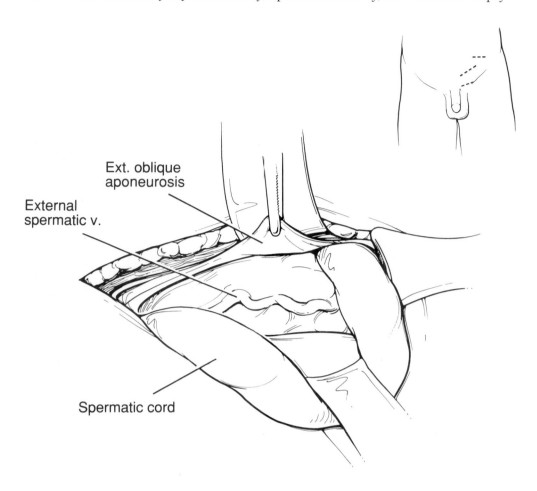

Figure 82–1. The floor of the inguinal canal may be inspected for incompetent external spermatic venous channels after delivery of the spermatic cord when the inguinal approach for varicocelectomy is used. The site of the skin incision for the retroperitoneal, inguinal, and subinguinal approaches for varicocelectomy is shown (*inset*).

over the spermatic cord, with care being taken not to damage the ilioinguinal nerve, which is frequently adherent to the underside of this fascia. The spermatic cord is delivered into the wound by simultaneously retracting the conjoined tendon cranially with the index finger of one hand and grasping the spermatic cord between the index finger and thumb of the other hand. Once the spermatic cord has been delivered, the floor of the inguinal canal is inspected for incompetent external spermatic veins (Fig. 82–1). If the external spermatic veins are prominent, they should be doubly ligated with 4-0 silk ties.

The cremasteric fibers are then dissected off the spermatic cord, which is now looped over either the index finger or a Penrose drain. The external spermatic fascia is incised to provide access to the vascular structures within. The vas deferens, along with its artery, vein, and lymphatic vessels, should be identified and protected from further dissection. At this point the internal spermatic artery or arteries should be identifiable by either visualization of pulsations (made easier by optical magnification with loupes) or intraoperative Doppler ultrasonography. Frequently, there is more than one branch of the internal spermatic artery present at this level. Spasm of the arteries secondary to dissection can be reversed by topical

administration of a vasodilator, such as papaverine or lidocaine (Fig. 82–2). Once the gonadal arteries have been identified, all of the remaining vascular structures may be ligated using 4-0 silk ties (Fig. 82–3).

The external oblique fascia is then closed with a

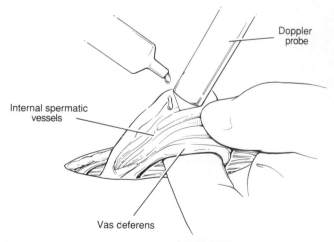

Figure 82–2. The gonadal arteries may be identified by visualization of arterial pulsations or by use of an intraoperative Doppler probe. Administration of topical vasodilators helps to combat vasospasm.

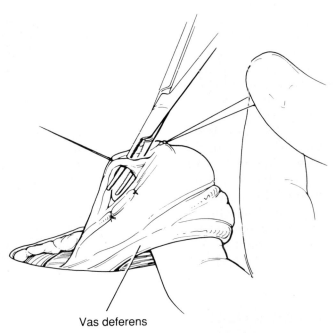

Vas deferens

Figure 82–3. Once the arteries have been identified, all the venous channels can be ligated. Care is taken to avoid dissection around the vas deferens.

running suture once it has been confirmed that the testis is in a dependent position within the scrotum. A long-acting local anesthetic may be administered at this time to assist with postoperative analgesia. The subcutaneous tissues and skin are closed with reabsorbable suture.

Retroperitoneal Approach

The internal spermatic veins may be ligated in the retroperitoneum just proximal to the internal ring of the inguinal canal using an open surgical or laparoscopic technique. In the open approach, a horizontal incision is made, starting two fingerbreadths medially and just inferior to the ipsilateral anterior superior iliac spine and extending medially. The external oblique fascia is incised in the direction of the fibers and the internal oblique muscle is retracted cranially. Placing the operating room table in a reverse Trendelenburg position will allow the gonadal vasculature to be identified more easily. Tilting the table to the opposite side of the varicocele is helpful in avoiding inadvertent incision of the peritoneum. Richardson retractors are used to maintain exposure within the retroperitoneal space, and long narrow Deaver retractors will improve exposure in obese patients. Blunt dissection with a moistened sponge stick may be necessary to identify the gonadal vessels, which are sometimes adherent to the undersurface of the peritoneum. Every effort should be made to spare the gonadal artery, but its ligation at this level will rarely result in testicular atrophy. The internal spermatic

veins should be doubly ligated with 3-0 silk ties. The incision is then closed in multiple layers with absorbable suture.

The laparoscopic approach is a minimally invasive alternative to the Palomo procedure for the retroperitoneal repair of a varicocele.[21] The initial patient preparation is similar to that for all laparoscopic procedures. A preoperative mechanical bowel preparation and antibiotic coverage are optional but encouraged. A Foley catheter is placed to drain the bladder and a nasogastric tube is placed to decompress the stomach. The patient is placed in the reverse Trendelenburg position and the peritoneal cavity is insufflated to a pressure of approximately 15 mm Hg with carbon dioxide through either a Veress needle or a Hasson cannula placed through the umbilicus. Secondary ports, either two to three, are placed in the midline just cranial to the symphysis pubis and laterally under direct vision to avoid injury to bowel or vascular structures. The peritoneal cavity is inspected and the gonadal vessels may be easily visualized in the retroperitoneum cranial to the internal ring of the inguinal canal. A peritoneotomy is created lateral to and parallel to the spermatic vessels and cranial to where the vas deferens joins these vessels. The incision through the peritoneum is made over the spermatic vessels, which can then be bluntly dissected away from other retroperitoneal structures. The internal spermatic artery may be easily identified by the presence of pulsations or by intraoperative Doppler examination. The venous vessels are carefully dissected from the artery or arteries and doubly ligated with hemaclips. The pneumoperitoneum is evacuated and the ports are removed. The Foley catheter and nasogastric tube can also be removed upon completion of the procedure.

There is considerable debate over which of these surgical techniques is superior in terms of efficacy, morbidity, and cost. The current literature suggests that there is less morbidity with the laparoscopic and subinguinal approaches over the other procedures and that the efficacy of these procedures are similar.[22] However, the retroperitoneal approach is preferable in a patient who has had previous inguinal surgery. The subinguinal approach has the decided advantage in cost and potential risk over the laparoscopic approach because it can be performed under local anesthesia with intravenous sedation. Despite all this, the inguinal approach remains the most popular technique used by urologists in the community. Randomized prospective studies are necessary to resolve these issues.

Postoperative Management and Complications

Most of these procedures can be performed using local, regional, or general anesthesia, depending on the patient's or the surgeon's preference, and are usually carried out on an outpatient basis. Postoperative pain is minimal and can be controlled with oral analgesics and an ice pack for the first 24 hours. The incisions should be re-examined 7 to 10 days postoperatively. Persistent venous dilatation is not unusual and does not necessarily indicate surgical failure. Examination of the patient in the standing position before and after he performs the Valsalva maneuver should confirm that the varicocele is gone. In patients who are being treated for infertility, the first semen analysis is performed 3 months postoperatively, and improvement, if it is to occur, should be observed within 6 months.

Complications of varicocelectomy are rare and are usually minor. Depending on the form of anesthesia used, there may be anesthetic complications. In one large series of 504 men treated surgically via an inguinal approach, 3 percent of patients developed hydroceles, 1 percent had wound infections, and only one patient had a recurrence.[23] Hydroceles should be preventable by preserving the lymphatic vessels. Complications specific to the laparoscopic approach include a low incidence of bowel, bladder, and vascular injury.

HYDROCELECTOMY

Indications

A hydrocele appears as an enlargement of the scrotum caused by an abnormal collection of fluid within the tunica vaginalis. Although this collection of fluid in an adult may be associated with testicular disease, such as infection or tumor, it is more commonly idiopathic. Hydroceles are generally asymptomatic and rarely require treatment. However, those that are quite large may cause discomfort or may become unsightly and embarrassing, and hydrocelectomy is then indicated.

Pediatric hydroceles may be associated with a patent processus vaginalis and an indirect hernia. This type of hydrocele requires a different surgical approach from hydroceles in adults: the hernia sac should be dissected and ligated high at the internal inguinal ring.

Preoperative Management

Most patients with hydroceles have chronic asymptomatic enlargement of the scrotum, which is usually easily differentiated from inguinal hernia. The acute presentation of a hydrocele may be associated with epididymitis, testicular torsion, or, rarely, testicular tumor. Treatment in any of these situations should

be directed toward the underlying cause. Palpation should be used to identify and examine the testis within the hydrocele sac to rule out testicular disease. An uncomplicated hydrocele is easily transilluminated. Auscultation of the scrotum may reveal bowel sounds, which helps differentiate a hernia from a hydrocele.

If the diagnosis is still in doubt, scrotal ultrasonography is helpful in differentiating a hydrocele from either a hernia or a tumor of the spermatic cord. A preoperative scrotal ultrasonogram should always be obtained in a patient in whom palpation has not provided satisfactory testicular assessment. The unexpected diagnosis of testicular tumor following a scrotal incision for hydrocele is easily avoided with the diagnostic tools currently available.[24]

Treatment Options

In a high-risk patient, scrotal aspiration of a hydrocele, with or without injection of sclerosing agents such as tetracycline, may be considered.[25] Aspiration alone, however, is rarely effective, and injection of sclerosing agents has been associated with high retreatment rates and occasional severe scrotal complications.[26] Surgical therapy is a simple, effective, and safe form of treatment and continues to be the therapeutic procedure of choice.

Numerous procedures are employed for the surgical treatment of hydroceles. These procedures can be divided into two categories on the basis of the extent of dissection within the scrotum and the amount of the hydrocele sac excised. The procedures with more limited dissection have lower complication rates (scrotal hematoma) and appear to be just as successful as more extensive procedures.

Jaboulay Procedure

The Jaboulay procedure[27] requires full dissection of the hydrocele sac and delivery of the intact sac through the wound. A transverse scrotal incision is made through the skin and dartos muscle. Dissection is carried out in the loose areolar tissue surrounding the hydrocele, and the sac is delivered through the wound, opened along its anterior surface, and drained. If the hydrocele is large, part of the sac may be excised. A running absorbable suture is then placed along the edge of the remaining sac to evert the tunica vaginalis behind the testis in such a way that the serous lining faces outward (Fig. 82–4). This running suture also helps maintain hemostasis. The scrotal incision is then closed in two layers with absorbable suture.

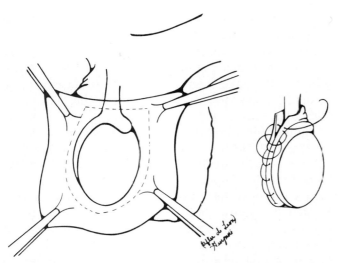

Figure 82–4. Jaboulay procedure. Part of the hydrocele sac can be excised and the free edges everted around the testis with a running suture. (From Glenn JF, ed. Urologic Surgery. Philadelphia, JB Lippincott, 1983.)

Lord Procedure

The Lord procedure[28] was first described in 1964 as a bloodless operation for the radical cure of idiopathic hydrocele. Its advantage is the need for little or no dissection within the scrotum. Therefore, the risk of postoperative hematoma is reduced. A transverse incision is made through the skin and dartos muscle, and the wound edges are grasped with Allis clamps. The hydrocele sac is incised on its anterior surface, and the testis is delivered through the opening in the sac. The tunica vaginalis is plicated with multiple radial absorbable stitches, which imbricate from the edge of the sac to the juncture of the testis and epididymis to prevent recurrence (Fig. 82–5). This maneuver forms a collar of everted tunica vaginalis around the testis, which, together with the testis, is placed back into the scrotum. Frequently, the incision needs to be stretched to allow the testis to be placed back into the scrotum. The wound is then closed in two layers with absorbable suture.

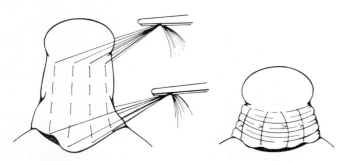

Figure 82–5. Lord procedure. The testis is delivered through an incision in the sac and the sac is then plicated with multiple radial sutures. (From Glenn JF, ed. Urologic Surgery. Philadelphia, JB Lippincott, 1983.)

Postoperative Management and Complications

Hydrocelectomy is performed on an outpatient basis using local, regional, or general anesthesia. The wound is dressed with antibiotic ointment, and a scrotal support is placed. Ice is applied to decrease pain and swelling for the first 24 hours postoperatively. Oral analgesics are usually sufficient to control postoperative pain. A drain is not necessary because of the limited dissection involved but can be left indwelling overnight in a patient who has an increased risk of bleeding. The patient should return within 2 weeks for wound examination.

Complications of this procedure are usually self-limiting and include edema, hematoma, wound infection, scrotal abscess, and recurrent hydrocele. In one series of 87 patients, the complications resulting from four different procedures for hydrocelectomy, performed by the same surgeons, were compared: 10 percent of patients developed hematomas, 7 percent had wound infections, and only one patient developed a scrotal abscess.[29] None of these complications occurred in patients undergoing the Lord procedure.

SPERMATOCELECTOMY

Indications

Spermatoceles are cystic cavities containing fluid and sperm arising from the rete testis, efferent ducts, or epididymis. The prevalence of spermatoceles has been estimated to be 1 percent.[30] Most are found near the head of the epididymis and are rarely symptomatic. Indications for excision include discomfort, size sufficient to cause embarrassment, and inability to confirm the diagnosis.

Treatment Options

Options in therapy are similar to those for a hydrocele. Aspiration, with and without injection of sclerosing agents, has been successful,[31] but surgical excision remains the primary form of therapy for the rare patient who requires it. The spermatocele can be approached through a transverse scrotal incision. Small spermatoceles may be removed by simple ligation and sharp excision. Large spermatoceles require more extensive dissection and prevention of recurrence by careful suture ligation at the site of communication with the epididymis.

Postoperative Management

Postoperative management includes use of a scrotal supporter and ice packs for 24 hours. Complications, including hematoma and wound infection, are rare and usually self-limited.

TESTICULAR BIOPSY

Indications

Testicular biopsy, once a routine test in the evaluation of an infertile man, is now limited to the evaluation of azoospermia. Azoospermia may be caused by pretesticular conditions, such as endocrinopathy; testicular disorders, such as germinal cell aplasia; or post-testicular conditions, such as ductal obstruction. A testicular biopsy is necessary to differentiate between obstruction and an intrinsic testicular abnormality. In an azoospermic patient with gonadotropin levels within two times the normal range and at least one testis of normal size, a testicular biopsy is necessary to differentiate between an obstruction and an intrinsic testicular abnormality.[32] In addition to the azoospermic patient, the pediatric patient with leukemia sometimes undergoes testicular biopsy for staging purposes. Testicular biopsy is rarely performed in an adult with an intratesticular mass because radical orchiectomy is the procedure of choice.

Operative Technique

Testicular biopsy may be performed on an outpatient basis using local, regional, or general anesthesia. Local anesthesia can be achieved with a short-acting anesthetic injected into the skin and subcutaneous tissues. A longer-acting anesthetic is used for a spermatic cord block. The cord block may be administered by trapping the spermatic cord near the pubic bone close to the external inguinal ring and infusing it with 10 ml of anesthetic through a 25-gauge needle, carefully aspirating before injection. This method will effectively block pain sensation in both the testis and the epididymis. Clinicians concerned about possible trauma to the gonadal vasculature with this maneuver prefer to use general anesthesia for testicular biopsy.

In an azoospermic patient, a testicular biopsy establishes the presence of normal spermatogenesis. Vasography is then used to determine the site of obstruction. Unfortunately, differentiation of normal spermatogenesis from late spermatogenic maturation arrest may be difficult on the basis of a frozen section, and permanent sections are often required for the final diagnosis. For this reason, it is better to stage the procedures, performing a testicular biopsy at one time and postponing vasography until reconstructive surgery is performed. Vasography should be performed only at the time of reconstruction to avoid damaging the vas at a site separate from that of the original pathological condition.

Extensive intrascrotal dissection, particularly within the tunica vaginalis, may produce adhesions, which will make later reconstructive surgery more difficult. Therefore, it is best to use the "window" testicular biopsy technique[33] because it limits the amount of intrascrotal dissection. In patients who are undergoing a testicular biopsy for reasons other than diagnosis of infertility, the entire testis may be delivered through an opening in the tunica vaginalis.

The window testicular biopsy technique is performed through a small, transverse scrotal incision. It is extremely important that the epididymis be held posteriorly away from the incision site and maintained in that position throughout the procedure to avoid inadvertent epididymal damage. The small incision is made through the tunica vaginalis, and an eyelid retractor is used to maintain exposure of the tunica albuginea (Fig. 82–6). Examination of the intragonadal vascular patterns has demonstrated that the major arterial branches maintain a superficial course beneath the tunica albuginea and thus may be severed with incision of the tunica albuginea.[34] The medial and lateral surfaces of the superior pole of the testis are least likely to contain one of these arteries and are therefore the safest sites for biopsy. A single stay suture should be placed through the tunica albuginea at one end of the proposed tunica incision to help maintain the testis in proper position beneath the window; the needle is left on the suture. The tunica albuginea is then incised with a scalpel. The extruded testicular tissue should be excised with either sharp scissors or a scalpel, using a no-touch technique.

The testicular tissue should then immediately be placed in a suitable fixative, such as Bouin's, Zenker's, or buffered glutaraldehyde. Formalin is not a proper fixative for testicular tissue. In addition to tissue obtained for permanent sections, a touch preparation of exfoliated germ cells can be helpful in the final interpretation of a testicular biopsy specimen. This preparation can be obtained by taking a second piece of tissue, smearing it over a sterile glass slide, and immediately spraying the slide with cytofixative. Alternatively, a portion of testicular tissue can be placed on a slide and examined as a wet mount for the presence of motile sperm.[35] Testicular tissue handled in this fashion is usually not suitable for permanent sections.

The incision through the tunica albuginea is closed with the previously placed stay suture. Hemostasis should be achieved before the wound is closed to avoid formation of a hematocele. The tunica vaginalis, dartos muscle, and skin are closed in multiple layers with absorbable suture.

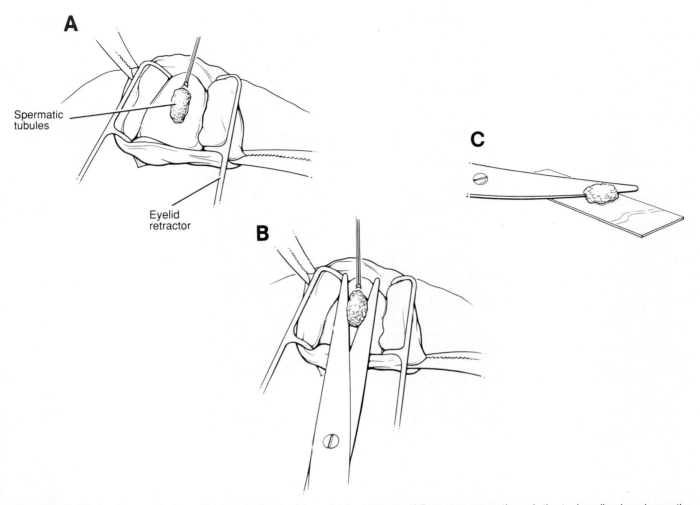

Figure 82–6. Window biopsy. *A,* An eyelid retractor is used to maintain exposure while a stay suture through the tunica albuginea keeps the testicular incision site in view. *B,* Testicular parenchymal tissue is excised, using a no-touch technique, and placed into an appropriate fixative. *C,* Another piece of tissue is taken for a touch preparation on a glass slide. This specimen is immediately sprayed with a cytofixative before it dries.

Postoperative Management and Complications

The postoperative care following testicular biopsy is simple, because complications are rare and discomfort is minimal. A scrotal support is suggested, and ice packs may be used during the first 24 hours to reduce pain and swelling. If bleeding from the vessels beneath the tunica albuginea has not been properly controlled, a large hematocele may develop. When a great deal of blood is lost into the scrotum, postoperative healing will be accelerated if the scrotum is re-explored, hemostasis achieved, and the hematocele drained.

Summary

Varicocelectomy, hydrocelectomy, spermatocelectomy, and testicular biopsy can all be performed on an outpatient basis using local anesthesia. By this means, the patient experiences significant savings in cost, time lost from work, and separation from family. Regardless of the type of anesthesia, the mortality rate should be zero and the morbidity less than 5 percent. These results are particularly important, considering the elective nature of these procedures.

REFERENCES

1. Saypol DC, Lipshultz LI, Howards SS. Varicocele. In Lipshultz LI, Howards SS, eds. Infertility in the Male. New York, Churchill Livingstone, 1983.
2. Laven JSE, Maans LCF, Mali WPT, et al. Effects of varicocele treatment in adolescents: A randomized study. Fertil Steril 58:756, 1992.
3. Dubin L, Amelar RD. Etiologic factors in 1294 consecutive cases of male infertility. Fertil Steril 22:469, 1971.
4. Greenberg SH, Lipshultz LI, Wein AJ. Experience with 425 subfertile male patients. J Urol 119:507, 1978.
5. Rodriguez-Rigau LJ, Weiss DB, Zukerman Z, et al. A possible mechanism for the detrimental effect of varicocele on testicular function in man. Fertil Steril 30:577, 1978.
6. MacLeod J. Seminal cytology in the presence of varicocele. Fertil Steril 16:735, 1965.

7. Nilsson S, Edvinsson A, Nilsson B. Improvement of semen and pregnancy rate after ligation and division of the internal spermatic vein: Fact or fiction? Br J Urol 51:591, 1979.

8. Pryor JL, Howards SS. Varicocele. Urol Clin North Am 14:499, 1987.

9. World Health Organization. Comparison among different methods for the diagnosis of varicocele. Fertil Steril 43:575, 1985.

10. Yarborough MA, Burns JR, Keller FS. Incidence and clinical significance of subclinical scrotal varicoceles. J Urol 141:1372, 1988.

11. McClure RD, Hricak H. Scrotal ultrasound in the infertile man: Detection of subclinical unilateral and bilateral varicoceles. J Urol 135:711, 1986.

12. Wheatley JK, Fajman WA, Witten FR. Clinical experience with the radioisotope varicocele scan as a screening method for the detection of subclinical varicoceles. J Urol 128:57, 1982.

13. Netto NR Jr, Lemos GC, Barbosa EM. The value of thermography and of the Doppler ultrasound in varicocele diagnosis. Int J Fertil 29:176, 1984.

14. Nadel SN, Hutchins GM, Albertsen PC, White RI Jr. Valves of the internal spermatic vein: Potential for misdiagnosis of varicocele by venography. Fertil Steril 41:479, 1984.

15. Coolsaet BLRA. The varicocele syndrome: Venography determining the optimal level for surgical management. J Urol 124:833, 1980.

16. Palomo A. Radical cure of varicocele by a new technique: Preliminary report. J Urol 61:604, 1949.

17. Bach D, Bahren W, Gall H, Altwein JE. Late results after sclerotherapy of varicocele. Eur Urol 14:115, 1988.

18. Berkman WA, Price RB, Wheatley JK, et al. Varicoceles: A coaxial coil occlusion system. Radiology 151:73, 1984.

19. Kaufman SL, Kadir S, Barth KH, et al. Mechanisms of recurrent varicocele after balloon occlusion or surgical ligation of the internal spermatic vein. Radiology 147:435, 1983.

20. Goldstein M, Gilbert BR, Dicker AP, et al. Microsurgical inguinal varicocelectomy with delivery of the testis: An artery and lymphatic sparing technique. J Urol 148:1808, 1992.

21. Jarow JP, Assimos DG, Pittaway DE. Effectiveness of laparoscopic varicocelectomy. Urology 42:544, 1993.

22. Lynch WJ, Badenoch DF, McAnena OJ. Comparison of laparoscopic and open ligation of the testicular vein. Br J Urol 72:796, 1993.

23. Dubin L, Amelar RD. Varicocelectomy as therapy in male infertility: A study of 504 cases. Fertil Steril 26:217, 1975.

24. Roy CR, Peterson NE. Positive hydrocele cytology accompanying testis seminoma. Urology 39:292, 1992.

25. Shokeir AA, Eraky I, Hassan N, et al. Tetracycline sclerotherapy for testicular hydroceles in renal transplant recipients. Urology 44:96, 1994.

26. Badenoch DF, Fowler CG, Jenkins BJ, et al. Aspiration and instillation of tetracycline in the treatment of testicular hydrocele. Br J Urol 59:172, 1987.

27. Jaboulay M. Chirurgie des centres nerveux, des visceres et des membres. Lyon, Storck, 1902, (second volume) p. 192.

28. Lord PH. A bloodless operation for the radical cure of idiopathic hydrocele. Br J Surg 51:914, 1964.

29. Rodriguez WC, Rodriguez DD, Fortuno RF. The operative treatment of hydrocele: A comparison of four basic techniques. J Urol 125:804, 1981.

30. Rolnick HC. The etiology of spermatocele. J Urol 19:613, 1928.

31. Bullock N, Thurston AV. Tetracycline sclerotherapy for hydroceles and epididymal cysts. Br J Urol 59:340, 1987.

32. Jarow JP, Espeland MA, Lipshultz LI. Evaluation of the azoospermic patient. J Urol 142:62, 1989.

33. Coburn M, Wheeler T, Lipshultz LI. Testicular biopsy: Its use and limitations. Urol Clin North Am 14:551, 1987.

34. Jarow JP. Clinical significance of intratesticular arterial anatomy. J Urol 145:777, 1991.

35. Jow WW, Steckel J, Schlegel PN, et al. Motile sperm in human testis biopsy specimens. J Androl 14:194, 1993.

Chapter 83

Microsurgical Vasovasostomy

Marc Goldstein

PREOPERATIVE EVALUATION

Physical Examination

Several aspects of the physical examination have an impact on vasovasostomy and its outcome:

1. Testis: Small or soft testes suggest impaired spermatogenesis and predict a poor outcome.

2. Epididymis: An indurated irregular epididymis often predicts secondary epididymal obstruction, necessitating vasoepididymostomy.

3. Sperm granuloma: A sperm granuloma at the testicular end of the vas means sperm has been leaking at the vasectomy site. This vents the high pressures away from the epididymis and improves the prognosis for restored fertility, regardless of the time interval since vasectomy.

4. Vasal gap: When a very destructive vasectomy has been performed, most of the scrotal straight vas may be absent or fibrotic, and the patient should be advised that inguinal extension of the scrotal incision may be necessary to enable a tension-free anastomosis.

5. Scars from previous surgery: Operative scars in the inguinal or scrotal region should alert the surgeon to the possibility of vasal obstruction at a site remote from the vasectomy. If two vasovasostomies are performed simultaneously in the same vas, devascularization of the intervening segments could result, with subsequent fibrosis and failure.

Laboratory Tests

Semen analysis with centrifugation and examination of the pellet for sperm should be performed preoperatively. The presence of even rare sperm means microrecanalization has occurred. Under these circumstances, sperm are certain to be found in the vas on at least one side, improving the prognosis for restored fertility.[1] Men with a low semen volume should undergo a transrectal ultrasound examination for possible ejaculatory duct obstruction.

Serum antisperm antibody studies should be performed. The presence of serum antisperm antibodies corroborates the diagnosis of obstruction. Also, men with small, soft testes should have serum concentrations of follicle stimulating hormone (FSH) measured. An elevated FSH level is a predictor of impaired spermatogenesis and carries a poorer prognosis.

ANESTHESIA

Light general or regional anesthesia is preferred. In cooperative patients, local anesthesia with sedation can be used if the time interval since vasectomy is short, the vasal ends are easily palpable, or if a sperm granuloma is present, which decreases the likelihood of secondary epididymal obstruction. Slight movements are greatly magnified by the operating microscope and make anastomosis difficult. When large vasal gaps are present, extensions of the incisions high into the inguinal canal may be necessary. Furthermore, if vasoepididymostomy is necessary, the operating time could exceed 4 or 5 hours. Local anesthesia limits the options available to the surgeon. Hypobaric spinal anesthesia with long-acting agents such as bupivacaine (Marcaine) can provide 4 to 5 hours of anesthesia time and has the advantage of eliminating lower body motion. Epidural anesthesia with an indwelling catheter can be equally effective.

With local anesthesia and cord block there is a small risk of inadvertent injury to the testicular artery.[1] If the vasal artery has been disrupted by previous vasectomy, testicular artery injury could result in testicular atrophy.

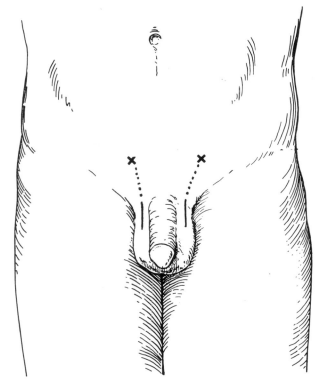

Figure 83–1. Preferred incisions for vasectomy reversal allow extension to the external inguinal ring (x) when the abdominal vas is short. (From Goldstein M. Vasovasostomy surgical approach, decision making, and multilayer microdot technique. In Goldstein M, ed. Surgery of Male Infertility. Philadelphia, WB Saunders, 1995, pp 46–60.)

SURGICAL APPROACHES

Scrotal

Bilateral high vertical scrotal incisions provide the most direct access to the obstructed site in cases of vasectomy reversal. The location of the external inguinal ring is marked (Fig. 83–1). If the vasal gap is large or the vasectomy site is high, this incision can easily be extended inguinally toward the external ring. If the vasectomy site is low, it is easy to pull up the testicular end. This incision should be made at least 1 cm lateral to the base of the penis. The testis should be delivered with the tunica vaginalis left intact. This provides excellent exposure of the entire scrotal vas deferens and, if necessary, the epididymis.

Inguinal Incision

An inguinal incision is the preferred approach in men with suspected obstruction of the inguinal vas deferens from prior herniorrhaphy or orchiopexy. Incision through the previous scar usually leads directly to the site of obstruction. If the obstruction turns out to be scrotal or epididymal, it is a simple

matter to deliver the testis through the inguinal incision or through a separate scrotal incision.

PREPARATION OF THE VASA

The vas is grasped above and below the site of obstruction with two Babcock clamps. These are replaced with Penrose drains, which facilitate the dissection. The vasal vessels and periadventitial tissue are included. Enough vas is mobilized to allow a tension-free anastomosis. To preserve a good blood supply, the vas should not be stripped of its sheath. The obstructed segment and, if present, the sperm granuloma at the vasectomy site should be dissected out. The vasal ends usually remain in continuity. This allows serial sectioning beginning at the obstructed segment and ensures preservation of a maximal length of healthy vas. If the vasectomy site or sperm granuloma involves the internal spermatic vessels, the vas is cut as close to the obstruction as possible and the defunctionalized stumps tied with a 2-0 Vicryl suture ligature. This avoids the risk of injuring the testicular artery. Injury to adjacent cord structures, especially the testicular artery, is likely to result in testicular atrophy because the vasal artery has usually been interrupted at the vasectomy site.

When large vasal gaps are present, a gauze-

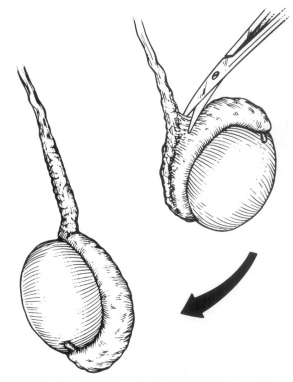

Figure 83–2. A convoluted vas dissected off the epididymal tunic provides additional length on the testicular side. (From Goldstein M. Vasovasostomy surgical approach, decision making, and multilayer microdot technique. In Goldstein M, ed. Surgery of Male Infertility. Philadelphia, WB Saunders, 1995, pp 46–60.)

wrapped index finger is used to separate the cord structures away from the vas. Blunt finger dissection through the external ring will free the vas to the internal inguinal ring if additional abdominal length is necessary. These maneuvers leave all the vasal vessels intact. When the vasal gap is extremely large, additional length can be achieved by dissecting the entire convoluted vas free of its attachments to the epididymal tunic, allowing the testis to drop upside down. These maneuvers can provide an additional 4 to 6 cm of length (Fig. 83–2). To maintain the integrity of the vasal vessels, this dissection is best performed with the aid of magnifying loupes or the operating microscope. If the amount of vas removed is so large that even these measures fail to allow a tension-free anastomosis, the incision can be extended to the internal inguinal ring, the floor of the inguinal canal cut, and the vas rerouted under the floor as in a difficult orchiopexy. An additional 4 to 6 cm of length can be obtained by dissecting the epididymis off the testis from the vasoepididymal junction to the caput epididymidis (Fig. 83–3). The superior epididymal vessels are left intact and provide adequate blood supply to the testicular end of the vas. With this combination of maneuvers, 15-cm gaps can be bridged.

After the vas has been freed up, its testicular end is sharply cut. An ultrasharp knife drawn through a slotted 2- to 3-mm diameter nerve clamp yields a perfect 90-degree cut (Fig. 83–4). The cut surface of the testicular end of the vas deferens is inspected under 8- to 15-power magnification. A healthy white

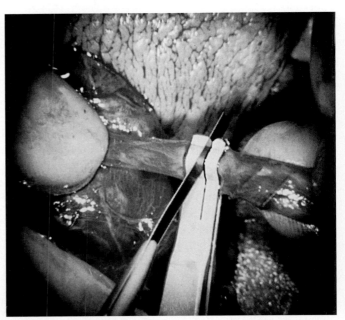

Figure 83–4. An ultrasharp knife drawn through a 2- to 3-mm slotted nerve-holding clamp (from Accurate Surgical and Scientific Instrument Corp., Westbury, NY) produces a perfect 90-degree cut. (From Goldstein M. Vasovasostomy surgical approach, decision making, and multilayer microdot technique. In Goldstein M, ed. Surgery of Male Infertility. Philadelphia, WB Saunders, 1995, pp 46–60.)

mucosal ring that springs back immediately after gentle dilation should be seen. The muscularis should be smooth and soft, not gritty. The cut surface should look like a bull's eye with the three vasal layers distinctly visible. Healthy bleeding should be noted from both the cut edge of the mucosa and the surface of the muscularis. If the blood supply is poor or the muscularis is gritty, the vas should be recut until healthy tissue is found. The vasal artery and vein are then clamped and ligated with 6-0 Prolene. Small bleeders are controlled with a bipolar microforceps set at low power. Once a patent lumen has been established on the testicular end, the vas is milked and a clean glass slide touched to its surface. The vasal fluid is immediately mixed with a drop or two of saline and preserved under a cover slip for microscopical examination. The abdominal end of the vas deferens is prepared in a similar manner, and the lumen is gently dilated with a microvessel dilator and cannulated with a 24-gauge angiocatheter sheath. Injection of saline or lactated Ringer's confirms its patency. A minimum of instrumentation of the mucosa should be performed.

After preparation, the ends of the vasa are stabilized with a Goldstein Microspike approximating clamp to remove all tension before the anastomosis is performed. A sterile tongue blade is slipped inside a Penrose drain and placed beneath the ends of the vasa. This provides an excellent platform on which to perform the anastomosis. Isolating the field through a

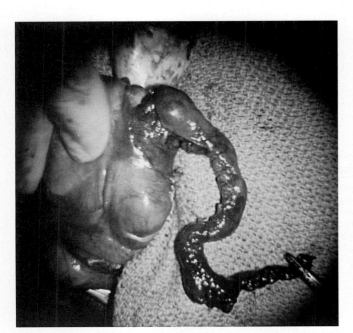

Figure 83–3. The entire vasoepididymal complex dissected to the caput epididymidis to bridge massive vasal gaps. (From Goldstein M. Vasovasostomy surgical approach, decision making, and multilayer microdot technique. In Goldstein M, ed. Surgery of Male Infertility. Philadelphia, WB Saunders, 1995, pp 46–60.)

slit in a rubber dam prevents microsutures from sticking to the surrounding tissue.

WHEN TO PERFORM VASOEPIDIDYMOSTOMY

The gross appearance of fluid expressed from the testicular end of the vas is usually predictive of findings on microscopical examination (Table 83–1). If microscopical examination of the vasal fluid reveals the presence of sperm with tails, vasovasostomy is performed. If no fluid is found, a 24-gauge angiocatheter sheath is inserted into the lumen and barbitage with 0.1 ml of saline performed while the convoluted vas is vigorously milked. Men with large sperm granulomas often have virtually no dilation of the testicular end of the vas, and little or no fluid may be noticed initially. The barbitage fluid is expressed onto a slide and examined. Invariably, when sperm granulomas are present, sperm are found in this scant fluid. If the vas is absolutely dry and spermless after multiple samples are examined, vasoepididymostomy should be performed. If the fluid expressed from the vas is found to be thick, white, water insoluble, and toothpaste-like in quality, examination rarely reveals sperm. Under these circumstances, the tunica vaginalis is opened and the epididymis inspected. If clear evidence of obstruction is found, e.g., an epididymal sperm granuloma with dilated tubules above and collapsed tubules below, vasoepididymostomy is performed. When in doubt, or if one is not very experienced with vasoepididymostomy, vasovasostomy should be performed. About 30 percent of men with bilateral absence of sperm in the vasal fluid have sperm return to the ejaculate. When copious, clear, water-like fluid squirts out of the vas and no sperm are found in this fluid, a vasovasostomy is performed, because the prognosis is good that sperm will return to the ejaculate.

MULTIPLE VASAL OBSTRUCTIONS

If saline injection reveals that the abdominal end of the vas deferens is not patent, a 2-0 nylon suture is gently passed to determine the site of obstruction. If the obstruction is within 5 cm of the original vasectomy site, the abdominal end of the vas deferens may be dissected to this site and excised. The incision should then be extended inguinally to extensively free up the vas toward the internal inguinal ring. The testicular end should also be freed up to the vasoepididymal junction. If the site of the second obstruction is so far from the vasectomy site that two vasovasostomies are necessary, the distance to the inguinal obstruction is measured and recorded for future reference. A vasovasostomy is then performed at the vasectomy site. The patient is re-explored at a later date for an inguinal vasovasostomy after the vasal segment beyond the original vasovasostomy site has been allowed to become well vascularized. Simultaneous vasovasostomies at two separate sites are risky and may lead to devascularization of the intervening segment with fibrosis and necrosis.

VARICOCELECTOMY AND VASOVASOSTOMY

When men who are to undergo vasovasostomy or vasoepididymostomy are found to have significant varicoceles on physical examination, it is tempting to repair the varicoceles at the same time. This temptation should be resisted. When varicocelectomy is properly performed, all spermatic veins are ligated and the only remaining avenues for testicular venous return are the vasal veins. In men who have had vasectomy and are to undergo reversal, the vasal veins are likely to be compromised from either the original vasectomy or the reversal itself. Furthermore, the integrity of the vasal artery in those men is also

TABLE 83–1. Relationship Between Gross Appearance of Vasal Fluid and Microscopical Findings

Vasal Fluid Appearance	Most Common Findings on Microscopical Examination	Surgical Procedure Indicated
Copious, clear, watery	No sperm in fluid	Vasovasostomy
Copious, cloudy, thin, water soluble	Usually sperm with tails	Vasovasostomy
Copious, creamy yellow, water soluble	Usually many sperm heads, occasional sperm with tails	Vasovasostomy
Copious, thick, white, toothpaste-like, water insoluble	No sperm	Vasoepididymostomy
Scant, white, thin fluid	No sperm	Vasoepididymostomy
Dry, spermless vas—no granuloma at vasectomy site	No sperm	Vasoepididymostomy
Scant fluid, granuloma present at vasectomy site	Barbitage fluid reveals sperm	Vasovasotomy

From Goldstein M. Vasovasostomy: Surgical Approach, Decision Making, and Multilayer Microdot Technique. In Goldstein M, ed. Surgery of Male Infertility. Philadelphia, WB Saunders, 1995, p 46.

likely to be compromised. Varicocelectomy in such men requires preservation of the testicular artery as the primary remaining testicular blood supply as well as preservation of some avenue for venous return.

Microsurgical varicocelectomy[3] can ensure preservation of the testicular artery in most cases. Deliberate preservation of the cremasteric veins provides venous return. Of 407 men examined for vasectomy reversal, 14 had large varicoceles (ten left, four bilateral). Microsurgical varicocelectomy was performed at the same time as vasovasostomy. The cremasteric veins and the fine network of veins adherent to the testicular artery were left intact for venous return and to minimize the chances of injury to the testicular artery. Postoperatively, four of 18 varicoceles recurred (22 percent) and two testes atrophied (11 percent). This compares with a recurrence rate of 0.6 percent and no cases of atrophy in 640 varicocelectomies performed by the author in nonvasectomized men in which the vasal vessels were intact and the cremasteric veins and periarterial venous network were ligated.

Because of the significantly increased risk of testicular atrophy and varicocele recurrence, varicocelectomy should never be performed at the same time as vasovasostomy or vasoepididymostomy. The vasovasostomy or vasoepidymostomy should be done first. The semen quality is then determined postoperatively. If necessary, varicocelectomy can be safely performed 6 months or more later, when venous and arterial channels have formed across the anastomotic line. This two-stage delayed approach has been completed a dozen times with no atrophy or recurrence. The varicocelectomy should be done microscopically to preserve the testicular artery, since atrophy can occur after testicular artery ligation even when the vasal blood supply to the testis is intact. Interestingly, the marked increase in recurrences when the cremasteric veins and periarterial venous network were left intact suggests that these veins contribute to a significant proportion of varicocele recurrences.

ANASTOMOTIC TECHNIQUES: KEYS TO SUCCESS

All successful vasovasostomy techniques depend on adherence to surgical principles that are universally applicable to anastomoses of all tubular structures. These include the following:

1. Accurate mucosa-to-mucosa approximation. In human vasovasostomy, the testicular side lumen is often dilated to diameters three to six times that of the abdominal side lumen. Techniques that work well with lumina of equal diameters may be less successful when applied to lumina of markedly discrepant diameters.

2. Leakproof anastomosis. Sperm are highly antigenic and provoke an inflammatory reaction when they escape from the normally intact lining of the excurrent ducts of the male reproductive tract. Extravasated sperm adversely influence the success of vasovasostomy.[4, 5] Unlike blood vessel anastomoses, where platelets and clotting factors seal the gaps between sutures, vasal and epididymal fluid contain no platelets or clotting factors, so the watertightness of the anastomosis is entirely dependent on the mucosal sutures.

3. Tension-free anastomosis. When an anastomosis is performed under tension, sperm may appear in the ejaculate for several months after surgery. Ultimately, sperm counts and motility will decrease and azoospermia may ensue. At re-exploration, only a thin fibrotic band is found at the anastomotic site. This can be prevented by adequately freeing up the end of the vasa and placing reinforcing sutures in the periadventitia (sheath) of the vas.

4. Good blood supply. If the cut vas exhibits poor blood supply, it should be recut until healthy bleeding is encountered. If extensive resection is necessary, additional length should be obtained using the techniques described earlier.

5. Healthy mucosa and muscularis. If the mucosa or cut surface of the vas exhibits poor distensibility after dilation or easily peels away from the underlying muscularis or shreds easily, the vas should be cut back until healthy mucosa is found. If the muscularis is found to be fibrotic or gritty, the vas must be recut until healthy tissue is found.

6. Good atraumatic anastomotic technique. If multiple surgical errors occur during the procedure, such as cutting of the mucosa with needles, tearing through of sutures, or backwalling of the mucosa, the anastomosis should be immediately resected and redone.

MICROSURGICAL TECHNIQUE

Set-up

An operating microscope providing variable magnification from 6 to 32 power is used. A diploscope providing identical fields for both surgeon and assistant is preferred. Foot pedal controls for a motorized zoom and focus leave the hands free.

Both surgeon and assistant should be comfortably seated on well-padded stools to stabilize the lower body. I prefer a simple rolling stool with a round beanbag (meditation pillow) taped on top for padding. Two arm boards placed on either side of the surgeon and built up to the correct height with folded blankets taped to the board provide excellent arm support and dramatically improve stability and accu-

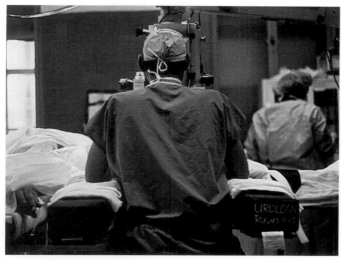

Figure 83–5. Two arm boards, placed on either side of the surgeon and assistant and built up to the right height with folded blankets taped to the board, provide excellent arm support and dramatically improve stability and accuracy.

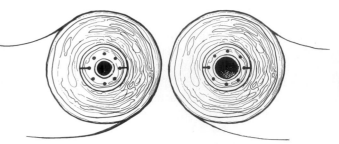

Figure 83–6. Use exactly eight mucosal sutures.

racy (Fig. 83–5). This set-up is flexible and maneuverable and can be obtained at a fraction of the cost of cumbersome electric microsurgery chairs. The surgeon should sit on the patient's right side so that the forehand stitch is always on the smaller, more difficult abdominal side lumen.

Multilayer Microdot Method

The multilayer microdot method of vasovasostomy can be used for lumina of markedly discrepant diameters in the straight or convoluted vas. Monofilament 10-0 Prolene sutures, double-armed with 70-μm diameter taper-point needles bent into a fishhook configuration, are used.

Precision placement of sutures is facilitated by dry-

ing the cut surface of the vas with a Weck cell and using a microtip marking pen to map out planned needle exit points (Fig. 83–6). Lines are drawn on the 3 o'clock and 9 o'clock dots to help match them up. This mapping prevents dog-ears and leaks when the lumen diameters are discrepant. Exactly eight mucosal sutures are used for all anastomoses. Dots are made at 3, 9, 12, and 6 o'clock and then exactly between each pair (Fig. 83–7A). If the mucosal rings are not sharply defined, the cut surfaces of the vasal ends are stained with indigo carmine to highlight the mucosa (Fig. 83–7B). Double-armed sutures allow inside-out placement (Fig. 83–8), eliminating the need for manipulation or dilation of the mucosa and the possibility of backwalling. The anastomosis is begun with the placement of four 10-0 monofilament Prolene sutures in the mucosa (Fig. 83–9). If the mucosal edges of the small abdominal side lumen are not clearly visualized, the lumen should be gently and momentarily dilated with a microvessel dilator just before placement of the sutures. The mucosa and about one third of the thickness of the muscularis should be included in the suture. Exactly the same amount of tissue should be included in the bites on each side. After these four mucosal sutures are tied, three 9-0 monofilament Prolene sutures are placed

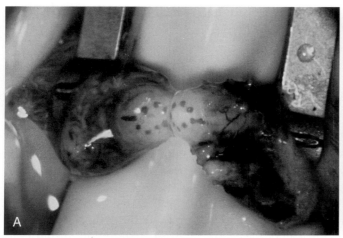
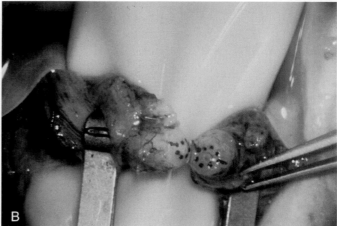

Figure 83–7. *A,* An indigo carmine stain highlights the vas mucosal ring. *A* and *B,* Precision placement of sutures is facilitated by drying the cut surface of the vas with a Weck cell and using a microtip marking pen to map out planned needle exit points. Lines are drawn at 3 and 9 o'clock dots to help match them up. This mapping prevents dog-ears and leaks when the luminal diameters are discrepant.

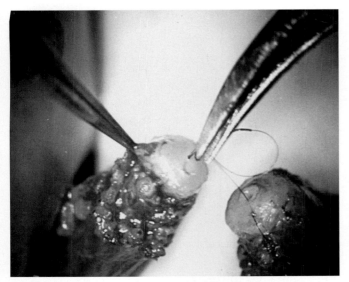

Figure 83–8. Inside-out placement of mucosal sutures using double-armed, fishhook-shaped needles (Sharpoint microdots facilitate accurate suture placement). (From Goldstein M. Vasovasostomy surgical approach, decision making, and multilayer microdot technique. In Goldstein M, ed. Surgery of Male Infertility. Philadelphia, WB Saunders, 1995, pp 46–60.)

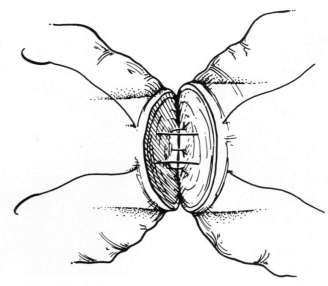

Figure 83–10. Deep muscularis sutures placed between mucosal sutures. (From Goldstein M. Vasovasostomy surgical approach, decision making, and multilayer microdot technique. In Goldstein M, ed. Surgery of Male Infertility. Philadelphia, WB Saunders, 1995, pp 46–60.)

deep in the muscularis exactly between the previously placed mucosal sutures, just above, but not through the mucosa (Fig. 83–10), and then tied. These sutures seal the gaps between the mucosal sutures (Fig. 83–11) without trauma to the mucosa from the larger 100-μm diameter cutting needle required to

penetrate the tough vas muscularis and adventitia. If the space between these two deep 9-0 sutures is such that the underlying 10-0 mucosal suture is visible, a superficial adventitial 9-0 suture is placed between these two muscularis sutures (covering the underlying mucosal suture) to provide additional strength

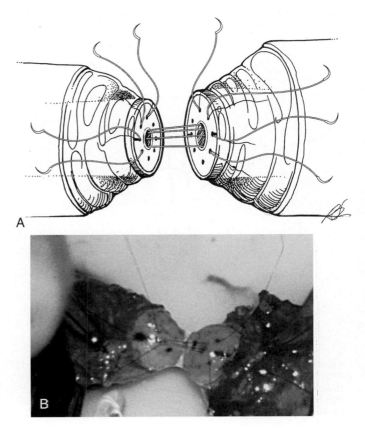

Figure 83–9. *A,* Scheme for placement of the first four mucosal sutures. *B,* First three mucosal sutures placed. Note that sutures exit through microdots. (From Goldstein M. Vasovasostomy surgical approach, decision making, and multilayer microdot technique. In Goldstein M, ed. Surgery of Male Infertility. Philadelphia, WB Saunders, 1995, pp 46–60.)

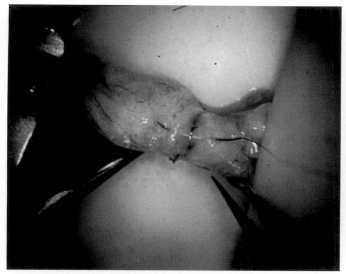

Figure 83–11. 9-0 sutures placed just above but not through the mucosa to seal the gaps between mucosal sutures. (From Goldstein M. Vasovasostomy surgical approach, decision making, and multilayer microdot technique. In Goldstein M, ed. Surgery of Male Infertility. Philadelphia, WB Saunders, 1995, pp 46–60.)

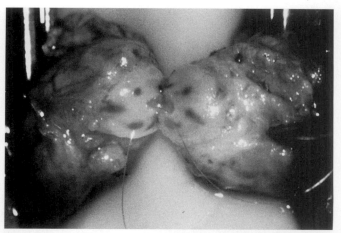

Figure 83–13. Appearance of the anastomosis after the vas is rotated 180 degrees.

(Fig. 83–12). The vas is then rotated 180 degrees (Fig. 83–13), and four additional 10-0 sutures are placed to complete the mucosal portion of the anastomosis (Figs. 83–14 and 83–15). Just before the last mucosal suture is tied, the lumen is irrigated with heparinized Ringer's solution to prevent the formation of clot in the lumen. After the mucosal layer is completed, 9-0 sutures are placed deep in the muscularis exactly in between each mucosal suture, just above but not

penetrating the mucosa. Each 9-0 suture should be placed and cut long and the next one placed and cut long before the previously placed suture is tied. The previously placed 9-0 suture is left untied until the next 9-0 suture is placed. This facilitates more accurate placement. If needed, superficial adventitial 9-0 sutures are then placed exactly between each of the previously placed deep muscularis sutures to seal the muscularis and adventitia over the underlying mucosal sutures (Fig. 83–16). The anastomosis is finished by approximating the vasal sheath with four to six sutures of 6-0 Prolene (Fig. 83–17). This layer completely covers the anastomosis and relieves it of all tension.

ANASTOMOSIS IN THE CONVOLUTED VAS

Vasovasostomy performed in the convoluted portion of the vas deferens is technically more de-

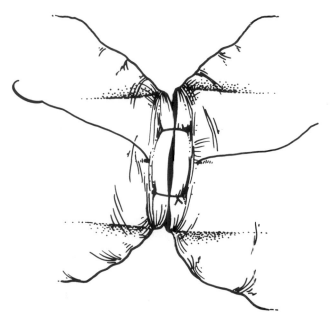

Figure 83–12. 9-0 superficial adventitial sutures are placed only if necessary. (From Goldstein M. Vasovasostomy surgical approach, decision making, and multilayer microdot technique. In Goldstein M, ed. Surgery of Male Infertility. Philadelphia, WB Saunders, 1995, pp 46–60.)

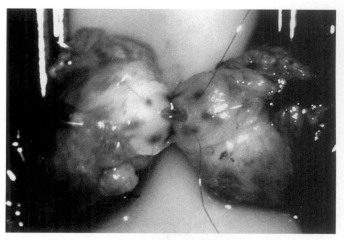

Figure 83–14. Placement of additional 10-0 mucosal sutures, which exit through microdots.

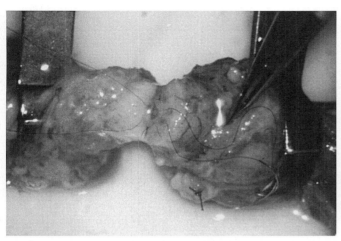

Figure 83–15. Mucosal layer nearing completion. Note the absence of dog-ears.

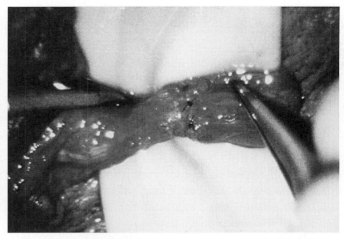

Figure 83–17. Approximation of the vasal sheath with 6-0 Prolene.

manding than anastomosis in the straight portion. Fear of cutting back into the convoluted vas to obtain healthy tissues may lead surgeons to complete an anastomosis in the straight portion when the testicular end of the vas has a poor blood supply, unhealthy or friable mucosa, or gritty, fibrotic muscularis. Adherence to the following principles will enable an anastomosis in the convoluted vas to succeed equally as often as one in the straight portion.

1. A perfect transverse cut yielding a round ring of mucosa and a lumen directed straight down is essential (Fig. 83–18*A*). A very oblique lumen with a thin flap of muscle and mucosa on one side is not acceptable (Fig. 83–18*B*). The vas should be recut at 0.5-mm intervals until a perfect cut with a good blood supply and healthy tissue is obtained. A slotted nerve clamp 2.5 or 3 mm in diameter and an ultrasharp knife facilitate this part of the procedure (see Fig.

83–4). Often the vas must be recut two or three times before the right cut is obtained.

2. The convoluted vas should not be unraveled. This disturbs the blood supply at the anastomotic line.

3. The sheath of the convoluted vas may be carefully dissected free of its attachments to the epididymal tunic (see Fig. 83–2). This will minimize disturbance of its blood supply and provide the necessary length to perform a tension-free anastomosis.

4. Care must be taken to avoid taking large bites of the muscularis and adventitial layers on the convoluted side to prevent inadvertent perforation of adjacent convolutions.

5. The anastomosis is reinforced by approximating the vasal sheath of the straight portion to the sheath of the convoluted portion with multiple 6-0 Prolene sutures. This will remove all tension from the anastomosis.

CROSSED VASOVASOSTOMY

A crossed vasovasostomy is a useful procedure that often provides an easy solution for otherwise difficult

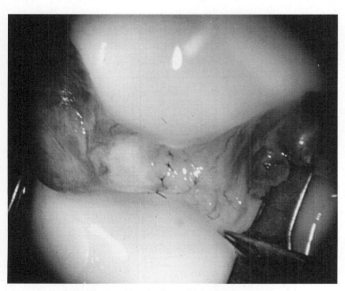

Figure 83–16. Completed 9-0 layer.

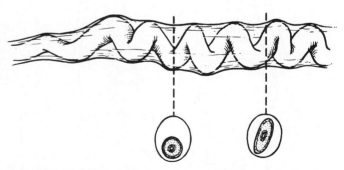

Figure 83–18. A round lumen (*left*) essential for success in convoluted anastomoses. An oblique cut (*right*) is not acceptable. (From Goldstein M. Vasovasostomy surgical approach, decision making, and multilayer microdot technique. In Goldstein M, ed. Surgery of Male Infertility. Philadelphia, WB Saunders, 1995, pp 46–60.)

problems.[6, 7] Cross-over is indicated in the following circumstances:

1. Unilateral inguinal obstruction of the vas deferens associated with an atrophic testis on the contralateral side.

2. Unilateral obstruction or aplasia of the inguinal vas or ejaculatory duct and contralateral obstruction of the epididymis. It is preferable to perform one anastomosis with a high probability of success (vasovasostomy) rather than two operations with a much lower chance of success, e.g., unilateral vasovasoepididymostomy and contralateral transurethral resection of the ejaculatory ducts.

3. In general, one should opt for one good anastomosis instead of two mediocre ones: opt for one good vasovasostomy rather than a unilateral vasoepididymostomy and contralateral mediocre vasovasostomy.

To perform a crossed vasovasostomy, transect the vas attached to the atrophic testis at the junction of its straight and convoluted portion and confirm its patency with a saline or methylene blue vasogram (Fig. 83–19). Dissect the contralateral vas toward the inguinal obstruction. Clamp it as high up as possible with a right-angled clamp. Transect it and cross it through a capacious opening made in the scrotal septum and proceed with vasovasostomy as described above. This procedure is much easier than trying to find both ends of the vas within the dense scar of a previous inguinal operation.

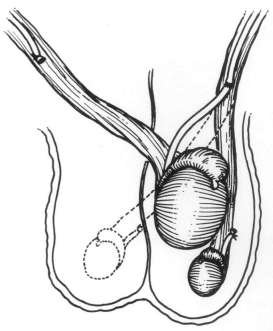

Figure 83–20. Testicular transposition. (From Goldstein M. Vasovasostomy surgical approach, decision making, and multilayer microdot technique. In Goldstein M, ed. Surgery of Male Infertility. Philadelphia, WB Saunders, 1995, pp 46–60.)

TRANSPOSITION OF THE TESTIS

Occasionally, when vasal length is critically short, a tension-free crossed anastomosis can best be accomplished by testicular transposition (Fig. 83–20).

WOUND CLOSURE

If the dissection was extensive, Penrose drains are brought out of the dependent portion of the right and left hemiscrota and fixed in place with sutures and safety pins before the anastomosis is begun. This prevents any possible disturbance of the anastomosis engendered by attempts at drain placement. The dartos is loosely approximated with interrupted absorbable sutures and the skin with subcuticular sutures of 5-0 monocryl. This closure promotes drainage from the wound, thereby minimizing hematoma formation. The wound heals with a fine scar and none of the "railroad tracks" associated with through-and-through skin closures. Most of our procedures are performed on an ambulatory basis. If drains were placed, the patients are given detailed instructions (with explicit drawings) on how to remove the drains the next morning.

Postoperative Management

Sterile fluffs are held in place with a snug-fitting scrotal supporter. Only perioperative antibiotics are

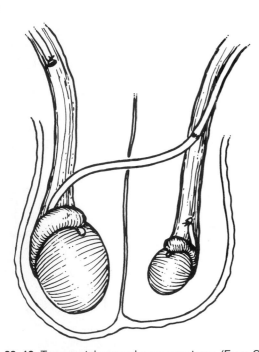

Figure 83–19. Transseptal crossed vasovasostomy. (From Goldstein M. Vasovasostomy surgical approach, decision making, and multilayer microdot technique. In Goldstein M, ed. Surgery of Male Infertility. Philadelphia, WB Saunders, 1995, pp 46–60.)

used. Patients are discharged with a prescription for acetaminophen (Tylenol) with codeine. They may shower 48 hours after surgery. They must wear a scrotal supporter at all times (except in the shower), even when sleeping, for 6 weeks postoperatively. Desk work can be resumed in 3 days. No heavy work or sports are allowed for 3 weeks. No intercourse or ejaculation is allowed for 4 weeks postoperatively. Semen analyses are performed at 1, 3, and 6 months postoperatively and every 6 months thereafter. If azoospermia persists at 6 months, the vasovasostomy is redone or vasoepididymostomy is performed.

Postoperative Complications

The most common complication is hematoma. In 1300 operations, seven small hematomas occurred. None required surgical drainage. Most were walnut sized and perivasal. They take 6 to 12 weeks to resolve. No wound infections have occurred. Late complications include sperm granuloma at the anastomotic site (about 15 percent). This is usually a harbinger of eventual obstruction. Late stricture and obstruction are dissappointingly common (see below). Loss of motility followed by decreasing counts indicates stricture. Our recent switch to Prolene sutures (which are less reactive than nylon as shown in rat studies),[8] use of the microdot system to prevent leaks, and minimizing disturbance of the vasal blood supply may reduce this incidence.

Long-term Follow-up Evaluation After Vasovasostomy

When sperm were found in the vasal fluid on at least one side at the time of surgery, the anastomotic technique described resulted in the appearance of sperm in the ejaculate in 99 percent of our last 100 men treated.[9] Late obstruction, after initial patency, will occur in 13 percent of men by 14 months postoperatively. Pregnancy has occurred in 63 percent of couples followed for at least 2 years when female factors are excluded, and sperm were found in the vas on at least one side at the time of vasovasostomy.

Editorial Comment
Fray F. Marshall

Microsurgical techniques have produced excellent results with vasovasostomy. An accurate lumen-to-lumen anastomosis is essential. Double-armed needles that allow inside-out placement are expensive but helpful, especially in the performance of a vasoepididymostomy. A transvasovasostomy is sometimes a useful technique, especially in the presence of vasal injury from an inguinal herniorrhaphy. We rarely leave scrotal drains.

REFERENCES

1. Lemack GE, Goldstein MD. Presence of sperm in the prevasectomy reversal semen analysis: Incidence and implications. J Urol (in press).
2. Goldstein M, Young GPH, Einer-Jensen N. Testicular artery damage due to infiltration with a fine gauge needle: Experimental evidence suggesting that blind cord block should be abandoned. Surg Forum 24:653, 1983.
3. Goldstein M, Gilbert BR, Dicker A, et al. Microsurgical varicocelectomy: An artery and lymphatic sparing technique. J Urol 148:1808, 1992.
4. Hagan KF, Coffey DS. The adverse effects of sperm during vasovasostomy. J Urol 118:269, 1977.
5. Silber S. Microsurgical aspects of varicocele. Fertil Steril 31:230, 1979.
6. Lizza EF, Marmar JL, Schmidt SS, et al. Transseptal crossed vasovasostomy. J Urol 134:1131, 1985.
7. Hamidinia A. Transvasovasostomy—an alternative operation for obstructive azoospermia. J Urol 140:1545, 1988.
8. Chen L-E, Seaber AV. Comparison of 10-0 polypropylene and 10-0 nylon sutures in rat arterial anastomosis. Microsurgery 14:328, 1993.
9. Matthews GJ, Schlegel PN, Goldstein M. Patient following microsurgical vasoepididymostomy and vasovasostomy: Temporal considerations. J Urol (in press).

Chapter 84

Vasoepididymostomy, Epididymal Sperm Retrieval, and In Vitro Techniques for Male Factor Infertility

Peter N. Schlegel

For men with obstructive azoospermia, the standard therapy has been microsurgical reconstruction of the obstructed reproductive tract. Because a chronically obstructed male reproductive tract contains sperm of abnormal quality and reconstruction is possible in many cases, microsurgical reconstruction has been the optimal approach. For men with primary epididymal obstruction or epididymal obstruction after vasectomy, vasoepididymostomy with an accurate microsurgical anastomosis is the recommended procedure. Recent advances with in vitro fertilization (IVF) have allowed for dramatically increased pregnancy rates despite very poor sperm quality. With the expanded role of IVF for sperm of severely abnormal quality, it is evident that sperm should now be retrieved and cryopreserved during any complicated attempt at reconstruction, including vasoepididymostomy. The overall low (20 to 30 percent) pregnancy rate for couples in which the man has undergone vasoepididymostomy suggests that some consideration should also be given to primary sperm retrieval with IVF instead of a reconstruction. In this chapter, the techniques of microsurgical vasoepididymostomy and epididymal sperm retrieval are presented. The advances in IVF and their impact on contemporary approaches to and pregnancy success rates for men with reproductive tract obstruction are also discussed.

Until recently, men with bilateral congenital absence of the vas deferens (BCAV) or other surgically unreconstructable reproductive tract obstructions have had only anecdotal success at achieving fertility.

The technique of retrieving sperm from alloplastic spermatoceles, processing it, and using it for intrauterine insemination has resulted in rare live births.[1] In 1984, Pryor reported the first pregnancy with surgically aspirated sperm in conjunction with in vitro fertilization. Other authors have reported pregnancies or live births for men with BCAV after failed vasoepididymostomy or with an ejaculation in anecdotal reports. Asch and Silber[2] first reported a consistent success rate using surgical sperm retrieval in conjunction with IVF.

The general trend in the management of men with surgically unreconstructable obstructions has been toward the recognition of the importance of assisted reproductive technologies, including IVF and related micromanipulation procedures, for treatment of surgically retrieved sperm. These technologies have resulted in pregnancy rates of up to 50 percent per attempt in the management of these previously infertile men.[3, 4]

MICROSURGICAL VASOEPIDIDYMOSTOMY

Indications

Microsurgical vasoepididymostomy is indicated for the repair of reproductive tract blockage within the epididymis. Epididymal obstruction may be congenital, resulting from a malformation of the connections of the efferent ducts to the main body of the epididymis, or secondary to epididymitis or long-term vasal obstruction, as may occur after vasectomy. I have also seen iatrogenic injuries to the epididymis from orchiopexy, hydrocelectomy, or other scrotal surgery that cause epididymal obstruction and can be repaired by vasoepididymostomy. Men should have a fructose-positive, normal-volume, azoospermic ejaculate before being considered for reconstructive surgery of the epididymis. Sperm production can and should be suggested by the presence of normal-volume testes with epididymal fullness. However, these findings on physical examination are inadequate to guarantee normal sperm production. If sperm production has not been documented by paternity before vasectomy, a testicular biopsy to demonstrate normal sperm production should be performed before exploration for vasoepididymostomy.

The decision to proceed to microsurgical vasoepididymostomy during a vasectomy reversal is more difficult. For a surgeon who is inexperienced with vasoepididymostomy, a primary vasovasostomy should be performed at the time of attempted vasectomy reversal, almost regardless of any intraoperative vasal fluid findings. For an experienced microsurgeon who finds no fluid in the testicular end of the vas deferens or thick and pasty fluid in the vas with no sperm, epididymal exploration is recommended in preparation for vasoepididymostomy. The risk of finding intravasal azoospermia at the time of vasectomy reversal increases if the vasectomy was performed 10 years or more before reversal is attempted.

For both experienced and inexperienced surgeons, the choice of performing a vasovasostomy or a vasoepididymostomy is dependent on the chances of the patient having sperm in the ejaculate after either reconstruction. The chances of finding sperm in the ejaculate postoperatively are poor if the surgeon attempting vasoepididymostomy is inexperienced, and such intervention may adversely affect the chances for a subsequent reconstruction. However, men with copious, watery, azoospermic fluid in the testicular end of the vas may have a better chance of having sperm return to the ejaculate after primary vasovasostomy than the 70 percent chance of patency after a vasoepididymal anastomosis, even if performed by an experienced microsurgeon.[5] Therefore, if the surgeon is in doubt about the approach (vasoepididymostomy vs. vasovasostomy) during vasectomy reversal, primary vasovasostomy is recommended.

Vasoepididymostomy: Technique

The two most popular contemporary approaches to vasoepididymostomy involve either anastomosis of the end of the vas deferens to the side of the epididymis (end to side) or to the end of the cut epididymis (end to end). Individual preference usually determines the choice of technique for a surgeon, but anatomical considerations are also of importance. The end-to-side technique is generally faster because less dissection is necessary. However, vasal length may limit the ability of a surgeon to complete a vasoepididymal anastomosis with the end-to-side approach. If the prepared vas deferens is short, an end-to-side anastomosis may be performed only to the caput epididymidis without tension. Otherwise, the distal epididymis or testis may have to be mobilized into the high scrotum. Dissection of the distal epididymis away from the testis may provide greater functional length of the vas deferens, facilitating a vasoepididymal anastomosis with a short vas deferens to the distal epididymis with an end-to-end approach (Fig. 84–1). The disadvantages of the end-to-end approach include difficulty in isolating the prominent epididymal tubule that effluxes sperm, blood contaminating the field of the microsurgical anastomosis because of the rich blood supply of the epididymis, and the more extensive dissection necessary.

Although the end-to-end specific tubule approach was the first successful microsurgical technique to be described, the end-to-side technique has gained popularity because of its ease of application. One problem has been the difficulty in determining the level of epididymal obstruction by means of visual and tactile evaluation. An incorrect estimate of the

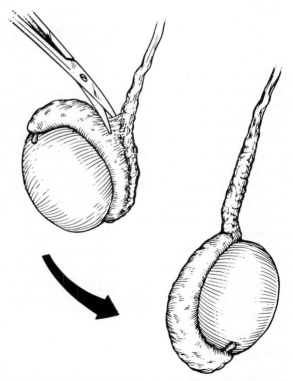

Figure 84–1. Dissection of the distal epididymis off the testis allows for a longer functional length of the epididymis to obviate the effects of a short vas deferens.

level of epididymal obstruction may lead to securing the vas to the epididymal tunic at an inappropriate level and then finding that there are no sperm present in the selected epididymal tubule. The anastomosis so initiated would then need to be taken apart and repeated at a higher level. A detailed description of the techniques for vasoepididymal anastomosis now follows.

Vasal Evaluation

The first maneuver in a vasoepididymostomy is to confirm the diagnosis of epididymal obstruction. This is done by isolating the vas deferens and performing a hemivasotomy. The latter is optimally performed under direct vision with a 15-degree ultrasharp knife under the operating microscope. At least 20-power magnification is necessary to visualize the mucosa and lumen of the vas. Intravasal fluid is obtained and evaluated under a microscope by an experienced examiner. The absence of spermatozoa in the intravasal fluid, in the presence of normal sperm production documented by testicular biopsy, confirms the presence of epididymal obstruction.

The patency of the distal vas deferens should be confirmed with a saline vasogram. The abdominal lumen of the vas deferens is cannulated with a 24-gauge angiocatheter, and it should be possible to inject 5 to 7 ml of saline without backpressure. If any question exists about the patency of the abdominal vas deferens, a 16 Fr. Foley catheter is passed into the bladder. The balloon is inflated with 10 cm³ of air to provide contrast with the bladder in case a formal vasogram is needed. Methylene blue–tinged saline can then be injected through the vas. The presence of blue fluid draining from the bladder confirms the patency of the system. If a question still exists about the patency of the vas, a formal x-ray vasogram is performed. Optimal visualization of the vas, the ejaculatory ducts, and the seminal vesicles with x-ray vasography is obtained by (1) tilting the x-ray camera down from the head of the patient and (2) using air in the Foley balloon, as described. Tilting the x-ray camera helps move the pubic symphysis off the region of the ejaculatory ducts, as occurs with a pelvic inlet/outlet view. The air in the Foley balloon allows identification of the bladder neck. Slight tension of the Foley balloon against the bladder neck prevents reflux of contrast into the bladder, which can obscure the details of the seminal vesicles and ejaculatory ducts.

Preparation of the Vas Deferens

After the vas has been confirmed to be patent on its abdominal end, a clean cut is made through the vas at a 90-degree angle to its course. This is obtained with a 2- to 2.5-mm slotted nerve clamp and a sharp knife. The two sets of vasal vessels are each ligated with nonreactive sutures. I prefer 6-0 or smaller monofilament nylon for this purpose. The small vessels on the cut adventitial edge of the vas are cauterized with a bipolar forceps. As much periadvential tissue as possible is preserved with the vas deferens to optimize the blood supply to the vas and to facilitate anastomosis of the vas to the epididymis. Extensive mobilization of the vas should be avoided to prevent devascularization that could lead to scarring and fibrosis of the vas. An accurate anastomosis, without tension, of well-vascularized vas deferens to a single epididymal tubule is the goal of the procedure.

Specific Anatomical Considerations for Reconstruction

Reconstruction of one reproductive tract with good sperm production is preferable to reconstruction of two marginal systems. For example, consider the case of a patient with an atrophic testis with poor sperm production and an intact vas deferens and contralateral extensive vasal obstruction. Transseptal crossover reconstruction of the normal testis and epididymis to the contralateral intact vas deferens by vasovasostomy is far more likely to be successful than difficult bilateral reconstructions.

End-to-end Anastomosis

After confirmation of intravasal azoospermia, the epididymis is dissected off the testis, beginning near the vasoepididymal junction and extending well above the site of suspected obstruction. The epididymis is serially sectioned with a slotted nerve clamp and ultrasharp knife (Fig. 84–2) until a continuous flow of cloudy fluid is seen effluxing from a single epididymal tubule. If many sperm with tails are present in this fluid, the single effluxing tubule is outlined with a drop of methylene blue on the cut surface of the epididymis. Meticulous hemostasis is important at this stage to prevent formation of a hematoma near the vasoepididymal anastomosis, which potentially could block this connection in the perioperative period. The epididymis and vas deferens can be stabilized with a Microspike approximating clamp so that the mucosa of the vas and the single epididymal tubule are adjacent to each other. The anastomosis is initiated by placement of two posterior mucosal sutures of 10-0 monofilament nylon or polypropylene with 70-μm fishhook-shaped taper-point needles into the mucosa of the epididymis and the mucosa and muscularis layers of the vas (Fig. 84–3). Inside-out placement and the fishhook configuration of the needle help to prevent backwalling of the mucosa. Addi-

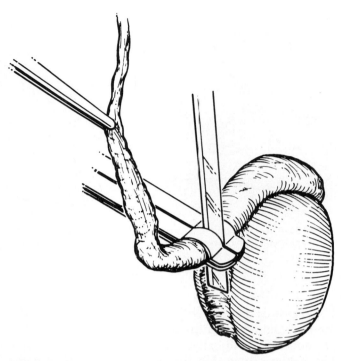

Figure 84–2. Serial sectioning technique for dividing the epididymis, in preparation for end-to-end microsurgical vasoepididymostomy.

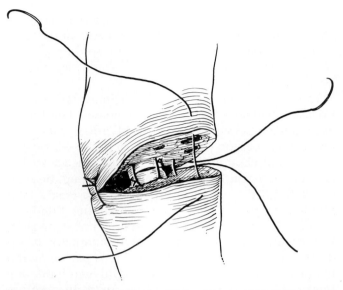

Figure 84–4. Placement of adventitial and muscularis sutures during end-to-end vasoepididymostomy.

bules and to keep the mucosal anastomosis exactly aligned in a watertight fashion (Fig. 84–4).

End-to-side Anastomosis

The end-to-side anastomosis provides several potential advantages in addition to its rapid and relatively simple performance. When vasoepididymostomy is performed at the same time as varicocelectomy or inguinal vasovasostomy, the continuity of the perivasal vessels must be maintained to provide

tional sutures (up to a total of five) are placed on the anterior surface of the anastomosis.

After completion of the mucosal anastomosis, 15 to 20 interrupted sutures of 9-0 monofilament nylon are used to approximate the sheath and muscularis of the vas to the epididymal tunic. The sutures must be placed to avoid obstructing any epididymal tu-

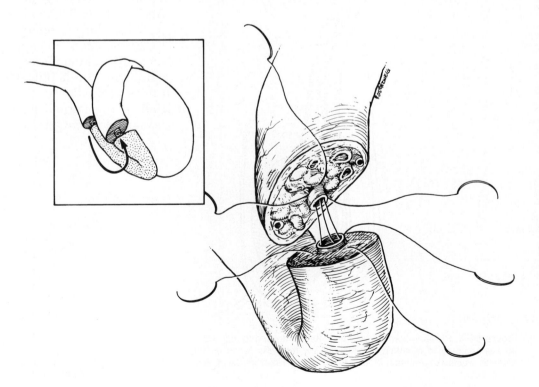

Figure 84–3. Initial performance of an end-to-end vasoepididymostomy; the mucosal sutures are placed.

venous outflow of the testis and preserve the vasal blood supply (Fig. 84–5). If prominent epididymal tubule dilation and a clear level of epididymal obstruction are evident, a rapid end-to-side vasoepididymal anastomosis is possible.

The end-to-side vasoepididymostomy is initiated by vasal evaluation, as described above. The tunica vaginalis is opened and the epididymis is examined under the operating microscope at 15 to 20 power. The level of vasal obstruction is determined visually, and a 2- to 3-mm incision is made in the epididymal tunic. Blunt dissection is used to free a single loop of dilated epididymal tubule. When the tubule is sitting freely in the tunical incision, a linear incision is fashioned in the epididymal tubule with a 15-degree ultrasharp knife. A glass slide is placed on the tubule to obtain a sample of the epididymal fluid; this is examined under a microscope. With an absolute minimum of blood contamination, sperm are aspirated from within the lumen of the epididymal tubule and processed for cryopreservation. Motile sperm should be sought for optimal results after freezing.

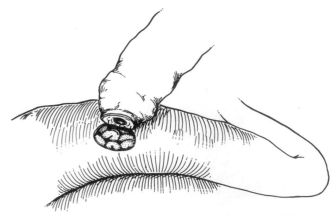

Figure 84–6. The vas deferens is secured to the edge of the incision in the epididymal tunic as a first step in an end-to-side vasoepididymostomy.

The region is painted with methylene blue to identify the mucosal edges of the cut epididymal tubule. The presence of sperm is determined under a microscope. The testis is placed in its natural position, and the optimal course of the vas deferens to the region of epididymal anastomosis is determined. The vas deferens can then be brought through the tunica vaginalis to allow the vas to follow a straight course. The vas is then tacked to the tunical layer of the epididymis with three 9-0 monofilament nylon sutures through the muscular and adventitial layers of the vas (Fig. 84–6).

At least four to six 10-0 monofilament nylon or polypropylene sutures are placed through the mucosal layers of the vas and the epididymis (Fig. 84–7). Again, 70-μm fishhook needles are used for the anastomosis. The anastomosis is completed by placing 15 to 20 9-0 monofilament nylon sutures through the remaining circumference of the vas deferens into the epididymal tunic (Fig. 84–8). With this approach, the tunica vaginalis can then be closed to allow restoration of the normal anatomical relationships of the testis and its coverings.

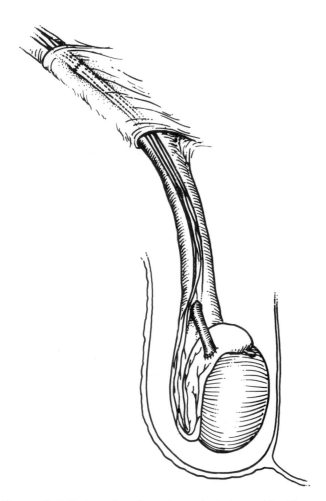

Figure 84–5. Preservation of vasal vessels during end-to-side vasoepididymostomy to maintain venous outflow from the testis by this route as well as to maintain blood supply to the vas from the testicular vessels.

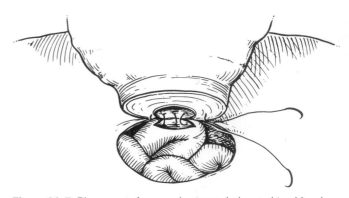

Figure 84–7. Placement of mucosal sutures during end-to-side microsurgical vasoepididymostomy.

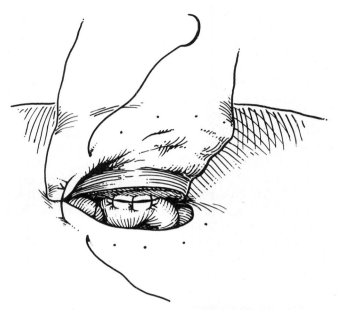

Figure 84–8. Later stages of end-to-side vasoepididymostomy.

Follow-up

Semen analyses are performed 1 and 3 months postoperatively, and subsequently every 3 months. Once patency has been established, the sperm quality and the interests of the couple will determine whether natural intercourse, intrauterine insemination, or in vitro fertilization are considered for conception. If sperm were not cryopreserved during the reconstructive procedure, cryopreservation of any postoperative ejaculated sperm with good motility should be considered, since more than 10 percent of all vasoepididymal anastomoses will close off after patency is established.[5]

Results of Vasoepididymostomy

Despite improvements in patency rates with a microsurgical approach to vasoepididymostomy, overall results are less than optimal. The best pregnancy rates are often seen only in patients who have been followed for more than 2 years and when optimal findings were present at epididymal exploration. It is inappropriate to quote these results to a couple considering vasoepididymostomy, since (1) they may not apply to that couple, if the preoperatively expected sperm production is not found at exploration; and (2) the couple typically expects that early pregnancy will be achieved after the problem is "fixed." In other words, superficial review of postoperative patency and pregnancy results usually leaves a patient with the expectation of a 70 percent chance of achieving a pregnancy within several months of surgery. Patency cannot be equated with success,

since patients consider a successful result to be delivery of a baby. My results with microsurgical reconstruction reflect patency rates very similar to those of previously published series. However, the actual pregnancy rate was only 27 percent in my series when all patients who underwent surgery were considered in the outcome analysis. The results of several published series are summarized in Table 84–1. However, it is necessary to read the primary articles in some cases to determine the denominator for pregnancy rates.

EPIDIDYMAL SPERM RETRIEVAL

Indications and Preoperative Evaluation

Men with bilateral congenital absence of the vas deferens or other unreconstructable obstructions who are interested in fertility are candidates for epididymal sperm retrieval in conjunction with IVF for their female partner. One question that has arisen for men with BCAV or other long-term obstructions is whether sperm production is present. If a man has no sperm in his ejaculate, sperm production can be documented inferentially by testicular biopsy. Since congenital absence of the vas deferens can be diagnosed on physical examination, testicular biopsy is unnecessary if sperm production is highly likely to be present. Previous studies have documented that men have continued sperm production after vasectomy. My experience, as well as that of a U.S. multicenter study of treatment results from sperm microaspiration, has indicated that over 99 percent of men undergoing attempted sperm retrieval have adequate sperm numbers if serum follicle stimulating hormone (FSH) levels and testicular volume are normal.[3, 6] Therefore, men with BCAV do not require testicular biopsy to diagnose sperm production if testicular volume and serum FSH levels are normal.

For men with BCAV, several other medical conditions need to be considered. These include the frequent association of cystic fibrosis gene mutations

TABLE 84–1. Results of Microsurgical Vasoepididymostomy Compiled from Several Series

Primary Surgeon	Year	No. of Patients	Patency (%)	Pregnancy (%)
Fogdestam	1986	41	85	37
Silber	1988	139	78	56
Fuchs	1991	39	60	36
Goldstein	1993	107	70	27
Thomas	1992	137	78	47

with BCAV, the infrequent (11 percent) association of BCAV with unilateral renal agenesis, and the potential formation of antisperm antibodies in men with BCAV. Men with cystic fibrosis typically have no vas deferens. These patients have defects in both copies of the cystic fibrosis transmembrane conductance regulatory (CFTR) gene. This finding raised the question of whether men with BCAV may carry gene defects associated with the development of cystic fibrosis. Intensive study of the CFTR gene mutations in men with BCAV as well as their parents and offspring has been proposed by several sets of investigators. A review of these data by Oates and Amos[7] indicated that a single CFTR gene defect is detectable in 82 percent of all patients tested, including 18 percent who are found to be compound heterozygotes (two different CFTR gene defects on the two copies of the CFTR gene).[4] These findings clearly suggest an increased probability of children having the disease of cystic fibrosis if the father has BCAV. The critical information needed for couples interested in fertility is the CFTR gene mutation status of the wife. Since not all CFTR gene mutations have been documented, the chance of having a child with cystic fibrosis cannot be brought to zero. However, CFTR mutation testing is critical for all couples interested in fertility in which the man has BCAV. The lack of detectable CFTR gene mutations in the female partner minimizes the risk of having a child with cystic fibrosis. Since not all CFTR gene mutations have been identified, the risk of a man with BCAV having a child with cystic fibrosis is never less than 0.6 percent.

Men with BCAV also have an increased risk of having renal agenesis, so we recommend renal ultrasound evaluation of all men for the anatomical presence of kidneys. Because antibodies may be present in some men and I have observed spontaneous sperm agglutination after epididymal retrieval despite the absence of detectable antibodies, I pretreat men with prednisone for 3 months before epididymal aspiration. These men are given 20 mg/day prednisone for 10 days a month after a careful informed consent is obtained regarding the risks of prednisone therapy.

Sperm Quality in an Obstructed Reproductive Tract

In the normal male reproductive tract, sperm exiting the testis have minimal motility and limited capacity for fertilizing eggs. Sperm attain the potential for progressive motility and improved fertilizing capacity during epididymal transit. Therefore, one would expect to find optimal sperm quality in the most distal segments of the unobstructed epididymis. In the obstructed epididymis, a very different pattern of sperm quality is seen. Very poor sperm quality (as

evaluated by percentage of motile cells) is found in the most distal epididymis. Careful histological evaluation of sperm aspirated from the distal epididymis reveals extensive contamination of the sperm specimen with macrophages and sperm fragments. Only rare intact or motile sperm are present. Progressively better sperm quality is found in the more proximal epididymis (Fig. 84–9). These findings have led surgeons to begin sperm retrieval in the middle portion of the obstructed reproductive tract and to proceed more proximally. In some cases, optimal sperm quality is actually found in the efferent ducts. In addition, motile sperm can be retrieved from the testis from testicular biopsy specimens.

The seemingly contradictory findings of epididymal sperm quality in obstructed and unobstructed men can be easily explained. Sperm production continues in the obstructed reproductive tract. Sperm that are not ejaculated or lost in urine must be removed by intraluminal macrophages in the reproductive tract. The distal segment of the obstructed reproductive tract will therefore be filled with dead and dying sperm that are being removed by intraluminal macrophages. This results in the very poor sperm quality seen in the distal epididymis of these patients. The intraluminal resorption of senescent sperm from the distal epididymis results in the "inversion of motility" seen in the reproductive tract of chronically obstructed men.

Importance of Assisted Reproduction

Assisted reproduction involves IVF and associated techniques. IVF is the insemination of eggs (oocytes) with sperm outside the body. A cycle of IVF replaces one menstrual cycle. Stimulation of oocyte production, insemination of oocytes with sperm, and transfer of fertilized oocytes (embryos) constitute one IVF cycle. Induction of ovulation is obtained by ovarian stimulation with FSH analogues or FSH-stimulating agents such as clomiphene citrate. Typically, pituitary control of the ovulatory process is prevented by pretreatment of the woman with gonadotropin releasing hormone agonists during the second half (luteal phase) of the preceding menstrual cycle. Multiple follicles of the ovaries (containing oocytes) are followed with transvaginal ultrasound studies and serial monitoring of serum estrogen and progesterone levels. Oocytes are subsequently retrieved by needle aspiration under transvaginal ultrasound guidance. Fertilized oocytes are then transferred back to the female partner's uterus. Recent advances in sperm preparation techniques have resulted in improved pregnancy rates for male-factor infertility with IVF. Fertilization of oocytes by even severely abnormal sperm is now possible with micromanipulation.

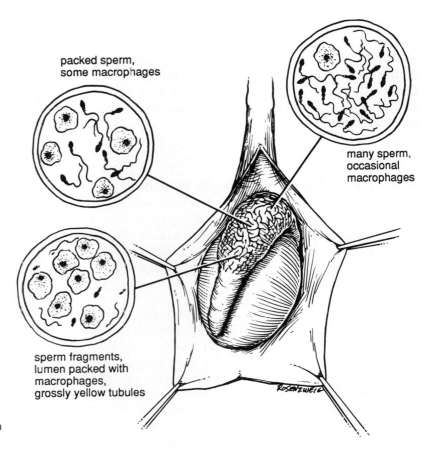

packed sperm,
some macrophages

many sperm,
occasional
macrophages

sperm fragments,
lumen packed with
macrophages,
grossly yellow tubules

Figure 84–9. Intraluminal contents of the epididymis in men with congenital absence of the vas deferens.

Sperm micromanipulation significantly improves fertilization and pregnancy rates in cases of very severe male-factor infertility.[8] Micromanipulation techniques successfully applied to human gametes include partial zona dissection, subzonal insertion of sperm, and intracytoplasmic sperm injection. Partial zona dissection (PZD) is the process of mechanically (or chemically) opening the zona pellucida, the natural surface around the oocyte. Subzonal insertion (SuZI) involves injection of three to 15 sperm under the zona pellucida surrounding the oocyte. Early micromanipulation techniques using SuZI or PZD provided clinical pregnancy rates of up to 21 percent using ejaculated sperm in the least favorable male-factor cases. However, not all centers have achieved these results.

An additional form of micromanipulation, intracytoplasmic sperm injection (ICSI), has been instituted by many centers with excellent results in cases of extreme male-factor infertility. ICSI involves direct injection of a single sperm into the cytoplasm of an oocyte during an IVF cycle. It is the quantitatively most efficient micromanipulation technique practically implemented to date, since only a single sperm is required to fertilize each egg. A review of micromanipulation procedures for severe male-factor infertility supports the achievement of clinical pregnancy

rates of up to 35 percent per attempt with ICSI.[8] This clinical pregnancy rate translates into a chance of actually having a baby per IVF cycle of better than one in four.

The importance of micromanipulation to improve the fertilization potential of ejaculated sperm is well established. Several reports also support the importance of micromanipulation for sperm surgically retrieved from the epididymis. I reported 51 IVF cycles of epididymal sperm retrieval in which 11 couples had cohort eggs treated with either micromanipulation (SuZI or PZD) or standard insemination; fertilization was achieved only with micromanipulation.[6] Analysis of an additional cohort of men with surgically retrieved sperm treated with IVF and ICSI compared with IVF/PZD/SuZI indicates that fertilization rates improved with ICSI. Fertilization rates per oocyte were 45 percent (84 of 187) using IVF and ICSI versus 21 percent with IVF/PZD/SuZI.[9] Clinical pregnancy rates were 27.5 percent with IVF/PZD/SuZI versus 56 percent (10 of 18) per cycle of sperm and egg retrieval with ICSI. Ongoing pregnancies or deliveries have occurred in 24 percent (12 of 51) of cycles using IVF/PZD/SuZI and in 48 percent (13 of 27) with IVF/ICSI. Silber et al.[4] compared pregnancy results for men with congenital absence of the vas from one institution where IVF was used with those obtained at another institution with IVF/ICSI. They reported that the ongoing pregnancy and delivery rate was only 4.5 percent with IVF alone and 30 percent with IVF/ICSI. These findings, in addition to the quantitatively very small numbers of sperm needed for ICSI, have led us to abandon all other micromanipulation techniques except for ICSI in the management of surgically retrieved sperm.

Procedure of Surgical Sperm Retrieval

Sperm retrieval is most commonly performed as a microsurgical procedure in which individual epididymal tubules or the vas deferens are opened under direct vision and epididymal or vasal fluid retrieved as it flows out of the opened tubule, as described by Asch and Silber et al.[2] Contamination of sperm samples with blood cells is common if the luminal contents are allowed to spill out of the epididymal tubule before they are collected. Blood cells, especially white cells, are known to adversely affect sperm function. I described a micropuncture apparatus to collect sperm directly from within the epididymal lumen to limit contamination.[6] This micropuncture was adapted from the laboratory apparatus used for study of the epididymis. Briefly, glass micropipettes with a tip width of 250 to 350 μm are attached to medical grade silicone tubing, a 1-ml plastic syringe, and a very clean 10-ml glass syringe (Fig. 84–10). The glass syringe allows very accurate control of the aspiration process. The 1-ml plastic syringe is available for collection of large volumes of fluid and to flush collected sperm out of the collection apparatus. Typically, only microliter quantities that fill less than the length of the glass micropipette are needed, since sperm concentrations in the epididymis are typically in the range of 10^9 sperm/ml.

Marmar et al. (cited in Schlegel[3]) have used both the micropuncture approach as well as simple aspiration and reported better results with intraluminal (micropuncture-type) retrieval. In summary, micropuncture retrieval of sperm seems to limit contamination with blood cells and is conceptually attractive, but it has not yet been proved to improve fertilization or pregnancy rates for epididymal sperm.

Initial reports have described epididymal sperm retrieval on the same day as oocyte retrieval to optimize sperm retrieval. The results of ICSI appear to be independent of sperm quality. This finding has allowed Tournaye et al (cited in Schlegel[3]) to perform epididymal sperm retrieval 1 day before oocyte retrieval. Experience with ICSI has encouraged me to perform sperm retrieval with cryopreservation of sperm during all epididymal retrieval cycles, as well as difficult reconstructions, including epididymovasostomies. Pregnancy rates with fresh versus frozen

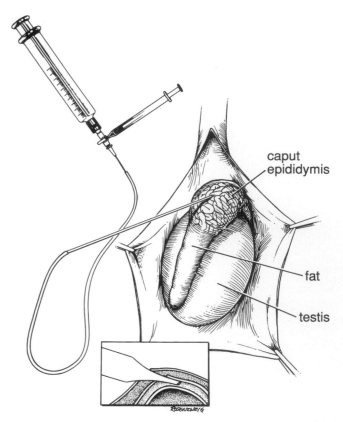

Figure 84–10. Overview of apparatus used for micropuncture retrieval of epididymal sperm. *Inset*, Magnified view of the pipette entering an epididymal tubule through the visceral layer of the tunica vaginalis.

epididymal sperm appear to be similar but have not yet been directly compared.

Sperm retrieval should begin at the middle portion of the obstructed reproductive system and proceed proximally, toward the testis. If the entire epididymis is present without vas, retrieval is initiated in the corpus epididymidis. Often, an approach to the efferent ducts is necessary. A surgical approach that exposes the efferent ducts but avoids exposure of and the potential for injury to the testicular vessels is shown in Fig. 84–11. When sperm are not retrievable from the epididymis, testicular sperm retrieval is attempted.

Fertilizing Capacity of Testicular Sperm

Since testicular sperm in an unobstructed system have limited oocyte fertilizing ability, some question has existed regarding the utility of sperm retrieved from the testis for assisted reproductive technologies. Craft et al[10] first reported fertilization using sperm retrieved from the testis with the assistance of IVF and ICSI. It appears that ICSI is needed to provide optimal results with testicular sperm. In addition, testicular sperm are much more difficult to isolate

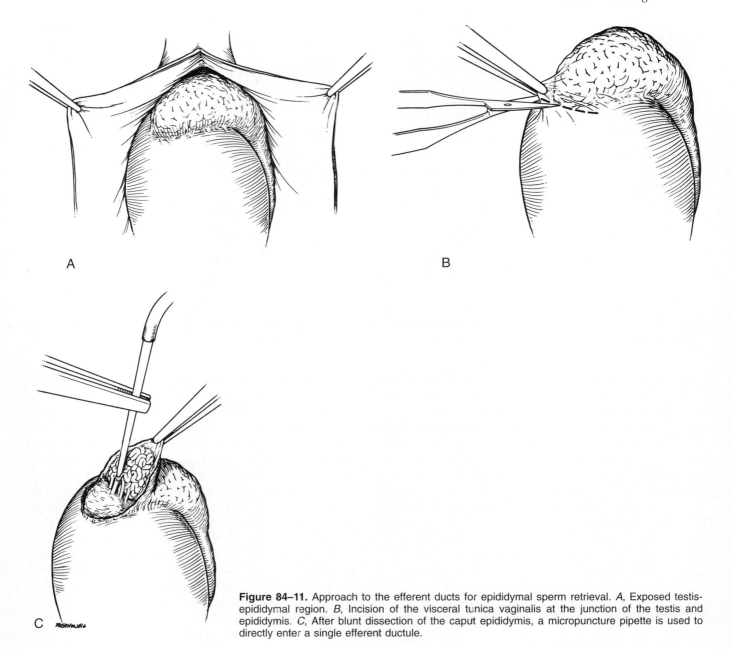

Figure 84–11. Approach to the efferent ducts for epididymal sperm retrieval. *A*, Exposed testis-epididymal region. *B*, Incision of the visceral tunica vaginalis at the junction of the testis and epididymis. *C*, After blunt dissection of the caput epididymis, a micropuncture pipette is used to directly enter a single efferent ductule.

from testicular tissue, and testicular sperm cannot usually be frozen for subsequent IVF cycles, as is possible with epididymal sperm.[3]

Results of Sperm Retrieval with IVF

Previously published results of epididymal sperm retrieval are summarized in Table 84–2. Only series with ten or more cycles or attempts are presented.

Predictors of Success Using Epididymal Sperm

Several factors have been proposed that may influence the likelihood of fertilization and subsequent pregnancy in IVF cycles with surgically retrieved sperm. Epididymal length appears to affect sperm quality and fertilization and pregnancy rates. Several investigators have reported improved sperm quality in men with a longer length of epididymis.[3] A longer epididymis allows for greater separation of recently produced sperm and the degenerating sperm that mix with macrophages in the most distal segment of the obstructed epididymis. Sperm of better quality, including a higher percentage of motility, are more likely to fertilize a higher proportion of eggs, allowing more embryos for transfer and a higher pregnancy rate. These findings may be abrogated by ICSI, because with ICSI, fertilization and pregnancy rates are independent of sperm quality,[9] as long as the sperm are viable.

TABLE 84–2. Results of Treatment Series for Couples in Whom the Man had Surgically Retrieved Sperm

Authors	Clinical Pregnancy/ Sperm Retrieval		Assisted Reproduction	Findings
Southwick and Temple–Smith	1/30	(3%)	IVF	Low fertilization and pregnancy rates
Asch and Silber[2]	15/54	(28%)	TET, IVF	IVF pregnancy rate 12%
Mathieu et al	2/14	(14%)	IVF	
Marmar et al	3/25	(12%)	IVF	Improved pregnancy rate with Lupron suppression, intratubular aspiration of sperm and mini-Percoll with pentoxifylline
SMART Study Group	21/219	(10%)	IVF, GIFT, ZIFT	U.S. pooled experience
Schlegel et al[6]	14/51	(27%)	IVF/PZD/SuZI	Micropuncture retrieval of sperm and egg micromanipulation enhanced pregnancy rates
Tournaye et al	5/14	(36%)	ICSI	ICSI is highly efficient in achieving fertilization and pregnancies, despite grossly abnormal epididymal sperm
Schlegel et al[9]	10/18	(56%)	ICSI	ICSI is the optimal micromanipulation technique with epididymal sperm
Silber et al[4]	6/67	(9%)	IVF	ICSI is mandated for all future epididymal sperm retrieval cycles
	8/17	(47%)	ICSI	

TET, tubal embryo transfer; GIFT, gamete intrafallopian tube transfer; ZIFT zona intrafallopian tube transfer.

One group reported that the presence of the ΔF508 CFTR mutation will adversely affect sperm function as reflected by decreased sperm motility and fertilization and pregnancy rates. My experience with epididymal sperm from men with BCAV indicates that CFTR gene mutations do not affect fertilization or pregnancy rates.[3] The discrepancy between my results and those of Patrizio et al (cited in Schlegel[3]) may be because we enhanced sperm-egg interaction with micromanipulation, including ICSI,[11] whereas Patrizio et al used only standard insemination with IVF. Initial sperm quality is not predictive of fertilization or subsequent pregnancy rates with micromanipulation.

Summary

Surgical retrieval of sperm from men with obstructive or functional azoospermia in conjunction with IVF is now feasible with ongoing pregnancy and delivery rates per attempt ranging up to 50 percent per cycle. Advances in assisted reproductive techniques, including ICSI, allow high pregnancy rates for cases with fewer sperm retrieved even with very poor sperm quality. Cryopreservation of sperm from a single surgical retrieval procedure further enhances the chance of achieving a pregnancy for a couple in which the man has surgically uncorrectable reproductive tract obstruction.

MICROSURGICAL RECONSTRUCTION VERSUS EPIDIDYMAL SPERM RETRIEVAL

The excellent results being reported with epididymal sperm retrieval and IVF are now dramatically better than the pregnancy rates after vasoepididymostomy. Since it may take several years to achieve the pregnancy after microsurgical reconstruction, a couple is more likely to achieve an early pregnancy if they initially choose epididymal sperm retrieval rather than vasoepididymostomy for fertility treatment of the obstructed epididymis. However, epididymal sperm retrieval requires the application of IVF and ICSI, which may cost up to $12,000 per attempt, in addition to the costs of surgical sperm retrieval. Probably the best of all options is to retrieve good-quality sperm from one epididymis and bilaterally perform a vasoepididymostomy. This is my current approach for men with bilateral epididymal obstruction. It preserves all options for the couple and gives a reasonable chance of achieving pregnancy from the microsurgical reconstruction alone.

Editorial Comment

Fray F. Marshall

In vitro fertilization techniques have expanded greatly. Even with poorer-quality sperm, it is most impressive that patients with vasal agenesis or proximal vasal obstruction can still achieve significant pregnancy rates with intracytoplasmic sperm injections. With this capability come new concerns. Bilateral vasal agenesis is associated with the cystic fibrosis gene, so that it becomes important to test the wife as a potential carrier.

REFERENCES

1. Belker AM, Jimenez-Cruz DJ, Kelami A, Wagenknecht LV. Alloplastic spermatocele: Poor sperm motility in intraoperative fluid contraindicates prosthesis implantation. J Urol 136:408, 1986.

2. Asch RH, Silber SJ. Microsurgical sperm aspiration and assisted reproductive techniques. Ann NY Acad Sci 626:101, 1991.
3. Schlegel PN. Sperm retrieval and in vitro fertilization. Curr Opin Urol 4:328, 1994.
4. Silber SJ, Nagy ZP, Liu J, et al. Conventional in-vitro fertilization versus intracytoplasmic sperm injection for patients requiring microsurgical sperm aspiration. Hum Reprod 9:1705, 1994.
5. Schlegel PN, Goldstein M. Microsurgical vasoepididymostomy: Refinements and results. J Urol 150:1165, 1993.
6. Schlegel PN, Berkeley AS, Goldstein M, et al. Epididymal micropuncture with in vitro fertilization and oocyte micromanipulation for the treatment of unreconstructable obstructive azoospermia. Fertil Steril 61:895, 1994.
7. Oates RD, Amos JA. The genetic basis of congenital bilateral absence of the vas deferens and cystic fibrosis. J Androl 15:1, 1994.
8. Schlegel PN. Micromanipulation of gametes for male factor infertility. Urol Clin North Am 21:477, 1994.
9. Schlegel PN, Palermo GD, Alikani M, et al. Micropuncture retrieval of epididymal sperm with IVF: Importance of in vitro micromanipulation techniques. Urology 46:238, 1995.
10. Craft I, Bennett V, Nicholson N. Fertilising ability of testicular spermatozoa. Lancet 342:864, 1993.
11. Schlegel PN, Cohen J, Goldstein M, et al. Cystic fibrosis gene mutations do not affect sperm function during in vitro fertilization with micromanipulation for men with congenital absence of vas deferens. Fertil Steril 64:421, 1995.

Chapter 85

Penile Prosthesis Implantation

Drogo K. Montague, Kenneth W. Angermeier, and Milton M. Lakin

PREOPERATIVE EVALUATION

Treatment Options for Erectile Dysfunction

Today, in contrast to one or two decades ago, there are many treatment options for erectile dysfunction. Sex therapy continues to be the preferred initial treatment for psychogenic erectile problems. Erectile dysfunction secondary to hypogonadism or hyperprolactinemia can usually be effectively treated with hormone replacement or dopamine agonists. For other forms of organic erectile failure, standard therapy includes the use of a vacuum constriction device, intracavernous injection therapy, or penile prosthesis implantation. For selected patients in an investigational setting, penile vascular surgery may be appropriate.

Penile prosthesis implantation is appropriate in men with organic erectile dysfunction if treatment with a vacuum constriction device or intracavernous injection therapy is unsuccessful or not accepted by the patient and his partner. Penile prosthesis implantation is not appropriate for men with temporary or potentially reversible erectile dysfunction. In men with long-standing psychogenic erectile dysfunction that is refractory to sex therapy, penile prosthesis implantation may be appropriate if the patient receives clearance from his psychologist or psychiatrist.

Patient Evaluation

The evaluation of the man with erectile dysfunction is designed to identify the cause and help select appropriate therapy. A complete medical and sexual history is still the single most important element in this evaluation. This is followed by physical examination and blood studies to assess the general state of health; screen for hypogonadism and hyperprolac-

tinemia; and identify diabetes, liver, or kidney disease. Nocturnal penile tumescence testing can help separate psychogenic from organic causes of erectile dysfunction. Intracavernous injection of a vasoactive drug combined with duplex ultrasound examination of the penile arteries often provides additional information regarding penile vasculature that is useful diagnostically and therapeutically. Other more specialized studies, such as cavernosometry, cavernosography, and penile arteriography, are generally reserved for men who are possible candidates for penile vascular surgery.[1]

Prosthesis Types

Penile prostheses can be divided into two general types: rod or nonhydraulic devices and hydraulic or inflatable devices. Hydraulic prostheses can be subdivided into one-, two-, and three-piece devices. One-piece hydraulic devices consist of paired cylinders that are implanted entirely within the corpora cavernosa. The AMS Dynaflex (American Medical Systems, Minnetonka, MN) is currently the only available one-piece device. After inflation the AMS Dynaflex produces penile rigidity similar to that produced by nonhydraulic rod prostheses. After deflation it loses a portion of this rigidity. Two-piece hydraulic devices consist of paired cylinders connected by tubing to a scrotal component. In the Mentor Mark II (Mentor Corporation, Goleta, CA) device, this scrotal component is both a pump and a fluid reservoir. In the AMS Ambicor device, this scrotal component is a pump and the fluid reservoir is located in the rear of each cylinder. Three-piece inflatable prostheses consist of paired cylinders connected by tubing to a scrotal pump, which in turn is connected to an abdominal fluid reservoir. Mentor Corporation produces a three-piece device, the Alpha I; American Medical Systems produces the following three-piece devices: the AMS 700CX, AMS 700CXM, AMS Ultrex, and AMS Ultrex Plus.

Selecting a Penile Prosthesis

The ideal penile prosthesis should have a low incidence of erosion through tissue and a low incidence of mechanical failure. The penis containing the ideal prosthesis should feel normal when palpated. Finally, the ideal prosthesis should produce penile flaccidity and erection resembling that which occurs naturally.

Rod penile prostheses have higher erosion rates than hydraulic devices, are constantly rigid, and are not palpably normal. Today's hydraulic penile prostheses have reasonably low mechanical failure rates; consequently, implantation of their nonhydraulic, semirigid rod counterparts is done less often than in the past.

To produce optimal penile flaccidity and erection requires the presence of a large-volume abdominal fluid reservoir. American Medical System's three-piece product line makes available the greatest number of choices for a variety of implantation considerations. The cylinders of the AMS product line have a triple-ply construction (Fig. 85–1). The inner silicone tube expands as fluid is pumped into it. The expansion of this inner tube is controlled by the middle woven fabric layer. The outer silicone layer prevents tissue growth into the middle layer.

The AMS 700CX cylinder has a deflated diameter of 12 mm and an inflated diameter of 18 mm. No length expansion occurs with this cylinder. The AMS Ultrex cylinder also has a deflated diameter of 12 mm and an inflated diameter of 18 mm; however, it expands 20 percent or more in length as the device is inflated. The AMS 700CXM device has a deflated

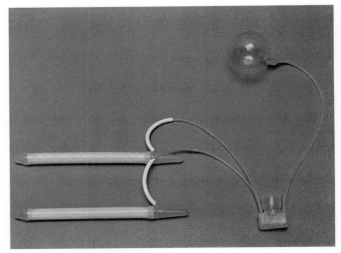

Figure 85–2. The AMS Ultrex penile prosthesis.

diameter of 9.5 mm and an inflated diameter of 14.2 mm; no length expansion occurs with this cylinder. The AMS 700CX, AMS 700CXM, and AMS Ultrex devices all have separate paired components that are filled with normal saline in the operating room before implantation. Three tubing connectors unite the various components of each of these prostheses. The AMS Ultrex Plus device is prefilled with normal saline, and the paired cylinders and the pump are a single unit. The reservoir is implanted separately and then filled with normal saline. Only one tubing connection is required with this device.

The small-diameter AMS 700CXM device is useful for implantation in men with small penises and in men with cavernosal fibrosis, as might occur after priapism or after removal of an infected penile prosthesis. This device and the standard-diameter AMS 700CX prosthesis do not lengthen with inflation. The AMS 700CX device is useful for implantation in men whose penises are not straight, e.g., in men with Peyronie's disease. It is also useful for implantation in men who have a long, narrow penis and in men who have had a previous prosthesis associated with either distal cylinder cross-over or urethral erosion. The AMS Ultrex (Fig. 85–2) and AMS Ultrex Plus devices, which provide both controlled girth and length expansion, are indicated for most other implant recipients.

Two-piece hydraulic prostheses produce some compromise in penile flaccidity and erection quality in comparison with their three-piece counterparts. Nevertheless, these devices (the Mentor Mark II and the AMS Ambicor) are useful in situations in which it is advantageous to avoid an abdominal fluid reservoir. This includes men who have had cystectomy and men with abdominal hernias that have been repaired with mesh.

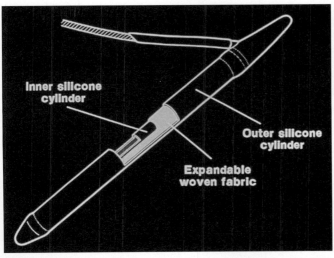

Figure 85–1. Triple-ply cylinders of the AMS three-piece inflatable penile prosthesis product line. (Courtesy of American Medical Systems, Minnetonka, MN.)

OPERATIVE TECHNIQUE

Patient Preparation

The man who is to undergo penile prosthesis implantation should have sterile urine and should not have any dermatitis or open skin lesions in the operative area. Antibiotics providing both gram-negative and gram-positive coverage, such as gentamicin and vancomycin, are given 1 hour before the incision is made. One or more doses of these antibiotics are given postoperatively; however, there is probably no rationale for extending prophylactic antibiotic coverage longer than 24 or 48 hours after the operation.

After administration of spinal, epidural, or general anesthesia, the patient is placed in the supine position and the operative area is shaved. The operative field is then scrubbed for 10 minutes. During the implantation procedure, traffic into and out of the operating room should be limited. The prosthesis should not be removed from its sterile package until just before implantation. Throughout the procedure the operative field should be irrigated with an antibiotic solution, and this solution should be used to irrigate each implanted prosthetic component before tissue is closed over it.

Implantation of the AMS Ultrex Penile Prosthesis

Cylinder Implantation

A Foley catheter is inserted into the urethra and then plugged. A 3-cm transverse incision is made in the upper scrotum approximately 1 cm below the penoscrotal junction. The dartos and Buck's fasciae are divided transversely, exposing the urethra and

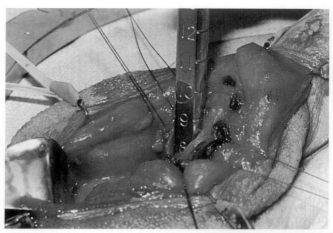

Figure 85–4. The proximal measurement is made from the proximal edge of the corporotomy to the insertion of the crus on the pelvis.

both corporeal bodies. Two-centimeter corporotomies parallel to the urethra are made on each side. Horizontal mattress sutures of 2-0 PDS (polydioxanone) are placed; these will be used first as stay sutures during corporeal dilation and measurement and then as closure sutures after cylinder implantation[2] (Fig. 85–3). The corpora are dilated with Hegar dilators to 16 mm proximally and 14 mm distally.

The proximal corporeal measurement (Fig. 85–4) is from the proximal end of the corporotomy to the end of the crus as it attaches to the bone. The distal corporeal measurement (Fig. 85–5) is from the distal end of the corporotomy to the end of the corporeal body under the middle glans penis. This technique of determining total corporeal length and thus correct cylinder size tends to overestimate the corporeal length. For this reason the 2-cm corporotomy is not included as part of the measurement. To determine the correct cylinder size for an Ultrex or Ultrex Plus device, these measurements are added and then 1 cm

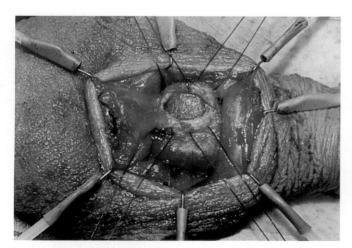

Figure 85–3. A 2-cm corporotomy with four horizontal mattress sutures to be used as stay sutures during corporeal dilation and then as closure sutures after cylinder implantation.

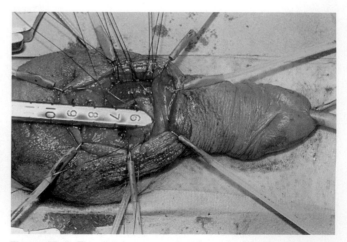

Figure 85–5. The distal measurement is made from the distal edge of the corporotomy to the distal end of the corpus cavernosum under the glans.

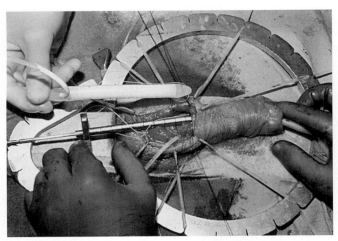

Figure 85–6. A Furlow cylinder inserter is used to help place the distal portion of the cylinder.

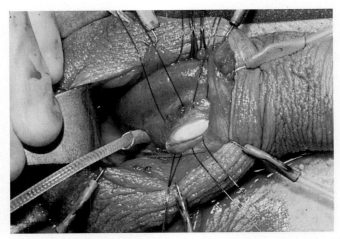

Figure 85–8. The proximal portion of the cylinder has been placed, and the tubing exits through the stab incision.

is subtracted. Because the Ultrex cylinder lengthens, slight undersizing is not harmful. On the other hand, slight oversizing is harmful since the length-expanding Ultrex cylinder will exaggerate this measurement error and an S-shaped cylinder deformity will result. Ultrex cylinders come in the following sizes: 12, 15, 18, and 21 cm. Adjustments between sizes are made by the addition of 1-, 2-, or 3-cm rear-tip extenders.

Silicone is a semipermeable material, and therefore silicone prostheses must be filled with isotonic fluid. Normal saline is recommended for this purpose. All components of the Ultrex device are filled in the operating room after removal from their sterile packages.

The saline-filled cylinder is implanted in the distal corpus cavernosum with the aid of the Furlow cylinder inserter (American Medical Systems) (Fig. 85–6). If needed, rear-tip extenders are applied to adjust cylinder length. A stab incision is then made for the input tubing (Fig. 85–7); this incision is approxi-

mately half the distance from the base of the penis to the attachment of the crus. After the input tubing is brought out through the stab incision, the proximal portion of the cylinder is inserted into the crus (Fig. 85–8). The corporotomy is then closed by tying the preplaced horizontal mattress sutures.

Pump Implantation

A dartos pouch for the pump is made in the septum of the scrotum (Fig. 85–9). After the pump is placed in this pouch, the two cylinder tubings and the reservoir tubing are routed through the back wall of the dartos pouch (Fig. 85–10). After cutting off excess tubing, connections to each cylinder are made with the sutureless connector system (Fig. 85–11).

Reservoir Implantation

The Foley catheter is unplugged and the bladder emptied. The surgeon's index finger is placed inside

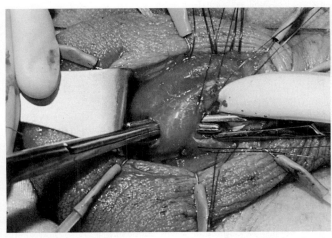

Figure 85–7. A right-angled clamp creates a stab incision for the exiting of the cylinder tubing.

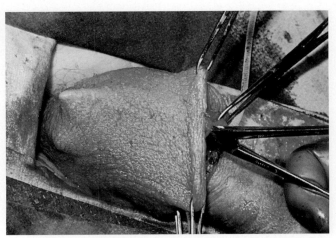

Figure 85–9. A dartos pouch for the pump is created in the scrotal septum.

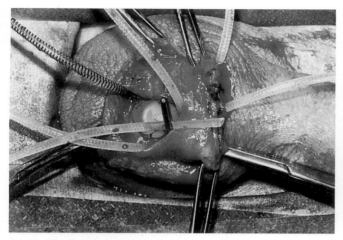

Figure 85–10. Right-angled clamps are used to bring the pump tubing through the back wall of the dartos pouch.

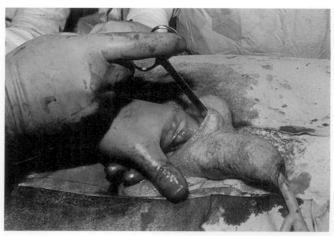

Figure 85–12. The surgeon inserts an index finger through the incision into the external inguinal ring and then uses long Metzenbaum scissors to perforate the transversalis fascia in the floor of the ring.

the incision and then moved up until it is in the external inguinal ring. Long Metzenbaum scissors are used to perforate the transversalis fascia in the floor of the ring (Fig. 85–12), and the surgeon then inserts a finger through this defect. Correct entry into the retropubic space is confirmed by palpation of the back of the symphysis pubis and the Foley balloon in the empty bladder. A long-blade nasal speculum is inserted through the fascial defect and spread to hold it open. The empty reservoir is inserted through this defect (Fig. 85–13). The reservoir is then filled with normal saline and palpation confirms its correct placement in the retropubic space. Fluid is then removed from the reservoir until the pressure is zero. For 12- and 15-cm cylinders a 65-ml reservoir is used; for 18- and 21-cm cylinders, a 100-ml reservoir. A 65-ml reservoir holds approximately 55 ml of fluid at zero pressure and a 100-ml reservoir holds approximately 90 ml of fluid at zero pressure. After excess tubing is removed, a connection between reservoir and pump is made with a sutureless connector.

Prosthesis Testing

The prosthesis is then fully inflated and deflated several times to check cylinder placement and the quality of the erection. The pubis to midglans distance is then measured with the prosthesis deflated (Fig. 85–14) and the prosthesis inflated (Fig. 85–15). The difference between these measurements has ranged from 1 to 4 cm (mean 2 cm).[3]

Wound Closure and Dressing

Throughout the procedure the prosthetic components are irrigated with an antibiotic solution before tissue closure over each component. The opening in the dartos fascia through which the pump was inserted is closed with running 3-0 Dexon (polyglycolic acid) suture. A 7-mm Blake drain (Johnson & Johnson Medical, Inc., Arlington, TX) is placed through a stab incision above and lateral to the external inguinal

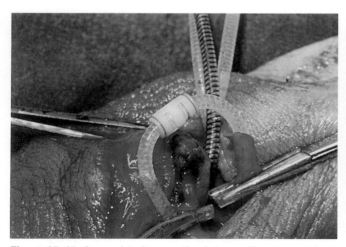

Figure 85–11. A completed connection between the pump and one of the cylinders.

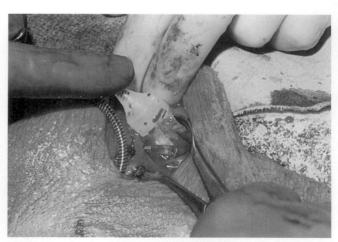

Figure 85–13. A long-blade nasal speculum is used to hold the fascial incision open while the empty reservoir is inserted into the prevesical space.

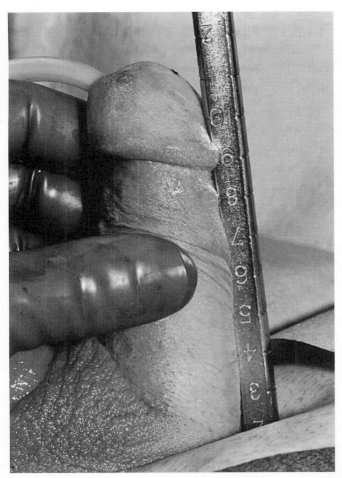

Figure 85–14. The pubis to midglans length is determined with the prosthesis deflated.

ring on the side of the reservoir insertion. This drain is then brought down into the scrotum and placed on top of the cylinder tubing connections in front of the urethra. The dartos fascia beneath the scrotal incision is then closed with running 3-0 Dexon suture. The skin is closed with a running 4-0 Vicryl (polyglactin 910) subcuticular suture.

The prosthesis is left fully deflated and the penis is placed up on the lower abdomen. A dressing is applied to the wound, and the dressing and penile position are maintained with mesh briefs (Scott Health Care Products, Rosemont, IL). A Davol (Cranston, R.I.) 100-ml silicone closed wound suction evacuator is attached to the Blake drain.

Implantation of the AMS 700CX and AMS 700CXM Prostheses

The implantation of the AMS 700CX prosthesis is identical to that described above except that when determining cylinder size, 1 cm is not subtracted from the combined proximal and distal corporeal measurements. Cylinder sizes are the same as for the

Ultrex device, and a 65-ml reservoir is used for all cylinder sizes. There is no need to measure the pubis to midglans length deflated and inflated, as this measurement does not change when the CX cylinders are used.

The AMS 700CXM prosthesis has smaller cylinders (12, 14, 16, and 18 cm), a smaller pump, and a smaller (50-ml) reservoir. The implantation of this device is identical to that of the AMS 700CX prosthesis except that the distal corpora need to be dilated to only 10 mm, and the proximal corpora to only 12 mm. The 50-ml reservoir holds approximately 40 ml of normal saline at zero pressure.

Implantation of the AMS Ultrex Plus Penile Prosthesis

This device is identical to the AMS Ultrex prosthesis except that the cylinders and pump are connected and prefilled with normal saline. Because of this, the cylinder tubing must be brought out through the rear of the corporotomy, with the first corporotomy closure suture placed just in front of the tubing. To avoid

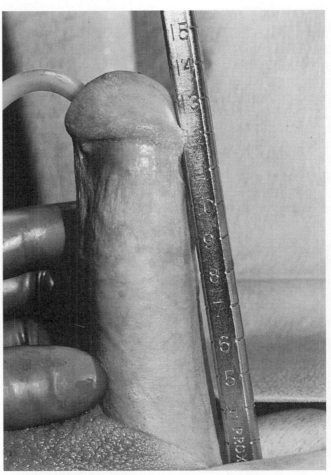

Figure 85–15. The pubis to midglans length is determined with the prosthesis inflated.

having palpable tubing at the base of the penis, the corporotomy should be placed more proximally. Also, the pump needs to be placed directly into the dartos pouch, and it is not possible to route the pump tubing through the back wall of the pouch as was done for the Ultrex device. The reservoir for the Ultrex Plus device is implanted separately, and only one connection (between the pump and the reservoir) is necessary.

Implantation of the AMS Ambicor Penile Prosthesis

This two-piece device is prefilled with normal saline and has paired cylinders preconnected to a scrotal pump. The corporotomy placement and sizing considerations are the same as for the AMS 700CX prosthesis. The cylinder and pump implantation are the same as for the Ultrex Plus prosthesis. After cylinder implantation, the Ambicor device is shown deflated (Fig. 85–16) and inflated (Fig. 85–17).

POSTOPERATIVE MANAGEMENT

The urethral catheter is removed on the first day, the drain is removed on the second day, and the patient is discharged from the hospital. It is important that the penis be kept up on the lower abdomen for the first month. The body reacts to silicone by forming a fibrous pseudocapsule around it. If the penis is worn down in briefs during the healing process, a permanent ventral curvature may result. The prosthesis should be maintained in the deflated state for the first month to help avoid subsequent autoinflation.

Most men can be instructed on device inflation and deflation at the 1-month postoperative visit. If

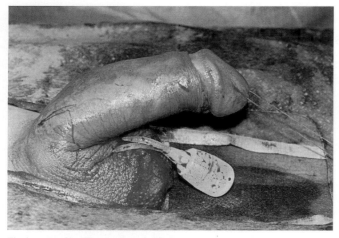

Figure 85–16. The deflated AMS Ambicor penile prosthesis after cylinder implantation.

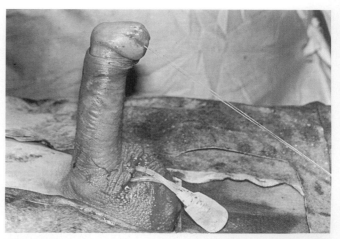

Figure 85–17. The inflated AMS Ambicor penile prosthesis after cylinder implantation. Traction on the cylinder guy sutures demonstrates excellent penile rigidity.

tenderness around the pump prevents this, instruction can be delayed until the tenderness resolves. The implant recipient is instructed to begin having coitus when he is pain free. Because the couple may be anxious during initial coital attempts, it is helpful to instruct them to use a water-soluble lubricant.

A man with a penile prosthesis is able to initiate coitus without being sexually aroused. When this happens, men can exhaust themselves and their partner without reaching orgasm. For this reason, adequate sexual stimulation before vaginal intromission is important not only for the woman but also for the man.

POSTOPERATIVE COMPLICATIONS

Infection is a complication inherent in all surgical procedures. In prosthetic surgery, infection has special significance, since elimination of the infection usually requires removal of all prosthetic material. Prosthesis reimplantation at a later date is not difficult as far as the pump and reservoir are concerned; however, the fibrosis within the corpora that results from infection usually makes the penis smaller and cylinder reimplantation difficult. The small-diameter AMS 700CXM cylinders are particularly useful in these circumstances.

Erosion is often associated with infection; when it is, the entire prosthesis should be removed. Erosion of a cylinder into the urethra often occurs because the urethra was damaged during corporeal dilation. If this damage is recognized during the implant procedure, it is usually wise to abandon the procedure and return for implantation after the urethra has healed.

Cylinder sizing errors occur because of measurement errors and also because of incomplete corporeal dilation. Cylinders that are too short result in poor glans support. Cylinders that are too long produce asymmetrical inflation (an S-shaped cylinder deformity), especially in the case of the Ultrex and Ultrex Plus devices.

Pump malposition occurs during healing when the pump leaves its dependent scrotal position and assumes a position in the upper scrotum, often impinging on the base of the penis. Reservoir malposition occurs when the reservoir is displaced from the prevesical space.

Early experience with these newer prostheses indicates a degree of mechanical reliability far exceeding that of earlier versions of these devices.[4–7] When failure of a component does occur, it is often several years after the device was implanted, and under these circumstances it is often preferable to replace the entire device rather than just the failed single component.

Editorial Comment

Fray F. Marshall

With the use of vacuum devices and injection therapy, there may be less indication for a penile prosthesis.

This chapter carefully outlines the reasons to consider different devices and the small nuances of technique that may be very important in achieving a successful result.

REFERENCES

1. Lakin MM, Montague DK. Surgical treatment of the patient with erectile dysfunction: Clinical evaluation and diagnostic techniques. Atlas Urol Clin North Am 1:9, 1993.
2. Montague DK. Penile prosthesis corporotomy closure: A new technique. J Urol 150:924, 1993.
3. Montague DK, Lakin MM. Early experience with the controlled girth and length expanding cylinder of the AMS Ultrex penile prosthesis. J Urol 148:1444, 1992.
4. Furlow WL, Motley RC. The inflatable penile prosthesis: Clinical experience with a new controlled expansion cylinder. J Urol 139:945, 1988.
5. Knoll LD, Furlow WL, Motley RC. Clinical experience implanting an inflatable penile prosthesis with controlled-expansion cylinder. Urology 36:502, 1990.
6. Mulcahy JJ. Use of CX cylinders in association with AMS 700 inflatable penile prosthesis. J Urol 140:1420, 1988.
7. Quesada ET, Light JK. The AMS 700 inflatable penile prosthesis: Long-term experience with the controlled expansion cylinders. J Urol 149:46, 1993.

SECTION III

FEMALE UROLOGY

Chapter 86

Periurethral Injections in the Treatment of Intrinsic Sphincteric Dysfunction

J. Christian Winters and Rodney A. Appell

In the evaluation of the incontinent patient, it is essential to identify the cause or causes of the incontinence in order to administer appropriate therapy. Urinary incontinence may originate at the level of the bladder or the level of the urethra. When incontinence occurs at the level of the urethra, this is due to either anatomical displacement of a normally functioning proximal urethra (genuine stress urinary incontinence) or intrinsic incompetence of the urethral closure mechanism (intrinsic sphincteric dysfunction, ISD). Patients exhibiting ISD generally have had a previous surgical procedure on or near the urethra, sympathetic neurological injury, or myelodysplasia. Patients exhibiting incontinence resulting from anatomical displacement benefit from a bladder neck suspension procedure, whereas patients with ISD require procedures to increase outflow resistance. These patients are candidates for pubovaginal sling procedures, artificial urinary sphincters, or periurethral injections. Patients with concomitant lack of anatomical support and urethral dysfunction should generally undergo artificial urinary sphincters or pubovaginal sling procedures. Patients with a fixed, well-supported urethra in association with ISD are excellent candidates for periurethral injections to eradicate urinary incontinence. Injectables are designed to increase the urethral resistance to the flow of urine by augmenting intraurethral pressure. However, a well-supported urethra is necessary if periurethral injections are to be used in the treatment of ISD.

PREOPERATIVE EVALUATION

A history of previous surgery or underlying neurological disorder is sought in all patients. A urologist's neurological examination is performed to identify occult causes of incontinence (Table 86–1). In females, the physical examination is essential to ascertain whether concomitant prolapse and urethral hypermobility are present. The Q-tip test is employed with women in the lithotomy position: an angle of greater than 30 degrees from the horizontal signifies urethral hypermobility.[1] A urinalysis is performed in all patients and a culture obtained, if indicated. Urodynamic studies are performed to ascertain whether associated detrusor causes of incontinence are present, as well as to demonstrate poor or absent urethral function. The urodynamic studies may be performed simultaneously with radiographical assessment of the

---

TABLE 86–1. Urologist's Neurological Examination

Saddle anesthesia
Anal reflex (wink)
Bulbocavernosus reflex
General sensation (pattern of loss, e.g., stocking–glove in peripheral neuropathy)
Presence of hemiparesis, paraparesis, tremor
General mental status

---

bladder and urethra. The presence of an open bladder neck in the absence of a detrusor contraction suggests ISD. Also, leak point pressures are obtained to determine the urethral opening pressure. Low urethral opening pressure signifies minimal urethral resistance and suggests poor or absent urethral function. The simplest and most reproducible leak point pressure is the abdominal or Valsalva leak point pressure. An abdominal leak point pressure is obtained with the patient straining while the bladder is filled to 150, 200, 250, and 300 ml, with the pressure recorded when urine leaks through the urethral mechanism. Abdominal pressures of less than 60 cm H_2O imply poor resistance and low urethral opening pressures, signifying poor or absent urethral function. These measurements have been known to correlate with the urethral pressure profiles, are less variable, and are easier and cheaper to perform.[2]

Patients who exhibit poor urethral function, lack of detrusor instability, and good anatomical support are considered good candidates for injectables. Contraindications to this therapy include an active urinary tract infection, untreated detrusor instability, and known hypersensitivity to the injected agent. For this reason, patients undergoing transurethral injection of collagen undergo skin testing 1 month before the procedure to determine whether hypersensitivity to the material is present.

INJECTABLE MATERIALS

The ideal material for periurethral injection is one that is easy to inject, is biocompatible, and causes little or no inflammatory reaction. Also, the substance should elicit no immunogenic response. There should be no migration of the injected material, and it should maintain its bulking effect for a long time. Many agents have been used as injectables for urinary incontinence, ranging from sclerosing agents to autologous blood. Currently, the three most widely used agents are polytetrafluoroethylene (PTFE) paste, cross-linked bovine collagen, and autologous fat. PTFE paste had received Food and Drug Administration (FDA) approval for the treatment of male postprostatectomy incontinent patients, but has recently been removed from the marketplace because of concerns over its safety. Collagen has received FDA approval for the treatment of ISD in both males and females. Autologous fat is gaining acceptance as an alternative injectable, particularly in patients who have shown hypersensitivity to the collagen skin test. Autologous blood can be used for a demonstration of efficacy, but the duration of response is too short to recommend this as a substance for long-term treatment.

Polytetrafluoroethylene Paste

Urethrin and Teflon (PTFE, polytef) are proprietary names for a paste consisting of a sterile mixture of PTFE micropolymer particles (ranging in size from 4 to 10 μm), glycerin, and polysorbate. These particles stimulate an ingrowth of fibroblasts at the injection site, eventually becoming encapsulated and producing a permanent bolstering effect.[3] The particles, although ostensibly inert, do elicit a chronic foreign body reaction leading to granuloma formation. This may result in long-term fibrosis and possibly carcinogenesis, as related polymers of PTFE have been shown to be carcinogenic in rats.[4] Documented evidence of particle migration and granuloma formation have raised concerns about the use of this material in younger patients.[5] Despite these reports, there is a large experience with periurethral injections of PTFE, and no adverse reactions have been documented in human subjects.

Collagen

Glutaraldehyde cross-linked collagen is both biocompatible and biodegradable. It is a sterile, nonpyrogenic purified bovine dermal collagen that has been cross-linked with glutaraldehyde and dispersed in a phosphate-buffered physiological saline. This cross-linking process improves the integrity of the material for injection, resulting in a substance having a longer duration of existence when injected into humans while simultaneously reducing the immunogenicity of the substance. This reduction in immunoreactivity and cytotoxicity of the implant results in this substance eliciting no foreign body reaction. A minimal inflammatory response has been associated with the injection of collagen, but no granuloma formation is present. Collagen begins to degrade in 12 weeks. In this time, however, neovascularization and the deposition of fibroblasts and collagen occur within the implant.[6] The collagen completely degrades within 19 months and there are no reports of particle migration of the collagen material.[7]

Autologous Fat

As a periurethral bulking agent, autologous fat has several advantages: it is readily available, biocompatible, and reasonably easy to obtain. Autologous fat integrates at a graft, but a significant portion of the injected material is reabsorbed and replaced by inflammation, fibrosis, and connective tissue meant to produce the final bulking effect.[8] The high degree of reabsorption, with up to 50 to 70 percent absorbed, is the major limitation in using fat as an injectable

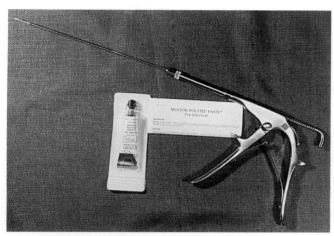

Figure 86–1. Bruning's device used for injection of PTFE paste (Storz Instrument Co, St. Louis, MO).

agent. There has been no evidence of migration of injected fat particles.

TECHNIQUE OF INJECTION

PTFE Paste

PTFE paste is a very thick material requiring the use of injection under pressure. The Bruning's otolaryngological device (Storz Instrument Company, St. Louis, MO), which resembles a caulking gun, or other devices such as the Lewy syringe or a metal piston syringe, can all be used to inject the PTFE paste (Figs. 86–1 and 86–2). These devices commonly require an assistant to activate the injecting device.

Most patients require general or regional anesthesia because the pressure during accumulation of this material may be discomforting. Selected patients may be administered local anesthesia employing periurethral 1 percent lidocaine (Xylocaine) and transurethral 2

percent lidocaine jelly. The transurethral or periurethral approach may be used in both male and female patients. The periurethral approach in females has the advantage of minimizing bleeding and extrusion of the injected substance. The transurethral approach in males has the advantage of optimizing needle placement under direct vision.

PTFE Injection in Females

Preoperatively, all patients receive a prophylactic dose of a cephalosporin chosen for a spectrum to include anaerobic coverage, and a povidone-iodine (Betadine) douche. The patient is prepared and draped in the lithotomy position, and the vulva is anesthetized topically with 2 percent lidocaine jelly. In the transurethral approach, a 16-gauge cystoscopic injection needle (Fig. 86–3) is inserted into the periurethral tissues at the level of the midurethra and advanced to the bladder neck under cystoscopic visualization. Injections are performed in the 3 and 9 o'clock positions, creating suburothelial cushions of material to compress the urethral lumen. During each injection, an obvious bleb is created in the urethral wall, gradually occluding the lumen of the urethra. As this cushion reaches the midline, a similar procedure should be performed on the opposite side. When complete urethral coaptation is achieved, creating an appearance of obstructing prostatic lobes, the end result is reached. Additional injections may be performed at the 6 o'clock position if necessary. When an injection is performed at the 6 o'clock position, digital guidance of needle placement may be performed transvaginally. It is best to minimize the number of puncture sites in order to prevent extravasation of the material.

In the periurethral approach, in addition to topical lidocaine jelly, the 4 and 8 o'clock positions in the periurethral tissue are infiltrated with 1 percent lidocaine using 2 to 4 ml on each side. Cystoscopy with a 0- or 30-degree lens is employed and the injection

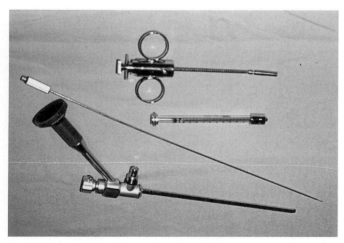

Figure 86–2. Metal piston syringe system for injection of PTFE paste.

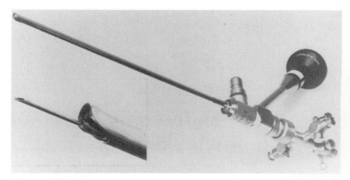

Figure 86–3. A 16-gauge transcystoscopic injection needle used during transurethral injection of PTFE paste.

needle is inserted periurethrally at the 4 o'clock position. The needle is advanced slowly while the surgeon visualizes the tip of the needle against the lining of the urethra so that proper positioning of the needle just below the bladder neck is visualized (Fig. 86–4). The surgeon stabilizes the cystoscope with one hand, and the needle with the other. The assistant then injects the material to create a periurethral cushion advancing to the midline of the urethra. As the needle is withdrawn, additional material is injected. The procedure is then repeated on the opposite side and at the 6 o'clock position if necessary. Regardless of the approach chosen, the end result is the same: coaptation and closure of the urethra (Fig. 86–5). Approximately 10 to 15 ml of material again are used to achieve this result.[3]

An important aspect of this procedure is the depth of penetration of the needle. If the material is injected into the immediate suburothelial plane, the bleb created may burst, causing extravasation of the injected material. Therefore the needle is inserted at a 45-degree angle to add approximately 1 cm depth of penetration. In contrast, collagen injection, as discussed later, is best performed within the suburothelial space within the lamina propria in order to more effectively create urethral coaptation with the collagen material.

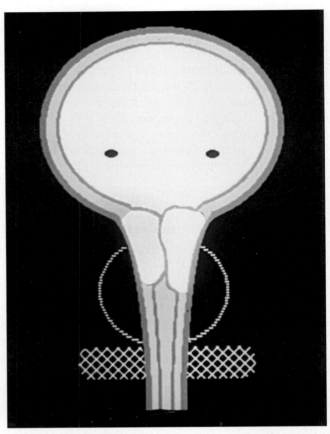

Figure 86–5. Coaptation and closure of the urethra after injection. (From Appell R. Use of collagen injections for the treatment of incontinence and reflux. Adv Urol 5:145, 1992.)

PTFE Injection in Males

Just as in females, a periurethral or transurethral approach may be chosen. The lithotomy position is assumed and the external genitalia and perineum are prepared with a povidone-iodine solution. Two percent lidocaine is injected intraurethrally for 10 minutes, and the perineum puncture site may be infiltrated with 5 ml of 1 percent lidocaine solution if a periurethral approach is chosen. A cystoscope is positioned in the urethra, and a 17-gauge needle is

inserted in the perineum and advanced toward the prostatic apex. With a gentle rocking motion, the needletip can be identified in proximity to the external sphincter. When the proper position is obtained, material is injected to produce closure of the urethra. The needle is repositioned in several sites around the urethra, and sequential injections are performed to achieve urethral coaptation.[9]

In postprostatectomy patients, more accurate placement of the needle is achieved by way of a transurethral approach. The cystoscope is advanced into the bladder, and the needle is extended until the tip of the needle is visualized. The cystoscope is then withdrawn to the level of the external sphincter, and the needle is inserted at a 45-degree angle in the 4, 8, 10, and 2 o'clock positions. Insertion of the needle at the level of the sphincter with proximal advancement ensures placement of the material proximal to the external sphincter. After the desired cushion is created, additional material is injected as the needle is withdrawn. The injection is systematically carried out in a four-quadrant fashion, creating urethral coaptation. Approximately 5 ml is required in each quadrant to achieve closure of the urethra, using 15 to 20 ml to complete urethral closure.[10]

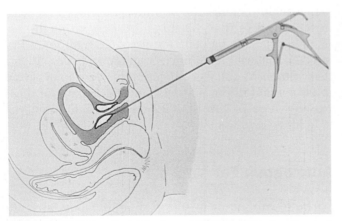

Figure 86–4. Periurethral injection of PTFE paste using Bruning's device. (Courtesy of Tulane Medical Center.)

Collagen

Although the techniques of injection are similar to PTFE, the material required for periurethral injection of collagen is only a 20- or 22-gauge spinal needle or a 20 Fr. cystoscope with an injection needle (Fig. 86–6). The collagen is supplied in a 3-ml plastic Luer-Lok syringe, containing 2.5 ml of collagen. The material is easily injected and therefore these injections can be performed without the use of an assistant.

In females a periurethral approach is almost universally chosen, as it appears to minimize the possibility of bleeding and extravasation of the injected material. The preparation and positioning of the patient is identical to the periurethral approach chosen for PTFE paste. The spinal needle is advanced under cystoscopic guidance from the 4 and 8 o'clock periurethral positions, as previously described. It is important to note, however, that positioning of the needle should be within the suburothelial plane. The needle should not purposely be positioned in the muscular wall of the urethra. This will not allow appropriate molding of the collagen and will result in the use of excessive material. Figures 86–7, 86–8, and 86–9 illustrate proper positioning of the needle in the suburothelial plane for injection of collagen. The figures demonstrate the material accumulating during injection and the end result of urethral coaptation.

In male patients the transurethral approach is almost universally chosen, as it allows more accurate placement of the injection material. The four-quadrant approach, similar to that previously described for PTFE paste, is used. However, the needle is not inserted at a 45-degree angle as for PTFE. The needle is inserted into the suburothelial plane so as to optimize accumulation of collagen required to coapt the urethra (Fig. 86–10). There is less chance of perfora-

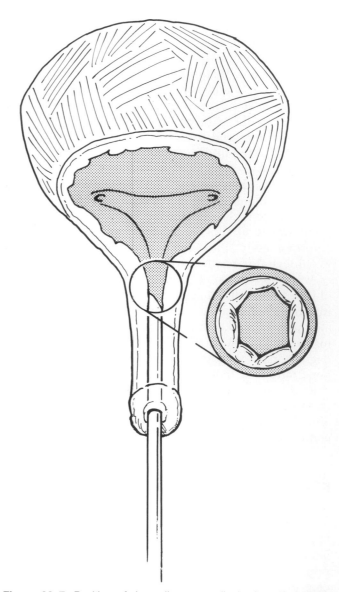

Figure 86–7. Position of the collagen needle in the suburothelial plane before injection (note the open urethral lumen).

tion of the mucosa and therefore deeper needle penetration is not desired.[11]

In female patients the volume of collagen material injected is less than 30 ml in 90 percent of the patients, and 65.8 percent require less than 20 ml of injected material to achieve dryness. In male patients the volume of collagen injections is less than 36 ml in 90 percent of the patients, and 58 percent of these patients require less than 20 ml of injected material to achieve dryness.[12]

Autologous Fat

The technique of injection of autologous fat is divided into two phases: first, harvesting the fat, and second, periurethral injection of the fat. Both proce-

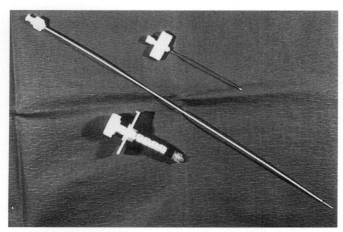

Figure 86–6. Collagen injection system for periurethral and transurethral use.

cause injury to intra-abdominal organs. Approximately 250 ml of lactated Ringer's solution with 10 ml lidocaine with 1:1000 epinephrine are injected through the injection cannula into the lower abdomen to prepare the fat for harvesting. This solution provides local anesthesia and also decreases bleeding from the harvested fat. After this, the 2.1-mm cannula is inserted with a 60-ml syringe attached. The syringe is locked into a suction position. With a gentle rocking motion to and through the infiltrated lower abdomen, 20 to 30 ml of fat is obtained. A 60-ml transferring adapter is then used to add additional saline to the syringe. With a rocking motion, the fat is cleaned with the saline. The bloody saline is discarded and the process is repeated until the saline is clear. This leaves pellets of golden-brown fat. The syringe is placed upright and the fat allowed to settle. The excess saline is discarded and the fat is then trans-

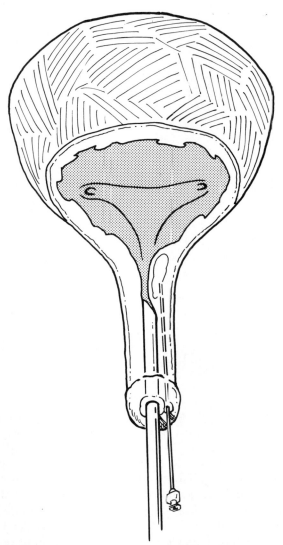

Figure 86–8. Injection of collagen material and formation of a suburothelial collection of collagen.

dures may be performed with the use of local anesthesia. The patient is placed in the lithotomy position and the preparation is done as previously described. The lower abdomen is prepared with povidone-iodine scrub and solution.

Harvesting Fat

The Tulip fat harvesting and injection system (Tulip Co., San Diego, CA) is used for this procedure (Fig. 86–11). The skin puncture site chosen on the lower abdomen is infiltrated with 5 ml of lidocaine solution. The puncture trocar is advanced through the site to facilitate cannula placement. After this, the 3-ml injection cannula is used to inject the fat preparation solution into the abdominal wall between the layers of Camper's and Scarpa's fasciae. Placement of the injection cannula too superficially will cause skin dimpling; placement too deeply may

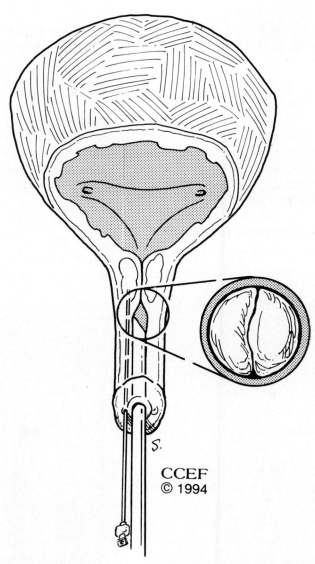

Figure 86–9. Completed collagen injection (note the urethral coaptation).

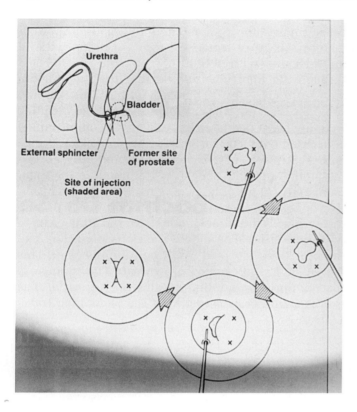

Figure 86–10. Four-quadrant closure of the prostatic urethra with collagen (note the needle placement within the suburothelial plane). (From McGuire EJ, Appell RA. Collagen injection for the dysfunctional urethra. Contemp Urol 3:11, 1991.)

ferred to a Luer-Lok syringe for periurethral injection through an 18-gauge needle.

The technique of periurethral injection of fat is similar to that used for collagen procedures in both preparation and needle placement. Again, the end result is similar, with coaptation of the urethra. Successful fat injections have not been reported in male patients to date.

Autologous Blood

In selected patients a temporary trial of periurethral injection may be performed with autologous blood.

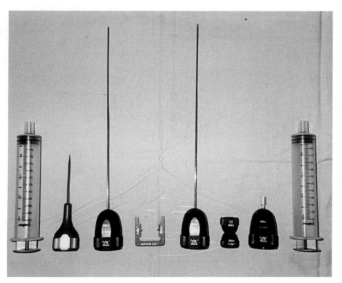

Figure 86–11. Tulip fat harvesting and injection system.

Approximately 20 ml of blood is collected in two preheparinized 10-ml syringes. The syringes are manually preheparinized by rinsing 3 ml of heparin flush solution within the syringe and then discarding it. Commercially available preheparinized syringes contain too much heparin and do not allow the desired blood clotting. After collection, as the material is injected into the periurethral tissues, a distinct blue bleb is created. This signifies proper placement of the material.

Postoperative Care

Perioperative antibiotic coverage is continued for 3 days after the procedure. If transient retention develops, clear intermittent catheterization is begun. Indwelling Foley catheters are to be avoided in patients undergoing collagen and fat injection, as these promote molding of the material around the catheter. Minimal periods of Foley placement (24 to 48 hours) have been described by authors using PTFE injections. If long-term catheterization is needed, suprapubic cystotomy should be performed in these patients.

Patients are contacted 1 to 2 weeks after injection to assess continence status. For patients undergoing collagen and fat injection, repeat injections are scheduled 1 month later as necessary. It is preferable to wait 4 to 6 months before repeating PTFE injections, as continence may improve late with developing inflammation and capsule formation around the PTFE particles.

RESULTS

In evaluating the results of periurethral injection in the treatment of ISD, these procedures are compared with pubovaginal sling procedures and artificial urinary sphincters. Patients are considered improved if "social continence" (wetting controlled with the use of tissues or a small minipad) is obtained. They are considered cured if rendered completely dry by treatment. Patients rendered socially continent or dry are considered to have successful results. Pubovaginal sling surgery is successful in approximately 81 to 98 percent of patients, and sphincter surgery in over 90 percent of patients. PTFE injections are successful in 70 to 95 percent of women, and the injection of collagen is successful in 64 to 90 percent of female patients.[13] In an early experience with fat injections, 70 to 90 percent of patients appeared to be improved.[14] These procedures have success rates comparable with those of surgery. They have not gained universal acceptance, however, owing to questionable factors: (1) the inability to quantify the amount of material needed for injection in the particular patient and (2) their long-term safety.[13]

In male patients, PTFE particles have been shown to achieve improvement or dryness in 88 percent after transurethral resection of the prostate and in 67 percent after radical prostatectomy.[15] In treating postprostatectomy patients with collagen, approximately 80 percent of patients after transurethral resection of the prostate are cured or improved. However, after radical prostatectomy, only 25 to 40 percent of patients are cured or improved. In patients receiving prior irradiation for prostate cancer, the results are even worse, with only 10 to 20 percent of patients achieving improvement.[16]

COMPLICATIONS

The complications associated with periurethral injections are minimal. The rate of urinary retention in patients undergoing PTFE injections is approximately 35 percent. These patients may undergo a transient period of Foley catheter drainage and should undergo intermittent catheterization as feasible. Approximately 20 percent of these patients have developed irritative voiding symptoms that resolve after several days of conservative treatment with antibiotics.[3] Few patients experience perineal discomfort, which also resolves with sitz baths. After PTFE injection, patients have been noted to develop fever with both negative blood and urine cultures. This also resolves after a few days and indicates a probable mild allergic response.

In the multicenter clinical trial of collagen injections, transient urinary retention developed in approximately 15 percent of patients. Urinary tract infection was observed in approximately 5 percent, and 2 percent of patients experienced transient hematuria that resolved conservatively. Urinary urgency, pain at the injection site, and urethritis occurred in less than 1 percent of patients.[12] The clinical experience with autologous fat is small, yet the complication rate appears minimal and similar to that of collagen implants.

Summary

In the properly selected patient, injectables offer excellent treatment results for intrinsic sphincteric dysfunction. PTFE paste may be used in elderly men after radical prostatectomy and in women over the age of 65. However, concerns of granuloma formation and particle migration limit its use in younger patients. Collagen injections have been shown to be both biocompatible and biodegradable. There are no reports of particle migration of this material and at present it is the most widely used injectable. Repeated injections are frequently necessary, yet are safely performed under local anesthesia. Autologous fat is gaining acceptance as an alternative periurethral injectable, particularly in patients who have positive skin tests to collagen.

The treatment responses with these procedures are similar to surgical procedures to correct ISD, and the complications appear to be minimal. Therefore, the use of periurethral injections for ISD certainly has a role in the treatment of properly selected patients.

Editorial Comment
Fray F. Marshall

Initially, polytef was used as an injectable material, but because of migration it is not typically used in the United States. Autologous fat has the advantage of being safe with readily available material, but its permanence remains questionable. At this time, collagen appears to be the most attractive alternative, at least in males. It remains quite expensive. With lesser amounts of incontinence, small changes in resistance may produce significant improvement in urinary control.

REFERENCES

1. Chrystle C, Charmel S, Copeland W. Q-tip test for stress urinary incontinence. Obstet Gynecol 38:313, 1971.
2. Appell R. Valsalva leak point pressure (LPP) vs urethral pressure profile (UPP) in the evaluation of intrinsic sphincteric

deficiency (ISD) (abstract). Presented at the American Urogynecology Society Annual Meeting, Toronto, Canada, 1994.

3. Politano V. Periurethral polytetrafluoroethylene injection for urinary incontinence. J Urol 127:439, 1982.

4. Oppenheimier B, Oppenheimier E, Stout A. The latent period in carcinogenesis by plastic in rats and its relation to the presarcomatous stage. Cancer 11:204, 1958.

5. Malizia A, Reiman J, Myers R, et al. Migration and granulomatous reaction after periurethral injection of polytef (Teflon). JAMA 251:3277, 1984.

6. Stegman S, Chu S, Bensch K, Armstrong R: A light and electron microscopic evaluation of Zyderm and Zyplast implants in aging human facial skin. A pilot study. Arch Dermatol 123:1644, 1987.

7. Remacle M, Marbaix E. Collagen implants in the human larynx. Pathologic examination of two cases. Arch Otorhinolaryngol 245:203, 1988.

8. Sanatarosa R, Blaivis J. Building continence with periurethral fat injections. Contemp Urol 5:96, 1993.

9. Politano V. Periurethral Teflon injection for urinary incontinence. Urol Clin North Am 5:415, 1978.

10. Stanisic T, Jennings C. Miller J. Polytetrafluoroethylene injection for post-prostectomy incontinence: Experience with 20 patients during 3 years. J Urol 146:1575, 1991.

11. Appell R. Collagen injection therapy for urinary incontinence. Urol Clin North Am 21:177, 1994.

12. CR Bard Co. PMAA submission to US Food and Drug Administration for IDE 6850010, 1990.

13. Appell R. Periurethral injections. In Hurt W, ed. Urogynecologic Surgery. Gaithersburg, MD, Aspen, 1992, p 139.

14. Ganabathi K, Leach G. Periurethral injection techniques. Atlas Urol Clin North Am 101, 1994.

15. Politano V. Transurethral polytef injection for post-prostatectomy urinary incontinence. Br J Urol 69:26, 1992.

16. McGuire E, Appell R. Transurethral collagen injections for urinary incontinence. Urology 43:413, 1994.

Chapter 87

Urethral Reconstruction for Urinary Incontinence

Brett A. Trockman and Gary E. Leach

Defects in the female urethra resulting in urinary incontinence present a challenging urological problem. The degree of urethral defect spans a spectrum from a small urethral fistula causing vaginal voiding to loss of the entire urethra and bladder neck causing total incontinence. These anatomical defects are usually complications of previous gynecological or urological surgery.[1, 2] Fortunately, modern obstetrical care has made birth trauma a rare cause of urethral loss in the United States.[2]

Many different techniques for urethral reconstruction have been described,[1-6] and most use some form of bladder or vaginal flap. Both bladder and vaginal flap urethral reconstruction have a high rate of postoperative incontinence unless a simultaneous anti-incontinence procedure is performed.[1] Accurate preoperative assessment of the extent of urethral loss, as well as identification of any concomitant urethral hypermobility or intrinsic sphincter deficiency, is critical to planning a successful urethral reconstruction. The utility of the vaginal approach for urethral reconstruction has been well described.[1, 7, 8] Thus, this chapter is limited to description of the vaginal approach for female urethral reconstruction.

PREOPERATIVE EVALUATION

In patients who are not totally incontinent, a complete voiding history will help identify components of stress or urge incontinence. A history of multiple previous vaginal or pelvic surgeries increases the chance of severe scarring and intrinsic sphincter deficiency secondary to periurethral fibrosis. A thorough physical examination is needed to assess the extent of urethral loss, the location and size of any urethrovaginal fistula, the degree of urethral support during straining, and the quality of the surrounding vaginal tissue. The presence of atrophic vaginitis should be noted and treated with vaginal estrogen cream before reconstruction.

Careful urethroscopy with a 20 Fr. female cystoscope usually confirms the diagnosis of urethrovaginal fistula. When confirmation is difficult, simultaneous vaginal exposure with a speculum may aid in visual identification of the fistula.[7] Cystoscopy is essential to assess any involvement of the bladder neck or trigone. When the trigone is involved, upper tract screening with a renal ultrasound or intravenous pyelography is recommended. A voiding cystourethrogram performed under fluoroscopic control, with the patient in the standing position with adequate voiding views, may be useful to identify the urethral defect, exclude a vesicovaginal fistula, and demonstrate urethral hypermobility or leakage of contrast across the bladder neck with stress. Urodynamic studies may be used selectively to assess bladder function or document evidence of intrinsic sphincter deficiency.

In general, patients with symptomatic, small to moderately sized urethrovaginal fistulas can be managed with urethrovaginal fistula repair, assuming a tension-free closure can be obtained. Vaginal flap urethral reconstruction is required for patients with very large urethrovaginal fistulas or extensive urethral loss. The results of the preoperative evaluation will determine the need for a simultaneous anti-incontinence procedure.

Patients are usually admitted on the morning of surgery. Any urinary tract infections are treated before admission. Patients perform a povidone-iodine scrub of the genitalia and vaginal douche at home the evening before surgery. Parenteral antibiotics are administered preoperatively.

OPERATIVE TECHNIQUE

Urethrovaginal Fistula Repair

The patient is placed in the lithotomy position and a 14 Fr. urethral catheter and a 20 to 24 Fr. suprapubic Foley catheter are placed using the modified Lowsley tractor.[7] After infiltrating the anterior vaginal wall with plain saline, an inverted-U incision is made with the apex just proximal to the urethrovaginal fistula (Fig. 87–1). An anterior vaginal wall flap is raised with the wide base of the flap at the bladder neck. The dissection should be performed in the relatively avascular plane below the vaginal epithelium on the shiny white interior surface of the vaginal wall. If the dissection is carried too deeply, excessive bleeding or bladder perforation may occur. At this point, if treatment of symptomatic urethral hypermobility or intrinsic sphincter deficiency is needed, the vaginal dissection may be carried laterally and the endopelvic fascia perforated laterally in preparation for a bladder neck suspension or pubovaginal sling. Full descriptions of bladder neck suspension and pubovaginal sling procedures are found in Chapters 88, 89, and 93.

The fistula is circumscribed but not excised because the scarred margins are used to provide a secure closure of the fistula tract (Fig. 87–2). Excision of the tract only increases the the size of the fistula and may decrease the strength of the closure. The margins of the fistula are freed from surrounding scar tissue to allow tension-free closure. Just distal to the

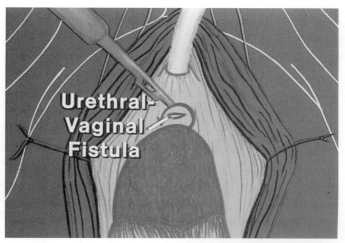

Figure 87–2. Circumferential incision around the fistula without actually excising the fistula tract. (From Leach GE. Urethrovaginal fistula repair with Martius labial fat pad graft. Urol Clin North Am 18:409, 1991.)

fistula, a portion of the vaginal epithelium is removed to allow adequate vaginal wall flap advancement and avoid overlapping suture lines during closure. The fistula is closed with a running locked 4-0 absorbable suture (Fig. 87–3). A second layer of closure is accomplished with interrupted Lembert-type sutures of 3-0 absorbable material in the periurethral fascia. These two layers should result in a watertight closure without tension.

If there is any concern about the quality of vaginal tissues or integrity of the closure, a Martius labial fat pad graft can be used to reinforce the fistula closure.[9] A Martius graft is obtained by making a vertical incision over the labia majora, exposing the deep labial fat pad. The fat pad is mobilized starting anteriorly, preserving the pudendal vascular supply that enters posteriorly (Fig. 87–4). After completely mobilizing

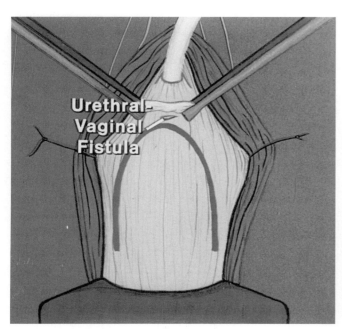

Figure 87–1. Anterior U-shaped vaginal incision with the apex adjacent to the urethrovaginal fistula. (From Leach GE. Urethrovaginal fistula repair with Martius labial fat pad graft. Urol Clin North Am 18:409, 1991.)

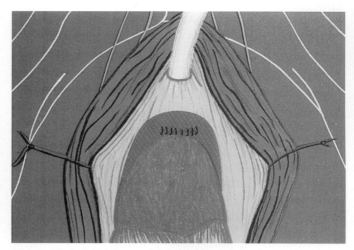

Figure 87–3. Initial layer of fistula closure with a running locked absorbable suture. (From Leach GE. Urethrovaginal fistula repair with Martius labial fat pad graft. Urol Clin North Am 18:409, 1991.)

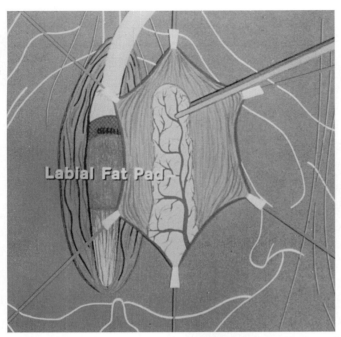

Figure 87–4. Mobilized labial fat pad with careful preservation of inferior blood supply. (From Leach GE. Urethrovaginal fistula repair with Martius labial fat pad graft. Urol Clin North Am 18:409, 1991.)

the fat pad on its posterior vascular pedicle, a tunnel is made medially from the labia to the vagina. The Martius graft is then carefully passed through the tunnel without tension and secured over the fistula repair site with absorbable sutures (Fig. 87–5).

The anterior vaginal flap is the final layer of closure. The vaginal wall flap can be advanced over the Martius graft, avoiding overlapping suture lines (Fig. 87–6). The vaginal closure is completed with a running locked absorbable suture. A small Penrose drain is placed deep in the labial wound, and the labial incision is closed in layers. Both the urethral and suprapubic catheters are placed to drainage and an antibiotic-soaked vaginal pack is inserted.

Vaginal Flap Urethral Reconstruction

The patient is placed in the lithotomy position. A 20 to 24 Fr. suprapubic Foley catheter is placed using the modified Lowsley tractor.[7] A 14 Fr. urethral Foley catheter is placed and the balloon overinflated enough to prevent passage through the bladder neck. In most cases, an inverted-U vaginal incision is used with its apex just proximal to the meatus of the damaged urethra and its base at the bladder neck[1] (Fig. 87–7A). The flap is sharply mobilized posteriorly. If indicated, lateral dissection in preparation for a simultaneous anti-incontinence procedure can be performed at this time, as discussed in the previous description of urethrovaginal fistula repair (Fig. 87–7B). When required, the pubovaginal sling is now passed beneath the bladder neck and proximal

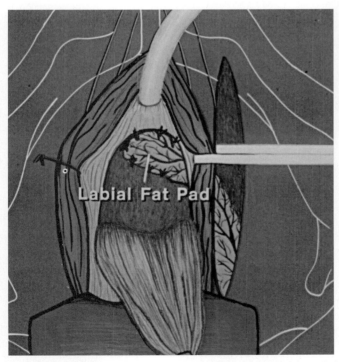

Figure 87–5. Martius labial fat pad graft passed through the medial tunnel and fixed over the fistula closure site with an absorbable suture. (From Leach GE. Urethrovaginal fistula repair with Martius labial fat pad graft. Urol Clin North Am 18:409, 1991.)

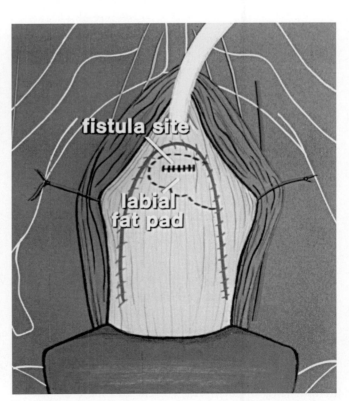

Figure 87–6. Final advancement of a vaginal wall flap over the fistula repair site and a Martius labial fat pad graft, avoiding overlapping suture lines. (From Leach GE. Urethrovaginal fistula repair with Martius labial fat pad graft. Urol Clin North Am 18:409, 1991.)

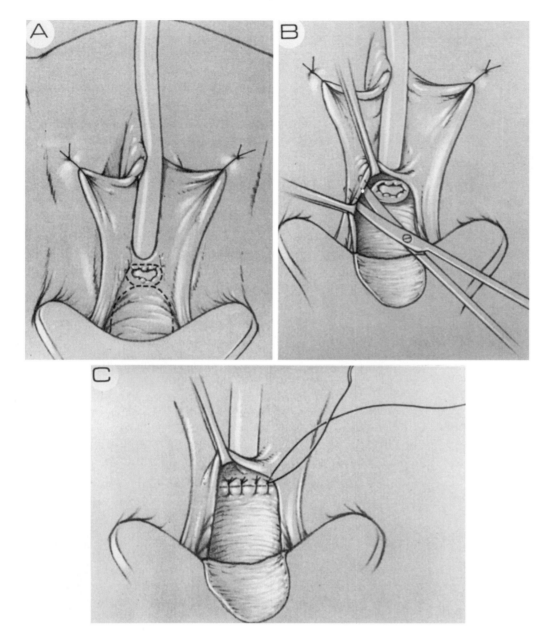

Figure 87–7. *A,* Anterior U-shaped vaginal incision. The fistula is circumscribed but not excised. *B,* A lateral dissection is performed if concomitant bladder neck suspension or a pubovaginal sling is planned. *C,* The fistula site is closed with absorbable sutures. (From Blaivas JG. Vaginal flap neourethra: An alternative to bladder flap urethral reconstruction. J Urol 141:542, 1989.)

urethra. Any urethral fistula is closed at this time using the technique previously described (Fig 87–7*C*).

The neourethra is then created by making two parallel incisions starting on each side of the meatus and extending distally (Fig. 87–8*A*). Flaps are then mobilized laterally to medially, allowing tubularization of the mobilized flaps around the 14 Fr. catheter. The flaps are approximated in the midline with 4-0 absorbable suture, forming the neourethra (Fig. 87–8*B*). The suture line is then reinforced with a Martius graft as described for the repair of urethrovaginal fistulas (Fig. 87–8*C*). The vagina and labia are closed with absorbable sutures (Fig. 87–8*D*). If a pubovaginal sling has been used, it should be secured with minimal tension to the abdominal fascia or pubic tubercle

before closing the vagina.[10] The suprapubic and urethral catheters are placed to drainage and an antibiotic-soaked vaginal pack is inserted.

As in all reconstructive surgery, anatomical considerations may make modifications of the usual technique necessary. A modified vaginal flap urethral reconstruction utilizing a meatal-based vaginal flap rotated distally has also been successful (Fig. 87–9).[1] Alternative means of suture line reinforcement include gracilis- and perineal artery–based flaps.[2, 3, 11] In cases with severe tissue loss, the neourethra can be constructed from the cutaneous portion of a gracilis- or perineal artery–based myocutaneous flap. In some severely debilitated patients with extensive tissue loss, the most practical alternative may be transvaginal closure of the bladder neck with creation of

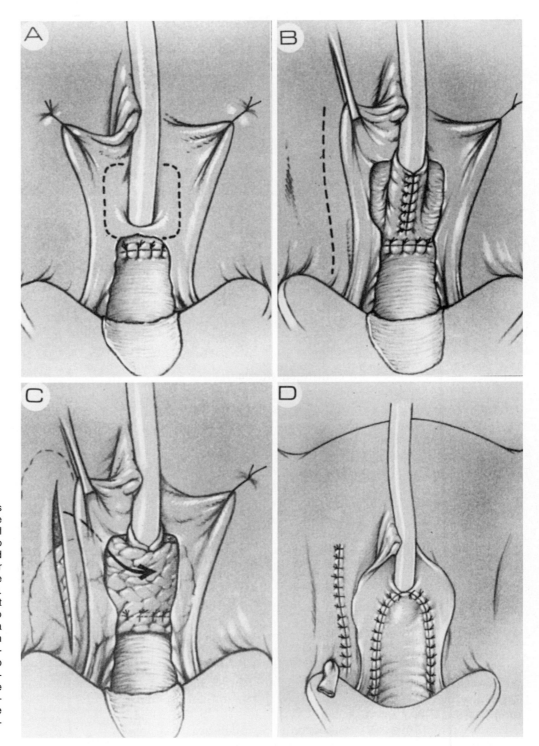

Figure 87–8. *A,* Parallel incisions are made on either side of the urethral catheter, and vaginal flaps are mobilized from lateral to medial. *B,* Vaginal flaps are rolled into a tube over a 14 Fr. catheter and approximated in the midline with absorbable suture material. *C,* A Martius labial fat pad graft is mobilized, tunneled medially to cover the neourethra and fistula site, and secured in position with absorbable sutures. *D,* The vaginal wall U flap is advanced to cover the entire neourethra. Closure is completed with absorbable sutures. (From Blaivas JG. Vaginal flap neourethra: An alternative to bladder flap urethral reconstruction. J Urol 141:542, 1989.)

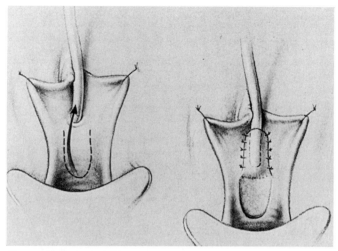

Figure 87–9. A rotated anterior vaginal wall flap to create a neourethra and advance the meatus. (From Blaivas JG. Treatment of female incontinence secondary to urethral damage or loss. Urol Clin North Am 18:355, 1991.)

a continent catheterizable stoma to the bladder or placement of a suprapubic tube.[12]

Postoperative Management

Parenteral antibiotics are continued for 24 hours. The vaginal pack and Penrose drain are removed 1 day postoperatively. Oral anticholinergics such as oxybutynin or propantheline bromide are used to prevent bladder spasms. Catheter drainage is maintained for 7 to 10 days, after which the urethral catheter is removed and a voiding cystourethrogram is performed via the suprapubic catheter. Anticholinergics should be discontinued 24 hours before performing the voiding cystourethrogram. If any extravasation is noted, the urethral catheter is not replaced and the suprapubic tube is placed to drainage. A repeat study is then performed in 1 to 2 weeks.

Complications

Excessive perioperative bleeding is rarely a problem during urethral reconstruction. Wound infection or vaginal abscess is an uncommon complication of vaginal surgery when there is proper preoperative preparation.

Urinary retention or elevated postvoid residuals are a more common problem after urethral reconstruction, especially if a simultaneous anti-incontinence procedure was performed. When the patient is unable to void or when elevated postvoid residuals are noted on the postoperative voiding cystourethrogram, the suprapubic catheter is not removed but is intermit-

tently opened to drain the residual urine. Intermittent catheterization through the reconstructed urethra should be avoided in the early postoperative period. Within a few weeks, most patients are able to void adequately and the suprapubic catheter is removed. When long-term intermittent catheterization is needed, it should not be initiated until healing of the reconstructed urethra is complete.

Urinary incontinence after urethral reconstruction may be secondary to stress incontinence, detrusor instability, or urethral fistula formation. As previously mentioned, careful preoperative evaluation helps select patients requiring a simultaneous anti-incontinence procedure, minimizing the risk of postoperative stress incontinence. However, if stress incontinence occurs, it should be evaluated and treated in the standard fashion. Periurethral injections may be useful for treatment of selected cases of postoperative stress incontinence.[13, 14] Persistent urge incontinence may be related to outlet obstruction and should be fully evaluated. Blaivas[8] reported restoration of continence in nine of ten patients undergoing vaginal flap urethral reconstruction. Six patients underwent one procedure, two patients required a subsequent pubovaginal sling for intrinsic sphincteric deficiency, and one patient needed a subsequent vesicovaginal fistula closure.[8]

Any new or recurrent urethrovaginal fistula identified in the immediate postoperative period is managed conservatively with suprapubic drainage and observation. Should the fistula persist, fistula repair may be undertaken after allowing at least 2 to 3 months for resolution of postoperative inflammation.

Editorial Comment
Fray F. Marshall

Complete evaluation of the patient for fistula, stress incontinence, neurological status, and anatomical defects is essential for appropriate therapy. In severe urethral trauma, a posterior-based buttock flap can also provide a large, well-vascularized pedicle of tissue for repair of a large defect.

REFERENCES

1. Blaivas JG. Vaginal flap urethral reconstruction: An alternative to the bladder flap neourethra. J Urol 141:542, 1989.
2. Patil U, Waterhouse K, Laungauni G. Management of 18 difficult vesicovaginal and urethrovaginal fistulas with modified Ingelman-Sundberg and Martius operations. J Urol 123:653, 1980.
3. Hendren WH. Construction of female urethra from vaginal wall and a perineal flap: J Urol 123:657, 1980.
4. Flocks RH, Boldus R. The surgical treatment and prevention of urinary incontinence associated with disturbance of the internal urethral sphincter mechanism. J Urol 109:279, 1973.
5. Tanago EA. Bladder neck reconstruction for total urinary incontinence: 10 years of experience. J Urol 125:321, 1981.

6. Leadbetter, GW Jr. Surgical correction of total urinary incontinence. J Urol 91:261, 1964.

7. Leach GE. Urethrovaginal fistula repair with Martius labial fat pad graft. Urol Clin North Am 18:409, 1991.

8. Blaivas JG. Treatment of female incontinence secondary to urethral damage or loss. Urol Clin North Am 18:355, 1991.

9. Martius H: Die operative Wiederherstellung der vollkommen fehlenden Harnröhre und Schliessmuskels derselben. Zentralbl Gynakol 52:480, 1928.

10. Sirls L, Leach GE. Pubovaginal sling procedures. Atlas Urol Clin North Am 2:61, 1994.

11. Nolan JF, Stillwell TJ, Barttelbort SW, Sands JP. Urethrovaginal reconstruction using a perineal aretery axial flap. J Urol 146:843, 1991.

12. Zimmern PE, Hadley HR, Leach GE, et al. Transvaginal closure of the bladder neck and placement of a suprapubic catheter for destroyed urethra after longterm indwelling catheter. J Urol 134:554, 1985.

13. Lockhart JL, Walker RD, Vorstman B, Politano VA. Periurethral polytetrafluoroethylene injection following urethral reconstruction in female patients with urinary incontinence. J Urol 140:51, 1988.

14. Ganabathi K, Leach GE. Periurethral injection techniques. Atlas Urol Clin North Am 2:101, 1994.

Chapter 88

Stress Incontinence in the Female

Victor F. Marshall

PREOPERATIVE EVALUATION

Stress incontinence is common and can be corrected by retracting the sphincteric mechanism from the introitus towards the umbilicus. Well-performed preliminary testing can determine whether such placement can succeed. Without this testing, a corrective program is as likely to be unsuccessful as successful. All vesical problems may not be corrected by surgery.

The objective of the stress or Marshall test is to observe the effect of temporarily elevating the vesical base from the introitus toward the umbilicus.[1, 2] Catheterization for residual urine is followed by instillation of 250 ml of fluid into the bladder and removing the catheter. The patient coughs and strains in supine and standing positions so that the examiner can make needed observations. Normally, no leakage is seen. Next, the vesical base is elevated transvaginally, with care taken to curve the finger so as not to compress the urethra to produce a falsely favorable examination (Fig. 88–1A and B). The displacement should restore control and eliminate leakage, giving a favorable test.

A general indication of the degree of displacement needed for control is provided. Inserting a vaginal pack (usually three or four rolled 4 × 4-inch gauze pads) may confirm the effect over the next 12 hours (Fig. 88–1C). If no previous attempts at surgical correction have been made, a cystoscopic examination is usually not required, but one is advisable after any previous attempts. The usual general preoperative examinations are, of course, mandatory.

In borderline diagnostic cases, repeated testing is often necessary, especially regarding the differentiation of stress incontinence from urgency-frequency syndrome. This syndrome is often called the urethral syndrome. A patient with urgency-frequency syndrome classically has a warning, at least momentarily, that leakage is about to occur before she gets wet. A patient with uncomplicated stress incontinence does not have this heralding. Often a trial of hot sitz baths twice a day for 20 minutes; mild urinary antiseptic (such as nitrofurantoin or sulfisoxazole); correction of any vaginitis; and, for the postmenopausal patient, an estrogen such as diethylstilbestrol, will reduce urgency-frequency syndrome in a week, so that the irritative symptoms can be assayed.

Our operation originated from a study of adults with excised rectums and not from a study of women with stress incontinence.[1] We discovered several patients with perineal hernias that could be reduced by manual pressure to improve vesical emptying and lessen stress incontinence. In fact, the first Marshall-Marchetti-Krantz (MMK)[3] procedure was successfully performed on a man by suturing the freed-up prostate to the back of the symphysis. The perineal postoperative hernia was thus overcome by displacement toward the umbilicus. This operation is almost never successful in overcoming postprostatectomy incontinence, because this type of incontinence is caused by intrinsic damage to the sphincter mechanism and not by simple lack of mechanical advantage due to poor support. The object is to end stress incontinence (as revealed by the stress test) and not to cure all vesical problems. However, some incidental improvements often occur because of improved emptying.

OPERATIVE TECHNIQUE

The incision should provide wide access to the space of Retzius. We usually prefer a vertical one well down into the mons veneris. After the muscles are retracted, the space on top of the vagina and urethra down within 1 cm of the external meatus (the approximate thickness of the vagina) is opened with a sponge on ring forceps with about 1 pound of pressure.

The veins are skeletonized by carefully picking fat away from them. Just wiping out the entire space

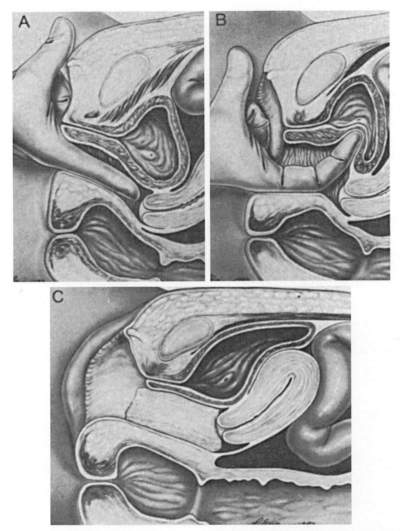

Figure 88–1. *A,* The stress test temporarily supports the sphincteric mechanism away from the introitus toward the umbilicus. *B,* Notice the curved finger is not compressing the urethra. *C,* The extended Marshall stress test utilizes a vaginal gauze tampon for several hours. (From Marshall VF, Vaughan ED Jr, Parnell JP. Urinary incontinence in the female. In Walsh PC, Gittes RF, Perlmutter AD, Stamey TA. Campbell's Urology, 5th ed. Philadelphia, WB Saunders, 1986, p 2712.)

produces too much bleeding. If any inadvertent tears in the veins occur, a pack usually controls bleeding while the operator cleans the opposite side of fat.

The main effect of the Trendelenburg elevated position for this procedure is that the pelvic cavity is made more accessible, more shallow in effect.[4] Trendelenburg did not describe the shock position! Significant arterial bleeders are rarely encountered in the space of Retzius, but if so, they obviously should be controlled in the usual manner. Excessive handling and stretching can produce major hemorrhage. However, transfusion is rarely necessary except under unusual circumstances, such as with reoperations in which the vagina must be separated sharply from the symphysis or in cases of extreme obesity.

Chromic 2-0 catgut sutures are placed on Mayo needles with double bites into the vagina close to, but not into, the urethra (a preoperatively placed catheter easily identifies the urethra) (Fig. 88–2). These sutures are placed on each side, beginning barely above the external urethral meatus, which an assistant may palpate from outside, if desirable. It is important to tag each progressive echelon with distinctive clamps to identify the sutures. A fourth-echelon suture is placed into the vagina on each side where the vesical neck flares toward the urethra proper. If there are any sagging areas in the upper vagina, sutures are applied there also.

These sutures are next inserted on Mayo needles serially and as single bites into the cartilage and perineum of the symphysis posteriorly so that when tied the space of Retzius is closed, thereby retracting the sphincteric mechanism away from the introitus toward the umbilicus (Fig. 88–3), as preoperatively shown by the stress test. Having an assistant support the urethra and vagina from below with fingers in the vagina facilitates closure while tying.

Closure is routine. A small split drain is left on either side of the suturing. The drain is usually removed about the third postoperative day. The Foley catheter remains on straight drainage, and adhesive is applied to it and the thigh, leaving the catheter slack to prevent downward displacement of the bladder (Fig. 88–4). The catheter can usually be removed in 3 days, but residual urine should be tested in 8 or 10 hours. If the residual is over 100 ml, the catheter is replaced overnight. Intermittent catheterization is initiated until good spontaneous voiding occurs. The patient may actually have overflow incontinence if not corrected by catheterization. Bethanechol chloride is occasionally useful for a few days if difficulty in emptying persists. A standard mild urinary antiseptic should be given for at least 10 days. The patient should be mobilized out of bed in about 6 hours. Heavy lifting is prohibited for a month, otherwise the patient may return to her regular activities progressively.

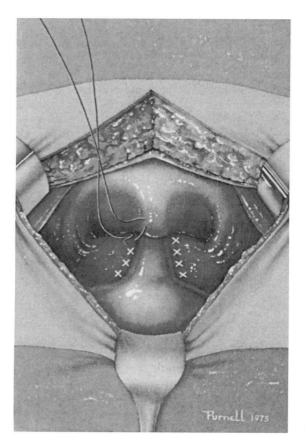

Figure 88–2. Downward view in the space of Retzius showing the sites of placement of the catgut sutures. (From Marshall VF, Vaughan ED Jr, Parnell JP. Urinary incontinence in the female. In Walsh PC, Gittes RF, Perlmutter AD, Stamey TA. Campbell's Urology, 5th ed. Philadelphia, WB Saunders, 1986, p 2714.)

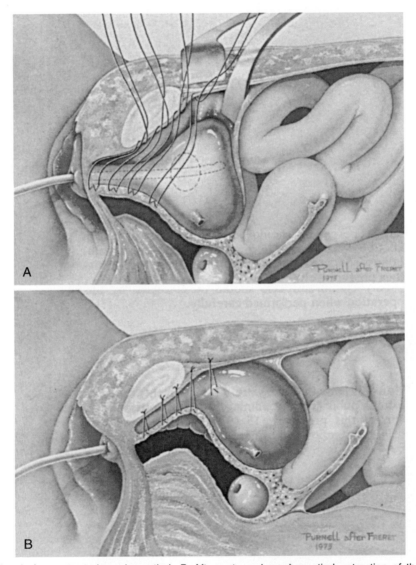

Figure 88–3. *A*, Sagittal view before sutures have been tied. *B*, After sutures have been tied, retraction of the urethra is drawn from the introitus toward the umbilicus. Actually, the space of Retzius is snugly closed and not "strung across" as illustrated here. (From Marshall VF, Vaughan ED Jr, Parnell JP. Urinary incontinence in the female. In Walsh PC, Gittes RF, Perlmutter AD, Stamey TA. Campbell's Urology, 5th ed. Philadelphia, WB Saunders, 1986, p 2715.)

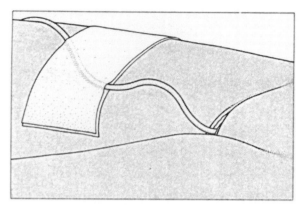

Figure 88–4. The transurethral catheter has been attached postoperatively to an adhesive on the thigh to forestall undue traction counter to the purposes of the operation. (From Marshall VF, Vaughan ED Jr, Parnell JP. Urinary incontinence in the female. In Walsh PC, Gittes RF, Perlmutter AD, Stamey TA. Campbell's Urology, 5th ed. Philadelphia, WB Saunders, 1986, p 2716.)

Any cystourethrocele should be corrected by this operation when it is performed carefully.

RESULTS

In 239 cases, there were 14 (6 percent) cases of osteitis pubis (prompt administration of cortisone will correct this problem); 15 (6 percent) of prolonged urinary retention; no urinary fistulas; 6 (3 percent) of pulmonary embolus; 2 (0.8 percent) of myocardial infarcts; 2 (0.8 percent) of failure to improve control at all; and no deaths.[6] We have never ligated a ureter or urethra, but we have heard of such complications.

Our operation, and its stress test, opened a new vista for the correction of stress incontinence.[5, 6] General surgeons can readily perform it without special instruments. Actually, this correction is fundamentally the same as the older transvaginal procedures and slings under the urethra. Adequate retraction away from the introitus toward the umbilicus to restore mechanical efficiency to an intrinsically intact sphincteric mechanism is accomplished rather than a new sphincter.

Editorial Comment
Fray F. Marshall

Although a number of new procedures have been used for stress incontinence, particularly transvaginal procedures, a place still exists for the "pinup operation." This operation has been very successful, as indicated in the author's experience of 239 cases. Both the short- and long-term success has been excellent with a minimum of complications. If stress incontinence is present and another abdominal procedure is contemplated, this operation can certainly be done in conjunction with it.

REFERENCES

1. Marshall VF, Pollock RS, Miller C. Observations on urinary dysfunction after excision of the rectum. J Urol 55:409, 1946.
2. Macleod D, Hawkins J, eds. Bonney's Gynecological Surgery, 7th ed. London, Cassell, 1964.
3. Marshall VF, Marchetti AA, Krantz KE. The correction of stress incontinence by simple vesicourethral suspension. Surg Gynecol Obstet 88:509, 1949.
4. Trendelenburg F. Medical Classics 2:566, 1940.
5. Burch JE. Urethrovaginal fixation to Cooper's ligament for the correction of stress incontinence. Am J Obstet Gynecol 81:281, 1961.
6. Parnell JP II, Marshall VF, Vaughan ED Jr. The management of recurrent stress incontinence by Marshall-Marchetti-Krantz vesicourethropexy. J Urol 132:912, 1984.

Chapter 89

Burch Colposuspension

Jacek L. Mostwin

Before the development of the retropubic urethropexy by Marshall, Marchetti, and Krantz (the MMK procedure) in 1949,[1] the only widely known methods for the treatment of stress urinary incontinence associated with vaginal prolapse were the pubovaginal sling and the Kelly plication. The MMK procedure introduced a new and rapidly accepted technique for the treatment of genuine stress urinary incontinence in women. As originally described, the operation required the placement of suspensory sutures in paraurethral vaginal tissue that were then carried to the periosteum of the symphysis pubis and along the anterior abdominal wall fascia.

Burch first developed the colposuspension that now bears his name during attempts to perform the MMK procedure.[2] He found that sutures often would not hold in the periosteum. He tried other structures. He tried and abandoned the obturator fascia (later developed as the paravaginal repair[3] and the obturator shelf repair) and eventually chose the iliopectineal line, known as Cooper's ligament.

Anyone who sees this structure cannot fail to be impressed by its thickness and strength, even in patients in whom other fascial structures (such as the abdominal wall fascia) may be attenuated. It is easy to gain access to Cooper's ligament through the retropubic approach, and a novice surgeon can comfortably identify and place sutures into the structure.

The simplicity of the approach and the impressive immediate cure rates have made the Burch colposuspension one of the most popular operations in the world for the treatment of women with stress urinary incontinence associated with vaginal prolapse.

INDICATIONS

Since the development of the Burch operation, advances in classification and understanding of pathophysiology have refined the indications for the operation. The ideal candidate is a mature woman with classical symptoms of stress urinary incontinence associated with physical findings of prolapse of the anterior vaginal wall during increases of intra-abdominal pressure. Intrinsic urethral function should be normal as measured either by Valsalva leak point pressure (the intra-abdominal pressure required to produce leakage, which should be >60 cm H_2O) or by urethral pressure profiometry (maximal closure pressure should be >20 cm). There should be a clear association of the incontinence with the presence of vaginal prolapse in the form of cystourethrocele (Green type II, Blaivas type II, Raz hypermobile type). Patients in whom intrinsic sphincteric deficiency is the primary cause of incontinence and who do not have evidence of vaginal prolapse are unlikely to benefit from colposuspension. Similarly, patients whose incontinence is caused primarily by bladder dysfunction—instability, overflow associated with loss of sensation, motor power or compliance—have a much higher risk of remaining incontinent after the operation. Previous failure of anti-incontinence surgery is not an absolute contraindication to Burch colposuspension.

RELATIONSHIP OF URETHRAL CLOSURE AND VAGINAL MOBILITY

Urinary continence in women depends on the proper integration of three factors: normal bladder function, intrinsic urethral closure, and vaginal support of the subpubic urethra. In discussions of genuine stress incontinence, it is assumed that bladder function is normal enough to provide stable and compliant storage of urine and voluntary, complete, and effective emptying of urine. The critical factors to consider in discussing stress urinary incontinence are vaginal mobility, urethral closure, and the effect of the former on the latter.

Investigators of stress incontinence in women have long drawn attention to the relationship of urethral closure and vaginal mobility.[4, 5] Rotational descent of the urethrovesical junction is associated with a loss of the posterior vesicourethral angle with consequent opening of the urethra during stress. Recent sonographic studies of urethral mobility have extended some of these earlier observations and provided new insights into anatomical mechanisms underlying this familiar observation.[6]

Vaginal prolapse produces leakage of urine by facilitating rotational descent of the otherwise normal proximal urethra and urethrovesical junction during increases in intra-abdominal pressure. The critical segment of the urethra affected by this movement is at the apex of the urogenital diaphragm. It is composed of well-developed internal longitudinal and smaller outer circular layers of smooth muscle, which contribute to the intrinsic closure mechanism. The longitudinal layers are continuations of detrusor muscle bundles from the bladder. Coaptation of the lumen of the proximal urethra is facilitated by a spongy endothelium and lamina propria, both of which are rich in estrogen receptors and are sensitive to estrogen stimulation.

The proximal urethra at the apex of the urogenital diaphragm is surrounded by a rhabdosphincter, which is the continuation of a cone of striated muscle forming the urogenital diaphragm musculature[7] (Fig. 89–1). This sphincteric area is the area of high pressure of the urethra as well as the area of maximal urethral closure pressure and cough transmission pressure.[8] The rhabdosphincter and the remainder of the urogenital diaphragm are covered by a dense layer of endopelvic fascia, which forms the floor of the space of Retzius in the midline behind the pubis and keeps these structures hidden from view during retropubic surgery.[9] Bilateral paired condensations of this endopelvic fascia are seen as the posterior pubourethral ligaments, which identify this portion of the urethra. The posterior pubourethral ligaments (analogous to the puboprostatic ligaments in the male) are the visible intrapelvic portion of a dense subpubic suspensory complex that continues underneath the pubis to become the anterior pubourethral ligament, analogous to the suspensory ligaments of the penis in the male.[10] This subpubic suspensory fascial complex anchors the urethra tightly to the undersurface of the pubis. The densest fascial attachments can be seen along the anterior surface of the proximal urethra. The precise description of this anatomy assumes critical importance when events occurring during stress incontinence are analyzed in detail.

The rhabdosphincter is composed of type I slow twitch tonic skeletal muscle innervated by perineal branches of the pudendal nerve. The pudendal nerve is tightly stretched between Alcock's canal where it enters the pelvis through the lesser sciatic foramen and is susceptible to crush or traction injuries during labor or episodes of prolapse. Such injuries have been demonstrated after childbirth[11] and also during vaginal prolapse.[12] Both factors probably contribute to ineffective tonic or reflex closure of the sphincter at rest and during prolapse. The apex of the urogenital diaphragm containing this critical portion of the ure-

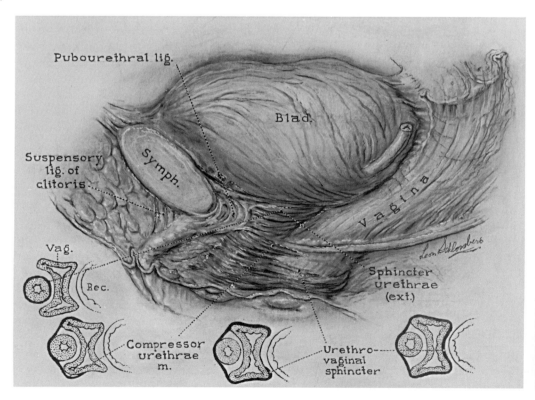

Figure 89–1. Parasagittal view of the urogenital diaphragm on the vaginal wall, passing through the levator hiatus. Transverse sections at various levels of the vaginal wall indicate the degree to which the urogenital diaphragmatic muscles surround the urethra. At the apex, the urethra is completely encircled by the rhabdosphincter, innervated by perineal branches of the pudendal nerve. This is the true external sphincter of the female urethra.

thra passes through a well-defined hiatus in the levator ani plate.[13] The levator ani, consisting of pubococcygeal and other groups, provides active support to all pelvic structures. In passing posteriorly from the pubis to form the puborectalis, the pubococcygeal muscle also gives off slips of muscle that insert onto the lateral apex of the urogenital diaphragm and the lateral superior vaginal sulcus beneath the endopelvic fascial coverings. These insertions contribute to the ability to interrupt voiding by elevating the urethrovesical junction. These are type II fast twitch muscles. They are not responsible for intrinsic urethral function and do not provide tonic closure. (This appears to explain why after radical prostatectomy some men can interrupt their urinary stream but remain incontinent at rest.) Some schematic depictions of the urogenital diaphragm in women often display the bladder as a spinning top balanced on a flat plane of muscle meant to represent an "external sphincter." This is misleading. A more accurate interpretation of the anatomy is to visualize the urogenital diaphragm as a sleeve pulled over the urethra, closed and tightly grasping the proximal urethra, widening in diameter as the vaginal introitus is approached. The combination of urethra and urogenital diaphragm then fits through the levator hiatus in modular fashion. The pubococcygeal fibers at the hiatus are only laterally inserted onto the urethra. They do not pass around circumferentially or form a sheet through which the urethra passes.

The anterior vaginal wall provides critical support to the proximal urethra, permitting it to remain stable during increases in abdominal pressure. Axial section at this level shows the vaginal wall to be shaped like a crescent, with its convex surface toward the vaginal lumen and its concave surface toward the urethra (Fig. 89–1). The lateral vaginal sulci are supported by slips of levator and connective tissue to the pelvic side wall, beginning at the level of the arcus tendineus levator ani, a dense almost cartilaginous structure originating at the medial insertion of the superior ramus of the pubis and extending toward the ischial spine. This structure is not normally seen during retropubic surgery because it is covered by the overlying levator muscles. The vaginal wall can be avulsed from its intrapelvic attachments or overstretched in its circular diameter during childbirth. It may never recover from these injuries. In addition, childbirth may stretch the levator hiatus in both length and width and avulse and overstretch pubococcygeal and levator muscle fibers. The effect of these injuries is loss of active support to the mesenchymal attachments of the vaginal wall, which are afterward subjected to greater gravitational stresses with time. Menopausal involution of mesenchymal structures further weakens support. The net result is a spectrum of predictable patterns of pelvic prolapse, two types of which are associated with stress incontinence: loss of vaginal attachments to the pelvis, and overstretching and attenuation of the subpubic urethra (Fig. 89–2). Either type of injury permits proximal urethral displacement away from its normal location during stress.

Sonographic examination of incontinent women with vaginal prolapse has permitted detailed consideration of the events that occur at the proximal urethra during vaginal prolapse. Initially, the entire urethra begins to rotate as a single unit away from the retropubic position and out of the pelvis. Eventually a point is reached at which the anterior portion of the urethra becomes arrested in its rotational movement, while the posterior wall of the urethra, in close contact with the vaginal wall, which has lost its lateral attachments or its midline wall strength, continues to

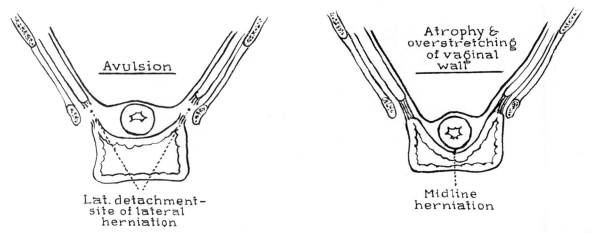

Figure 89–2. Types of anterior vaginal wall defects resulting in stress incontinence. *Left,* Lateral detachment of the superior vaginal sulcus on one or both sides gives rise to a cystourethrocele, which results in incontinence when the urethra descends to a threshold level (cf. fig. 3). The lateral type of defect can be repaired by Burch colposuspension. *Right,* A central defect may also result in urethral herniation. It may be a primary defect or may develop after previously successful repair of lateral defects. Long-term favorable results of central defects by Burch repair are less likely, and anterior vaginal reconstruction or direct sling support should be considered.

descend. This point of descent can be called the *incontinence threshold* (Fig. 89–3). Beyond it, there appears to be a shearing effect on the urethra produced by countertraction between the pubourethral complex, which prevents the anterior urethral segment from further rotational descent, and the vaginal wall, which facilitates it with its further downward momentum. To summarize, in addition to neurological factors, such as weakness of the rhabdosphincter or impairment of pudendal nerve function, there appear to be mechanical factors by which vaginal prolapse facilitates opening of the internal urethral meatus by a shearing force. The overall result, whether viewed with sonography or fluoroscopy, is a funnelling of the urethra with loss of urine.

Based on the above discussion, it becomes clear that the purpose of Burch colposuspension (as well as other suspensory operations) is to prevent the urethra from reaching the incontinence threshold. This is done by restoring vaginal support and preventing its descent to the point of the threshold. These more recent anatomical insights permit us to refine our surgical thinking and reinterpret the old paradigm: "place the urethra in a high retropubic position."

PREPARATION

Evaluation should include baseline urodynamic studies to ensure that stress incontinence and not overflow or bladder instability are the primary causes of urinary loss and that the incontinence is caused by hypermobility and not intrinsic sphincteric deficiency. A careful physical examination is necessary to determine the degree of prolapse, the presence of other forms of vaginal relaxation (enterocele, rectocele, uterine descensus), and the quality of vaginal tissue and its mobility. A thin, overstretched vaginal wall can be easily pulled into too high a retropubic position with resulting urinary retention, and thin postmenopausal tissue may be too weak to hold suspensory sutures for more than a few years or even months. Cystoscopy is desirable for evaluating the internal appearance of the bladder and urethra, as well as the location and number of the urethral orifices, which are at risk during the placement of the sutures in the paravesical and paraurethral vaginal wall.

Informed consent should list the indications for the surgery and the risks, which include bleeding, injury to bowel or ureter, and development of de novo instability in up to 15 percent of patients and resulting in urge incontinence. Postoperative urinary retention may occur, requiring intermittent catheterization. Preoperatively teaching the patient methods of clean intermittent self-catheterization may be considered in selected cases. The patient should be informed that alternatives to Burch suspension include physiotherapy and biofeedback, which can be expected to provide 50 percent improvement in 50 percent of pa-

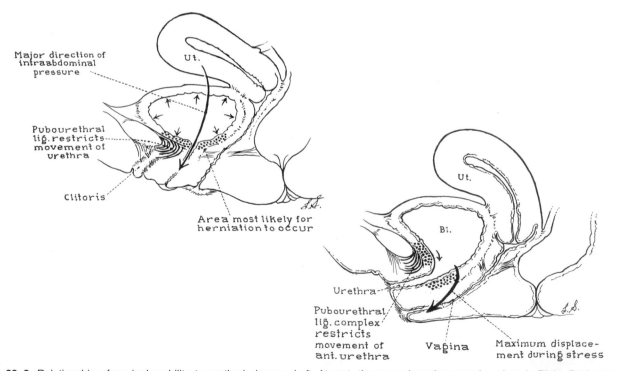

Figure 89–3. Relationship of vaginal mobility to urethral closure. *Left,* At rest, the normal urethra remains closed. *Right,* During rotational descent of the prolapsing vaginal wall, the anterior portion of the urethra is arrested in its movement by the subpubic suspensory ligament complex, while the posterior wall of the urethra continues to descend in continuity with the vaginal wall, producing urethral opening and loss of urine.

tients. Periurethral injection is not a satisfactory alternative to colposuspension in a patient with clearly identified vaginal prolapse. Pubovaginal sling may be considered a higher-risk alternative to colposuspension in patients in whom the vaginal wall is thin or weak, or if there have been previous suspensory failures.

The patient may receive an enema before surgery to evacuate the rectum. Preoperative antibiotics are used at the discretion of the surgeon, although the procedure to be described may be considered a clean, uncontaminated operation for which antibiotics are not essential to reduce the risk of wound infection, urinary infection, or pelvic abscess.

Instruments particularly helpful for this operation include a Balfour or similar self-retaining abdominal retractor, sponge sticks to facilitate exposure and traction in deep narrow spaces, long straight retractors such as Trimble or Heney, and a fiberoptic headlight. To prevent injury to the surgeon's hand when elevating and placing needles into the vagina, a blunt atraumatic steel instrument such as stapling rectal sizers or even a sterilized sewing thimble may be considered.

OPERATIVE PROCEDURE

After regional or general anesthesia is induced, the patient is placed in a supine position with thighs and knees slightly flexed and abducted to permit vaginal access during suspensory suture placement. A frog-leg position with heels together should be avoided because this stretches the femoral nerve at the level of the inguinal ligament and risks injury.[14] Both the abdomen and vaginal vault are prepared with sterile solution and draped to permit access from the umbilicus to the perineal body.

The space of Retzius may be entered through a vertical midline or transverse Pfannenstiel incision. Urological surgeons must remember that the female pelvis is more horizontal than the male and the bladder has a lower peritoneal reflection. Thus, to enter the space of Retzius, one should expect to identify the insertion of the rectus sheath at the level of the pubis, incising the transversalis fascia at this level and making the initial development of the space of Retzius lower than they would in a male.

The space of Retzius does not need to be developed extensively. Small friable veins on the periosteal surface of the pubic rami and symphysis are easily torn and should be avoided. It is helpful to free enough fat from the surface of the endopelvic fascia anterior to the urethra and on the sides of the bladder to permit visualization of four key anatomical features: the pubourethral ligaments, the endopelvic fascial covering of the bladder and the paravaginal reflec-

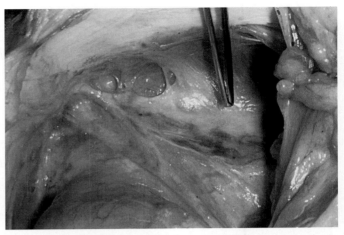

Figure 89–4. Surgeon's view of the space of Retzius in a fresh cadaver specimen. The instrument points to the right arcus tendineus fasciae pelvis (ATFP). The arcus courses left across the picture to blend into the right pubourethral ligament inserting at the pubis. The vaginal veins demarcating the lateral margin of the bladder are clearly visible.

tions, the arcus tendineus fasciae pelvis (ATFP), and the vaginal veins (Figs. 89–4 and 89–5). The pubourethral ligaments identify the position of the proximal urethra and delineate the inferior extent of suture placement; the vaginal veins identify the reflection of the endopelvic fascia over the lateral aspect of the bladder, delineating the medial limits of suture placement; and the ATFP identifies the lateral extent of vaginal reflection, aiding in the placement of vaginal sutures.

Cooper's ligament is most easily identified by finding the superior ramus of the pubis where the lacunar ligament can be seen or felt (Fig. 89–5). The horizontal ligamentous fibers can be seen better when the

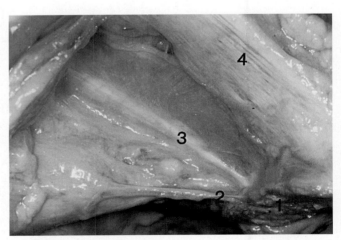

Figure 89–5. View of a resected portion of left lateral side wall from a fresh cadaver specimen. 1, Symphysis pubis; 2, the superficial dorsal clitoral vein overlies the proximal urethra; 3, the ATFP, particularly strong and well developed in this specimen; 4, Cooper's ligament on the surface of the superior pubic ramus. The vaginal wall beneath point 3 is to be connected by suspensory sutures to point 4. In this specimen, any attempt to make the two points connect would result in gross distortion of the anatomy.

superficial fat that normally covers them is teased away. Attention must be directed to possible aberrant or accessory obturator vessels forming the corona mortis ("circle of death"), which is present in up to 15 percent of patients, to avoid unnecessary bleeding.

A small Foley catheter (14 to 16 Fr.) may be placed in the bladder to empty it, permitting a roomier operative field, and to provide postoperative drainage. Suprapubic drainage with a 14-gauge Bonano catheter or a small Malecot catheter may be considered if prolonged urinary retention is anticipated. In many cases, simple Burch suspension should not produce retention, and the use of short-term Foley drainage is preferable.

Permanent sutures should be used for the repair, although there is little direct evidence in the literature to support this recommendation. Reports of erosion and infection associated with permanent sutures leave this an unresolved issue.[15] The needle should be a one-half or five-eighths circle taper to permit easy turning in a deep and narrow wound; it must be strong enough to pass through all layers of the vaginal wall and also the strong fibers of Cooper's ligament. The suture size should permit unquestionable strength (0 or 1).

Once the operative field has been developed and prepared, the goal of the operation is to establish a connection between the periurethral vaginal wall and Cooper's ligament on both sides of the pelvis by means of suspensory sutures. The suspension is designed to permit fixation and stabilization of the urethra during increases in intra-abdominal pressure. The goal of the operation is thus to prevent the vaginal wall from descending to the incontinence threshold (Figs. 89–6 and 89–7).

It is easiest to place the sutures into the vaginal wall first by identifying the point of insertion with a gloved hand or another instrument such as a rectal sizer or a sterile thimble elevating the vaginal wall, toward which the needle can be directly passed. Much has been said about avoiding passage of these sutures through the full thickness of the vaginal wall, penetrating into the vaginal cavity from within the pelvis. The experience of Gittes and Loughlin,[16] Loughlin et al,[17] and more recently Benderev,[18] however, would suggest that full-thickness suture bites should be safely tolerated and eventually overgrown by vaginal epithelium. It is certainly much easier to pass the needle through the full thickness without having to worry about whether or not the vaginal epithelium will be included.

There is no established way to place sutures into

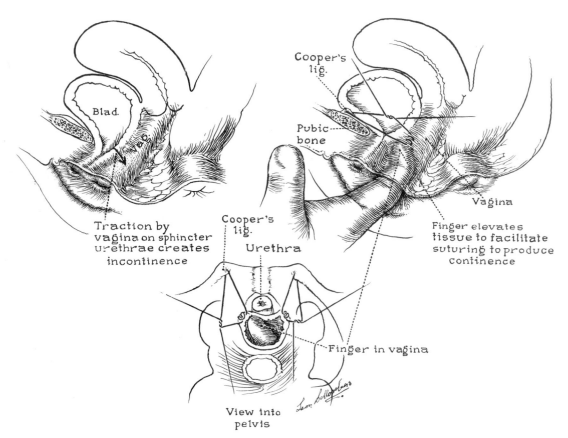

Figure 89–6. *Left,* The detached portion of vaginal wall is identified. *Right,* With a gloved hand, the surgeon identifies the point of suture placement: the lateral superior sulcus of the vaginal wall. *Bottom,* Sutures connect the lateral superior sulcus of the vaginal wall to Cooper's ligament.

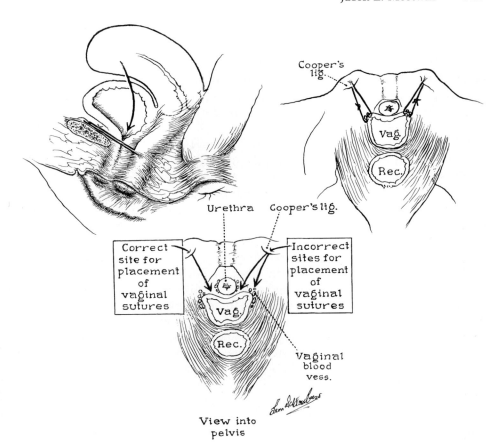

Figure 89–7. *Left,* The desired position of the vaginal wall in sagittal view after suspensory sutures have been tied. Sutures are tied loosely. Only a very redundant or overstretched vaginal wall can be expected to reach Cooper's ligament. Distortion and retention are otherwise potential complications. In the upright position, the sutures exert an anteroposterior direction of force. *Right,* The vaginal wall is supported to the level of the pubis. *Bottom,* Sutures should be placed lateral to the vaginal veins but medial to the ATFP to obtain good purchase of the vaginal wall and avoid injury to structures in the urogenital diaphragm.

the vaginal wall. A figure-of-eight or running helical suture of two or three passes is likely to produce a firm purchase. In the end, it is the amount of tension on vaginal tissues and the overall quality of these tissues that determines whether the sutures will remain in place beyond the immediate postoperative period. The earliest Burch suspensions were performed with absorbable sutures and relied on the development of scar along the suture lines to produce support. There have been few controlled studies to establish which technique is better.

The exact position of the suture line in the vaginal wall is worth considering in detail. It is important that the surgeon understand where the urethrovesical junction is located and where the vaginal wall and endopelvic fascia diverge laterally at the ATFP. The sutures need to be placed between these two points. If placed too medially, sutures run the risk of urethral penetration, inadvertent urethral closure, and injury to the periurethral autonomic nerves, which can be found in this location. If placed too laterally, sutures may pass through the endopelvic fascia and miss the vaginal wall entirely. If sutures are placed too laterally, they may also result in an excessively wide suburethral portion of vagina for urethral support. This may result in inadequate urethral stabilization or early failure of the operation. If the sutures are placed too superficially into the endopelvic fascia

and miss the remaining layers of vaginal wall below, the result may be excessive anterior fixation without adequate posterior fixation, easier opening of the urethra during stress, and possible worsening of the stress incontinence postoperatively.

Once sutures have been secured into the vaginal wall, they are carried to Cooper's ligament. Sutures should be placed as medially as possible in the ligament to maximize the anteroposterior direction of support that will be produced when the patient stands up. They should then be tied without excessive tension, just enough to stabilize the position of the vaginal wall against the surface of the inferior pubic ramus. Although the operation is performed with the patient in the supine position, it is important to remember that the effect of the operation will be experienced when the patient is in the upright position. Mentally rotating the patient's pelvis 90 degrees into a standing position reveals that the Burch suspensory sutures do not elevate the vaginal wall, but rather create anteroposterior support, permitting the vaginal wall to resist rotational descent down and out of the chute bordered anteriorly and superiorly by the pubis. The lines of support provided by the suspensory sutures from their insertion at Cooper's ligament thus resemble the direction of the fibers of the pubococcygeal muscle, i.e., they support the vaginal wall by providing anterior as well as superior traction. The Burch sutures, when tied, nearly always appear to be dangling, but in the upright position they are draped across the upper surface of the pubis, which is nearly horizontal with respect to the ground. Previsualizing the final effect of the suspensory sutures in this manner is a helpful way to determine where the sutures are to pass.

There is no agreement on whether one or more sutures should be used for each side of the Burch suspension. Two sutures provide some degree of assurance that at least one of the two will hold but produce a problem of more suture burden at the urethrovesical junction.

Injury to the ureters can be avoided if the vaginal suture passes are kept lateral to the vaginal veins seen at the lateral reflection of the bladder beneath the endopelvic fascia. The normal ureter is always medial to this reflection and is unlikely to be injured if no suture passes medial to the veins. The surgeon should resist the temptation to enter this plane to get a "better bite" of vaginal wall to avoid the possibility of ureteral injury. If the medial vaginal wall is so redundant that this kind of reefing maneuver is considered, it may mean that the patient requires midline repair or direct support such as a pubovaginal sling. These considerations should be made preoperatively during examination.

Several methods are available to evaluate ureteral patency when injury is suspected or must be excluded. Indigo carmine, 5 ml intravenously, administered by the anesthesiologist will appear in the urine within 5 minutes. Its appearance can be determined by using a flexible fiberoptic cystoscope introduced per urethram, a rigid Wappler cystourethroscope with a 70-degree lens introduced per urethram, or by opening the dome of the bladder to view the ureteral orifices directly. Techniques of passing the cystoscope through the anterior bladder wall have been described. Single-layer watertight closure afterward is desirable, and Foley or suprapubic drainage may be required for 4 to 5 days to ensure watertight healing before voiding is attempted.

Wound drainage is optional. If the procedure has gone well, venous bleeding has been minimal, there is no risk of urinary leak, and the wound is dry at completion, then no drainage is required. Closed sterile suction drainage is preferable to open rubber drains.

The wound layers are closed in a standard manner. A subcuticular absorbable suture permits earlier discharge of the patient without the need for return for suture removal.

POSTOPERATIVE MANAGEMENT

If only simple Foley drainage has been used postoperatively and the Burch suspension is performed for stabilization of the urethra as described above, the patient should be able to void as early as the first postoperative day. If not, clean intermittent self-catheterization may be used for drainage. Because there is no vaginal incision, it is well tolerated. Our practice has been to allow the patient out of bed the day after surgery, remove the Foley, determine whether voiding is comfortable, then discharge the patient home on the same day for convalescence.

A suprapubic tube limits the patient more and emphasizes a dependent state. When necessary, we have preferred the small Bonano tube because it is easy to insert and secure to the skin and easy to remove without pain several days or weeks after the surgery. It rarely causes bleeding from the bladder puncture site.

The patient should have complete pelvic rest for 6 to 8 weeks after surgery. There should be no strenuous lifting, exercise, or sexual activity. Straining at stool should be avoided by the use of laxatives and stool softeners. A combination of 15 to 30 ml of milk of magnesia and mineral oil daily in separate doses provides excellent prevention of constipation and can be modified as needed. The patient should be warned to expect a small amount of vaginal drainage or spotting for 1 to 2 weeks if the sutures have passed into the vaginal vault. Prophylactic postoperative oral antibiotics to prevent urinary infection may be considered.

RESULTS

The 1992 Treatment Guideline Panel of the Agency for Health Care and Policy Research reviewed available literature on retropubic urethropexy; 31 studies incorporating 2788 patients were reviewed.[19] The overall cure rate was 78 percent, with 5 percent improved and 18 percent overall complications. The Burch repair is the most widely used, and most recent studies of retropubic urethropexy have used this procedure. The findings of 19 reviews are summarized in Table 89–1.

Urodynamic and radiographic studies after retropubic urethropexy or colposuspension suggest that success or failure is due primarily to restoration of position, improvement of cough transmission pressures, and prevention of hypermobility. Resting changes in urethral pressure are usually unchanged. The results of seven of these studies are worth citing in detail.

Urodynamic studies of 25 women who underwent Burch 3 months earlier were performed. In this group the objective cure rate was 88 percent. The operation does not induce any significant change in resting urethral profile variables. The stress profile showed accentuation in pressure transmission ratios, most marked in the proximal urethra. Twenty-seven patients were studied after colposus-

TABLE 89–1. Long- and Short-term Results of Burch Colposuspension: Results of 19 Studies

Author	Year	No. of Patients	Results	Comments
Krahulec et al[35]	1992	69	94% subjective cure	Mailed questionnaire
Kiilholma et al[36]	1993	186	91% cured at 2 yr	95% primary cured; 84% recurrence cured; 12% enterocele
Vinagre et al[37]	1991	227	90.3% cured at 3.5 yr	
Antal et al[38]	1989	55	51/55 cured at 3.5 yr	
Enzelsberger et al[39]	1993	52	85% recurrent SUI	Half randomized to Lyodura sling; 88% success
Enzelsberger et al[40]	1991	31	87% recurrent SUI	
Irani et al[41]	1991	199	90% at 14 mo	Half had hysterectomy without affecting results
Guerinoni et al[25]	1991	173	95% cure at 4.5 yr	Postoperative bladder instability 22%; enterocele 10%
Lim et al[42]	1990	113	89% cure at 2 yr	
Penders et al[43]	1990	86	71% with stable bladder cured at 5 yr:, 57% with SUI and DI cured	
Korda et al[44]	1989	177	87.5% over 5 yr cured	
Stanton and Cardozo[45]	1979	180	87% at 6 mo, 87.5% at 1 yr, and 86% at 2 yr objectively cured	
Gillon et al[46]	1992	40	87.5% cure	22% associated DI preoperatively
Langer et al[47]	1990	122	88.4% of 69 premenopausal women, 66% of 53 postmenopausal group, dry	
Zuluaga-Gomez et al[48]	1992	61	95%: 3 mo; 85.7%: 1 yr; 77.1%: 5 yr	Decreasing long-term efficacy
Vierhout and Mulder[49]	1992	396	64–98% average cure in pooled review	17% associated DI
Pigne et al[50]	1988	370	95.4% success at 5 yr	75% technical failures occur in first year postoperatively
Galloway et al[51]	1987	50	84% postoperative continence; only 64% with recurrent SUI continent	
Bergman et al[52]	1991	48	90% dry at 1 yr	Burch-Ball modification for recurrent SUI

SUI, stress urinary incontinence; DI, detrusor irritability.

pension with lateral bead-chain urethrocystography. Successful operation, compared with unsuccessful operation, repositioned the bladder neck significantly closer to the posterosuperior surface of the symphysis pubis, though not significantly higher. After successful colposuspension, the proximal urethra was exposed to compression against the symphysis pubis by the momentary descent of the pelvic viscera during physical effort.[20]

Neither surgical anterior vaginal repair nor Burch colposuspension affected the resting variables of the urethral sphincter mechanism. After Burch colposuspension the transmitted intra-abdominal pressure to the urethra significantly increased in all recording positions in all women who were successfully treated. The impact of successful surgery for stress incontinence is the enhancement of transmission of the intra-abdominal pressure rise to the proximal urethra. This is achieved primarily by anatomical alterations rather than by altering urethral sphincter function.[21]

The operation does not induce any significant change in resting urethral profile variables. The stress profile showed accentuation in pressure transmission ratios, most marked in the proximal urethra.[22]

The operation significantly elevated the bladder neck and reduced its mobility during acute stress. The urethral inclination angle and the posterior urethrovesical angle also became smaller at rest and on straining. A significant negative correlation was found between the postoperative mobility of the bladder neck and the postoperative pressure transmission ratio (PTR).[23]

The functional urethra length and urethral closure pressure at rest were unchanged. The urethral pressure under stress, depression quotient, and transmission factor increased significantly.[24]

The mechanism of action consists in improving the abdominal pressure transmission ratio ($+29$ percent) with only a little decrease of the postoperative mean maximal urethral closure pressure (-8.8 cm H_2O).[25]

Studies of cough transmission pressure ratios in recurrent stress incontinence show the same loss of transmission in recurrent operated patients as [in] those with genuine stress urinary incontinence who never underwent surgery.[26] The results suggest that stress incontinence operations fail because to failure to provide urethral support more commonly than because of new onset detrusor hyperactivity.

Complications after Burch suspensions include ureteral obstruction,[27–30] urethral obstruction,[31] and the onset of de novo instability.[29] It is important to recognize that up to 25 percent of patients with genuine stress urinary incontinence may have bladder instability, and approximately 75 percent of these will be relieved of their symptoms after relief of the genuine stress urinary incontinence.[32–34]

Summary

The Burch colposuspension is the most widely used reconstructive operation for the treatment of genuine stress urinary incontinence associated with cystourethrocele affecting the proximal urethra. The anatomical and surgical concepts required to understand the operation and perform it well are straightforward and can be mastered by urological or gynecological surgeons of moderate experience. A well-performed examination before surgery will help to identify patients who are suitable candidates. Burch suspension should not be the procedure of choice in a patient with intrinsic sphincteric deficiency or in recurrent prolapse when the vaginal wall is severely attenuated. Careful attention to details of suture placement in the periurethral vagina will avoid problems of ureteral injury, obstruction, or inadequate suspension. Obstruction can be avoided by permitting the suspensory sutures to drape without tension over the inner surface of the pubis. Extensive experience and reports in the literature support the long-term efficacy of the operation in at least 60% of patients and suggest that the operation succeeds because it provides stabilization and improved support to the proximal urethra during stress, increasing cough transmission pressures to the urethra and preventing descent beyond the continence threshold.

Editorial Comment
Fray F. Marshall

Burch colposuspension represents a modification of the Marshall-Marchetti procedure. As pointed out, the sutures are more secure if placed in Cooper's ligament. In addition, if the sutures are not drawn too tight, there is a reduced likelihood of urinary retention. It can be performed through a smaller suprapubic incision that is usually well tolerated.

REFERENCES

1. Marshall VF, Marchetti AA, Krantz KE. The correction of stress incontinence by simple vesicourethral suspension. Surg Gynecol Obstet 88:509, 1949.
2. Burch JC. Urethrovaginal fixation to Cooper's ligament for correction of stress incontinence, cystocele, and prolapse. Am J Obstet Gynecol 81:281, 1961.
3. Richardson AC, Edmonds PB, Williams NL. Treatment of stress urinary incontinence due to paravaginal fascial defect. Obstet Gynecol 57:357, 1981.
4. Green TH Jr. Urinary stress incontinence: Differential diagnosis, pathophysiology, and management. Am J Obstet Gynecol 122:368, 1975.
5. Hodgkinson CP. Relationship of the female bladder and urethra in urinary stress incontinence. Am J Obstet Gynecol 65:560, 1953.
6. Sanders RC, Genadry R, Yang A, Mostwin JL. Imaging the female urethra. Ultrasound Q 12:167, 1994.
7. Oelrich TM. The striated urogenital sphincter muscle in the female. Anat Rec 205:223, 1983.
8. Constantinou CE, Faysal MH, Rother L, Govan DE. The impact of bladder neck suspension on the mode of distribution of abdominal pressure along the female urethra. Prog Clin Biol Res 78:121, 1981.
9. Mostwin JL. Current concepts of female pelvic anatomy and physiology. Urol Clin North Am 18:175, 1991.
10. Milley PS, Nichols DH. The relationship between the pubourethral ligaments and the urogenital diaphragm in the human female. Anat Rec 170:281, 1971.
11. Snooks SJ, Badenoch DF, Tiptaft RC, Swash M. Perineal nerve damage in genuine stress urinary incontinence. An electrophysiological study. Br J Urol 57:422, 1985.
12. Benson JT. Electrodiagnosis. In Benson JT, ed. Female Pelvic Floor Disorders: Investigation and Management. New York, Norton Medical Books, 1992.
13. Zacharin RF. Pelvic Floor Anatomy and the Surgery of Pulsion Enterococele. New York, Springer-Verlag, 1985.
14. Wang Y, Mitchell D, Hadley HR. Anatomical basis for femoral neuropathy due to procedures performed in the modified lithotomy position. J Urol 145:373A, 1991.
15. McIntosh LJ, Mallett VT, Richardson DA. Complications from permanent suture in surgery for stress urinary incontinence. A report of two cases. J Reprod Med 38:823, 1993.
16. Gittes RF, Loughlin KR. No-incision pubovaginal suspension for stress incontinence. J Urol 138:568, 1987.
17. Loughlin KR, Whitmore WF III, Gittes RF, Richie JP. Review of an 8-year experience with modifications of endoscopic suspension of the bladder neck for female stress urinary incontinence see comments. J Urol 143:44, 1990.
18. Benderev TV. Anchor fixation and other modifications of endoscopic bladder neck suspension. Urology 40:409, 1992.
19. U.S. Department of Health and Human Services, Public Health Service. Urinary Incontinence in Adults. Clinical Practice Guidelines. Washington, DC, Agency for Health Care Policy and Research, 1992.
20. Hertogs K, Stanton SL. Lateral bead-chain urethrocystography after successful and unsuccessful colposuspension. Br J Obstet Gynaecol 92:1179, 1985.
21. van-Geelen JM, Theeuwes AG, Eskes TK, Martin CB Jr. The clinical and urodynamic effects of anterior vaginal repair and Burch colposuspension. Am J Obstet Gynecol 159:137, 1988.
22. Hilton P, Stanton SL. A clinical and urodynamic assessment of the Burch colposuspension for genuine stress incontinence. Br J Obstet Gynaecol 90:934, 1983.
23. Penttinen J, Lindholm EL, Kaar K, Kauppila A. Successful colposuspension in stress urinary incontinence reduces bladder neck mobility and increases pressure transmission to the urethra. Arch Gynecol Obstet 244:233, 1989.
24. Schurmann R, Ralph G. Urodynamic results of Burch colposuspension. Zentralbl Gynakol 112:577, 1990.
25. Guerinoni L, Treisser A, Klein P, Renaud R. Functional and urodynamic results of Burch's colpopexy. A series of 173 cases. J Gynecol Obstet Biol Reprod 20:231, 1991.
26. Bump RC, Fantl JA, Hurt WG. Dynamic urethral pressure profilometry pressure transmission ratio determinations after continence surgery: Understanding the mechanism of success, failure, and complications. Obstet Gynecol 72:870, 1988.
27. Maulik TG. Kinked ureter with unilateral obstructive uropathy complicating Burch colposuspension. J Urol 130:135, 1983.
28. Ferriani RA, Silva-de-Sa MF, Dias-de-Moura M, et al. Ureteral blockage as a complication of Burch colposuspension: Report of 6 cases. Gynecol Obstet Invest 29:239, 1990.
29. Delaere KP, Strijbos WE, Zandvoort JA. Perirenal urinary extravasation complicating Burch colposuspension. Urol Int 44:119, 1989.
30. Applegate GB, Bass KM, Kubik CJ. Ureteral obstruction as a complication of the Burch colposuspension procedure: Case report. Am J Obstet Gynecol 156:445, 1987.
31. Lose G, Jorgensen L, Mortensen SO, et al. Voiding difficulties after colposuspension. Obstet Gynecol 69:33, 1987.
32. Langer R, Ron-el R, Newman M, et al. Detrusor instability following colposuspension for urinary stress incontinence. Br J Obstet Gynaecol 95:607, 1988.
33. Langer R, Ron-El R, Bukovsky I, Caspi E. Colposuspension in patients with combined stress incontinence and detrusor instability. Eur Urol 14:437, 1988.
34. Eriksen BC, Hagen B, Eik-Nes SH, et al. Long-term effectiveness of the Burch colposuspension in female urinary stress incontinence. Acta Obstet Gynecol Scand 69:45, 1990.
35. Krahulec P, Rovny F, Matysek P, et al. Personal experience with colpoureteral suspension using the Burch method. Cesk Gynekol 57:197, 1992.

36. Kiilholma P, Makinen J, Chancellor MB, et al. Modified Burch colposuspension for stress urinary incontinence in females. Surg Gynecol Obstet 176:111, 1993.

37. Vinagre M, Pardo H, Roa E, de-la-Fuente S. Colposuspension in the treatment of stress urinary incontinence: Long-term yield. Rev Chil Obstet Ginecol 56:284, 1991.

38. Antal H, Attila T, Nagy F. Surgical colpo-suspension (Burch's method) in the management of female stress incontinence. Orv Hetil 130:781, 1989.

39. Enzelsberger H, Kurz C, Seifert M, et al. Surgical treatment of recurrent stress incontinence: Burch versus lyodura sling operation—a prospective study. Geburtshilfe Frauenheilkd 53:467, 1993.

40. Enzelsberger H, Kurz C, Adler A, Schatten C. Effectiveness of Burch colposuspension in females with recurrent stress incontinence—a urodynamic and ultrasound study. Geburtshilfe Frauenheilkd 51:915, 1991.

41. Irani J, Dore B, Ruscillo MM, et al. Burch's procedure. Value of association with fixation to the promontorium and colpoperineorrhaphy. J Urol 97:123, 1991.

42. Lim PH, Brown AD, Chisholm GD. The Burch colposuspension operation for stress urinary incontinence. Singapore Med J 31:242, 1990.

43. Penders L, Lombard R, Jehaes C. Reinforced colposuspension (modified Cukier's operation). Immediate results, complications, indications. Acta Urol Belg 58:59, 1990.

44. Korda A, Ferry J, Hunter P. Colposuspension for the treatment of female urinary incontinence. Aust NZ J Obstet Gynaecol 29:146, 1989.

45. Stanton SL, Cardozo LD. Results of the colposuspension operation for incontinence and prolapse. Br J Obstet Gynaecol 86:693, 1979.

46. Gillon G, Engelstein D, Servadio C. Risk factors and their effect on the results of Burch colposuspension for urinary stress incontinence. Isr J Med Sci 28:354, 1992.

47. Langer R, Golan A, Ron-El R, et al. Colposuspension for urinary stress incontinence in premenopausal and postmenopausal women. Surg Gynecol Obstet 171:13, 1990.

48. Zuluaga-Gomez A, Nogueras-Ocana M, Martinez-Torres JL, et al. Stress urinary incontinence. Our results with the Burch's technique. Arch Esp Urol 45:609, 1992.

49. Vierhout ME, Mulder AF. De novo detrusor instability after Burch colposuspension. Acta Obstet Gynecol Scand 71:414, 1992.

50. Pigne A, Keskes J, Maghioracos P, et al. Clinical and urodynamic results of the Burch colposuspension operation in the treatment of female urinary stress incontinence. A study apropos of 370 cases. J Gynecol Obstet Biol Reprod 17:922, 1988.

51. Galloway NT, Davies N, Stephenson TP. The complications of colposuspension. Br J Urol 60:122, 1987.

52. Bergman A, Koonings PP, Ballard CA. The Ball-Burch procedure for stress incontinence with low urethral pressure. J Reprod Med 36:137, 1991.

Chapter 90

Paravaginal Repair

Jacek L. Mostwin

In 1981, Richardson advanced the thesis that "the physical findings of pelvic relaxation, such as cystourethrocele, are the results of isolated defects in the pelvic fascia rather than the results of generalized stretching or attenuation of the supporting structures."[1] While this thesis remains a subject of considerable debate among prominent gynecological anatomists and surgeons, it has given rise to both an operation (the paravaginal repair) and an entire school of thought[2] regarding the management of pelvic prolapse. Clinical results from paravaginal repair for stress incontinence have been sufficiently encouraging to justify serious consideration of the anatomical basis and the surgical method.

ANATOMICAL BASIS

Urinary continence in women depends on the integration of three factors: bladder function, urethral closure, and vaginal support. Vaginal support arises from active muscular contraction provided by the levator ani diaphragm and passive mesenchymal support assigned to three levels called by DeLancey levels I, II, and III.[3] Level I supports are the firm attachments of the urogenital diaphragm at the level of the pubis. Here, the lateral vaginal sulcus is firmly tucked behind the pubis, where it is connected by elastic and fibrous connective tissue and supported by slips of pubococcygeal muscle en passant as it continues in its course to encircle the rectum as the puborectal muscle. The upper supports, level III, consist of the mesenchymal supports of the cervix and uterus, the cardinal and uterosacral ligaments. There is general agreement that the upper and lower levels provide strong support to the two ends of the vaginal wall. It is above level I that the vaginal axis turns from 45 degrees from the vertical to a more nearly horizontal axis, which it maintains until reaching the cervix. As Nichols and Randall have emphasized, the vagina is slung like a hammock between these two firm points

of attachment.[4] Controversy arises over the role of mid-vaginal level II support and the functional interpretation of the arcus tendineus fasciae pelvis (ATFP). Level II supports are the paravaginal supports, the attachments of the vaginal wall to the pelvic side wall between the two firm areas of support at the urogenital diaphragm and the cardinal-uterosacral ligament complex. It is the general experience of most surgeons and anatomists that, with the exception of the endopelvic fascial condensation forming the ATFP, the midvagina is quite loosely attached to the lateral pelvic wall. Incision into the endopelvic fascia along the ATFP from the space of Retzius permits easy access around the lateral vaginal wall. The functional interpretation of this anatomical area remains unresolved. It is Richardson's hypothesis, based on clinical observation and cadaver dissection, that

> The most frequently encountered defect resulting in cystourethrocele with stress urinary incontinence [is] a paravaginal break in the pubocervical segment of the endopelvic fascia between the lateral edge of the vagina and the pelvic side wall.[1]

Although these conclusions are intuitively appealing to a growing number of gynecological surgeons, a problem has arisen because there has been no accepted method for demonstrating these breaks. The significance of Richardson's observations lies in the attention they have directed toward lateral vaginal support and the observation that stress incontinence is frequently seen in association with cystocele in which the midline of the vagina and its rugae are well preserved but the vagina appears detached from the lateral wall. Other types of defects in vaginal support are recognized, including midline, central, and transverse defects, which are hypothesized to give rise to the most commonly seen patterns of cystocele.[5] Provided that there is good intrinsic sphincteric function, stress incontinence only will occur if there are lateral or central defects.

Richardson has described the typical paravaginal defect[5]:

. . . the lateral attachment of the pubocervical fascia separates from its attachments to the fascial coverings of the obturator internus and the levator muscles. This separation may be unilateral or bilateral. It usually yields a combination urethrocystocele. Because the vagina is attached to the pubocervical fascia, when the break is in this area, the lateral superior vaginal sulcus descends, the bladder neck becomes hypermobile, and often there is SUI [sic]. When the superior sulcus is supported on each side, the cystourethrocele disappears. If the defect is unilateral (more often on the right), then support of the sulcus on that side alone corrects the cystourethrocele. It is in the correction of this defect (and only this defect) that the paravaginal repair is appropriate.

The operation of paravaginal repair was originally designed to correct what were seen as these isolated defects in lateral vaginal support. Richardson acknowledged that in 1909 White described an operation for the transvaginal repair of cystocele by reattaching the lateral superior sulcus of the vagina to the arcus tendineus (the white line) of the pelvic fascia.[6]

INDICATIONS

The operation should be selected and performed by a surgeon who understands the subtleties of vaginal anatomy and prolapse and their relationship to stress incontinence. It is important to be able to distinguish among the various kinds of anterior vaginal wall defects, and to determine the stability and position of the cervix or the vaginal cuff and its contribution to the entire spectrum of pelvic prolapse in a given patient.

The ideal candidate for the operation is an adult woman in whom unilateral or bilateral vaginal detachment gives rise to cystocele with or without incontinence (Figs. 90–1 and 90–2). To result in incontinence, the cystocele must involve the proximal urethra and result in opening during prolapse (see Chapter 89 on Burch Colposuspension for discussion of pathophysiology). Not all patients with stress in-

continence are candidates for paravaginal repair, and certainly not patients with intrinsic sphincteric deficiency. Similarly, patients with cystocele in whom there is considerable attenuation of the anterior vaginal wall, many of whom will not have stress incontinence, are better served by anterior colporrhaphy.

It is essential to perform a careful physical examination with the patient at rest and during straining. In fact, in no other current method for the treatment of stress incontinence is more emphasis placed on the physical findings. The vaginal wall should be healthy and well preserved despite lateral detachment and should be expected to provide urethral and bladder support for many years after the repair. Stress incontinence, if present, should occur only during vaginal wall descent. Urodynamic studies may be required if there is doubt about the stability, sensation, or storage capabilities of the bladder or if there is doubt that the bladder will empty properly after surgery.

In obtaining informed consent, the patient should be counseled that less invasive methods such as physiotherapy and behavioral conditioning may be considered, but that their success may be no more than 50 percent improvement in 50 percent of patients.[7] Although the reported incidence of operative injuries and postoperative complications after paravaginal repair has been minimal, patients should be warned that there are risks of urinary retention, ureteral injury, obturator nerve injury, irritative symptoms, and de novo bladder instability until widespread experience shows otherwise.

OPERATIVE PROCEDURE

The approach is transabdominal retropubic, similar to the Marshall, Marchetti, and Krantz (MMK) or Burch procedures. Regional or general anesthesia is administered. The patient is placed supine with slight abduction and flexion of the thighs and knee flexion. A frog-leg position risks injury to the femoral nerve in its course out of the femoral canal.[8] The

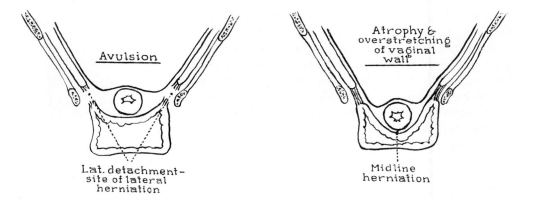

Figure 90–1. Urethral prolapse may occur as a result of detachment of the lateral superior sulcus (lateral detachment with preservation of midline integrity) or midline attenuation with preservation of lateral attachments. Only lateral detachments (*left*) are suitable for paravaginal repair. Midline defects require anterior colporrhaphy or sling repair.

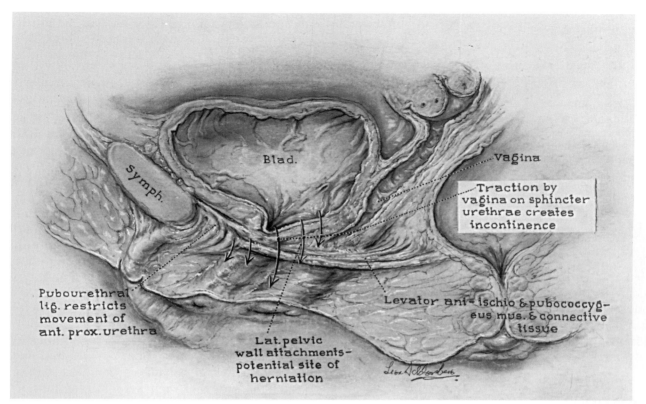

Figure 90–2. Effect of vaginal herniation at the level of the lateral superior sulcus on urethral mobility. When abdominal pressure is increased, the anterior portion of the urethra is arrested in its rotational movement by the subpubic suspensory complex, while the posterior portion is pulled further by the vaginal wall, producing a shearing action. Paravaginal repair prevents descent of the vaginal wall by fixing the superior lateral sulcus to the obturator fascia along the inner side wall of the pelvis.

space of Retzius is entered through a Pfannenstiel incision, but other incisions may be used, depending on the surgeon's preference. The space of Retzius is developed to permit identification of the key landmarks for the operation (Figs. 90–3 and 90–4): the posterior pubourethral ligaments (which may be partially obscured by fat and may be recognized only by palpation unless the fat is cleared away), the ATFP, the vaginal veins (identifying the lateral extent of the bladder on the surface of the vaginal wall), and the ischial spine (recognized by palpation). The obturator nerve and vessels are considerably anterior to the ATFP and should not be injured or even encountered during the operation (Fig. 90–5). However, if there is doubt, the structures can be identified within the obturator fossa or at their entry through the obturator foramen.

The goal of the repair is reattachment of the lateral superior vaginal sulcus to the obturator fascia at the level of the ATFP from the pubourethral ligaments to the ischial spine, using small permanent sutures at 1-cm intervals, that connect tissue directly to tissue and are not left dangling. In contrast to the Burch colposuspension, the weight of the vaginal wall is distributed over a much greater length, and the apex of the attachment is much lower on the pelvic side wall in contrast to dangling Burch sutures to Cooper's ligament. Small sutures such as 2-0 or 3-0 may be used, permitting smaller, more delicate needles.

One side is reattached at a time (Fig. 90–6). The abdominal fascia is elevated near the side wall with a Richardson or similar retractor, and the bladder is retracted medially with a sponge stick or a deep

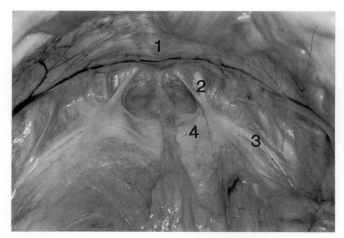

Figure 90–3. Floor of the space of Retzius as seen during retropubic surgery. 1, pubis; 2, right posterior pubourethral ligament; 3, arcus tendineus fasciae pelvis (ATFP); 4, endopelvic fascia firmly condensed over the proximal urethra. This is the medial edge of suspensory sutures placement for paravaginal repair as well as for colposuspension.

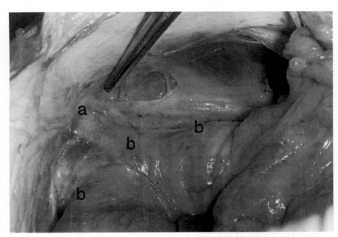

Figure 90–4. The vaginal wall as seen from the space of Retzius in a fresh cadaver specimen. The vaginal wall is covered by endopelvic fascia; the pubourethral ligament is clearly seen. *A,* The proximal urethra is within the pelvis. *B,* The curve of the partially full bladder is demonstrated; and the vaginal veins mark the lateral boundary of the bladder.

straight retractor such as a Trimble or Heney. One hand may be placed in the vagina to provide digital counterpressure and help elevate the wall for the placement of the sutures. The view will be similar to that in Figure 90–4. Sutures are placed through all layers of the vaginal wall except for the endovaginal epithelium. The sutures should engage the vaginal wall just lateral to the vaginal veins, which mark the lateral border of the bladder. Richardson described the first suture to be placed as the "key suture," the one that creates the apex of the vaginal elevation. This suture should be carried from the lateral sulcus of the vagina to the lateral pelvic side wall at the level of the ATFP. It is placed but not tied until the

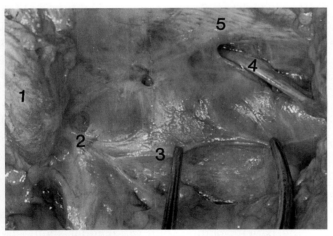

Figure 90–5. Right lateral pelvic wall in a fresh cadaver specimen. 1, pubis; 2, pubourethral ligament; 3, ATFP demonstrated by instrument traction; 4, obturator vessels entering the obturator foramen (5). The levator ani fibers can be seen just below the layers of endopelvic fascia at and above the line of the ATFP. The ATFP is the structure to which the detached lateral sulcus must be reattached during paravaginal repair.

remaining sutures are placed both proximal and distal to it at intervals of 1 cm. Closer to the pubis, the obturator fascia overlying the levator muscles is firmer and has a sinewy quality below the surface that holds sutures well. Deep bites at this level are likely to penetrate through the levator ani muscles and into the arcus tendineus levator ani, which lies on the surface of the obturator internus muscle. The arcus tendineus levator ani cannot be seen during standard retropubic exposure but is very strong and fully capable of supporting weight (Fig. 90–7). Such bites would give additional strength but were not specifically mentioned in Richardson's previous descriptions. As the sutures are placed along the side wall toward the vaginal apex, the overlying fascia becomes progressively more attenuated and may not hold sutures as well. The distalmost suture should be at the level of the pubourethral ligaments, which is the approximate level of the junction of the proximal and medial two thirds of the urethra, and should be continued along the vaginal veins until the ischial spine is reached. This approaches the cardinal ligaments. Thus, approximately one half to two thirds of the middle and upper vagina are held by sutures. At the level of the ischial spine, the fascia is thinnest and may vanish. The final repair will consist of six or more sutures on either side of the pelvis. One can visualize the final result as a restoration of the lateral superior vaginal sulcus, the so-called plis du chat.

The bladder may be drained at the start of the operation with a Foley catheter, which can be left in place until the patient recovers from anesthesia or the following morning. Richardson's practice has been to drain the bladder by needle puncture and to leave the bladder undrained after the operation without a catheter.

If performed in the manner described, paravaginal repair should not damage the ureters, which are located in the vesicovaginal space, medial to the vaginal veins from the level of the cervix to the bladder. If there is doubt about ureteral patency, indigo carmine, 5 ml intravenously, may be given and can be seen within 5 minutes with a flexible fiberoptic or 70-degree rigid cystoscope. If necessary, the bladder may be opened to examine the ureteral orifices, but if this is done, postoperative urethral catheter drainage and closed sterile suction drainage of the wound will be required.

The wound is closed in a standard manner. If the wound is dry and there has been no significant urinary leak, drainage should not be required. Subcuticular skin closure permits quick discharge from the hospital without the need for outpatient suture removal. If a catheter has been left in place, it may be removed as soon as the patient has recovered from anesthesia, because the operation does not produce urethral obstruction if properly performed.

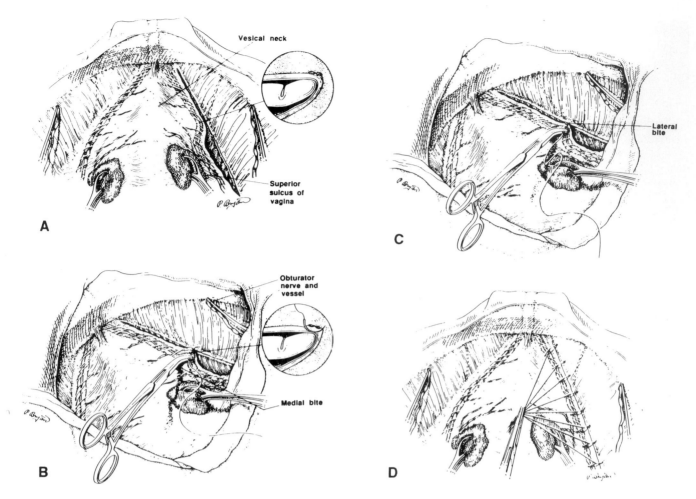

Figure 90–6. Steps of paravaginal repair. *A,* The superior vaginal sulcus is elevated by vaginal palpation at the lateral border of the bladder, indicated by the vaginal veins. A sponge stick facilitates medial countertraction on the empty bladder. *B,* The first "key" suture is placed through the vaginal wall at the lateral sulcus. *C,* The suture is carried (but not tied) through the obturator fascia to reattach the sulcus in an anatomical position. *D,* The remaining sutures are placed at 1-cm intervals along the lateral pelvic wall to distribute the load. After all sutures have been placed, they are tied. (From Youngblood JP. Paravaginal repair. Contemp OB/GYN 35:28, 1990.)

Like the Burch suspension and the MMK urethropexy, paravaginal repair provides indirect support to the urethra to prevent stress incontinence. Like the Burch suspension, paravaginal repair focuses attention on the urethrovesical junction, but suspensory sutures are not left dangling. Burch, in fact, mentioned in his original description that he attempted placing suspensory sutures into the obturator fascia but was dissatisfied with the strength of the tissue and elected to use Cooper's ligament.[9] One can draw an imaginary, almost straight line extending the vector of support from the obturator fascia to Cooper's ligament, where all the strength of the Burch support is concentrated. In significant contrast to the Burch suspension, paravaginal repair distributes the weight-bearing suture line along a much greater length of vaginal wall. While this difference may be theoretically appealing, there is no objective way at present to determine whether it is significant. Paravaginal repair also bears some resemblance to MMK urethropexy because the urethrovesical angle is attached by direct contact to supporting structures. Instead of angulation at the symphysis pubis, however, which runs the risk of stretching and elevating the urethra too tightly, paravaginal repair reconstructs the plis du chat, the lateral superior vaginal sulcus, to its original location on the pelvic side wall with much less risk of retention, obstruction, and deformity. As should be evident, all three operations attempt reconnection of the lateral vaginal wall to bridge the gap between the vaginal wall and the pelvis that has given rise to prolapse and stress incontinence.

POSTOPERATIVE MANAGEMENT

If the patient cannot void, the bladder should be catheterized in a sterile manner in the hospital. If the patient is still unable to void after several attempts, clean intermittent catheterization should be instituted. If the operation is done properly, there should be no obstruction. The patient should have complete

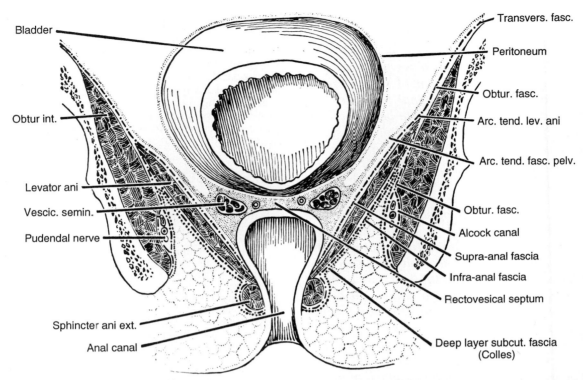

Figure 90–7. Schematic representation of layers of pelvis in coronal section. Note that the ATFP is the *visible* condensation of endopelvic fascia on the surface of the obturator internus. The arcus tendineus levator ani (deep arcus) from which the levator ani muscles arise is higher than the ATFP and covered by both the endopelvic fascia and the levator musculature that arise from it. (From Goss CM, ed. Gray's Anatomy of the Human Body, 29th American ed. Philadelphia, Lea & Febiger, 1973, p 715.)

pelvic rest for 6 to 8 weeks after surgery, with no strenuous lifting, exercise, or sexual activity. Straining at stool should be avoided by the use of laxatives and stool softeners. A combination of 15 to 30 ml of milk of magnesia and mineral oil daily in separate doses provides excellent prevention of constipation and can be modified as needed. If the sutures have passed into the vaginal vault, the patient should be warned to expect a small amount of vaginal drainage or spotting for 1 to 2 weeks Prophylactic postoperative oral antibiotics to prevent urinary infection may be considered.

COMPLICATIONS

The use of paravaginal repair for the treatment of stress incontinence has been confined to a small number of experienced gynecological groups, in whose hands complications have been few. However, as other surgeons begin performing the procedure, and unintentional modifications develop, complications may occur that cannot be predicted at this time. Ureteral and obturator nerve injury, the two most likely injuries, have been rare, as has significant hemorrhage from sutures placed near or through the vaginal veins. Obstruction of the urethra has been rare. New-onset instability, although theoretically as much a

potential complication as after the Burch or MMK procedures, has not been specifically considered in most reports.

RESULTS

Richardson reported 800 patients who had undergone paravaginal repair with 95 percent "satisfactory" results, which he defined as correction of cystourethrocele, elimination of stress incontinence, and normal voiding function without new voiding dysfunction.[5] Richardson claimed no new onset of bladder instability after these procedures. The absence of de novo instability is in sharp contrast to other standard operations such as Burch, MMK, Stamey, and Raz, in which de novo instability has approached 15 percent. More detailed reports of smaller subsets of patients have presented successful results with follow-up periods of up to 8 years.[1] Other reports have described the appearance of other postoperative problems, possibly indicating a difference in the way patients were selected preoperatively. Shull et al reported 149 patients seen over a 6-year period[10]: 97 percent were reported to have excellent results with no postoperative complaints of stress incontinence, 6 percent showed evidence of vaginal cuff prolapse, and 5 percent developed enterocele.

Summary

Paravaginal repair is the most recent procedure to be developed for the treatment of stress urinary incontinence associated with vaginal prolapse. The operation is based on what appear to be sound anatomical principles gained from both clinical observation and cadaver dissection. The author of the operation has made it clear that it is designed only for the repair of lateral defects of support of the lateral superior sulcus of the vagina, the critical portion that supports the urethra during stress. The successes claimed for this operation are in no small measure related to the ability of the surgeon to perform careful physical examination and select patients carefully. The results reported by a handful of practitioners appear favorable when compared with other operative procedures for the treatment of stress incontinence. The relatively low incidence of retention and de novo instability is a potentially attractive feature, although the exact reasons for this cannot be determined. There has been little radiographical or urodynamic data to support the reported successful outcome of the procedure. The operation has not yet gained widespread popularity, and no doubt many new insights can be expected in the future if it does.

The paravaginal repair is an anatomical operation for the repair of a specific anatomical defect associated with stress incontinence. It challenges us to refine our concepts and to explain and confirm its reported success.

Editorial Comment

Fray F. Marshall

The paravaginal repair popularized by Richardson is attractive because it anatomically corrects a common defect in lateral vaginal support. The incidence of complications appears low, and there are few instances of urinary retention. Patient selection remains important, but this repair is one that can be considered in the appropriately evaluated patient.

REFERENCES

1. Richardson AC, Edmonds PB, Williams NL. Treatment of stress urinary incontinence due to paravaginal fascial defect. Obstet Gynecol 57:357, 1981.
2. Baden WF, Walker T. Surgical Repair of Vaginal Defects. Philadelphia, JB Lippincott, 1992.
3. DeLancey JOL, Richardson AC. Anatomy of genital support. In Benson JT, ed. Female Pelvic Floor Disorders: Investigation and Management. New York, WW Norton, 1992, pp 19–26.
4. Nichols D, Randall C. Vaginal Surgery. Baltimore, Williams & Wilkins, 1989.
5. Richardson AC. Paravaginal repair. In Benson JT, ed. Female Pelvic Floor Disorders. New York, WW Norton, 1992, pp 280–288.
6. White GR. Cystocele; a radical cure by suturing lateral sulci of vagina to white line of pelvic fascia. JAMA 53:1707, 1909.
7. U.S. Department of Health and Human Services, Public Health Service. Urinary Incontinence in Adults. Clinical Practice Guidelines. Washington, DC, Agency for Health Care Policy and Research, 1992.
8. Wang Y, Mitchell D, Hadley HR. Anatomical basis for femoral neuropathy due to procedures performed in the modified lithotomy position. J Urol 145:373, 1991.
9. Burch JC. Urethrovaginal fixation to Cooper's ligament for correction of stress incontinence, cystocele, and prolapse. Am J Obstet Gynecol 81:281, 1961.
10. Shull BL, Baden WF. A six-year experience with paravaginal defect repair for stress urinary incontinence. Am J Obstet Gynecol 160:1432, 1989.

Chapter 91

Vaginal Surgery for Female Incontinence and Vaginal Wall Prolapse

Shlomo Raz, Lynn Stothers, and Ashok Chopra

Urinary incontinence in women can result from either detrusor or sphincteric dysfunction. Sphincteric incompetence can originate either from anatomical malposition of an intact sphincteric unit (anatomical incontinence) or from intrinsic sphincteric dysfunction secondary to multiple surgical procedures, neurogenic disease, or radiation therapy. The goal of surgery for anatomical incontinence is to reposition the bladder neck and urethra in a high fixed retropubic position. However, when the sphincter is intrinsically damaged, mere restoration of position may fail to cure the problem. In such a case the goal of surgery is to provide increased urethral resistance by improving urethral coaptation and compression. This can be achieved by means of either an artificial urinary sphincter, a sling procedure, periurethral injection, or bladder outlet reconstruction.

Because urinary incontinence in women is often one manifestation of vaginal wall prolapse, preoperative consideration should include, in addition to the type of incontinence, assessment of any degree of anterior vaginal wall prolapse or coexisting findings such as an enterocele, a rectocele, perineal laxity, or uterine prolapse. A concurrent cystocele should be corrected at the time of any anti-incontinence procedure. Failure to do so may result in urinary obstruction caused by a valvular mechanism at the bladder neck after surgery. On the other hand, if only the cystocele is repaired, urinary incontinence may appear or worsen. It is prudent to restore the normal vaginal axis and to correct any concomitant vaginal wall prolapse. If only the anterior vaginal wall is supported, any coexisting enterocele, rectocele, or uterine prolapse may be aggravated. One advantage of a vaginal surgical approach to cure incontinence is that it allows simultaneous correction of associated pelvic prolapse.

ETIOLOGY OF INCONTINENCE AND PELVIC PROLAPSE

Many patients with minor degrees of pelvic prolapse are asymptomatic, and only a small subset have stress incontinence. The reason for this is that continence is determined by a combination of factors, of which anatomical malposition is only one.

The etiology of incontinence and pelvic prolapse is frequently multifactorial in any one patient. Childbirth, hysterectomy, menopause, pelvic denervation, and weakened pelvic support are contributory factors in the genesis of incontinence and prolapse. Chronic intra-abdominal pressure (physical exertion or chronic cough), birth trauma, and pelvic surgery constitute the most common types of physical injury. Hormonal deprivation that accompanies menopause results in atrophy of muscular and connective tissue elements critical to pelvic support. Denervation secondary to myelomeningocele, cauda equina injury, or pelvic surgery results in relaxation of the pelvic musculature. Congenital weakness of the pelvic supports and inflammatory diseases can also predispose the pelvic organs to prolapse. Loss of pelvic support affects the position and function of the urethra, bladder, vagina, uterus, cervix, small bowel, and large bowel.

Specific injuries may affect one or more supporting structures. Although hormonal changes have a generalized effect, second-stage labor injuries may affect the middle vaginal support (cardinal and uterosacral ligaments), anterior vaginal support (pubourethral ligaments and vesicopelvic fascia), posterior vaginal support (rectovaginal fascia), or perineal support. The urologist who treats a woman with urinary incontinence must be aware of the possibility of coexisting cystocele, uterine prolapse, enterocele, or rectocele.

PATHOPHYSIOLOGY OF PELVIC SUPPORT AND CONTINENCE

Conceptually there are four important factors that contribute to pelvic support and continence: (1) intact anatomical muscular and fascial supports, (2) a normal functioning sphincteric unit, (3) adequate functional and anatomical length of the sphincteric unit, and (4) proper response of the normal compensatory mechanisms of urethral competence during stress. Continence results from a balance of these factors.[1] For example, many patients have anatomical changes (prolapse) of the anterior vaginal wall but only some will have stress incontinence. Furthermore, excision of the distal urethra for carcinoma will not lead to incontinence if the proximal urethra is well coapted and supported. In the following section we will individually discuss these factors.

Anatomical Considerations

The bony pelvis provides the framework for support of all the pelvic organs, while the pelvic diaphragm and perineal musculature add inferior support to these organs (Table 91–1). The pelvic diaphragm is composed of the levator ani (pubococcygeus, iliococcygeus, and ischiococcygeus) and coccygeus muscles. The pubococcygeus is closely associated with the inferior support of the urethra, vagina, and rectum via the corresponding subdivisions (pubourethralis, pubovaginalis, and puborectalis), which, by contributing large muscle slings, hold the intrapelvic organs like a hammock. This hammock

provides support as well as stabilization during increases in intra-abdominal pressure. The levator muscle with its overlying fascia takes origin at the tendinous arch of the obturator fascia, extends from the inner part of the pubic bone lateral to the symphysis anteriorly, and continues to the ischial spine posteriorly. The anatomical descriptions of the levator fascia in the current literature are confusing. Numerous terms for the same anatomical structure are not uncommon. As an alternative, we propose a simplified, more conceptual approach to the various structures in the pelvis that are clinically relevant to physicians interested in the correction of incontinence and pelvic prolapse. The following descriptions are based on surgical experience and review of magnetic resonance images of the pelvis in patients with a wide range of pelvic pathology. They represent a personal interpretation of the anatomy by the authors.

The pelvic diaphragm is a muscular layer that provides support for the pelvic organs. It is formed by the levator ani muscle, which is shaped structurally like a hammock extending anteriorly from the pelvic brim to its posterior attachments at the sacrum and coccyx. Covering the levator musculature is a strong fascial layer. There appear to be four condensations of the levator fascia that play an important role in vaginal and vesicourethral support: (1) the pubourethral ligaments, (2) the urethropelvic ligaments, (3) the pubocervical (vesicopelvic) ligaments, and (4) the sacrouterine and cardinal complex. These condensations are not separate anatomical structures. They fuse to each other, forming a continuous fascial support for the pelvic organs.

Pubourethral Ligaments and Midurethral Complex

The pubourethral ligaments support the midurethra to the inferior rami of the symphysis. The pubourethral ligaments prevent hypermobility and inferior movement of the midurethra. Anatomically, the pubourethral ligaments divide the urethra into three segments: (1) a proximal intra-abdominal third, which is responsible for passive continence, (2) a midurethral complex, and (3) a distal third, serving only as a conduit without a true continence function. The midurethral complex is formed by not only the pubourethral ligaments but also the external sphincter. The external sphincter area consists of fibers from the levator musculature that increase urethral coaptation by three basic mechanisms: (1) basic tone, (2) voluntary activity of the external sphincter, and (3) reflex activity.

There is clinical evidence to suggest that the midurethral complex is the most important area of continence: It is known that 30 to 50 percent of postmenopausal *continent* women have an open bladder neck.

TABLE 91–1. Pathophysiological Classification of Stress Incontinence

Intrinsic urethral mechanisms	Coaptation	Mucosa Submucosa
	Compression	Submucosa Smooth muscle Skeletal muscle Neural stimuli
Anatomical support	Configuration	Bladder neck mechanisms Intra-abdominal pressure transmission Efficient intrinsic mechanism function
Mixed		

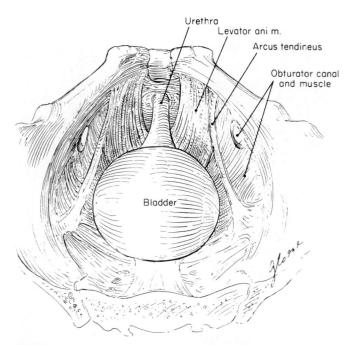

Figure 91–1. A view of the lower pelvis illustrates the spatial relationship between the bladder and urethra and the pelvic floor muscles. The origin of the levator ani from the arcus tendineus is demonstrated. The latter overlies the obturator muscle and extends from the inner part of the pubic bone anteriorly to the ischial spine posteriorly.

Furthermore, Y-V plasty does not invariably produce incontinence. Female patients with myasthenia gravis may develop incontinence despite a closed bladder neck. These data support the role of the midurethral complex in normal continence. However, this area of the urethra is still poorly understood and more investigation will be necessary.

Urethropelvic Ligaments

The fascial structures supporting the bladder neck and urethra play an important role in normal conti-

URETHRAL SUPPORT

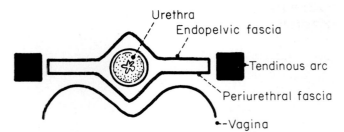

Figure 91–3. Schematic illustration of the major components of urethral support.

nence (Figs. 91–1 to 91–3). The proximal urethra and bladder neck are attached to the side wall of the pelvis by fascial layers that act as a unit to support the urethra and bladder neck and increase urethral closure during cough and strain. Vaginal dissection around the urethra clearly demonstrates a well-defined fascial layer covering the urethral wall. This extends laterally, underneath the pubic bone, toward the side wall of the pelvis. Retropubic dissection will reveal a distinct fascial layer covering the dorsal part of the urethra extending laterally toward the side wall of the pelvis. Both the retropubic and vaginal (periurethral) fascial layers cover on two sides, as a sandwich, the urethral wall. Both layers fuse together laterally and anchor the urethra to the tendinous arc of the obturator muscle. We have termed this fascial complex the urethropelvic ligament. The bladder neck and proximal urethra are primarily supported by this structure, which maintains their normal anatomical position (Figs. 91–4 and 91–5). Contraction of the levator muscles creates tension on the urethropelvic fascia, thereby elevating and compressing the urethra. Relaxation produces descent and downward rotation of the proximal urethra and bladder neck

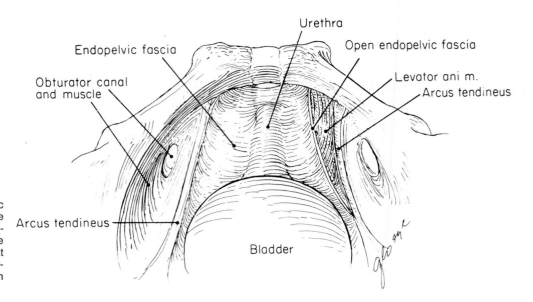

Figure 91–2. The urethropelvic fascia extends laterally from the urethra, inserting into the tendinous arch. The opening in the urethropelvic fascia was made at the location where the fascial perforation is usually performed in Raz bladder neck suspension.

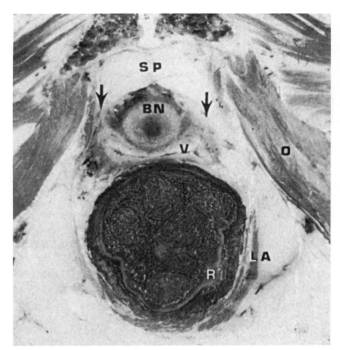

Figure 91–4. A transverse cut in a frozen autopsy specimen at the level of the bladder neck demonstrates well the obturator muscle (O), the levator ani muscle sling (LA), the bladder neck (BN), and the urethropelvic fascia *(arrows)* surrounding the urethra and extending toward the junction of the levator ani with the obturator muscle. R, rectum; V, vagina; SP, symphysis pubis.

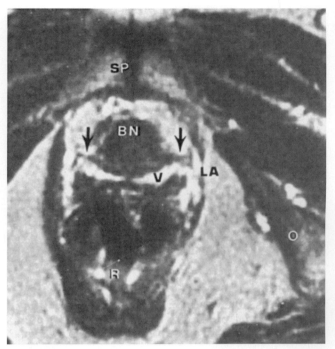

Figure 91–5. Magnetic resonance imaging (MRI) in a transverse view at the level of the bladder neck illustrates the urethropelvic fascia *(arrows)* as related to the neighboring structures. O, obturator muscle; LA, levator ani muscle; BN, bladder neck; V, vagina; R, rectum; SP, symphysis pubis.

around the midurethral anchor (the pubourethral ligaments). During cough or strain, there is a reflex contraction of the pelvic floor that increases urethral resistance. The urethral supports are elastic and thus allow motion of the urethra during contraction of the pelvic floor. This mobility allows the urethra to adapt to changes in intra-abdominal pressure.

It is of clinical interest to note that on fluoroscopy many patients with anatomical stress incontinence demonstrate an increase in the distance between the symphysis and the midurethra. In many of these patients the urethra appears to slide under the symphysis. Most current surgical repairs suspend the bladder neck without restoring midurethral support.

Pubocervical (Vesicopelvic) Ligaments

The pubocervical fascia is a direct extension of the urethropelvic ligament. At the level of the bladder the levator fascia splits into two leaves: the vaginal side or pubocervical fascia, and the abdominal side or endopelvic fascia. These leaves fuse laterally and are attached to the tendinous arc of the obturator. The pubocervical fascia lends support to the bladder. Because of its physiological function, we prefer to call this portion of the levator fascia the vesicopelvic fascia as opposed to pubocervical fascia. The vesicopelvic fascia extends from its continuation with the urethropelvic fascia to the cervix along the posterior

surface of the urethra and bladder. This fascia supports the anterior vaginal wall (Figs. 91–6 and 91–7). The attachment of the pubocervical fascia at the level of the cervix establishes anterior continuity between the lower pelvic support and the middle support (cardinal and sacrouterine ligaments). The vesicopelvic fascia provides support that contributes to the prevention of both urethral hypermobility and cystocele formation.

Clinically, a defective vesicopelvic fascia results

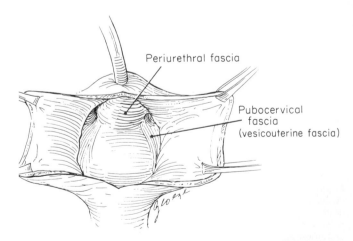

Figure 91–6. After lateral dissection of the anterior vaginal wall, the pubocervical fascia is exposed, extending from the pubic bone to the cervix, anterior to the urethra and bladder base.

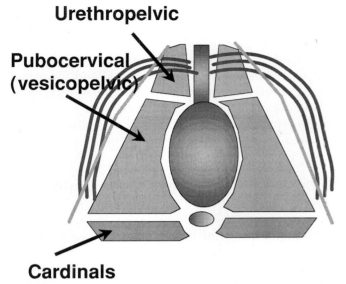

Figure 91–7. Diagram outlining the rectangular support of the bladder base and bladder neck.

in two main defects. A central defect exists when weakness, separation, or elongation of the middle segment of the fascia is found, singly or in combination, but the lateral support is intact. A lateral defect exists when the fascial attachment to the tendinous arc is compromised. Lateral defects result in a sliding hernia of the bladder base. In the clinical setting, patients most frequently have a combination of lateral and central defects with subsequent anterior vaginal wall prolapse.

Sacrouterine and Cardinal Complex

The sacrouterine ligaments are true ligaments of musculofascial consistency that run from the upper part of the cervix to the sides of the sacrum. As they approach the uterus, they merge with the posterior aspect of the cardinal ligaments. The cardinal ligaments are composed of condensed fibrous tissue and some smooth muscle fibers. They extend from the lateral aspects of the uterine isthmus toward the pelvic wall and insert into the obturator and superior fascia of the pelvic diaphragm. Medially and inferiorly, they merge with the uterovaginal and vesicopelvic fascia. These structures are the main suspensory complex that supports the cervix and upper vagina over the levator plate.

In the normal vagina, support of the cuff and levator plate maintains the proximal vaginal axis at approximately 110 degrees and the distal vaginal axis at approximately 45 degrees to vertical. This horizontal orientation is able to protect the dome of the vagina and the cervix from prolapse. Any change in the vaginal axis to the vertical, such as after bladder neck suspension and cystocele repair, may entail a higher risk of superior and posterior vaginal wall prolapse.

Potential spaces exist within the layers of pelvic fascia that provide valuable natural surgical cleavage planes (Fig. 91–8). The urethral fascia and the vaginal fascia are fused in the region of the distal and mid-urethra and form the periurethral fascia, with no potential space available in this region. At the level of the proximal urethra and bladder neck, the vaginal and vesical fasciae can be surgically separated to develop the vesicovaginal space. At the lateral borders of the vesicovaginal space, the fusion of the vaginal and vesical fasciae forms the vesicopelvic and vesicouterine ligaments.

The rectovaginal fascia extends posteriorly from the perineal body to the pouch of Douglas, establishing continuity of support in the posterior plane. The posterior vaginal fascia is fused with the perianal fascia in the perineum but can be surgically separated from the prerectal fascia for entrance into the rectovaginal space. This space is bordered laterally by the rectal pillars (rectal septa), which are two fibrous structures extending from the vagina to the lateral surface of the rectum and then to the sacrum. The rectal pillars separate the rectovaginal space from the pararectal space (Fig. 91–8). Development of the rectovaginal space is essential for adequate repair of rectocele.

Last, there exists a layer more superficial to the levator ani that provides additional pelvic support. The perineal musculature, the urogenital diaphragm (which consists of superior and inferior fasciae and the deep transverse perineal muscle), the superficial perineal muscles (bulbocavernosus, ischiocavernosus, and superficial transverse perineal muscle), and the external anal sphincter are all important contributing factors in total pelvic support. The perineal

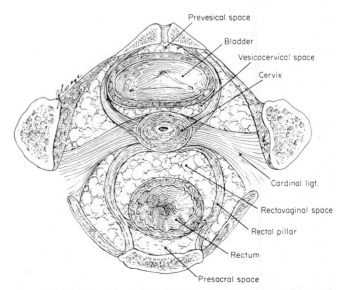

Figure 91–8. Transverse view of the pelvis illustrating the middle supports of the cervix and upper vagina (cardinal and uterosacral ligaments) and the natural cleavage planes.

body is in the midline between the rectum and vagina at the level of the ischial tuberosities. The superficial and deep transverse perineal muscles, the inferior fusion of the rectovaginal fascia, and the fibers of the levator ani converge at this central point. This natural anatomical landmark is the central point of the perineum and provides a common point of attachment for the many superficial perineal supports.

Intrinsic Sphincteric Unit

The female urethra consists of an outer envelope of fibroelastic and muscular tissue, an inner spongy layer, and mucosal and submucosal layers. The submucosa consists of very loosely woven connective tissue with scattered smooth muscle bundles and an elaborate vascular plexus. The mucosal lining of the urethra is thrown into numerous folds. These anatomical features act in concert to provide continence. The smooth muscle coat directs submucosal expansion forces inward toward the mucosa. The mucosa is under estrogenic hormonal influence. Estrogens have been shown to promote proliferation and maturation of atrophic epithelium of the urethra and trigone, to widen the vascular lumen, and to increase vascular pulsations in the urethral bed.

Complete apposition of the urethral surface is promoted by the elasticity of the mucosa. Mucous secretions enhance the development of surface tension.

Numerous factors can lead to secondary malfunction of the intrinsic sphincter mechanism. Estrogen deficiency may lead to atrophy and replacement of the vascular tissue by fibrous elements, thereby contributing to a decrease in urethral closure pressure. Surgical trauma and radiation can create a rigid urethra. The normal aging process causes neuronal loss and poor sphincter coaptation. Neuronal dysfunction is also found in patients with myelomeningocele. Several factors frequently coexist in any one patient that contribute to the clinical entity known as intrinsic sphincteric dysfunction.

Urethral Length

Urethral length can be approached either as an anatomical measurement or as a functional value. The anatomical length of the urethra is approximately 3 to 4 cm. The average functional length is 2.8 cm. The impact of anatomical length is controversial. Many patients with shortened anatomical length (after distal urethrectomy for benign or malignant diseases) are continent as long as the remaining urethral continence mechanism is well supported and capable of supplying adequate resistance to flow. Functional urethral length is defined as the length of the urethra along which urethral closing pressure exceeds bladder pressure. It is shortened in most patients with anatomical stress urinary incontinence. In general, surgical correction of anatomical incontinence restores the normal anatomical and functional length of the urethra. There is no clinical correlation between continence and functional or anatomical length. However, there is a critical urethral length required for normal continence.

Compensatory Changes of the Urethra During Stress

A crucial factor for maintaining continence is the ability of the urethra to compensate for increases in intra-abdominal pressure. In a normal urethra this is the result of several effects.

1. *Valvular effect.* The normal urethra is in a well-supported retropubic position, and increases in pressure generated by coughing are transmitted to both the bladder and the urethra. The location of the bladder neck in a nondependent position and the force generated with an increase in intra-abdominal pressure will not be experienced at the bladder neck but at the bladder base (the most dependent structure). This causes a valvular effect that decreases the chance of incontinence.

2. *Coaptation effect.* Reflex contraction of the midurethra and contraction of the obturator and levator increase the tensile forces across the urethropelvic ligament, thereby increasing coaptation.

3. *"Back-board" effect.* The impact of pelvic floor support is very important in maintaining continence during strain maneuvers. For example, with coughing, a reflex contraction of the pelvic floor occurs, increasing urethral resistance. Under normal circumstances, the well-supported pelvic floor will act as a "back-board" to the bladder. Transmission of forces without damping will occur. When pelvic floor relaxation exists, ineffective force transmission occurs, and decreased coaptation forces to the urethra result. This concept relates to the importance of posterior vaginal wall repair, when indicated, at the time of surgery for stress incontinence.

In summary, in contemplating surgical correction of incontinence and pelvic prolapse, the extent of the anatomical defect is a critical factor. A different treatment plan is applied when there is only urethral and bladder neck hypermobility compared with anatomical incontinence combined with various degrees of cystocele. It should be noted that physical examination of the bladder with the patient in the supine position may not provide complete anatomical data. A properly performed voiding cystourethrography is an excellent adjunctive tool for assessing anatomical defects objectively. We feel that this imaging study is the equivalent of the physical examination of the bladder in the erect position.

SURGICAL TREATMENT OF ANATOMICAL STRESS URINARY INCONTINENCE

The Kelly plication,[2] described in 1914, historically was the most common procedure performed for stress urinary incontinence. The procedure involves an anterior vaginal wall incision, dissection of the vagina from the bladder neck, and placement of two or three vertical mattress sutures to buttress the periurethral tissues. This procedure may correct mild degrees of prolapse but has only a 50 percent success rate for the correction of incontinence. Failure to correct stress incontinence occurs because of a failure to restore the bladder neck into a high, supported retropubic position without causing obstruction.

In 1942, Aldridge[3] popularized the "fascial sling" technique proposed by several German gynecologists (the Goebel-Frangenheim-Stoeckel technique) in the early 1900s. A rectus fascial strip left attached to the midline was used to suspend and sling the bladder neck, taking advantage of the favorable anatomical relationship of the rectus muscle to the urethra. This procedure was devised to repair typical anatomical postpartum stress urinary incontinence, but it is also of clinical utility for incontinence caused by intrinsic sphincteric damage.

In 1949, Marshall, Marchetti, and Krantz[4] described the retropubic suspension operation for the treatment of stress incontinence. After retropubic dissection to mobilize the urethra and bladder neck, several pairs of No. 1 chromic sutures are used to anchor the upper wall of the vagina and lateral wall of the urethra (extraluminally) to the pubic periosteum. When tied, the retropubic space is obliterated. Additional sutures are placed in the muscle of the bladder, which is tacked to the rectus muscle. A distinct disadvantage is the potential for urethral obstruction by the sutures in the periurethral tissues. Other disadvantages are the inability to correct a cystocele by this approach, the need for a laparotomy, and the potential occurrence of osteitis pubis by sutures placed in the pubic periosteum.

In 1961, Burch[5] reported a retropubic suspension procedure in which three pairs of No. 2 chromic sutures were used to anchor the perivaginal fascia and vaginal wall, excluding the epithelium, to Cooper's ligament (Fig. 91–9). This is facilitated by a finger in the vagina, which elevates the perivaginal fascia. Advantages of the Burch colposuspension include lateral placement of the suspension sutures, thus obviating urethral obstruction; the ability to cor-

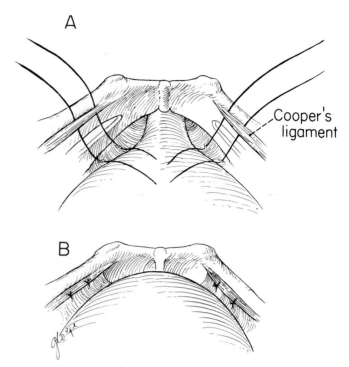

Figure 91–9. *A,* Burch colposuspension, anchoring the vaginal wall at the level of the proximal urethra and bladder neck to Cooper's ligament bilaterally, thus achieving bladder neck suspension *(B).* The urethra is free in the retropubic space and is suspended by the vaginal wall and urethropelvic fascia.

rect a mild cystocele; and the reliability of Cooper's ligament as a strong anchoring tissue. The short-term success rate of the Burch suspension has been over 80 percent. In clinical series of patients undergoing Burch suspension, 54 percent of patients were completely cured and 30 percent significantly improved.[6] The disadvantages of this procedure include the need for a laparotomy incision, the inability to correct more severe coexisting degrees of cystocele, and potential enterocele formation.

Pereyra first described the original needle suspension technique in 1959.[7] He used a pair of No. 30 stainless steel wires to suspend the paraurethral tissues to the abdominal fascia. He introduced a special cannula to permit suture insertion, which required only a stab wound in the suprapubic area and avoided an extensive abdominal incision. This cannula is passed blindly from the suprapubic stab wound through the retropubic space and paraurethral tissues 2 to 3 cm posterior to the urethral meatus to emerge through the anterior vaginal wall. A trocar component of the cannula is then advanced through the anterior vaginal wall at the level of the bladder neck. The cannula and trocar tips are then threaded with the steel wire, transferred to the suprapubic area, disengaged, and clamped. After the contralateral side is approached in a similar fashion, the suspension wires are tied. The paraurethral tissues are cauterized at several points along the proximal urethra, about 1 cm lateral to the urethra, so that support would be rendered by fibrous tissue long after the wires cut through the soft paraurethral tissues.

Each subsequent modification of the original Pereyra procedure has resulted in the progressive evolution of the technique. Harer and Gunther,[8] in 1965, modified the technique by introducing a vaginal incision to achieve mobilization of the urethra and approximation of the paraurethral tissues across the midline. In addition, they performed the suspension with No. 1 chromic sutures and transferred the sutures in such a way as to create a sling on each side of the bladder neck, which is tied across the rectus fascia.

In 1967, Pereyra in conjunction with Lebherz[9] introduced the concept of entering the retropubic space by opening the lateral paraurethral tissue. This allowed for fingertip guidance for passage of the cannula, which avoided blind passage of the device from the suprapubic to the vaginal region with its attendant risks of penetration of the bladder and urethra. They also adopted the vertical vaginal incision for mobilization, the paraurethral plication, and the use of absorbable sutures as described by Harer and Gunther. The surgery was not widely accepted because of complications such as bleeding, obstruction, and recurrent incontinence.

Tauber and Wapner,[10] in 1967, described placement of the suspension sutures under direct visual control. A midline anterior vaginal wall incision is made to expose the pubocervical fascia, and a pair of No. 0 nonabsorbable sutures are placed in the pubocervical fascia at the level of the bladder neck under direct vision. The free end of each suture is tied, forming a loop around the encircled portion of the fascia. The sutures are than transferred to the suprapubic area by means of a special needle and tied to each other over the rectus fascia, after which the vaginal incision is closed.

In 1973, Stamey[11] contributed several novel concepts to needle suspension. He introduced the idea of cystoscopic control, which allowed for accurate suture placement at the bladder neck and visualization of bladder neck closure with elevation of the suspension sutures. In addition, Stamey used bolsters to support the bladder neck. A T-shaped anterior vaginal wall incision is made and the vaginal wall dissected off the urethra. The Stamey needle is introduced through the anterior rectus fascia via a stab wound, and directed through the retropubic space and out the vaginal incision at the level of the bladder neck. The Foley catheter is removed, and cystoscopy confirms movement of the bladder neck with motion of the needle and lack of penetration of the bladder lumen by the needle. A No. 2 nylon suture is threaded through the needle and transferred suprapubically. The needle is then passed through the same stab wound about 1 cm lateral to the original entry in the rectus fascia, through the

retropubic space, exiting the vaginal incision about 1 cm distal to the nylon suture. Cystoscopy is repeated, and before the suture is transferred, it is passed through a 1-cm tube of 5-mm Dacron arterial graft to buttress the vaginal loop. The same procedure is repeated on the contralateral side of the bladder neck. Endoscopic examination while traction is applied on the nylon sutures will demonstrate vesical neck closure. After placement of a suprapubic tube, the vaginal incision is closed before the nylon sutures are tied with tension. The suprapubic tube is generally clamped on the fourth postoperative day and removed on the following day.

In 1976, Winter[12] reported a modification of the Pereyra procedure, with a no–vaginal incision approach, in which a straightened 3-inch curved needle with a swaged No. 2 plastic suture is passed from the vagina alongside the bladder neck to the lower abdominal wall adjacent to the symphysis, and the tip grasped with a clamp. The needle attached to the other end of the suture is passed in a similar fashion 1 cm parallel to the first. The contralateral side is approached in identical fashion. A small suprapubic incision is made between the needles and carried down to the rectus fascia, after which the sutures are tied snugly.

Cobb and Ragde[13] introduced in 1978 the double-pronged ligature carrier, which minimized the number of passes necessary for suspension and allowed for a sufficient fascial bridge to support the suspension sutures. They also contributed the concept of a barrel knot tied in a nylon suture to support the paraurethral tissues as an alternative to the Dacron graft buttress described by Stamey. The double-pronged needle is passed from a suprapubic stab wound through the retropubic space and allowed to exit through the anterior vaginal wall adjacent to the bladder neck. Cystoscopy is performed to rule out needle penetration, after which the vaginal epithelium between the needle shafts is incised, the needles are threaded with a No. 2 nylon suture with a centrally tied barrel knot, and the sutures are transferred suprapubically. The contralateral side is approached similarly. The vaginal incision is closed, and the nylon sutures are tied snugly while the assistant elevates the vagina toward the symphysis.

In 1981[14] and 1985,[15] Raz presented another modification of the needle suspension technique. In the Raz procedure, an inverted-U incision is made in the anterior vaginal wall, and the plane between the vagina and the glistening periurethral fascia is entered while dissection is directed laterally toward the pubic bone. The retropubic space is entered either bluntly or sharply between the pubic bone and the urethropelvic fascia (Fig. 91–10). The urethropelvic fascia is freed from its lateral attachments from the level of the pubic bone to the ischial tuberosity, which allows for ade-

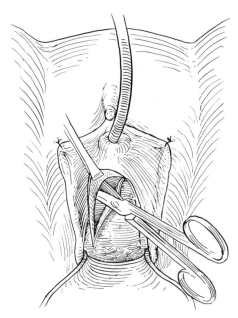

Figure 91–10. Raz bladder neck suspension: an inverted-U incision in the anterior vaginal wall. The plane between the vaginal wall and the periurethral fascia is sharply dissected and the retropubic space is entered.

most important and reliable structure for suspension. A potential complication of other suspension procedures, including the Marshall-Marchetti-Krantz, the original Pereyra, and the Stamey, is urethral obstruction secondary to the close proximity of the suspending sutures to the urethra itself, which prevents satisfactory funneling and shortening of the bladder neck during voiding. The principle of the Raz procedure is similar to that of the Burch colposuspension in that the sutures are placed laterally, obviating obstruction. We feel that it is important to enter the retropubic space, not merely to facilitate fingertip control of the ligature carrier, but also to mobilize the urethra and bladder neck sufficiently from adhesions and scars before the suspension is performed. This is a sine qua non in a patient who has had previous procedures, either retropubic or vaginal, to reposition the bladder neck and proximal urethra in a high retropubic position. We routinely use cystoscopy after administration of intravenous indigo carmine to ensure bilateral ureteral efflux, lack of suture penetration of the urethra and bladder, and adequate suspension of the bladder neck when minimal traction is placed on the suspension sutures. Contrary to the

quate mobility of the urethra, bladder neck, and vaginal wall. A No. 1 Prolene suture is placed in a helical fashion in the vaginal wall (excluding the epithelium), the pubocervical fascia, and the medial edge of the urethropelvic fascia (Fig. 91–11). Traction on the suture tests the integrity of the anchoring tissue. The contralateral side is approached similarly. The anterior rectus sheath is exposed through a 3-cm suprapubic incision, and a double-pronged ligature carrier is guided through the retropubic space by the surgeon's finger and out through the vaginal incision (Fig. 91–12). The sutures are threaded and transferred suprapubically. After cystoscopic examination, the vaginal incision is closed with a running No. 2-0 polyglycolic acid suture, and the Prolene suspension sutures are tied without undue tension. Suprapubic and urethral Foley catheters are left indwelling. The urethral catheter and vaginal packing are removed on the first postoperative day, and the suprapubic tube is removed when voiding resumes and urine residuals become negligible.

Several principles were introduced with the Raz bladder neck suspension. The inverted-U vaginal epithelial incision was devised to allow the dissection to be lateral to the urethra and bladder neck, thus avoiding dissection directly beneath the urethra and bladder neck and facilitating entrance into the retropubic space. The pubocervical and urethropelvic fasciae are conveniently approached from the limbs of the inverted-U incision. We believe that the medial edge of the urethropelvic fascia, detached from the tendinous arch when the retropubic space is entered, is the

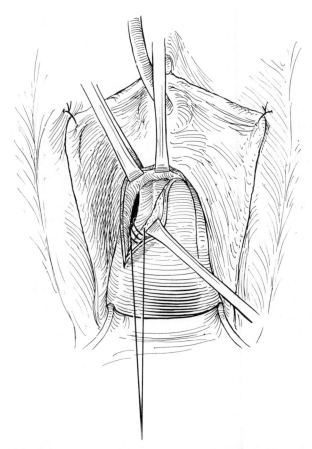

Figure 91–11. Raz bladder neck suspension *(continued)*. A No. 1 Prolene suture is placed in a helical fashion, incorporating the vaginal wall (except for epithelium), the pubocervical fascia, and the medial edge of the urethropelvic fascia.

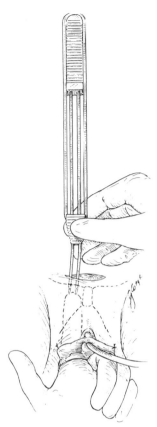

Figure 91–12. Raz bladder neck suspension *(continued)*. A double-pronged ligature carrier, introduced through a small suprapubic incision, is finger guided through the retropubic space and out through the vaginal incision for later transfer of the suspension sutures to the suprapubic region.

Stamey procedure, in which the purpose of cystoscopy is to observe proper placement of the sutures at the level of the bladder neck, the Raz procedure does not rely on cystoscopy for suture placement because the sutures are placed under direct observation.

In 1987, Gittes and Loughlin[16] described a no-incision modification of the Pereyra technique. Without making a vaginal incision, a Stamey needle is passed from a suprapubic stab wound through the retropubic space and out the anterior vaginal wall at the level of the bladder neck. A heavy nylon or Prolene suture is threaded and withdrawn suprapubically; a second pass of the needle is made and advanced out the anterior vaginal wall about 2 cm from the first puncture site, and before the suture is threaded, a full-thickness helical bite of the vaginal wall is taken between the first and second vaginal perforations. The suture is threaded and transferred, and after the contralateral side is approached in the same manner and cystoscopy performed, the sutures are tied down with tension to bury the knots in the fat of the suprapubic stab wound. This procedure relies on the suspension sutures breaking through the vaginal epithelium and becoming incorporated in the underlying tissues.

Since the development of the needle bladder neck suspension, Raz has reported on the development of the vaginal wall sling for anatomic incontinence (AI) and intrinsic sphincter dysfunction (ISD). This procedure has evolved to incorporate the benefits of the vaginal bladder neck needle suspension with the support and compression of the midurethra found with sling procedures. As discussed earlier, it is our impression that the midurethra is a vital component of the continence mechanism. One frequent radiological finding is the presence of significant degrees of separation of the midurethra from the symphysis. It is our impression that support of this area may contribute to success of the repair. Bladder neck suspension alone will not achieve this goal. The technique of our current procedure, incorporating midurethral support, is shown in Figures 91–13 and 91–14 and described later in this chapter.

With such a multitude of different procedures from which to choose, all with practically similar reported cure rates, ranging between 87 and 96 percent, what is a reasonable approach for the clinician? Is a vaginal approach superior to a retropubic approach? Is a no-incision technique better than a procedure that requires a vaginal incision? The answers to these questions can be approached by a comparative analysis of the results, advantages, and disadvantages of the individual techniques. Clearly, if similar results can be achieved with retropubic and vaginal approaches, it would be in the best interest of the patient to undergo the procedure that results in less pain, morbidity, and risk and that entails the shortest hospital stay and the most rapid return to a normal life style. In this regard, the vaginal needle suspension procedures confer a distinct advantage. Additionally, the ability to simultaneously correct concomitant vaginal pathological conditions (cystocele, rectocele, enterocele, uterine prolapse, and perineal laxity) favors the vaginal approach. In the final analysis, however, the best operation is usually the one that works best in the hands of the individual surgeon.

SURGICAL TREATMENT OF INTRINSIC SPHINCTERIC INCOMPETENCE

Bladder Neck Reconstruction

Reconstruction of the bladder neck is one method of restoring sphincteric continence in a patient with a fixed, open bladder outlet. It was first introduced by Young[17] and was subsequently modified by Leadbetter and Fraley.[18] Procedures utilizing the Young-Dees principle involve construction of a neourethra from the posterior surface of the bladder wall and trigone. The Leadbetter modification involves proximal reimplantation of the ureters to allow more ex-

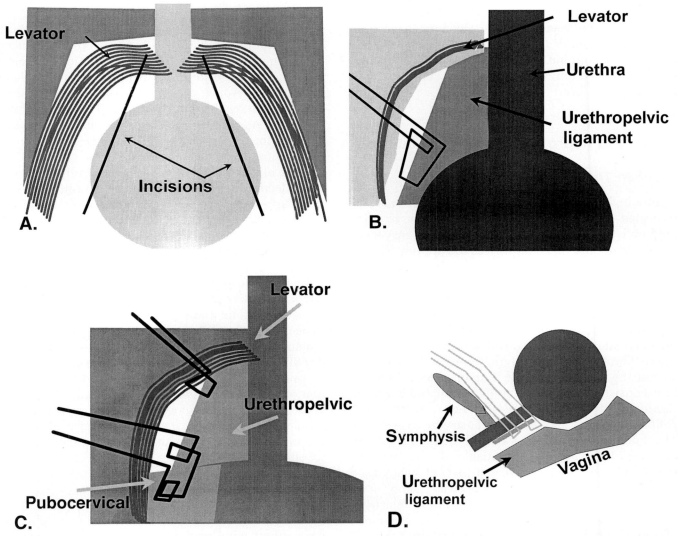

Figure 91–13. Vaginal wall sling for anatomic incontinence (AI) and intrinsic sphincter dysfunction (ISD). *A,* Two longitudinal incisions are made extending to the area of the vaginal cuff. *B,* No. 1 Prolene sutures are placed to encompass the pubocervial fascia, the vaginal wall without epithelium, and the urethropelvic ligament. *C,* The second sutures encompass the levator musculature and the anterior vaginal wall without epithelium at the level of the midurethra. *D,* The four sets of sutures are transferred to the suprapubic area with the Raz needle.

VAGINAL WALL SLING

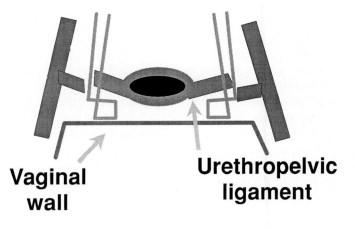

Figure 91–14. Schematic diagram of a vaginal wall sling for AI and ISD after suture transfer.

tensive tubularization of the trigone. Long-term success rates of between 60 and 70 percent have been achieved. Tanagho[19] described a procedure based on a similar concept but using the anterior bladder neck to create a functioning neourethra. A success rate of 70 percent has been reported.

Surgery to Improve Urethral Coaptation

Injection Therapy

Intraurethral injections of inert materials may be indicated in cases where urethral resistance to urine outflow is impaired and aim at increasing resistance by an added bulk that compresses the urethra. Materials used for such injections have included collagen, autologous fat, and polytetrafluoroethylene (Teflon).

Teflon was one of the first materials chosen for periurethral injection. The particles, measuring 50 to 100 μm, stimulate an ingrowth of fibroblasts at the injection site and are encapsulated by fibrous tissue. These fibroblasts may aid in holding the particles within the tissues, and the implant thus achieves a firm consistency and retains its shape and position. Carrion and Politano reported their results with Teflon injections for various causes in 51 women. The number of injections ranged from one to four (average 1.8). Fifty-one percent of the patients achieved an excellent result, 20 percent had a good result, and in 29 percent the result was poor.[20]

A major drawback of periurethral Teflon injections is the possible migration of particles. This phenomenon has been demonstrated experimentally.[21] The issue, however, is whether the particles that migrate produce any harm. During the more than 20 years that Teflon injections have been used, no significant clinical complication secondary to distal embolization has been reported. Particle migration has led to the virtual abandonment of the use of Teflon for periurethral injection today.

More recently, cross-linked bovine collagen has been used for periurethral injection. This material is suspended in glutaraldehyde to add physical stability. The technique is shown diagrammatically in Figure 91–15. Utilizing endoscopic visualization of the bladder neck area, the implant is injected under sterile technique into the urethral spongy tissue underlying the periurethral fascia. The volume injected varies with each patient. The end point is that volume which provides occlusion of the urethra under visualization and is judged appropriate by personal experience of the surgeon. Total volumes needed to achieve or maintain continence vary and have ranged from 2.5 to 85 ml.[22]

Clinical studies in children undergoing ureteral reimplantation after failed collagen injection for reflux indicate that there is some neovascularization and fibroblastic ingrowth into the implants at between 3 and 19 months.[23] Skin testing must be performed before injection to rule out the possibility of allergic reaction to bovine collagen. In a series of 162 patients reported by Appel et al,[24] 1.9 percent of patients had positive results on skin testing. Potential clinical complications of the procedure include urinary retention, urethritis, urinary tract infection, bladder neck contracture, and hemorrhage.

Clinical case series report varying results for collagen injection depending upon the definition of success. Appel[25] reported in 1990 that 95 percent of 115 women with sphincteric incontinence achieved 12 months of persistent dryness after two injections of periurethral collagen. Goldenberg reported 132 patients treated with periurethral collagen injection, noting that 36 percent remained completely dry and 48 percent were improved. Most patients required repeat injections to either achieve or maintain continence.[26] The manufacturer's literature indicates that women have about a 40 percent chance of remaining dry after one or two collagen injections.[27]

Autologous fat injection is an alternative method that may be used in patients with an allergy to collagen. The patient's adipose cells are harvested with a specialized suction device and then injected into the periurethral area in a fashion similar to that for collagen injection.[28]

Artificial Urinary Sphincter

Candidates for insertion of an artificial sphincter are patients who have incontinence related to pelvic trauma; previous radical pelvic surgery; congenital abnormalities; neuropathic sphincter dysfunction; or multiple, previously failed anti-incontinence procedures. Patients with postradiation damage to the external sphincter have also undergone successful implantation procedures. The urological work-up of potential candidates should be designed to exclude patients who have underlying disease that would result in a high risk of device failure or who would be at risk for upper tract deterioration once the device was implanted. The work-up should therefore include urine culture and sensitivity, excretory urography, voiding cystourethrography, cystourethroscopy, and a urodynamic evaluation. The detailed surgical technique is discussed elsewhere and is beyond the scope of this review.

Scott reported his results in 139 women with the transabdominal insertion of sphincter models 791/792 and AMS 800 between the years 1978 and 1984.[29] Ninety-one percent of the patients were rendered socially continent and 66 percent became completely dry. Four of the 139 devices (3 percent) were removed because of infection. A total of five erosions occurred

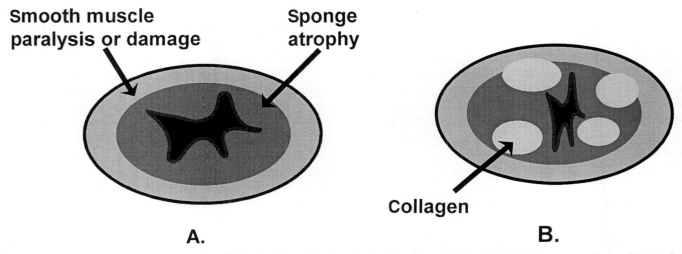

Figure 91–15. Diagrammatic technique of periurethral collagen injection. *A,* The injection needle is placed into the spongy tissue of the urethra via a perineal approach. Injection of collagen is continued until a unilateral bulging under the mucosa is noted endoscopically. *B,* Injection into the contralateral side results in closure of the urethra endoscopically.

in 139 patients, and most of them were delayed. No mechanical failures were reported.

Appel[30] reported his experience with implantation of the artificial urinary sphincter by a vaginal approach in 34 women with type III stress incontinence. The follow-up period for 19 patients was at least 3 years. All patients were reported to be dry; however, three underwent reoperation for mechanical complications. No infections or erosions occurred. It seems from this report that transvaginal dissection of the urethra is as safe as transabdominal dissection with a similar success rate.

Whereas some patients with small preoperative bladder capacity may experience expansion after insertion of an artificial sphincter, this is not universally true. Up to 30 percent of patients may require subsequent augmentation cystoplasty.[31] The potential complications of this procedure have drastically decreased as mechanical improvements in the implants have developed through the years. Erosion or infection is currently experienced by approximately 10 percent of patients. Simultaneous placement of an artificial urinary sphincter and bladder augmentation has been reported and may be successful if meticulous technique and antibiotic coverage are employed.[31]

Sling Procedures

Although several inorganic materials have been used to create a sling (e.g., Marlex mesh, nylon, Mersilene, Silastic), most slings do not incorporate a prosthetic material and achieve external urethral compression by applying autologous tissues in a hammock-like support around the urethra. The surgical procedures vary in the choice of the tissue used to apply the compression and the tissues to which it is anchored.

PUBOVAGINAL SLING. The operative technique for a pubovaginal sling, as reported by Blaivas,[32] uses a combined abdominal-vaginal approach. A low transverse abdominal incision is made and the rectus sheath is divided, ensuring that the inferior fascial flap is at least 4 to 5 cm above the symphysis. A 1 × 12-cm long strip of rectus and external oblique fascia is cut from the lower margin of the fascial incision. An incision is then made in the anterior vaginal wall, and the vaginal mucosa is reflected laterally off the posterior urethra and bladder neck. Sutures are attached to the fascial sling. Next, a clamp is used to puncture the rectus fascia, and the sutures are passed anteriorly. Finally, these sutures are secured to the fascia, and the bladder is drained by a suprapubic cystostomy tube.

McGuire and associates[33] reported their experience with a fascial sling in 81 female patients treated between the years 1983 and 1986. The sling was done in conjunction with undiversion and bladder augmentation in three patients and with augmentation cystoplasty in five other patients. Most of the patients had previously undergone at least one operation for stress incontinence. After the surgery, initial success occurred in 67 patients, with 15 failures. Of these failures, seven were related to urethral dysfunction and four were rendered continent by either another sling procedure (two) or medication (two). A total of eight patients suffered detrusor-related incontinence postoperatively; of these, two required augmentation cystoplasty. In long-term follow-up 78 patients (95 percent) were reported continent, with 12 being on a planned intermittent self-catheterization program.

VAGINAL WALL SLING. Through a better understanding of the anatomy of the pelvic floor and bladder neck, we have improved the vaginal sling procedure, which previously involved the creation of a vaginal flap and burying of vaginal wall. The modified anterior vaginal wall sling is now our procedure of choice for stress incontinence caused by anatomical changes as well as ISD. It involves the creation of a sling using vaginal wall and underlying fascial structures, which provide both compression and support for the midurethra.

Vaginal Wall Sling for AI and ISD

In recent years a new technique for creating a sling without burying vaginal epithelium has been developed. The principles that led to its development included (1) a need to correct a defect of midurethral support, (2) a better understanding of the anatomy of the levator musculature as it envelops the urethra just distal to the pubourethral ligaments, and (3) evidence to suggest that the bladder neck is not the most important mechanism of continence. Most bladder neck suspension procedures elevate the bladder neck, creating a valvular effect, but do not have an impact on the midurethral area. Like any new procedure, the sling for AI and ISD should be easy to perform, produce minimal morbidity, and require a short hospital stay. The Raz vaginal wall sling for AI and ISD involves construction of a sling from the vaginal wall and underlying fascia that provides both compression and support for the urethra. The technique is demonstrated in Figures 91–13 and 91–14.

The patient is placed in the dorsal lithotomy position. A weighted vaginal speculum and labial retraction sutures are used for exposure. A suprapubic tube and urethral catheter are placed. After the tissues have been infiltrated with saline to facilitate dissection, two incisions are made in the anterior vaginal wall. A rectangular segment of anterior vaginal wall and fascia underlying the urethra and bladder neck is developed. No. 1 Prolene sutures are applied to the bladder neck area. These sutures encompass the urethropelvic ligaments, the pubocervical fascia, and the vaginal wall without epithelium. The midurethra is supported by a second set of sutures. These encompass the levator musculature as it enters and envelops the midurethral segment, the urethropelvic ligament, and the vaginal wall without epithelium. A Raz double-pronged needle carrier is used to transfer the sutures to a suprapubic location. No vaginal flaps are created and no transverse incision is made over the urethral area or the area of the bladder neck. No vaginal tissue is buried. The advantage of this technique lies in its simplicity, the avoidance of a laparotomy, short hospital stay, lateral placement of permanent nonreactive sutures, and the ability to correct

cystocele. The technique relies on healthy, well-vascularized supporting tissues.

The results of this technique have recently been reviewed in 86 patients with intrinsic sphincteric dysfunction resulting from failed stress incontinence surgery or patients with significant stress incontinence regardless of the anatomical position of the bladder neck and urethra. Fifty-six percent of patients underwent two to six previous procedures for urinary incontinence. Eighty-one of 86 patients denied any stress incontinence and were not wearing protection. Fifty-eight percent of the 86 patients had associated urgency incontinence preoperatively. Postoperatively the preoperative urgency incontinence had resolved in 60 percent. De novo instability was found in 7 percent. No patient required permanent self-catheterization. The results of short-term follow-up are encouraging; however, long-term follow-up is required.

VAGINAL WALL ISLAND SLING. Before the advent of the vaginal wall sling for AI and ISD, a technique utilizing an island of vaginal wall was employed at the University of California at Los Angeles (UCLA). In this technique a rectangular island of vaginal wall was buried under normal vaginal epithelium after the creation of a vaginal flap.[34] This provided a mechanism to increase urethral compression. This technique has been replaced by the sling for AI and ISD at our center.

SURGICAL TREATMENT OF VAGINAL WALL PROLAPSE

Surgery for vaginal wall prolapse pertains to corrective measures for repair of uterine prolapse, cystocele, enterocele, rectocele, and perineal floor laxity. A pelvic surgeon who is involved in the surgical treatment of female urinary incontinence should also be able to recognize and treat the various types of pelvic prolapse. Awareness of proper surgical technique will facilitate correction of all significant pelvic pathological conditions with one combined surgical procedure, in cooperation with our gynecological colleagues when appropriate.

Anterior Vaginal Wall Prolapse

Anterior vaginal wall prolapse is the most common type of pelvic prolapse. Structures adjacent to the anterior vaginal wall that may be involved in the prolapse include the urethra, bladder neck, and bladder base. With the patient in the dorsal lithotomy position, vaginal examination with the lower portion of the vaginal speculum exposes the anterior vaginal wall. It is examined with the patient at rest and while straining. Significant descent of the proximal urethra and bladder neck with straining is usually identified in women with stress urinary incontinence, and this is effectively treated with transvaginal needle suspension, as already discussed.

In addition to urethral descent into the anterior vagina with stress, the bladder may also herniate through the anterior vaginal wall because of attenuated and defective pubocervical fascia. On careful examination of the anterior vaginal wall (with a full bladder), a significant bulge through the anterior vaginal wall proximal to the area of the bladder neck indicates the presence of a cystocele. Cystoceles may be categorized into one of four groups: minimal hypermobility of the bladder base (grade I), bladder base descent to the introitus (grade II), bladder base descent outside the introitus with straining (grade III), and herniation of the bladder base outside the introitus at rest (grade IV). A voiding cystourethrogram in the standing position is an important adjunct to physical examination in evaluating the degree of cystocele. This radiographical study gives an objective evaluation of bladder position in an upright patient, information that is very difficult to obtain on physical examination with the patient in the standing position.

When grade I cystocele is present, it usually can be corrected at the time of needle bladder neck suspension (as previously described). If there is a moderate cystocele (grades II and III), we correct it by performing six-corner bladder and bladder neck suspension. We reserve the technique of formal cystocele repair for severe (grade IV) cystocele (Table 91–2).

Six-Corner Bladder and Bladder Neck Suspension

We have designed a bladder and bladder neck suspension procedure that corrects moderate bladder prolapse and repositions the bladder neck in a high retropubic position without the need for dissection and reapproximation of the attenuated pubocervical fascia. As one would expect, this procedure is particularly well suited for patients with isolated lateral defects. In this technique the bladder base and bladder neck are resuspended by permanent sutures that anchor the urethropelvic fascia, the pubocervical fascia, the cardinal ligaments, and the vaginal wall.

With the patient under general or regional anesthesia and in a dorsal lithotomy position, a weighted vaginal retractor is positioned and the labia are retracted laterally with stay sutures. A suprapubic tube and a urethral Foley catheter are placed. The bladder neck is identified by placing traction on the Foley catheter and palpating the balloon. Two parallel incisions are made in the anterior vaginal wall with their distal ends at the level of the middle urethra. The base of the incision extends farther posteriorly beyond the bladder neck to the bladder base and toward the level of the cardinal ligaments. If the uterus is still present, the incision is carried lateral to the cervix. The vaginal epithelium is dissected laterally toward the pubic bone at the level of the bladder neck, and the retropubic space is entered. Next, the urethropelvic fascia is detached from its attachment to the pelvic side wall and the urethra is bluntly and sharply freed up from any adhesions. Three pairs of No. 1 Prolene sutures are placed on each side. The two distal sutures are placed at the level of the mid-urethra and incorporate the levator muscle, the urethropelvic ligament, and the tissue of the anterior vaginal wall (minus the epithelium). The middle sutures are placed at the level of the bladder neck, incorporating the full thickness of the vaginal wall except for epithelium, the vesicopelvic (or pubocervical) fascia, and the lateral edge of the urethropelvic fascia in a helical fashion. The two proximal sutures are placed at the level of the bladder base, incorporating the full thickness of the vaginal wall except for epithelium, the pubocervical fascia, and the anterior extension of the cardinal ligaments in a helical fashion. The strength of the anchor is tested by pulling on the sutures and virtually moving the patient on the table. The three sets of sutures are transferred to the suprapubic position with a double-pronged ligature carrier, under finger guidance, through a small suprapubic incision. Cystoscopy is performed after indigo carmine is injected intravenously to verify proper suspension of the bladder and the patency of the ureters and to rule out penetration of suture material into the bladder. After the vaginal wall is closed, the suspension sutures are tied individually and then to each other across the midline over the rectus fascia.

Between 1984 and 1988, 120 patients with grade II and grade III cystoceles underwent four-corner bladder and bladder neck suspension at UCLA. A total of 107 patients were available for follow-up that ranged from 6 months to 5 years, with an average follow-up of 2 years. Eighty-four of 89 (94 percent) patients

TABLE 91–2. Surgery for Anterior Vaginal Wall Prolapse

Grade	Definition	Therapy
I	Bladder neck hypermobility	Bladder neck suspension
II	Bladder base reaching introitus with strain	Four-corner bladder and bladder neck suspension
III	Bladder neck bulging through introitus with strain	Four-corner bladder and bladder neck suspension
IV	Bladder base outside introitus at rest	Bladder neck suspension and classical cystocele repair

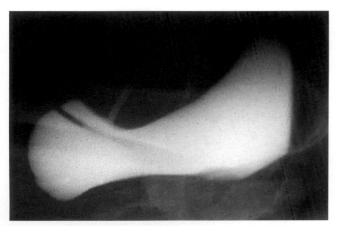

Figure 91–16. Cystogram revealing a grade IV cystocele. Marked descent of the bladder with hourglass appearance is noted. The intraureteric ridge can be clearly seen.

with preoperative incontinence were cured of incontinence or greatly improved, and cure of the cystocele (no cystocele or a mild degree) was seen in 105 of 107 cases (98 percent).[35]

Surgical Repair of Grade IV Cystocele

Grade IV cystocele, with or without stress urinary incontinence, results from severe weakness of the pubocervical fascia with large herniation of the bladder base in the midline (Fig. 91–16). Repair of a grade IV cystocele requires attention to the status of the urethra. If only cystocele repair is performed, de novo incontinence may ensue after the change of the urethral axis and anatomical position. On the other hand, if only bladder neck suspension is performed, the patient may develop obstructive symptoms and urinary retention secondary to creation of a valvular mechanism at the bladder neck. Urethral hypermobility in the presence of a cystocele is an example of combined loss of anterior support (urethropelvic ligaments, pubourethral ligaments, and pubocervical fascia), and all of these anatomical features need to be corrected to result in cure.

Three distinct goals are addressed in the repair of grade IV cystoceles:

1. Support and coaptation of the urethra. Evaluation of the urethra in this group of patients can be difficult and de novo incontinence may follow surgical repair. We use the vaginal wall sling for AI and ISD to address these concerns.

2. Repair of the lateral defect is accomplished by supporting the cardinal/uterosacral complex and the pubocervical fascia with suspension Prolene sutures.

3. Repair of the central defect is achieved through reapproximation of the cardinal/sacrouterine complex and the pubocervical fascia in the midline.

After induction of anesthesia, the patient is placed

in a dorsal lithotomy position. A weighted speculum is inserted, the labia are retracted laterally with stay sutures, and a suprapubic tube and urethral Foley catheter are introduced. A circular self-retaining retractor is positioned. While traction is placed on the Foley catheter, the bladder neck is identified by palpating the balloon. If the uterus is present, we perform the vaginal hysterectomy first. We do not close the cuff at this time and we leave tags on the sacrouterine/cardinal complex. A goalpost incision is then made in the anterior vaginal wall with the two arms extending distally toward the middle urethra and the center post extending toward the level of the sacrouterine/cardinal ligament complex (Fig. 91–17). The vaginal wall is dissected laterally in the avascular plane between the vaginal wall and pubocervical fascia, and the herniated bladder base is freed up. The edges of the pubocervical fascia are identified. The dissection is carried posteriorly to the peritoneal fold. At that stage the urethral hypermobility is corrected with a vaginal wall sling, as previously described, with the suspension sutures anchoring the inner part of the anterior vaginal wall, the levator musculature, and the edge of the urethropelvic fascia in a helical fashion. The lateral defect is repaired by using Prolene sutures to incorporate the medial edge of the urethropelvic ligaments, the sacrouterine/cardinal ligament complex, and the pubocervical fascia (Fig. 91–18). A small puncture in the suprapubic area is made, and the suspension sutures are transferred with a double-pronged ligature carrier. During passage the carrier should scratch the symphysis to minimize mobility and avoid postoperative pain. These sutures are left untied temporarily. The cystocele is then reduced with a Dexon mesh. The central defect is repaired by placing mattress sutures of 2-0 polyglactin to reapproximate the pubocervical fascia and

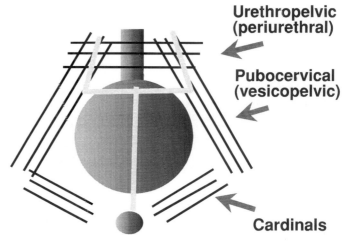

Figure 91–17. Schematic drawing of a patient with a grade IV cystocele. Note the divergence of the pubocervical fascia and cardinal ligaments. The goalpost incision is superimposed.

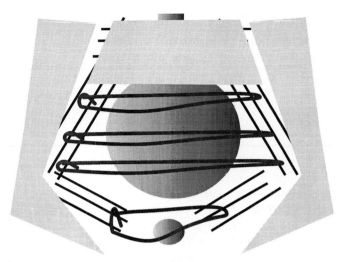

Figure 91–18. Repair of the lateral defect. The pubocervical (vesico-pelvic) fascia and the cardinal ligaments are supported with sutures that will be passed anteriorly to a suprapubic stab wound and secured to the rectus fascia. Note too the sutures in the urethropelvic fascia, which will also be passed to the suprapubic incision.

the cardinal ligaments in the midline (Fig. 91–19). Once cystoscopy confirms adequate suspension of the bladder neck and the patency of the ureters and that no suture material traverses the bladder, the vaginal incision is closed after the excess vaginal wall is trimmed, and the suspension sutures are tied as described.

This technique of repair has been used at UCLA for approximately 2 years. Six-month to 1-year results are available for 29 of 31 patients who underwent repair in 1993. Preoperative evaluation included lateral cystography, videourodynamics studies, and cystoscopy. Preoperative and postoperative scores of 0 to 3 were assigned using the SEAPI incontinence classification method (0, cure; 1, mild symptoms; 2,

moderate symptoms; 3, severe symptoms). The variables included S for activity-related incontinence, E for emptying ability, A for degree of anatomical defect, P for use of protection, and I for instability.

Subjective stress results showed 17 patients with preoperative stress urinary incontinence (SUI). Postoperatively, four patients had subjective SUI. Only one patient developed de novo stress incontinence (S-1). With regard to emptying ability, 28 of 29 patients emptied the bladder with clinically insignificant residuals (scores 0 to 1) and one patient had preoperative and postoperative retention requiring intermittent straight catheterization. Regarding the correction of the anatomical defect, 27 of 29 had excellent repair of the severe cystocele with scores 0 to 1, and two patients developed recurrent asymptomatic cystoceles. Protection results showed two patients with a rare need for pads (S-1) and two patients requiring daily use of pads for occasional incontinence (S-2). Preoperative instability was present in 20 of 29 patients and resolved in 17 patients. Four patients developed de novo instability. Only one patient had progression of inhibition score by more than one point.

Enterocele Repair

An enterocele is defined as a true hernia at the apex of the vagina. The major supporting structures for the uterus and vagina are the uterosacral ligaments and the cardinal ligaments. When there is wide separation of these structures (either before or after hysterectomy), a potential space is created. Peritoneum, with its contents, can herniate inferiorly into this space, forming an enterocele. The two major types of enteroceles are traction enteroceles and pulsion enteroceles. Traction enteroceles are found in association with prolapse of the uterus. Pulsion enteroceles are most commonly found after hysterectomy secondary to separation of the sacrouterine complex and enlargement of the cul-de-sac. Urologists should be aware of the incidence of enterocele after Burch colposuspension (5 to 17 percent) and anterior bladder neck suspension (3 percent).

The clinical manifestation of an enterocele is a vaginal mass causing increasing pain and discomfort and, depending on its size, rarely leading to bowel obstruction. On pelvic examination, the enterocele appears as a bulge high in the vagina, either posterior to the cervix (if it is present) or at the apex of the vaginal vault after hysterectomy (most commonly). Because an enterocele is frequently associated with a rectocele (see below), the enterocele bulge may appear as a high continuation of the bulge in the posterior vaginal wall. The enterocele sac may contain bowel, which is visible through the attenuated vagi-

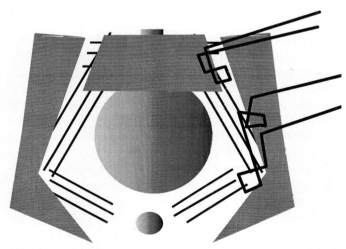

Figure 91–19. Repair of the central defect is demonstrated. The pubocervical (vesicopelvic) fascia is plicated and the cardinal ligaments are reapposed.

nal wall. With a finger in the rectum, the impulse of the enterocele hernia sac may be felt against the fingertip during coughing (analogous to the impulse felt during examination for an inguinal hernia). When performing a bimanual vaginal-rectal examination, an increased thickness of the rectal-vaginal septum high in the vagina at the level of the enterocele will be noted. Physical examination with the patient in the standing position will reveal a hernia into the vagina from posterior to the cervix (or emerging from the vaginal vault after hysterectomy). A voiding cystourethrogram is always performed to verify that the bladder is not part of the bulging mass.

After induction of anesthesia the patient is placed in a dorsal lithotomy position. The rectum is packed with Betadine-impregnated lubricated gauze and isolated from the surgical field. A weighted posterior vaginal retractor is placed in the vagina, and the labia are retracted laterally with stay sutures. The bladder is emptied with a Foley catheter, and a Scott retractor is positioned. The enterocele bulge is grasped with two Allis clamps, and a vertical incision is carried out in the vaginal epithelium over the bulge. The peritoneal hernia sac is identified and dissected away from the vaginal wall, bladder, and rectum using sharp and blunt dissection. The sac is opened and its contents are reduced. The uterosacral and cardinal ligaments are identified laterally, and two sets of interrupted No. 1 polyglycolic acid sutures are placed in the uterosacral and cardinal ligaments on each side. These are secured with a clamp to be tied later. We use a modified McCall culdoplasty for vaginal cuff support. In our technique a suture is passed from outside to inside the open sac. This stitch should incorporate the sacrouterine/cardinal complex. This suture then incorporates the prerectal fascia and the contralateral sacrouterine/cardinal complex. The suture exits on the ipsilateral side (Fig. 91–20). An identical suture is placed on the contralateral side. These sutures will generally provide good cuff sup-

TABLE 91–3. Classification of Posterior Lacerations of the Fourchette

Grade	Extent of Laceration
I	Involving only the mucosa
II	Involving the bulbocavernosus and superficial and deep transverse perineal muscles
III	Involving the rectal sphincter
IV	Involving the rectal mucosa

port. However, in cases of severe prolapse, sacrospinalis fixation of the vault may be required. After completion of the culdoplasty, two pursestring sutures of No. 1 polyglycolic acid are placed more proximally, incorporating prerectal fascia posteriorly, the cardinal and uterosacral ligaments laterally, and the vesicopelvic ligaments and perivesical fascia anteriorly. A Haney retractor is used to hold the trigone upward so that the ureters will be avoided. The sutures are then tied in a proximal-to-distal direction, thus obliterating the space of Douglas. The remaining peritoneal sac is suture ligated at its base and excised. The redundant vaginal epithelium is excised and the vaginal incision closed, incorporating the peritoneal stump in the closure to eliminate the space.

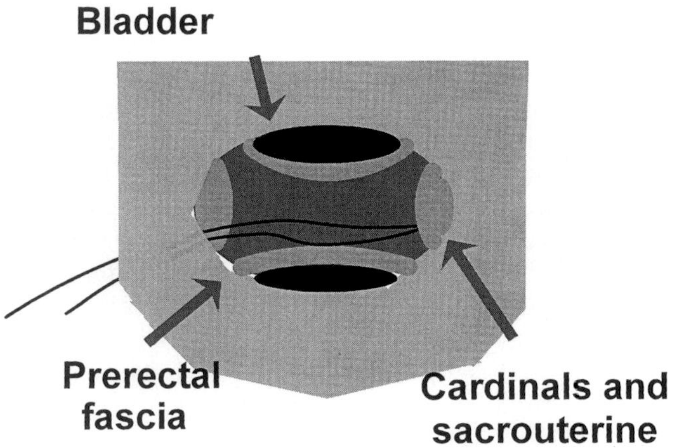

The technique of enterocele repair must be amended when concurrent vault prolapse is found. In these cases the vault must be addressed to ensure success of the procedure. When vault prolapse is found with a cystocele, we perform vaginal vault suspension with the enterocele repair. When vault prolapse is found without cystocele, we repair the enterocele and perform sacrospinous fixation of the vaginal vault.

Posterior Vaginal Wall Prolapse—Rectocele and Perineal Laxity Repair

A rectocele is defined as a herniation of the anterior rectal wall through the prerectal fascia into the posterior vagina. This develops when the prerectal fascia is insufficient to support the rectum. Because perineal laxity caused by attenuation and laceration of the perineal muscles (Table 91–3) usually accompanies a rectocele, perineal reconstruction is also carried out at the time of rectocele repair.

The diagnosis of rectocele is made when the patient complains of a bulging mass through the vagina. This usually occurs with straining and may be accompanied by difficulties in evacuation of stool during defecation. On pelvic examination the rectocele appears as a bulge in the posterior vaginal wall. Occasionally there may be a coexistent enterocele, which appears as a bulge high in the posterior vaginal wall

Bladder

Prerectal fascia   Cardinals and sacrouterine

Figure 91–20. Schematic diagram of a modified McCall culdoplasty.

or at the vaginal apex. Preoperative appreciation of both of these types of herniation is essential so that proper surgical measures can be taken. On rectal examination the anterior rectal wall is palpated, and the extent of the rectal herniation into the posterior vagina is readily demonstrated. As already mentioned, when a large symptomatic rectocele is present, there is usually associated laxity and attenuation of the perineum, which on examination appears as a large gaping introitus.

Surgical repair of rectocele incorporates three components: (1) plication of prerectal and pararectal fascia, (2) reapproximation of the relaxed levator hiatus, and (3) perineal repair.

After induction of anesthesia, the patient is placed in a dorsal lithotomy position. The rectum is packed with Betadine-impregnated lubricated gauze and then isolated from the operative field. The labia are retracted laterally with stay sutures and the bladder is drained with a Foley catheter. The introitus is inspected, and if significant perineal and introital weakness is present (as is usually the case), two Allis clamps are applied to the mucocutaneous junction at the 5 and 7 o'clock positions of the posterior introitus. These clamps are placed so that when they are brought together in the midline, a normal-sized introitus is created. The mucocutaneous junction is then excised between these two clamps. A circular self-retaining retractor is positioned. Two Allis clamps are applied to the rectocele bulge, and a triangular incision is made in the posterior vaginal wall with the apex of the triangle at the apex of the vault and the base of the triangle along the previously made perineal incision. A plane is developed between the herniated rectal wall and the vaginal epithelium with careful sharp dissection on the vaginal wall itself, staying as close to vaginal epithelium as possible to avoid injury to the rectum. The dissection is continued laterally to expose the prerectal and pararectal fascia. The isolated triangle of vaginal epithelium is excised, as is the excessive vaginal wall on both sides of the dissected rectocele. Obliteration of the rectocele defect in the posterior vaginal wall is done with a single layer of running, locking No. 2-0 polyglycolic acid suture, starting at the apex of the vault. The sutures incorporate the edge of the vaginal epithelium and a generous bite of the prerectal and pararectal fascia. The fascia is thus approximated in the midline over the reduced rectocele. The levator musculature is then reapproximated (Fig. 91–21). Finally, the perineal laxity is corrected by using two or three No. 2-0 polyglycolic acid sutures, placed in a horizontal mattress fashion to reapproximate (in the midline) the weakened and separated perineal muscles. This maneuver will reinforce the perineal floor and central perineal tendon. The perineal skin is closed with a running No. 4-0 polyglycolic acid suture.

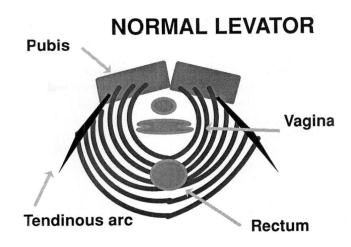

A

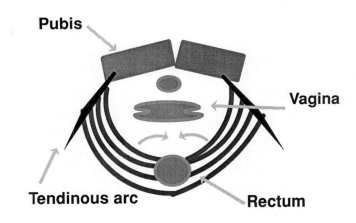

B

Figure 91–21. *A* and *B*, Schematic diagram of normal and relaxed levator musculature.

POSTOPERATIVE CARE FOR VAGINAL SURGERY

In addition to the standard postsurgical care, vaginal surgery has its own routine for immediate postoperative management of diet, medications, catheters, vaginal packing, and physical activity.

The patient is permitted to take food and medications orally as soon as tolerated. Prophylactic antibiotics are continued intravenously for one or two doses, and then the patient is switched to an oral agent, usually a cephalosporin or quinolone. In uncomplicated vaginal surgery for incontinence or prolapse, the urethral catheter and vaginal packing are removed on the first postoperative day, and the suprapubic tube, if present, is plugged. The patient is instructed in the use of this tube to measure residuals and to drain the bladder until adequate emptying is achieved. The patient is usually told to restrict fluid intake (1000 ml/day) and is discharged home on the first or second postoperative day. Oral stool softeners are prescribed. There are no limitations on physical activity. The suprapubic catheter is removed once the postvoid residual is less than 2 ounces. If by 2 weeks after surgery the patient is still unable to void, the suprapubic catheter is removed and the patient is started on an intermittent self-catheterization program until satisfactory bladder emptying ensues.

Editorial Comment

Fray F. Marshall

This chapter demonstrates the total approach to female incontinence and vaginal wall prolapse. The management approaches to stress incontinence, cystocele, enterocele, and rectocele are reviewed. A detailed description of the female anatomy helps the understanding of its management. Although many nonsurgical changes are occurring in urology, surgical management of stress incontinence and prolapse in female patients will likely be necessary for some time.

REFERENCES

1. Staskin DR, Hadley HR, Leach GE, et al. Anatomy for vaginal surgery. Semin Urol 4:2, 1986.
2. Kelly HA, Dumm WM. Urinary incontinence in women, without manifest injury to the bladder. Surg Gynecol Obstet 18:444, 1914.
3. Aldridge AH. Transplantation of fascia for relief of urinary stress incontinence. Am J Obstet Gynecol 44:398, 1942.
4. Marshall VF, Marchetti AA, Krantz KE. The correction of stress incontinence by simple vesicourethral suspension. Surg Gynecol Obstet 88:509, 1949.
5. Burch JC. Urethrovaginal fixation to Cooper's ligament for correction of stress incontinence, cystocele, and prolapse. Am J Obstet Gynecol 81:281, 1961.
6. Cardozo LD, Kelleher CJ, Khullar V. Gauging the success of surgery for genuine stress incontinence: Can we improve on the colposuspension? Published abstracts of the Proceedings of the International Continence Society. Neurourol Urodyn 13:1994.
7. Pereyra AJ. Simplified surgical procedure for the correction of stress incontinence in women. West J Surg 67:223, 1959.
8. Harer WB, Gunther RE. Simplified urethrovesical suspension and urethroplasty. Am J Obstet Gynecol 91:1017, 1965.
9. Pereyra AJ, Lebherz TB. Combined urethrovesical suspension and vaginourethroplasty for correction of urinary stress incontinence. Obstet Gynecol 30:537, 1967.
10. Tauber R, Wapner P. Surgical repair of severe and recurrent urinary incontinence. Obstet Gynecol 30:741, 1967.
11. Stamey TA. Endoscopic suspension of the vesical neck for urinary incontinence. Surg Gynecol Obstet 136:547, 1973.
12. Winter CC. Unilateral and bilateral bladder neck suspension operation for stress urinary incontinence. J Urol 116:47, 1976.
13. Cobb OE, Ragde H. Simplified correction of female stress incontinence. J Urol 120:418, 1978.
14. Raz S. Modified bladder neck suspension for female stress incontinence. Urology 17:82, 1981.
15. Hadley HR, Zimmern PE, Staskin DR, Raz S. Transvaginal needle bladder neck suspension. Urol Clin North Am 12:291, 1985.
16. Gittes RF, Loughlin KR. No-incision pubovaginal suspension for stress incontinence. J Urol 138:568, 1987.
17. Young HH. An operation for the cure of incontinence of urine. Surg Gynecol Obstet 28:84, 1919.
18. Leadbetter GW, Fraley FE. Surgical correction of total urinary incontinence. Five years after. J Urol 97:869, 1967.
19. Tanagho EA. Bladder neck reconstruction for total urinary incontinence: 10 years of experience. J Urol 125:321, 1981.
20. Carrion HM, Politano VA. Periurethral polytef (Teflon) injection for urinary incontinence. In Raz S, ed. Female Urology. Philadelphia, WB Saunders, 1983, p 293.
21. Malizia AA Jr, Reiman HM, Myers RP, et al. Migration and granulomatous reaction after periurethral injections of Polytef (Teflon). JAMA 251:3277, 1984.
22. Kursh E, McGuire E, eds. Female Urology. Philadelphia, JB Lippincott, 1994.
23. Leonard MP, Canning DA, Epstein JI, et al. Local tissue reaction to the subureteral injection of gluteraldehyde cross-linked bovine collagen in humans. J Urol 143:1209, 1990.
24. Appel RA. Periurethral collagen injection for female incontinence. Probl Urol 5:134, 1991.
25. Appel RA. Injectables for urethral incompetence. World J Urol 8:208, 1990.
26. Goldenberg SL. Periurethral collagen injection for patients with stress urinary incontinence. Presented at the annual meeting of the Canadian Urological Association, Montreal, Canada, 1993.
27. CR Bard Inc. Contigen Bard Collagen Implant: Important patient information supplement. Educational publiclication, 1993.
28. Raz S, ed. Atlas of Transvaginal Surgery. Philadelphia, WB Saunders, 1992.
29. Scott FB. The use of the artificial sphincter in the treatment of urinary incontinence in the female patient. Urol Clin North Am 12:305, 1985.
30. Appel RA. Techniques and results in the implantation of the artificial urinary sphincter in women with type III stress urinary incontinence by a vaginal approach. Neurourol Urodyn 7:613, 1988.
31. Adams MC, Mitchell ME, Rink RC, et al. Gastrocystoplasty: An alternative solution to the problem of urological reconstruction in the severely compromised patient. J Urol 140:1152, 1988.
32. Blaivas JG. Pubovaginal Sling. Kursh ED, McGuire E, eds. Female Urology. Philadelphia, JB Lippincott, 1994.
33. McGuire EJ, Bennet CJ, Konnak JA, et al. Experience with pubovaginal slings for urinary incontinence at the University of Michigan. J Urol 138:525, 1987.
34. Raz S, Siegel AL, Short JL, Synder JA. Vaginal wall sling. J Urol 141:43, 1989.
35. Klutke CG, Golomb J, Raz S. Four corner bladder and urethral suspension for moderate cystocele. J Urol 142:712, 1989.
36. Raz S, et al. Vaginal wall sling. Presented at the annual meeting of the American Urologic Association, San Antonio, TX, 1993.
37. Strawbridge LR, et al. Augmentation cystoplasty and the artificial geniturinary sphincter. J Urol 142:297, 1989.

Chapter 92

Management of Voiding Dysfunction Following Incontinence Surgery

George D. Webster

Cystourethropexy for the correction of stress urinary incontinence is a commonly performed urological and gynecological procedure, and a successful outcome is anticipated in 80 to 90 percent of cases. Perhaps because of the relative simplicity of most of these procedures, an adverse outcome is rarely anticipated by the surgeon and may not be discussed with the patient. However, clinical experience and review of the literature prove that these procedures are of suspect durability and certainly have a significant incidence of postoperative problems. The patient's preoperative expectation may be that her incontinence will be permanently cured by surgery, whereas in reality an excellent early success rate is often followed by relatively early return of incontinence.[1] These long-term failures are not procedure specific, and unfortunately, because of the variations in groups treated, comparison of one procedure with another is not possible.

This chapter does not specifically address late recurrent stress urinary incontinence but focuses on the problem of iatrogenic outlet obstruction leading to voiding dysfunction. This may result in obstructive symptoms with inefficient bladder emptying or even total urinary retention, or it may result in the emergence of postoperative bladder instability symptoms such as urinary frequency, urgency, and urge incontinence. Recurrent infections are also common in this scenario. The incidence of this problem after anti-incontinence surgery is not well documented but is estimated to be between 2.5 and 24 percent for the variety of procedures performed.[2–6]

The procedures for correction of stress urinary incontinence in women include anterior colporrhaphy, a variety of retropubic suspensions, endoscopic needle suspensions, and sling cystourethropexy.[7–13] Although, in reality, procedure selection seems to be primarily based on the individual surgeon's philosophy and preference, other factors that should influence procedure selection include the need for simultaneous repair of other vaginal pathology such as prolapse; the patient's age and body habitus, which may render a vaginal approach more appropriate; any history of previous repairs and the resultant anatomical changes; and the possible need for simultaneous abdominal surgery such as hysterectomy. In addition to these considerations regarding procedure selection, it is probable that no technique is exempt from complication, and some procedures may lend themselves more readily to resultant obstruction than others. Historically, the sling procedure carried a high risk of obstruction, but current techniques render this complication rare.[14] Needle suspension procedures, whether performed by the Raz, Stamey, or Gittes technique, all have the potential to cause obstruction. The Raz technique carries a lesser risk, the sutures being placed distant from the urethra; while the Stamey and Gittes procedures, relying on endoscopic suture placement, may more commonly have such adverse outcomes. The Marshall-Marchetti-Krantz (MMK) procedure has been singled out as a cause of postoperative urinary obstruction.[15, 16] Parnell and colleagues reported a 28.5 percent incidence of emergent bladder "irritative" symptoms after the MMK suspension, most of which are likely due to outlet obstruction. It is my opinion that the procedure least likely to cause obstruction is the paravaginal fascial repair.[9] Even the Burch colposuspension, purported to avoid obstruction by avoidance of overcorrection or distortion of the urethral axis, carries a high reported incidence of emergent bladder instability.[6]

Most patients have a period of voiding dysfunction during the initial days and even weeks after cystourethropexy, but with the resolution of surgical trauma, voiding should become efficient and urgency symptoms should resolve. During the immediate postoperative procedure, some physicians rely on suprapubic catheter drainage, and others teach clean intermittent self-catheterization. Neither technique appears to have an advantage over the other. Because the time to return of efficient emptying and resolution of instability symptoms is so variable, there is no absolute postoperative time at which concern should register. Total persistent retention 1 month after surgery and persistence of bladder instability symptoms with urge incontinence 3 months after surgery, particularly if associated with voiding problems, indicate a need for concern and investigation.

Bladder instability symptoms are common in women with stress incontinence, occurring in up to 50 percent of patients presenting for surgery. In most these symptoms resolve after cystourethropexy, and their preoperative presence should have been identified and the patient counseled regarding their likelihood of resolution, or their management, should they persist.[18] De novo or emergent bladder instability symptoms have been reported in a small percentage of women as a natural consequence of the perivesical dissection of bladder neck suspension surgery.[17] However, in my opinion, in most cases they result from relative outlet obstruction. Preexisting bladder instability symptoms may be of congenital origin, in which case their history will be of long standing; may be anatomical because of the pelvic floor relaxation phenomenon that is to be corrected by suspension surgery; may be due to aging phenomena; or may be idiopathic.

Persistent voiding problems after bladder neck suspension surgery may have their basis in preexisting poor detrusor contractility. This may be preoperatively identified by a history of voiding symptoms with hesitancy and poor flow, a history of previous retention, or the identification of significant postvoid residual urine. Preoperative urodynamics should be performed in such cases; important evidence would be features such as bladder hyposensitivity, large bladder capacity, poor detrusor contractility during the voiding study, the absence of an isometric contraction, and an intermittent flow pattern with inefficient emptying. Preoperative pressure flow studies are not always performed in women undergoing surgery for stress urinary incontinence but certainly are indicated when there are these warning signs. Many women with stress urinary incontinence void with a negligible detrusor contraction, presumably because of low outlet resistance, and identification of adequate detrusor contractility or of an isometric contraction during the "stop flow test" may be difficult.[2]

In most women with postcystourethropexy voiding problems, preexisting poor detrusor contractility is not the cause. Outlet obstruction may result from the surgery itself because of a variety of events. Regardless of the procedure performed, the urethral axis may be overcorrected and the urethra obstructed against the retrosymphysis. Predisposing to this outcome is the overtightening of suspension sutures or the placement of suspension sutures too close to the urethra. The original description of the MMK procedure actually described suture placement through the urethral wall, a technique modified in later descriptions. The urethra may be distorted because of the inappropriate location of sutures. This is exemplified by suspension sutures placed at the midurethra, leaving the urethra to "hinge" and obstruct at this location. In patients in whom there is significant vaginal wall hypermobility, a MMK procedure, although adequately suspending the urethra, may leave the cystocele to rotate around the well-supported vesical neck, causing a valvular-like obstruction. Fibrosis of the urethra due to multiple repairs may also cause obstructive changes.

EVALUATION OF THE PATIENT WITH POSTCYSTOURETHROPEXY VOIDING DYSFUNCTION

Patient History

The diagnosis may be strongly suggested by the patient's history. Patients generally report preoperative stress urinary incontinence with no voiding symptoms or bladder irritative/instability symptoms. After cystourethropexy they experience delayed return of voiding function; once this is established, flow is generally intermittent and slow, the stream is often misdirected, and emptying is incomplete. Symptoms of bladder instability are present, including frequency and nocturia, urgency, and urge incontinence. Frequently the magnitude and unpredictability of urge incontinent episodes exceed the problem created by the original stress incontinence! Inefficient voiding and mild bladder instability symptoms are very common during the early postoperative period but generally resolve within 3 to 4 weeks. Voiding problems or even urinary retention are not uncommon even for 1 to 4 weeks after bladder neck suspension, and there is no agreement over when concern should be expressed that these symptoms are not going to resolve. In general, concern is registered only 6 to 12 weeks after surgery. If the diagnosis is made earlier, and if a needle suspension has been performed, the situation may be resolved by simply cutting the suspension sutures on one or both sides; this can be performed under local anesthesia, even in the office setting. However, the diagnosis is rarely made in such a timely fashion, and by the time it is certain that symptoms are going to persist, there is generally so much retropubic fixation from surgical adhesions that simply cutting the sutures does not release the urethra.

Physical Examination

Physical examination suggests the diagnosis in most cases. In my initial reported series, an overcorrected urethral axis was evident in all 15 cases.[19] In some cases the obstruction appears to be distortional as a result of urethropexy performed in the face of significant anterior vaginal wall hypermobility. In this event, while the urethra is pexed, the cystocele is left free to descend posterior to the vesical neck. This appears to be a more common event after MMK procedures. Identification of associated vaginal prolapse is important in planning the revision surgery.

Endoscopy

While urethral obstruction cannot be identified by urethroscopy, the fixed retropubic angulation of the urethra is generally demonstrated. In patients obstructed by a pubovaginal sling, the site of sling support may be evident and in some cases is seen to be distal to the bladder neck, in which event urethral distortion may occur as the proximal urethra may rotate around this fixed point. The appearance of the urethral mucosa may help determine whether intrinsic sphincter deficiency is present and whether incontinence is likely to recur after urethrolysis. An unhealthy-appearing urethra may dictate a need for sling procedure at the time of revision surgery.

Urodynamic Studies

Urodynamics is generally performed in all cases, although a number of reports comment on the difficulty such studies have in defining obstruction.[20] Customarily, provocative filling cystometry and a pressure flow micturition study are performed. Video urodynamics offers the best means for evaluating the obstructed bladder, because it allows anatomical localization of the site of obstruction.

Bladder irritative/instability symptoms of urinary frequency, nocturia, urgency, and urge incontinence are evaluated by filling cystometry; however, it is recognized that in some cases involuntary bladder contractions will not be identified. In a series previously reported by me, 13 of the 15 patients had bladder instability symptoms, but only five demonstrated involuntary contractions on provocative cystometry.[19] These patients are classified as having motor urge incontinence or bladder instability. The remaining eight patients by current terminology are classified as having sensory urgency. It is evident, however, that these patients are on a spectrum of the same disorder and perhaps in the laboratory setting were able to inhibit involuntary detrusor activity. In the series reported by Nitti and Raz, 30 of 41 patients (73 percent) had clinical instability symptoms, including 16 (39 percent) with urgency incontinence. However, urodynamic evidence of detrusor instability was documented in only 14 (34 percent).[20]

Bladder outlet obstruction is best defined by pressure flow micturition studies, but there is some controversy regarding the standardized definition of outlet obstruction in female patients. Massey and Abrams proposed that two or more of four parameters should be present for the diagnosis.[21] These include a flow rate of less than 12 ml/sec, a detrusor pressure at peak flow of greater than 50 cm water, urethral resistance (detrusor pressure at maximal flow rate divided by the square of maximal flow rate) greater than 0.2, and significant residual urine in the presence of high pressure or resistance. Using these criteria, these authors identified 2.74 percent of 5948 women undergoing urodynamic evaluation for a variety of complaints as having obstruction. Farrar et al used only flow rates to diagnose obstruction because they believed that low flow in the presence of normal or low detrusor pressure may be an indication of relative obstruction, defined as a maximal flow rate of less than 15 ml/sec with a volume of 200 ml or more.[22] Bass and Leach used a peak flow rate of greater than 15 ml/sec with a voided volume of greater than 100 ml, a normal uroflowmetry curve configuration, and no significant residual volume as exclusionary criteria for outlet obstruction.[23] Accepting that there is no consensus regarding hard criteria for the diagnosis of outlet obstruction in women, it is appropriate to consider Blaivas' philosophy that obstruction is to be considered in any case in which there is low flow in the face of a detrusor contraction that is adequate in force, speed, and duration.[24]

Notwithstanding this dilemma, pressure flow study results are reported from a number of series of postcystourethropexy patients with voiding dysfunction. Nitti and Raz, reporting a series of 41 obstructed women, comment that the strength of detrusor contraction preoperatively and pressure flow analysis did not predict outcome (Table 92–1).[20] They did, however, report that the preoperative postvoid residual was statistically significant in predicting outcome. The greater the postvoid residual, the more likely it was that urethrolysis would not be successful. Of their 41 patients, 29 percent (71 percent) had

TABLE 92–1. Preoperative Voiding Dynamics and Outcome of Urethrolysis

Maximum Detrusor Pressure (cm water)	No. Successful (%)	Maximal Flow Rate (ml/sec)	Total No. Patients (%)
30 or more	12 or less	23 (56)	16 (70)
	> 12	7 (17)	4 (57)
< 30	12 or less	5 (12)	3 (60)
	> 12	2 (5)	2 (100)
Acontractile	—	4 (10)	4 (100)

From Nitti VW, Raz S. Obstruction following anti-incontinence procedures: Diagnosis and treatment with transvaginal urethrolysis. J Urol 152:93, 1994.

a postvoid residual of 100 ml or more (mean 236 ml), while 12 (29 percent) had symptoms only without a significant postvoid residual (mean 50 ml). Overall, 29 of their patients (71 percent) were successfully managed by urethrolysis and resuspension of the vesical neck. Of these, 19 (66 percent) had initial postvoid residuals of greater than 100 ml (reducing significantly to a mean of 30 ml) postoperatively, and 10 of 12 (83 percent) had low preoperative postvoid residuals but severe voiding and irritative symptoms, in whom symptoms resolved. Only eight of the 41 patients still required clean intermittent catheterization after urethrolysis. Leach's group also reported pressure flow data in this condition, but unlike Raz they noted that preoperative postvoid residuals were not predictive of postoperative failure.[27]

Reviewing 32 patients with bladder instability and obstruction symptoms after bladder neck suspension, Mark and Webster found that 90 percent of patients presented with instability symptoms, 52 percent had urge incontinence, and 48 percent required self-intermittent catheterization.[25] These patients were categorized into different urodynamic groups after a videourodynamic pressure flow study (Table 92–2). After this evaluation, all patients underwent urethrolysis by a retropubic approach, and 30 of 32 were subsequently able to void satisfactorily, only two requiring self-catheterization. Bladder instability symptoms resolved in seven of ten. Our conclusion was that urodynamics was unable to predict those patients in whom urethrolysis would be unsuccessful, and that surgery for such de novo symptoms after cystourethropexy should be indicated by patient history, physical examination, and endoscopic findings.[25]

MANAGEMENT

This is an iatrogenic problem, the implication being that it may be avoidable. I have already addressed those issues most likely to result in obstruction: primarily misplaced sutures, overcorrection of the urethral axis by excessively tight sutures, periurethral or vaginal wall fibrosis resulting in extrinsic obstruction, and distortion due to vaginal prolapse (particularly cystocele) in the face of a normally pexed vesical neck. To be successful, vesical neck suspension procedures, whether by cystourethropexy or by pubovaginal sling, require only correction of the urethrovesical axis to an anatomical one. Particularly in the case of the pubovaginal sling procedure, the end point of sling tightening is one at which the sling abuts upon the vesical neck without occluding it, and this is easily ascertained endoscopically. Endoscopy at the termination of cystourethropexy is an invaluable adjunct to avoid these complications, for it allows one to judge the urethrovesical axis and ensure that there are no per urethral sutures. In an anesthetized woman with the bladder filled, a suprapubic Credé maneuver should be able to express urine from the urethra. The end point of cystourethropexy should not prevent this phenomenon.

TABLE 92–2. Outcome After Urethrolysis in 32 Women with Postcystourethropexy Voiding Dysfunction

		No. of Patients (%)	Successful Outcome	Failure Voiding Dysfunction	Instability	Genuine Stress Incontinence
Group A						
↑ Pressure (> 50 cm H₂O)	↓ Flow (< 12 ml/sec)	12 (38)	10	—	1	1
Group B						
↑ Pressure (> 50 cm H₂O)	↑ Flow (> 12 ml/sec)	9 (27)	7	1	1	1
Group C						
↓ Pressure (≤50 cm H₂O)	↓ Flow (≤ 12 ml/sec)	4 (13)	3	—	1	—
Group D						
Acontractile		7 (22)	6	1	—	—
Total		32*	26	2	3†	2

*Ten patients had preoperative detrusor instability.
†All three "failures" with persistent instability had detrusor instability or preoperative urodynamics, but seven out of 10 had complete resolution of symptoms.

To some degree, some women may be primed to develop postoperative voiding dysfunction and bladder instability symptoms. This group has been identified as those women with preexisting voiding dysfunction by history, postvoid residual urine estimation, or urodynamic study. Additionally, in women with preexisting bladder instability of long standing, those symptoms are unlikely to resolve after cystourethropexy. All women should be counseled preoperatively about these possibilities.

Conservative Management

The issue of initial expectant management has already been addressed: many women improve their voiding efficiency and have resolved bladder instability symptoms within the first 3 months after surgery. If retention or inefficient bladder emptying persist, the use of clean intermittent self-catheterization will temporize, and the frequency of catheterization will be dictated by the magnitude of the residual urine. Anticholinergic medications to reduce bladder instability symptoms may be helpful but may also reduce voiding efficiency. Urinary infection is not uncommon, and prophylactic antibacterial agents are given.

Urethral dilation has been advised but has limited success. Otis urethrotomy has also been used but may cause further harm because of damage to the intrinsic sphincter mechanism. Cutting the suspension sutures is rarely successful, as by the time a decision has been made that it is necessary, retropubic adhesions will have fixed the urethral and vaginal wall and a more formal surgical takedown will be required.

Surgical Urethrolysis

Three approaches to urethrolysis are described: transvaginal, abdominal/retropubic, and infrapubic. Each has its proponents, and probably each has its specific role.

Transvaginal Urethrolysis

The transvaginal approach has been reported by Nitti and Raz, McGuire et al, and Dmochowski et al.[20, 26, 27] Nitti and Raz suggest that it allows for complete mobilization of the urethra from the pubic bone; facilitates repair of any associated vaginal prolapse, which they identified in a significant number of their patients; and allows for the performance of a resuspension procedure. Cystocele, enterocele, or rectocele required repair in 15 of 41 (38 percent) of their patients. They addressed the issue of recurrent adherence of the urethra to the symphysis, suggesting that a Martius labial fat pad may be interposed. Nitti and

Raz also comment on the resuspension of the vesical neck using the Raz technique, which they found necessary in 18 of 19 patients who had persistent or recurrent stress urinary incontinence despite obstruction. McGuire et al, reporting urethrolysis in 13 women, noted only two patients who required resuspension and cystocele repair, and one with type III stress incontinence who underwent pubovaginal sling repair.[26]

TECHNIQUE. The vaginal procedure is performed with the patient in the lithotomy position. Anterior vaginal wall epithelial incisions are made on each side of the vesical neck from the midurethra cephalad for approximately 4 cm (Fig. 92–1). Scissor dissection of the epithelium from the underlying periurethral fascia is accomplished on each side until the vaginal wall structures are penetrated and the retropubic space entered quite laterally. This entering hiatus is enlarged and the retropubic space then dissected bluntly and sharply, freeing the urethra from the retrosymphysis. This dissection may be tedious but can be accomplished safely without penetration of urethra or bladder. A urethral Foley catheter aids in this dissection. Intraoperative endoscopy helps confirm an absence of injury and also confirms that lysis has been adequate and urethral mobility restored. Resuspension using the Raz technique consists of placement of a No. 1 Prolene helical suture through the medial edge of the urethropelvic ligament, bilaterally. The sutures are transferred across the retropubic space using a ligature carrier and tied over the rectus fascia. Generally, a suprapubic catheter is placed to facilitate the postoperative voiding trial.

Abdominal Urethrolysis

Webster and Kreder reported a series of women managed by abdominal urethrolysis.[19] This approach is advisable for surgeons lacking expertise for or experience of the more difficult vaginal dissection. Ideally the surgery is performed with the patient supine but with the legs abducted on leg supports so that the vagina is also accessible. A midline abdominal or Pfannenstiel incision is used and the retropubic space is carefully lysed with sharp dissection. By limiting the dissection to the region of the urethra, rather than including lateral pelvic lysis, the obstructing adhesion may be released but vaginal support preserved. To prevent readhesion to the retrosymphysis, an omental pedicle may be brought into the retropubic space. Once again, suprapubic catheter drainage is optimal.

Infrapubic Urethrolysis

The infrapubic procedure is performed using an inverted-U incision, the apex of which is between the

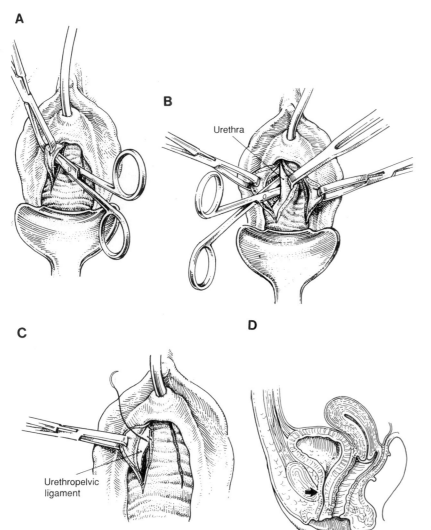

Figure 92–1. *A*, Inverted-U incision in the anterior vaginal wall and entrance into the retropubic space. *B*, The urethra is sharply dissected off the undersurface of the pubic bone. The urethropelvic ligament, periurethral fascia, and vaginal wall are retracted medially to expose the urethra in the retropubic space. *C*, Resuspension of the bladder neck by the Raz technique. *D*, Sagittal view shows the urethra fixed to the undersurface of the pubic bone (*arrow*). The urethra is completely freed after urethrolysis. (From Nitti VW, Raz S. Obstruction following anti-incontinence procedures: Diagnosis and treatment with transvaginal urethrolysis. J Urol 152:93, 1994.)

urethral meatus and clitoris. The anterior urethral surface is then dissected, separating the urethra posteriorly from the symphysis anteriorly. The dissection continues cephalad to just above the vesical neck, and laterally as far as is needed to reproduce urethral mobility. Once again, a Martius fat pad can be introduced to prevent readhesion. I have used this approach in patients in whom abdominal and vaginal access are poor. The primary indication has been a morbidly obese patient.

RESULTS

The significant success achieved by urethrolysis in resolving obstructive and irritative symptoms has been suggested earlier. Mark and Webster, reporting 15 women with this syndrome, noted resolution of bladder instability symptoms in 13; of seven patients who were in urinary retention, efficient voiding was restored in six, and only one continued to require clean intermittent catheterization. In two patients, stress urinary incontinence occurred after urethrolysis but was successfully managed by an artificial urinary sphincter implanted at a further surgical procedure in one and by Contigen injection in the second. An updated series from Webster has comparable results, as shown in Table 92–2.[25]

McGuire et al noted that ten of 13 obstructed patients were able to void after retropubic urethrolysis, three continuing to perform self-catheterization.[26] None of their patients developed new-onset incontinence. Nitti and Raz reported 41 patients undergoing a transvaginal urethrolysis together with resuspension, and noted that overall 33 patients (80 percent) benefited from surgery.[20]

Summary

All patients with voiding problems and new-onset bladder instability symptoms after bladder neck suspension should be considered for urethrolysis after sufficient time (more than 3 months) has been given for spontaneous resolution. Patient selection is based primarily on the chronology of events and the physical and endoscopic findings. Persistent de novo or emergent bladder instability symptoms after bladder neck suspension should always be suspected as being of obstructive origin, and when combined with inefficient bladder emptying and recurrent infections are generally sufficient evidence to justify urethrolysis. Urodynamic findings are not always diagnostic, as many women do not respond to obstruction with typical high-pressure, low-flow features. Patients in total retention, who on preoperative urodynamics appear acontractile, are the group in whom the outcome is most in question. However, even women with seemingly poor detrusor contractility may benefit from surgical revision. Urethrolysis may be performed vaginally, infrapubically, or abdominally, depending on the surgeon's choice, and the outcome is probably comparable in each. The question of whether to resuspend the vesical neck must be addressed at the time of surgery; certainly in patients in whom urethrolysis results in the recurrence of significant vesical neck hypermobility, suspension would seem appropriate. There is always a possibility that urethrolysis may unmask incontinence due to intrinsic sphincter deficiency, the obstruction having protected against it. There is no preoperative way to foresee this event, but if it is suspected, a pubovaginal sling or vaginal wall sling procedure should certainly be performed at the time of lysis. Alternatively, the problem may be addressed postoperatively with a periurethral Contigen injection.

REFERENCES

1. Trocman BA, Leach GE, Hamilton J, et al. Modified Pereyra bladder neck suspension: Mean 10 year following in 125 patients. Presented at the Urodynamic Society, 17th Annual Meeting, Las Vegas, April 1995.
2. Juma S, Sdrales L. Etiology of urinary retention after bladder neck suspension. J Urol 149:401A, 1993.
3. Spencer JR, O'Conor VJ Jr, Schaeffer AJ. A comparison of endoscopic suspension of the vesical neck with suprapubic vesicourethropexy for treatment of stress urinary incontinence. J Urol 137:411, 1987.
4. Rost A, Fiedler U, Feeter C. Comparative analysis of the results of suspension-urethroplasty according to Marshall-Marchetti-Krantz and of urethrovesicopexy with adhesive. Urol Int 34:167, 1979.
5. Mundy AR. A trial comparing the Stamey bladder neck suspension with colposuspension for the treatment of stress incontinence. Br J Urol 55:687, 1983.
6. Cardozo LD, Stanton SL, Williams JE. Detrusor instability following surgery for genuine stress incontinence. Br J Urol 51:204, 1979.
7. Marshall VF, Marchetti AA, Krantz KE. The correction of stress incontinence by simple vesicourethral suspension. Surg Gynecol Obstet 88:509, 1949.
8. Burch JC. Urethrovaginal fixation to Cooper's ligament for correction of stress incontinence, cystocele and prolapse. Am J Obstet Gynecol 81:281, 1961.
9. Shull BL, Baden WF. A six-year experience with paravaginal defect repair for stress urinary incontinence. Am J Obstet Gynecol 160:1432, 1989.
10. Pereyra AJ. A simplified surgical procedure for the correction of stress incontinence in women. West J Surg 67:223, 1959.
11. Raz S, Sussman EM, Erikson DB, et al. The Raz bladder neck suspension: Results in 206 patients. J Urol 148:845, 1992.
12. Stamey TA. Endoscopic suspension of the vesical neck for urinary incontinence in females. Report on 203 consecutive patients. Ann Surg 192:465, 1980.
13. Gittes RF, Loughlin KR. No-incision pubovaginal suspension for stress incontinence. J Urol 138:568, 1987.
14. McGuire EJ, Bennett CJ, Konnak JA, et al. Experience with pubovaginal slings for urinary incontinence at the University of Michigan. J Urol 138:525, 1987.
15. Zimmern PE, Hadley HR, Leach GE, Raz S. Female urethral obstruction after Marshall-Marchetti-Krantz operation. J Urol 138:517, 1987.
16. Parnell JP, Marshall VF, Vaughn ED. Primary management of urinary stress incontinence by the Marshall-Marchetti-Krantz vesicourethropexy. J Urol 127:679, 1982.
17. Turner-Warwick R, Brown ADG. A urodynamic evaluation of urinary incontinence in the female and its treatment. Urol Clin North Am 6:203, 1979.
18. McGuire EJ. Bladder instability in stress incontinence. Neurourol Urodyn 7:563, 1988.
19. Webster GD, Kreder KJ. Voiding dysfunction following cystourethropexy: Its evaluation and management. J Urol 144:670, 1990.
20. Nitti VW, Raz S. Obstruction following anti-incontinence procedures: Diagnosis and treatment with transvaginal urethrolysis. J Urol 152:93, 1994.
21. Massey JA, Abrams PH. Obstructed voiding in the female. Br J Urol 61:36, 1988.
22. Farrar DJ, Osborne JL, Stephenson TP, et al. A urodynamic view of bladder outflow obstruction in the female: Factors influencing the results of treatment. Br J Urol 47:815, 1976.
23. Bass JS, Leach GE. Bladder outlet obstruction in women. Probl Urol 5:141, 1991.
24. Chancellor MB, Blaivas JG, Kaplan SA, Axelrod S. Bladder outlet obstruction versus impaired detrusor contractility: The role of outflow. J Urol 145:810, 1991.
25. Mark SD, Webster GD. The assessment and surgical management of an obstructive cystourethropexy. Presented at the Société International Urologie meeting, Sydney, Australia, 1994.
26. McGuire EJ, Letson W, Wang S. Transvaginal urethrolysis after obstructive urethral suspension procedures. J Urol 142:1037, 1989.
27. Dmochowski RR, Leach GE, Zimmern PE, et al. Urethrolysis to relieve outlet obstruction after prior incontinence surgery. J Urol 151:420A, 1994.

Chapter 93

Pubovaginal Slings

Edward J. McGuire

HISTORY

Sling procedures have been used since the early 1900s for both stress and neurogenic incontinence. German surgeons in the early 1900s described the construction of periurethral slings utilizing fascia, or a combination of fascia and muscle.[1-3] English workers described the use of rectus fascia and fascia lata for slings somewhat later.[4] American, Canadian, and European surgeons have described the use of lyophilized dura mater, bovine fascia, and various synthetic materials, including Marlex and Gore-Tex, as material for slings.[5-8] Although most surgeons who use slings do so only after a previous operative procedure has failed, slings were used occasionally by Germans very early in this century as a primary operation for certain types of neurogenic incontinence.[3] Slings were later used as a primary operation for certain kinds of stress incontinence after these had been definitively identified.

DEVELOPMENT OF THE INDICATIONS FOR PUBOVAGINAL SLINGS

In the 1970s, several surgeons independently noted patients who demonstrated a well-supported urethra after a retropubic operative procedure but who nevertheless leaked urine with effort.[9] Robertson[10] called this kind of urethra a "stovepipe," referring to the characteristic endoscopic appearance of the organ. Green[11] and Hodgkinson[12] independently described systems for the classification of stress incontinence based on the degree of urethral mobility, and the position of the urethra vis-à-vis the bladder and fixed pelvic anatomical locations. Both surgeons recognized the problem of a persistent incontinence due to a lack of urethral function despite a previous technically faultless operation that fixed the urethra in its proper anatomical position. Both Hodgkinson and Green used slings for these latter patients. The slings

were somewhat different from those in common use today and they used different materials, but they had basically the same purpose.

The identification of patients who might benefit from sling operations was at first primarily by virtue of failure of a retropubic operation to resolve a problem of stress incontinence.[11] In the 1970s, gynecologists were struggling to define the place of anterior colporrhaphy in the treatment of urinary stress incontinence.[11] The various methods used to classify and stratify patients with stress incontinence were primarily designed to select individuals for a retropubic suspension as opposed to those suitably repaired by a vaginal procedure. This situation occurred because the failure rate after a standard Kelly plication was very high.[9-11] Slings were used as a last resort only when a retropubic operation, which typically followed a previously unsuccessful vaginal operation, failed. Since the failure rate after Kelly plication approached 60 to 70 percent and the failure rate for a retropubic suspension was approximately 7 to 10 percent, the major focus of gynecological interest was in the area of Kelly suspensions and retropubic procedures and not on slings, which were rarely required.

However, with time, and the gradual increase in retropubic suspensions by gynecological surgeons as compared with transvaginal procedures the number of patients who failed well-performed retropubic procedures also grew. When these patients were studied with a video urodynamic technique, it became obvious that there were two mechanisms for urethral leakage during stressful maneuvers.[9, 13] The most common finding in women with primary stress incontinence was urethral hypermobility. In this condition the urethra is driven by abdominal pressure to a position where it seems to be less effective in resisting abdominal pressure.

Gynecologists were interested in the degree of mobility as an indicator of possible success or failure after a Kelly plication.[11, 12] Urologists who performed only retropubic suspensions were not interested in the degree of mobility, but both groups encountered a few patients with leakage apparently unrelated to mobility. Although this was not a large group of patients, studies ultimately led to the identification of patients with type III stress incontinence.[14, 15] That kind of incontinence, type III, particularly if it persisted after a retropubic operation, was associated with a nonfunctional proximal urethral sphincter mechanism. Although the urethra was well supported and immobile with stress, it nevertheless leaked profusely. The observation that this condition occurred in association with an open internal sphincter led directly to the use of a sling in an effort to close that specific area of the urethra.[15–17] Although the procedure cured stress incontinence, sling tension was often too great, and prolonged or permanent urinary retention, as well as exacerbation of inhibited or unstable bladder contractility, often occurred. These two problems were enough to discourage the use of slings as primary procedures.

RAPID CLINICAL ASSESSMENT OF URETHRAL SPHINCTER FUNCTION

With time and better urodynamics, it became obvious that the function of the urethra was more complicated and dynamic than originally thought and that more subtle varieties of urethral dysfunction existed besides pure urethral hypermobility and total loss of proximal urethral function. The elucidation of urethral function required the development of measurements that determined the extent of the loss of function by direct assessment of the ability of the urethra to resist the forces acting against it.[16, 17] These forces consist of the sum of detrusor and abdominal pressures, or total bladder pressure. Abdominal pressure is the result of muscular activity and of gravity in the upright position. Detrusor pressure is the sum of the weight of the urine bolus, which is quite small; the mural tension of the detrusor muscle; and the additional composite elements of the bladder wall that act on the urinary bolus, known as the viscoelastic component. Normally, the detrusor components are relatively small because the storage mode of bladder activity is associated only with very small increases in pressure despite large changes in volume. Detrusor pressure is directed at the internal urethral meatus and will open it and induce leakage when the resistance of the urethra is exceeded. This is a linear relationship. The detrusor pressure required to induce leakage is equal, or nearly equals, to the maximal urethral closing pressure. That is not true for abdominal pressure. A normal urethra will resist, at the internal meatus, virtually any abdominal pressure. The ability of the urethra to resist abdominal pressure is not defined by urethral closing pressure. A very bad urethra, which leaks in association with minimal effort, can be made to resist any abdominal pressure excursion by a sling procedure, by a suspension operation, or in some instances by the injection of materials like collagen. None of these treatments change maximal urethral closing pressure at all and none improve the ability of the external, volitional sphincter to contract. Despite a dramatic effect on the abdominal pressure required to induce leakage engendered by these treatments, the same treatments change detrusor pressure required to induce leakage only slightly, if at all. It is possible then to induce a profound change in the ability of the female urethra to resist abdominal pressure without producing any change in urethral closing pressure or the detrusor pressure required to produce urinary flow.[19–21]

Bladder Compliance as a Factor in Incontinence

The choice of procedure depends first on accurate identification of the precise force that causes leakage in any given case, abdominal or detrusor pressure. This is particularly important when bladder compliance is known to be abnormal. If a gradual gain in bladder pressure occurs during filling, leakage, apparently induced by changes in abdominal pressure, is the result. The real problem here, however, is the gradual incorporation of the urethra into the bladder with the gain in detrusor pressure. At some volume, any poorly compliant bladder will produce type III incontinence, in which the bladder and proximal urethra become isobaric. In any circumstance where this could occur (e.g., after radiation therapy or extirpative pelvic surgery, in neurological disease, or after failure of multiple operations to cure incontinence), a cystometrogram should be taken to prove, at a minimum, that the bladder stores urine at normally low pressures. If the detrusor pressure component is excessive, which could be defined as a pressure more than 20 cm H_2O at normal bladder capacity, a urethral procedure is unlikely to resolve the patient's incontinence problem. If, on the other hand, the bladder stores urine normally, assessment of urethral resistance to abdominal pressure as the most important force of expulsion should be made for accurate comparative data.

CLINICAL TESTING OF URETHRAL FUNCTION

For comparison of data, zero pressure is by convention that value recorded with the subject supine, the bladder empty, and, if a fluid flow system is used, with the transducer localized at the level of the symphysis. The bladder is filled to 200 ml and the patient is placed in the upright position. At this point, measured pressure in the bladder (P_{ves}) results from the volume increment, gravity, and weight of the abdominal contents and the fluid bolus. The patient is at this point asked to strain until leakage occurs. The total bladder pressure required to induce leakage is noted. The most dramatic component of the expulsive force, provided that the detrusor component is minimal, is abdominal pressure, but total P_{ves} is the actual expulsive force. The abdominal pressure component required to induce leakage is inversely proportional to the deficiency in urethral sphincter function. In cases in which the detrusor contribution to total bladder pressure is small, most of the expulsive force is abdominal pressure. If leakage occurs at pressures less than 60 cm H_2O, poor intrinsic (internal) sphincter function is present. Leakage at pressures above 90 cm H_2O usually indicates hypermobility of the urethra or the presence of a cystocele. In cases in which leakage occurs at pressures between 60 and 90 cm H_2O, both elements of urethral dysfunction, hypermobility and lack of internal sphincter closure, are usually present.

SELECTION OF SURGERY

Once the leak point pressure is known, a careful pelvic examination with the patient first supine and then standing is important. The presence and extent of urethral mobility with maximal straining should be noted. If the urethra is immobile, or nearly so at pressures known to be associated with leakage, there is a possible role for injectable agents.[22] If, on the other hand, the urethra does move and leakage is produced at a low pressure of 60 cm H_2O or less, a standard suspension operation will have a fairly high failure rate and a sling is the preferred operation. Leak point pressures are totally unreliable in the presence of significant bladder prolapse. Opinions vary about the cause of this relationship, but it is true that women with large cystoceles show very high leak point pressures, often higher than those normally associated with good urethral function. This occurs even when a given urethra can be shown to be very mobile or very poorly closed. When the cystocele is reduced, the urethra will be found to leak at much lower pressures. For these reasons, selection of an operative procedure by symptoms, or by reported grade of incontinence, or even by leak point pressure, is likely to be inaccurate in many patients with incontinence. Considerable other information, including that obtained from pelvic examination and a determination of the ability of the bladder to store urine at low pressure, is essential before a decision can be made on operative indications and the type of operation best suited for a given patient.

SELECTION FACTORS FOR THE USE OF SLINGS

Patients who have failed a previous operation for stress incontinence, as, for example, a retropubic procedure, or a needle suspension, often do better with a sling. Women who engage in extremely vigorous athletic activity are probably better off with a primary sling procedure. Women with myelodysplasia, those with poor proximal urethral function after urethral diverticulectomy, and those with asthma or chronic obstructive pulmonary disease are better served by a sling procedure than by a suspension. As long as some care is taken to adjust sling tension, the procedure is not more likely to induce retention or bladder instability than any other operation for stress incontinence, with the exception of an anterior vaginal repair (or Kelly plication). That operation, although not associated with retention, is totally unsuited for the conditions enumerated above and for most women without those specific more difficult conditions who have type II hypermobility.

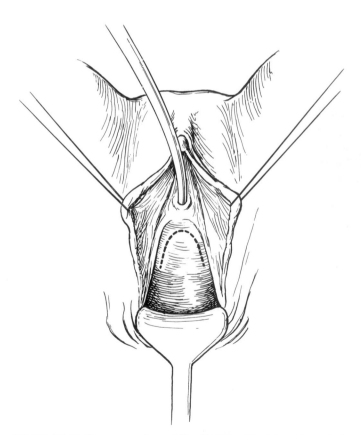

Figure 93–1. General outline of the U-shaped incision. A vertical incision can also be used.

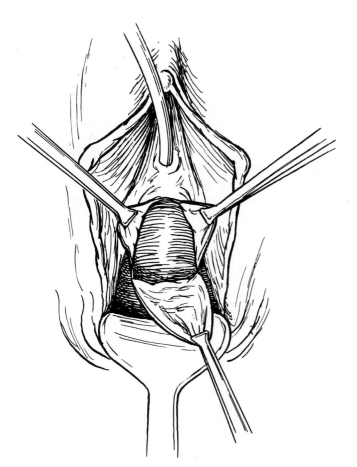

Figure 93–2. Development of a vaginal flap. The most important part of this aspect of the procedure is to stay superficial to white glistening periurethral fascia, which lies deep to the vaginal epithelial lining. Generally, sharp dissection is used here and a knife dissection is often superior to scissors dissection, at least to begin the plane.

OPERATIVE TECHNIQUE

The patient is placed in a modified dorsal lithotomy position with the feet supported by Allen-type stirrups. Care is taken to avoid pressure on the lateral surface of the calf. The legs need be only moderately flexed at the hip, which allows for simultaneous vaginal and retropubic approaches to the urethra. An 18-Fr. Foley catheter is inserted to outline the urethra and to provide for bladder drainage during the procedure. Preoperative antimicrobial agents are given in sufficient time to achieve a blood level when the skin incision is made. Either a midline or inverted-U vaginal incision can be made overlying the urethra (Fig. 93–1). The vaginal epithelium is sharply dissected off the underlying periurethral fascia, which is white and somewhat reflective of light. This fascia is a definite layer and every effort must be made to stay superficial to it (Fig. 93–2). There are instances when the periurethral fascia has been damaged or lost or when the fascia is fused to the vagina and underlying urethra. This occurs after urethral diver-

ticulectomy, sometimes after anterior colporrhaphy, and occasionally after needle suspension procedures, but very rarely after a retropubic suspension. When there is difficulty with the very first part of the dissection, great care must be taken to stay as close to the inner layer of the vaginal lining as feasible until the lateral extent of the scarring or tissue loss is reached before one attempts to enter the retropubic space. The periurethral fascia should be identified before the scissors are advanced, parallel to the perineum, well lateral to the urethra, and always superficial to the periurethral fascia. That places the entry point of the instrument into the retropubic space at the point where the endopelvic fascia inserts on the inferior margin of the ischium, lateral to the urethra at or near the plane of the bladder outlet (Fig. 93–3). This is a safe entry point even in those patients who have failed a prior retropubic operation. Once the retropubic entry has been made, the scissors, closed, are gently advanced in the same direction (as when the penetration was made), laterally and slightly upward, for 1 to 2 cm. At this point the instrument is opened and a tissue plane is created by spreading the tissue fairly vigorously. The vaginal wound can be packed for a few minutes while the retropubic part of the procedure is done.

A transverse suprapubic incision is made 2 fingerbreadths above the symphysis, or via any transverse suprapubic scar. The dissection is carried to the rectus fascia, which is incised in the direction of the

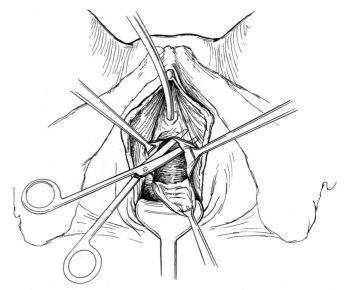

Figure 93–3. Entry to the retropubic space is performed on both sides. Keeping the scissors parallel to the plane of the perineum, the retropubic space is entered immediately adjacent to the ischial ramus, freeing the end of pelvic fascia at that point from its attachment to the bony structure. This direction of the scissors is lateral and slightly anterior, but not at this point pointed in the direction of the bladder: rather away from the bladder and the urethra. Generally, sharp dissection is used to enter the retropubic space; once this is accomplished, blunt finger dissection is also useful.

incision (Fig. 93–4). Usually the inferior leaf of fascia is the sling source, but the upper leaf can also be used. To permit easy closure of the fascia after sling removal, mobilization of the upper and lower leaves is done for 4 to 5 cm to gain freedom from the rectus muscles. The sling should measure 1.5 to 2.0 cm in its center diameter and 0.5 cm at either end. It can vary in length from 8 cm to 11 or 15 cm. Once the sling is harvested, it is oversutured at either end with 0 sutures, taking several bites and making two or more ties to secure all the fibers. Sling tensile strength is longitudinal rather than lateral, and each end should be secured to the suture very firmly.

The lateral border of each rectus muscle is then retracted toward the midline one at a time. There is a triangular defect or partial defect in the fascia and muscle at the point just lateral to where the rectus muscle inserts into the symphysis (Fig. 93–5). At this site, sharp and blunt dissection is used to enter the retropubic space immediately in contact with the symphysis. That maneuver, in conjunction with finger dissection from below, should result by bimanual contact. If that does not occur, further dissection from below, more laterally, is often required. If direct contact is not made and there is intervening tissue between the two examining fingers, some care is required, because this tissue may well be the bladder. If the intervening tissue is low at the level of the pelvic floor or at the level of entry into the retropubic space by the vaginal operator through the endopelvic fascia, penetration is safe. If, on the other hand, the intervening tissue is higher, it is usually bladder

pinned to the back of the symphysis. This can be negotiated by carefully advancing a sharp-nosed clamp (a tonsil or Crawford clamp) or dissecting scissors, either in an upward or downward direction through the tissue, but with the tip of the instrument in constant direct contact with the posterior surface of the symphysis. Once the clamp is in place, traversing the retropubic entry points above and below, it can be opened safely, and the tissue gently spread, to create a passageway for the sling.

At this point the urethral catheter is withdrawn and a 70-degree lens is used to visualize the interior of the bladder with both clamps still in position traversing the retropubic space. Leaving the clamps in place greatly facilitates inspection of the tracks of the clamps, and if an inadvertent injury to the bladder has occurred, it will be obvious. This is most likely to occur at the 11 and 2 o'clock positions well up toward the bladder dome. If the bladder is intact, the sling sutures are grasped in the clamps and pulled up into the retropubic space (Fig. 93–6). This results in seating of the broadest part of the sling just at and spread out below the bladder neck. The sling is sutured in place to the periurethral fascia with a single 3-0 absorbable suture so that it cannot move, and continues to be broadly seated at the point of contact with the urethra. The position of the sling vis-à-vis the urethra and ureters is controlled by the entry points made by the vaginal operator into the retropubic space from below. Since these are at the level of the vesical outlet, the sling goes where is designed to go, i.e., the bladder neck, without any special precautions.

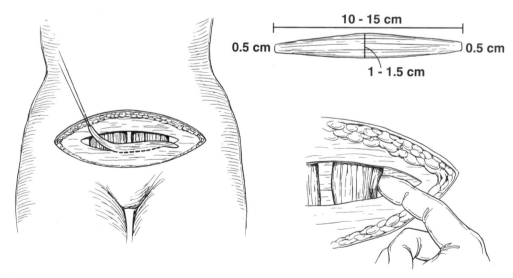

Figure 93–4. Detail of the transverse suprapubic abdominal incision and harvesting of the sling. Generally, the fascia is mobilized off the underlying bellies of the rectus muscles superiorly and inferiorly. The sling is taken from the interior leaf of the rectus fascia. The middle portion of the sling is usually 1 to 2 cm in transverse width, and may be somewhat narrower at the end. Although it is easier to work with a sling 10 to 15 cm in length, one as short as 8 cm can certainly be used. Approach to the retropubic space, from above, in patients who have had previous needle suspension procedures or retropubic suspension procedures is depicted at the bottom right-hand corner. There is a defect in the fascia immediately lateral to the rectus muscle where that structure inserts on the superoposterior surface of the symphysis pubis. At exactly that point, minimal sharp dissection opens a plane into the retropubic space that provides easy access to the entry point in the retropubic space made by the vaginal operator.

tween are circumstances in which somewhat more tension is required. In general, the lower the leak point pressure and the higher the grade of incontinence, the more tension needs to be applied. In the final analysis, the objective of the procedure is to make the urethra able to resist abdominal pressure but not bladder pressure. Thus, filling the bladder and compressing it, while at the same time adjusting tension on the sling, represents massive overkill. No sling need be, or should be, tight enough to resist bladder pressure as an expulsive force. There are, however, limits to what a sling will do to a urethra without inducing some degree of obstructive uropathy to the detrusor as an expulsive force. The sling is only a vector force, unlike the artificial sphincter, which is a circular (or nearly so) compressive force. A very wide patulous urethra, destroyed by prolonged catheter drainage, may not be completely closed by the posterior vector force imposed by the sling without inducing at the same time bladder outlet obstruction and imposing the need for intermittent catheterization.

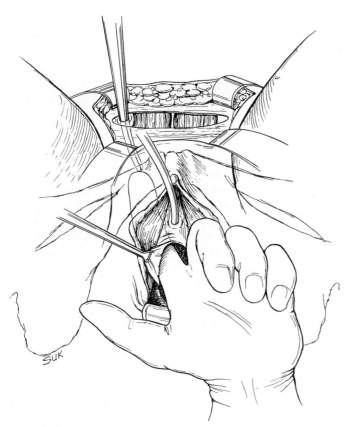

Figure 93–5. The instrument, generally a thoracic-type Crawford clamp with a relatively sharp nose, is passed from above toward the vaginal wound, the approach being lateral to the medial and inferior. The vaginal operating finger is kept immediately behind the nose of the clamp, with the nose of the clamp in contact with the inferior surface of the pubic symphysis. There may be some residual tissue at the pelvic floor on the pelvic fascia, but generally the passageway is completely clear of an obstruction if the lateral entry point from above has been used in the proper plane and direction of the scissors has been employed from below. After passage of the clamp on both sides, the instrument is left in situ while endoscopy of the bladder is performed to make sure there has been no inadvertent injury to that structure. If an injury occurs, it will be superior and lateral when visualized cystoscopically at the dome of the bladder, or almost at the dome of the bladder.

The vaginal incision is first closed and then the rectus fascia is closed at the same time. The sling sutures are then tied together over the closed rectus fascia (Fig. 93–7). Blunt dissection is used to create a tunnel for both sling sutures on either side of the midline. Adjustment of sling tension takes some practice, and the amount of tension applied has some relationship to the condition being treated. A patient with neurogenic urethral failure and a neurogenic bladder emptied by intermittent catheterization should have a very tight sling. The only caution in this case would be to allow for intermittent catheterization. A patient with recurrent stress incontinence due to hypermobility needs a sling tight enough to prevent urethral motion. In practical terms, after the sling is tied, particularly in the latter circumstance, a finger should slide easily under the suture. In be-

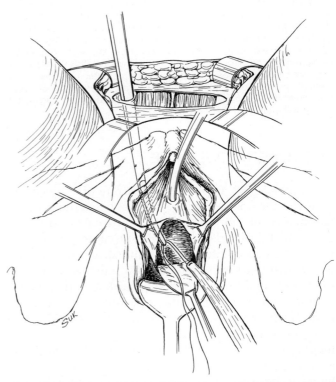

Figure 93–6. The sling is oversutured with 0 absorbable or nonabsorbable suture, involves several bites of that material into the sling, and then a secure knot so that as many of the longitudinal fibers of the sling as possible are trapped in the suture. The sutures are then grasped by the Crawford clamps and pulled up, traversing the retropubic space. This seats the sling securely behind the urethra, where it is sutured in place with a single suture of 3-0 Vicryl. The sling sutures are then tunneled through the rectus muscle fascia above while the vaginal epithelium is reclosed. After closure of the vaginal epithelium the rectus fascia is closed and the sling is tied down over the rectus fascia.

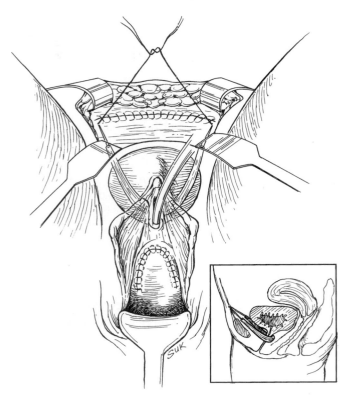

Figure 93–7. After closure of the rectus fascia in the vaginal epithelium, the sling is adjusted for tension by tying down the sutures over the closed rectus fascia. The sutures should not be tied very tightly: generally, an examining finger can easily slide underneath the knot, between the knot and the rectus fascia. However, this sling should be seated in a position behind the urethras with sufficient tension so that when traction is placed on the Foley catheter from below the urethral access does not change: i.e., the urethra will not rotate posteriorly and inferiorly into the potential space of the vagina because of the effect of the sling.

POSTOPERATIVE CARE

A vaginal pack is placed on the day of surgery and removed the next morning. In most cases the catheter is removed on the second day, but this can often be done on the first day. Intermittent catheterization is instituted immediately after removal of the catheter on an every-4-hours and as-required basis. All patients are taught to perform intermittent self-catheterization. When they can do intermittent catheterization easily or can empty the bladder well, and sometimes both, they are discharged. The average length of stay for a simple sling is 3.2 days. The average operating time is 40 minutes and the average blood loss 50 ml. The major problem with slings is, in the early period, resumption of normal voiding, which can take a long time. This is completely unpredictable and is not correlated with sling tension.

Another problem is the tendency for some patients who are in the process of re-establishment of normal voiding to develop urge incontinence. Whereas treatment of that problem with anticholinergic agents is often successful, these drugs delay the onset of nor-

mal bladder voiding. About 10 percent of patients complain of intermittent sharp pain on one side or the other, which seems to be due to sling tension. That supposition is supported by successful relief of pain and symptoms upon complete removal of the sling sutures 10 to 12 weeks after the sling procedure.

PERSISTENT RETENTION

As with any suspension procedure, slings carry a risk of prolonged retention. When this problem persists beyond 8 weeks, release of sling tension is practical and does not result in recurrent stress incontinence. The procedure involves a vaginal incision with deliberate incision of the sling in the midline, and then dissection laterally into the retropubic space on both sides to free the urethra. This generally takes only 10 minutes, and though it is possible to use local anesthesia, the exposure and mobilization are much better with general or regional anesthesia.

LONG-TERM OUTCOME

Slings are durable and reliable. Failure of a sling to resolve a problem of stress incontinence is distinctly unusual. More commonly, slings fail to resolve problems associated with the bladder or to effect full closure of the urethra, so that leakage still occurs is some circumstances. Those outcomes, although unusual, are associated with a fairly typical symptom complex. The patient complains of incontinence with certain movements or with the assumption of certain positions, but denies leakage with coughing or straining. Video urodynamic studies demonstrate good function of the sling with coughing or straining, but leakage is visible at rest, when abdominal pressure is not elevated, when certain positions appear to splint the sling and result in transient loss of urethral closure. These patients leak at low abdominal pressures but not at much higher pressures, at which the sling works as it is designed to do.

Combining all results from slings from three institutions where 3-year follow-up is possible suggests that slings cure recurrent type III stress incontinence in about 92 percent of patients. In patients with other problems, including poor bladder function, vesicovaginal and urethra vaginal fistulas, and urethral diverticula or urethral erosion and reconstruction, the sling will resolve incontinence approximately 82 percent of the time.[23–25]

Editorial Comment
Fray F. Marshall

Pubovaginal slings may help patients who have failed previous operations for stress incontinence. The slings may stabilize an existing sphincter to allow it to function more effectively, and they reduce movement of bladder neck during physical activity. As Dr. McGuire states, slings do not have to be performed with significant tension to prevent hypermobility. These procedures have undergone a significant resurgence since their introduction by the Germans in the early 1900s.

REFERENCES

1. Goebel R. Zur operativen Beseitigung der angeborenen Incontinentia vesicae. Zentralbl Gynakol 2:187, 1910.
2. Stoeckel W: Über die Verwendung der Musculi pyramidalis bei der operativen Behandlung der Incontinentia vesicae. Zentralbl Gynakol 41:11, 1917.
3. Frangenheim P. Zur operativen Behandlung der Incontinenz der männlichen Harnröhre. Verh Dtsch Ges Chir 43:149, 1914.
4. Aldridge AH. Transplantation of fascia for the relief of urinary stress incontinence. Am J Obstet Gynecol 14:398, 1942.
5. Morgan TE. A sling operation using Marlex polypropylene mesh for treatment of recurrent stress incontinence. Am J Obstet Gynecol 106:369, 1970.
6. Faber P, Beck L, Heidenveich J. Treatment of urinary stress incontinence with the Lyodura sling. Urol Int 33:117, 1978.
7. Stauton SC, Brindley GS, Holmes DM. Silastic sling for urethral sphincter incontinence in women. Br J Obstet Gynaecol 92:747, 1985.
8. Sauel PH, Bower LW, Pariganisam, et al. The low pressure urethra as a factor in foiled retropubic urethropexy. Obstet Gynaecol 69:399, 1987.
9. McGuire EJ. Urodynamic findings in patients after failure of stress incontinence operations. In Zinner NR, Sterling AM, eds. Female Incontinence, New York, Alan R Liss, 1985, p 351.
10. Robertson JR. Ambulatory gynecologic urology clinic. Obstet Gynecol 17:261, 1974.
11. Green TH Jr. Development of a method for the diagnosis and treatment of urinary stress incontinence. Am J Obstet Gynecol 83:632, 1962.
12. Hodgkinson CP. Stress urinary incontinence. Obstet Gynecol 47:255, 1976.
13. McGuire EJ, Lython B, Pepe V, Kohnn EI. Stress urinary incontinence. Obstet Gynecol 47:255, 1976.
14. Blaivas JG: A modest proposal for the diagnosis and treatment of urinary incontinence in women. J Urol 138:597, 1987.
15. McGuire EJ, Lytton B. Pubovaginal sling procedure for stress incontinence. J Urol 119:82, 1978.
16. Blaivas JG. Treatment of female incontinence secondary to urethral damage or loss. Urol Clin North Am 18:355, 1991.
17. Gardy M, Kozminski M, DeLanuces, JOL, et al. Stress incontinence and cystoceles. J Urol 145:1211, 1991.
18. Blaivas JG, Salinas Lupe J III: Stress incontinence: The importance of proper diagnosis and treatment. Surg Forum 35:472, 1984.
19. McGuire EJ, Wang C, Usetalo H, Savastauo JA. Modified pubovaginal sling in female children with myelodysplasia. J Urol 135:94, 1986.
20. Wan J, McGuire EJ, Bloom DA, Ritchey M. Stress leak point pressure: A diagnostic tool for incontinent children. J Urol 150:700, 1993.
21. McGuire EJ, Fitzpatrick CC, Wan J, et al. Clinical assessment of urethral sphincter function. J Urol 150:1452, 1993.
22. McGuire EJ. Active and passive factors in urethral continence function. Int Urogynecol. 3:54, 1992.
23. Norbeck JC, McGuire EJ. The use of pubovaginal and puboprostatic slings. Dialog Pediatr Urol 14:2, 1991.
24. Key D, Wan J, Brainer R, et al. Urinary tract reconstruction: Applied biodynamics. Neurourol Urodyn 9:509, 1990.
25. McGuire EJ, Bennett CS, Konssak J, et al. Experience with pubovaginal slings for urinary incontinence at the University of Michigan. J Urol 138:525, 1987.

Chapter 94

Artificial Sphincter in the Treatment of Female Urinary Incontinence

Eduardo Kleer and David M. Barrett

PREOPERATIVE EVALUATION

The incontinent female patient most likely to benefit from placement of an American Medical Systems 800 artificial genitourinary sphincter (AGUS) is the one with type III stress urinary incontinence, characterized by a noncoapting proximal urethra and bladder neck. Type III stress urinary incontinence may result from spinal cord and pelvic trauma, radiation, neurological diseases such as myelomeningocele, and scarring to the bladder neck area after previous urethral suspension procedures. Unlike male urinary incontinence, for which the AGUS is generally the best treatment option to achieve dryness secondary to sphincteric incompetence, several other effective treatment options exist for the female with type III stress urinary incontinence. These include sling procedures as well as injection of periurethral bulking agents. The goal of these treatment options is to achieve a constant compression of the proximal urethra and bladder neck region, thus mimicking a functional bladder neck sphincter.[1]

The AGUS has been used effectively in the treatment of type III stress urinary incontinence with a rate of success ranging from 80 to 100 percent.[1, 2] Most urologists use the AGUS only in patients who have failed more conservative surgical procedures. On the other hand, dissection in virgin areas with abundant blood supply gives the patient the best chance to avoid cuff erosion. The advantage of the AGUS in the treatment of type III stress urinary incontinence in females is that in women with normal bladder function, the risk of retention and need for lifelong clean intermittent catheterization is decreased.[3]

In general, the same preoperative evaluation that was discussed for the male patient with urinary incontinence before AGUS implantation also applies to the female incontinent patient. All female patients should be instructed in the need for clean intermittent catheterization before sphincter implantation. This is important in case they develop postoperative urinary retention or require pharmacotherapy and clean intermittent catheterization to optimize continence.

The possibility of future pregnancies must also be discussed with the patient before AGUS implantation. She must be forewarned that although an implanted AGUS is not a contraindication to pregnancy, an elective cesarean section should be performed at the time of delivery to decrease the possibility of any damage to the bladder neck and its surrounding cuff. In addition, deactivation of the AGUS is recommended for the last trimester of pregnancy to reduce pressure on the cuff and bladder neck region and thus decrease the possibility of subsequent erosion.[4] Patients with previous vesicovaginal fistula repair and rectal pullthrough procedures should be cautioned that cuff placement may not be technically possible.[5]

OPERATIVE TECHNIQUE

Patients are advised to undergo an antiseptic shower the night before surgery as well as a standard vaginal preparation on the morning of surgery. Urine sterility must be ensured. Hair removal is carried out just before surgery, and broad-spectrum parenteral antibiotics are administered on call to the operating room. After the patient is positioned in a dorsal lithotomy position with knees at the level of the abdomen, a full 10-minute iodophor skin scrub should be performed of the lower abdomen, vagina, and perineum. An iodoform-impregnated gauze is used to pack the vagina, and a 16 Fr., 5-ml Foley catheter is introduced per urethra.

A Pfannenstiel or lower abdominal midline incision is made and carried down into the retropubic space toward the bladder neck area. The dissection should be extraperitoneal. After palpation of the vaginal pack and Foley catheter, a plane is created between the urethra and vagina (Fig. 94–1). The vesicovaginal plane is next established at a point superior to the endopelvic fascia, below the insertion of the ureters into the bladder (Fig. 94–2). This plane may be difficult to establish, especially in patients with a history of retropubic or bladder neck surgery, as well as in girls around the age of puberty. Occasionally, the bladder may have to be opened to define the plane of dissection. In such cases the bladder incision must be made in the anterior midline, away from the bladder neck, to avoid the risk of erosion through the suture lines. A finger placed in the vagina or rectum may help better define the plane.

After circumferential dissection of the bladder neck is achieved, the bladder is filled with a methylene blue–antibiotic solution. Leakage points should be

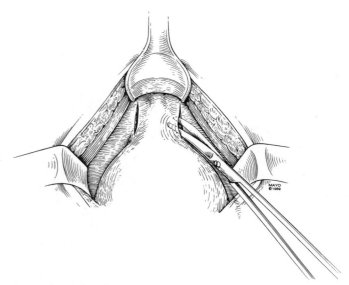

Figure 94–2. The vesicovaginal plane is established at a point superior to the endopelvic fascia, below the insertion of the ureters into the bladder. (By permission of Mayo Foundation.)

closed watertight in two layers with absorbable suture. Any tears in the vagina should also be closed in two continuous layers with absorbable suture. The established circumferential plane should be approximately 2 cm in width to allow unrestricted placement of the cuff. The bladder neck is circumferentially measured with the calibrated measuring strap after the Foley catheter is removed (Fig. 94–3). In most women a 6- to 8-cm cuff is chosen.[5] The properly sized cuff is then passed underneath the bladder neck and snapped in place (Fig. 94–4A and B). The tubing from the cuff is passed through the belly of one rectus muscle and through the anterior abdominal wall fascia, near the internal inguinal ring on the side of the patient where the pump will be placed. A curved

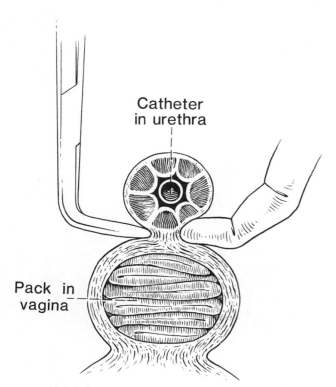

Figure 94–1. The catheter in the urethra and the vaginal pack help to identify the plane that must be established between the urethra and vagina. (From Furlow WL. Artificial sphincter. In Stanton SL, Tanagho EA, eds. Surgery of Female Incontinence, 2nd ed. New York, Springer-Verlag, 1986, pp 155–172. Copyright, Springer-Verlag.)

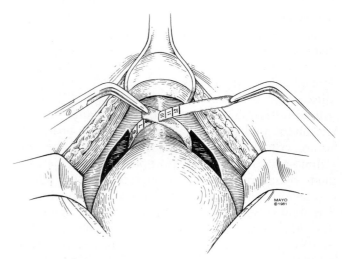

Figure 94–3. The bladder neck is circumferentially measured with the calibrated measuring strap. (By permission of Mayo Foundation.)

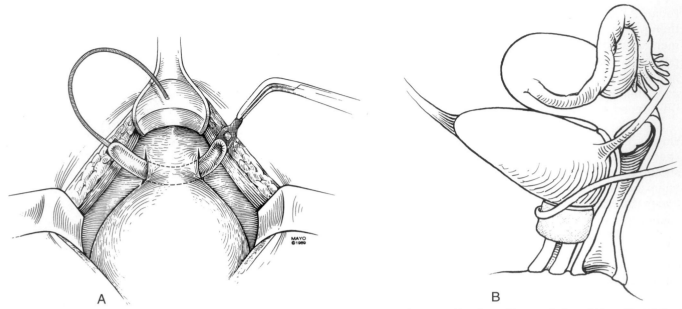

Figure 94–4. *A,* The properly sized cuff is passed underneath the bladder neck and snapped in place. (By permission of Mayo Foundation.) *B,* A sagittal view of the cuff around the bladder neck. (From Furlow WL. Artificial sphincter. In Stanton SL, Tanagho EA, eds. Surgery of Female Incontinence, 2nd ed. New York, Springer-Verlag, 1986, pp 155–172. Copyright, Springer-Verlag.)

shod clamp is used on the end of the cuff tubing, closed with only one click.

The pressure balloon reservoir is then placed in the prevesical space. Its tubing penetrates the rectus muscle next to the tubing of the cuff. A straight shod clamp closed with only one click is left on the end of the reservoir tubing. A 61- to 70-cm H_2O reservoir is routinely used in most patients and filled with 22 ml of isosmotic contrast medium (Fig. 94–5).

With a Hegar dilator, a pocket is developed in the subcutaneous tissue of the labia majora for the control assembly (Fig. 94–5). The pump is placed in an optimally dependent position with the activation/deactivation button laterally. Once a satisfactory position for the pump has been ensured, a Babcock clamp is placed around it and the labial skin to prevent its proximal migration when the tubing connections are made. A curved shod clamp should be on the control tubing to the cuff and a straight shod clamp on the control tubing to the reservoir, each with only one click.

Before the tubing connections are made, the anterior abdominal wall fascia is closed with absorbable suture. A Jackson-Pratt drain may be left in the retropubic space if needed. Appropriate connections are made between the AGUS components using straight connectors tied in place with 2–0 Prolene (nonabsorbable) suture. Connections may also be made with the quick-connect connectors. The remainder of the incision is closed in layers with absorbable suture. After the device has been tested and cycled, the cuff is left in an open deactivated position (Fig. 94–6).

POSTOPERATIVE MANAGEMENT

The patient should have ice packs to the perineum for the first 24 hours postoperatively to minimize edema and hematoma formation. The Foley catheter is left indwelling for the first 48 hours. The patient

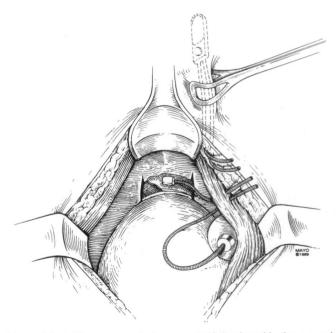

Figure 94–5. The pressure balloon reservoir is placed in the prevesical space, its tubing penetrating the rectus muscle next to the tubing of the cuff. The pump is placed in a pocket in the subcutaneous tissue of the labia majora and held in place with a Babcock clamp. (By permission of Mayo Foundation.)

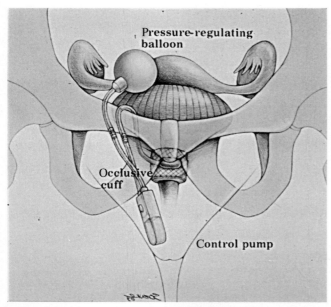

Figure 94–6. The implantation of the artificial genitourinary sphincter (AGUS) has been completed. (From Furlow WL. Artificial sphincter. In Stanton SL, Tanagho EA, eds. Surgery of Female Incontinence, 2nd ed. New York, Springer-Verlag, 1986, pp 155–172. Copyright, Springer-Verlag.)

usually voids without difficulty. Some patients may experience a transient postoperative continence secondary to tissue edema around the cuff. If indicated, a postvoid residual should be checked, and if it is greater than 150 ml, clean intermittent catheterization should be instituted with a small-caliber catheter until postvoid residuals decrease. Postoperative oral antibiotics should be continued for 10 to 14 days.

Activation of the AGUS is recommended at 6 weeks postoperatively. Activation is performed by firm compression of the pump. The deactivation button will switch into the activated configuration, allowing fluid to circulate through the control assembly. Activation can be monitored by deflate and inflate radiographs, which confirm filling of the cuff after activation.

Patients unable to completely empty their bladders, such as those with neurogenic bladders or bladder augmentations, should use self-intermittent catheterization. The sphincter cuff must be deflated before catheter insertion into the bladder. Patients who have diminished flow rates may require a second pumping to allow enough time to adequately empty the bladder before cuff recompression occurs. Patients who are dry at night in a recumbent position are instructed to deactivate the AGUS once in bed to reduce the risk of ischemia to the underlying urethra or bladder neck.

A transvaginal approach to placement of the AGUS in the female patient has also been described and appears to be successful.[2, 6] These authors recommend the application of an estrogen cream postoperatively to the vagina as well as anaerobic antibiotic coverage perioperatively.

POSTOPERATIVE COMPLICATIONS

Postoperative complications have been reviewed in Chapter 74 on the use of the AGUS in the treatment of male incontinence. One additional consideration in the female patient who presents with continuous incontinence after AGUS implantation is the possibility of a vesicovaginal fistula that could have resulted from injury to the vagina or bladder during bladder neck dissection. Iatrogenic fistula as the cause of postoperative incontinence needs to be ruled out.

Editorial Comment
Fray F. Marshall

Urethral slings (see Chapter 93) have been used in place of sphincters to provide additional outlet resistance and improve urinary continence in the female. Another option in the female includes the placement of an artificial sphincter around the bladder neck. Although drains are sometimes placed, it may be reasonable to try to avoid a drain unless there is bleeding or some other reason to consider it. Drains may provide a potential source for infection. Dissection around the urethra is more difficult as the dissection moves distally. It is usually easier to develop the plane somewhat higher at the most proximal portion of the urethra. Care must also be taken to avoid injury to the ureters if the dissection is made at a higher level.

REFERENCES

1. Parulkar BG, Barrett DM. Application of the AS-800 artificial sphincter for intractable urinary incontinence in females. Surg Gynecol Obstet 171:131, 1990.
2. Appell RA. Techniques and results in the implantation of the artificial urinary sphincter in women with type III stress urinary incontinence by a vaginal approach. Neurourol Urodynamics 7:613, 1988.
3. Petrou SP, Barrett DM. The use of artificial genitourinary sphincter (AGUS) in female urinary incontinence. In Webster G, Kirby R, King L, Goldwasser B, eds. Reconstructive Urology, 1st ed. Boston, Blackwell, 1993, p 915.
4. Barrett DM, Parulkar BG. The artificial sphincter (AS-800): Experience in children and young adults. Urol Clin North Am, 16:119, 1989.
5. Barrett DM, Goldwasser B. The artificial urinary sphincter: Current management philosophy. American Urological Updates, Vol 5, lesson 32, 1986.
6. Abbassian A. A new operation for insertion of the artifical urinary sphincter. J Urol 140:512, 1988.

SECTION IV

SURGERY AFTER UROLOGICAL TRAUMA

Chapter 95

Renal Trauma: Evaluation and Surgical Treatment

Jack W. McAninch

INDICATIONS

The indications for renal surgery are based primarily on clinical conditions, but the radiographical findings complement the urological surgeon's knowledge by better defining the extent of injury. Absolute indications for renal exploration after trauma are related to active bleeding and include an expanding retroperitoneal hematoma or pulsatile hematoma. Relative indications are urinary extravasation, nonviable renal tissue associated with a parenchymal laceration, and arterial injury. Renal exploration may be prompted by a combination of these indications.[1] In certain situations the trauma surgeon may choose to perform a laparotomy to manage an associated abdominal organ injury. This procedure provides the urological surgeon with the opportunity to repair major renal injuries that might otherwise be managed nonoperatively. This repair can be done with minimal risk of renal loss and can reduce the potential for late complications.

PREOPERATIVE MANAGEMENT

Resuscitation of an acutely injured patient is essential and initially includes control of hemorrhage and shock. Careful examination of the chest and abdomen is essential. Penetrating injuries of the upper abdo-men, flank, and back should immediately prompt suspicion. Flank contusions and lower rib fractures suggest renal injury from blunt trauma.[2]

Blood in the urine is the best indicator of renal injury. Any patient sustaining a penetrating injury of the upper abdomen, flank, or back should undergo renal imaging studies. The presence of red blood cells, 5 per high-power field (RBC/HPF), in the urine strongly suggests injury and mandates renal imaging. Adult patients with *blunt* trauma can undergo imaging selectively based on the following criteria (Fig. 95–1): patients with gross hematuria or shock (systolic blood pressure <90 mm Hg) and microscopical hematuria (5 RBC/HPF) should have imaging studies, and patients without shock and with only microscopical hematuria can be followed expectantly without renal imaging.[3] Any patient in whom the clinician has a high suspicion of renal injury on the basis of the physical examination should undergo imaging despite the aforementioned guidelines. Pediatric patients with any degree of hematuria should also undergo imaging studies.

The process of defining the extent of a renal injury is termed "staging."[4] This process begins with high-dose (2 ml/kg) excretory urography or intravenous pyelography (IVP). Should the patient require immediate abdominal exploration, the IVP can be obtained in the operating suite. This study is essential to localize the site of injury and establish the presence of

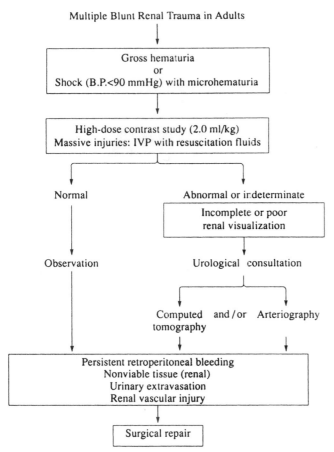

Figure 95–1. Algorithm for diagnosis and treatment of multiple blunt traumatic renal injuries. IVP, intravenous pyelogram.

aortic bifurcation, superior to the inferior mesenteric artery, and extend superiorly to the ligament of Treitz. The aorta may on occasion be impalpable as a result of large retroperitoneal hematomas. In such a case, the inferior mesenteric vein becomes a key landmark in determining the site of the incision. By placing the incision just medial to the inferior mesenteric vein, one can safely dissect in this avascular plane down to the anterior surface of the aorta. Once the aorta is identified, its anterior surface should be dissected superiorly.

The dissection is continued superiorly on the anterior surface of the aorta to the left renal vein as it crosses the aorta anteriorly. This vein is an anatomical landmark for locating the remaining renal vessels (Fig. 95–3). The left renal artery lies just superior and posterior to the left renal vein as it exits the aorta to the left kidney; the right renal artery is superior and medial to the left renal vein as it exits the aorta. The right renal vein can be isolated through this incision and usually enters the vena cava at about the same level as the left renal vein. An alternative approach is to mobilize the second portion of the duodenum off the vena cava to expose the right renal vein. Vessel loops are used to isolate the individual renal vessels of the involved kidney. If bleeding is heavy, the ves-

two kidneys. In some instances in which the patient is hemodynamically stable after resuscitation, the trauma surgeon may wish to evaluate the abdominal injury by computed tomography (CT). In such cases, renal CT should be performed in lieu of IVP. Renal CT or arteriography should be performed when the injury is not clearly defined on IVP.

OPERATIVE TECHNIQUE

A transabdominal midline incision provides complete access to the intra-abdominal viscera and vasculature. Major abdominal bleeding should be controlled with laparotomy packs, followed by surgical control and repair. The liver, spleen, bowel, and pancreas should be carefully inspected.

The surgical approach to the kidney is shown in Figure 95–2. The transverse colon is lifted from the abdomen superiorly and placed on moist laparotomy packs. The small bowel is then lifted on its mesentery superiorly and to the right to expose the retroperitoneum. A vertical incision is made in the retroperitoneum over the aorta just medial to the inferior mesenteric vein. This incision should begin just above the

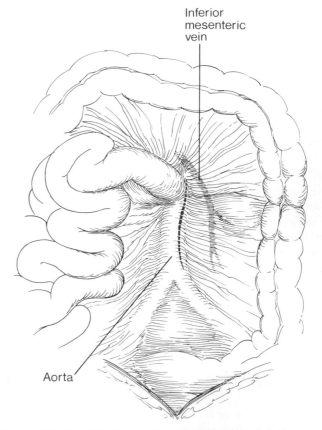

Figure 95–2. Initial incision in the retroperitoneum over the aorta. Note the medial location of the incision with respect to the inferior mesenteric vein.

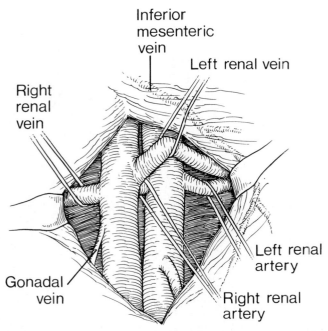

Figure 95–3. Anatomical relationship of the renal vasculature. Note the landmark location of the left renal vein.

sels should be occluded immediately by tightening the loops. Otherwise, vascular control will be adequate until the kidney is completely exposed and the full extent of injury determined. By not clamping the vessels, renal perfusion is continuous and warm ischemia is avoided.

Once vascular control is obtained, the colon is reflected medially by an incision just lateral to it. The hematoma is exposed, Gerota's fascia opened, and the kidney completely exposed. The entire renal surface and vasculature must be exposed to detect multiple renal injuries. Rumel tourniquets can be applied to the vessel loops for vascular occlusion should heavy bleeding be encountered.

Once the kidney is exposed, the site of injury will be obvious. Major polar parenchymal lacerations are best treated by partial nephrectomy. The injured area should be sharply dissected and debrided (Fig. 95–4). The segmental artery to the involved area, but not the renal vein, can be occluded if necessary to control bleeding. If warm ischemia is expected in excess of 30 minutes, the kidney should be cooled in ice slush. After removal of all nonviable tissue, points of bleeding are individually ligated with 4-0 chromic sutures. The collecting system is closed in a watertight manner with running 4-0 chromic sutures. Hemostasis may be improved by application of a gelatin sponge (Gelfoam) or microcollagen hemostatic material to the parenchymal surface. When sufficient capsule is present, it is closed over the defect with a running suture. A pedicle flap of omentum can be used for defect coverage in a case with insufficient capsule (Fig. 95–4C).

The omentum can be brought through a window in the colon mesentery or brought over the colon laterally. The omentum is sutured into place with interrupted 4-0 chromic sutures, which should draw up only small amounts of parenchyma and any existing capsule. The omental flap provides defect coverage with viable vascular tissue that has excellent lymphatic drainage to promote wound healing. In addition, it aids improved hemostasis and reduced urinary extravasation.

Major injuries to the midportion are more difficult to repair (Fig. 95–5). The area must be completely debrided and all nonviable tissue removed. Sites of bleeding should be ligated individually with 4-0 chromic suture and the collecting system securely closed. Gelfoam and microcollagen hemostatic agents are again used to control vascular oozing. When sufficient capsule is present, Gelfoam should be used as a bolster to the 3-0 polydioxanone sutures that are placed in the capsule. As individual sutures are tied, the bolster secures the reconstruction and effectively seals the parenchymal defect to prevent bleeding and extravasation. If the defect is so extensive that the bolster method will not effect closure, an omental pedicle flap can be used.

Injuries to the vasculature are the major causes of renal loss.[5] Penetrating injuries that transect the main renal artery and vein cause massive hemorrhage. Reconstruction is seldom possible. In certain situations in which the kidney appears viable and is not contaminated by fecal spillage, one could choose to preserve it by autotransplantation or ipsilateral repair with hypogastric autograft of splenic artery grafts. These same techniques could be applied to renal artery thrombosis occurring from blunt trauma.

Partial laceration of the main renal artery can be

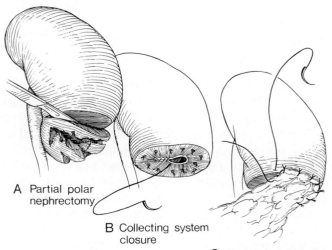

Figure 95–4. A, Debridement and excision of nonviable parenchyma. B, Watertight closure of the collecting system. C, Pedicle flap of the omentum to cover the defect.

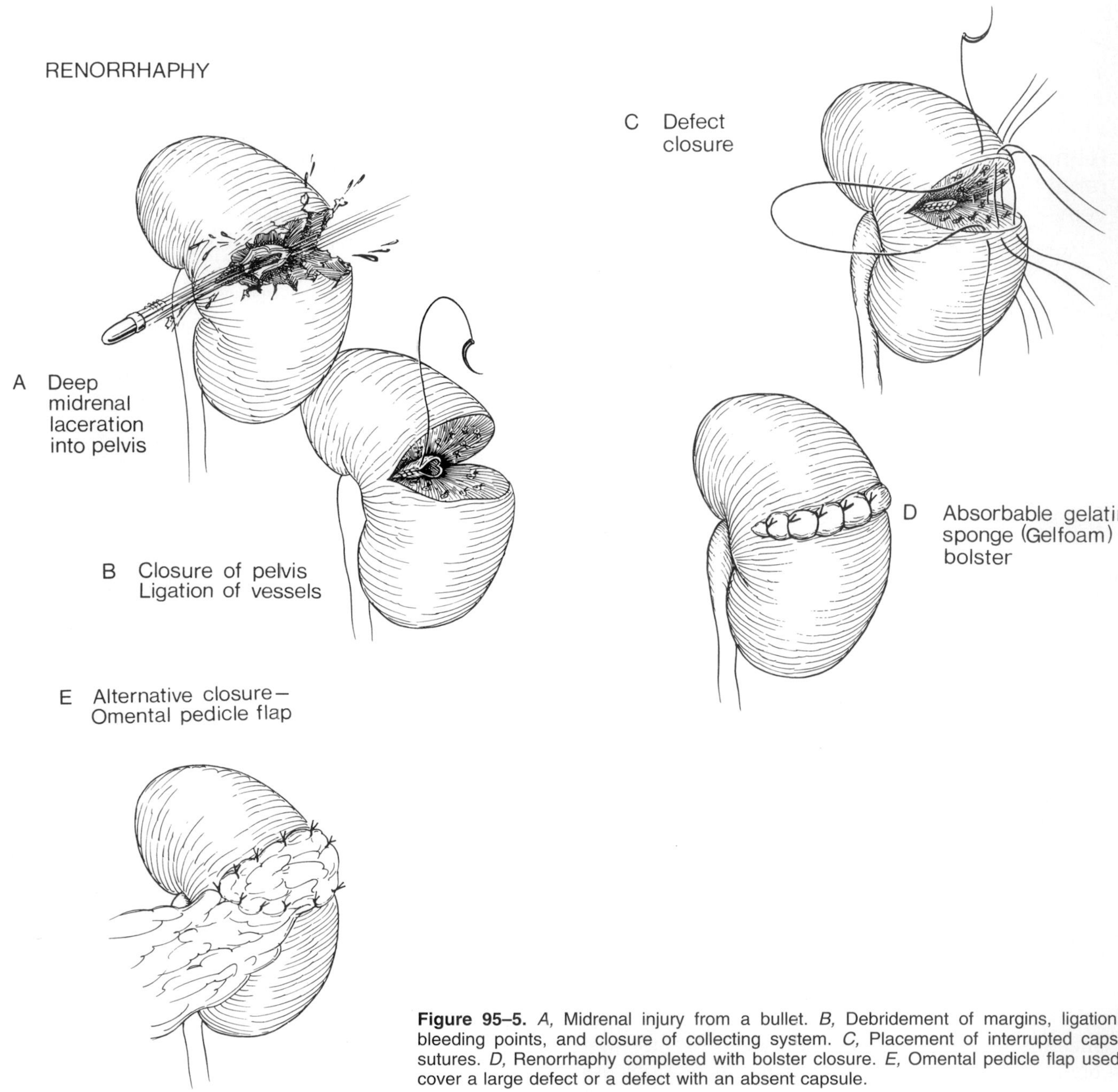

RENORRHAPHY

A Deep midrenal laceration into pelvis

B Closure of pelvis Ligation of vessels

C Defect closure

D Absorbable gelatin sponge (Gelfoam) bolster

E Alternative closure— Omental pedicle flap

Figure 95–5. *A,* Midrenal injury from a bullet. *B,* Debridement of margins, ligation of bleeding points, and closure of collecting system. *C,* Placement of interrupted capsule sutures. *D,* Renorrhaphy completed with bolster closure. *E,* Omental pedicle flap used to cover a large defect or a defect with an absent capsule.

repaired with interrupted 5-0 vascular sutures. Proximal vascular control by arterial clamps is necessary. Local intraluminal irrigation with heparin solution will aid in preventing clot formation. Segmental arteries become thrombosed by blunt trauma. When this problem is associated with parenchymal laceration, a partial nephrectomy should be done. When no parenchymal laceration is present and when the capsule remains intact over the nonviable tissue, expectant management is recommended. These patients so affected are at low risk for hypertension.

Partial transections of the main renal vein require proximal and distal vascular clamps as well as renal artery occlusion by a Rumel tourniquet. The vein can be closed with running 5-0 vascular sutures. Segmental venous injuries can be managed by ligation, which can be done without ischemic damage to the kidney because of the internal collateral circulation of the venous system.

POSTOPERATIVE MANAGEMENT

Gross blood usually clears from the urine within 24 hours. Output should be monitored closely. Retroperitoneal drainage should be checked for creatinine—a level equal to that of serum suggests peritoneal fluid rather than urine. Persistent urinary drainage through the flank drains is unlikely. These drains can usually be removed within 48 to 72 hours. When left in place for a longer period, they offer a source of infection to the retroperitoneal hematoma.

Functional evaluation of the kidney is usually made at 10 days and 3 months by radionuclide renal scan. An IVP is usually obtained at 3 months and 1 year. Frequent blood pressure monitoring ensures that the rare complication of hypertension is detected.

Summary

Total nephrectomy from renal injuries is seldom necessary. In approximately 88 percent of kidneys requiring exploration, sufficient renal tissue can be preserved to avoid dialysis should the opposite kidney be lost. The principles of renal reconstruction after major trauma presented here provide the bases by which renal salvage can be successful.

Editorial Comment
Fray F. Marshall

The management of renal trauma has changed significantly. In an adult with blunt trauma, the absence of shock and fewer than 5 red blood cells per high-power field in the urine are infrequently associated with major injuries requiring surgery. If any clinical suspicion is aroused, I would still have a low threshold for some form of investigation.

Children may present a different clinical situation. If hematuria is present, investigation is generally indicated. Penetrating injuries also usually require investigation. In surgical exploration of the kidney, especially on the right side, occlusion of both the renal vein and renal artery may sometimes be necessary, because significant back-bleeding from the renal vein can occur.

REFERENCES

1. McAninch JW, Carroll PR. Renal exploration after trauma: Indications and reconstructive techniques. Urol Clin North Am 16:203, 1982.
2. Cass AS. Immediate radiologic and surgical management of renal injuries. J Trauma 22: 361, 1982.
3. Mee SL, McAninch JW, Robinson AL, et al. Radiographic assessment of renal trauma: 10-year prospective study of patient selection. J Urol 141:1095, 1989.
4. Carroll PR, McAninch JW. Staging of renal trauma. Urol Clin North Am 16:193, 1989.
5. Cass AS. Renovascular injuries from external trauma: Diagnosis, treatment, and outcome. Urol Clin North Am 16:213, 1989.

Chapter 96

Surgical Repair of Ureteral Injuries

Jack W. McAninch

Injuries to the ureter can result from a variety of causes, including gunshots, stab wounds, surgery, blunt trauma, and radiation. Recognition of these injuries is perhaps the greatest challenge to the clinician. Once ureteral injury is established, surgical repair is required in most cases.

PREOPERATIVE MANAGEMENT

Gunshot and stab wounds to the abdomen are the major causes of ureteral injury from external violence.[1] Patients often have a low level of microhematuria, rarely gross hematuria. In up to 30 percent of these patients, no hematuria can be detected.

Blunt abdominal trauma rarely results in injuries to the ureter. When noted, the injury is most often avulsion at the ureteropelvic junction.[2] Microhematuria is usually present.

Iatrogenic injuries occur during complex retroperitoneal procedures, particularly those in the pelvis. The ureter may be transected, ligated, or partially transected. If the injury is not recognized immediately, delay in diagnosis may create problems in management.[3] If it is recognized within 7 days and immediate re-exploration takes place, repair is usually still possible.

Preoperative imaging of the ureter should be done when suspicion of injury is aroused.[4] Excretory urography is the best initial study. Transected ureters show extravasation of opacified urine; ligated ureters, delayed visualization (occasionally nonvisualization) and hydronephrosis. Retrograde ureterography should be performed in most instances to establish the exact location of injury and provide valuable information regarding the distal ureter.

Intraoperative recognition of injury is best accomplished by exploration and visual inspection of the ureter. Intravenous indigo carmine or methylene blue will begin to appear in the urine within 7 minutes and is helpful in establishing the diagnosis of partial ureteral transection. Exploration of retroperitoneal hematomas, particularly in the pelvis, may be undesirable as a means of establishing the diagnosis. We have applied the technique of opening the bladder, observing the efflux of urine from the ureteral orifice, and passing a catheter to indicate that the ureter has been spared injury.

OPERATIVE TECHNIQUE

The principles of surgical repair of the injured ureter should be applied to each injury: (1) debridement of the nonviable tissue, (2) spatulated or oblique ureteral margins, (3) tension-free anastomosis, (4) watertight anastomosis, and (5) absorbable sutures. A transabdominal approach is best.

Ureteroureterostomy

Ureteroureterostomy is particularly appropriate for injuries to the upper and middle portions of the ureter (Fig. 96–1). The ends of the ureter should be debrided back to viable tissue, established by active bleeding at the margins (Fig. 96–1A).[5] Each end should be spatulated for 5 mm or cut cleanly at an oblique angle. The proximal and distal ureteral ends should be mobilized to make the anastomosis tension free. Optical loupe magnification is desirable and gives the greatest accuracy for suture placement. Interrupted 6-0 absorbable sutures are generally used (Fig. 96–1B). Chromic, polyglycolic acid, or a similar absorbable material is selected. An internal ureteral stent is recommended and can be inserted before

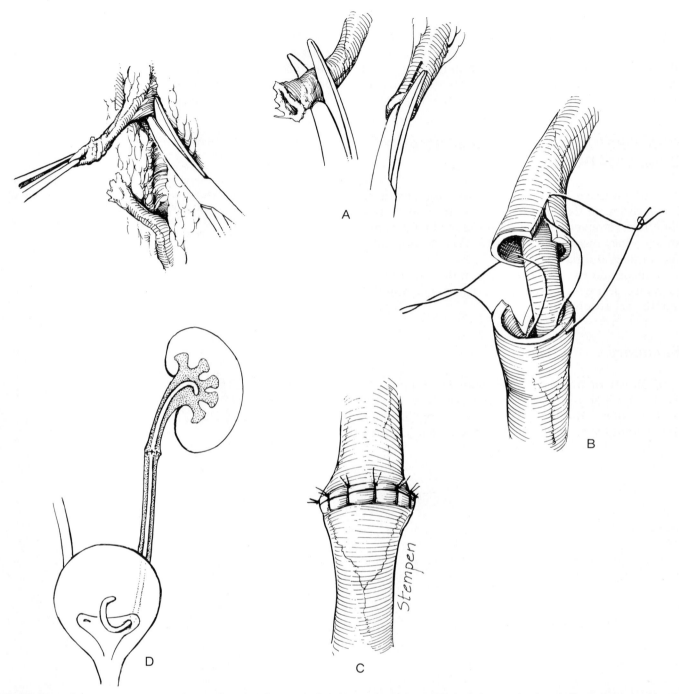

Figure 96–1. Typical ureteral injury from external violence. *A,* Debridement and spatulation of the proximal and distal ureteral ends. *B,* Interrupted anastomosis with an absorbable suture over an internal stent. *C,* Watertight anastomosis completed. *D,* Completed repair with stent in place.

closure to provide proper alignment of the anastomosis and urinary diversion. The anastomosis should be watertight when the procedure is complete (Fig. 96–1*C* and *D*). A Penrose or closed system drain should be used in the area of repair. The stenting catheter should be left in place until the major associated injuries have been stabilized, usually 2 weeks at a minimum. Stents left in place for longer than 3 months risk becoming obstructed from calcium deposit.

Transureteroureterostomy can be used when a segment of ureter is missing and an adequate length cannot be obtained for a tension-free anastomosis.

Injuries to the lower ureter in the pelvis are often best managed by reimplantation into the bladder. An antireflux technique should be used when possible. Tension on the ureteral anastomosis in the bladder can be lowered by using the psoas hitch technique. These repairs are best left with internal stents in place.

Surgical ureteral ligation without transection by sutures can cause ischemia and tissue death. Deligating and observing the area of injury is reassuring, but at the minimum an internal stent should be placed. In the pelvis, ureteral reimplantation should be performed if ureteral viability is uncertain.

POSTOPERATIVE MANAGEMENT AND COMPLICATIONS

Fluid drainage should be checked for creatinine. When drainage has been absent for 48 hours, drains should be removed. Before stent removal (at 2 weeks), an excretory urogram will ensure that the anastomosis is intact and patent.

Stenosis and stricture can occur at the site of repair; therefore, follow-up excretory urograms at 3 and 12 months are recommended.

Summary

Diagnosis of ureteral injury may be difficult, but excretory urography should be performed for any suspected injury. Microscopical or gross hematuria is highly variable and may be absent in some instances. Ureteroureterostomy for the upper and midureteral injury provides excellent and predictable results. Lower ureteral injuries are best managed by ureteral reimplantation into the bladder with an antireflux technique. Early recognition and surgical repair will prevent significant major complications.

Editorial Comment
Fray F. Marshall

After ureteroureterostomy, either a double-J catheter or a stent draining the kidney brought out through the bladder can be temporarily used. Double-J catheters left in place for more than 3 months can calcify at either end and create technical problems during removal.

REFERENCES

1. Presti JC Jr, Carroll PR, McAninch JW. Ureteral and renal pelvic injuries from external trauma: Diagnosis and management. J Trauma 29:370, 1989.
2. Drago JR, Wisna LG, Palmer JM, Link DP. Bilateral ureteropelvic junction avulsion after blunt trauma. Urology 17:169, 1981.
3. Dowling RA, Corriere JN Jr, Sandler CM. Iatrogenic ureteral injury. J Urol 135:912, 1986.
4. Guerriero WG. Ureteral injury. Urol Clin North Am 16:237, 1989.
5. Cass AS. Ureteral contusion with gunshot wounds. J Trauma 24:59, 1984.

Chapter 97

Rupture of the Bladder: Surgical Treatment

Jack W. McAninch

Rupture of the bladder most commonly (8 to 10 percent incidence) occurs in association with pelvic fractures. The blastlike effect of the injury is thought to be the major force rather than penetration of the bladder wall by bony fracture spicules.[1] Multiple injuries are associated. In most cases, soft tissue and intra-abdominal organ injuries and bony fractures are involved. Their repair initially takes precedence over that of the bladder, but simultaneous management is accomplished without difficulty.

PREOPERATIVE MANAGEMENT

Gross hematuria is invariably present in the initial bladder urine of patients who sustain blunt trauma and bladder rupture. Cystography is essential to establish the diagnosis. The bladder must be filled with at least 300 ml of contrast fluid and an abdominal film obtained. The contrast fluid is allowed to drain completely and a postevacuation film is taken. Cystography is very accurate—approximately 15 percent of bladder ruptures are found only on the postevacuation film.[2]

Extraperitoneal bladder rupture can be managed nonoperatively by urethral catheter drainage.[3] This should be maintained for 14 days and a cystogram obtained to confirm healing before catheter removal. In patients undergoing abdominal exploration for associated injuries, bladder repair should be performed.

Intraperitoneal bladder rupture requires operative repair.[4] To avoid the possibility of peritonitis, nonoperative management with urethral catheter drainage should not be undertaken.

OPERATIVE TECHNIQUE

Extraperitoneal Rupture

A midline lower abdominal incision should be made. The large pelvic hematoma, often present, is to be avoided, lest heavy blood loss ensue. This step is best performed by entering the extraperitoneal space over the anterior bladder surface and gently sweeping away the hematoma to expose the anterior bladder surface. Any extensive dissection lateral to the bladder will produce violation of the hematoma, with resultant blood. The bladder wall is lifted superiorly by two stay sutures and incised in the midline. The vertical incision exposes the bladder lumen.

Careful inspection will demonstrate the laceration, most often on the lateral wall. The laceration is closed with interrupted 3-0 chromic sutures, making certain that muscularis and mucosa are included in each stitch (Fig. 97–1). Trigonal laceration near the ureteral orifices or extending into the bladder neck

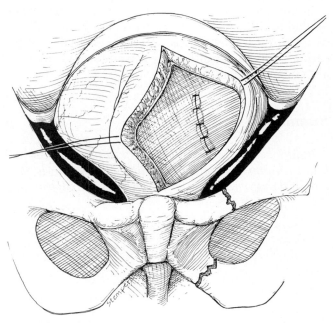

Figure 97–1. Repair of extraperitoneal bladder rupture.

requires special attention. Closure with fine absorbable 4-0 sutures in two layers provides more precise anatomical reconstruction. Ureteral orifices may require temporary catheterization during repair. A cystostomy catheter is left in place.

Intraperitoneal Rupture

The midline incision extends from the symphysis pubis to above the umbilicus. The abdomen is opened and fully explored to detect associated injuries. The margins of the bladder at the rupture site are grasped with Allis clamps, the bladder lumen is inspected for other injury, and the margins are debrided. Closure is made in two layers with continuous 3-0 chromic sutures (Fig. 97–2). The inner layer includes bladder mucosa and muscularis; the outer layer gathers bladder muscle, serosa, and peritoneum. A small extraperitoneal opening is made in the bladder for placement of a cystostomy catheter, which should avoid the peritoneal cavity.

To prevent pelvic hematoma infection, retropubic drains are not placed.

POSTOPERATIVE MANAGEMENT AND COMPLICATIONS

The cystoscopy catheter should remain in place for 7 to 10 days or until the associated injuries are stabilized and the patient can void. Gross hematuria clears within a few days. Bladder recovery allows spontaneous voiding at the time of catheter removal. The cystostomy site will close quickly. The initial urinary frequency slowly subsides, and most patients void normally within 4 to 6 weeks. Patients are prone to bladder infection—prophylactic antibiotics should be given for 6 weeks after catheter removal. Complications of fistula, voiding dysfunction, and infection are uncommon.

Summary

Bladder rupture usually occurs in association with blunt trauma and pelvic fracture. Hematuria is present, and cystography is essential to establish the diagnosis. Extraperitoneal bladder rupture can be managed nonoperatively, although surgical repair can be undertaken if exploratory laparotomy is being performed. All intraperitoneal ruptures should be surgically repaired. Complications are few, and recovery of full bladder function is usual.

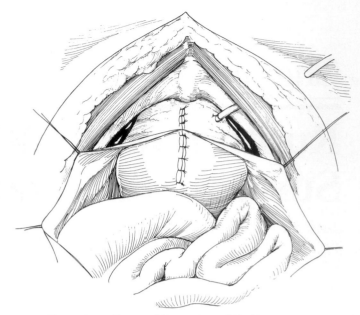

Figure 97–2. Repair of intraperitoneal bladder rupture.

Editorial Comment

Fray F. Marshall

It is emphasized that intraperitoneal ruptures should be closed because of the possibility of continued contamination. Care should be taken on exposure of the retroperitoneal portion of the bladder so that the tamponade of a large pelvic hematoma is not disrupted.

REFERENCES

1. Corriere JN Jr, Sandler CM. Mechanisms of injury, patterns of extravasation and management of extraperitoneal rupture due to blunt trauma. J Urol 139:43, 1988.
2. Carroll PR, McAninch JW. Major bladder trauma: The accuracy of cystography. J Urol 130:887, 1983.
3. Corriere JN Jr, Sandler CM. Management of the ruptured bladder: Seven years with 111 cases. J Trauma 26: 830, 1986.
4. Carroll PR, McAninch JW. Major bladder trauma: Mechanisms of injury and unified method of diagnosis and repair. J Urol 132:254, 1984.

Chapter 98

Membranous Urethral Stricture: Use of Pubectomy in Repair

Jack W. McAninch

Removal of the pubic bone has been used as an aid in the visualization of the prostatomembranous area.[1, 2] This is done particularly in traumatic prostatomembranous urethral disruption, in which the formation of scar tissue prevents easy access for repair. Initial cystostomy drainage of traumatic rupture of the posterior urethra will allow fractures to heal and rehabilitation to begin. Delayed repair of the resulting stricture should be undertaken when the patient is ambulating and the physical condition is stable, but not within 3 months of injury. The major indication for pubectomy is to provide increased exposure so that the anastomosis may be precise.

PREOPERATIVE MANAGEMENT

Complete stricture at the prostatomembranous junction will result after initial treatment with cystostomy drainage for traumatic urethral rupture. There is little reason to evaluate the area radiographically before 3 months, because repair should not be undertaken until then.[3] As the bladder reaches capacity, the patient is asked to void in an attempt to open the bladder neck and fill the prostatic urethra. Simultaneously, retrograde urethrography is performed and the stricture length and location are determined. Fistulous cavities and diverticula can be detected with this technique. At times, flexible cystoscopy of the bladder is useful to inspect the bladder neck and prostatic urethra preoperatively. The verumontanum can be noted, and the site of the obliterating stricture and level of transection determined. The primary indications for pubectomy in prostatomembranous stricture reconstruction are to (1) improve visualization of the anastomosis, (2) remove fistulous tracts and cavities, (3) allow complete excision of scar tissue at the prostatic apex, and (4) allow a tension-free anastomosis between the bulbar urethra and the distal prostatic urethra.[4] Preoperative antibiotics should be given to ensure sterile urine.

OPERATIVE TECHNIQUE

A lithotomy position is preferable, with the buttocks supported by a Vac-Pac (Olympic Medical Corp. Seattle, WA) to help maintain the position and prevent stretch on the sciatic nerves. The goals of this repair are to remove all scar tissue and to direct urethrourethral anastomosis.

An initial midline incision is made in the perineum. The bulbar urethra is mobilized completely and the stricture exposed proximally. A catheter placed in the urethra will detect the exact site where the obliterating stricture begins; intraurethral sounds should be avoided. The urethra with its surrounding corpus spongiosum can be transected at this point. Dissection and repair can be completed through this incision if vision is adequate.

To excise the pubis, a lower abdominal midline incision is made and extended inferiorly down to the base of the penis. The bladder is opened and the prostatic urethra located. The anterior pubis is exposed down to the periosteum and the penile suspensory ligament released. The entire anterior pubis is exposed by lateral dissection. The dorsal penile nerve may be exposed during this dissection and should be carefully preserved.

Attention is given to the posterior aspect of the pubis, which has the underlying densely adherent prostate. The dissection is performed along the posterior pubic symphysis adjacent to the periosteum. Inferior and lateral dissection is required. Bleeding can be minimized by dissection on the periosteum, but subperiosteal dissection is not necessary. At the inferior margin of the pubis, the dissection will communicate with the anterior dissection. Gigli saws are placed laterally and the symphysis is removed (Fig. 98–1). An exposure width of 2.5 to 3.5 cm over the prostate and 4.0 to 5.0 cm anteriorly can be expected.

Hemostasis is carefully obtained. Bone wax is applied to the bone margin. The anterior surface of the prostate is exposed, and the apex identified by placing a sound through the prostatic urethra from inside the bladder. It is important not to attempt any mobilization of the prostate.

All scar tissue surrounding the prostatic apex should be excised and the prostatic urethra calibrated to the diameter of a 30 Fr. catheter. The excellent visualization simplifies this dissection. A short (0.5-cm) spatulation on the anterior surface of the prostate is desirable.

The bulbar urethra is dissected distally from its attachment to the erectile bodies until the urethral ends can be approximated with ease. A 1-cm spatulation is made on the inferior surface of the bulbar urethra and calibrated to the diameter of a 28 Fr. catheter. A direct mucosa-to-mucosa anastomosis of the anterior urethra to the prostatic urethral apex is made with interrupted 5-0 absorbable sutures (Fig. 98–2). Excellent visualization provides the opportunity to place eight to 12 sutures to ensure a watertight anastomosis.

A stenting silicone urethral catheter (18 Fr.) is left in place, and a cystostomy catheter is left in the bladder at closure. A closed suction drain should remain in the pubectomy space for 4 to 5 days. I have not attempted to fill the space with omentum or other material.

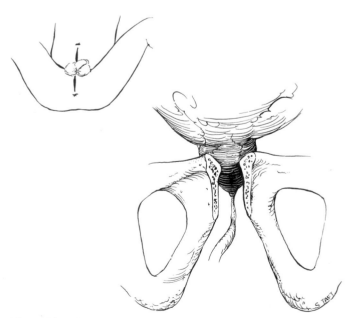

Figure 98–1. A combined perineal/lower abdominal approach is used. The pubis is removed to expose the prostatic apex and stricture.

POSTOPERATIVE MANAGEMENT

Antibiotics should be maintained in the postoperative period. Mean blood loss, in my experience of over 30 patients, has been 800 ml. In most patients with normal preoperative hematocrit values, transfusion can be avoided. Ambulation is begun on the first postoperative day. No patient in our experience has had gait problems or any evidence of an unstable pelvis. Wound infections are uncommon.

The urethral catheter is removed in 3 to 4 weeks. Urine should be sterile. A voiding cystourethrogram should be obtained at this time via the suprapubic cystostomy. In the absence of extravasation or obstruction, the cystostomy is clamped and the patient allowed to void spontaneously for 48 hours. This technique assures the patient that, after not voiding for several months, the surgery has been successful and the bladder is functional. The catheter is removed.

Urine should be kept sterile with antibiotics for several months to permit infection-free healing of the anastomosis. Flow rates should be evaluated regularly. Urethrography should be repeated at 3 and 12 months.

COMPLICATIONS

Incontinence will not occur as a result of the procedure as described. However, incontinence (usually partial) is noted in association with nerve injury to the pelvic and hypogastric plexuses.

Stricture can recur at the anastomotic site (in approximately 10 percent of patients in my experience). This problem is initially managed by visual urethrotomy. Repeated dilation of the urethra should not be required if the procedure is a success.

Potency should not be affected by the operative procedure. Approximately 50 percent of patients will be potent before urethroplasty and will maintain potency postoperatively. The overall impotence rate for this injury, managed as described, is 16 percent.[4] Many patients note return of erectile function only after urethroplasty. The longest delay has been approximately 2 years in our experience. Most patients are temporarily impotent for several weeks immediately after the operative procedure. Ejaculation should be normal in neurologically normal patients.

Summary

Rupture of the posterior urethra is a devastating injury to anyone, particularly the young. Complications of impotence, incontinence, and lifelong stricture disease can create a major disability. Initial cystostomy drainage without attempting repair allows

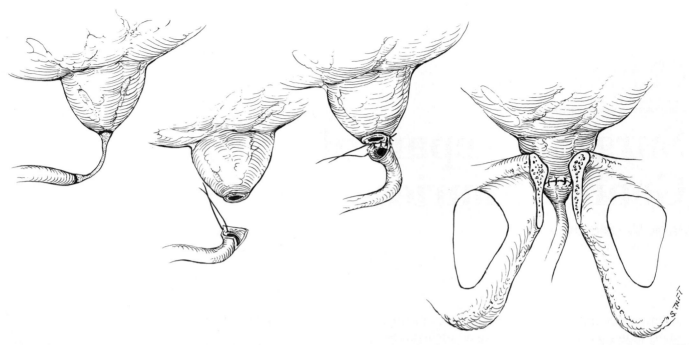

Figure 98–2. The stricture must be completely excised. The bulbar urethra is mobilized distally and spatulated on the inferior surface. Urethrourethral anastomosis is accomplished at the prostatic apex.

the numerous associated injuries to be corrected and healed before urethral reconstruction of the resulting stricture.

Many techniques for repair of the posterior urethral stricture have been described, but complete excision of the scar tissue and direct anastomosis of the urethral ends provide excellent results with few complications. Removal of the pubis during this repair is merely an aid to more complete visualization during reconstruction.

Editorial Comment

Fray F. Marshall

Although we have performed endoscopic reconstruction of total membranous urethral transections, some patients have long defects, fistulas, diverticula, or bone fragments that may preclude this repair. Resection of the symphysis may aid in the operative repair of these patients, as described by Dr. McAninch.

REFERENCES

1. Waterhouse K, Abrahams JJ, Gurber H, et al. The transpubic approach to the lower urinary tract. J Urol 109:486, 1973.
2. Middleton RG, Sutphin MD. Pubectomy in urological surgery. J Urol 133:635, 1985.
3. McAninch JW. Traumatic injuries to the urethra. J Trauma 21:291, 1981.
4. McAninch JW. Pubectomy in repair of membranous urethral stricture. Urol Clin North Am 16:297, 1989.

Chapter 99

Surgical Repair of Genital Injuries

Jack W. McAninch

Genital trauma is very common, but fortunately major injury is rare. Specific anatomical areas are discussed in this chapter to provide for a better description of management.

GENITAL SKIN LOSS

Loss of genital skin can result from avulsion injuries, burns, and infection. Other associated injuries should be stabilized. For infection, drainage, debridement, and antibiotics are indicated. Most wounds require local care to control infection, which can best be accomplished by alternating wet saline dressings with dry dressings and by intermittent debridement of nonviable tissue.

Localized areas of penile or scrotal skin loss can be covered with adjacent skin flaps. Genital skin is very elastic and provides excellent tissue for coverage of large defects.

Total loss of penile and scrotal skin requires an alternative approach—most often, free skin grafts to this area.[1] Split-thickness grafts (0.014 to 0.018 inches thick) taken from the thigh or abdomen are excellent for penile coverage. A very high percentage will take, because the penis has excellent vascularity. Hair does not grow on these grafts and the cosmetic result is excellent.

Total scrotal skin loss can also be managed by grafts. The testicles and spermatic cords are approximated with sutures. Split-thickness grafts are taken and meshed in a 3:1 ratio. These meshed grafts are applied to the testes and cords in sheets. Excellent graft take usually occurs. The resultant healing of the meshed areas leaves the scrotum with a rugation that is similar to normal. The weight and shape of the testicles keep the neoscrotum well expanded and dependent as healing occurs.

PENILE RUPTURE

Rupture of the tunica albuginea occurs with the penis in the erect state. This injury most often occurs during intercourse or other sexual activity but can occur from a direct blow. A loud "cracking" sound is often reported. The patient has immediate pain and detumescence. The penile skin enlarges diffusely from the developing hematoma and darkens with the appearance of a severe contusion. A urethrogram should be obtained, because approximately 20 percent of patients have associated urethral rupture.

Surgical repair provides the best results.[2] A circumferential incision is made in the subcoronal area and the skin is retracted back to the penile base. The laceration is usually near the base of the penis and extends through the tunica albuginea transversely. Should the tear extend around to the ventral penile surface, the urethra is likely to be injured. Margins of the lacerations can be lightly debrided and approximated with interrupted absorbable 2-0 polyglycolic acid sutures.

The functional result is excellent: erections are straight and pain free. Normal sexual activity can be resumed within 3 months.

TESTICULAR RUPTURE

Blunt trauma to the scrotum is the major cause of testicular rupture. Patients often have large scrotal hematomas, and examination is extremely painful. Sonography of the testicles may aid in establishing the diagnosis.

Surgical repair provides drainage of the hematoma and reconstruction of the testicle.[3] Exposure of the testicle via a transscrotal incision will reveal a transverse laceration of the tunica albuginea with extruding testicular parenchyma. The nonviable parenchymal fragments are debrided with preservation of the tunica albuginea, which is approximated with running 4-0 absorbable sutures. The area is usually drained for 48 hours.

The testicle maintains excellent viability and size in most cases. Testosterone secretion should not be affected. However, scar tissue may interrupt drainage of the seminiferous tubules, preventing sperm from leaving the testicle.

Summary

Genital injuries can be devastating if damage is extensive. With appropriate diagnostic tests and reconstructive techniques, a high percentage of patients will have excellent cosmetic and functional results.

Editorial Comment
Fray F. Marshall

Usually, reconstruction can be accomplished satisfactorily. Dr. Lowe has described management of extensive cases of genital injuries and infections, such as Fournier's gangrene, in Chapter 79. Care must be taken to ensure that no concomitant urethral injury is present that deserves repair.

REFERENCES

1. McAninch JW. Management of genital skin loss. Urol Clin North Am 16:387, 1989.
2. Orvis BR, McAninch JW. Penile rupture. Urol Clin North Am 16: 369, 1989.
3. Fournier GR Jr, Laing FC, McAninch JW. Scrotal ultrasonography and the management of testicle trauma. Urol Clin North Am 16:377, 1989.

Chapter 100

Total Penile Construction/ Reconstruction

Gerald H. Jordan, Steven M. Schlossberg, and Charles J. Devine, Jr.

Total penile reconstruction is a therapeutic option for both trauma patients and for young males born with congenital anomalies. Fortunately, the penile amputation patient is rarely encountered in our culture. The ability to successfully reconstruct the penis in these patients has been well documented; however, when a penile amputation patient presents with his amputated organ, all attempts should be made to replant it.

In the case of a patient born with a micropenis/microphallus, three options should be presented to the parents: sex reassignment, eventual phallic construction, or allowing the child to mature without intervention. In the United States, sex reassignment at birth has been the most common choice. While the issue of gonadal labeling of the brain remains controversial, it is accepted that castration should be accomplished in the immediate postbirth period, and vaginal construction performed at puberty. Historically, it was accepted that when sex reassignment was not accomplished early in life, phallic construction was an absolute necessity later on. However, in 1989, Reilly and Woodhouse[1] evaluated a group of micropenis patients in their second and third decades who were allowed to mature without intervention. Despite the fact that these patients reported embarrassing remarks made during adolescence, their data showed that all these patients were sexually active and enjoyed well-balanced sexual identity as adults. Not all patients who persist with their micropenis anomaly into adulthood are happy and sexually active, however, and for this subset of patients, phallic construction for the purpose of enhanced sexual identity is appropriate.

MICRONEUROVASCULAR TECHNIQUES FOR PHALLIC CONSTRUCTION/ RECONSTRUCTION

State-of-the-art total penile construction/reconstruction involves microneurovascular techniques. Basic to the understanding of penile reconstructive techniques is a knowledge of graft and flap techniques, the unique vascular anatomy of the genitalia, and the ischemic tolerance of penile tissues.

Today, the most commonly employed flaps for penile reconstruction and total phallic construction are forearm flaps. Forearm flaps are fasciocutaneous flaps, vascularized via either the ulnar or radial artery. In the upper forearm, the radial artery lies beneath the belly of the brachioradial muscle and is the continuation of the brachial artery. The brachial artery profuses the skin of the forearm via perforators to the fascial plexuses, and has a predictable and well-defined cutaneous vascular territory that encompasses almost its entire circumference. This cuticular vascular territory is more reliable the more closely centered it is to the path of the radial artery. The ulnar artery also arises as a distal continuation of the brachial artery, and like the radial artery, provides a vascular supply via the fascia to most of the circumference of the forearm skin. Its cuticular vascular territory is rotated toward the ulnar aspect and is therefore predictably more reliable over the path of the ulnar vessel.

The forearm flap includes the cephalic, basilic, and medial antebrachial veins. In some patients, these veins predictably provide the dominant venous system. In others the venae comitantes are the dominant system. At the time of flap transfer, it is imperative to evaluate which venous system is providing the venous runoff and to ensure that this system is anastomosed to the recipient veins.

The lateral and medial antebrachial cutaneous nerves are included beneath the fascia of the forearm. The lateral antebrachial cutaneous nerve arises at the elbow as an arborization of the musculocutaneous nerve, providing sensation to both the volar and dorsal radial aspects of the forearm. The medial antebrachial cutaneous nerve arborizes, providing sensation to the ulnar aspect of the forearm.

As with all flaps, there are disadvantages to the forearm flap. Most disadvantages are related to donor site morbidity: unattractive donor site and the development of cold intolerance. Although there is a theoretical possibility of the development of cold intolerance in the donor site caused by the sacrifice of a portion of the arm's arterial blood supply, cold intolerance in the donor site has not been a problem in our series, despite the fact that reconstruction of the radial/ulnar artery is not performed.

Flap Elevation

The forearm flap is elevated from the nondominant arm. Every effort is made to center the urethral portion of the flap in the nonhirsute forearm skin. As stated above, it can be elevated on either the ulnar or radial artery. Neither of these arteries give off necessary branches into the deep tissues of the forearm proper. Elevation of the dominant artery with the flap or elevation of the flap on an inadequate artery would predictably provide a poor outcome. Our patients are carefully screened preoperatively for evidence of insufficiency of the forearm arteries or lack of communication distally through the superficial and deep palmar arches. The Allen screening test is one used to check for sufficiency of the forearm arteries; it allows detection of a patient in whom one artery is clearly dominant. When doubt exists, angiography of the upper extremity is recommended. At our center, we have adopted almost uniform use of flaps based on the ulnar artery.

Flap Application

After the flap is elevated on the forearm, profusion is left intact and the flap is configured into a phallus. A number of modifications for the sculpture of the forearm flap into a phallus have been proposed (Fig. 100–1). As described by Chang and Hwang,[2] shaft coverage is accomplished using the radial aspect of the flap, with a section of de-epithelialized skin separating the shaft from the urethra. The flap is thus a

tube within a tube, with the ulnar aspect (urethra) and the radial aspect (shaft) wrapped around the neourethra, and the urethral portion on the lateral extent of the cuticular vascular territory. A limitation to the use of this design is the occurrence of ischemic stenosis of the urethral portion of the flap. This phenomenon is seemingly more common in white patients than in Asians.

In the modification of Farrow et al,[3] the flap is configured in the shape of a "cricket bat." The wide section of the upper forearm portion of the flap provides shaft coverage, and the urethral portion is a narrow extension centered over the selected artery. The phallus is configured by transposing and inverting the tubed urethral portion into the center of the shaft coverage. This flap design allows the urethral portion to be centered over the respective artery, and we have not observed ischemic stenosis of the urethral portion of the flap using this design. In some patients, the phallus may be quite short and thick, depending on the body habitus of the patient.

Biemer's modification also centers the urethra over the desired forearm artery.[4] In this configuration the urethral tube is central in the flap. Two lateral skin islands, separated from the midline urethral strip by adjacent de-epithelialized strips, are used for shaft coverage. Although the portions of the flap providing shaft coverage may be rather distant to the cuticular vascular territory with this design, the urethra is centered over the artery and consequently reliable. We have, however, observed some spotty areas of ischemia in the shaft coverage portions of this flap.

As stated, we have preferentially shifted to the use of ulnar elevated flaps at our center. The flap design that we use incorporates a number of modifications that have been individually described by a number of others (Fig. 100–2). The urethral and shaft design is Biemer's modification.[4] However, the end of the flap is extended to allow a paddle to be elevated and diverted over the tip of the shaft, creating a cosmetically convincing glans penis. This innovation was used by Puckett and Montie,[5] who used groin flaps to construct phalluses.

All the forearm flaps described in this section create a neourethra that is anastomosed to the patient's native urethra, allowing him to void in a standing position. These forearm flap designs also include superficial sensory nerves, and therefore microcoaptation of the flap cuticular nerves to recipient nerves allows for the development of flap sensibility.

After preparation of the recipient site, the flap is prepared for transfer by meticulous marking and dividing of the respective vessels and nerves. The flap is then immediately transferred to the recipient site, arterial anastomosis is accomplished, two to four venous anastomoses are performed, and urethral anastomosis is achieved. Full-thickness stitches of absorba-

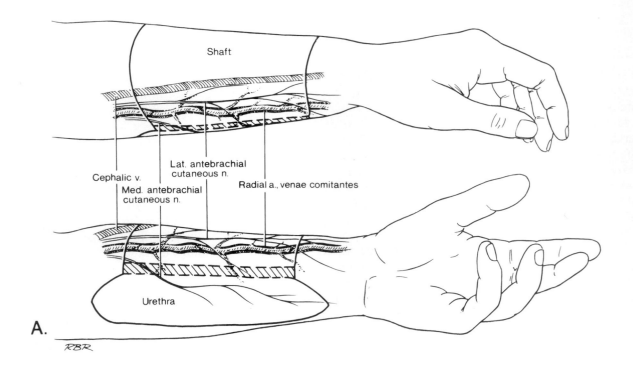

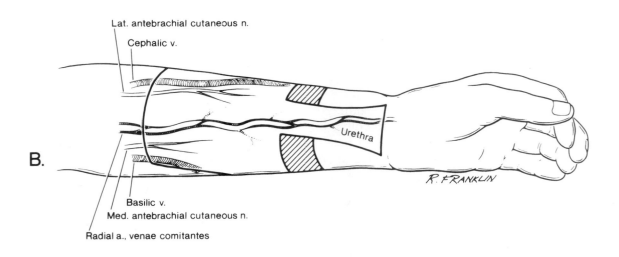

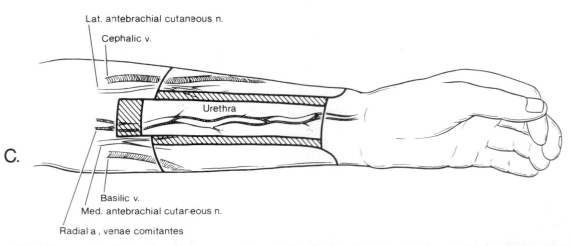

Figure 100–1. Free forearm flap designs for phalic construction. *A,* Chinese flap. *B,* Cricket bat flap. *C,* Biemer design. (From Jordan G. Penile reconstruction. In McAninch JW, ed. Traumatic and Reconstructive Urology. WB Saunders, in press.)

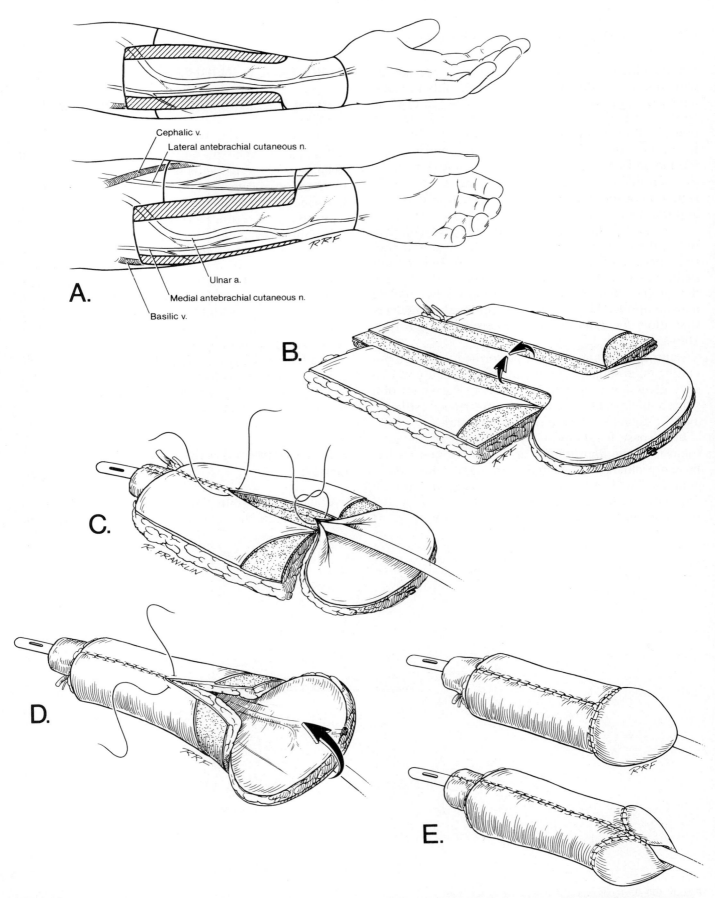

Figure 100–2. Modified Biemer design. Note that the central portion of the flap is centered over the ulnar artery (A). In B the flap is elevated with the midportion of the paddle tubularized to form the urethra. The lateral shaft skin islands are sutured in the ventral midline (C) and then sutured in the dorsal midline (D). The distal extension is flipped over the tip, forming the neoglans and coronal margin (E). (From Jordan G. Penile reconstruction. In Libertino JA, ed. Reconstructive Urologic Surgery. Philadelphia, Mosby-Year Book, in press.)

Labels in A:
Cephalic v.
Lateral antebrachial cutaneous n.
Ulnar a.
Medial antebrachial cutaneous n.
Basilic v.

ble monofilament are used for epithelial apposition, and an outer buttressing layer of absorbable monofilament sutures provide a second layer of the urethral closure. An operating microscope and 9-0 or 10-0 nylon or Prolene sutures are used for the microvascular anastomoses. After the arterial anastomosis is performed and unclamped, the flap veins are examined to determine which ones are providing the dominant runoff, to ensure that those veins are anastomosed to appropriate recipient veins.

After the flap has demonstrated good revascularization without signs of vasospasm, the "glans definition" portion of the procedure is undertaken, if glans definition is not inherently achieved with the flap design (i.e., the modification proposed by Puckett and Montie[5]). There are several optional maneuvers that allow for definition of the coronal margin (Fig. 100–3).

Neurocoaptations are then performed using the operating microscope and 9-0 monofilament suture. Urinary diversion is accomplished with placement of a suprapubic cystostomy tube. A soft, ribbed, silicone 14 Fr. catheter is used to stent the urethra.

In the past, fistula formation at the site of the anastomosis of the flap urethra to the native urethra has been a problem. The switch to monofilament suture, combined with the mobilization of a gracilis muscle flap, appears to have had a favorable impact on the incidence of fistula and/or anastomotic strictures.

AMPUTATION INJURIES

Patient Presents Without an Amputated Organ

The patient who presents without the amputated distal portion of his penis is clearly at a disadvantage in terms of reconstruction. The initial concerns in these patients are hemorrhage and wound management. Because of the marked elasticity of the penile skin, however, amputations often remove more skin than actual penile shaft structures. In many cases, therefore, the shaft can be covered primarily with a split-thickness skin graft, as opposed to being buried, and the distal urethral stump can be managed with the creation of a widely spatulated neomeatus. The neomeatus is constructed in the same manner as one after partial penectomy. In a patient who is left with an inadequate length of penis, the result is not unlike that of someone with a congenital micropenis. For these patients, delayed reconstruction can be performed as described above.

Patient Presents with an Amputated Organ

Whenever possible, the amputated organ should be transported to the treatment facility. To extend the

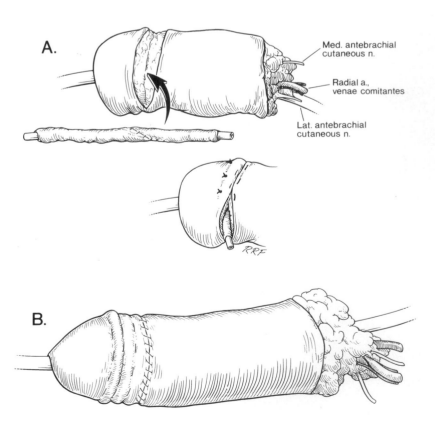

Figure 100–3. Techniques of coronoplasty for free flaps. *A,* Buried split-thickness skin graft technique. *B,* Skin graft with plication technique. (From Jordan G. Penile reconstruction. In Libertino JA, ed. Reconstructive Urologic Surgery. Philadelphia, Mosby-Year Book, in press.)

ischemia time, the organ should be transported using the bag-within-a-bag preservation technique (Fig. 100–4).

Microsurgical replantation techniques have been demonstrated to be superior and are now considered to be the state-of-the-art method of replantation. However, it should be emphasized that if microsurgical techniques are not possible because of the lack of an adequate facility or technical expertise, or if the patient's overall condition is not suitable for a lengthy microvascular-microneural replantation procedure, the replantation can be accomplished by corporeal reapproximation and microvascular penile reattachment, as described by McRoberts et al.[6]

Microsurgical replantation begins with exploration of both ends of the amputated organ, identifying the structures necessary for reanastomosis (Fig. 100–5). When necessary, debridement is judiciously accomplished. Mechanical stabilization of the penis is achieved by stenting the urethra, followed by a two-layer spatulated urethral reanastomosis. I approximate the mucosa with either 6-0 polydioxanone or 6-0 chromic sutures, the adventitia and spongy erectile tissue with either 4-0 or 5-0 PDS suture, and the corpora cavernosa with alternating interrupted 4-0 and 5-0 monofilament sutures.

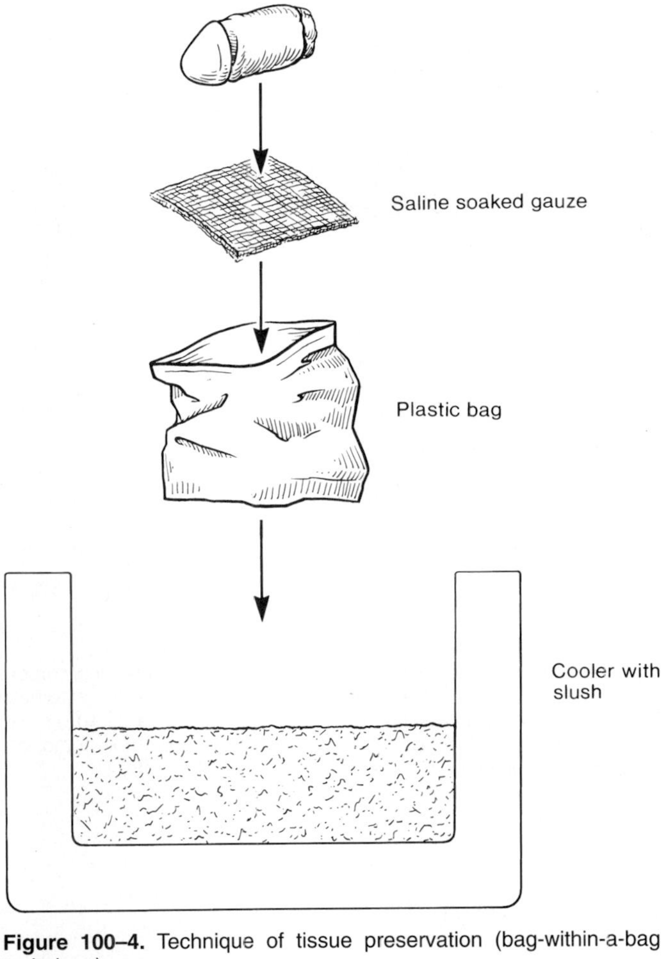

Attention is then directed to the dorsoneurovascular structures. Both arteries are reanastomosed using the operating microscope and 11-0 monofilament suture. Depending on its size, the dorsal vein can be reanastomosed with either 9-0 or 10-0 monofilament suture. After the vascular anastomoses are accomplished, the nerves are coapted with 9-0 monofilament suture. In most cases, an epineural coaptation is applicable.

The skin of the penis should be closed and preserved, even in a circumcised patient. The dartos fascia is closed with absorbable monofilament suture, and the skin can be approximated with either absorbable monofilament suture or small braided absorbable sutures.

The urine should be diverted with a suprapubic cystostomy catheter, and the urethral anastomosis stented with a soft silicone tube. These patients require the same postoperative monitoring as other patients undergoing microvascular surgical procedures: they should be kept well hydrated, and body temperature should be kept normal. Heating lamps, heating blankets, and a heated recovery room are all appropriate. Although anticoagulants are indicated in some cases, we do not routinely use these. However, we do begin our patients on aspirin as soon as they can tolerate oral feedings.

Summary

The success of microvascular transfer techniques for phallic construction, combined with the data of Reilly and Woodhouse,[1] should make one strongly reevaluate the place of sex reassignment in a male born with an inadequate penis. The parents of these children should be made aware not only that the surgical procedures involved with sex reassignment are technically simple, but that their reassigned female child may confront them during adolescence with the fact that she does not want to live the rest of her life under these conditions. There are also many unknowns concerning the long-term effects of phallic construction, and many opportunities for complications with each of the multiple surgeries involved with phallic construction in a prepubertal child, that should be taken into consideration by involved families.

Sex reassignment is not an option in a patient who has had a traumatic penile amputation. The unique vascular properties of the penis, however, have allowed for excellent results with both microsurgical and macrosurgical replantation procedures. Today, total phallic construction and aggressive reconstruc-

Figure 100–4. Technique of tissue preservation (bag-within-a-bag technique).

Saline soaked gauze

Plastic bag

Cooler with slush

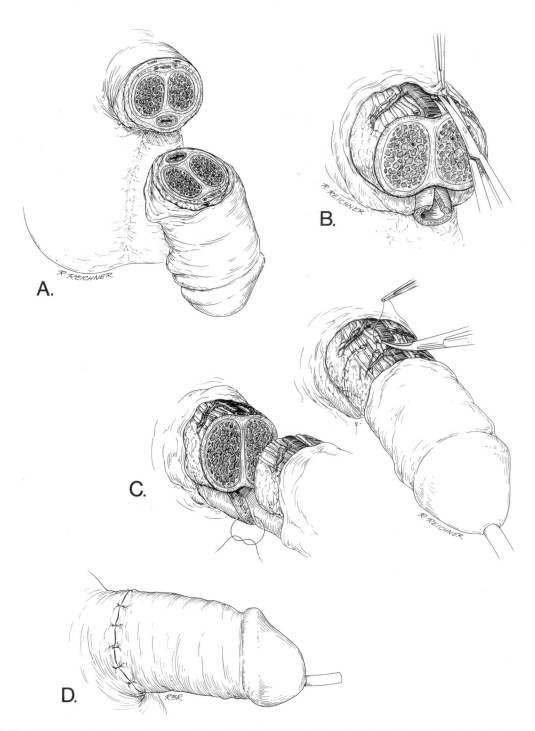

Figure 100–5. *A*, Typical appearance after penile amputation. *B*, The dorsal neurovascular elements are dissected and identified, the corporal stumps are debrided, the corpus spongiosum is mobilized, and the urethral stump is spatulated. *C*, A two-layer spatulated urethral anastomosis is completed. The dorsal vein, both dorsal arteries, and dorsal neural structures are anastomosed/coapted with small (9-0, 10-0, 11-0) monofilament suture. *D*, The skin is approximated (even in the circumcised patient), an SP tube is placed, and the urethral anastomosis is stented. Technique of penile replantation. (From Jordan G. Management of amputation injuries. Urol Clin North Am 16:365, 1989.)

tion are a reality that has improved patients' life styles in even the most difficult of cases.

Editorial Comment

Fray F. Marshall

The cosmetic features of total penile reconstruction have improved. In addition, cutaneous sensation can be produced with microsurgical neural anastomosis. As more of these procedures are carried out, it will be interesting to ascertain the sensation and later sexual activity with this reconstructed type of phallus.

REFERENCES

1. Reilly JM, Woodhouse CR. Small penis and the male sexual role. J Urol 142:569, 1989.
2. Chang TS, Hwang WY. Forearm flap in one-stage reconstruction of the penis. Plast Reconstr Surg 74:251, 1984.
3. Farrow GA, Boyd JB, Semple JL. Total reconstruction of a penis employing the "cricket bat flap" single stage forearm free graft. AUA Today 3:2, 1990.
4. Biemer E. Penile construction by the radial arm flap. Clin Plast Surg 15:425, 1988.
5. Puckett CL, Montie JE. Construction of the male genitalia in the transsexual using a tubed groin flap for the penis and a hydraulic inflative device. Plast Reconstr Surg 61:523, 1978.
6. McRoberts JW, Chapman WH, Ansell JS. Primary anastomosis of the traumatically amputated penis. Case report and summary of literature. J Urol 100:751, 1968.

SECTION V

PEDIATRIC UROLOGICAL SURGERY

Part I
Kidney

Part II
Ureter/Bladder

Part III
Genitalia/Urethra

Part IV
Miscellaneous

Part I

KIDNEY

Chapter 101

The Correction of Ureteropelvic Junction Obstruction

Terry W. Hensle and Andrew J. Kirsch

Obstruction at the ureteropelvic junction (UPJ) is most frequently diagnosed in infancy and childhood but can be diagnosed in all age groups. Initial presenting symptoms may vary widely, but prenatal ultrasonography is the most common form of presentation in the totally asymptomatic newborn. Older children usually present with abdominal pain, urinary tract infection, or hematuria. UPJ obstruction occurs twice as often in males, and in most reports the left kidney is more frequently involved than the right. The incidence of bilaterality varies in different series but is considered generally to be about 20 percent.[1-7]

The dilated collecting system in the neonate has become a widely debated issue. It is clear that dilation does not always represent obstruction. Mild or moderate neonatal hydronephrosis may be associated with a low risk of causing renal damage and often can be managed nonoperatively.[8]

PATHOGENESIS

Obstruction at the UPJ can be related to either extrinsic or intrinsic lesions of the collecting system. Regardless of the cause, the end result is poorly propelled urinary bolus across the UPJ that results in hydronephrosis. True obstruction may lead to varying degrees of renal parenchymal destruction. In the most severe form, seen with proximal ureteral atresia, the result is the development of a multicystic kidney. The association of UPJ obstruction in the contralateral kidney of an infant with unilateral multicystic kidney suggests that the cause is often a bilateral ureteral bud defect.[3-7]

In most instances a congenital intrinsic lesion is responsible for the UPJ obstruction. The histopathology of the obstruction has been shown to be very similar to that of primary obstructive megaureter. An abundance of intracellular ground substance and collagen is present within the ureter as well as smooth muscle cell dysplasia, which is most striking at the point of maximal obstruction, decreasing in severity proximal to the obstruction (Fig. 101–1). This finding has been convincingly demonstrated in electron microscopic and histochemical studies by Hanna and co-workers[9, 10] and Gosling and Dixon.[11]

Other conditions, such as aberrant lower pole vessels, ureteral bands, kinks, high insertions of the ureteral ostium on the renal pelvis, intraluminal polyps, and ureteral valves, have been proposed as causes of some UPJ obstructions. The controversy over whether polar vessels are primarily responsible for UPJ or whether the redundant hydronephrotic renal pelvis merely drapes over the vessel is long-standing.[9, 12] Most investigators agree that the primary lesion is intrinsic and that the ballooning of the renal pelvis over the polar vessels is usually secondary to the intrinsic lesion.[13]

UPJ obstruction may also be encountered in association with vesicoureteral reflux.[14] Whether the upper ureteral obstruction is a concomitant anomaly or a direct result of the reflux is often difficult to determine. When significant UPJ is found in the presence of low grades of reflux, the obstruction is usually an independent lesion. When UPJ obstruction is associated with massive degrees of reflux, however, it is usually caused by tortuosity and kinking of the upper ureter from the reflux.[14] In either case the degree of obstruction should be quantified before antireflux surgery is performed. In most instances, if the ob-

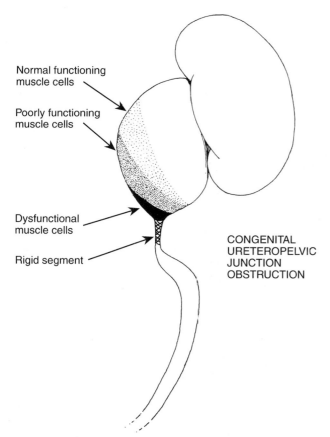

Normal functioning
muscle cells

Poorly functioning
muscle cells

Dysfunctional
muscle cells

Rigid segment

CONGENITAL
URETEROPELVIC
JUNCTION
OBSTRUCTION

Figure 101–1. Pathophysiology of a ureteropelvic junction obstruction demonstrating both a distal rigid segment and more proximal dysfunctional tissue that extends up into the renal pelvis itself.

struction at the UPJ is mild, it will subside once the reflux has been corrected. If, however, significant obstruction coexists with significant reflux, it should be corrected before undertaking antireflux surgery. The resultant edema at the ureterovesical junction may further compromise renal drainage.

PRESENTATION AND DIAGNOSIS

Prenatal screening with ultrasonography has radically changed the mode of presentation of UPJ obstruction. With increasing frequency, hydronephrosis is found in an otherwise normal fetus on routine prenatal ultrasonographic screening. This screening has shifted the average age group of the patients being evaluated for UPJ obstruction from older children to neonates. Our own data indicate that in most infants undergoing surgery for UPJ obstruction, the initial diagnosis was made with prenatal ultrasound screening. In our series, 79 percent of infants having pyeloplasty were discovered prenatally, while only 11 percent had an abdominal mass and 10 percent presented with urinary tract infection.[15]

In older children and adults, the presenting symptoms are most often abdominal or flank pain, urinary tract infection, and hematuria. Gross hematuria can occur in the adolescent with UPJ obstruction after minor flank or abdominal trauma.[1–7] Vague abdominal symptoms mimicking gastrointestinal disorders have frequently been recognized to be caused by UPJ obstruction alone in children.[2] Many of the symptoms of UPJ obstruction may be intermittent and occur only during rapid diuresis. In suspected cases of intermittent obstruction, a diuretic excretory urogram or radionuclide scan may not only reproduce the symptoms but also simultaneously confirm the obstruction.[13, 14]

Ultrasonography and isotope scanning have largely replaced the excretory urogram as the primary diagnostic tools for evaluation of UPJ obstruction in neonates and infants. In older children and adults, however, the excretory urogram probably remains the cornerstone of diagnosis. High-grade obstruction may cause marked delay in the excretion of contrast material, and delayed films are often necessary. The renal pelvis may not be visualized, and high-dose intravenous drip infusion urography and nephrotomography improve the diagnostic yield. Alternatively, we prefer the technetium 99m diethylenetriamine pentaacetic acid (DTPA) diuretic renogram, as popularized by Koff and associates and others,[16–18] which provides an objective assessment of renal parenchymal function as well as a quantification of the degree of obstruction.

The antegrade pressure perfusion studies originally described by Whitaker[19, 20] often give wonderful pictures but are cumbersome to perform and often add little to solving a diagnostic dilemma. We tend to reserve antegrade studies for patients in whom a preoperative percutaneous nephrostomy tube might be indicated.

Voiding cystourethrography has traditionally been carried out in all patients with UPJ obstruction to determine the 10 to 13 percent of these patients with concurrent vesicoureteral reflux, but there is some sentiment against this. The routine use of retrograde pyelography as a diagnostic tool is not indicated except as a confirmatory study just before pyeloplasty. Retrograde pyelography in the presence of an obstructed renal pelvis may precipitate urosepsis and should be carried out only immediately before surgery.[21]

SURGICAL OPTIONS

Historically, the surgical correction of UPJ obstruction has been approached in many ways. In 1937, Foley[22] reported his technique of Y-V plasty that remains a useful operation for high insertion of the ureter on the renal pelvis. Davis[23] first described intubated ureterostomy in 1943. In 1949, Anderson and

Hynes[24] introduced the dismembered pyeloplasty that remains popular today. In the 1950s, a variety of pyeloplasties using renal pelvic flaps were introduced. Scardino and Prince[25] advocated a vertical flap technique, for which Culp and DeWeerd[26] suggested a spiral flap. Both these techniques are extremely useful in long, proximal ureteral strictures where dismembered pyeloplasty cannot be accomplished without tension.

The Dismembered Pyeloplasty

In our opinion, the dismembered pyeloplasty is the most versatile of the ureteropelvic reconstructive procedures. Dismembered pyeloplasty allows removal of the primary pathology and the creation of a dependent, funnel-shaped pelvis, which can initiate a strong enough peristaltic wave to carry a urinary bolus across the reconstructed UPJ. Hanley[27] described a normal funnel-shaped renal pelvis and a boxlike abnormal renal pelvis obstruction noted during diuresis. His data indicate that the creation of a dependently draining, funnel-shaped renal pelvis is likely to result in a favorable outcome after plastic repair.

Surgical Technique

Adherence to rigid principles in surgical technique offers the best chance of obtaining favorable results in UPJ reconstruction, no matter what technique is selected. We attempt to employ the operation that best fits the patient's anatomical defect. However, the Anderson-Hynes dismembered pyeloplasty, because of its simplicity, has become our preferred procedure, as it has at most medical centers around the world.[24]

The patient is placed in a supine position with a sandbag under the flank. The table is flexed modestly to facilitate the anterior approach to the renal pelvis. An incision is made from the tip of the twelfth rib and carried medially in a transverse fashion to a point 2 fingerbreadths lateral to the rectus abdominis muscle and 2 fingerbreadths above the umbilicus (Fig. 101–2). This incision allows the surgeon direct access to the renal hilum and UPJ. The tip of the twelfth rib may be resected if additional exposure is needed, but we have not found this step necessary in most pediatric patients.

The external and internal oblique muscle incision is in the direction of the skin incision. Laterally, the latissimus dorsi is incised just enough to provide sufficient relaxation of the wound. The transversus abdominis is split in the direction of its fibers, and the lumbodorsal fascia is sharply incised (Fig. 101–3). The peritoneum is bluntly displaced medially and Gerota's fascia incised. At this point, the Denis

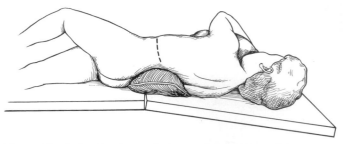

Figure 101–2. Position for pyeloplasty using a subcostal transverse muscle-splitting incision.

Browne self-retaining ring retractor is placed in the wound for maximal exposure (Fig. 101–4).

Great care must be taken to minimize trauma to the upper ureter. The blood supply of this region is segmental (Fig. 101–5) and is best maintained by minimal dissection of the upper ureter and pelvis in situ.[28]

Once the area of obstruction is exposed, attention is directed toward designing the repair. Stay sutures are placed in the superomedial and inferolateral renal pelvis as well as the adventitial layer of the upper ureter. Methylene blue is useful for marking the line of resection once the pelvis is decompressed (Fig. 101–6).

The upper ureter is transected obliquely and spatulated ventrally for about 2 cm, leaving the medial blood supply undisturbed. The reanastomosis of the ureter and resected renal pelvis is accomplished using 5-0, 6-0, or 7-0 absorbable sutures, depending on the size of the patient. The suture line can be either interrupted or continuous with knots tied outside the lumen (Fig. 101–7).

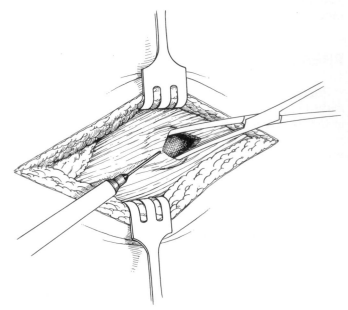

Figure 101–3. Incision in the external oblique muscle utilizing electrocautery.

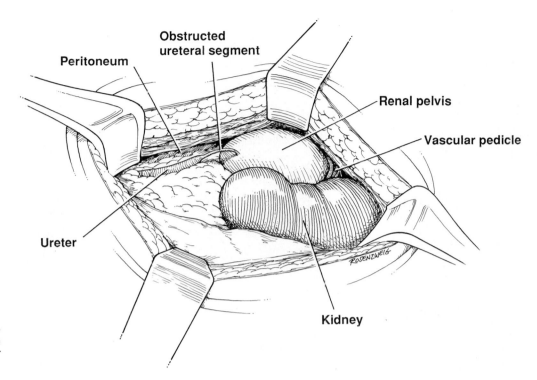

Figure 101–4. Anatomy of the exposed ureteropelvic junction with the Denis Browne ring retractor in place.

After several sutures have been secured, a nephrostomy tube can be placed in the lower pole if indicated. In most instances we prefer to perform the pyeloplasty without a nephrostomy tube in place unless there is a contraindication, such as tissue inflammation, renal calculi, or reoperation. We use a small feeding tube (5 Fr.) or red rubber catheter of appropriate size as a temporary stent to facilitate the anastomosis (Fig. 101–8).

The stent must be removed before the anastomosis is completed and the tapered renal pelvis is closed (Fig. 101–9). The anastomosis can be tested for patency and leakage either through the nephrostomy tube, if one is in place, or through a small butterfly

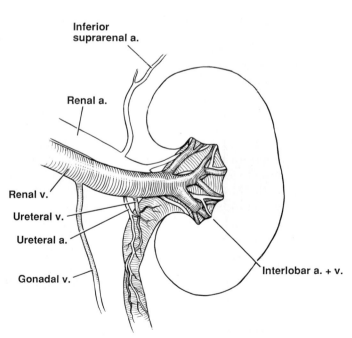

Figure 101–5. Vascular anatomy of the kidney and upper ureter demonstrating the segmental blood supply to the upper ureter from the ureteral artery.

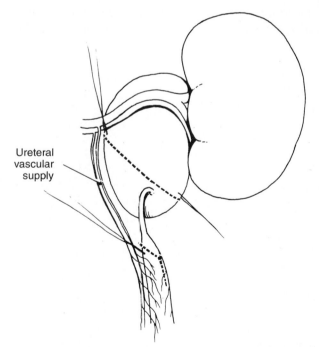

Figure 101–6. Design of a dismembered pyeloplasty showing traction sutures in place in both the renal pelvis and upper ureter to help maintain anatomical symmetry.

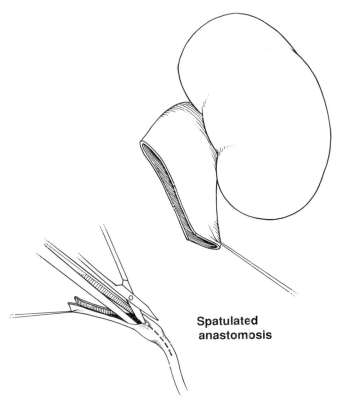

Figure 101–7. Beginning of the ureteropelvic anastomosis with the renal pelvis attached to the most distal portion of the spatulated ureter on its medial border.

needle placed into the renal pelvis. A leak can be closed with additional sutures. The repair is drained postoperatively with a soft Penrose drain, which is placed dependently and brought out through the posterior aspect of the incision. Wound closure is accom-

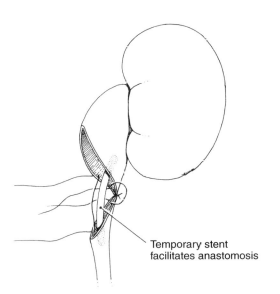

Figure 101–8. Beginning of a running suture for the ureteropelvic anastomosis with a temporary plastic stent in place to help identify the exact lumen of the spatulated ureter.

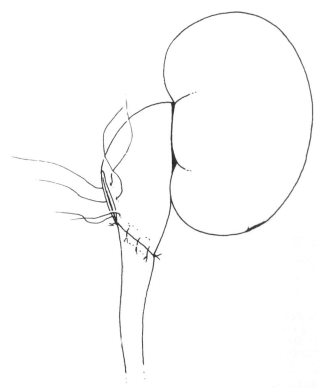

Figure 101–9. Anastomosis being completed after the temporary stent has been removed.

plished in layers, using continuous absorbable suture, and the bladder is drained with a Foley catheter.

Whether stenting a ureteropelvic anastomosis is beneficial or not remains controversial. Evidence from several investigators suggests that fewer long-term problems are encountered in dismembered pyeloplasty done without stenting catheters passing through the anastomosis.[28] However, a strong case for proximal urinary diversion after pyeloplasty can be made from data provided by Caine and Hermann,[29] who demonstrated in cineradiographical studies that normal ureteral peristalsis does not return for about 3 weeks after anastomosis. If a nephrostomy is created, the tube is left to gravity drainage for 3 to 4 days postoperatively and clamped intermittently. Residuals are measured. In most instances the patient is discharged on the fifth postoperative day with the tube clamped. At 10 days a nephrostogram is performed with fluoroscopy. If the renal pelvis drains well, the nephrostomy or pyeloplasty tube is removed. If contrast is retained in the renal pelvis, the patient may be sent home again with the tube in place and re-examined in a similar manner after several weeks. The nephrostomy tract can on rare occasions be used for endoscopy of the anastomosis if persistent obstruction is present.

Other Pyeloplasty Techniques

Each of the major types of nondismembering pyeloplasty techniques has specific advantages and applications that allow maximal surgical results when these operations are applied to a particular pathological anatomy. For example, the Foley Y-V plasty is particularly helpful in reconstructing the high insertion type of UPJ obstruction.[22]

The surgical technique in all the nondismembering operations is the same as in the Anderson-Hynes procedure described, until the point where the UPJ is approached.

In the Foley Y-V plasty a widely based V-flap is designed from the inferolateral aspect of the renal pelvis and carefully outlined with a tissue marker or methylene blue (Fig. 101–10A). The ureter, which is best left in situ, is spatulated laterally. The apex of the V-flap is brought down and anastomosis is performed to the lowest point of spatulation (Fig. 101–10B and C).

A very similar procedure has been described that is particularly helpful in a high-insertion UPJ obstruction and in a horseshoe kidney with an anteriorly placed renal pelvis (Fig. 101–11).

The various flap procedures are similar in principle to the Foley Y-V plasty in that a wide-based flap of redundant pelvis is rotated inferiorly, and anastomosis is beyond a spatulated, narrowed UPJ. The two most popular flap procedures have been the Culp-DeWeerd spiral flap[24] and the Scardino-Prince procedure.[25]

The Culp-DeWeerd operation involves creation of a long flap of pelvis, which when rotated laterally and inferiorly will oppose the spatulated, narrowed segment or proximal ureter. The spatulation is generally performed on the anteromedial aspect of the ureter and should extend just beyond the narrowed segment (Fig. 101–12). This procedure and the Scar-

dino-Prince flap procedure have particular application to long proximal ureteral strictures. The Scardino-Prince operation differs from the Culp-DeWeerd procedure only in that a vertical flap of redundant pelvis is rotated inferiorly and anastomosis is to the spatulated proximal ureteral stricture (Fig. 101–13).

Nephrectomy

Nephrectomy is rarely necessary as a form of primary therapy in the pediatric patient with UPJ obstruction. In 1968, Uson and co-workers[30] reported a 36 percent primary nephrectomy rate in a series of 136 kidneys. Kelalis and associates[31] described a nephrectomy rate of 24 percent. In the late 1970s, fewer reports of primary nephrectomies appeared. In Great Britain, Williams and Kenawi[4] and Johnston and colleagues[6] described a 4.8 and 10 percent primary nephrectomy rate, respectively. In the United States, Hendren and co-workers[1, 32] reported a primary nephrectomy rate for UPJ obstruction of only 5 percent. This improvement is consistent with better surgical technique, as well as earlier diagnosis.

POSTOPERATIVE MANAGEMENT

After successful surgical correction of UPJ obstruction, patients are maintained on antibiotics for 3 months. Radioisotope scanning or excretory urography is performed at 3 months to assess the patency of the pyeloureteral anastomosis and level of renal function of the affected renal unit.

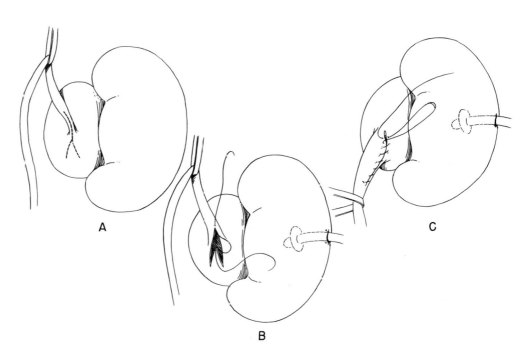

Figure 101–10. Foley Y-V pyeloplasty. *A,* Inverted Y incision from the ureter into the dilated renal pelvis. *B,* Advancement of the tip of the Y incision up into the ureteral incision. *C,* Anastomosis being completed.

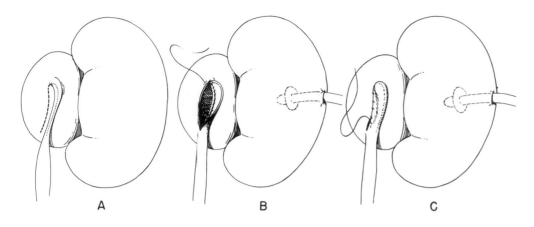

Figure 101–11. Repair of a high-insertion ureteropelvic junction obstruction. *A,* Inverted U incision extending from the dilated renal pelvis into the ureter. *B,* Anastomosis of the ureter itself into the incised renal pelvis. *C,* Completion of the anastomosis.

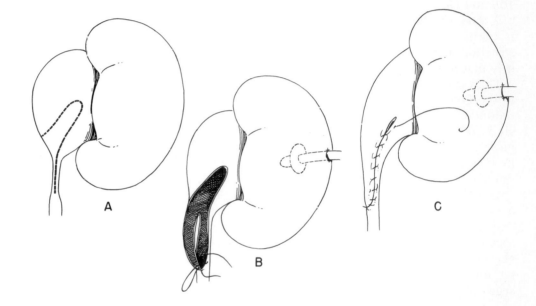

Figure 101–12. Culp-DeWeerd flap pyeloplasty. *A,* Outline of a U flap designed in the renal pelvis and extended into the stenotic portion of the ureter. *B,* Advancement of the U flap into the opened spatulated ureter. *C,* Completion of the anastomosis.

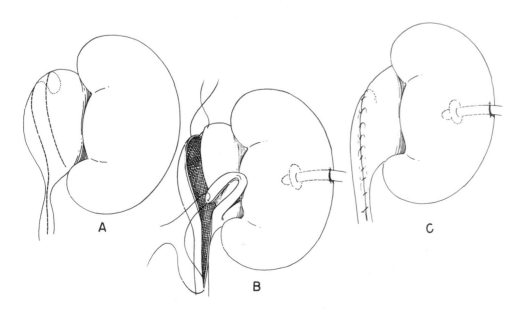

Figure 101–13. Scardino-Prince vertical flap pyeloplasty. *A,* Design of a spiral flap on the renal pelvis. *B,* Mobilization of the flap advanced into the spatulated ureter. *C,* Completion of the anastomosis.

Editorial Comment
Craig A. Peters

Management of the infant with a presumed UPJ obstruction remains highly controversial. The surgical management, however, is well defined as outlined in this chapter. Retrograde pyelography remains part of my evaluation when the ureter has not been visualized by an intravenous pyelogram. Although the likelihood of identifying a separate process is low, the benefit of finding it preoperatively is significant. The lumbodorsal incision has proved to be a very useful approach for pyeloplasty in both infants and older children. There is no real compromise in exposure, crossing vessels are readily managed, and patients seem to recover more quickly from the non–muscle-cutting incision. Tubes or stents are not part of my routine surgical management of a UPJ obstruction at present.

Repeat surgery for pyeloplasty is difficult, yet open surgery remains the most certain means of treatment. Recent investigation into the use of endopyelotomy for secondary obstructions suggests this as a possible alternative, the effectiveness of which remains to be proved in children.

REFERENCES

1. Hendren WH, Radhakrishnan J, Middleton AW. Pediatric pyeloplasty. J Pediatr Surg 15:133, 1980.
2. Zincke H, Kelalis PP, Culp OS. Ureteropelvic obstruction in children. Surg Gynecol Obstet 139:873, 1974.
3. Robson WJ, Rudy SJ, Johnston JH. Pelvic ureteric obstruction in infancy. J Pediatr Surg 11:57, 1976.
4. Williams DI, Kenawi MM. The prognosis of pelviureteric obstruction in childhood: A review of 190 cases. Eur Urol 2:57, 1976.
5. Smith P, Roberts M, Whitaker RH, Garousche AR. Primary pelvic hydronephrosis in children: A retrospective study. Br J Urol 177:97, 1977.
6. Johnston JH, Evans JP, Glassberg KI, Shapiro SR. Pelvic hydronephrosis in children: A review of 219 personal cases. J Urol 177:97, 1977.
7. Williams DI, Karlaftis CM. Hydronephrosis due to pelviureteric obstruction in the newborn. Br J Urol 38:138, 1969.
8. Koff SA, Campbell KD. The nonoperative management of unilateral neonatal hydronephrosis: The natural history of properly functioning kidneys. J Urol 152:593, 1994.
9. Hanna MK. Some observations on congenital ureteropelvic junction obstruction. Urology 12:151, 1978.
10. Hanna MK, Jeffs RD, Sturgess JM, Baskin M. Part II: Congenital ureteropelvic junction obstruction and primary obstructive megaureter. J Urol 116:725, 1976.
11. Gosling JA, Dixon JS. Functional obstruction of the ureter and renal pelvis: A histological and electron microscopic study. Br J Urol 50:145, 1978.
12. Flashner SC, King LR. Ureteropelvic junction. In Kelalia PP, King LR, Belman AB, eds. Clinical Pediatric Urology, 3rd ed, Vol 2. Philadelphia, WB Saunders, 1992, p 693.
13. Johnston JH. The pathogenesis of hydronephrosis in children. Br J Urol 41:724, 1969.
14. Lebowitz RL, Johan BG. The coexistence of ureteropelvic junction obstruction and reflux. Am J Radiol 140:231, 1982.
15. Landman J, Kirsch AJ, Hensle TW. Ureteropelvic junction obstruction in infancy: Trends in diagnosis and treatment (unpublished data).
16. Koff SA, Thrall JH, Keyes JW Jr. Diuretic radionuclide urography: A noninvasive method of evaluating nephroureteral dilation. J Urol 122:451, 1989.
17. Koff SA, Thrall JH, Keyes JW Jr. Assessment of hydroureteronephrosis in children using diuretic radionuclide urography. J Urol 123:531, 1989.
18. O'Reilly PH, Testa HJ, Lawson RS, et al. Diuresis renography in equivocal urinary tract obstruction. Br J Urol 50:76, 1978.
19. Whitaker RH. Investigating wide ureters with ureter pressure flow studies. J Urol 116:81, 1976.
20. Whitaker RR. The Whitaker test. Urol Clin North Am 6:529, 1979.
21. Rushton HG, Salem Y, Belman AB, et al. Pediatric pyeloplasty: Is routine retrograde pyelography necessary? J Urol 152:604, 1994.
22. Foley FB. A new plastic operation for stricture at the ureteropelvic junction. J Urol 38:643, 1937.
23. Davis DM. Intubated ureterstomy—a new operation for ureteral and ureteropelvic stricture. Surg Gynecol Obstet 76:513, 1943.
24. Anderson JC, Hynes W. Retrocaval ureter: A case diagnosed preoperatively and treated successfully by plastic operation. Br J Urol 21:209, 1949.
25. Scardino PL, Prince CL. Vertical flap ureteropelvioplasty. South Med J 46:325, 1953.
26. Culp OS, DeWeerd JH. A pelvic flap operation for certain types of ureteropelvic obstruction: Observations after 2 years' experience. J Urol 71:523, 1954.
27. Hanley HG. The pelviureteric junction: A cinepyelographic study. Br J Urol 31:377, 1959.
28. Nguyen D, Albabodi H, Ercole C, et al. Non-intubated Anderson-Hynes repair of ureteropelvic junction obstruction in 60 patients. J Urol 142:704, 1989.
29. Caine M, Hermann G. The return of peristalsis in the anastomosed ureter. Br J Urol 42:164, 1970.
30. Uson AC, Cox LA, Lattimer JK. Hydronephrosis in infants and children. JAMA 205:75, 1968.
31. Kelalis PP, Culp O, Strickler GB, et al. Ureteropelvic obstruction in children: Experience with 109 cases. J Urol 106:418, 1971.
32. Crooks KK, Hendren WHH, Pfister RC. Giant hydronephrosis in children. J Pediatr Surg 14:844, 1979.

Chapter 102

Partial Nephrectomy and Ureteropyelostomy

James Mandell

The anatomical abnormalities for which the operative procedures of polar partial nephrectomy and/or ureteropyelostomy are indicated include duplex anomalies with either an ectopic ureter or ectopic ureterocele. Both are congenital in origin and arise in association with a completely duplicated collecting system with two separate ureteral orifices. In both instances the lower pole collecting system enters the bladder in a normal or laterally placed position on the trigone. The upper ureter may enter within the bladder or entirely outside its confines.

PREOPERATIVE EVALUATION

Ureterocele

A ureterocele arises from a cystic dilation of the terminal ureter, usually associated with the upper renal moiety of a duplex collecting system. It can be less commonly associated with a single collecting system, but these are rarely symptomatic in childhood. If located entirely within the bladder, the ureterocele is termed intravesical; if it extends into the bladder neck or distally into the urethra, it is called extravesical or ectopic.

Previously, the most common clinical presentation of a duplex abnormality with ureterocele was with urinary tract infection. Rarely, in neonatal girls, prolapse of the ureterocele into the urethra can present as an introital mass. With the advent of widespread maternal-fetal ultrasound examinations, the most common current scenario is an asymptomatic neonate seen for follow-up of a prenatal ultrasound diagnosis of hydronephrosis.

The initial evaluation of the symptomatic or asymptomatic child should be renal and pelvic ultrasonography. At the renal level, this study most often

shows a longer kidney on the duplex side, polar separation of renal sinus echoes, a dilated upper pole ureter, and varying degrees of upper pole parenchymal echogenicity. The lower collecting system may also be dilated from reflux or secondary obstruction from the dilated upper ureter or ureterocele. Occasionally, the upper pole parenchyma may be so atrophic that it cannot be visualized by ultrasound examination. This is termed ureterocele disproportion.[1]

The next study performed is a voiding cystourethrogram (VCUG) to evaluate the presence of reflux, both ipsilaterally and contralaterally, and to assess the degree of distortion of trigonal muscle. To assess the degree of relative function of the upper renal segment and to evaluate obstructive changes (compared with the lower pole), a renal scan or intravenous pyelogram (IVP) should be obtained.

Ectopic Ureter

The insertion of an ectopic ureter is distal (caudal) to the trigone. In female patients the ureteral meatus may enter in the urethra, vaginal vestibule, vagina, or uterus. In male patients it can drain into the bladder neck, urethra, seminal vesicles, vas deferens, or epididymis. The initial symptoms of girls with an ectopic ureter include continuous wetting with otherwise normal voiding patterns, vaginal discharge, and/or urinary tract infection. Boys may have urinary tract infections, epididymitis, or a seminal vesical mass.

The evaluation and diagnosis of this abnormality is similar to that of the ectopic ureterocele. At the time of definitive surgery, the position of the ectopic ureter's orifice is sought by direct examination with cystoscopy and vaginoscopy, although it often remains elusive. In those unusual cases in which the history strongly suggests an ectopic insertion, but because the upper segment is diminutive the ultrasound scan and IVP do not show it, cross-sectional imaging with computed tomography (CT) or magnetic resonance imaging (MRI) may be necessary.

OPERATIVE TECHNIQUES

The type of incision used for either the upper pole heminephrectomy or the ureteropyelostomy remains at the surgeon's discretion. The anterior extraperitoneal approach, with the child rotated to a 45 to 60 degree flank position and the incision made from the tip of the twelfth rib forward, allows rapid and wide exposure. It requires division of the oblique muscles, however, and in older children this may lead to postoperative splinting and discomfort. Care should be taken to retract the twelfth intercostal neurovascular bundle so as to maximize muscle function return.

I have found the posterior lumbodorsal approach quite satisfactory in this setting. An exaggerated flank position with the patient rotated anteriorly can be used, but the prone position provides the best exposure for stability of the patient. Two rolls are placed lengthwise, laterally under the abdomen, and an incision is made from the angle of the twelfth rib to above the iliac crest. The lumbodorsal fascia is incised and the sacrospinalis bluntly dissected medially. Beneath the anterior lamella of the lumbodorsal fascia is Gerota's fascia, and the kidney is easily approached.

Heminephrectomy

The first step in the renal dissection is to identify the ureters as arising from either the upper or lower segment and to delicately dissect the upper ureter free just caudal to the hilum. The upper ureter is then transected and carefully passed posterior to the lower pole vessels cranially. Using this ureteral end as a handle will help facilitate dissection of the hilum and the upper pole.

The upper pole of the kidney is exposed with blunt and sharp dissection. The vessels supplying the most cranial aspect of the upper moiety usually enter superiorly. However, near the line of demarcation with the lower moiety, small arteries may arise from the main renal artery or one of its branches, partially supplying the lower segment. *Care must be taken to avoid traction on the lower pole hilum during this dissection.* If the vascular supply is in doubt, the vessel in question may be occluded temporarily to observe the effect on the renal parenchyma. If one is using pedicle clamps, atraumatic instruments should be used, and administration of an intravenous osmotic diuretic (i.e., mannitol) before and after the

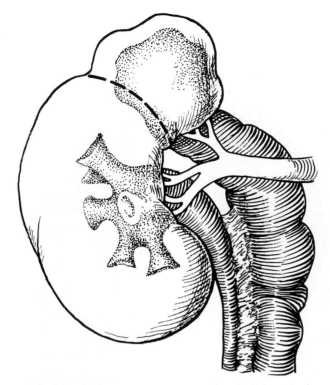

Figure 102–1. Duplex system with abnormal upper pole parenchyma and dilated upper ureter. Note the line of demarcation between the two segments. (From Retik AB, Colodny AH, Bauer SB. Pediatric urology. In Paulson DF, ed. Genitourinary Surgery, Vol 2. New York, Churchill Livingstone, 1984.)

renal vessels are occluded is advisable. Also, topical vasodilating agents (i.e., papaverine) after unclamping may help relieve vascular spasm.

After the feeding vessels are ligated, the renal capsule is incised at the apex or above the line of demarcation on the anterior and posterior aspects (Fig. 102–1). Sharp and blunt dissection is used to dissect the capsule off the parenchyma. The general rules on excising the upper segment relate to the critical importance of maintaining the integrity of the vascular and collecting system of the lower pole. Sharp dissection is needed to separate the upper and lower poles and can be done with knife, scissors, or delicate cautery (Fig. 102–2). It is advisable to dissect above the line of demarcation, leaving the most inferior aspect of the upper moiety with a portion of the calices behind. These are then carefully trimmed off along with some remaining upper parenchyma.

Bleeding vessels on the cut surface of the exposed renal parenchyma are next carefully ligated with fine absorbable sutures. Vertical mattress sutures of slightly larger size are then used to approximate the remaining upper parenchyma, picking up the dissected capsule and some perinephric fat and taking extra care not to injure the hilum (Fig. 102–3). These are tied gently so that they will not tear out (Fig. 102–4).

In rare instances, only the lower pole segment of a

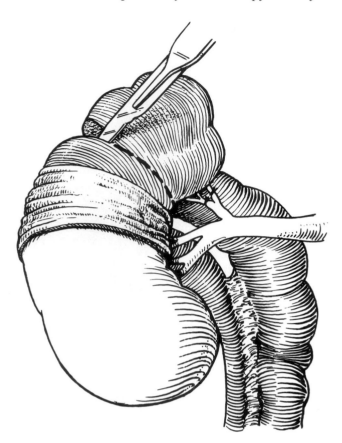

Figure 102–2. After ligation of the upper pole vessels, incision and dissection of the overlying renal capsule is carried out. The upper pole parenchyma is being transected sharply. (From Retik AB, Colodny AH, Bauer SB. Pediatric urology. In Paulson DF, ed. Genitourinary Surgery, Vol 2. New York, Churchill Livingstone, 1984.)

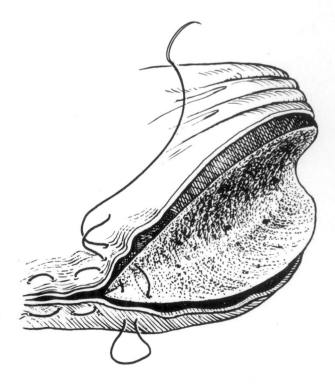

Figure 102–3. Closure of the remaining lip of parenchyma is carried out using mattress sutures and redundant capsule. Note the slight inward beveling of the parenchyma to allow tensionless approximation. (From Retik AB, Colodny AH, Bauer SB. Pediatric urology. In Paulson DF, ed. Genitourinary Surgery, Vol 2. New York, Churchill Livingstone, 1984.)

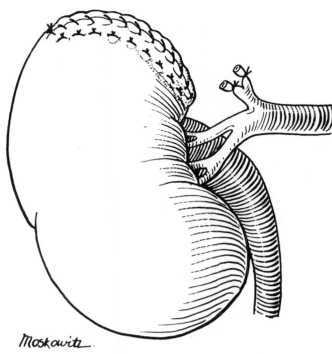

Figure 102–4. Final closure of the renal capsule. (From Retik AB, Colodny AH, Bauer SB. Pediatric urology. In Paulson DF, ed. Genitourinary Surgery, Vol 2. New York, Churchill Livingstone, 1984.)

duplex system may be nonfunctioning in association with high-grade vesicoureteral reflux. In these cases, a lower pole partial nephroureterectomy is performed. The principles of the renal mobilization and dissection are the same as for the upper pole nephrectomy. Extreme caution must be exercised in ligating the lower pole vascular supply to preserve the upper segment viability. The ureter must be excised all the way to the bladder hiatus.

The kidney is again inspected for bleeding or leakage and returned to its normal position. A Penrose drain is brought through a separate skin incision, through the muscle, and left in the perirenal space. The incision is closed with absorbable sutures, usually 4-0 or 5-0 PDS in infants.

Ureteropyelostomy

The exposure for a ureteropyelostomy is similar to that for heminephrectomy, but is limited by the need to expose only the upper pole ureter crossing near the lower pole pelvis and to identify the hilar vessels. The upper moiety does not need to be as extensively dissected, so retraction of the kidney is minimized.[2] The upper ureter is transected at a point where no traction is needed for it to be anastomosed to the lower pole pelvis or ureter, but where there is little redundancy and a straight path from above. A generous incision is made in the lower pelvis with extension down into the ureter if necessary. If the lower

pelvis is diminutive and/or intrarenal, the proximal ureter is incised longitudinally (Fig. 102–5).

The anastomosis between the end of the upper ureter and the lower collecting system is performed with a small absorbable suture (6-0 or 7-0 PDS) and an atraumatic needle. The apices are approximated and then the posterior and anterior suture lines are closed, using a running technique, either locking or not (Fig. 102–6). A small feeding tube can be left in place until the last few sutures are sewn, to protect the back wall and to irrigate the pelvis free of any clots.

Ureterectomy

The distal ureter is excised toward the bladder in a similar manner regardless of whether the upper segment is salvaged. The lower ureter should be identified but not directly manipulated at any time. The periureteral adventitia of the dilated upper segment is dissected away, leaving all this tissue remaining with the lower ureter. If the upper segment is nonrefluxing, the back wall of the most distal portion of this ureter can be left attached to the lower ureter to preserve its blood supply. In cases of ectopic ureterocele, it is important to remember to aspirate the ure-

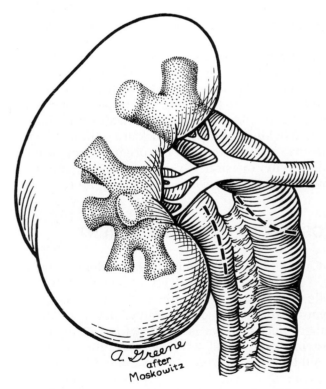

Figure 102–5. The incisions are outlined for transection of the upper pole ureter and opening of the lower ureter in preparation for ureteroureterostomy. (From Retik AB, Colodny AH, Bauer SB. Pediatric urology. In Paulson DF, ed. Genitourinary Surgery, Vol 2. New York, Churchill Livingstone, 1984.)

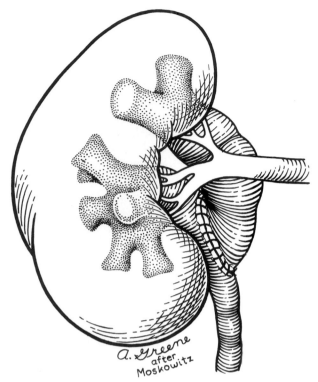

Figure 102–6. The completed watertight anastomosis. Note the fairly straight direction of the upper pole ureter without tension. (From Retik AB, Colodny AH, Bauer SB. Pediatric urology. In Paulson DF, ed. Genitourinary Surgery, Vol 2. New York, Churchill Livingstone, 1984.)

terocele before releasing control of the distal remaining ureter. This is usually done using a soft red catheter to avoid puncturing the ureterocele.

If the upper ureter is refluxing, the remaining end must be dissected free and suture ligated with absorbable suture. In cases of ectopic ureter, extra care should be taken to excise the upper ureter as far toward the bladder as possible, while avoiding dissection behind the bladder neck or urethra. In infants, this may be done through the original flank or dorsal lumbotomy incision. In older patients, a second, lower abdominal incision may be required.

POSTOPERATIVE MANAGEMENT

Catheter decompression of the bladder may be used for 1 to 3 days postoperatively, especially if there was reflux into the resected ureter. The Penrose drain is removed if dry by postoperative day 2 or 3. With either upper pole partial nephrectomy or ureteropyelostomy and distal ureterectomy, the ureterocele should decompress. Any obstruction of the ipsilateral or contralateral collecting system should resolve quickly. Resolution of any ipsilateral lower pole reflux may occur, depending on the degree of mechanical distortion of the trigone by the ureterocele.

If a second procedure is eventually required, it can

be performed on an elective basis with less distortion by the decompressed ureterocele. This usually involves excision of the ureterocele, reimplantation of the lower pole ureter, and reconstruction of the bladder floor muscle, if necessary. In one group of patients treated by this approach, three of 14 (21 percent) required reoperation for persistent lower pole reflux or failure of the ureterocele to decompress.[3] In another series, seven of 36 patients treated by either upper nephrectomy or ureteropyelostomy underwent a second procedure.[4]

POSTOPERATIVE COMPLICATIONS

The major complications of upper pole nephroureterectomy or pyeloureterostomy remain vascular compromise of the lower pole; urinary leakage; failure to decompress the ectopic ureterocele; and leaving the distal ureter too long, leading to urinary infections. We have not seen injury to the lower ureter, but this has been reported. All of these are avoidable by handling the kidney delicately, carefully oversewing any caliceal openings, watertight anastomosis of the collecting system, adequate dissection and excision of the distal ureter, and aspiration of the ureterocele. Persistence of reflux of the lower segment or development of reflux of the contralateral ureter is not a complication, but rather the natural history of this complex disorder.

Editorial Comment
Craig A. Peters

Partial nephrectomy of a dilated and atrophic system may be facilitated by using the dilated pelvis as the line of dissection between the two poles and dissecting outward to separate the rim of parenchyma. This is a natural plane and avoids entry into the collecting system of the pole to be left in place. The maneuver of using the dilated ureter as a traction handle works well with this approach.

Determination of whether an upper pole nephrectomy or a ureteropyelostomy is appropriate is often made at the time of exploration and based on the appearance of the upper pole. A very thick pole would be more difficult to remove and may have more potential function than a thin-rimmed shell of tissue that would be readily removed.

REFERENCES

1. Share JC, Lebowitz RL. Ectopic ureterocele without ureteral or calyceal dilation (ureterocele disproportion): Findings on urography and sonography. AJR 152:567, 1989.
2. Huisman TK, Kaplan GW, Brock WA, et al. Ipsilateral ureteroureterostomy and pyeloureterostomy: A review of 15 years experience with 25 patients. J Urol 138:1207, 1987.
3. Mandell J, Colodny AH, Lebowitz RL, et al. Ureteroceles in infants and children. J Urol 123:921, 1980.
4. Caldamone TA, Snyder HM III, Duckett JW. Ureteroceles in children: Follow-up of management with upper tract approach. J Urol 131:1130, 1984.

Chapter 103

Pediatric Nephrectomy

David B. Joseph

INDICATIONS

The need for nephrectomy in the pediatric patient is relatively rare. As with most problems in children, the preservation of tissue is of utmost importance. There are, however, pathological lesions that require surgical extirpation of the kidney. With the availability of growth hormone and erythropoietin, bilateral nephrectomy is playing a greater role in children with renal failure, particularly when that failure is associated with chronic infections, hypertension, and the nephrotic syndrome. An end-stage obstructive process may also benefit from nephrectomy when identified before the onset of hypertension or an upper urinary tract infection. Blunt and penetrating trauma can result in significant renal damage. The need for surgical intervention and possible nephrectomy is dependent on the clinical stability of the child and any associated injuries.

Nephrectomy to treat a multicystic kidney is controversial. Early intervention is suggested by some experts because of concern for the onset of hypertension or malignant transformation of the dysplastic tissue. This is supported by the fact that removal of the multicystic kidney in an infant carries little morbidity, the hospitalization period is short, and the recovery is rapid. The true incidence of hypertension or tumors due to a multicystic kidney is unknown but likely to be very low. Therefore, other surgeons support a nonoperative approach to the child with a multicystic kidney. It is to be hoped that information gained from the Multicystic Kidney Registry will help resolve these issues.[1]

PREOPERATIVE MANAGEMENT

The preoperative management of a child undergoing a nephrectomy is limited and directed by the underlying pathologic renal condition. Children who are to receive a unilateral nephrectomy require an imaging study documenting the function of the contralateral kidney. This is essential in the face of renal trauma.

Most children are admitted on the day of surgery, their NPO status adjusted according to their age. It is important to communicate with the nephrology service when bilateral nephrectomies are to be undertaken. Children can be dialyzed the morning of the operative procedure, with the use of heparin closely monitored.

It is helpful to determine the size of the kidney and location of the renal hilum. This can be accomplished by renal sonography with the child in the prone position. This is particularly important if a dorsal approach is considered.

OPERATIVE TECHNIQUE

The most important aspect of an operative procedure is the need to obtain adequate surgical exposure. Several approaches allow for adequate exposure during a pediatric nephrectomy. Operative approaches can be broadly classified as intraperitoneal or extraperitoneal. The former is important for neoplasms and renal trauma, particularly when renal trauma is associated with other internal injuries. Bilateral nephrectomies can be undertaken through a single transperitoneal approach, but this prevents early peritoneal dialysis when this is deemed appropriate. An extraperitoneal approach to the kidney should be taken whenever possible to avoid the increased morbidity associated with entering the peritoneal cavity.

Laparoscopic techniques of pediatric nephrectomy have been described, but it remains debatable whether this minimally invasive technique will be beneficial.[2] It is difficult to improve upon the single small incision, minimal operative time, and limited postoperative course incurred by most children undergoing simple nephrectomy by an open technique.

Personal preference most often determines which

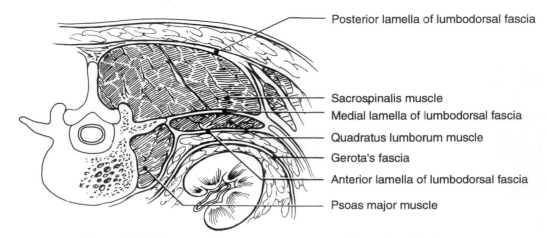

Posterior lamella of lumbodorsal fascia

Sacrospinalis muscle
Medial lamella of lumbodorsal fascia
Quadratus lumborum muscle
Gerota's fascia
Anterior lamella of lumbodorsal fascia
Psoas major muscle

Figure 103–1. The transverse anatomy encountered with the dorsal lumbotomy.

approach is used for nephrectomy. It is important that the surgeon become comfortable with several approaches allowing for effective management of any given clinical situation. Two extraperitoneal approaches (dorsal lumbotomy and subcostal) and an intraperitoneal approach (anterior transperitoneal) are presented here. These three provide excellent access for nephrectomy when the renal unit is in an orthotopic position.

Dorsal Lumbotomy

The dorsal lumbotomy has gained respect in the United States as an ideal approach to the kidney for various surgical procedures (Fig. 103–1). A dorsal approach is appropriate for simple nephrectomy, especially when the kidney is hydronephrotic or multicystic. An incision of less than 4 cm is made. The renal pelvis or cysts may be decompressed to decrease the size of the specimen and facilitate removal. A dorsal approach is beneficial for bilateral nephrectomy because of minimal postoperative discomfort and decreased morbidity. However, the operative field and exposure to the kidney are limited in a dorsal lumbotomy as compared with other approaches. For this reason, an alternative to the dorsal approach should be undertaken when the kidney is large, or when previous surgery or infection is ex-

pected to have resulted in perirenal fibrosis. These conditions inhibit dissection and limit the mobility of the kidney.

After anesthetic induction, the patient is placed in the prone position. A bolster is positioned horizontally under the pelvis and a second bolster under the thorax. This will straighten the spine and drop the peritoneal contents to a dependent location (Fig. 103–2). The horizontal chest roll elevates the cervical spine to an anatomical position with the head gently resting on a cushion. The axilla will also be elevated and free of compression. The horizontal chest roll will not compromise respiration when positioned appropriately.

The location of the dorsal incision is critical for exposure. When maximal exposure is required, particularly in an older child, the incision should be made obliquely. It starts at the lateral third of the twelfth rib and extends to the posterior iliac crest. It is important to place the incision in line with the lateral border of the sacrospinal muscle. If the incision is made too close to the spine, it will be difficult to mobilize the sacrospinal and quadratus lumborum muscles (Fig. 103–3).

An incision following Langer's lines is more appealing and cosmetic in infants and young children. It is placed one third of the distance between the twelfth rib and the crest of the iliac spine. The medial limit of the incision begins over the middle of the

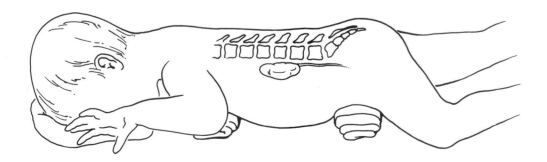

Figure 103–2. The prone position used for the dorsal approach. Note that the spine and neck are straight. The abdominal compartment is dependent and the head rests on a cushion. Appropriately placed, the horizontal chest roll will not compromise respirations.

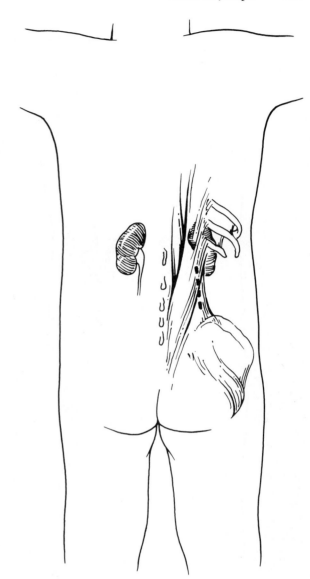

Figure 103–3. For maximal exposure, an oblique dorsal incision should be made. The incision is in line with the lateral aspect of the sacrospinal muscle, allowing for medial retraction.

sacrospinal muscle and is continued 3.5 to 4 cm laterally (Fig. 103–4). The plane between the subcutaneous tissue and the posterior lamella of the lumbodorsal fascia is easily developed, creating superior and inferior skin flaps.

The posterior lamella of the lumbodorsal fascia is opened using cutting current from the twelfth rib extending to the posterior iliac spine. On occasion, slips of the latissimus dorsi will be encountered, particularly if the incision is located too laterally. Opening this portion of the latissimus dorsi will lead to the posterior lamella of the lumbodorsal fascia (Fig. 103–5).

The sacrospinal muscle is mobilized medially by rotating it off the fascia with a blunt dissector. Perforating vessels are cauterized, allowing for full mobility. It may be necessary to incise the costispinal ligament of the twelfth rib in order to maximize the exposure gained by mobilization of the sacrospinal muscle. Care should be taken not to injure the twelfth

subcostal nerve and vessels located in this region (Fig. 103–6).

The medial lamella of the lumbodorsal fascia is visualized and opened the full extent of the incision, exposing the quadratus lumborum muscle. The latter is mobilized medially, again fulgurating perforating vessels. The anterior lamella of the lumbodorsal fascia will be encountered with medial retraction of both muscles. An incision is made in the anterior lamella of the lumbodorsal fascia, avoiding the ilioinguinal and iliohypogastric nerves (Fig. 103–7). Gerota's fascia is often poorly defined in neonates and will be entered when the anterior lamella of the lumbodorsal fascia is opened. The lower pole of the kidney is palpated but not mobilized. It is helpful to place a retractor within Gerota's fascia inferiorly before mobilizing the lower pole. Gentle traction will facilitate access to the upper pole and renal hilum. After the renal hilum is secured, the lower pole is mobilized and the ureter transected. The specimen is finally removed.

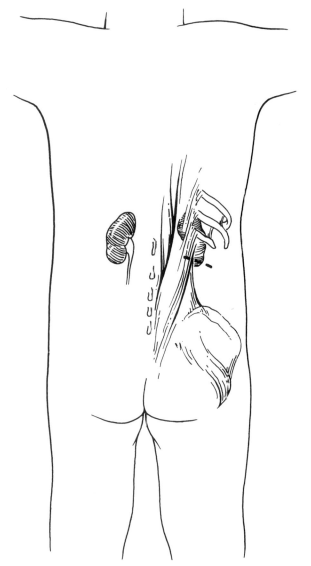

Figure 103–4. A dorsal incision following Langer's lines is more cosmetically appealing in children. Superior and inferior skin flaps are easily created, resulting in appropriate exposure.

The wound is closed by reapproximating the medial and posterior lamella of the lumbodorsal fascia with independent running sutures of appropriately sized Vicryl or Monocryl. The subcutaneous tissue and skin are reapproximated in a subcuticular technique.

Subcostal Approach

The subcostal incision can be in either a posterior flank or anterior position. The subcostal flank exposure provides appropriate access for most pediatric nephrectomies. The transcostal incision, performed in adults by removing the twelfth rib, is rarely required to enhance exposure for a pediatric nephrectomy.

After anesthetic induction, the child is placed in the flank position. A roll is placed under the opposite flank in a child too small to benefit from the kidney rest, in order to expand the distance between the twelfth rib and iliac spine. The flank is then rotated 15 degrees posteriorly (Fig.103–8). The contralateral leg is flexed and the ipsilateral leg extended. Padding is used to prevent ischemic compression of the lower extremities. An axillary support is positioned and the child is secured.

A line is marked approximately 1 cm beneath the twelfth rib following a gentle curve extending downward to the lateral aspect of the rectus muscle. The curve of the line is parallel to the expected course of the twelfth subcostal nerve. A 4-cm incision is then made on the course of this line, beginning posteriorly beneath the midportion of the twelfth rib. Cheek retractors can be placed in each corner of the skin incision and provide excellent exposure of the muscles. With cutting current the lateral aspect of the latissimus dorsi is incised, exposing the dorsal portion of the external oblique muscle. The latter is then opened, followed by the internal oblique muscle. The twelfth subcostal nerve and vessels will be encountered after opening the internal oblique muscle and are gently retracted superiorly without injury. The lumbodorsal fascia is opened next. With blunt dissection the retroperitoneal fat and peritoneum are mobilized from the underside of the transversalis fascia (Fig. 103–9). Finally, the transversus abdominis muscle and transversalis fascia are opened the full extent of the incision. Aggressive lateral dissection beneath the transversalis fascia does not improve exposure and can lead to an inadvertent entrance into the peritoneum. Gerota's fascia is mobilized bluntly from the psoas muscle and opened posteriorly. A retractor is placed inferiorly before mobilization of the lower pole, allowing for downward mobility of the kidney and access to the upper pole of the kidney and the renal hilum. The latter may be approached anteriorly or posteriorly. After the hilar vessels are secured, the lower pole is freed and the ureter transected.

The wound is closed by reapproximating the transversalis fascia, the internal oblique and the external oblique fascia, as independent layers using appropriately sized Vicryl or Monocryl. Subcutaneous tissue and skin are reapproximated with a subcuticular technique.

Anterior Transperitoneal (Chevron) Approach

Malignant neoplasms in children mandate maximal surgical exposure owing to the large size of the tumor and the need for contralateral renal exposure (see Chapter 125). The anterior transverse incision pro-

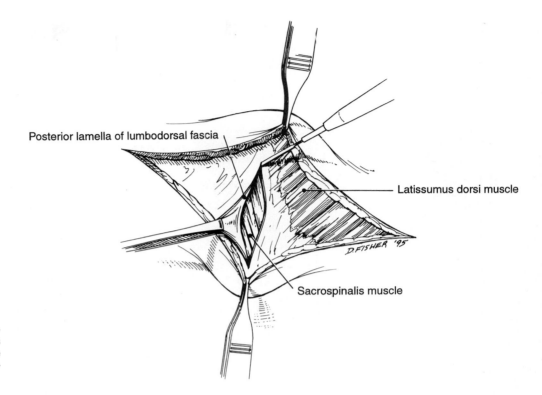

Posterior lamella of lumbodorsal fascia

Latissumus dorsi muscle

Sacrospinalis muscle

Figure 103–5. The posterior lamella of the lumbodorsal fascia is opened from the twelfth rib to the posterior iliac crest. The sacrospinal muscle resides beneath.

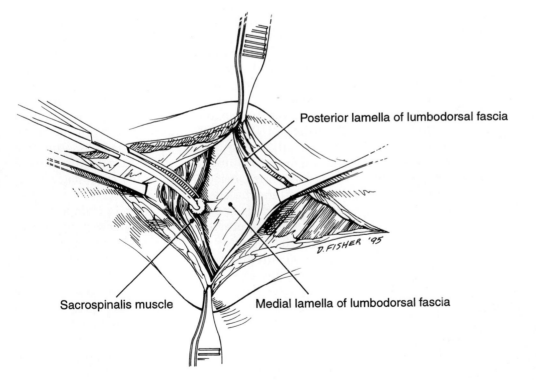

Posterior lamella of lumbodorsal fascia

Sacrospinalis muscle

Medial lamella of lumbodorsal fascia

Figure 103–6. Lateral elevation of the posterior lumbodorsal fascia along with medial retraction of the sacrospinal muscle exposes the medial lamella of the lumbodorsal fascia.

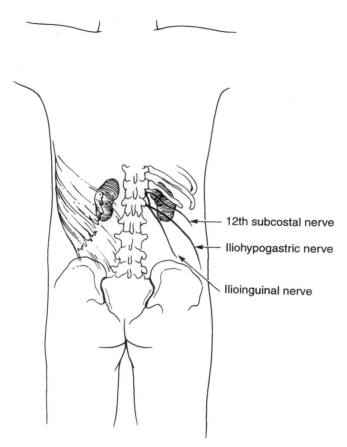

Figure 103–7. The course of the ilioinguinal, iliohypogastric, and twelfth subcostal nerves.

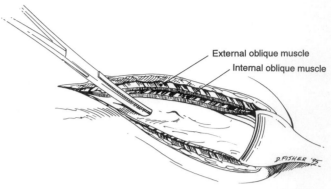

Figure 103–9. The posterior lamella of the lumbodorsal fascia has been entered and the transversus abdominis and transversalis fascia elevated. Care is taken to sweep the preperitoneal fat and peritoneum from the underside.

vides access for nephrectomy and abdominal exploration superior to the exposure obtained from a midline transperitoneal approach.

After appropriate anesthetic administration, the flank and pelvis of the involved side is elevated 10 degrees with the ipsilateral leg extended and the contralateral leg flexed. Padding of the lower extremities is undertaken to prevent ischemic pressure injury (Fig. 103–10). A line is marked 1 cm below the twelfth rib of the involved side and curved anteriorly an equal distance below the costal margin, xiphoid, and contralateral costal margin. A skin incision is

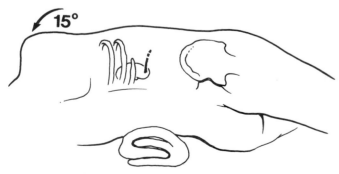

Figure 103–8. Positioning for the flank approach and location of the subcostal incision.

initiated off the tip of the eleventh rib and continued two thirds of the way across the contralateral rectus. The ipsilateral anterior rectus sheath is then incised and the rectus mobilized. An Army-Navy retractor is placed beneath the rectus and gently elevated for transection of the muscle and identification of perforating vessels. The superior epigastric artery is ligated (Fig. 103–11). The posterior rectus sheath is grasped with forceps and sharply opened along with the transversalis fascia and the peritoneum. Two fingers are inserted into the peritoneal cavity, elevating the abdominal wall. The oblique muscles and transversus abdominis are then opened with the cautery. Elevation of the abdominal wall prevents potential injury of the underlying renal tumor. The anterior sheath of the contralateral rectus is opened next, and approximately half of the contralateral rectus is incised. Excellent exposure can often be obtained without completely transecting the contralateral rectus. If greater exposure is needed, the incision can be continued through the full extent of the rectus. The terminal branches of the eighth, ninth, and tenth subcostal nerves will be disrupted. This may lead to atrophy of the rectus and numbness of the skin, particularly if the incision is carried lateral to the contralateral rectus and along the costal margin.

The round ligament of the liver is clamped, transected, and suture ligated after opening the peritoneum. The retractor of choice is placed. Exposure of the renal hilum may be difficult with large tumors. To reach the right renal vessels, dissection can be initiated on the caudal aspect of the inferior vena cava and taken superiorly until the renal hilum is encountered. On occasion, a Kocher maneuver will be required to directly approach the right renal hilum. This is performed by incising the posterior peritoneum lateral to the second portion of the duodenum and reflecting the duodenum medially. Care must be taken to prevent injury to the pancreas.

The left renal hilum may be approached by incising

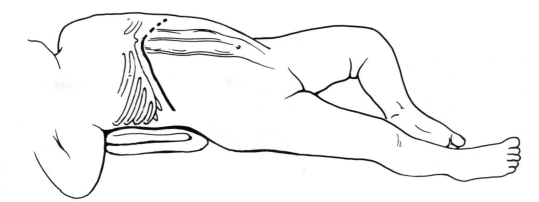

Figure 103–10. Positioning for an anterior transperitoneal nephrectomy. The involved side is elevated 10 degrees.

the posterior peritoneum caudal to the ligament of Treitz, adjacent to the fourth portion of the duodenum. This exposes the ventral surface of the aorta where the left renal vein most often crosses anteriorly.

The wound is closed by reapproximating the linea alba with a figure-of-eight suture. The peritoneum, transversalis fascia, and posterior rectus sheath are all closed with a continuous suture of appropriately sized Vicryl or Monocryl. The fascia of the internal oblique, external oblique, and anterior rectus sheath are also reapproximated with independent layers of a similar running suture. Subcutaneous tissue and skin are secured in a subcuticular fashion.

POSTOPERATIVE MANAGEMENT

The postoperative management depends on the approach taken. Children who have undergone a dorsal approach have minimal discomfort even when a bilateral procedure is performed, owing to the lack of muscle transection and nerve damage. They are allowed a clear liquid diet later on the day of surgery or on the morning of the first postoperative day. Their intake is quickly liberalized. Postoperative ileus sec-

ondary to a dorsal approach is rarely encountered. Total hospital stay is 1 to 3 days. An infant undergoing a dorsal approach for nephrectomy of a multicystic kidney can be discharged on the same day as surgery.

Children who have undergone an extraperitoneal subcostal incision remain on NPO status through the first postoperative day. If clinical signs of bowel activity are then present, they are started on a clear liquid diet and advanced as tolerated. Most children are on a general diet by the second or third postoperative day. Total hospitalization is usually 2 to 4 days.

Children who have had an anterior transperitoneal incision remain NPO until signs of bowel activity return, usually within 2 to 4 days of surgery. Total hospitalization is 5 or 6 days.

COMPLICATIONS

The most common intraoperative complication relates to blood loss, often because of poor hilar exposure and large tumors. Injury to the superior mesenteric artery may occur if this is not identified before ligating hilar vessels, particularly with a large left renal tumor. Bulging of the flank postoperatively is

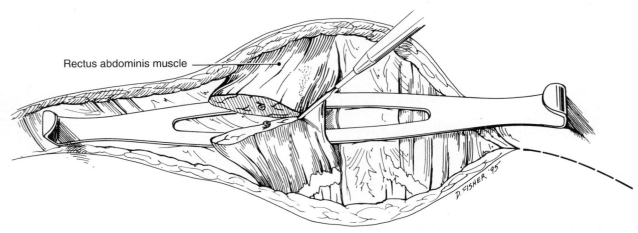

Rectus abdominis muscle

Figure 103–11. The rectus is elevated with an Army-Navy retractor, which enhances identification of vessels and limits blood loss.

encountered most often from a subcostal flank approach with injury to the nerves. This flank weakness will improve over several months.

Any transperitoneal procedure carries the risk of postoperative bowel obstruction. This has been documented as being as high as 6.9 percent in children undergoing radical nephrectomy for Wilms tumor.[3] The risk of bowel obstruction is a strong deterrent to a transperitoneal approach for a simple unilateral or bilateral nephrectomy.

Few studies have evaluated the long-term effect of hyperfiltration on children who have undergone a unilateral nephrectomy. Proteinuria, renal insufficiency, and hypertension have been reported to occur in 27, 30, and 10 percent of children, respectively.[4] Because of these findings, it is recommended that children with a single kidney have an annual evaluation, including blood pressure measurement and urinalysis with quantification of urinary protein.[4]

Summary

Multiple approaches to a pediatric nephrectomy are available. It is important for the surgeon to become comfortable with several alternatives. The exact approach will be dictated by the underlying patholog- *ical process, the size of the child, and the size and location of the kidney.*

Editorial Comment
Craig A. Peters

Nephrectomy remains a basic, although now uncommonly performed, operation in children. The details of the surgical exposure of the kidney described by Dr. Joseph are fundamental to any renal surgery in children. The dorsal lumbotomy exposure is extremely effective and produces less morbidity than the standard flank approaches. There seems a reluctance on the part of some surgeons to use this approach until they become familiar with it. This description is clear and succinct and should encourage those not using the technique to try it.

REFERENCES

1. Wacksman J, Phipps L. Report of the Multicystic Kidney Registry: Preliminary findings. J Urol 150:1870, 1993.
2. Peters CA. Laparoscopy in pediatric urology. Urology 41:33, 1993.
3. Ritchey ML, Kelalis PP, Breslow N, et al. Surgical complications after nephrectomy for Wilms' tumor. Surg Gynecol Obstet 175:507, 1992.
4. Argueso LR, Ritchey ML, Boyle ET, et al. Prognosis for children with solitary kidney after unilateral nephrectomy. J Urol 148:747, 1992.

Part II

URETER/BLADDER

Chapter 104

Noncontinent Urinary Diversion

Michael A. Keating

Not every child with severe bladder dysfunction or recalcitrant urinary incontinence is a candidate for continent reconstruction of the native bladder or creation of an enteric continent diversion. Some are too small or too ill to tolerate definitive urinary reconstruction and others are mired in unacceptable social settings. Continent reconstructions, which are typically emptied by intermittent catheterization, demand *active* participation on the part of the affected patient and family or caretakers. Careful selection is critical to long-term efficacy. Simply put, some children are best served by creating noncontinent urinary diversions. These are easier to construct, require less care, and allow the patient and family to assume a *passive* role in urinary tract drainage, at least for the time being.

A variety of different alternatives in noncontinent diversion are available (Table 104–1), but the criteria for selection in children differ from those for adults. Many of the latter have intractable urinary disease, and diversions provide an effective panacea for the remainder of shortened lives. In contrast, pediatric diversions are planned with an eye to the future when undiversion or definitive continent reconstruc-

tion becomes an option in management. The long-term efficacy of noncontinent diversions is guarded, and diapers or appliances become socially and psychologically unacceptable for most older children or young adults. As a consequence, the choice in diversion should not only protect the urinary tract but also preserve as many options as possible in its subsequent reconstruction if and when undiversion becomes a possibility (see Chapter 112, Continent Diversion).

EVALUATION

The reasons for any type of diversion must be understood to avoid misapplication or overextension in usage. Each primary cutaneous urinary diversion has a defined role in the management of an ill child. Proximal diversions of the collecting system (ureterostomy, pyelostomy) are typically used to treat obstructive causes of hydroureteronephrosis. Most secondary causes of hydronephrosis (reflux, neurogenic dysfunction, and urethral valves) that do not respond to other measures can be effectively managed by venting the affected bladder with a vesicostomy. Standard radiological studies that help make this differentiation include voiding cystourethrography and ultrasonography. A functional study (renal scintigraphy and/or excretory urography) is also indicated, especially in cases in which the salvageability of a kidney comes into question, but may be of equivocal value in the face of immature renal function or severe obstruction. When this is the case, percutaneous drainage is recommended to vent the affected system and provide anatomical detail if need be. Percutaneous drainage also provides a useful means of temporarily decompressing the urinary tract of a septic or unstable child who is too ill to undergo even the simplest surgery.

TABLE 104–1. Noncontinent Urinary Diversions

Endourological
    Percutaneous nephrostomy tube
    Suprapubic tube
Primary cutaneous
    Loop cutaneous ureterostomy
    End cutaneous ureterostomy
    Pyelostomy
    Vesicostomy
Enteric diversions
    Ileal conduit
    Colon conduit
    Ileocecal conduit

Noncontinent enteric conduits are usually created on a less urgent basis and are typically meant to provide a longer duration of diversion. The interposition of bowel between the abdominal wall and urinary tract can sometimes eliminate the direct route of entry for bacteria provided by other forms of diversion. It also offers improved fitting of urinary appliances. However, conduits require more complex reconstructions and bring their own acute and chronic morbidity. Again, the indications for diversion are defined using standard radiological and, where indicated, urodynamic studies. Unlike the situation in the past, enteric diversions are rarely constructed for incontinence or hydronephrosis in children. Our broadened understanding of many urological disorders, including neurogenic bladder, has resulted in improved medical management. When this is unsuccessful, better surgical options are now available that either restore the desired capacity and compliance of the native bladder or offer continent enteric replacements in its stead.

CUTANEOUS URETEROSTOMY

Indications and Selection

The simplicity of cutaneous ureterostomies offers their greatest benefit. They provide effective drainage of the upper urinary tract and can be created in even the smallest and most critically ill infants with a high likelihood of success. Ureterostomies are usually reserved for disorders that produce ureteral obstruction when primary reconstructions cannot be performed or where other methods of diversion are contraindicated. Percutaneous drainage, ureteral stents, and dialysis have largely abolished the role of ureterostomies as a means of acutely decompressing the urinary tract, but in the chronic setting these diversions are more effective than intubated procedures, presumably because of the absence of a foreign body. Ureterostomies, however, are not regarded as permanent in most children. Diapers can be worn over the stoma in infants, but appliances are difficult to fit in older children. As a result, the diversion is not as well tolerated as other options that utilize bowel, especially with bilateral disorders, although the absence of bowel does offer one major metabolic advantage.[1, 2]

Two methods continue to be used occasionally, the end (low) ureterostomy and the loop (high) ureterostomy. With either procedure, a ureteral diameter of at least 1 cm should be present to minimize problems with stomal stenosis. Midureteral ureterostomies limit the options in undiversion and have been abandoned. More complex modifications that create a single stoma by constructing a transureteroureterostomy or by joining both ureters in the midline, have higher complication rates and should also be avoided in children. End ureterostomies are used to decompress systems with proven distal obstructions (e.g., ectopic ureter, ureterocele) that are too large for primary reconstruction. Undiversion by simple circumferential mobilization and reimplantation can be done at a later date through the same incision. In contrast, reconstruction with the more proximal loop ureterostomy requires separate incisions and, in most cases, a ureteroureterostomy after takedown of its stoma. Despite this drawback, when the site of obstruction cannot be defined radiologically, the higher loop diversion should be created, erring on the side of maximal decompression. In addition to their role in supravesical obstruction, the more widely used loop ureterostomies are advocated by some clinicians as the primary treatment for posterior urethral valves. In theory, affected systems are maximally decompressed by proximal diversion, but whether an actual advantage is provided over cutaneous vesicostomy or even primary valve ablation remains open to debate. An occasional boy with valves will be seen whose renal function and drainage fail to improve despite initial catheter decompression of the obstructed bladder. When the kidneys appear salvageable, high ureterostomies should be created to circumvent unyielding ureteral kinks or a functional ureterovesical junction obstruction.

Loop Ureterostomy—Operative Technique

POSITIONING. A flank incision provides the best exposure, but bilateral diversions will require repositioning (Fig. 104–1). The child is placed in a modified semilateral position with the upper leg extended and the lower leg flexed. A pillow is placed between the two, and other pressure points are padded. Elevation of the kidney rest and flexion of the table facilitate the subsequent dissection.

INCISION AND EXPOSURE. A small (4- to 5-cm) transverse subcostal skin incision is planned so that the stoma will be ultimately positioned at its middle along the anterior axillary line. When necessary, additional exposure can be gained by incising the underlying musculature in both directions. Cautery is used to separate the subcutaneous fat and oblique muscles. The transversus abdominis is spread bluntly initially to help identify and avoid entering the peritoneum, which extends far laterally in infants. Gerota's fascia is defined by retracting the peritoneum and retroperitoneal viscera medially and dissecting along the bloodless plane anterior to the retroperitoneal musculature with a Kitner (peanut) dissector.

URETERAL MOBILIZATION. After Gerota's fascia

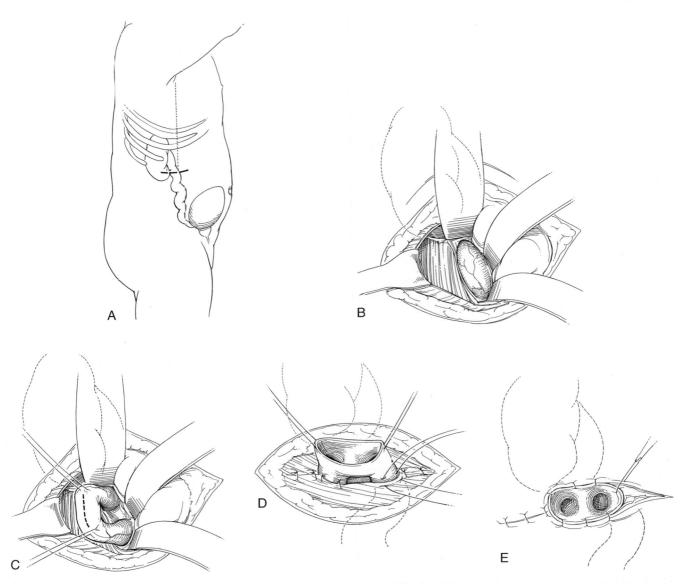

Figure 104–1. Loop cutaneous ureterostomy. *A,* Subcostal incision planned to position the stoma along the axillary line. *B,* Dilated ureter exposed after retracting the peritoneum medially and opening Gerota's fascia. *C,* Dilated ureter mobilized with traction sutures from the retroperitoneum. The proposed longitudinal ureterotomy is shown. *D,* Ureter opened and anastomosed to the fascia. The proximal ureteral ostium is placed posteriorly. *E,* Ureteral stoma matured.

is opened vertically, the dilated ureter is identified. Infant intestine can mimic a megaureter. When doubt exists, aspiration with a 25-gauge needle helps identify the structure in question. A Denis Browne retractor provides excellent exposure during this portion of the procedure. The ureter is gently handled with fine traction sutures (5-0 chromic); it should not be grasped with forceps or encircled with vessel loops or clamps. This helps preserve the medially based blood supply so that ureteral vascularity is intact when later undiversion with excision of the ureterostomy and ureteral anastomosis is performed. Two sutures are placed at the site of the proposed stoma and the proximal ureter is mobilized to permit a tension-free anastomosis with the skin. Proximal patency is assessed by intermittently passing an 8 Fr. red rubber

catheter or feeding tube. Redundant kinks must be straightened by lysing fibrous tethers, but periureteral dissections are meant to preserve the adventitia to avoid devascularization. In addition the distal ureter must not be excessively mobilized. This causes upward tethering and can lead to problems with length at future reimplantation or reconstruction.

MATURING THE STOMA. A 1.5-cm longitudinal ureterotomy is made between the traction sutures that avoids larger blood vessels. The segmental and longitudinal distribution of the blood supply of the ureter is well recognized but becomes variable in the face of ureteral dilation and tortuosity. Fortunately, most megaureters are highly vascular and not easily compromised by these techniques when correctly handled. By convention, the ostium of the proximal ureter is positioned posteriorly to permit identification after surgery. Ureteral adventitia is circumferentially anchored to the fascia of the transversalis and oblique muscles, 1 cm below the level of the ureterotomy, with interrupted 4-0 polyglycolic acid sutures. Closing muscle behind the ureter can cause obstruction and is unnecessary. After the remaining fascia is closed on each side up to the ureter, the stoma is matured to the skin with fine (6-0) interrupted polyglycolic acid sutures. Catheter-proved patency must be present at completion of the procedure. No drains are left or dressings applied.

End Ureterostomy—Operative Technique

POSITIONING. The patient is placed in the supine position and the bladder emptied to facilitate subse-

quent exposure of the pelvis. Flexion of the lower abdomen can also be helpful.

INCISION AND EXPOSURE. A lower abdominal transverse incision is made just below McBurney's point that extends from a point 3 cm inferomedial from the anterior superior iliac spine to the lateral border of the rectus abdominis (Fig. 104–2). The layers of the abdominal wall musculature are divided along the direction of their fibers, but division of the rectus muscle or inferior epigastric vessels is unnecessary. Upon retraction of the bladder medially and the peritoneal envelope superiorly, the obliterated hypogastric artery will be encountered as it exits the retroperitoneum. Dividing the vessel and following it proximally serves as a useful guide to the ureter at the bifurcation of the iliac vessels.

URETERAL MOBILIZATION. After a chromic traction suture is placed, the ureter is mobilized as far

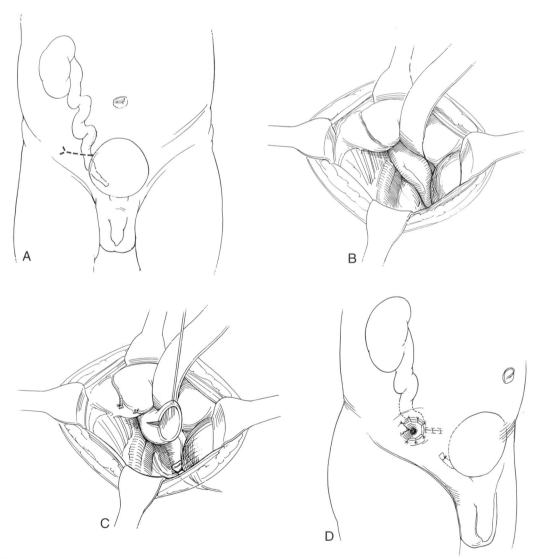

Figure 104–2. End cutaneous ureterostomy. *A,* A transverse lower abdominal incision allows extraperitoneal perivesical access to the lower ureter. *B,* The bladder and peritoneum retracted medially aid in exposure. *C,* Distal ureter ligated and the proximal ureter mobilized from the pelvis. Spatulation of its end will receive a V flap from the lateral aspect of the skin incision. *D,* Ureteral stoma matured.

distally as possible and transected near the bladder. The small stump that remains rarely presents a problem, but it should be ligated if reflux is present or is suspected. Care is taken to avoid disruption of the blood supply to the uterus or vas. Duplex ureters present a special problem. Creating double-barreled ureterostomies should be avoided unless both ureters are enlarged (greater than 1 cm in diameter). Distally, duplex ureters share a common blood supply but their vascularity is not shared above the level of the iliacs. By beginning above this level, the megaureter of a duplication can be mobilized without compromising an adjacent normal-sized partner. Proximal patency by retrograde catheterization is sometimes difficult to confirm, but no effort is made to straighten a significantly tortuous ureter.

MATURING THE STOMA. The proximal ureter is carried through the lateral aspect of the wound. One centimeter below its end the adventitia of the ureter is circumferentially anchored to the transversalis fascia and obliques with interrupted polyglycolic acid (4-0) sutures. The remainder of the muscular defect is closed with similar sutures. To minimize the risk of stenosis, a small V-shaped skin flap is fashioned at the lateral extent of the incision that is advanced into a counterincision made in the lateral aspect of the ureter. The ureteral stoma is then matured with fine interrupted sutures (as above). Stenting of the ureter is unnecessary and no drains are left.

Complications

The performance of ureterostomies in historical series, especially those composed largely of adults, was equivocal at best.[3–5] Stomal stenosis and ischemia are common complications when these diversions are constructed with ureters that are of normal size or are only acutely dilated, lacking redundancy and accessory blood supply. In addition, freeing the length of ureter necessary to traverse the abdominal wall of many adults risks devascularization. The congenitally dilated ureters of infancy do not suffer these drawbacks and stomal stenosis, retraction, and blockage can usually be avoided with delicate handling and adherence to the techniques discussed above. Most obstructed megaureters drain effectively. In rare cases, intrinsic myopathy or scarring impair peristalsis. In others, a proximal kink or angulation can cause secondary obstruction. If these are suspected beforehand, a high ureterostomy or even pyelostomy should be created.

Chronic bacteriuria is usually present, but full-blown urinary infections in the face of low-pressure drainage are unusual. Nevertheless, the long-term implications of ascending infections to renal function are real, and undiversion should be considered as soon as it becomes technically feasible. The other disadvantages of ureterostomies are indigenous to all noncontinent diversions. Ammoniacal and monilial dermatitis are common but respond to urinary acidification and antifungal creams.

PYELOSTOMY

Indications

The only real advantage pyelostomy offers over ureterostomy is that undiversion can be done without completing the formal ureteroureterostomy required of a loop ureterostomy. The procedure can be performed only in kidneys having a large extrarenal pelvis that allows tension-free extension and anastomosis to the skin, greatly limiting its application. Otherwise, retraction and stomal stenosis are inevitable.

Operative Technique

Exposure and mobilization can done through the same incision and technique as a loop ureterostomy, although an alternative approach can be offered by the posterior lumbotomy incision. Obstructed kidneys are often malrotated by their distorted collecting systems. If a pyelostomy is being considered, a retrograde study can help decide the proper approach. In either instance, the pelvis is exposed by following the ureter proximally, and stay sutures are placed transversely 2 cm apart on its posterolateral aspect. It is usually necessary to mobilize the pelvis somewhat, but twists of the collecting system or tension on the vascular pedicle must be avoided. Maturation of the pelvis to the skin is done in a fashion similar to that for ureterostomy. Stomas should not be made too large, to avoid prolapse of a floppy renal pelvis and even part of the kidney.

CUTANEOUS VESICOSTOMY

Indications

Cutaneous vesicostomy offers an effective panacea for a variety of neuropathic conditions of the bladder that pose a threat to the upper tracts but cannot be managed effectively with medication and intermittent catheterization or surgery. The spectrum includes those bladders that empty incompletely (prune belly syndrome, lower motor neuron lesions, massive reflux) to others that are small and noncompliant (posterior urethral valves, upper motor neuron lesions). Vesicostomies of the latter tend to drain more completely than their more capacious counterparts, perhaps as a consequence of better tonus, but inefficient drainage is rarely a problem in either case. By venting the bladder, most kidneys in these settings are protected from ascending infections through the creation of low-pressure drainage and resolution of secondary reflux.[6] Common applications of vesicostomy include newborns with massive refluxing megaureters whose size does not allow reconstruction, neonates with urethral valves and small-caliber urethras that do not allow a venue for primary ablation, and any child with a neurogenic bladder in whom augmentation cystoplasty is not an option in management.

Operative Technique

Although a number of different techniques have been described for creating vesicostomies, Blocksom's is the most effective.[7]

POSITIONING. The patient is placed in the supine position and prepared to allow access to the urethra and intermittent filling of the bladder.

INCISION AND EXPOSURE. A modified Pfannenstiel incision offers excellent exposure (Fig. 104–3). Filling the bladder is also very helpful. A small (3- to 4-cm) transverse incision is made midway between the umbilicus and symphysis pubis. After the rectus fascia is opened transversely, the underlying muscle is cleared away with blunt dissection, creating small fascial flaps. The recti are divided, the transversalis fascia is opened in the midline, and the peritoneum is swept superiorly with a finger. A Denis Browne or baby Balfour retractor is positioned to expose the prevesical space and bladder.

BLADDER MOBILIZATION. Any tendency to use the initial bladder encountered should be avoided. Instead, a 4-0 chromic holding suture is used to gently mobilize the bladder by pulling it inferiorly.

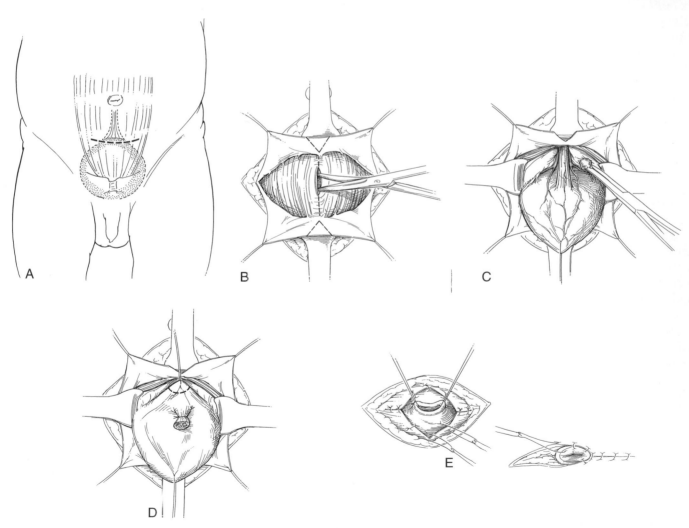

Figure 104–3. Cutaneous vesicostomy. *A,* Transverse incision made midway between the umbilicus and symphysis pubis. *B,* Modified Pfannenstiel approach. Fascial flaps are raised and the rectus muscles separated in the midline. *C,* Urachal remnant, dome, and posterior bladder gradually accessed by progressively retracting the bladder inferiorly and sweeping away the peritoneum. *D,* Site for cystostomy selected behind the ligated urachus. *E,* Detrusor circumferentially anastomosed to the fascia below the cystostomy. The mucosa is matured to the skin with interrupted sutures.

This allows successive sutures to be gradually placed in more superior positions as the peritoneum is swept away from the anterior dome of the bladder with a dissector or moist sponge. As the urachus and obliterated hypogastric vessels are approached, the peritoneum becomes more adherent and sharp dissection is often necessary to avoid peritoneal tears. The cystostomy site on the bladder's posterior dome is marked with a suture placed 2 cm behind the urachus after that structure and the adjacent umbilical vessels are divided.

MATURING THE STOMA. A small triangular wedge (0.5-cm sides) is removed from both fascial flaps in the midline, and the bladder is pulled into the wound. Detrusor 1 cm proximal to the proposed cystostomy is circumferentially matured to the fascial defect with interrupted 3-0 or 4-0 polyglycolic acid sutures, and the remaining fascia on both sides of the bladder is closed with the same suture. At the skin level, detrusor is incised until mucosa is encountered and opened. The walls of an extremely thickened bladder can coapt and impair the drainage of a simple incisional cystostomy. To avoid this, it is sometimes necessary to shave away muscle adjacent to the cystostomy. After maturing the bladder mucosa to the skin with fine, interrupted chromic sutures, the remainder of the skin is closed with subcutaneous stitches. The vesicostomy should allow the easy passage of a 20 Fr. catheter and is tested by filling the bladder and noting the free outflow of saline. Drains and dressings are unnecessary.

Complications

Bladder prolapse represents the most significant complication of vesicostomy.[8] Prolapse occurs if the diversion is created with anterior bladder rather than its dome, thus allowing the mobile posterior wall to evert through the defect in the abdominal wall. Manual reduction to temporarily alleviate obstruction is usually possible, but revision using the technique described above is inevitable. This is done by taking down and closing the existing stoma and creating a new vesicostomy with a more superiorly based cystostomy. Other complications occur less acutely and are not as serious. Bladder mucosa exhibits proliferative tendencies when not constantly bathed by urine. Granulation tissue and stomal stenosis result. Periodic dilation with a catheter or sound will sometimes resolve the stenosis, but a simple stomal revision becomes necessary when drainage is impaired. This is done by incising the fibrous ring and advancing a small triangular flap of healthy tissue into the defect in the cicatrix. Periodic checks for residual urine with a catheter or ultrasound provide useful measures of the completeness of bladder emptying.

Despite its effectiveness, vesicostomy is typically regarded as a temporary diversion.[9] The position of the stoma makes fitting an appliance extremely difficult in older children when diapers are no longer acceptable. In addition, prolonged drainage and the chronic bacterial colonization that is often present can potentially lead to intrinsic fibrosis of the detrusor and permanent alteration of its dynamics. Although the frequency of this complication and the duration until its occurrence remain undefined, it seems prudent to undivert at the earliest possible age.

ILEAL AND COLONIC URINARY DIVERSIONS

Indications—Diversion Selection

The introduction of Bricker's ureteroileal conduit in 1950 permanently altered the field of urology.[10] This novel technique represented a significant advancement over then-available methods of urinary diversion, including those cited above. Widespread and sometimes overextended application followed. After the initial furor, realistic follow-up allowed identification of the diversion's shortcomings and a better definition of its indications. Metabolic derangements, stomal stenosis, and progressive renal deterioration became well-recognized complications of so-called ileal loops. The nonrefluxing colon conduit with its larger stoma and antirefluxing ureteroenteric anastomoses was subsequently offered as a means of minimizing the last two and may have made some difference in this regard. Nevertheless, these drawbacks, coupled with the alteration of body image caused by a stoma and its appliance, and the evolution of continent urinary reservoirs and enteric substitutes of the native bladder, have left ileal and colon conduits with a limited role in pediatric urological management.

The price now being paid for continence is unknown, and only extended follow-up will determine whether the long-term benefits of continent reconstructions outweigh their potential risks. We do know that noncontinent enteric diversions provide effective, low-maintenance drainage of the urinary tract. This is an important consideration when compliance in the care required of continent urinary reconstructions is suspect or when catheterization cannot be performed. Conduits should also be considered for children with a limited life expectancy or who are unable to undergo the prolonged surgery required of continent reconstruction. Other candidates are those who have a paucity of bowel, massively dilated upper urinary tracts, or such severe nephrogenic diabetes insipidus that continent reconstruction is an impossibility because of excessive urinary output.

It is important to remember that creating a noncontinent diversion does not condemn a child to a stoma for life. Undiversion and continent reconfiguration can be considered at an older age if other negating factors can be controlled or corrected. Colon conduits are preferred in children when preservation of the upper tracts is a prime consideration. The diversion and its nonrefluxing ureterocolonic anastomoses can also be easily incorporated into secondary reconstructions and should be created if later undiversion is planned. In contrast, the technical benefits of the more simply constructed ileal loop are desirable in occasional cases. In others, the selection of an enteric diversion is dictated by the patient's history or anatomical variation. For example, ileal conduits are avoided in children with Crohn disease of the small intestine or radiation injury to the ileum or ureters, and colon conduits are contraindicated with a history of inflammatory disease of the large bowel.

Preoperative Evaluation and Preparation

RADIOGRAPHICAL STUDIES. Excretory urography provides a rough gauge of renal function as well as assessments of scarring, hydronephrosis, and the presence of calculi. Ureteral caliber becomes a factor when selecting a conduit. The creation of nonrefluxing subtenial tunnels for megaureters can be challenging at best. Tapering with implantation into colon conduits has been successful, but when the elimination of reflux is a primary concern, other options such as an ileal-cecal conduit (see below) should be considered.

RENAL STATUS. Renal failure is a relative contraindication to enteric diversion. Neither ileum nor colon offers an advantage in terms of the absorptive tendencies of bowel in the urinary tract. Some degree of hyperchloremic acidosis is expected after constructing any conduit, but the incidence of actual clinical manifestations is variable. Patients with normal kidneys typically handle the increased acid load without demonstrable metabolic alterations, although the depletion of buffer stores required to maintain hematological normalcy has raised some concerns with regard to growth and development in children. In contrast, significant alterations with conduits can result in the face of decreased renal function. A nadir creatinine clearance of 40 ml/min/m² has been proposed as a level below which urinary diversion should not be considered. Solute contact time and absorption can be lessened after surgery by avoiding conduit redundancy and encouraging frequent emptying of the appliance and adequate hydration.

STOMAL PLANNING. Preoperative consultation with an enterostomal therapist is recommended. The child's habitus and abdomen are examined in the supine, sitting, and upright positions and the stoma is created on a flat surface positioned away from skin creases, scars, or bony prominences. Consideration is also given to clothing, manual dexterity, and handedness if the patient is to assume self-care of the appliance. Having the patient wear an appliance for a few days is an invaluable aid to determining stomal position.

BOWEL PREPARATION, PROPHYLAXIS, AND OTHER FACTORS. An adequate bowel preparation is instrumental to minimizing postoperative wound infections. Polyethylene glycol electrolyte solutions are well tolerated by children and are hemodynamically safe and mechanically reliable, even in the face of chronic constipation. Enteral neomycin and erythromycin base are also given to further decrease bacterial flora. Finally, a broad-spectrum parenteral antibiotic having anaerobic coverage (e.g., cefoxitin) is also recommended. Intravenous hydration is begun the night before surgery to avoid problems with dehydration.

Ileal Conduit—Operative Technique

URETERAL MOBILIZATION. A midline approach offers the best exposure and greatest surgical flexibility in these cases. The right ureter is identified medial to the cecum where it crosses the common iliac artery (Fig. 104–4). The left ureter is exposed as it crosses the contralateral common iliac artery by incising the base of the sigmoid mesocolon at its junction with the parietal peritoneum. After opening the posterior peritoneum, each ureter is transected a few centimeters above the ureterovesical junction. During mobilization, care is taken to preserve periureteral vascularity. To minimize trauma and facilitate handling, 5 Fr. feeding tubes are placed and sutured to their ends. With smaller ureters, these feeding tubes can be clamped if dilation is desired to aid in their anastomosis. A tunnel across the mesosigmoid is created by joining the two peritoneotomies with blunt dissection. The left ureter must be mobilized enough to allow for an unobstructed, tension-free route along its new course. Angulation below the inferior mesenteric vessels and twisting are avoided as the ureter is passed to the other side.

HARVESTING THE CONDUIT. A segment of distal ileum is identified that is supplied by a branch of the ileocolic artery or terminal superior mesenteric artery. The arcade adjacent to the ileocecal valve is preserved to avoid problems with enterohepatic circulation and folate deficiency. Transillumination usually helps identify mesenteric vessels, but a Doppler flow probe can be helpful in the case of markedly

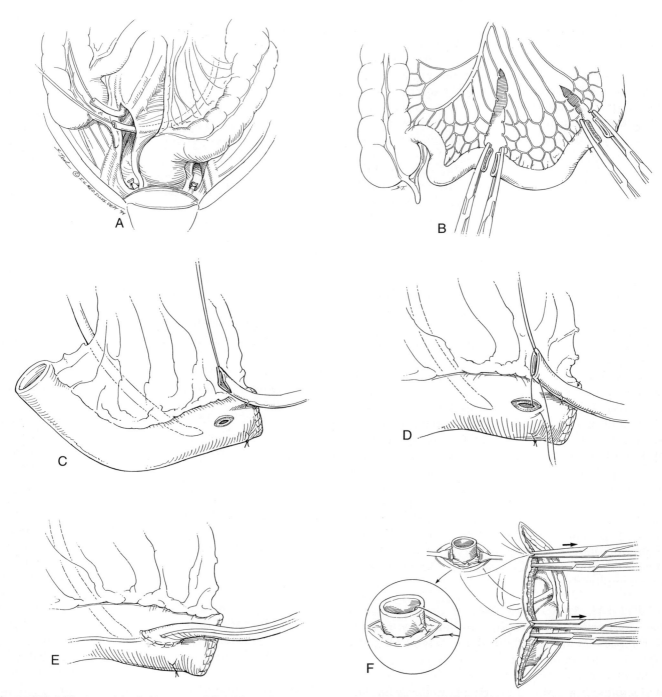

Figure 104–4. Ileal conduit. *A,* Ureters mobilized from the retroperitoneum after opening the posterior peritoneum. The left ureter crosses beneath the sigmoid colon with a gentle curve. *B,* Conduit harvest with the distal ileal arcade preserved. The distal mesenteric window of the selected segment is extended to the root of the mesentery to provide mobility. *C,* Ureter spatulated to match enterotomies that are staggered along the conduit. *D,* Watertight anastomosis of the ureter and ileum with interrupted sutures approximating full thicknesses of ureter and bowel. *E,* Ureteroileal anastomosis completed. *F,* Stomal maturation. Traction on the fascia and dermis aligns tissues and helps avoid shelves. Sutures to create a bud stoma *(inset)* approximate skin, the proximal conduit, and the conduit end.

thickened mesentery. A measurement is taken from the sacral promontory to the stomal site, and enough bowel is used to bridge the distance to just beyond the skin level (about 15 cm in most patients). Length and adequate mesenteric extension are checked with the bowel intact and straightened as much as possible. Redundancy should be avoided, although excess can be discarded during subsequent creation of the stoma. An ileal loop should remain isoperistaltic because of the unidirectional nature of its peristalsis. A stay suture is placed to identify the proposed proximal (butt) end of the loop and avoid later loop reversal.

A broadly based mesentery provides the mobility required of a tension-free stoma. This is created by making a long distal mesenteric window that is extended toward its root. Since the proximal mesenteric window is ultimately anchored in the retroperitoneum, it can be left relatively short. Vessel loops are placed that define the extent of the loop, the key vasculature, and its proposed mesenteric windows. The windows are created by sharply incising the mesentery and using clamps and ties to take down any crossing vessels. Kocher clamps are used to divide the bowel and, after the segment is isolated, one of the clamps is removed to allow for lavage with antibiotic solution using a bulb syringe and sump suction. The remainder of the field is covered with towels to avoid spillage. The proximal end of the loop is closed with a running Parker-Kerr stitch of 3-0 chromic reinforced with interrupted 4-0 silk Lembert sutures. A stapled or two-layer hand-sewn reanastomosis of the ileum is performed above the future conduit using standard techniques. Early results with synthetic absorbable staples that offer a means of harvesting the loop while simultaneously closing its butt have been encouraging. The mesenteric trap is closed at the completion of the procedure to avoid tearing the mesentery as the ureteroileal anastomoses and stoma are being completed.

URETERAL ANASTOMOSES. Meticulous care is given to creating watertight urothelium-to-mucosa anastomoses on either side of the proximal loop. An ellipse of ileal serosa and muscularis is taken with tenotomy scissors at the anastomosis site. A tiny nipple of submucosa and its underlying mucosa can then be extruded with fine forceps and excised. The end of the ureter is freshened by excision and spatulated to mirror the enterotomy. Placing a stay suture that approximates more proximal ureter and ileum a few centimeters away from the enterotomy minimizes handling of the tissues. Fine interrupted chromic sutures (5-0) that incorporate the full-thickness of the ureter and a cuff of ileal serosa and muscularis, but very little mucosa, complete the anastomosis. These are tied on the outside to evert the suture line. A 5

or 8 Fr. feeding tube is placed across the repair to aid in visualization and ensure patency. The stent is secured to the loop with chromic suture so that it does not become dislodged later in the procedure. After the anastomoses are completed, the base of the conduit is fixed to the area of the sacral promontory with absorbable sutures. Freed edges of peritoneum from the hiatus where the ureters exit can usually be tacked to the loop to blanket the anastomoses and reretroperitonealize the repair.

CONJOINED URETERAL ANASTOMOSES (WALLACE TECHNIQUE). When the ureters are significantly dilated, the conjoined technique of Wallace is ideal.[11] The proximal end of the loop is left open. Both ureters are spatulated medially for a distance equal to half the diameter of the ileum. After the spatulations are joined with fine interrupted chromic suture, the common ureteral end is approximated to the conduit's proximal end with a running absorbable stitch. A second layer can be used to reinforce the repair. Stents are usually unnecessary with this technique.

CREATING THE STOMA. A circular opening 2 cm in diameter is made in the skin at the site previously determined for the stoma. The subcutaneous fat is spread with scissors but little is actually excised, since removing too much fat can result in stomal inversion. The anterior fascia is opened with a cruciate incision 2 cm in length, and the underlying muscle is separated initially with a Kelly clamp followed by retractors. Parastomal herniation can be avoided by minimally dividing the muscle. Once the posterior fascia is exposed, a second cruciate incision is made that aligns directly beneath the first. Failure to do so can leave a shelf that obstructs the loop at the fascial level. The hiatus created should allow two fingers. Four 3-0 polydioxanone sutures that approximate the anterior and posterior fascia are placed at the extents of the cruciate and are left untied. After the conduit is pulled through the hiatus with a Babcock clamp, its distal end should lie without tension 2 to 3 cm above the skin to allow creation of an everted "nipple" stoma. If tension is present, Turnbull loop stoma should be considered instead (see below).[12] The four previously placed sutures are used to anastomose the conduit's serosa and muscularis to the fascia with care taken to avoid the blood supply of its mesentery. To create a nipple, a second quadrant of polyglycolic sutures (4-0) are placed sequentially through (1) the dermis of the skin, (2) the serosa of the loop at the dermal level, and finally (3) the end of the loop. Final maturation of stoma to skin is completed with fine interrupted chromic sutures. A large red rubber catheter should pass easily into the conduit at completion of the procedure.

ALTERNATIVE STOMA (TURNBULL LOOP). The

Turnbull loop is particularly useful in an obese patient whose conduit must negotiate a deep layer of fat to reach the skin level, causing its mesentery to be stretched.[12] Rather than bring its end to the skin and risk compromising the blood supply, a more proximal mobile portion of loop is brought through the hiatus in the abdominal wall. In some cases, it still becomes necessary to carefully undercut the mesentery to the conduit's distal end, preserving the arcade, to obtain adequate mobility. The muscularis of the loop stoma is secured to a cruciate incision in the fascia (as above) and the loop is opened transversely near its defunctionalized (distal) limb. Polyglycolic sutures (4-0) that approximate the subcuticular layer of the skin to the seromuscular and mucosa layers of the loop are used to evert the stoma.

COMPLETING THE REPAIR. The feeding tubes are anchored at the stomal level with chromic sutures, cut short, and allowed to drain freely into an appliance. Penrose drains that can sometimes be positioned entirely within the retroperitoneum are placed near the butt end of the loop. Finally, the mesenteric trap and midline incision are closed.

Colon Conduit—Operative Technique

Construction of a colon conduit is similar to that of an ileal loop, but some differences deserve emphasis.

HARVESTING THE CONDUIT. Typically, it is easiest to work with sigmoid colon in children. However, the vasculature of the descending, ascending, and transverse colonic segments is predictable and usually associated with adequate mesenteric length. Like ileum, the mesenteric incision of the end of the segment destined to become the stoma can be extended to the root of the mesentery to increase its mobility. Colon tends to contract during these operations, and it is wise to select a generous length of bowel initially, trimming what is not needed later when the stoma is being constructed. It is also notable that the colon empties readily by mass contraction rather than peristalsis and carries little residual. As a consequence, isoperistaltic orientation is probably unnecessary.

URETERAL ANASTOMOSES. After its proximal end is closed, the loop is left unanchored until the ureters are implanted. This aids in exposure and handling. A tenia on each side of the conduit is isolated for creation of a nonrefluxing ureteral anastomosis (Fig. 104–5). Tacking sutures placed 6 cm apart help define the proposed tunnels, which should be at least 4 cm long. If possible, the tunnels are staggered along the length of the conduit to minimize any compromise of bowel that might occur between tunnels created in parallel. Saline is injected beneath the tenia

to help define its plane with the underlying mucosa. After the tenia is incised longitudinally, this plane is developed with tenotomy scissors and a dissector. The dissection is largely directed laterally toward the mesentery to avoid devascularization of the strip of bowel between the tunnels. At the distal extent of each tunnel, an anastomosis between the spatulated ureter and colonic mucosa is completed with fine interrupted chromic sutures (as above). Feeding tubes are placed and the tenia is reapproximated over the ureters with interrupted Prolene sutures to aid in identification if reoperation becomes necessary. Care must be taken to avoid extreme angulation or twisting of the ureters at their entrance into the tunnels. If the hiatus is tight or sharply angulated, the proximal tenial suture(s) should be removed.

CREATING THE STOMA. The colonic stoma is only slightly larger than that of an ileal loop and is completed in a similar fashion after a circumferential skin incision 2 to 3 cm in diameter is made. Like ileum, stomas that protrude above the skin do a better job of preventing leakage by directing urine directly into collecting devices.

ILEOCECAL CONDUIT

Diversion can be difficult in a child with significantly dilated ureters if eliminating reflux is one of the goals. Conduits created from the ileocecal segment offer one effective option in management. The ileocecal valve plays a role in the antireflux mechanism, but to achieve long-term efficacy, valvular reconfiguration becomes necessary. In situ the valve is competent in most patients. Once incorporated in urinary reconstructions, however, progressive incompetence has been a common occurrence. A variety of different methods have been used to reinforce the valve, but a modification based on the work by Hendren appears to be the most effective. Here the intussuscepted ileal segment is fixed to the adjacent cecal wall, which, in effect, transforms it into a flap valve. This lessens the detrimental influence of intraluminal pressures that eventually efface and break down other valvular configurations that might be used instead, including an unaltered ileocecal nipple.

Ileocecal Conduit—Operative Technique

HARVESTING THE CONDUIT. The cecal segment forms the body of the conduit, and approximately 6 cm of terminal ileum is used to create its antirefluxing mechanism (Fig. 104–6). Conduit length, mesenteric mobilization, and loop harvest are completed using the techniques described previously.

MODIFYING THE VALVE. A small mesenteric win-

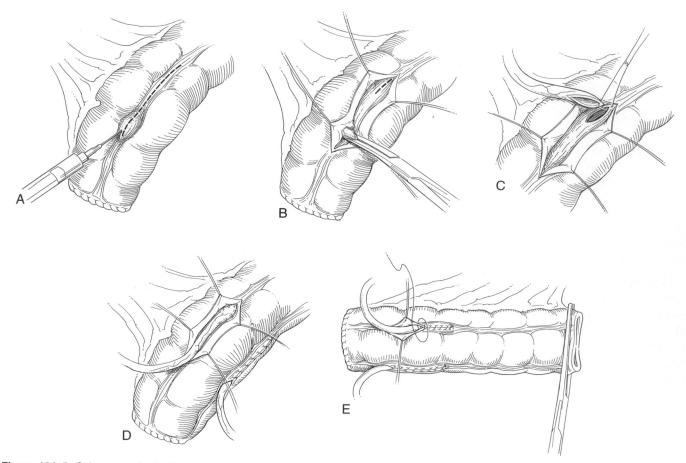

Figure 104–5. Colon conduit. *A,* After harvesting a segment, the sites proposed for subtenial tunnels and ureterocolonic anastomoses are marked. Saline injection defines the plane between the tenia and underlying mucosa. *B,* Tenia mobilized using a combination of blunt and sharp dissection. The site proposed for anastomosis is shown. *C,* Spatulated ureter anastomosed to the colon with interrupted sutures. *D,* Anastomosis complete. *E,* Tenia closed with running nonabsorbable suture to aid in future identification if necessary. The stoma is constructed as in an ileal conduit.

dow is created by taking down the blood vessels from the arcade that supply the distal segment of ileum. As much as 8 cm of small bowel can be isolated with this technique while still maintaining its viability by way of intrinsic vascularity. The mesentery to the end of the ileum is kept intact and open in anticipation of the ureteral anastomosis. The distal ileum is intusscepted across the ileocecal valve by grasping the segment with a Babcock clamp from within. An antimesenteric incision is made through the mucosal layer of the nipple of ileum, which is matched by a similar incision in the adjacent cecal wall. The ileum and cecum are then anastomosed by running two 4-0 polydioxanone sutures that approximate the two sides of the incisions.

COMPLETING THE REPAIR. The enlarged ureters are anastomosed to the end of the ileum using the Wallace technique, and the stoma is completed as above.

Postoperative Care and Follow-up

A 1-week hospitalization is anticipated. Nasogastric decompression is continued for 3 or 4 days until cessation of the postoperative ileus. Once oral intake is adequate, intravenous fluids can be discontinued. Hyperalimentation is maintained if the patient's nutritional status is deficient. Stentograms are obtained 5 days after surgery and the drains removed if no problems are seen. Prophylactic antibiotics (a cephalosporin) are continued until all drains are removed.

Other than examination, subsequent follow-up consists of periodic serum chemistry profiles and urine cultures. Loop cultures should be obtained by the double-catheter technique to maximize validity. An estimate of conduit residual is also provided. Most enteric conduits are chronically colonized with bacteria, but treatment is recommended only for symptomatic patients. When recurrent bouts of pyelonephritis occur, calculi and obstruction must be considered. An excretory urogram is obtained a few weeks after surgery to assess healing and rule out obstruction. Afterward, children with conduits should be followed at yearly intervals, even in the absence of symptoms. The anatomical correlate provided by ultrasound examination is used for serial surveillance of the upper urinary tract. Loopography

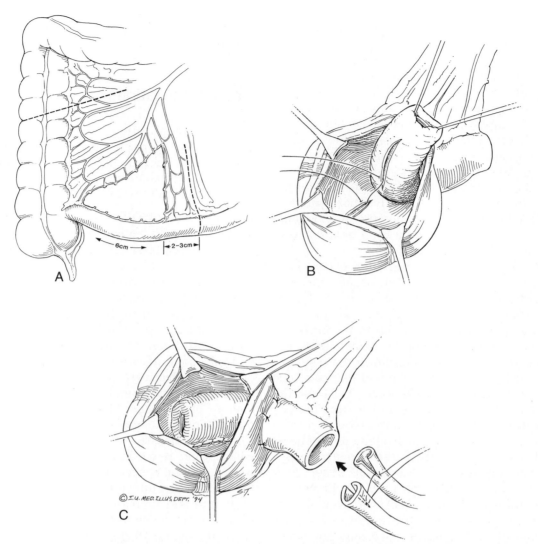

Figure 104–6. Ileocecal conduit. *A,* Proposed lines of harvest. A cecal segment is used to create a conduit. The mesentery of the distal ileum is taken down to allow reconfiguration of the valve. A length of 2 to 3 cm of intact proximal ileum maintains vascularity and serves as a recipient for the ureters. *B,* Distal ileum intussuscepted into the cecum. Counterincisions in the cecum and ileum are approximated with running sutures on each side of the wounds. *C,* Valve reconfiguration complete. The ileum is reinforced outside the cecum with interrupted sutures. A Wallace-type anastomosis of the ureters completes the repair.

becomes the initial study of choice when new or worsening hydronephrosis is noted. Conduits without tunneled ureters should freely reflux. Its absence is strongly suggestive of stricture. When problems exist, additional studies (e.g., excretory urography, nephrostogram) may become necessary to help formulate a treatment plan.

Early Complications

Noncontinent urinary diversions present the same perioperative complications generic to every major intra-abdominal surgical procedure. These include wound infection and dehiscence, intestinal obstruction, enteric fistula, and, of course, death. Concerns over the use of colon, the flora of which might carry a more significant threat of infection, rather than ileum

when constructing diversions are unfounded. Comparisons of the two from the literature show similar rates of wound infection, dehiscence, and fistula formation. There has also been no difference in mortality between the two diversions: an incidence of 2 to 5 percent has been noted in most series. Adequate bowel preparation and antibiotics appear to be instrumental in this regard. Although a review of the other complications generic to intra-abdominal surgery will be deferred, two complications, ureteroenteric anastomotic leaks and loop infarction, are unique to conduits and deserve additional attention.

ANASTOMOTIC LEAKS. Significant ureteroenteric anastomotic leaks reportedly occur at a frequency of 2 to 10 percent, although they can usually be avoided by careful surgical technique. A leak should be suspected in any patient whose urine output has suddenly diminished or who exhibits a rising blood urea nitrogen level despite aggressive hydration. Abdominal distention and prolonged ileus are common. Most occur early after surgery if a conduit is unstented or soon after stents have been removed. The debate over stents will continue, but the arguments of most critics are based on complications experienced before the era of soft, pliable, nonreactive tubes. Contemporary stents do not appear to cause problems at the anastomosis. When stents are used, the urinary diversion required as the antidote for most leaks is already in place, providing a form of pre-emptive management. If extravasation is seen on a postoperative stentogram, drainage should be continued for a week or two; most small leaks heal within this time.

These fistulas are similar to those that occur elsewhere in the body. Other than technical mishaps, the most common (and easily correctable) risk factor is distal loop obstruction. A large Foley catheter provides a simple and effective solution to the obstruction of flow caused by postoperative stomal edema or later stenosis. A loopogram will confirm the patency of a conduit or help define the site and degree of its disruption when this is not the case. Most minor leaks resolve once distal obstruction has been alleviated. Larger leaks, regardless of cause, require proximal diversion. Nephrostomy tubes alone are ineffective. Instead, indwelling stents placed percutaneously across the anastomosis are the best means of successfully dealing with a challenging problem. Extended conservative therapy (6 to 8 weeks or even more) is warranted unless urinary extravasation or sepsis cannot be controlled. Persistent leaks sometimes belie more formidable technical challenges, including slough of the distal ureter, anastomotic disruption, and a blowout of the end of the loop. Reoperations are difficult at best, and repeating the original operation is sometimes impossible. One option for unilateral ureteral problems is proximal diversion by transureteroureterostomy after the loop is closed. When the loop cannot be salvaged, a transverse colon conduit that employs more proximal virgin ureters is an ideal choice.

LOOP INFARCTION. A somewhat dusky and edematous stoma is common early after surgery. This appearance typically improves as venous congestion resolves. An ischemic appearance that persists, especially when coupled with signs of urinary leakage, is an ominous indicator of loop infarction. The potential for vascular compromise can usually be appreciated as the conduit is being constructed. Here, mesenteric tension and hematomas are well-known risk factors. Infarctions can be localized to the distal loop and stoma or involve the entire conduit. Looposcopy is done to define the extent of the mishap and aid in the planning of its surgical correction with solutions that range from simple stomal revision to complete loop replacement.

Late Complications

Overall complication rates of 30 to 80 percent underscore the shortcomings of enteric urinary conduits. These include renal deterioration, hydronephrosis, loop stenosis, ureteral strictures, stomal problems, calculi, and malignancy.

RENAL DETERIORATION. Renal deterioration has been noted with both colonic and ileal diversions, and the comparative efficacy in avoiding this complication remains a point of contention. A review of their respective performances is revealing, but caution must be exercised when drawing conclusions from the data of historical series. Although the techniques remain essentially the same, today's surgical milieu is different and indications have changed. For example, conduits are rarely constructed now in children. Retrospectively, loops could not have been expected to preserve function in kidneys when developmental insults had already occurred, which was possibly often the case.[13, 14]

Much of the early enthusiasm for ileal loops diminished when it became apparent that renal damage was a common consequence of the procedure. In fact, loss of function appears to be the rule rather than the exception and increases with the duration of diversion. An incidence as high as 61 percent was noted with an average follow-up of 15 years.[15] Unfortunately, the mechanisms that lead to renal deterioration cannot always be identified. The significance of chronic asymptomatic bacteriuria in low-pressure refluxing systems such as an ileal loop remains to be defined, but the implications of frank pyelonephritis, which occurs in 7 to 38 percent of patients, and hydronephrosis are widely recognized.[16]

Growing disenchantment with ileal loops caused other investigators to focus on the colon conduit after Mogg's initial report painted a very encouraging picture of its performance in children with neurogenic bladders.[17] Two advantages colon offered were nonrefluxing ureteral anastomoses and a larger-diameter stoma that could theoretically minimize stenosis. Extended follow-up of those same children, however, cited alarming rates of upper tract deterioration (48 percent) and reflux (58 percent).[18] It is notable that 73 percent of kidneys without reflux remained normal, but only 21 percent were preserved when reflux was present. This tendency was also noted in a more recent series of colon conduits in which none of 39 kidneys with normal nonrefluxing anastomoses developed renal scarring. In comparison, 5 of 11 kidneys (45 percent) with reflux or ureteral stricture developed scars.[19] These types of clinical data and experimental models suggest that a properly constructed colon conduit offers a protective advantage to the kidneys.[20]

HYDRONEPHROSIS. Transient hydronephrosis from anastomotic edema could be found with most conduits if studies were performed early enough after surgery. More than 90 percent resolve by 6 months. Persistent or late-onset hydronephrosis presents a different dilemma. Common causes include loop stenosis, ureteral stricture, and calculi. Stomal stenosis, reflux, and infrequent emptying of the appliance should also be considered.

LOOP STENOSIS. Enteric urinary conduits can develop segmental stenosis or complete stricturing at any time. This phenomenon occurs more commonly in ileum, the smaller diameter of which makes it more prone to manifest constriction, but it has also been described in colon. Transmural scarring from chronic infection and an altered immune response have been implicated. Once exposed to urine, ileum demonstrates progressive atrophy of Peyer patches and hypertrophy of its regional lymph nodes.[21] These same changes might also play a part in ureteroileal obstruction, stomal stenosis, and total conduit fibrosis. Loopography and looposcopy are used to confirm the diagnosis. When these obstructions become clinically significant, total loop replacement is usually warranted. A clinically evident cicatrix represents change that has probably affected the entire loop, and segmental resections with reanastomosis of adjacent bowel are usually only temporarily effective. One exception is distal stenosis, which can be managed by loop mobilization and advancement after unhealthy bowel is resected.

URETERAL STRICTURES. Ureteral strictures occur with ileal conduits at rates between 1 and 9 percent.[16] and may be more common in colon conduits. Causes include overt angulation of the left ureter as it passes through the sigmoid mesentery, periureteral fibrosis from urinary extravasation, and devascularization from traumatic ureteral mobilization. In the face of previous radiation therapy, ureters well above the field and nonirradiated bowel should be employed. The transverse colon conduit is an ideal diversion when this is the case.[22]

The presentation of strictures is variable. Those having a basis in technical error usually become evident soon after surgery and cause persistent hydronephrosis, flank pain, and urinary infection. Others may develop months and even years later if progressive scarring is the cause. Transureteroureterostomy is effective for unilateral strictures, although some clinicians have voiced concerns over further manipulating the contralateral ureter that has been similarly treated

and might be at an equal, although unknown, risk for obstruction. Despite this, complete loop revision is unnecessary unless bilateral change is present. Endourological management has not been encouraging. Balloon dilation usually provides an unsatisfactory solution to what is often a vascular insult, and the long-term efficacy of novel techniques such as endoscopic ureterotomy is undefined, especially in children.[23]

STOMAL PROBLEMS. The circular anastomosis of bowel to skin is prone to cicatricial contraction and causes stomal stenosis to be the most common complication of ileal diversion. Skin reconfiguration has done little to decrease stenosis, although the addition of the everted stoma has decreased its incidence from rates as high as 25 to 50 percent in some early series. Turnbull loop stoma is reportedly less prone to stenosis.[24] Colon conduits are also prone to these problems despite their larger diameters. Possible causes include retraction, lymphatic alteration, peristomal dermatitis, and compromised vascularity. Infected alkaline urine causes phosphatic encrustation, irritation, and epithelialization of the mucosa and is probably implicated in superficial stenosis. Proper stomal care and treatment of infections eliminate most local problems, but a protruding stoma and properly fitted appliance are the key to avoidance. The surgery for stenosis varies with the severity of the obstruction. Some can be treated by advancing a V-shaped skin flap into an incision made in the stomal cicatrix. In others, reconstruction of a new stoma with repositioning at another site becomes necessary.

Stomal complications can be avoided by using the principles of construction discussed above. Parastomal hernias and loop prolapse are caused by inadequate fixation of the conduit to the anterior abdominal wall. Hernias that develop early after surgery can cause abdominal distention and bowel obstruction. The appearance of peritoneal fluid from the lateral margins of a stoma is an ominous sign of incarceration and impending surgical emergency. Those that develop gradually can be managed less urgently and may not require correction unless large or symptomatic. Loop prolapse occasionally causes venous congestion and progressive ischemia that require surgical attention. Otherwise, most moderate degrees of prolapse can be managed expectantly for long periods.

CALCULI. Urinary calculi represent one of the more common complications of enteric diversions. A 5- to 10-percent incidence is generally cited, although rates as high as 30 percent have been described. Most are composed of magnesium ammonium phosphate and are associated with *Proteus* urinary tract infections. A component of calcium is also often present. The tendency to stone formation is probably related to a variety of factors, including dehydration, immobilization, and alkaline urine as a result of the bowel's chloride-bicarbonate exchange and the mobilization of calcium from bone to buffer acidosis.[25] Morphological abnormalities also probably contribute, with calculi occurring much less commonly in kidneys that are normal before diversion.[13] Finally, mucus may act as a nidus for stone formation in the presence of infected urine. Stone formation can be rapid and relatively innocuous. Surveillance and early treatment are the keys to management. The ureteral anastomoses of either colon or ileal conduits do not present an obstacle to the stone debris of extracorporeal shock wave lithotripsy unless the burden is excessive.

MALIGNANCY. The malignant potential of urinary conduits is unknown, but concerns have been voiced over the use of bowel in the urinary tract, even when fecal interaction such as that with ureterosigmoidostomy is not present. To date, three cases of carcinoma in colon conduits and one in an ileal conduit have been reported. Two instances of adenomatous polyps within ileal loops have also been seen.[26] Histological studies of ileal loops, many of which existed for more than 10 years, have shown nonspecific changes, including chronic inflammation, fragmentation, and thickening of the muscularis, and submucosal edema.[27] Colon loops exhibit more worrisome tendencies such as increased mitotic figures, metaplasia, altered nuclear-to-cytoplasmic ratios, and inflammatory infiltrate.[28] Not surprisingly, the severity of change appears to be proportional to the duration of diversion. On the basis of these findings, the risks of malignancy with any enteric diversion appear to be low but may be slightly higher with colon. Endoscopic follow-up is probably unnecessary unless the patient has been diverted for an extended period.

Editorial Comment
Craig A. Peters

While the emphasis in pediatric urology has been away from urinary diversion in favor of functional reconstruction or continent diversion techniques, temporary urinary diversion remains an important aspect of pediatric urological practice. The appropriate selection of technique and its effective use are critical, as they are so often used in patients with severe abnormalities or impaired renal function. It remains important to consider the temporary nature of the diversion and include a plan for refunctionalization in the formulation of the diversion strategy.

Colon conduit diversion has been the most useful means of temporary diversion in children with pelvic malignancy, in that these are consistently effective and may be readily integrated into subsequent definitive continent diversions.

REFERENCES

1. MacGregor PS, Kay R, Straffon RA. Cutaneous ureterostomy in children—long term follow-up. J Urol 134:518, 1985.
2. Kogan BA, Gohary MA. Cutaneous ureterostomy as a permanent external urinary diversion in children. J Urol 132:729, 1984.
3. Perlmutter AD, Patil J. Loop cutaneous ureterostomy in infants and young children. Late results in 32 cases. J Urol 107:655, 1972.
4. Hendren WH. Complications of ureterostomy. J Urol 120:269, 1978.
5. Burstein JD, Firlit CF. Complications of cutaneous ureterostomy and other cutaneous diversion. Urol Clin North Am 10:433, 1983.
6. Duckett JW Jr. Cutaneous vesicostomy in childhood: The Blocksom technique. Urol Clin North Am 1:485, 1974.
7. Blocksom BH. Bladder pouch for prolonged tubeless cystostomy. J Urol 78:398, 1957.
8. Hurwitz RS, Erlich RM. Complications of cutaneous vesicostomy in children. Urol Clin North Am 10:503, 1983.
9. Noe HN, Jerkins GR. Cutaneous vesicostomy in infants and children. J Urol 134:301, 1985.
10. Bricker EM. Bladder substitution after pelvic evisceration. Surg Gynecol Obstet 30:1511, 1950.
11. Esho JO, Vitko RJ, Freland GW, Cass AS. Comparison of Bricker and Wallace methods of ureteroileal anastomosis in urinary diversion. J Urol 111:600, 1974.
12. Turnbull RB Jr, Fazio V. Advances in the surgical technique and ulcerative colitis surgery. In Nyhus L, ed. Surgery Annual. New York, Appleton-Century-Crofts, 1975, p 315.
13. Richie JP. Intestinal loop urinary diversion in children. J Urol 11:687, 1974.
14. Pitts WR, Muecke EC. A 20-year experience with ileal conduits: The fate of the kidneys. J Urol 122:154, 1979.
15. Orr JD, Shand JE, Watters DA, et al. Ileal conduit urinary diversion in children. An assessment of the long-term results. Br J Urol 53:424, 1981.
16. Heath AL, Eckstein HB. Ileal conduit urinary diversion in children: A long-term follow-up. J Urol (Paris) 90:91, 1984.
17. Mogg RA. The treatment of neurogenic urinary incontinence using the colon conduit. Br J Urol 37:681, 1965.
18. Elder DD, Moisey CV, Rees RW. A long-term follow-up of the colonic conduit operation in children. Br J Urol 51:462, 1979.
19. Hussman DA, McLorie GA, Churchill BM. Nonrefluxing colonic conduits: A long-term life-table analysis. J Urol 142:1201, 1989.
20. Richie JP, Skinner DG. Urinary diversion: The physiologic rationale for nonrefluxing colonic conduits. Br J Urol 47:269, 1975.
21. Tapper D, Folkman MJ. Lymphoid depletion in ileal loops: Mechanism and clinical implications. J Pediatr Surg 11:871, 1976.
22. Schmidt JD, Buchsbaum HJ. Transverse colon conduit diversion. Urol Clin North Am 13:233, 1986.
23. Kramolosky EV, Clayman RV, Weyman PJ. Endourological management of ureteroileal anastomotic strictures: Is it effective? J Urol 137:390, 1987.
24. Noble MJ, Mebust WK. Creation of the Urinary Stoma. AUA Update Series. Lesson 13, Vol. 5, 1986.
25. Dretler SP. The pathogenesis of urinary tract calculi occurring after ileal conduit diversion: I. Clinical study. II. Conduit study. III. Prevention. J Urol 109:204, 1973.
26. Filmer RB, Spencer JR. Malignancies in bladder augmentations and intestinal conduits. J Urol 143:671, 1990.
27. Deane AM, Woodhouse CRJ, Parkinson MC. Histological changes in ileal conduits. J Urol 132:1198, 1984.
28. Moorcraft J, DuBoulay CEH, Isaacson P, et al. Changes in the mucosa of colon conduits with particular reference to the risk of malignant change. Br J Urol 55:185, 1983.

Chapter 105

Ureteral Reimplantation: Including Megaureter Repair

Craig A. Peters and Alan B. Retik

INDICATIONS

Ureteral reimplantation into the bladder is indicated for abnormalities of the ureterovesical junction that may cause renal damage. This includes both vesicoureteral reflux (VUR) and obstruction at the ureterovesical junction. Vesicoureteral reflux spontaneously resolves with time, depending on the grade of reflux. While 80 percent of grade I/II reflux will resolve, only 41 percent of reflux of grades III through V will do so.[1] Resolution has been seen to occur at a rate of 20 to 30 percent every 2 years.[2, 3] A trial of observational management on prophylactic antibiotics is therefore justified in most patients. The appropriate waiting period before surgery depends on several factors, including the age and sex of the patient, the grade of reflux, and parental wishes. There are contraindications to medical management. These include the presence of massive reflux with severe metabolic derangement, breakthrough infections, patient noncompliance, associated and contributing anatomical anomalies, impaired renal growth or function, significant renal scarring, and failure of reflux to subside after full linear somatic growth has been achieved. An obstructed ureter should be repaired. A dilated ureter is not always obstructed; the objective assessment of the degree of obstruction necessitating repair is controversial and spontaneous resolution has been documented.[4] Cases requiring repair may usually be discerned with careful imaging studies.

PREOPERATIVE MANAGEMENT

Aggressive treatment of urinary infection is necessary, as is sufficient time for the effects of cystitis to resolve. Bladder drainage is usually not required. In an infant with massive VUR, the megaureter/mega-cystis association[5] may present a clinical appearance of acute, life-threatening sepsis, including a biochemical picture of adrenal insufficiency. In general, we do not use preoperative catheter or vesicostomy drainage. Imaging of the upper urinary tract with ultrasound, an intravenous pyelogram (IVP), or an isotope renal scan is essential, as is imaging of the lower tract with a voiding cystourethrogram. Cystoscopy is generally of little value in terms of providing prognostic information.[6]

The assessment of obstruction may be conducted with isotope renal scans with a diuretic washout component or with a dynamically interpreted IVP. Urodynamic evaluation is appropriate in the setting of a neurogenic bladder or when there is evidence suggesting neuropathic changes, bladder outlet obstruction, or dysfunctional voiding.[7] Preoperative management of constipation and a mild bowel cleansing often avoid postoperative problems of spasm and refractory constipation.

TECHNIQUE

CYSTOSCOPY AND POSITIONING. Cystoscopy may be performed using the same anesthesia. Cystoscopic identification of definite anatomical abnormalities may aid in the surgical decision making during the procedure. For example, identification of a Hutch saccule associated with a nonrefluxing contralateral ureter is an indication for bilateral surgery. The bladder is left full and the patient is placed with a slight break in the table to raise the hips. The perineum is prepared with the operative field.

INCISION. Routine cases are performed through a low transverse incision (Pfannenstiel), preferably with a transverse fascial incision, although a vertical fascial incision is acceptable. Reoperations are best handled with a midline incision that can be extended superiorly if needed.

EXPOSURE. The prevesical space is developed by sweeping the transversalis fascia and peritoneum superiorly off the bladder. Minimal perivesical dissection is needed. The bladder is opened between stay sutures with electrocautery to within 1 cm of the bladder neck. The inferior bladder edges are sutured to the rectus fascia to protect the bladder neck and elevate the trigone. Ring retractor blades (Denis Browne) are placed laterally in the bladder. The dome of the bladder is gently packed with moist sponges, progressively elevating and stretching the trigone. A minimal amount of manipulation of the bladder mucosa will avoid edema and distortion of the operative field.

URETERAL MOBILIZATION. Chromic sutures (4-0) are placed above and below the ureteral orifice (Fig. 105–1). A fine infant feeding tube (3.5 or 5 Fr.) helps in the initial identification and ureteral dissection. The bladder mucosa is incised with electrocautery, providing an adequate cuff of tissue for subsequent anastomosis. Initial mobilization of the muscular attachments requires sharp dissection at the level of the ureteral wall. This is aided by identifica-

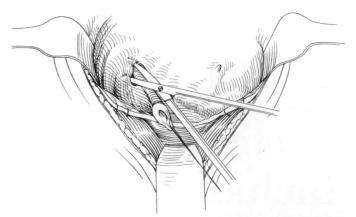

Figure 105–2. Tenotomy scissors are used to establish the correct plane inferiorly, which is then carried around the circumference of the ureter. (From Retik AB, Colodny AH, Bauer SB. Pediatric urology. In Paulson DF, ed. Genitourinary Surgery, Vol 2. New York, Churchill Livingstone, 1984, p 758.)

tion of the periureteral plane inferiorly, which is maintained as a point of reference to which the dissection may return. Sharp dissection with tenotomy scissors parallel to the ureter develops this plane, and the ureter is dissected from its intramural and extravesical attachments (Fig. 105–2). After the muscular attachments have been taken down, further mobilization progresses more readily. Attention should be paid to preservation of the periureteral adventitia with its essential blood supply. Hemostasis is essential, but cauterization directly on the ureter should be avoided.

The peritoneal edge is usually identified superiorly and laterally; in boys the vas deferens is also identified. A small vascular bridge that may kink the ureter is often seen near the peritoneal edge and should be divided. The infant feeding tube is removed for the final portion of the mobilization. At this point, the ureter should have an element of "spring" when gently stretched, usually after 6 to 8 cm of ureter has been mobilized. The appropriate length of ureteral mobilization is that which will provide a tunnel length approximately five times the diameter of the ureter.[8]

After the ureters are mobilized, the various techniques for ureteral reimplantation and megaureter repair differ. Each is described separately.

Politano-Leadbetter Technique

Described in 1958,[9] the Politano-Leadbetter method has been widely used with excellent results. Use of a lighted suction tip and careful exposure of the posterior bladder permits excellent exposure and complete control with few complications. We continue to use this method, with modification, in approximately one half of our patients. It is often the preferred method

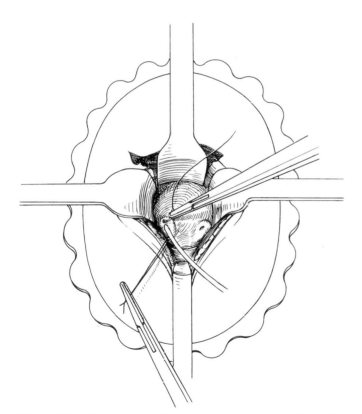

Figure 105–1. Fine chromic stitches are placed above and below the ureteral orifice for traction, and an infant feeding tube is placed as an aid in the initial dissection of the ureter. (From Retik AB, Colodny AH, Bauer SB. Pediatric urology. In Paulson DF, ed. Genitourinary Surgery, Vol 2. New York, Churchill Livingstone, 1984, p 757.)

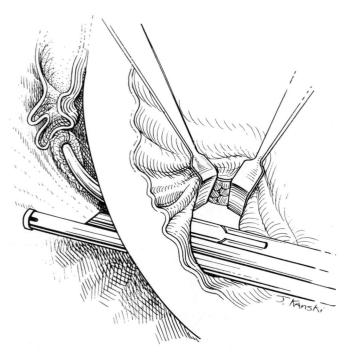

Figure 105–3. With visualization provided by the lighted suction tip and hiatal retractors, the peritoneum is swept from the posterior bladder wall with a fine gauze dissector ("peanut"). (From Keating MA, Retik AB. Management of failures of ureteroneocystostomy. In McDougal WS, ed. Difficult Problems in Urologic Surgery. Chicago, Year Book, 1988, p 121.)

for reimplantation of a unilaterally refluxing ureter or for reimplantation of duplex systems.[10]

EXPOSURE OF THE POSTERIOR BLADDER WALL AND NEOHIATUS. The ureteral hiatus is widened by spreading the musculature with a blunt right-angled clamp. With the aid of a lighted suction tip and hiatal retractors, a fine gauze dissector ("peanut")

is used to sweep the peritoneum from the posterior bladder wall (Fig. 105–3). This provides better visualization of the perivesical region and the site for the neohiatus. When an adequate distance has been cleared, the right-angled clamp is carefully guided behind the bladder wall, pushing the peritoneum away, to the position of the neohiatus (Fig. 105–4). This position is critical and ideally should be 2.5 to 3 cm superior and slightly medial to the original hiatus. Too lateral a placement risks ureteral kinking with bladder filling; too short a distance may yield a tunnel of inadequate length to prevent reflux.

CREATION OF THE NEOHIATUS. The bladder mucosa and muscle are incised over the right-angled clamp at the point of the neohiatus, allowing the clamp to be spread wide (Fig. 105–5). Another right-angled clamp is then passed from the neohiatus to the original hiatus (Fig. 105–6) and used to pull the ureter (Fig. 105–7) through the new opening (Fig. 105–8). The relocated ureter should be completely visualized behind the bladder after this maneuver. If it is not, the ureter may have been inadvertently passed through the peritoneum (Fig. 105–9). A fine feeding tube is passed up the ureter to confirm that obstruction is not present.

CLOSURE OF THE ORIGINAL HIATUS AND CREATION OF THE URETERAL TUNNEL. The original muscular hiatus is closed with interrupted absorbable sutures, 4-0 chromic or polyglycolic acid, to provide a solid muscular backing for the ureter and to avoid a diverticulum. The superior suture is helpful for traction in creation of the submucosal tunnel. Tenotomy scissors are useful in this maneuver and the tunnel should be of adequate caliber to easily accept

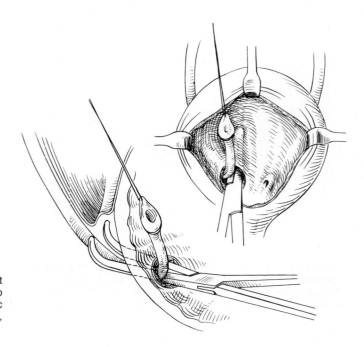

Figure 105–4. A blunt right-angled clamp indents the bladder wall at the new hiatus, approximately 2.5 cm superior and slightly medial to the original hiatus. (From Retik AB, Colodny AH, Bauer SB. Pediatric urology. In Paulson DF, ed. Genitourinary Surgery, Vol 2. New York, Churchill Livingstone, 1984, p 759.)

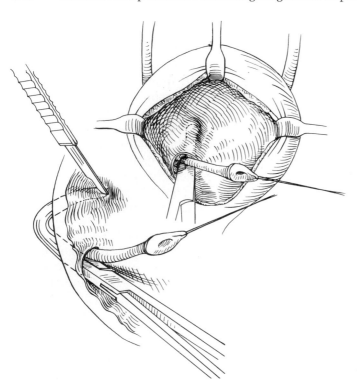

Figure 105–5. The clamp is incised upon from within the bladder and spread widely to make certain that the new hiatus is of adequate width. (From Retik AB, Colodny AH, Bauer SB. Pediatric urology. In Paulson DF, ed. Genitourinary Surgery, Vol 2. New York, Churchill Livingstone, 1984, p 759.)

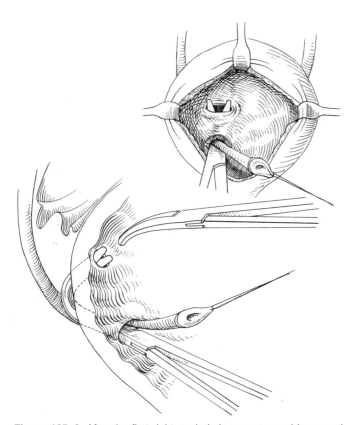

Figure 105–6. After the first right-angled clamp, a second is passed from within the bladder to the original hiatus. (From Retik AB, Colodny AH, Bauer SB. Pediatric urology. In Paulson DF, ed. Genitourinary Surgery, Vol 2. New York, Churchill Livingstone, 1984, p 760.)

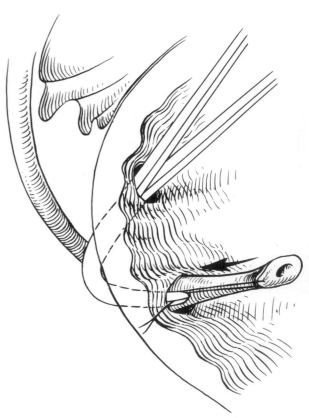

Figure 105–7. The inferior ureteral traction stitch is grasped by the right-angled clamp through the original hiatus. (From Retik AB, Colodny AH, Bauer SB. Pediatric urology. In Paulson DF, ed. Genitourinary Surgery, Vol 2. New York, Churchill Livingstone, 1984, p 761.)

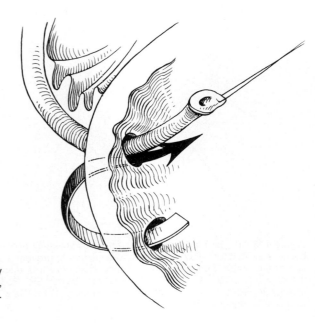

Figure 105–8. The ureter is guided into the bladder through the new hiatus by the traction suture and the right-angled clamp. (From Retik AB, Colodny AH, Bauer SB. Pediatric urology. In Paulson DF, ed. Genitourinary Surgery, Vol 2. New York, Churchill Livingstone, 1984, p 761.)

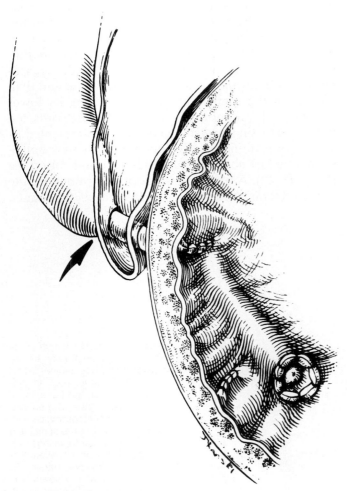

Figure 105–9. A ureter reimplanted through the peritoneum as it enters its new hiatus. (From Keating MA, Retik AB. Management of failures of ureteroneocystostomy. In McDougal WS, ed. Difficult Problems in Urologic Surgery. Chicago, Year Book, 1988, p 122.)

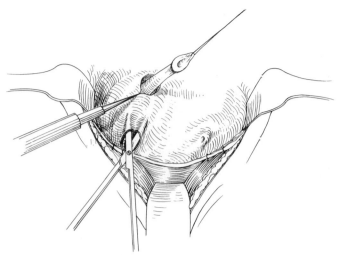

Figure 105–10. The bladder muscle on the lateral aspect of the new hiatus is divided for a few millimeters with cautery to prevent angulation of the ureter. Spreading the scissors widely ensures adequate tunnel width. (From Retik AB, Colodny AH, Bauer SB. Pediatric urology. In Paulson DF, ed. Genitourinary Surgery, Vol 2. New York, Churchill Livingstone, 1984, p 761.)

the ureter (Fig. 105–10). Mobilization of the mucosa around the neohiatus and the original hiatus is also performed, using sharp dissection. The ureter is then passed through the tunnel, with care taken to avoid twisting. Tunnel length may be extended up to 1 or 1.5 cm with an advancement toward the bladder neck. This is done by incising and mobilizing the bladder mucosa to accommodate the ureter or by tunneling and making a new mucosal hiatus (Fig. 105–11).

ANASTOMOSIS OF THE URETER INTO THE BLADDER. The ureteral cuff should be inspected and preserved if intact and healthy. If the orifice is narrow or the distal ureter has been damaged, the tip of the ureter is excised and the ureter spatulated. The ureter is anchored to the trigonal musculature with three chromic sutures (4-0), and the anastomosis is completed with 5-0 chromic sutures. The previously mobilized bladder mucosa is closed loosely over the ureter with running or interrupted 5-0 chromic suture. A final check of free passage with a fine infant feeding tube is performed and the ureter, in most instances, is left unstented (Fig. 105–11).

Cohen Transtrigonal Technique

This technique has been widely applied since it was introduced in 1975[11] and offers a simplified reimplantation technique. The transtrigonal method is particularly applicable when there is a wide trigone with laterally placed ureteral orifices, in the small bladder, or when bladder neck reconstruction is being performed.

CREATION OF THE TRANSTRIGONAL TUNNEL. Slightly less ureteral mobilization is needed for the transtrigonal than for the Politano-Leadbetter technique. After the ureters are mobilized, the mucosa surrounding the ureteral hiatus is sharply mobilized. Occasionally, the muscular ureteral hiatus needs to be closed slightly. When necessary, slightly more tunnel length may be obtained by extending the muscular hiatus in a superior and lateral direction and then narrowing the hiatus carefully by closing its lower portion. It is important not to make the hiatus too tight. When one ureter needs to be reimplanted, a submucosal tunnel is developed with its new mucosal hiatus just above the contralateral ureteral orifice (Fig. 105–12). A traction suture placed in the muscle of the ureteral hiatus is helpful in creating the tunnel.

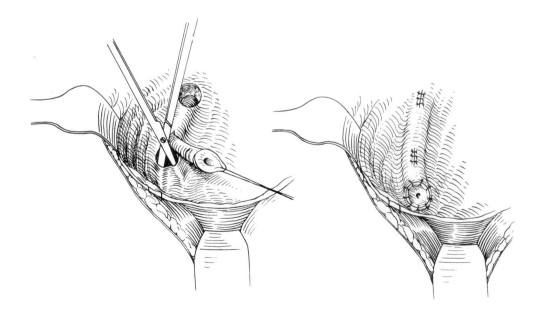

Figure 105–11. The length of the submucosal tunnel may be increased by making another tunnel toward the bladder neck for approximately 1 cm and creating a new mucosal hiatus. The anastomosis of the ureteral orifice with the bladder mucosa is completed and the mucosal openings are closed over the ureter. (From Retik AB, Colodny AH, Bauer SB. Pediatric urology. In Paulson DF, ed. Genitourinary Surgery, Vol 2. New York, Churchill Livingstone, 1984, p 763.)

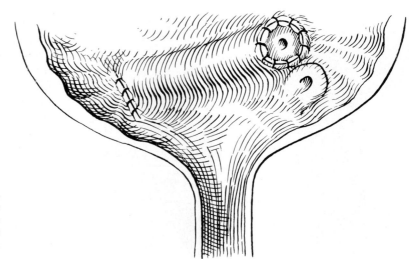

Figure 105–12. Unilateral transtrigonal ureteral reimplantation with the submucosal tunnel leading to the new mucosal hiatus just above the contralateral ureteral orifice. (From Retik AB, Colodny AH, Bauer SB. Pediatric urology. In Paulson DF, ed. Genitourinary Surgery, Vol 2. New York, Churchill Livingstone, 1984, p 764.)

If both ureters are to be reimplanted, a submucosal tunnel for the superiormost ureter is made with a new mucosal hiatus located above the contralateral orifice. The other tunnel is then developed so that the ureteral orifice is positioned at the inferior portion of the original contralateral hiatus (Fig. 105–13). If more length is required, the tunnel may sweep under the contralateral hiatus onto the side wall of the bladder.

ANASTOMOSIS OF THE URETER INTO THE BLADDER. The ureters are drawn through their widely created tunnels with the traction sutures. They are checked for kinks by passing a fine infant feeding tube through them. Anastomosis of the ureteral cuff is performed as in the Politano-Leadbetter procedure. The bladder mucosa over the original hiatus is loosely closed (Fig. 105–14). The ureters are checked one last time for kinks, and in most cases are left unstented.

Extravesical Ureteroplasty (Lich-Gregoir)

There has been a renewal of interest in the use of the extravesical technique, and several early reports have indicated that it is worthy of reappraisal. Originally described in the early 1960s[12, 13] as a technique to avoid opening the bladder to repair reflux, it fell into disfavor. This was largely because of reports of failure due to prolapse of the ureter through the tunnel and recurrence of the reflux. Hendren reported a 50 percent failure rate.[14]

Several reports have indicated better success in terms of resolution of reflux.[15–17] The distinction between these and previous reports is the use of an advancing stitch at the distal ureter securing it to the detrusor wall, which step was not included in the original descriptions of the technique. This addition is considered to prevent prolapse or "dessusception" of the ureter out of the bladder wall tunnel. The term *detrusorrhaphy* has been applied to this technique. The advantages of not opening the bladder in terms

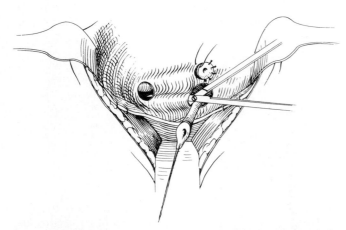

Figure 105–13. Bilateral transtrigonal ureteral reimplantation with the more superior ureter tunneled transversely to the new orifice just above the contralateral orifice. The inferior ureter is tunneled to the inferior edge of the contralateral mucosal hiatus. (From Retik AB, Colodny AH, Bauer SB. Pediatric urology. In Paulson DF, ed. Genitourinary Surgery, Vol 2. New York, Churchill Livingstone, 1984, p 765.)

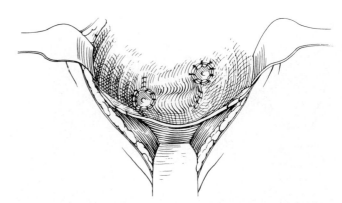

Figure 105–14. Appearance of completed bilateral transtrigonal ureteral reimplantation. (From Retik AB, Colodny AH, Bauer SB. Pediatric urology. In Paulson DF, ed. Genitourinary Surgery, Vol 2. New York, Churchill Livingstone, 1984, p 765.)

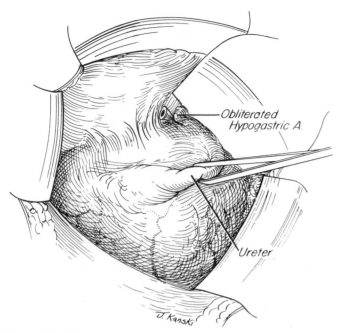

Figure 105–15. Exposure of the distal ureter in preparation for an extravesical antireflux procedure (Lich-Gregoir). The obliterated hypogastric artery is taken down to provide full exposure of the extravesical ureter.

of postoperative morbidity from bladder spasm and bleeding and the shortened hospital stay are attractive.

Of concern, however, has been the occurrence of urinary retention after bilateral extravesical ureteroplasties. The incidence has varied from 10 to 20 percent,[15] and while generally temporary, it represents a problem. The voiding dysfunction usually resolves spontaneously in a few weeks and the cause is unknown. It necessitates a period of intermittent self-catheterization. Some groups do not use the technique for bilateral repairs.

The technique involves a similar preparation of the patient as for the other antireflux methods, and a lower abdominal transverse incision is used. The ex-

travesical space is developed, sweeping the peritoneum superiorly. The critical landmark is the obliterated umbilical artery, below which will be found the ureter just before it enters the bladder wall. The obliterated umbilical artery is tied and divided (it is not always so obliterated), and the perivesical tissues are swept laterally until the ureter is identified (Fig. 105–15). The web of tissue between the ureter and bladder is cleared, and the bladder wall along the course of the ureter is stretched between traction sutures or clamps (Fig. 105–16). The muscle is divided with cautery to the depth of the bluish bladder mucosa, which everts through the muscular defect. This plane is extended around the ureter where it inserts into the bladder mucosa, which is maintained intact. The muscle is lifted away from the mucosa a sufficient amount to permit the ureter to be buried within the muscle layer, sandwiched between muscle and mucosa (Fig. 105–17). The tunnel should be of similar length to that obtained with an intravesical reimplantation, approximately five times the width of the ureter. The advancement sutures are then placed in a horizontal mattress fashion, bringing the distal edge of the ureter under the lip of the detrusor muscle (Fig. 105–18). This furls up the mucosa slightly. The muscle is closed over the ureter for the length of the new tunnel, with sufficient opening at the proximal portion of the tunnel to avoid constricting or kinking the ureter (Fig. 105–19). Interrupted sutures of absorbable material are used for the muscle closure. Ureteral stenting is not necessary unless there is concern regarding ureteral integrity. The bladder may be drained for 1 to 3 days or not at all. The wound is drained.

Megaureter Repair

The technique of megaureter repair is independent of its cause and is based on a reduction of the caliber

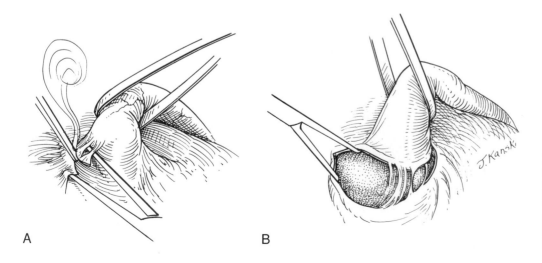

A   B

Figure 105–16. *A* and *B,* Exposure of the area surrounding the distalmost portion of the ureter as it attaches to the bladder mucosa. This area needs to be well exposed to permit accurate placement of the advancing/fixation stitch.

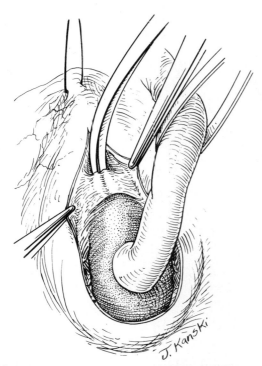

Figure 105–17. Creation of a muscular trough with exposure of the underlying bladder mucosa protruding into the trough. Care is taken to avoid cutting the mucosa, but small holes may be closed with fine absorbable suture.

of the ureter to permit successful reimplantation. A massively dilated ureter requires excisional tapering, while a smaller ureter may be managed with plication.

MOBILIZATION OF THE MEGAURETER. Initial mobilization is similar to that in a routine reimplantation, with particular attention paid to preservation of the accompanying adventitia. Loose connective tissue is swept toward the ureter. Occasionally a fibrous "peel" may be seen surrounding the ureter, and this should be excised because it lies outside the ureteral adventitia. If the ureter is not markedly tortuous or dilated, intravesical mobilization is adequate.

Extravesical dissection may be needed if the ureter is very large or tortuous, if there is difficulty with mobilization, or if there is any question regarding the origin of the ureteral blood supply. It is preferable to make the new hiatus before dissecting extravesically. The hiatus is widened and the peritoneal reflection swept from the back wall of the bladder, again using the lighted suction and hiatal retractors. The new hiatus is located using a right-angled clamp passed behind the bladder wall. The clamp is incised upon and spread to create the new hiatus, and a red rubber catheter, which will help guide the ureter through its new hiatus, is engaged and carried outside and back into the bladder, where it is clamped. Any lateral peritoneal attachments are swept superiorly. Dissection is performed away from the ureter, preserving the adventitia and blood vessels. The obliterated umbilical artery may be divided to facilitate mobilization. The ureter is often tortuous with multiple twists, but mobilization should be limited to straightening the portion of the ureter within the pelvis. Overzealous mobilization and straightening may compromise ureteral vasculature. A layer of redundant ureteral adventitia may be raised over the segment of ureteral wall to be excised and preserved to wrap over the line of closure.

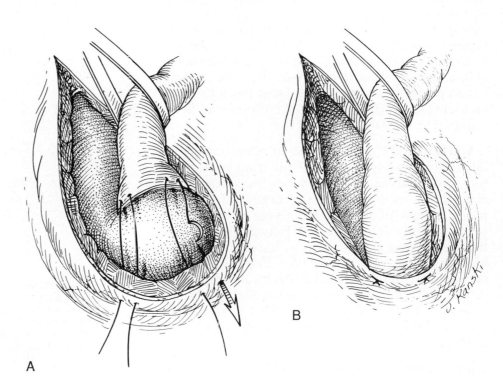

Figure 105–18. *A* and *B*, Placement of the advancing/fixation stitch is shown as paired horizontal mattress sutures.

A

B

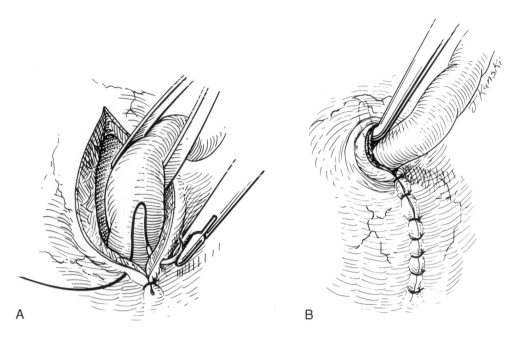

A   B

Figure 105–19. *A* and *B,* Closure of the muscular trough is shown with the ureter lying within. The length of the tunnel should be similar to what would be attained intravesically.

MEGAURETER TAPERING. The distal ureter to be tapered is held in position with stay sutures and a 12 Fr. catheter (10 Fr. in a baby) is placed. If the orifice is stenotic, the catheter is passed through a small incision near the tip of the ureter. If the ureter is snug over the catheter, tailoring is not necessary. The amount of ureteral redundancy is marked by applying baby Allis clamps laterally, leaving the medial vascular supply intact. Megaureter clamps are placed to mark the line of excision, leaving an adequate amount of ureter to close over the catheter.[18] It is important not to taper the ureter too far proximally. The proximal portion of the tailored ureter should remain just outside the bladder after reimplantation in both the tapered and plicated ureter. The redundant segment is excised and the ureter closed with running absorbable chromic suture (5-0 or 6-0) over the catheter. Interrupted sutures should be placed toward the distal aspect to allow the ureter to be trimmed to fit the tunnel (Fig. 105–20).

MEGAURETER PLICATION. In a moderately dilated megaureter (over 10 mm), plication is a satisfactory method of reducing ureteral caliber.[19] Megaureter clamps are used to mark the degree of plication needed over a 10 or 12 Fr. red rubber catheter. Starting proximally, interrupted 5-0 polyglycolic acid sutures are placed anteriorly in an imbricating fashion along the clamp impressions (Fig. 105–21). The catheter should continue to slide freely after plication. Severely dilated megaureters, particularly in babies, should be tapered because a plicated megaureter is bulky and difficult to reimplant in a satisfactory submucosal tunnel.

MEGAURETER REIMPLANTATION. After reduc-

tion of ureteral caliber, the megaureter is brought back into the bladder with the red rubber catheter through the new hiatus. The reimplantation is completed in the same way as with a routine reimplantation. Adequate tunnel length and caliber are essential. The ureters are checked for kinking with a fine feeding tube. The transtrigonal technique may also be used in megaureter repair, eliminating the need for a new hiatus. Extra tunnel length may be gained with a cutback of the ureteral hiatus superiorly and laterally and closure medially and inferiorly.

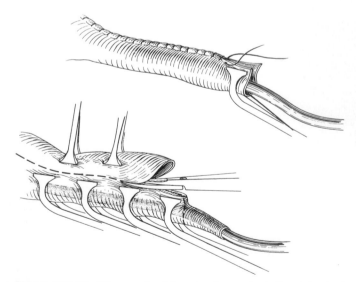

Figure 105–20. When ureteral tapering is required, the redundant ureter is clamped on the lateral aspect with baby Allis clamps, and atraumatic megaureter clamps are positioned on the ureter over a 12 Fr. red rubber catheter. The distal ureteral segment and the redundant lateral ureter is resected and the ureter closed with running absorbable suture. (From Retik AB, Colodny AH, Bauer SB. Pediatric urology. In Paulson DF, ed. Genitourinary Surgery, Vol 2. New York, Churchill Livingstone, 1984.)

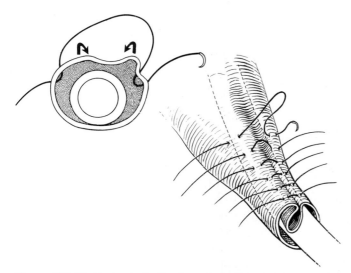

Figure 105–21. Ureteral plication is performed over the appropriate catheter with interrupted 5-0 Vicryl sutures placed in Lembert fashion. (From Keating MA, Retik AB. Management of failures of ureteroneocystostomy. In McDougal WS, ed. Difficult Problems in Urologic Surgery. Chicago, Year Book, 1988, p 131.)

STENTING. Routine stenting of reimplanted ureters is not necessary. Stenting is appropriate in a solitary ureter or if technical difficulties have been encountered. Tapered megaureters are stented for 5 to 7 days, whereas a plicated ureter does not require stenting in most cases. Radiographical contrast studies through the stent may be used to confirm the absence of leakage through the repaired ureter.

PSOAS HITCH. When an adequate tunnel length is not achievable with the usual techniques, a psoas hitch is a useful adjunct. A longer intravesical tunnel is provided as well as immobilization of the ureterovesical junction, giving a more effective antireflux mechanism (see Chapter 106).

BLADDER CLOSURE AND DRAINS. In girls a multiholed urethral catheter is held in place with a silk stay stitch run through the bladder and tied over a pledget on the abdomen. Boys are drained with a suprapubic tube or a Silastic Foley catheter if the period of drainage is to be short. Closure of the bladder is with two layers of running absorbable chromic suture and a third interrupted layer. A prevesical Penrose drain is placed.

POSTOPERATIVE MANAGEMENT

Parenteral antibiotics are given for 2 to 3 days in an uninfected patient and followed by an oral cephalosporin at a low dose. Preoperative oral prophylactic antibiotics are resumed at discharge. Prevesical drainage is maintained for 2 to 4 days. The bladder catheter is removed when no blood clots are seen or when the urine is clear, usually in 3 to 4 days. There is much latitude in this time because some children do not tolerate catheters and do well with only 2 or 3 days of drainage. In a megaureter repair, the bladder catheter is left until the stents are removed. Antispasmodics (oxybutynin, diazepam) are liberally used, often in the immediate postoperative period, to avoid a self-perpetuating cycle of bladder spasms. Constipation should be avoided. Postoperative continuous epidural analgesia has become a helpful element in the care of ureteral reimplantation patients, reducing the morbidity of the procedure and the need for antispasmodics and narcotics.

Oral antibiotics are continued until the absence of reflux is documented. An IVP or renal scan is obtained 4 to 6 weeks postoperatively to ensure adequate renal function without obstruction. A radionuclide cystogram is obtained 3 to 4 months postoperatively. At this point, further invasive studies are not warranted if these initial studies indicate a satisfactory result. Antibiotics are discontinued when the absence of reflux is confirmed. Renal ultrasonography is performed at 18 months, 3 years, and 5 years postoperatively, although we have not seen a documented late obstruction.

COMPLICATIONS

Early Obstruction

Obstruction is the principal complication of ureteral reimplantation within 2 to 3 weeks postoperatively. On occasion this may be entirely silent. Usually it is manifested as abdominal or flank pain, nausea, vomiting, fever, or (rarely) anuria. The underlying cause is usually edema, hematoma, kinking at the site of the reimplantation or nonviability of the ureter. Many of the transient obstructions appear to be due to mucous plugging or blood clots within the ureter, since they clear spontaneously with hydration in 48 to 72 hours. Assessment of the degree of obstruction may be achieved with an IVP or a diuretic renal scan. Parenteral antibiotics are included in supportive therapy. An observational approach may be guided by serial ultrasound examinations. Rarely, drainage is indicated in an ill patient with fever, azotemia, acidosis, or hyperkalemia. The facility and safety of percutaneous nephrostomy make it preferable to retrograde ureteral stenting. Often the obstruction resolves shortly after decompression from above.

Persistent Obstruction

Persisting obstruction may occur after reimplantation and may be entirely silent, leading to renal loss.[20]

The mechanism of this obstruction is usually ureteral ischemia, but it may be from kinking. Intermittent obstruction due to "J" hooking and occlusion of a laterally reimplanted ureter when the bladder fills may be seen. Percutaneous dilation of the area of obstruction is of unproven value but may be a worthwhile first step. Reoperative reimplantation is the definitive treatment, using transabdominal mobilization of the ureter and excising any fibrotic distal ureter. One must be prepared to perform a psoas hitch or even a transureteroureterostomy if necessary to obtain a nonrefluxing ureteral reimplantation.[21]

Persistent Reflux

Persistent reflux may be seen on follow-up cystograms secondary to an inadequate tunnel length, ureterovesical fistula, pull-out of the ureter, or ischemic fibrosis of the intravesical ureter. Beyond the technical reasons, one should be aware of the possibility of persistent reflux due to unrecognized dysfunctional voiding, bladder outlet obstruction, or a neuropathic bladder.[22] In general, a trial of observation is worthwhile, because many of the refluxing ureters detected on 4-month cystograms will not reflux 1 or 2 years later. Massive reflux or recurrent infections are best managed with earlier surgical repair, following the same principles as for an obstructed reimplant. On occasion, persistent reflux may be seen in patients with adequate submucosal tunnels who are cured with reoperative creation of "super-long" tunnels (approximately 8 cm). New contralateral reflux may be seen in up to 15 percent of the cases with unilateral ureteral reimplantation. This reflux resolves within 1 year in almost all cases. If contralateral reflux had been present preoperatively but resolved, it has been our practice to perform a reimplantation in the nonrefluxing ureter at the time of reflux correction.

Infection

The primary goal of ureteral reimplantation for reflux is prevention of chronic pyelonephritis. Successful ureteral reimplantation will not eliminate bladder infections, and parents should be forewarned of this.[23] When cure of reflux has been documented and antibiotics discontinued, episodes of cystitis should be treated acutely.

Retrograde Ureteral Access After Transtrigonal Reimplantation

The transtrigonal orientation of the ureter after the Cohen technique may make retrograde ureteral access

difficult. This is of concern only if such access is needed in the future. With flexible cystoscopes and patience, this is not an insurmountable problem,[24] and should not be a contraindication to this form of ureteral reimplantation.

RESULTS

In the carefully evaluated patient with uncomplicated VUR and the appropriate indications for surgical repair, ureteral reimplantation should provide a 99 percent cure rate.[25–29] Meticulous surgical technique, adequate exposure, delicate tissue handling, and complete ureteral visualization at all stages are essential in this procedure. Megaureter repair also demands an understanding of ureteral vascularity and wide mobilization of the dilated ureter. Success rates in all ages should reach 95 percent,[30] and in infants under 8 months a 90 percent rate may be anticipated.[31] Ureteral reimplantation remains a standard treatment for VUR, and new techniques to treat this condition must document a comparable record of safety and efficacy.

REFERENCES

1. Smellie JM, Normand ICS. Reflux nephropathy in childhood. In Hodson J, Kincaid-Smith P, eds. Reflux Nephropathy. New York, Masson, 1979, p 14.
2. Normand ICS, Smellie JM. Vesicoureteral reflux: The case for conservative management. In Hodson J, Kincaid-Smith P, eds. Reflux Nephropathy. New York, Masson, 1979, p 281.
3. Weiss R, Duckett J, Spitzer A. Results of a randomized clinical trial of medical versus surgical management of infants and children with grades III and IV primary vesicoureteral reflux (United States). The International Reflux Study in Children. J Urol 148:1667, 1992.
4. Keating MA, Escala J, Snyder HM III, et al. Changing concepts in the management of primary obstructive megaureter. J Urol 142:636, 1989.
5. Burbige KA, Lebowitz RL, Colodny AH, et al. The megacystis-megaureter syndrome. J Urol 131:1133, 1984.
6. Duckett JW. Vesicoureteral reflux: A conservative analysis. Am J Kidney Dis 3:139, 1983.
7. Koff SA, Murtagh DS. The uninhibited bladder in children: Effect of treatment on recurrence of urinary tract infection and on vesicoureteral reflux resolution. J Urol 130:1138, 1983.
8. Paquin AJ. Ureterovesical anastomosis: The description and evaluation of a technique. J Urol 82:573, 1959.
9. Politano VA, Leadbetter WF. An operative technique for the correction of vesicoureteral reflux. J Urol 79:932, 1958.
10. Weinstein AJ, Bauer SB, Retik AB, et al. The surgical management of megaureters in duplex systems: The efficacy of ureteral tapering and common sheath reimplantation. J Urol 139:328, 1988.
11. Cohen SJ. Ureterozystoneostomie. Eine Neue Antirefluxtechnik. Aktuel Urol 6:1, 1975.
12. Lich RJ, Howerton LW, Davis LA. Recurrent urosepsis in children. J Urol 86:554, 1961.
13. Gregoir W, VanRegemorter GV. Le reflux vésico-urétéral congénital. Urol Int 18:122, 1964.
14. Hendren WH. Reoperation for the failed ureteral reimplantation. J Urol 111:403, 1974.
15. Houle AM, McLorie GA, Heritz DM, et al. Extravesical nondis-

membered ureteroplasty with detrusorrhaphy: A renewed technique to correct vesicoureteral reflux in children. J Urol 148:704, 1992.

16. Wacksman J, Gilbert A, Sheldon CA. Results of the renewed extravesical reimplant for surgical correction of vesicoureteral reflux. J Urol 148:359, 1992.

17. Zaontz MR, Maizels M, Sugar EC, Firlit CF. Detrusorrhaphy: Extravesical ureteral advancement to correct vesicoureteral reflux in children. J Urol 138:947, 1987.

18. Hendren WH. Operative repair of megaureter in children. J Urol 101:491, 1969.

19. Starr A. Ureteral plication. A new concept in ureteral tailoring for megaureter. Invest Urol 17:153, 1979.

20. Weiss RM, Schiff M Jr, Lytton B. Late obstruction after ureteroneocystostomy. J Urol 106:144, 1971.

21. Hendren WH. Reoperation of the failed ureteral reimplantation. J Urol 111:403, 1974.

22. Noe HN. The role of dysfunctional voiding in failure or complication of ureteral reimplantation for primary reflux. J Urol 134:1172, 1985.

23. Willscher MK, Bauer SB, Zammuto PJ, Retik AB. Renal growth and urinary infection following antireflux surgery in infants and children. J Urol 115:722, 1976.

24. Argueso LR, Kelalis PP, Patterson DE. Strategies for ureteral catheterization after antireflux surgery by the Cohen technique of transverse advancement. J Urol 146:1583, 1991.

25. Ahmed S, Tan H. Complications of transverse advancement ureteral reimplantations: Divertivulum formation. J Urol 127:970, 1982.

26. Carpentier PJ, Bettink PJ, Hop WCJ, Schroder FH. Reflux—A retrospective study of 100 ureteric reimplantations by the Politano-Leadbetter method and 100 by the Cohen technique. Br J Urol 54:230, 1982.

27. Burbige KA. Ureteral reimplantation: A comparison of results with the cross-trigonal and Politano-Leadbetter techniques in 120 patients. J Urol 146:1352, 1991.

28. Duckett JW, Walker RD, Weiss R. Surgical results: International Reflux Study in Children—United States branch. J Urol 148:1674, 1992.

29. Hjalmas K, Lohr G, Tamminen MT, et al. Surgical results in the International Reflux Study in Children (Europe). J Urol 148:1657, 1992.

30. Retik AB, McEvoy JP, Bauer SB. Megaureters in children. Urology 11:231, 1978.

31. Peters CA, Mandell J Lebowitz RL, et al. Congenital obstructed megaureter in early infancy: Diagnosis and treatment. J Urol 142:641, 1989.

Chapter 106

Reconstruction of the Lower Ureter: Psoas Hitch, Boari Flap, and Transureteroureterostomy

Terry W. Hensle and William A. Kennedy II

Reconstruction of the lower ureter usually involves a loss of ureteral tissue. Procedures that are used to compensate for lost ureteral length vary widely. A surgical procedure is chosen on the basis of how much ureter needs to be replaced. Other variables include the condition of the ureter proximal to the damaged segment and the condition of the bladder. In general, provided that there is a loss of only the distal ureter and that there is a normal bladder, the primary choice for lower ureteral reconstruction or substitution is the psoas hitch and ureteral reimplantation.

Other options for dealing with lower ureteral loss, when there is more than just distal ureteral loss, include a vascularized bladder (Boari) flap or a transureteroureterostomy (TUU). Each of these techniques has distinct indications and contraindications, advantages and disadvantages, which must be defined, recognized, and understood.

PREOPERATIVE MANAGEMENT

The most important aspect of preoperative management in the patient with lower ureteral loss is a complete and thorough evaluation and understanding of the anatomical defect. The exact amount of ureteral tissue to be replaced must be understood clearly. The evaluation is best made by simultaneous imaging of both the affected ureter and the bladder. The studies can be done in either an antegrade or a retrograde fashion, to yield the maximal amount of information available at one sitting. In addition to radiographical studies, the patient should undergo urodynamic evaluation. Bladder function should be evaluated in

terms of volume, compliance, distensibility, and pressure. If the bladder has been defunctionalized previously, a period of preoperative hydrodistention may be necessary before a reliable urodynamic evaluation can be carried out. In addition, any history of stone disease should be thoroughly investigated. The patient's urine must be sterile before reconstruction of any kind is undertaken.

SURGICAL OPTIONS

Psoas Hitch and Ureteral Reimplantation

Most patients presenting for urinary tract reconstructions today have undergone previous diversion procedures, and most have lost at least the distal end of the ureter or ureters during the creation of the urinary diversion. When the tissue loss is limited to the distal ureter, an extended psoas hitch with a long ureter reimplantation is the procedure of choice.[1–3] It may be combined with a TUU if two renal units are present. A downward nephropexy can be performed if increased ureteral length is needed.[1] Bladder augmentation, utilizing an isolated segment of either small or large bowel, can also be done as part of the reconstruction if bladder capacity is a concern.

Operative Technique

The patient is placed on the table in the supine position. In children the frog-leg position is used, but in adults this position for a long surgical procedure can result in stretching of the lumbosacral plexus.

Stretching in turn can lead to postoperative anteromedial thigh pain, paresthesia, and hypesthesia. These problems are usually self-limited, but they can be distressing to both patient and surgeon when they occur.

In most instances a long midline incision extending from just below the xiphoid to the symphysis pubis is necessary to gain the kind of exposure and mobilization necessary for a reconstructive procedure, especially when there has been previous urinary diversion. When one is dealing with an isolated in situ lesion of the distal ureter, a more conservative lower abdominal or retroperitoneal approach is more reasonable (Fig. 106–1). In most cases, however, for an adequate operation, good exposure of the entire retroperitoneum on the affected side is necessary.

Once the peritoneal cavity has been entered, the colon and small bowel are reflected away from the ureter on one or both sides. The ureter is thoroughly mobilized, taking great care not to devascularize the ureter. Dissection can be carried out laterally. More attention must be given to the medial dissection to avoid damaging the remaining segmental blood supply of the middle and upper ureter. Once the ureter has been thoroughly mobilized and any abnormal or damaged tissue removed, the distance necessary for reconstruction can be better determined. A traction suture is placed in the ureter along with an 8 Fr. feeding tube for drainage.

In most instances, bladder mobilization in the patient who has had previous pelvic surgery is best done by entering the bladder in the midline and then mobilizing inferiorly and laterally toward the bladder neck (Fig. 106–2). When a psoas hitch is planned, the bladder must be thoroughly mobilized on the oppo-

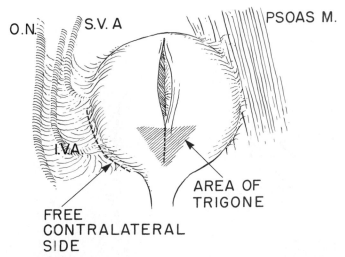

Figure 106–2. Incision and mobilization of the bladder. O.N., obturator nerve; S.V.A., superior vesical artery; I.V.A., inferior vesical artery.

site side to ensure enough bladder to reach the psoas muscle without tension. Once bladder mobilization has been accomplished, and after the psoas muscle and tendon are cleaned, two fingers can be placed within the dome of the bladder. The bladder is pushed upward and laterally toward the psoas tendon (Fig. 106–3). Three interrupted, heavy, nonabsorbable sutures are used to attach the bladder wall to the psoas tendon, taking great care to place the sutures into the detrusor muscle and not into the lumen of the bladder itself. The sutures are tied individually and can be reinforced, if necessary.

A point is then chosen for the ureter to be brought into the bladder. A peanut dissector can be placed against the bladder wall from the inside. Using electrocautery, a hiatus is created by cutting through the

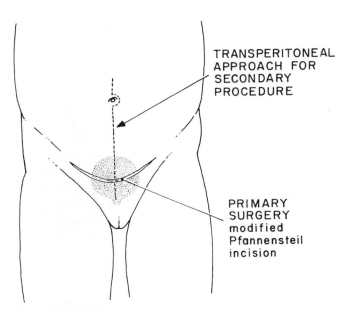

Figure 106–1. Midline incision and transperitoneal approach outlined for most reoperative patients.

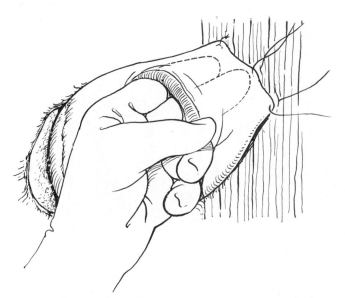

Figure 106–3. Psoas hitch made with heavy, nonabsorbable sutures.

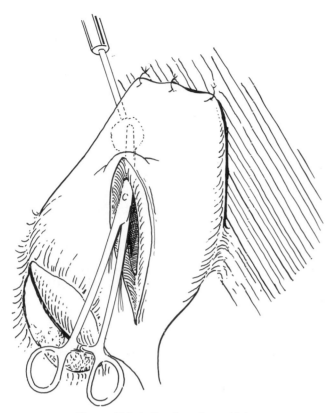

Figure 106–4. Creation of new hiatus.

bladder wall down into the dissection (Fig. 106–4). A clamp is passed through the new hiatus, and the ureter is brought into the bladder by its traction suture. Once proper orientation has been established and a point chosen for the new orifice, the ureter is removed and a suburothelial tunnel is created from the hiatus downward to the position chosen for the new orifice (Fig. 106–5).

If the caliber of the ureter is normal, a suburothelial tunnel of 3 to 5 cm in length is desired. After the tunnel has been created, the ureter can be pulled inferiorly, using the traction suture as a guide (Fig. 106–6). When the ureter lies comfortably within the tunnel, the cut edge of the ureter can be sutured to the urothelium with fine interrupted absorbable sutures (Fig. 106–7). Two tacking sutures are also placed outside the bladder to fix the ureter to the bladder wall as it enters through the new hiatus.

Once the reimplantation has been completed, an 8 Fr. feeding tube is placed as a drainage catheter and stent during healing. Extra holes are usually cut in the distal end to provide better drainage. The bladder is closed in a standard fashion with a Foley catheter placed for drainage.

Boari Flap

Another method available for lower ureteral substitution is the vascularized bladder flap. This procedure, which Casati and Boari described in 1894,[4] has gained wide clinical acceptance and can be selected to replace lost segments of the pelvic ureter that are too great for a psoas hitch and primary reimplantation.[5] The limiting feature of a vascularized bladder flap is a small, fixed-capacity bladder. In planning a bladder flap procedure, the ureter is mobilized as described for the psoas hitch and ureteral reimplantation. For best results, the bladder flap is usually combined with a psoas hitch to immobilize the base of the flap as well as to increase the length gained by

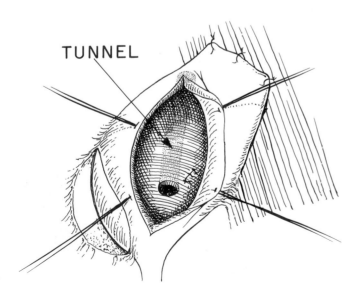

Figure 106–5. Creation of a new suburothelial tunnel.

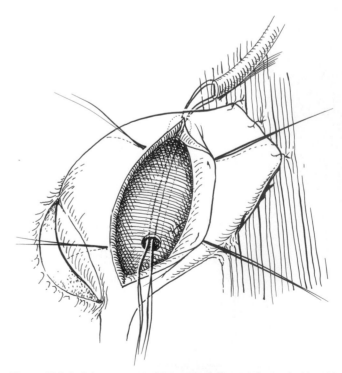

Figure 106–6. Advancement of the ureter into a newly created tunnel.

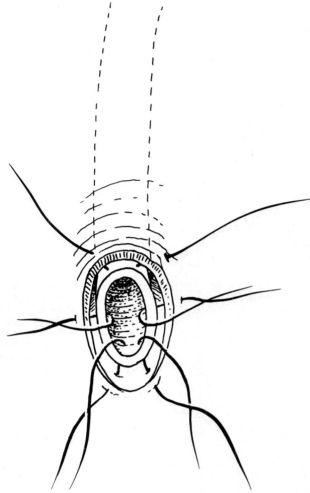

Figure 106–7. Vesicoureteral anastomosis.

the flap. In contrast to the standard psoas hitch, however, the bladder cannot be opened in the midline. Careful planning is necessary to isolate an adequate piece of anterior bladder wall to serve as a flap.

Operative Technique

The bladder is filled to capacity with a Foley catheter, and a flap is measured and outlined with a marking pencil (Fig. 106–8A). The width of the flap should be about 2 cm across, with the base slightly wider than the apex.[6] Adequate blood supply is not usually a problem. In patients with normal bladders, the flap should be well vascularized. The length of the flap depends entirely upon the amount of ureter to be replaced. Once the flap has been outlined, an incision is made into the distended bladder and the flap is elevated on traction sutures (Fig. 106–8B). With the bladder open, a psoas hitch can be carried out simply as described previously.

The ureter is then brought down to the flap, and if there is sufficient length, a suburothelial tunnel can be created (Fig. 106–9A).[7] The ureter is sutured in

place as in a standard ureteral reimplantation (Fig. 106–9B). After reimplantation, the bladder is closed in standard fashion using two layers of running nonabsorbable suture (Fig. 106–10).

When insufficient length on the ureter prevents a tunneled reimplantation, the cut end of the ureter can be attached directly to the urothelium. The muscle layer of the bladder is brought around the anastomosis as a cuff and outer layer. This maneuver is not as desirable as a tunneled reimplantation, but it can serve as a salvage procedure when options are limited.

Transureteroureterostomy

Like the vascularized bladder flap, TUU was described many years ago,[8] and its usefulness in replacing lost ureteral segments has been widely recognized.[9, 10] It is best employed to compensate for the loss of a major portion of the lower ureter. The major contraindication is any history of stone disease. When TUU is being considered, several technical points must be understood and adhered to[10]:

1. No tension must occur on angulation at the area where the two ureters join.
2. The ureter on the affected side must be thoroughly mobilized so that it is easily brought across the midline.
3. As the ureter is brought across the midline, it is important not to pass it under the inferior mesenteric vessels, which would result in trapping and angulation of the ureter.
4. The anastomosis should be made in a watertight fashion.

Operative Technique

After the ureter on the affected side has been thoroughly and widely mobilized, it is brought across the midline, avoiding angulation. The affected ureter is brought to a point on the recipient ureter that provides for a gentle and slightly downward course. A point on the recipient ureter should be chosen to avoid tension on the anastomosis. The anastomosis itself is made from the end of the affected ureter to the side of the recipient. This maneuver is best accomplished by rolling the recipient ureter laterally with traction sutures to ensure an end-to-side rather than an end-to-top suture line (Fig. 106–11), which could angulate the anastomosis. An incision is made in the recipient ureter corresponding to the diameter of the affected side (Fig. 106–12A). The anastomosis can be made with either a running or an interrupted suture line to provide a watertight closure (Fig. 106–12B). In most instances, placement of stenting cathe-

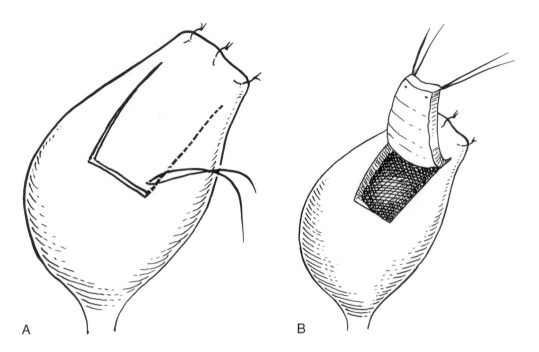

Figure 106–8. *A*, The anterior bladder flap is outlined, approximately 2 cm in width across the base. The length is adjustable, depending on the distance to be bridged. *B*, Evaluation of the bladder flap on traction sutures. The psoas hitch is in place.

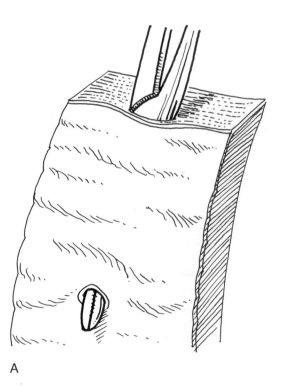

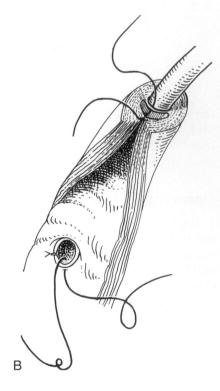

Figure 106–9. *A*, Creation of a suburothelial tunnel. *B*, Uretero-vesical anastomosis and closure of the bladder flap superiorly into a tube.

ters up each limb of the TUU is advisable to provide drainage and to allow healing without leakage.

POSTOPERATIVE MANAGEMENT AND COMPLICATIONS

In general, separate bladder and ureteral drainage is advisable in all forms of lower ureteral reconstruction. We usually employ 5 and 8 Fr. pediatric feeding tubes for ureteral stenting and upper tract damage during the healing process. The size of the stenting catheter depends on the size of the ureter involved. We use separate bladder drainage, usually in the form of a Foley catheter. The stenting catheters remain in place for 5 to 10 days, depending on the magnitude of the reconstruction.

Patients undergoing reconstruction are maintained on prophylactic antibiotics for the duration of hospitalization. Anticholinergics are usually given postop-

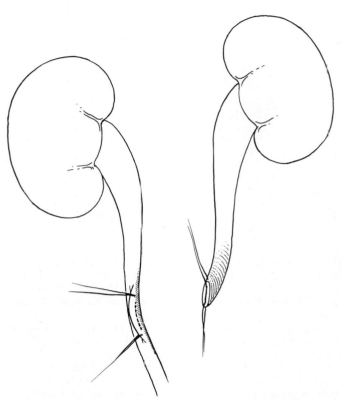

Figure 106–11. Downward direction of a donor-to-recipient ureter with traction sutures in place to roll the recipient ureter laterally.

eratively in an effort to suppress bladder spasms while the tubes are in place.

The complications of lower ureteral reconstruction involve both early and late problems. The early complications are bleeding and urinary leak. Late complications involve anastomotic stricture and persistent reflux. The stenting catheters aid greatly in avoiding persistent postoperative urinary leakage as well as in promoting good primary healing. Postoperative stricture formation can be largely avoided by preserving the vascularity of the ureter involved and by creating a meticulous anastomosis. Most reconstruction of the lower ureter should be feasible with very little morbidity in terms of either early or long-term complications.

Editorial Comment

Craig A. Peters

Psoas hitch and TUU have become essential tools in modern urological reconstructive surgery and should be familiar to anyone performing this sort of surgery. The psoas hitch provides extra length but, equally important, stabilizes the ureterovesical anastomosis to prevent reflux. This may be particularly important when large dilated ureters are present, or when a bowel ureter has been constructed. Extra length may be obtained by mobilization of the contralateral superior vesical pedicle to permit a more extreme movement of the bladder to the affected side. The steps in the operation are slightly different when performed by Dr.

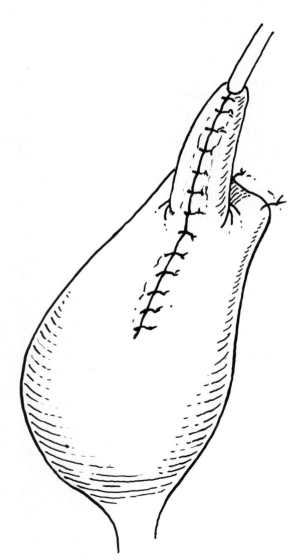

Figure 106–10. Bladder closure.

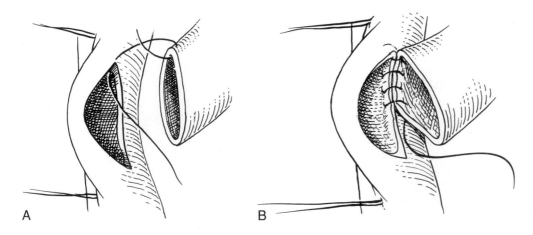

Figure 106–12. *A,* Incision in the recipient ureter to match the diameter of the donor ureter. *B,* Watertight closure.

W. H. Hendren. He performs the ureterovesical anastomosis first, with the bladder wall stretched up to its hitched position first. The hitching stitches are then placed to support this position, specifically adjusted to the ureteral anastomosis.

Both the TUU and the Boari flap received a bad name in the surgical literature that is largely undeserved. As emphasized in this chapter, adherence to basic principles of ureteral surgery will prevent the complications attributed to these reconstructive procedures. In particular, ureteral mobilization with an adequate amount of adventitia and vasculature will ensure a healthy ureter for anastomosis and function.

REFERENCES

1. Hensle TW, Burbige KA, Levin RK. Management of the short ureter in urinary tract reconstruction. J Urol 137:707, 1987.
2. Goldstein HA, Hensle TW. Urinary undiversion in adults. J Urol 128:43, 1982.
3. Hensle TW, Nagler HM, Goldstein HR. Longterm functional results of urinary tract reconstruction in childhood. J Urol 128:1262, 1982.
4. Casati E, Boari A. Contributo spermentale alla plastica dull uretere. Communicazione preventia. Atti Della Academia delle Scierze Mediche e Naturali in Ferrara, Anno 68, fasc 3, May 1894, p 149.
5. Kelami A, Fiedler U, Schmidt V, et al. Replacement of the ureter using the urinary bladder. Urol Res 1:161, 1973.
6. Boxer RJ, Johnson SF, Ehrlich RM. Ureteral substitution. Urology 78:398, 1978.
7. Gil-Vernet JM. Ureterovesicoplastie sous-muqueuse: Modification à la technique de Boari. J Urol Med Chir 65:504, 1969.
8. Sharpe NW. Transureteroureteral anastomosis. Ann Surg 44:687, 1906.
9. Hendren WH, Hensle TW. Transureteroureterostomy: Experience with 75 cases. J Urol 123:826, 1980.
10. Hodges CV, Moore RJ, Lehman TH, Behnam AM. Clinical experiences with transureteroureterostomy. J Urol 90:552, 1963.

Chapter 107

Lower Tract Surgery For Ureterocele and Duplication Anomalies

Edmond T. Gonzales, Jr.

A child with an anomaly of ureteral duplication incurs the possibility of a variety of surgically significant abnormalities, including ureteral ectopia, ureteroceles, ureteral obstruction, and vesicoureteral reflux. When the problem is simple ureteral ectopia without a ureterocele, the ureter may enter the genital system rather than the urinary system. In boys, the ureter drains directly into derivatives of the mesonephric structures. This particular anomaly is commonly associated with simultaneous abnormalities of the vasal/seminal vesicle system. In the development of girls, the ureter never directly enters the müllerian structures, although ectopic ureters can terminate in the vagina, uterus, or fallopian tubes. During female genitourinary development, remnants of the mesonephric system that would have formed the vas deferens in a boy remain in close apposition to the developing müllerian structures and are known as Gartner's duct, and an ectopic ureter would, embryologically, drain primarily into this structure. Subsequent absorption or rupture of Gartner's duct into the derivatives of the müllerian ducts allows for the finding of an ectopic ureteral orifice in the genital system of girls. When a ureterocele is present, distortion of the trigone and bladder neck can result in varying degrees of obstruction to the other ureters, or the ureterocele can cause bladder outflow obstruction. In other cases, reflux occurs into the other ureters.

In most cases, ectopic ureters, whether associated with a ureterocele or not, show changes associated with obstruction. In some cases, the orifice is truly stenotic; in others, the ureter appears to be obstructed where it passes through the urethral sphincter. Reflux is unusual in ectopic ureters, except when the orifice is positioned just at or slightly distal to the bladder neck. In this situation, reflux can occur when the bladder neck opens during voiding.

Abnormal development of the ureteral musculature and the renal parenchyma (dysplasia) is commonly associated with ureteral ectopia. Macki and Stephens first described an embryological theory of abnormal metanephric differentiation based on abnormal ureteral bud placement (believed to be the embryological cause for ectopia).[1] The more severe the ectopia, the more likely there is to be dysplasia. Any surgery to correct the anomaly at the level of the lower ureter and bladder must be preceded by a careful and thorough evaluation of the function of the affected renal segments.

INDICATIONS

Most children with ureteroceles or simple ureteral ectopia are seen because of urinary infection. When the ectopic ureter drains into the vagina, purulent vaginal drainage may be present rather than urinary infection. Older girls may have only paradoxical urinary incontinence—constant urinary dampness despite normal frequency of voiding without symptoms of detrusor instability. Ureteroceles may prolapse through the urethra and be mistaken for a periurethral cyst (Fig. 107–1).

Today, most of these lesions are being recognized on prenatal ultrasound scans because they are usually associated with some degree of hydronephrosis or an intravesical cystic mass. This early diagnosis allows for the prompt initiation of antibiotics to help control urinary infection and preserve renal tissue that other-

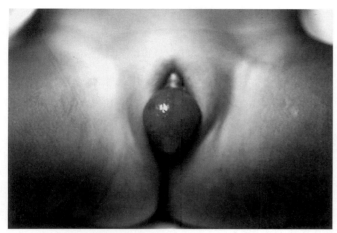

Figure 107–1. Prolapsed ureterocele. The mucosa is congested and edematous.

wise might have been lost while surgical management is planned.

PREOPERATIVE MANAGEMENT

The management of ureteroceles, with or without ureteral duplication, involves some of the most complex reconstructive problems seen in pediatric urology. Ureteroceles and ureteral ectopia occur with both single and duplex ureters, although these anomalies are about six times more common in duplicated systems. Ureteroceles can be very small and adversely affect only the unit they subtend, or they can be immense and distort the drainage of the other ureters and bladder neck. Perhaps one of the most complex anomalies to manage is bilateral single system ectopic ureters. In this situation, the bladder is often very rudimentary, and there may be no formation of or competence at the level of the bladder neck.

The anatomy of ureteroceles also varies greatly. They may be totally confined within the bladder or in an extravesical position. Detrusor musculature backing the ureterocele may be sufficient or deficient. In most cases, the orifice of the ureterocele is placed near the distal end, and in extravesical ureteroceles the orifice is usually found along the course of the urethra. Occasionally, however, the orifice is positioned within the bladder, but a blind, submucosal extension continues distally into the urethra—a so-called cecoureterocele (Fig. 107–2). The orifice of the ureterocele is often felt to be stenotic, but in more distal lesions the passage through the external sphincter may be the obstructing component.

Preoperative evaluation must include a thorough anatomical assessment (generally a renal/bladder ultrasound scan and cystogram) as well as a functional assessment by radionuclide renal scanning. Intravenous urography is used infrequently now but occa-

sionally may add additional information. The extent of function in all segments (but especially the parenchyma subtended by the ureterocele) is carefully noted. The presence and degree of reflux are assessed. The severity of dilation of other ureters (lower pole ipsilateral ureter and contralateral ureters) is recorded. Care is taken to evaluate whether there is good detrusor backing behind a ureterocele (does the ureterocele evert as a diverticulum during voiding?) and whether there is any obstruction to the bladder outlet. I believe cystoscopy adds a great deal to full assessment of the abnormal anatomy and provides some predictive value regarding a possible need for lower ureteral excision. All these variables are taken into consideration when planning the surgical approach.

Although ureteroceles and ectopic ureters are most often discussed in conjunction with duplication anomalies of the ureter, similar pathological conditions can be seen when only a single ureter is present. In general, the severity of renal parenchymal dysplasia correlates with the position of the ectopic orifice. When the orifice enters the genital system, the dysplasia is usually more severe than when the orifice enters just distal to the bladder neck. Similarly, extravesical single system ureteroceles can be just as obstructing to the bladder neck as an extravesical ure-

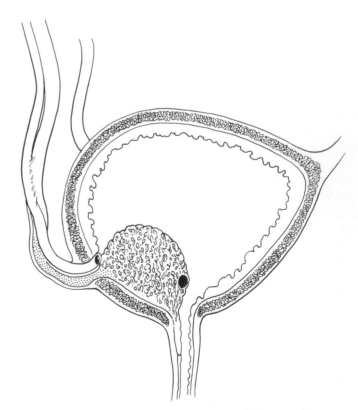

Figure 107–2. Anatomy of a cecoureterocele. The blind-ending mucosal extension into the urethra can function as an obstructing valve during voiding if the lumen of the ureterocele is not completely opened.

terocele involving the upper segment of a complete ureteral duplication.

OPERATIVE TECHNIQUE

Whereas there are many similarities in operative approach for ureteroceles or ectopia without a ureterocele, certain clear distinctions are present. This section is divided into the separate approaches one might consider when planning surgery for an individual patient. These include endoscopic decompression of ureteroceles, management of the lower segment of the ureter, and indications and techniques for excision of the ureterocele proper. Implicit in these decisions is the realization that one has already addressed the question of whether or not the renal parenchyma should be preserved. In cases of a duplication anomaly, it most likely will already have been decided whether a partial upper pole nephrectomy or ureteropyelostomy (upper pole ureter to lower pole pelvis) is preferred. With single system anomalies, a simple nephrectomy is all that may be necessary if no function is present in the affected kidney. These procedures are beyond the purview of this chapter but are frequently necessary as part of the complete management of a child with a ureteral duplication anomaly. Also not included is the technique of simple common sheath ureteral reimplantation, as might be done for management of primary reflux into a lower pole system of a completely duplicated system. On occasion, when the upper pole functions well and the ureter is not massively dilated, simple common sheath reimplantation is all that may be necessary here also.

Endoscopic Decompression of Ureteroceles

Decades ago, primary endoscopic "unroofing" of ureteroceles was frequently performed to relieve obstruction and drain infected segments. Although immediately effective in helping to control urosepsis, massive reflux universally resulted in dilated atonic systems. During that era, subsequent recurring urinary infections were such a significant problem that endoscopic unroofing was discarded.

In 1986, Tank reported a series of infants in whom he had performed endoscopic incision of the ureterocele.[2] In most instances, reflux resulted, but infection was much less of a problem with current programs of antimicrobial prophylaxis. Tank also demonstrated that some affected renal segments demonstrated improved function during the follow-up period (40 percent), and at times segments initially thought to require excision were later shown to be salvageable. This report stimulated a renewed interest in management of ureteroceles endoscopically. As surgeons became more familiar with the procedure, they were able, on occasion, to relieve obstruction without causing reflux. In some instances, this is sufficient to manage the problem. Endoscopic management as definitive therapy was first shown to be successful for single system ureteroceles,[3, 4] but its use has also been extended to duplex system ureteroceles.[5, 6]

Endoscopic decompression of a ureterocele, whether reflux results or not, will generally relieve obstruction to the other ureters and the bladder neck, and allow hydronephrosis to resolve. If one chooses to endoscopically decompress the ureterocele and wishes to avoid the development of vesicoureteral reflux, care must be taken regarding the location of the incision into the ureterocele. First, one should choose ureteroceles that have a firm detrusor backing as seen on cystourethrography. Second, the incision into the ureterocele should be medial and near the detrusor margin so that the roof of the ureterocele persists as an antireflux flap (Fig. 107–3). Duckett proposed simply puncturing the ureterocele with a small ball electrode (i.e., making a "neo-orifice"). If the opening from the ureterocele is seen in the proximal urethra, the incision can be made from the orifice proximally to a position just inside the bladder neck (Fig. 107–4).

The probability that endoscopic management of ureteroceles can be definitive therapy is best when the ureterocele is completely intravesical and there is no reflux into other ureters. However, endoscopic

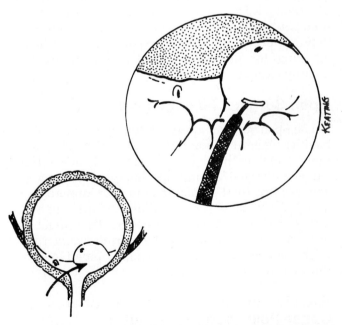

Figure 107–3. Location of incision into the ureterocele (medial and near the detrusor) when one hopes to achieve endoscopic decompression without vesicoureteral reflux. (From Rich MA, Keating MA, Snyder HM, Duckett LW. Low transurethral incision of single system intravesical ureteroceles in children. J Urol 144:120, 1990.)

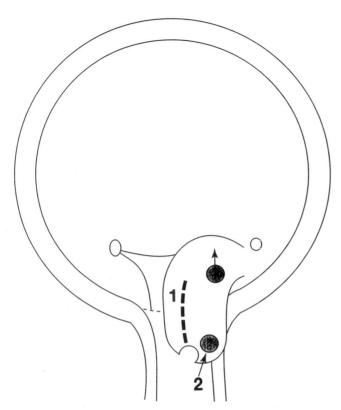

Figure 107–4. When the ureterocele has a significant urethral extension, the endoscopic surgeon must either incise the urethral extension to just within the bladder neck[1] or establish satisfactory openings at the distal end as well as within the bladder.[2] (From Blyth B, Passerini-Glazel C, Camuffo C, et al. Endoscopic incision of ureteroceles: Intravesical versus ectopic. J Urol 149:556, 1993.)

decompression appears to be beneficial in other cases, especially in neonates, by decreasing the risk of urinary infection while the patient is on chemotherapeutic prophylaxis, allowing hydronephrosis involving other ureters to resolve and ultimately allowing for elective reconstruction in an older, healthy child.[7]

Open Surgical Management

The open surgical approach to the lower ureter and bladder neck in anomalies of ureteral duplication or ureteroceles is through a Pfannenstiel incision. Any surgery directed at management of the upper pole abnormality (partial nephrectomy or ureteropyelostomy) would have been accomplished through a separate extraperitoneal flank approach. This might have been done previously or the entire reconstruction might be accomplished as a single operative session through two separate incisions.

Excision of the Distal Portion of an Upper Pole Ureter (Without a Ureterocele)

If the ureteral orifice of the ectopic ureter is identified in the distal urethra, on the perineum, or in the

vagina, elective excision of the distal portion of the ureter is generally not necessary. The remaining ureteral stump functions as a mucous fistula and is rarely a source of trouble. When the ureter drains into the proximal portion of the urethra, there is a greater likelihood of recurring urinary infection postoperatively, and these distal segments are best removed electively. In addition, correction of reflux into an ipsilateral lower pole ureter may be necessary and the remaining upper segment stump would then be excised simultaneously.

After appropriate exposure of the bladder through a Pfannenstiel incision, a transurethral catheter is placed to empty the bladder, and the duplex ureter is approached extravesically. The obliterated umbilical artery is identified, dissected free of the peritoneum, and transected. The proximal portion of the artery is then dissected into the true pelvis, reflecting the peritoneum cephalad until the ureters are identified. At this point, both ureters are mobilized widely and together within their adventitial sheath. A moment is taken to identify the ectopic upper pole ureter, usually more dilated and thick-walled than the lower segment ureter. If one cannot be sure which is the ureter to be excised, the bladder can be opened and a catheter passed into the lower pole ureter.

An incision is then made through the ureteral adventitia on the margin of the upper segment ureter opposite the lower segment ureter. At this point, all dissection compulsively sweeps the adventitia and its contained blood supply off the ureter to be discarded and toward the lower segment ureter. Special care is taken to preserve the delicate vessels that crisscross the common space between the two ureters. Initial dissection along the upper segment ureter proceeds cranially until the top of the remaining stump is found. If this has been a staged reconstruction, that portion of the ureter will be scarred, and special care must be taken not to injure the lower segment blood supply at this location.

Dissection along the upper segment ureter then proceeds distally. The unknown at this point is the length of the common sheath. When the ureter is significantly ectopic (in the perineum or vagina), a true "common sheath" may not be found. In this situation, the ureter is dissected deep near (or under) the bladder neck until the caliber begins to narrow. At this point, it is amputated and left open.

If a common sheath is encountered and the lower pole ureter does not require reimplantation, and additional circumferential dissection of the upper segment ureter would risk the vascularity of the lower ureter, the upper pole ureter can be excised obliquely, leaving a strip of ureter in continuity with the lower segment ureter along the margins of the common vascular sheath (Fig. 107–5).

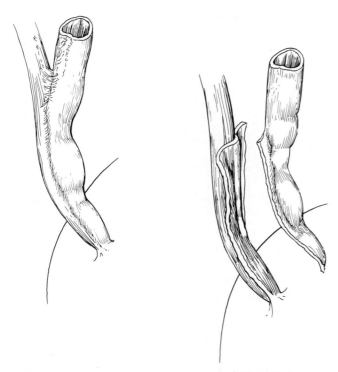

Figure 107–5. Technique for subtotal excision of the distal segment of ureter when a long common sheath is present. (Redrawn from Retik AB, Peters CA. Ectopic ureter and ureterocele. In Walsh PC, Retik AB, Stamey TA, Vaughan ED Jr, eds. Campbell's Urology, 6th ed. Philadelphia, WB Saunders, 1992, p 1750.)

Common Sheath Reimplantation or Ipsilateral Ureteroureterostomy (Upper Segment Ureter End to Side Into Lower Segment Ureter)

If upper pole function is satisfactory, reconstruction may be limited to correction of the lower ureteral anomaly only. Two surgical options are available: (1) common sheath reimplantation and (2) lower ureteroureterostomy.

The technique of common sheath reimplantation is no different from that employed to correct lower pole reflux. An intra- or extravesical approach may be chosen, although I find the latter preferable for duplication anomalies with ectopia. If the upper pole ureter is sufficiently dilated so that reduction ureteroplasty is necessary to achieve a successful reimplantation, ureteral tailoring, as described for megaureter repair, can be performed safely along the margin opposite the common sheath. Stenting is performed as is routine for reduction ureteroplasty (generally, in my practice, 10 days with a 7 Fr. Silastic ureteral catheter).

Lower ureteroureterostomy has not been the procedure of choice in most centers for managing duplication anomalies. Ureteropyelostomy has a long history of success and allows removal of a substantial length of dilated, poorly contractile ureter, reducing stasis

and eliminating the risk of developing "yo-yo" reflux. Lower ureteroureterostomy, however, has been preferred by some surgeons, who regard it as an option to avoid an upper abdominal incision and prefer not to simultaneously perform reduction ureteroplasty to the upper segment ureter during reimplantation.[8] The preferred location for the ureteroureterostomy is about at the level of the crossing of the obliterated umbilical artery. The artery is transected and the peritoneum mobilized cephalad. The ureters are mobilized just enough to allow a tension-free, mucosa-to-mucosa anastomosis. The upper pole ureter is transected, and the distal segment of the ureter is handled as described above for resection of a retained stump.

The site for the anastomosis is secured with two traction sutures of 6-0 chromic catgut placed about 2 cm apart along the anterolateral edge of the lower pole ureter. The ureteral lumen is entered with tenotomy scissors (my choice) or a No. 12 blade, and extended about 1.5 cm in length with Potts scissors. If the upper segment ureter is not of a large caliber, it is spatulated so as to accommodate the ureterotomy. The anastomosis is generally accomplished with 7-0 Vicryl or 7-0 PDS. A single suture is placed at each end of the ureterotomy. The sides are closed with a running, locking suture (Fig. 107–6). A Penrose drain is always left down to the anastomosis. Stenting is optional if a simultaneous ureteral reimplant has not been accomplished, but I believe it should be done if the lower pole ureter was reimplanted at the same session.

The main criticisms of lower ureteroureterostomy are that (1) the long segment of the upper pole ureter that is present may contribute to urinary stasis and an increased risk of infection and (2) there is a risk of devascularization of the lower portion of the lower

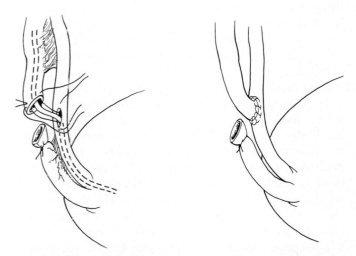

Figure 107–6. Technique for lower ureteroureterostomy, with the upper pole ureter end to side into the lower pole ureter. (Adapted from Amar AD. Ipsilateral ureteroureterostomy for single ureteral disease in patients with ureteral duplication: A review of eight years of experience with 16 patients. J Urol 119:472, 1978.)

pole ureter. Whereas these two complications are infrequent, I agree that these concerns are valid and have chosen this particular technique infrequently.

Excision of Ureterocele

When managing a child with a ureterocele, the question often arises of when to excise the ureterocele.[9] In some cases, simple decompression of the ureterocele by endoscopic incision or by upper pole nephrectomy (or ureteropyelostomy) can be definitive therapy.[10] This is more likely to be the case when the ureterocele is small and intravesical, when there is good detrusor backing behind the ureterocele, and when there is no reflux into associated ureters. In other cases, when the ureterocele is large, reflux is present, and bladder neck extension occurs, lower tract reconstruction is invariably necessary. Endoscopic decompression may help to control infection and improve hydronephrosis but is not likely to avert ultimate bladder reconstruction.

The choice of total excision versus marsupialization of the ureterocele has become a point of controversy.[11] However, the issue may be moot, since I believe most surgeons perform a combination of both procedures. The issue regarding successful reconstruction involves reapproximation of attenuated detrusor, incision or excision of any blind pockets of mucosa at the bladder neck or within the urethra, appropriate reimplantation, and re-epithelialization of the large mucosal defect. The large detrusor defect so often described in ureterocele surgery is more often iatrogenic than an inherent part of the anatomical anomaly.

I believe cystoscopy is an important part of the assessment of these children and is generally performed at the same time as the planned open procedure. The primary issue here is identification of the location of the ureteral orifice. If the orifice can be identified in the midurethra or more distally, it is very unlikely that a cecoureterocele is present.

Surgical management of a ureterocele is begun transvesically through a standard Pfannenstiel incision. The lower segment orifice is catheterized with a 5 Fr. feeding tube that is secured at the orifice with a 3-0 silk suture. An incision is then made through the mucosa around the medial, cranial, and lateral portions of the ureter (Fig. 107–7). This incision is then carried distally onto the ureterocele. At this location, the mucosa and lamina propria are generally thick and easy to separate from the ureterocele mucosa. Careful dissection of detrusor fibers will identify the lower segment ureter, and continued mobilization will free the two ureters within their common sheath. At this point, the dissection can be carried beneath the ureterocele at the junction with the ureters and the lower pole ureter can be separated, mobi-

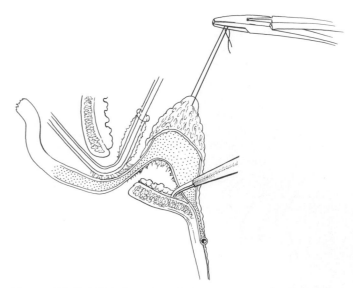

Figure 107–7. Initial dissection of the ureterocele and lower pole ureter. Dissection is begun intravesically and the remaining upper pole ureter is mobilized into the bladder. If the stump is relatively long, this portion of the mobilization may be completed extravesically.

lized, and placed aside for reimplantation (Fig. 107–8). Continued dissection along the upper segment ureter is then begun. If this is a staged procedure, dissection of the ureter will probably need to be completed extravesically, since it will be scarred in position after the first procedure. After the ureteral segment is freed, the upper pole ureter can be passed intravesically.

Dissection is then continued distally. Care is taken

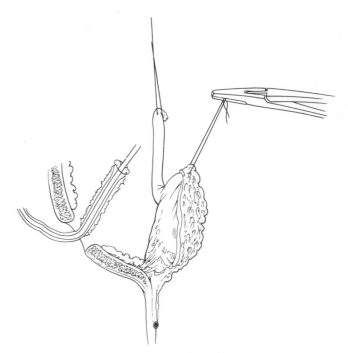

Figure 107–8. After separation of the two ureters, dissection of the ureterocele is continued toward the bladder neck.

to stay right on the mucosa of the ureterocele. Generally, this dissection is quite easy posteriorly and laterally. However, medially and anteriorly, especially as one approaches the bladder neck, the two separate mucosal layers become thin and difficult to separate. If it is known to extend through the bladder neck and terminate in the midurethra, I excise the ureterocele near the bladder neck. If a small catheter or probe passes easily through the urethral extension, I then slide the blade of a tenotomy scissors along the tract and open the thin mucosal membrane (Fig. 107–9). The back wall of the ureterocele mucosa is then used to re-epithelialize the region of the bladder neck and the distal trigone. I then make sure that a soft catheter can pass through the urethra antegrade without obstruction. The hiatal defect is approximated, attenuated detrusor is plicated with interrupted 4-0 chromic catgut, and transtrigonal reimplants are performed as needed. All mucosal defects are closed with 5-0 chromic catgut. Ureteral stents are not routinely left in place unless reduction ureteroplasty has also been necessary. A bladder catheter is left indwelling transurethrally in girls and suprapubically in boys.

COMPLICATIONS

Because ureteral reimplantation is commonly performed as part of any procedure to repair a uretero-

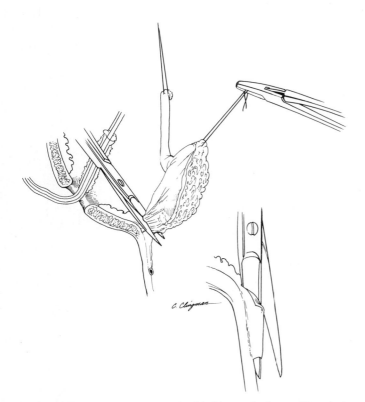

Figure 107–9. Just proximal to the bladder neck, the ureterocele is transected and the urethral extension incised completely. Antegrade catheterization is then performed to be sure no obvious distal flap remains.

cele or to excise the lower portion of an upper segment ureter, all the complications associated with ureteral reimplantation for correction of primary vesicoureteral reflux are likely to occur with surgical procedures to correct ureteroceles or ectopic ureters. These complications are thoroughly discussed in Chapter 105. In addition, three other complications are likely to occur as a result of surgery for these anomalies: injury to the bladder neck, injury to the vagina, and bladder outflow obstruction.

Ureteroceles and ectopic ureters tend to run for a distance submucosally through the bladder neck and proximal urethra before opening ectopically. Extravesical dissection along the ureter must stay compulsively on the adventitia of the ureter, and intravesical dissection on the mucosa of the ureterocele. A huge detrusor defect developing during the dissection is more often iatrogenic than a part of the anomaly proper. When an ectopic ureter is traced behind the bladder neck, it is appropriate to amputate it as soon as the caliber narrows substantially. When following a ureterocele, it is almost never necessary to dissect through the bladder neck. At that location, the ureterocele can be amputated and the luminal margin and intraurethral extension incised, leaving the urethral side of the ureterocele as the floor of the urethra.

Because ectopic ureters are often very large, they distort and displace the vagina. Aggressive dissection that does not stay right on the ureter may injure the vagina. Since the posterior bladder wall is often opened during this dissection also, a vesicovaginal or urethrovaginal fistula can result.

Finally, urethral extensions of ureteroceles may end blindly (cecoureteroceles). If this extension is not opened completely, postoperative urethral obstruction can result because of the presence of a flaplike valve of ureteral mucosa in the distal portion of the urethra. Preoperative assessment by cystoscopy may reveal the location of the ectopic orifice. Antegrade passage of a urethral catheter at the time of surgery may detect a residual flap that can be caught with the tip of fine tenotomy scissors. If postoperative obstruction does result, however, the obstructing lip is generally best managed endoscopically.

Editorial Comment

Craig A. Peters

Although two separate chapters discuss the surgical elements of management of duplication anomalies (Chapter 102 by Dr. Mandell and Chapter 107 by Dr. Gonzales), it is clear that the clinical decisions must be made in an integrated fashion, as discussed in this chapter. Specific indications and techniques for the various surgical approaches must be familiar to the surgeon to effectively manage individual patients.

Endoscopic management of ureteroceles has evolved in the last 10 years, from a practice that was considered inappropriate and generally condemned, to one that is widely used and recognized to have very specific and beneficial uses. It must be carefully chosen and applied. We have had good success with this method, but the incidence of reflux induced into the ureterocele is not trivial, even when the incision is low and small. This method is an excellent means of providing temporary drainage to prevent infection in complex ureteroceles, and permits a more effective definitive operation after decompression of the affected ureter.

In ureterocele excision, our preference is for careful detrusor reconstruction as outlined in this chapter, in that marsupialization of a ureterocele with less backing than anticipated may lead to complications of outlet obstruction. When the ureterocele extends into the urethra, great care must be taken to completely excise it, or (as specified in this chapter) to open it widely and completely, in order to prevent obstruction.

REFERENCES

1. Macki GG, Stephens FD. Duplex kidneys—a correlation of renal dysplasia with position of ureteral orifice. J Urol 114:274, 1975.

2. Tank ES. Experience with endoscopic incision and open unroofing of ureteroceles. J Urol 136:241, 1986.

3. Monfort G, Morrisson-Lancombe G, Coquet M. Endoscopic treatment of ureteroceles revisited. J Urol 133:1031, 1985.

4. Rich MA, Keating MA, Snyder HM, Duckett JW. Low transurethral incision of single system intravesical ureteroceles in children. J Urol 144:120, 1990.

5. Blyth B, Passerini-Glazel G, Camuffo C, et al. Endoscopic incision of ureteroceles: Intravesical versus ectopic. J Urol 149:556, 1993.

6. Monfort C, Guys JM, Coquet M, et al. Surgical management of duplex ureteroceles. J Pediatr Surg 27:634, 1992.

7. Smith C, Gosalbez R, Parrott TS, et al. Transurethral puncture of ectopic ureteroceles in neonates and infants. J Urol 152:2110, 1994.

8. Amar AD. Ipsilateral ureteroureterostomy for single ureteral disease in patients with ureteral duplication: A review of eight years of experience with 16 patients. J Urol 119:472, 1978.

9. Decter RM, Roth DR, Gonzales ET. Individualized treatment of ureteroceles. J Urol 142:535, 1989.

10. King LR, Koglowski JM, Schacht MJ. Ureteroceles in children: A simplified and successful approach to management. JAMA 249:1461, 1983.

11. Scherz HC, Kaplan GW, Parker MG, Brock WA. Ectopic ureteroceles: Surgical management with preservation of continence—review of 60 cases. J Urol 142:538, 1989.

Chapter 108

Prune-Belly Syndrome

John R. Woodard and Luis M. Pérez

The prune-belly syndrome, a term coined by Osler in 1901, refers to the triad condition of deficient abdominal wall muscles, dilation of the urinary collecting systems, and bilateral undescended testes.[1] Occurring predominantly in boys, the syndrome has an incidence of 1 per 35,000 to 50,000 live births.[2] The cause has not been determined. Because the urinary tract above the membranous urethra is dilated, some have theorized that temporary obstruction at the membranous urethra during fetal life results in either an extremely distended bladder or severe fetal ascites.[3] This in turn may compress the normal ventral mesenchyme, resulting in absence or deficiency of the abdominal wall musculature, and may prevent the gubernaculum from completing its role in aiding testicular descent. However, neither a floppy abdomen nor cryptorchidism occurs in patients with posterior urethral valves who truly suffer from urinary obstruction. A more logical explanation for prune-belly syndrome may be that of a partially hereditary condition resulting in a primary defect of the intermediate and lateral plate mesoderm, accounting for both an abdominal and a urinary tract dilation without obvious obstruction.[4] This theory allows for the fact that a few patients may also suffer from megalourethra and atypical posterior urethral "valves."[4]

Like most disease entities, there is a spectrum of severity for prune-belly syndrome. Patients with the most severe forms of the syndrome suffer from oligohydramnios, pulmonary hypoplasia, or pneumothorax and often are either stillborn or do not survive the neonatal period. A second group of patients have an intermediate condition and may or may not develop gradual renal failure and/or urosepsis. It is in this second group that significant benefit may be obtained from aggressive surgical intervention. In a third group of patients, the uropathy is mild and surgical intervention is deemed unnecessary.

Various disorders and congenital anomalies are not infrequently observed in prune-belly patients (Table 108–1). Aside from pulmonary abnormalities, intestinal malrotation is perhaps the most common nonurological congenital anomaly observed in these children. The intestinal malrotation tends to be benign, not requiring surgical intervention.

PREOPERATIVE EVALUATION

Clearly, the cardiopulmonary status of the neonate takes precedence over the urological evaluation. Initial chest x-ray and arterial blood gases are useful in documenting baseline pulmonary status. Initial urological evaluation should include physical examination, with special attention to the possibility of a dilated bladder and ureterohydronephrosis as well as a patent urachus. If possible, the quality of the newborn's urinary stream is noted. Other laboratory tests should include urinalysis, urine culture, serum electrolytes, and renal ultrasonography. Since most patients will have vesicoureteral reflux, it can be assumed to be present, and a voiding cystogram (VCUG) can be postponed initially. Significant ureteropelvic junction (UPJ) obstruction is also a possibility in these patients. If this is suspected from ultrasonography, a diuretic-assisted technetium 99m-

TABLE 108–1. Nonurological Conditions Associated with Prune-Belly Syndrome

Pulmonary	Pulmonary hypoplasia
	Pneumothorax
	Pneumomediastinum
	Pneumonia
Cardiac	Ventricular septal defect
	Atrial septal defect
	Tetralogy of Fallot
Gastrointestinal	Intestinal malrotation
	Gastroschisis
	Hirschsprung disease
	Constipation
Orthopedic	Clubfeet
	Congenital hip dislocation
	Skin dimple at knee or elbow

diethylenetetramine pentaacetic acid (DTPA) nuclear medicine scan is recommended in the first week of life after the newborn is well hydrated. Any DTPA scan to assess ureteral obstruction in this population should be performed with a catheter freely draining the bladder. Early cystourethroscopy is recommended if there is any suggestion of urethral valves. It is likely, however, that coexisting urethral valves are rare and that the typically wide prostatic urethra has led to misdiagnosis in some cases. Newborns who survive the neonatal period with stable renal status should be placed on antibacterial prophylaxis and followed on an outpatient basis with serial urine examinations and serum electrolyte evaluations.

Unless obtained earlier, a renal functional study in the form of a DTPA radioisotope scan should be performed at approximately 4 weeks of age. If upper tract drainage is adequate, a repeat renal ultrasound and/or radioisotope scan is performed at 3 months of age. If renal function and drainage remain stable, the child may undergo a radioisotope scan at 6 months of age and renal ultrasound at 9 months of age. Between 3 and 9 months of age, orchiopexy can usually be performed in a single stage without dividing the testicular vessels. Infants over about 9 months of age often require a Fowler-Stephens orchiopexy. A repeat ultrasound or radioisotope scan at 1 year of age is recommended. If anatomical detail of the upper collecting systems is needed, an intravenous urogram may be obtained rather than a radioisotope scan at about 1 year of age. If the child remains stable, studies may be spaced to every 6 months for the second year of life and yearly until age 5 years. Thereafter, periodic urinalyses, serum electrolyte tests, and radiological studies should be obtained no less often than every 2 years. Video-urodynamic studies should be obtained as indicated.

Although the prune-belly bladder typically has an irregular contour, is thick-walled, and is very voluminous, little trabeculation is present on cystoscopic examination. This is in contrast to patients with posterior urethral valves, whose bladder is severely trabeculated. The prune-belly trigone is very large, with laterally placed ureteral orifices. The bladder neck and prostatic urethra are quite patulous. While many patients show no urodynamic evidence of voiding dysfunction, others have dramatically elevated postvoid residual volumes and abnormal pressure flow studies, which have been reported to improve after internal urethrotomy of "apparent obstruction just below the verumontanum."[5]

If at any time urinary infections become a problem or the child's renal status deteriorates, a temporary form of diversion (cutaneous vesicostomy or pyelostomy) may be considered. Most often, a cutaneous vesicostomy provides for adequate drainage and avoids the risk of injuring the upper ureters, perhaps

the only portion of the patient's collecting system that is nearly normal in caliber and function. For this reason, loop cutaneous ureterostomies should be avoided. When considering a vesicostomy, one should be certain that there is no UPJ obstruction, otherwise a cutaneous pyelostomy would be more appropriate.

Whether patients with prune-belly syndrome should undergo extensive surgical remodeling of the urinary tract is controversial; although some do well with major reconstruction, others often appear to improve without any intervention. There is little question that poor bladder emptying, with resultant recurrent and chronic urinary tract infection, leads to upper tract deterioration in many of these patients. The large bladder capacity, abnormal bladder wall, and relative narrowing of the membranous urethra may all play some role. Although some efforts have been made to delineate this problem urodynamically, such data are sparse.[6, 7] On long-term follow-up of reduction cystoplasty in this population, the authors of one study determined that although the procedure "helped to improve voiding and minimize infection during early childhood . . . it does not seem to decrease bladder capacity or improve voiding dynamics in the long term."[7] Despite this single long-term study, it is likely that many surgeons, because of early improvement, will continue their efforts at remodeling these distorted urinary tracts. Before proceeding with surgical intervention in a patient without clear evidence of upper tract deterioration, one must realize that the surgery is difficult and that some patients have been harmed by unsuccessful surgical attempts at reconstruction.

OPERATIVE TECHNIQUE

The success of surgical reconstruction depends to a great extent on the use of the upper few centimeters of ureter, which are usually less dilated, less tortuous, and morphologically better than the distal ureter.[8] Meticulous surgical technique, with adherence to established principles of ureteral tailoring and reimplantation surgery, is required. Unfortunately, both the bladder and the ureter, by the very nature of this condition, are difficult structures with which to work. Despite these inherent difficulties, a reasonably high degree of success is possible with extensive reconstructive surgery in experienced hands, both in the neonate as a primary procedure and in the older infant or child as a primary or staged procedure.

Internal Urethrotomy: Ablation of Atypical "Valves"

In the past, some authors have found internal urethrotomy of the "apparent obstruction just below the verumontanum" a useful technique for improving voiding dysfunction in the prune-belly population.[5] Although this procedure has improved the upper tracts in some patients, it places them at risk for developing stress urinary incontinence, and should therefore not be considered unless combined cystometry-uroflowmetry documents functional obstruction, or unless endoscopic visualization reveals anatomical obstruction. Rather than using the Otis urethrotome in blind fashion, direct-vision internal urethrotomy of only the stenotic distal prostatic urethra or ablation of "prune valves" should be performed.

Ureteral Reconstruction and Reduction Cystoplasty

Surgical tailoring of the upper tracts as well as reduction cystoplasty may be performed along with abdominal wall reconstruction and orchiopexy as a single-stage procedure (Fig. 108–1). Through a midline or an abdominal wall–plasty incision, transperitoneal exploration is performed. The location and condition of the abdominal testes, spermatic vessels, and UPJs are noted after incision of the retroperitoneum and mobilization of the ureters at the pelvic brims. Once excision of the distal ureters is performed, tapering of the ureters over a 10 Fr. catheter is recommended if these are greater than 1 cm in width. Reimplantation of the ureters may then be performed using the technique of choice. Although bilateral nephrostomy tubes may be inserted for added protection during postoperative care, ureteral stents alone may suffice in most cases. We believe it is advantageous to perform a reduction cystoplasty and leave a Malecot suprapubic tube for drainage. If the bladder wall remaining is thin, which is unusual, a double-breasted bladder closure may be performed as described by Perlmutter[9] and Hanna.[10] In the senior author's experience (JRW), the prune-belly bladder has been thick in every case of reduction cystoplasty, and the double-layered closure has not been required. Ureteral catheters are left in place for approximately 5 to 10 days, depending on whether tapering of ureters is performed. If nephrostomy tubes are present, bilateral nephrostography may be performed a week later to make certain that an adequate reimplantation has been achieved. The suprapubic tube remains in place for about 2 weeks after a few days of voiding trials with the suprapubic tube clamped. A radioisotope scan may be obtained about 6 weeks postoperatively to make sure that upper tract drainage is adequate. VCUG may be performed 6 months postoperatively to evaluate for reflux.

Megalourethra Repair

The rare patient who suffers from megalourethra should undergo repair. Degloving of the penile skin is performed after a circumferential incision is made around the coronal sulcus. Usually only the penile urethra is dilated, making more feasible the excision of excess urethra and closure of the lumen over an appropriately sized catheter. The penile skin is then closed in usual fashion.

Orchiopexy

Paternity in men with prune-belly syndrome has not been reported. Prostatic hypoplasia and an incompetent bladder neck make retrograde ejaculation likely, adding to the complex fertility issue in these patients.[4] It is not clear whether early infant orchiopexy in affected patients will allow for fertility, but clearly the operation should be performed both because of the risk of testicular neoplasm and also to preserve normal hormonal production (Leydig cell function), which is possible in most patients. Usually, the testes are intra-abdominal and overlie the ureter at the pelvic brim (Fig. 108–1).[11] If orchiopexy is performed before the child is 6 to 9 months of age, transabdominal complete mobilization of the spermatic cord usually allows the testis to be positioned in the dependent portion of the scrotum without tension and without dividing the vascular portion of the spermatic cord (Fowler-Stephens technique). The orchiopexy is performed by tunneling bluntly through the abdominal wall at the external inguinal ring with a hemostat that slips easily into the scrotum. After creation of a dartos pouch, the testis is drawn into the scrotum and orchiopexy is performed in routine fashion. When the child is older, either a single- or two-stage Fowler-Stephens technique may be deemed necessary in some patients. Microvascular autotransplantation, although more cumbersome, has been successfully applied to the prune-belly population.[12]

Abdominal Wall Reconstruction

Electromyographic studies have demonstrated that the major functioning or recoverable muscle exists in the lateral and upper section of the abdomen; usually, little or no useful muscle is present in the more central and lower portion of the abdomen. Since the abdominal wall deformity in some patients seems to improve slightly with age, some authors have suggested that external support devices may offer a practical advantage over major surgical abdominal wall plication procedures.

The earlier abdominal wall reconstruction de-

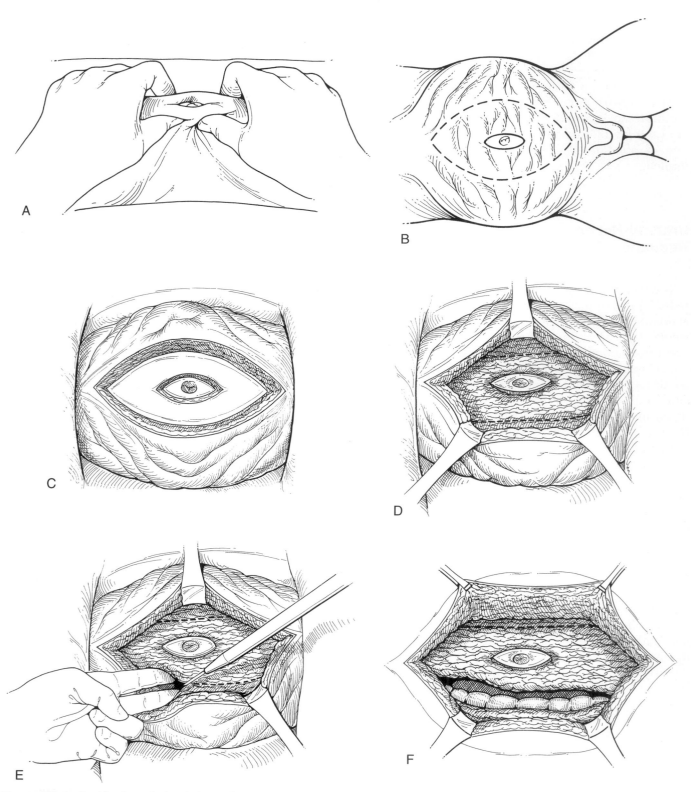

Figure 108–1. Combined surgical technique cf urinary tract reconstruction, orchiopexy, and abdominal wall reconstruction. *A* to *C*, Excess abdominal wall tissue is tented up and the umbilicus is isolated with a separate circumferential incision. *D*, Excess abdominal skin (dermis and epidermis only) has been excised with electrocautery. *E* and *F*, The abdominal wall musculature is then incised at the lateral border of the rectus muscles on either side, from the supericr epigastric to the inferior epigastric vessels, creating a central musculofascial plate.

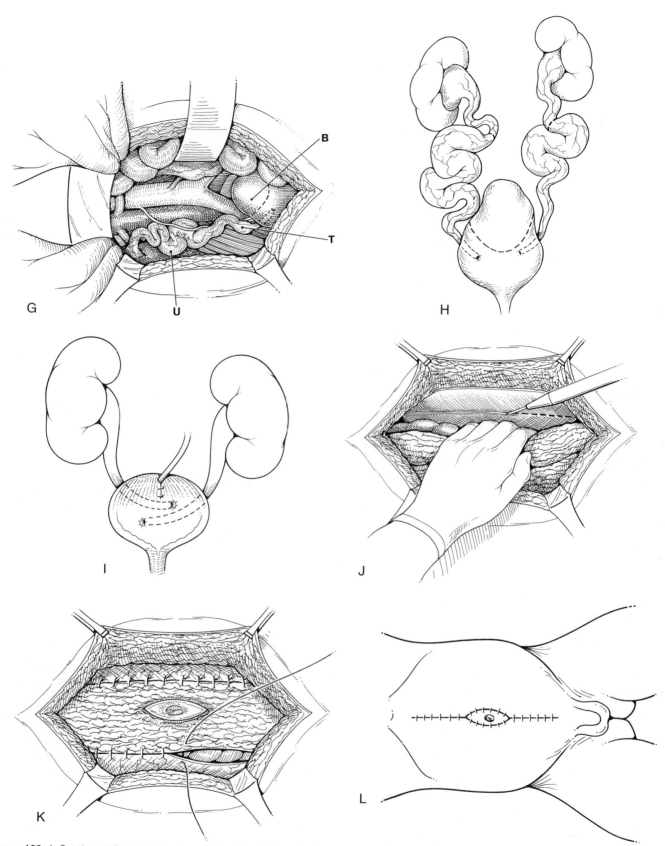

Figure 108–1 *Continued G* and *H*, A self-retaining retractor is placed unilaterally, providing adequate exposure of the intraperitoneal contents. After incision of the retroperitoneum and adequate dissection, the tortuous ureter is retracted on vessel loops. Note the abdominal testis (T) at the pelvic brim, the ureter (U), and the bladder (B). Dotted lines show the site of ureteral and bladder dome resection. *I*, The lower ureter and bladder dome have been excised and after tapering, the upper ureter has been reimplanted in cross-trigonal fashion. Orchiopexy has also been completed. A similar procedure is performed on the opposite side. *J*, Abdominal wall reconstruction is completed. Electrocautery is used to incise the peritoneum overlying the lateral abdominal wall musculature. *K*, The lateral border of the central musculofascial plate is sutured to the lateral abdominal musculature, which has been exposed by incising overlying peritoneum. *L*, The skin is then brought together in the midline, enveloping the umbilicus. Subcutaneous suction drains (not shown) are used for 2 to 3 days postoperatively.

scribed by Randolph and colleagues entailed the excision of a transverse elliptical portion of the lower abdominal wall; it did little to improve the waistline or physique.[13] In 1986, Ehrlich and associates reported one of the two currently used techniques for vertical abdominal wall reconstruction.[14] In 1991, Monfort and co-workers reported a technique they had used since 1970.[15] This is quite similar to the Ehrlich technique with some modifications, allowing preservation of the umbilicus and using the full thickness of the existing abdominal wall. Ehrlich and Lesavoy have subsequently modified their technique to preserve the umbilicus.[16] At our institution, the Monfort abdominal wall reconstruction technique has been used extensively with favorable results.[17] We have noted that most patients have improved voiding function after abdominal wall reconstruction secondary to an increased capacity to perform an adequate Valsalva maneuver.

POSTOPERATIVE COMPLICATIONS

The postoperative complications of ureteral tapering and reimplantation, particularly ureterovesical obstruction, persistent vesicoureteral reflux, and urinary tract infections, are discussed in Chapter 105 by Drs. Peters and Retik. Incisional problems after abdominal wall reconstruction have rarely occurred at our institution and have been limited to superficial wound separation, easily treated with local wound care and of no long-term consequence. In terms of persistent voiding dysfunction, the use of video-urodynamics has been a very important means of pinpointing the problem. Not infrequently, some patients may require temporary clean intermittent catheterization as long as pressure flow urodynamic studies document the lack of obstruction.

Summary

The urological evaluation and management of patients with prune-belly syndrome continue to be a challenge even in the most experienced hands. Herein we have illustrated a one-stage technique of performing the abdominal wall reconstruction, ureteral tapering and reimplantation, reduction cystoplasty, and bilateral orchiopexies. We again stress that aggressive surgical intervention remains a controversial issue that should be attempted only by experienced reconstructive surgeons.

Editorial Comment
Fray F. Marshall

The cause of prune-belly syndrome is still not totally understood. One hypothesis, however, that might explain this anomaly relates to an arrest of mesenchymal development at approximately 10 weeks of gestation. Mesenchyme can induce prostatic epithelium so that prostatic development may be affected. Deficiencies in mesenchymal development may also affect the maturation of the gubernaculum testes so that nondescent of the testes can occur. Deficiencies in mesenchyme could also be reflected in muscular deficiency of the abdominal wall, bladder, and lower ureters.[1]

Because abnormalities in the prostate may reflect a defect in stromal epithelial interaction, obstruction may not be a frequent cause of dilation in the prostatic urethra. Urethrotomies may not "correct" perceived obstruction. In addition, incontinence may be the result.

1. Marshall FF. Embryology of the lower urinary tract. Urol Clin North Am 5:3, 1978.

Editorial Comment
Craig A. Peters

Although it may seem counterintuitive to leave untouched the markedly abnormal urinary tract of children with prune-belly syndrome, Drs. Woodard and Pérez have shown the importance of careful selection of patients in whom reconstruction may be indicated. With time, many of these dilated systems will gradually improve without any evidence of functional deterioration. Careful monitoring is essential. Orchiopexy should not be deferred unnecessarily, however, as better results are obtained with early surgery. This may be feasible without a Fowler-Stephens approach in younger children, and more recently may be effectively accomplished with laparoscopy.

The Monfort abdominoplasty described in this chapter has provided excellent results in our hands also. Its basic strategy recognizes the pathological anatomy in prune-belly syndrome in which the lateral and superior musculature of the abdominal wall is better developed than the medial and inferior musculature. While it has been suggested that improving abdominal muscular tone may improve bladder emptying, this remains to be proved.

REFERENCES

1. Osler W. Congenital absence of abdominal muscles with distended and hypertrophied urinary bladder. Bull John Hopkins Hosp 12:331, 1901.
2. Woodard JR. Prune-belly syndrome. In Walsh PC, Retik AB, Stamey TA, Vaughan ED Jr, eds. Campbell's Urology, 6th ed. Philadelphia, WB Saunders, 1992, p 1851.
3. Rich MA, Duckett JW. The prune belly syndrome. AUA Update Series, Vol XI, lesson 17, 1992, p 130.
4. Stephens FD, Gupta D. Pathogenesis of the prune belly syndrome. J Urol 152:2328, 1994.
5. Snyder HM, Harrison NW, Whitfield HN, Williams DI. Urodynamics in the prune belly syndrome. Br J Urol 48:663, 1976.
6. Kinahan TJ, Churchill BM, McLorie GA, et al. The efficiency of bladder emptying in the prune belly syndrome. J Urol 148:600, 1992.
7. Bukowski TP, Perlmutter AD. Reduction cystoplasty in the prune belly syndrome: A long-term followup. J Urol 152:2113, 1994.
8. Woodard JR, Parrott TS. Reconstruction of the urinary tract in prune belly uropathy. J Urol 119:824, 1978.
9. Perlmutter AD. Reduction cystoplasty in prune belly syndrome. J Urol 116:356, 1976.
10. Hanna MK. Megaureter. In King LR, ed. Urologic Surgery in Neonates and Young Infants. Philadelphia, WB Saunders, 1988, p 160.

11. Woodard JR, Parrott TS. Orchiopexy in the prune belly syndrome. Br J Urol 50:348, 1978.
12. Silber SJ, Kelly J. Successful autotransplantation of an intra-abdominal testis to the scrotum by microvascular technique. J Urol 115:452, 1976.
13. Randolph J, Cavett C, Eng G. Abdominal wall reconstruction in the prune belly syndrome. J Pediatr Surg 16:960, 1981.
14. Ehrlich RM, Lesavoy MA, Fine RN. Total abdominal wall reconstruction in the prune belly syndrome. J Urol 136:282, 1986.
15. Monfort G, Guys JM, Bocciardi A, et al. Novel technique for reconstruction of abdominal wall in prune belly syndrome. J Urol 146:639, 1991.
16. Ehrlich RM, Lesavoy MA. Umbilicus preservation with total abdominal wall reconstruction in prune-belly syndrome. Urology 41:231, 1993.
17. Parrott TS, Woodard JR. Monfort operation for abdominal wall reconstruction in prune belly syndrome. J Urol 148:688, 1992.

Chapter 109

Surgical Repair of Exstrophy/ Epispadias

John P. Gearhart and Robert D. Jeffs

INDICATIONS

The surgical management of classical bladder exstrophy is one of the greatest reconstructive challenges for the urologist. Although many reconstructive techniques have been described, only in the past several years has a unified approach to the surgical management of this disorder evolved. The staged approach to functional closure of bladder exstrophy has also gained increasing success over the last few years.[1] The plan of treatment has consisted of bladder closure with or without penile lengthening and pelvic osteotomy, usually after birth or as soon thereafter as possible. Formerly, epispadias repair was completed when the patient reached 4 to 5 years of age, after bladder neck reconstruction. More recently, however, epispadias repair has been performed in patients 2 to 3 years of age before bladder neck reconstruction, because of the significant increase in capacity that comes from epispadias repair.[2]

Bladder neck reconstruction along with an antireflux procedure is usually performed when the patient is 4 to 5 years old, only after a satisfactory bladder capacity has been achieved and when the child is ready to accept toilet training.

PREOPERATIVE MANAGEMENT

Shortly after birth the exposed bladder needs to be protected from clothing, diapers, and physical injury. The best management is to cover the area with a large sheet of plastic wrap to allow urine to escape while providing a barrier between clothing and the delicate bladder mucosa. The old urine should be washed liberally with sterile water at body temperature at frequent intervals, usually at each diaper change.

It is important to prevent the umbilical clamp from gouging the surface of the exstrophied bladder. A tie can be substituted and the clamp removed shortly after birth to avoid this problem. If the closure is to be undertaken within the first 72 hours of life, little time should be wasted after delivery. Parents should be told the full nature of the problem and that it is possible to correct the urinary storage and reconstruct the genitalia so that sexuality and function approach normal. Referral to a surgical team experienced in the management of bladder exstrophy should be arranged. Basic investigation is undertaken to establish pulmonary and cardiac functions. Ultrasound examination can establish whether the urinary tract is undilated and therefore, presumably, draining well. If the ultrasound results are normal, showing no evidence of hydronephrosis and two normal kidneys, no further investigations are necessary.

At the time of initial closure, preoperative antibiotics are usually given in the form of ampicillin and gentamicin, which are continued for 10 days after surgery. Antibiotics are an important part of successful bladder closure, because all exstrophied bladders and surrounding tissues are contaminated areas. The local area is thoroughly washed and cleaned with povidone-iodine (Betadine) along with liberal soaking of the bladder and its interstices. The preparation at the initial closure involves the area from nipples to knees and from the base of the scapula, the buttocks, and the posterior aspect of the popliteal fossa. The entire area is draped into the operative field at the time of surgery. This allows access to the posterior body wall and hips when one is manipulating the pelvic ring to provide a stable anterior midline closure. An adhesive surgical dressing is applied over the anus to prevent stool contamination during the procedure.

INITIAL EXSTROPHY CLOSURE

The bladder often appears much smaller than expected for the gestational age of the child, so bladder size can only be judged adequately with the patient under anesthesia. A bladder that appeared small while the patient was in the newborn nursery may demonstrate an acceptable capacity, indenting easily into the pelvis when pushed inward by a gloved, sterile finger. If the initial bladder capacity is believed to be 5 ml or more after the closure, one can expect the bladder to develop a useful size and capacity after a successful closure. The bladder is turned in, removing it from irritation and repeated trauma so that it will enlarge and gradually increase its capacity over time.

Operative Techniques

The technique for initial primary bladder closure is described and diagrammed in Figure 109–1. The initial procedure is closure of the bladder, displacement of the bladder to a posterior position deep within the pelvis, approximation of the pubic symphysis, and provision of free urethral drainage. Penile lengthening, if required, should be performed at the same time. For later reconstruction and eventual production of continence, it is important to place the bladder and bladder neck within the pelvic ring so that the urethra can exit and drain between a well-closed pubic arch. This maneuver has the advantage of enabling the pelvic musculature to act on the urethra, and interruption of the stream may sometimes

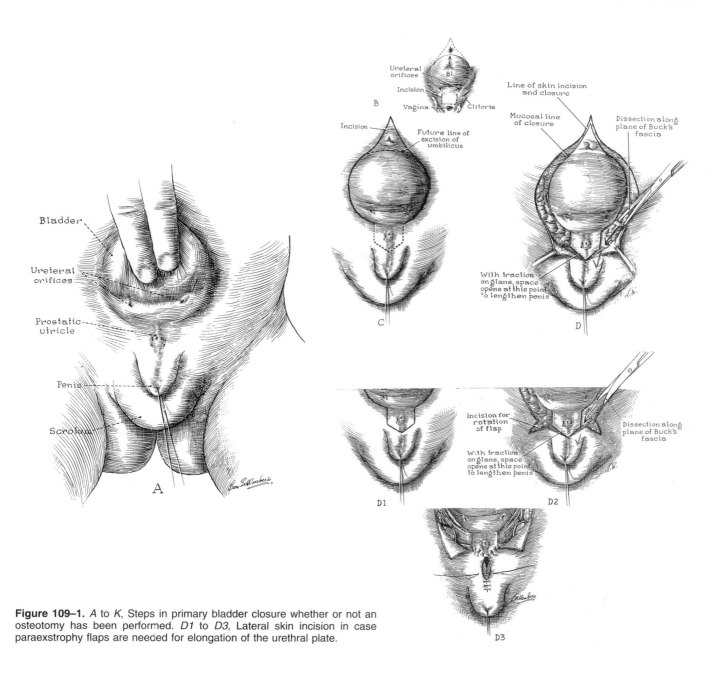

Figure 109–1. *A* to *K*, Steps in primary bladder closure whether or not an osteotomy has been performed. *D1* to *D3*, Lateral skin incision in case paraexstrophy flaps are needed for elongation of the urethral plate.

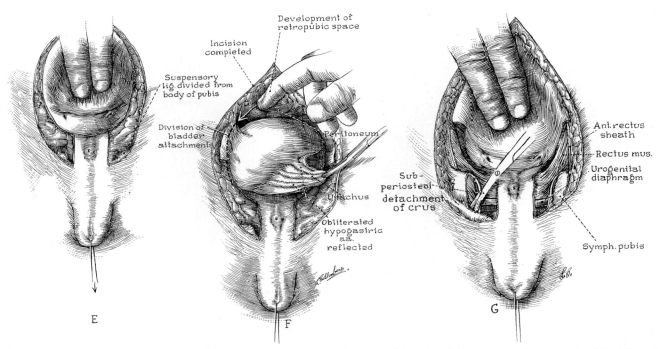

Figure 109–1 *Continued E*, The situation when flaps are not used. *F*, Development of the retropubic space from the area of umbilical dissection to facilitate separation of the bladder from the rectus sheath muscle. *G*, Medial fan of the rectus muscle attaching behind the prostate to the urogenital diaphragm. The diaphragm and anterior corpus are freed from the pubis in the subperiosteal plane.

Illustration continued on following page

be possible. Tailoring of the bladder neck and tension of the vesicoureteral angle are most easily achieved when the bladder neck is within the pelvic ring. They become more difficult when the bladder is merely covered by skin and fascial flaps and when continued mobility of tissue between the pubic bones is evidenced.

The distance from anal verge to umbilicus is shortened in exstrophy; thus, a deeper structure is crowded into a smaller space. By freeing the transverse bar of tissue, which represents the urogenital diaphragm, sharply from the pubic symphysis and inferior ramus of the pubis, one allows the urethra to take a more posterior exit from the pelvis (Fig. 109–1*G*). If the urogenital diaphragm is not separated completely from the urethra and pubis, the posterior urethra will be carried anteriorly when the pubic rami are brought together. At the same time, sectioning of the suspensory ligament tissue of the penis and the anterior attachments of the corpora cavernosa to the anterior ramus of the penis corrects a good deal of the dorsal chordee and allows the penis to gain length and a more dependent angle. In males, if significant chordee is present, the urethral groove is lengthened by transecting the mucosa distal to the prostatic urethra, allowing the bladder and bladder neck to recede into the pelvis (Fig. 109–1*C* to *D3*). The subsequent gap produced in the urethral groove is then filled with rotation flaps of paraexstrophy skin (Fig. 109-1*D*$_{1-3}$, 1 to 3). Care must be taken in the construction of any paraexstrophy skin flap so that ischemia and

subsequent stricture formation will not occur. Also, in a male patient who has a fairly straight penis and a deep urethral groove, the urethral mucosa maintained and not transected, thus reserving these tissues for later urethral reconstruction (Fig. 109–1*E* and *F*).

The bladder is then closed in two layers after placement of a suprapubic cystostomy tube (Fig. 109–1*H* to *J*). After bladder closure and after the pubic bones are brought together, the suprapubic tube and stents are brought out cephalad to the bladder through the neoumbilicus (Fig. 109–1*K*).

Pelvic Osteotomy

Closure within the first 48 to 72 hours of life should be considered and should be successfully achieved if one can easily bring the pubic bones into apposition with lateral pelvic compression.[1] However, some patients have a very wide diastasis and require osteotomy for a successful closure.[3] In patients who are not seen immediately after birth, osteotomy is necessary to obtain a secure midline closure. This is believed to be helpful in achieving continence in the subsequent bladder neck reconstruction. Osteotomy provides for a stable anterior midline wound closure in those patients who are not seen as newborns and who have less mobility of the pelvic ring.

In our experience, anterior innominate osteotomy is the preferred method of achieving apposition of the pubic rami.[3] The advantage of the anterior ap-

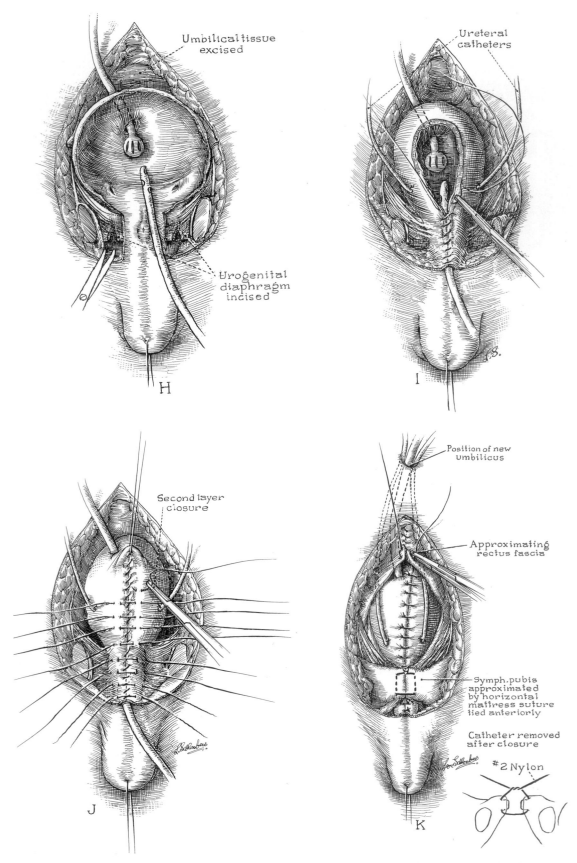

Figure 109–1 *Continued I*, Ureteral catheters are placed before bladder closure to provide renal drainage for 10 to 12 days. *J*, Second layer of urethral and bladder closure. The catheter is removed before symphyseal closure. *K*, A horizontal mattress suture is tied in the external surface of the symphysis. (Drawings by Leon Schlossberg.)

proach is that there is better pelvic mobilization, and both the osteotomy and bladder closure can be completed with the patient in the supine position. In addition, placement of interfragmentary stabilizing pins across the osteotomy fixes the bone fragments and allows excellent callus formation. The pins are held in place with an external fixator placed at the end of the abdominal closure. In patients in whom an osteotomy is not used and the pubic bones are simply brought together, modified Bryant traction is used instead of an external fixator.

Fixation of the wound is a very important part of the initial healing. An attempt is made to provide fixation of the coapted pubic bones by horizontal mattress sutures tied on the outside of the closure away from the posterior urethra. Once this is achieved, it is not difficult to place other heavy nylon sutures in the rectus fascia, which is now more near the midline. Nonreactive stitches of Dexon are used for the remainder of the closure, with nylon for the skin closure.

Other methods have been tried, but it is believed that distracting muscular forces are minimized more effectively by Bryant traction than by other measures. When an external fixating device or Bryant traction is used to provide stability of the pelvic closure, either of these necessitates a prolonged hospital stay, but they help to provide primary healing in a potentially contaminated wound, and the extra time is certainly worth it.

Control of the muscular activity of the child is important. This necessitates a team effort among physicians, nurses, and parents who must pamper the baby to make sure that pain, frustration, hunger, and muscular spasms do not produce undue or prolonged activity that defeats the other attempts to provide wound stability. In addition, analgesics, antispasmodics, and tranquilizers are provided liberally in an attempt to ensure a calm postoperative course.

POSTOPERATIVE MANAGEMENT AFTER BLADDER CLOSURE

Ureteral intubation is performed at the time of bladder closure. Normally, 3.5 Fr. pediatric feeding tubes are used as ureteral stents in an infant. These are routinely left in place for 10 to 14 days, after which drainage is by a suprapubic Malecot catheter. The stents, along with the suprapubic tube, are irrigated at regular intervals to ensure patency. No stents or catheters are left indwelling in the urethra to decrease the risks of prolapse or dehiscence.

When the child is removed from traction, an abbreviated intravenous pyelogram (IVP) is performed to check renal function and drainage. After the IVP, the suprapubic tube is routinely clamped and several

residual urine determinations are taken. Calibration of the posterior urethral outlet is also performed to ensure adequate patency and drainage. If both these measurements are satisfactory, the suprapubic tube is removed.

At the time of discharge, parents are cautioned about possible complications, particularly in relation to infection and urinary retention. They are also warned to be suspicious of a dry diaper after this initial closure, which would warrant immediate investigation.

Low-pressure drainage from the urinary tract is expected. Patients are placed on suppressive medication, such as ampicillin or nitrofurantoin (Furadantin), which is continued indefinitely. If the IVP reading looks relatively normal before discharge from the hospital, we simply perform renal ultrasound examination 4 to 6 months after the initial closure.

EPISPADIAS REPAIR

At one time, if the child had a bladder capacity that exceeded 60 ml at 3 years of age, a bladder neck reconstruction was performed. However, in a group of patients with relatively small bladder capacities after closure, an epispadias repair was performed before bladder neck reconstruction.[2] After epispadias repair, a mean increase in bladder capacity of at least 55 ml occurred. Thus, since 1990 the authors have routinely performed epispadias repair when the child is about 2 years of age, to enhance bladder capacity before bladder neck reconstruction.[1]

The goals of epispadias repair are to lengthen and straighten the penis. In addition, it should provide an adequate urethra for normal voiding. Along with the creation of a neourethra, the persistent dorsal chordee also needs to be addressed. Preoperatively, because of the short penile length, testosterone is given intramuscularly to help increase the corporeal length and availability of penile skin. Usually, testosterone enanthate in oil, 2 to 3 mg/kg, is given intramuscularly 5 weeks and 2 weeks before epispadias repair.

Many different procedures for creation of a neourethra have been proposed. In our experience, the Cantwell-Ransley has become the procedure of choice (Fig. 109–2) (see also Chapter 118).[4] The procedure is begun by placing a glans-holding suture. A strip along the urethral plate, approximately 1.5 cm in width, is then marked from glans to base of penis. A meatal advancement procedure may be performed at this point (Fig. 109–2B). The urethral plate is then incised along the axis of the markings (Fig. 109–2C and D). The ventral phallus is degloved in a manner similar to that of a hypospadias repair. However, care must be taken not to interrupt the leash of vessels in

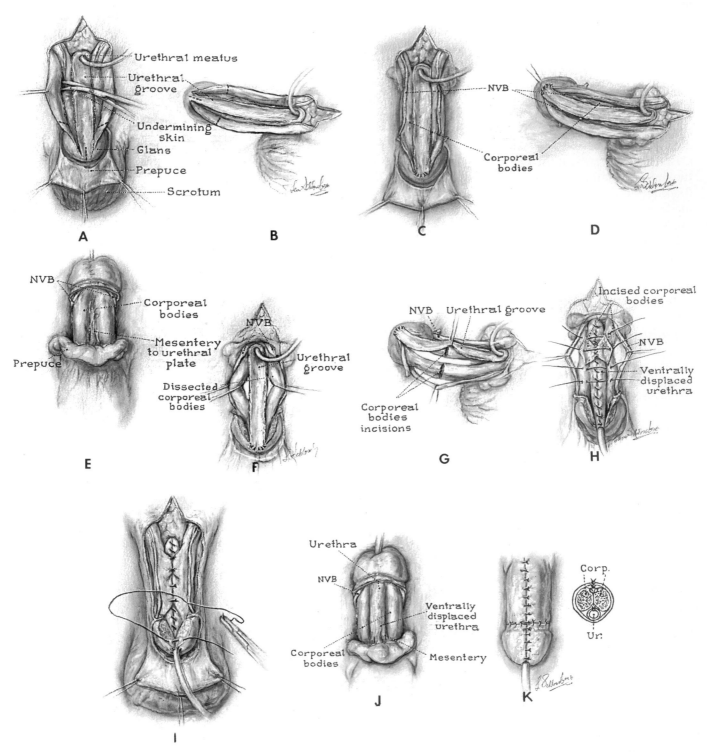

Figure 109–2. *A* to *K*, Modified Cantwell-Ransley epispadias repair. *B*, The meatal advancement manuever must be performed deeply to have a ventral meatus. *C* and *D*, Degloving of penile skin and exposure of neurovascular bundle. *E*, Mobilization of urethral plate begins from below, preserving the "mesentery" from below. *G*, Corporeal incisions to correct dorsal chordee (not always needed if previous maneuvers straighten and lengthen the penis adequately). *K*, Completed skin and glandular closure with an indwelling urethral stent for 10 to 12 days. NVB, neurovascular bundle. (Drawings by Leon Schlossberg.)

the midline that enter the urethral plate approximately between the corpora (Fig. 109–2E). The corporeal bodies and the urethral plate are widely mobilized (Fig. 109–2F). If needed to correct chordee, the corpora are incised for later reanastomosis over the neourethra (Fig. 109–2G and H). The urethral plate is then closed over a soft urethral stent with a running absorbable suture. After formation of the glandular wings, the neourethra is completed. The soft catheter is then sutured to the glans. By rotating the corporeal bodies medially, the urethra is allowed to assume a more normal position in the penis and dorsal chordee is corrected (Fig. 109–2H to K). The fistula rate has been markedly reduced by this procedure.[4]

BLADDER NECK RECONSTRUCTION

The purpose of bladder neck reconstruction is to allow for voluntary voiding with continence. The prerequisites for such reconstruction include the ability of the child to communicate, the desire to be dry, and a bladder capacity of at least 60 ml. Patience on the part of both physician and parents is imperative at this period as the child learns to recognize the sensation of a full bladder and learns to adequately empty the bladder when full. Initial or repeat osteotomy may need to be performed at the time of bladder neck reconstruction if there is a persistently wide pubic diastasis or a soft intrapubic bar.

A Young-Dees-Leadbetter reconstruction is next performed. The bladder is opened vertically with a transverse extension at the caudal end (Fig. 109–3A). In the exstrophy group, trigone tissue is employed to create a bladder neck and a posterior urethra approximately 3 cm in length, with sufficient double-breasted closure to provide resistance to the flow of urine. The tissue required for posterior urethral construction encroaches on the bladder floor, making it necessary to move the ureteral orifices cephalad by performing a transtrigonal reimplantation of the ureters, thus correcting reflux at the same time. Either a cephalotrigonal or a Cohen transtrigonal reimplant is typically used (Fig. 109–3B and C). The authors prefer the former because this allows a larger portion of the trigone to be incorporated into the bladder neck reconstruction. Optimally, a strip 30 mm long by 15 mm wide is outlined (Fig.109–3D to F). This strip is marked with a blue marking pen, beginning at the penile urethra and proceeding in a cranial direction. The epithelium lateral to the strip is excised. This mucosal strip is then rolled over an 8 Fr. catheter stent into a tube. In a vest-over-pants fashion, the deep layer of detrusor muscle is then closed over the tube (Fig. 109–3G and H). The final layers of suture of the superficial layer of detrusor muscle are left long so that a Marshall-Marchetti-Kranz suspen-sion of the bladder neck can be performed. The suprapubic catheter and ureteral stents are brought out of the bladder through a separate stab incision (Fig. 109–3I). The bladder is then closed in two layers, and a Penrose drain is placed. Again, as in initial bladder closure, no urethral stents or catheters are left in place postoperatively. This repair must be allowed to heal for 3 full weeks, using a suprapubic tube for drainage, before voiding trials are allowed.

POSTOPERATIVE MANAGEMENT AFTER BLADDER NECK CONSTRUCTION

Obstruction to the flow of urine occurring at the end of a 3-week period may be managed by continued suprapubic drainage or by gentle dilation of the urethra, passing an 8 Fr. catheter under anesthesia or sedation. If any difficulties are encountered, gentle cystoscopy under anesthesia will help. After the cystoscopy, a small 8 Fr. catheter is left in place. After 2 to 3 days of drainage, the catheter is removed, the suprapubic tube is again clamped, and a voiding trial is attempted. If further difficulty is encountered, after a period of urethral catheter drainage, the cystoscopy may need to be repeated and another catheter left indwelling for 2 to 3 days. A 3-hour dry interval and satisfactory control are usually obtained within 1 year of the bladder neck plasty, but nocturnal dryness may be delayed for a year or more.

Four months after the bladder neck plasty, a follow-up IVP and cystogram are performed to ensure freedom from reflux, satisfactory function, and drainage of the upper urinary tracts and to determine whether there is any residual infection. Patients are maintained on suppressive antibiotics until regular complete bladder emptying and no evidence of reflux are assured.

COMPLICATIONS

The main complications of bladder exstrophy closure are bladder prolapse, outlet obstruction, bladder calculi, renal calculi, and wound dehiscence.[5] However, our results have suggested a significant decline in these complications. Children who have experienced dehiscence of the bladder or significant bladder prolapse have had a failed initial closure. Dehiscence can occur because of infection, or more commonly as a result of pubic separation. Bladder prolapse can result from either partial wound separation or failure to create a tight enough bladder outlet. If bladder size is adequate, a second closure of the bladder can be performed 4 to 6 months after the

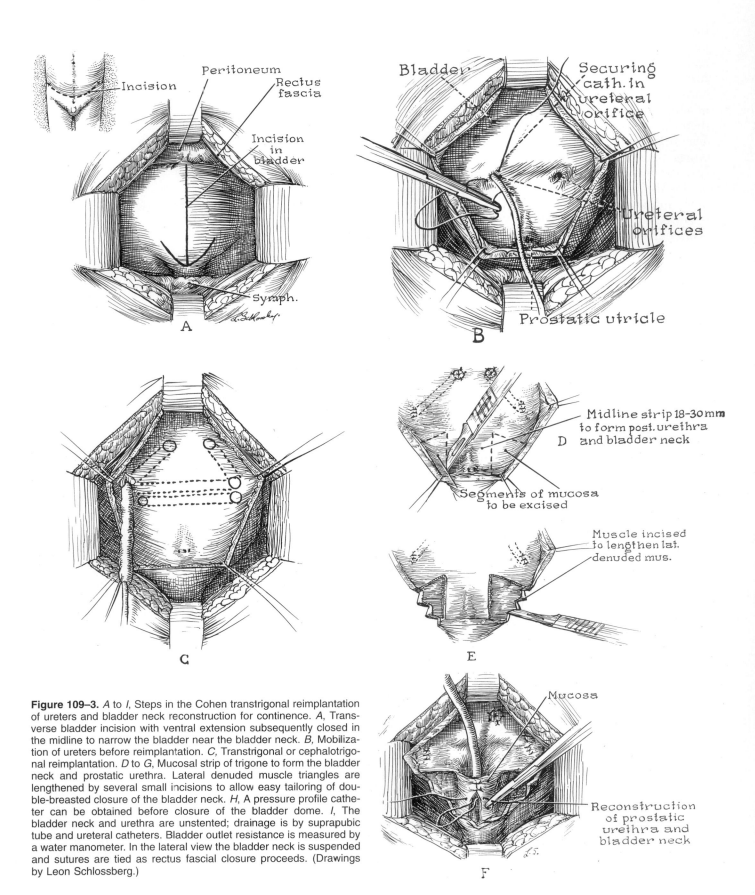

Figure 109–3. *A* to *I*, Steps in the Cohen transtrigonal reimplantation of ureters and bladder neck reconstruction for continence. *A,* Transverse bladder incision with ventral extension subsequently closed in the midline to narrow the bladder near the bladder neck. *B,* Mobilization of ureters before reimplantation. *C,* Transtrigonal or cephalotrigonal reimplantation. *D* to *G,* Mucosal strip of trigone to form the bladder neck and prostatic urethra. Lateral denuded muscle triangles are lengthened by several small incisions to allow easy tailoring of double-breasted closure of the bladder neck. *H,* A pressure profile catheter can be obtained before closure of the bladder dome. *I,* The bladder neck and urethra are unstented; drainage is by suprapubic tube and ureteral catheters. Bladder outlet resistance is measured by a water manometer. In the lateral view the bladder neck is suspended and sutures are tied as rectus fascial closure proceeds. (Drawings by Leon Schlossberg.)

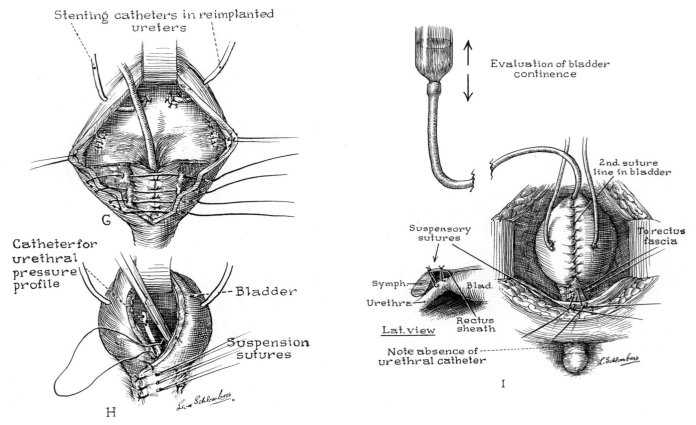

Figure 109–3 *See legend on opposite page*

initial attempt. Repeat closure should be performed with an osteotomy or repeat osteotomy. Since 1985, 38 patients with failed initial exstrophy closures have been seen at The Johns Hopkins Children's Center.[7] All these children underwent reclosure with an osteotomy. To date, there have been no complications from the repeat closures. However, despite the success of the repeat closure, the continence rate is less than in those with successful initial closures.

Complications of Epispadias Repair

Before routine use of the Cantwell-Ransley repair, urethrocutaneous fistulas occurred in approximately 30 percent of our patient population. However, since the advent of this repair, the persistent fistula rate has dropped to 8 percent.[4]

Complications of Bladder Neck Reconstruction

Complications after bladder neck reconstruction are rare. In a series of 25 consecutive operations, postoperative urinary retention developed in eight patients.[1] Bladder outlet obstruction resolved in all eight patients after dilation, prolonged suprapubic

catheterization, cystoscopy, or intermittent catheterization. The long-term complication from bladder neck reconstruction is persistent incontinence. If a continent interval does not develop in a 2-year period after bladder neck reconstruction, continence is a rare occurrence. Repeat bladder neck plasty can be performed in these patients if the capacity seems adequate. In addition to repeat bladder neck reconstruction, bladder augmentation or placement of an artificial urinary sphincter can be performed. Alternatively, bladder neck transection or creation of a continent urinary stoma with augmentation cystoplasty can be undertaken.[6]

Summary

In experienced hands, the surgical results after bladder closure, bladder neck reconstruction, and epispadias repair are quite acceptable. In a study of 144 exstrophy patients reviewed at our institution, those who underwent a successful initial closure without wound infection, dehiscence, or any degree of bladder prolapse had better overall courses.[7] These patients developed the largest bladders with time and had the shortest interval between primary closure and eventual bladder neck reconstruction. They also had the shortest intervals between bladder neck re-

construction and achievement of urinary continence (mean 1.5 years). These patients also experienced the highest urinary continence rate (92 percent) compared with another group whose initial repair was not successful.

In a recent review of 35 patients with failed staged bladder exstrophy reconstructions, all patients were doing well after bladder augmentation, bladder replacement, and/or continent stoma construction.[6] Therefore, although complications such as dehiscence, deterioration of renal function, and fistula occur, careful attention to surgical detail and frequent follow-up can salvage patients and help them become well-rounded children and later otherwise healthy adults.

Editorial Comment
Craig A. Peters

The staged functional reconstruction of patients with bladder exstrophy has been a major contribution to pediatric urology and to such patients. The importance of developing a close, supportive, long-term relationship with patient and family may not be explicitly stated in this chapter, but it is an essential part of day-to-day care. The role of postoperative behavioral management in attaining continence is substantial and cannot be ignored.

A recent tendency toward continent diversion for patients with exstrophy should be discouraged. While continence may be readily achieved with intermittent catheterization, we have also seen more cases with significant problems related to inadequate drainage of prostatic fluids after puberty, largely due to stricture of defunctionalized urethras. Fertility potential will also be affected.

REFERENCES

1. Gearhart JP, Jeffs RD. Exstrophy of the bladder, epispadias, and other bladder anomalies. In Walsh PC, Retik AB, Stamey TA, Vaughan ED Jr, eds. Campbell's Urology, 6th ed. Philadelphia, WB Saunders, 1992, p 1772.
2. Gearhart JP, Jeffs RD. Bladder exstrophy: Increase in capacity following epispadias repair. J Urol 142:525, 1989.
3. Sponseller PD, Gearhart JP, Jeffs RD. Anterior innominate osteotomy for failure or late closing of bladder exstrophy. J Urol 146:137, 1991.
4. Gearhart JP, Burgens J, Conrad M, Jeffs RD. The Cantwell-Ransley technique for repair of epispadias. J Urol 148:851, 1992.
5. Gearhart JP, Peppas DS, Jeffs RD. The failed exstrophy closure: Strategy for management. Br J Urol 71:217, 1993.
6. Gearhart JP, Peppas DS, Jeffs RD. The application of continent stomas to the failed exstrophy reconstruction. Br J Urol 75:87, 1995.
7. Oesterling JE, Jeffs RD. The importance of a successful initial bladder closure in the surgical management of classic bladder exstrophy: Analysis of 144 patients with bladder exstrophy treated at the Johns Hopkins Hospital from 1975 to 1985. J Urol 137:258, 1987.

Chapter 110

Cloacal Exstrophy

Michael E. Mitchell and Michael C. Carr

Cloacal exstrophy represents the severe end of a spectrum in which all the abnormalities associated with exstrophy, in addition to omphalocele, imperforate anus, and hindgut herniation, are present. Cloacal exstrophy was first described by Littre in 1709; however, it was not until 1960 that Rickham reported the first successful surgical reconstruction.[1] Before this time, most infants with this devastating complex malformation were allowed to die. Improvements in neonatal intensive care and nutritional support contributed to early successes. In a compiled series of patients treated before 1970, only six of 19 survived. At the Boston's Children's Hospital, 17 of 34 patients treated from 1968 to 1976 survived the correction. The latest review from that hospital now shows 100 percent survival.[2]

Cloacal exstrophy, also referred to as vesicointestinal fissure, ectopic cloaca, ectopia viscerum, complicated exstrophy of the bladder, and abdominal wall fissure, is the most severe form of ventral abdominal wall defect. The characteristic defects in cloacal exstrophy are illustrated in Figure 110–1. An omphalocele is seen superiorly along with exposed bowel and bladder inferiorly. The bladder is divided in the midline by a segment of intestinal mucosa, and each hemibladder contains a ureteral orifice. Often the terminal small bowel everts through the central hindgut. The general appearance is much like the face of an elephant with the bladder halves as the ears, the central hindgut as the face, the herniated small bowel as the trunk, and, sometimes, duplicated appendices as tusks and the hindgut as the mouth. The pubic symphysis is also widely separated. Genital abnormalities are found in all cases. In girls, the clitoris is divided and usually associated with a duplex vagina and bicornuate uterus. In boys, cryptorchidism is often present. The penis is usually bifid, with each half epispadiac and attached to widely separated pubic rami.

The upper urinary tract may include such anomalies as pelvic kidney, unilateral renal agenesis, multicystic dysplastic kidney, ureteral duplication, and crossed-fused ectopia. Gastrointestinal anomalies include malrotation, duplication, and anatomically short small bowel; duodenal atresia; and Meckel's diverticulum. Vertebral anomalies can occur, and central nervous system abnormalities include sacral agenesis and spinal dysrhaphism, most commonly lipomeningocele. The lower extremities may show dislocated hips, talipes equinovarus and dysmorphism, and agenesis of the lower limbs.

The human embryo does not pass through a stage that corresponds to exstrophy, and thus cloacal exstrophy is considered a manifestation of abnormal embryogenesis rather than an arrest in development. A grasp of the normal embryology of the cloacal region is essential to an understanding of the development of cloacal exstrophy. The cloaca is the expanded end of the hindgut, which received initially the allantoic diverticulum and later the mesonephric ducts. The cloaca is divided by the urorectal septum and/or by lateral mesenchymal folds into the primary

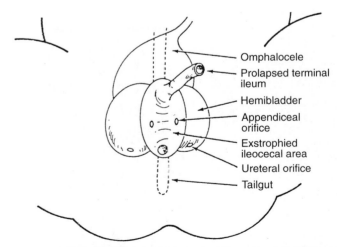

Figure 110–1. Classical cloacal exstrophy. The general appearance is much like the face of an elephant. (From Hurwitz RS, Manzoni GAM, Ransley PG, Stephens FD. Cloacal exstrophy: A report of 34 cases. J Urol 138:1060, 1987.)

Omphalocele
Prolapsed terminal ileum
Hemibladder
Appendiceal orifice
Exstrophied ileocecal area
Ureteral orifice
Tailgut

urogenital sinus ventrally and the (ano) rectum dorsally. Further subdivision of the primary urogenital sinus occurs with entry of the mesonephric ducts at the end of the fourth week. This results in formation of the vesicourethral canal (future bladder and urethra) cephalically and the definitive urogenital sinus caudally. The urogenital sinus at this point consists of a pelvic part proximally and a phallic part distally. The cloacal membrane eventually ruptures from urinary pressure (Fig. 110–2).

During the fifth week, the division between the dorsal (rectal) and ventral (urogenital) cloaca begins to appear. The division at the upper part of the cloaca becomes the urorectal septum, which grows caudad in a frontal plane by progressive fusion of lateral ridges to reach the cloacal membrane during the seventh week. The septum unites with the cloacal plate to form the perineal body. At about the same time, the cloacal plate (or membrane) ruptures, forming anal and urogenital orifices separated by the perineum.[3]

Cloacal exstrophy arises from failure of secondary mesoderm from the primitive streak to cover the infraumbilical wall. It differs from exstrophy of the bladder in that a midline herniation has occurred early (in the fifth week), preventing fusion of the

genital tubercles and the descent of the urorectal septum, which normally separates the cloaca into bladder and rectum. As the cloaca herniates ventrally, its central portion is the posterior wall of the gut, whereas its lateral portions receive the ureters and differentiate into bladder mucosa. This ventral rupture of the cloaca prevents medial migration of the abdominal wall (therefore, omphalocele develops) and closure of the pelvis (diastasis of symphysis) and failure of the normal tail curvature (spinal defects, renal defects). The exstrophic gut may lie caudal to the bladder. In such a case, cloacal rupture took place *after* the urorectal septum began to descend, but *before* its descent was complete. These cases represent a stage between classic exstrophy of the bladder and typical exstrophy of the cloaca. Thus, cloacal rupture early in the fifth week results in cloacal exstrophy with omphalocele in addition to spinal, renal, and bowel malformation. Herniation, however, in the seventh week results in bladder classic exstrophy only.[4]

Cloacal exstrophy may be detected at the time of prenatal ultrasonography. A bladder is not seen to fill and empty in spite of the presence of normal kidneys and amniotic fluid at the time of scanning. Because exstrophy and cloacal exstrophy are surgically correctable malformations, these findings (kidneys, nor-

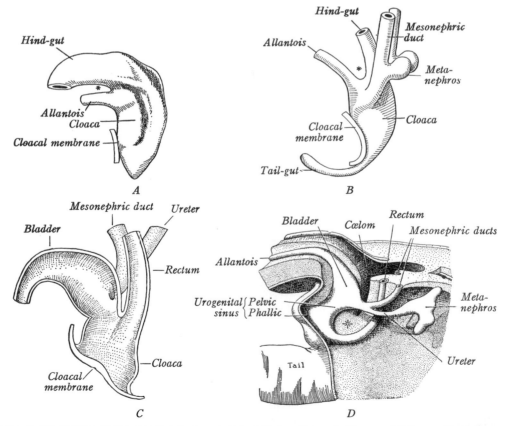

Figure 110–2. Stages in the division of the cloaca into dorsal and ventral portions. *A,* Cloaca at 3.5 mm. *B,* At 4 mm. The mesonephric (wolffian) ducts have joined the ventral cloaca. *C,* The ventral cloaca is enlarged to form the bladder at the 8-mm stage, and division of the cloaca has started. *D,* At 11 mm. The allantois has stopped growing and the cloaca is almost divided. An asterisk indicates the site of the caudad-growing cloacal septum. (From Arey LB. Developmental Anatomy, 7th ed. Philadelphia, WB Saunders, 1974, p 309.)

mal amniotic fluid, no bladder filling) should *not* be grounds for intervention. Cloacal exstrophy demands emergent assessment and treatment of the newborn, often by multiple services (pediatric urology, surgery, neurosurgery, orthopedics, and the gender assessment committee). Unlike a newborn with classic exstrophy, in whom renal ultrasound alone is adequate for preoperative assessment, a patient with cloacal exstrophy requires at the very least chest and abdominal films plus renal and spinal ultrasonography preoperatively. A radionuclide scan and/or intravenous urogram is also necessary, but not acutely. A 46,XY cloacal exstrophy patient represents a major challenge. Real debate and serious doubt now exist over whether all cloacal exstrophy patients should be raised as girls, regardless of genetic sex. Although it is theoretically easier to create a vagina than to reconstruct a phallus in some of these patients, intrauterine sex imprinting may preclude sexual reversal. Vaginal reconstruction in a patient with severe pelvic diastasis is often less than satisfactory because of the tendency for vaginal prolapse. We now have an experience with 16 46,XY cloacal exstrophy patients, eight of whom have been raised as boys and eight as girls. The advantage of sexual reversal has not necessarily been obvious. Such a decision should be individualized on the basis of surgical assessment of the anatomy, not the diagnosis alone.

In general, the strategy for treatment of a cloacal exstrophy patient consists of staged reconstruction, converting the more complex to the less complex. Therefore, a severe cloacal exstrophy patient will have an omphalocele closure, separation of the gastrointestinal tract from the bladder, and closure of the vesicointestinal fissure with the creation of a colostomy and a uniting of the two bladder halves. In patients with a large omphalocele, it may not be possible, and is unwise, to close the bladder during the initial surgical procedure. The patient's condition is thus converted from cloacal exstrophy to classical exstrophy. The second stage of the surgical reconstruction can be considered once the infant's pulmonary and nutritional status has been optimized. In some patients, particularly those with the liver outside the abdominal cavity, staged closure is absolutely necessary, usually with a Silastic silo to gradually reduce the omphalocele. The bladder is left open, but the halves are joined in the midline after the hindgut is closed and brought out as a colostomy. The hindgut will grow and develop. It must be remembered that its development was curtailed by early proximal diversion. It is a bad mistake to leave any portion of the hindgut with the bladder. Bladder closure may take place 4 weeks to several months after the initial surgical procedure, depending on the severity of the omphalocele. The situation is now analogous to classic exstrophy, with the variations relating to bladder size as well as pelvic and genital deformities. For purposes of clarity, correction of each of the defects is presented separately.

CLOSURE OF THE OMPHALOCELE

Initial surgical management of cloacal exstrophy involves closure of the omphalocele. This can usually be achieved primarily but may involve placement of prosthetic material, such as a Silastic silo. The inherent elasticity of the pubis in the first 24 to 48 hours of life facilitates closure during this time. Polydioxanone suture (PDS) can be used for approximation of the pubic symphysis. When the omphalocele is large the intact membrane may be left in place as a barrier for the potential staged reconstruction. A superior and inferior extension of the midline incision may be necessary to accomplish this (Fig. 110–3).

INTESTINAL TRACT

Preservation of the intestinal tract is of paramount importance in patients with cloacal exstrophy. Separation of the intestinal segment from the bladder halves with creation of an end-fecal colostomy should be performed. Failure to utilize the hindgut segment with creation of an ileostomy can lead to short bowel syndrome with fluid and electrolyte ab-

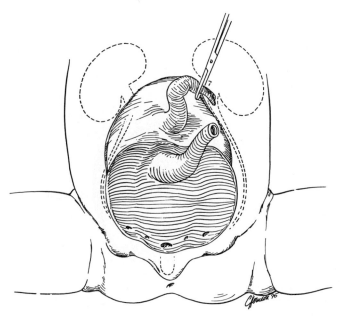

Figure 110–3. Incision for repair of cloacal exstrophy. The bladder halves are mobilized after dividing the vesicointestinal fissure. The abdominal cavity is entered to repair the omphalocele. A superior and inferior extension of the incision may be required. (Modified from Warner BW, Ziegler MM. Exstrophy of the cloaca. In Ashcraft KW, Holder TM, eds. Pediatric Surgery, 2nd ed. Philadelphia, WB Saunders, 1993, p 398.)

normalities and nutritional compromise, and is thus not recommended. Closure of the intestinal plate analogous to the cecum can be performed over a red rubber catheter. At times a Heineke-Mikulicz type of closure is necessary at the junction of the tubularized intestinal plate with the hindgut to prevent a functional obstruction. The stoma should be placed laterally to minimize contamination of the abdominal wall and allow placement of prosthetic material for closure if necessary. This small segment of bowel will expand greatly after refunctionalization (Fig. 110–4).

Thought may be given to preservation of the appendices for future use in the urinary reconstruction, although they usually remain disappointingly small. Similarly, duplicated segments of colon may be incorporated in the intestinal tract. The resultant extra colon may also prove useful for bladder augmentation during subsequent reconstruction.

Some authors have advocated a primary pull-through procedure if the length of hindgut is adequate at the time of the initial surgical procedure. In our experience, this should be considered *only* in those patients at the exstrophy end of the spectrum, i.e., with basically imperforate anus plus exstrophy without spinal abnormality. Intraoperative electrical stimulation of the perineum is necessary to assess the strength and location of the sphincter complex. There is often a spinal dysraphism that contributes to denervation of the pelvic musculature. This, plus the severe pelvic deformity with resultant abnormality in the pelvic diaphragm, usually precludes a successful pull-through procedure.

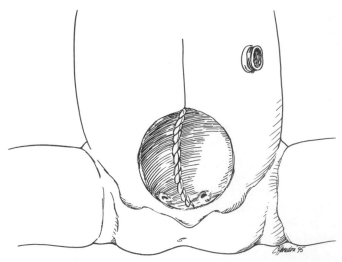

Figure 110–5. Staged bladder closure may be required, particularly with a large omphalocele closure. Iliac osteotomies are performed, followed by mobilization of the bladder and tubularization of the bladder neck. The repair is similar to closure of classical exstrophy. (Modified from Warner BW, Ziegler MM. Exstrophy of the cloaca. In Ashcraft KW, Holder TM, eds. Pediatric Surgery, 2nd ed. Philadelphia, WB Saunders, 1993, pp 398, 400.)

URINARY TRACT

Separation of the bladder halves from the vesicointestinal fissure, followed by bladder reapproximation posteriorly in the midline, converts the cloacal exstrophy to classical exstrophy (Fig. 110–5). Primary closure of the bladder may not be possible or wise at the time of the omphalocele closure and creation of the colostomy. It is often better to stage bladder closure, permitting the bladder to act as a "pop-off" mechanism, which also results in stretching of the bladder and abdominal wall, facilitating bladder closure. Pulmonary compromise, lower extremity ischemia, and loss of renal function can result from aggressive primary closure. Therefore, either anterior or posterior iliac osteotomies may be necessary to close the symphysis at the time of the subsequent bladder closure. The bladder may vary in size from large and floppy to a small plate. Usually the original size of the bladder provides a rough indication of the potential for the bladder to stretch to a useful capacity. This is not an absolute rule and should never limit consideration of primary or secondary closure. The trigone is usually obvious, as are the ureteral orifices, which can be observed to spout urine. Multiple polyps of mucosa may be evident. These should be excised at the time of bladder closure because they do not usually disappear and can serve as lead points for herniation through an open bladder neck after closure. Furthermore, the bladder polyps can occupy a considerable volume, occasionally making closure of a small bladder impossible without polyp excision. The trigone is broad and the ureters are lateral (they

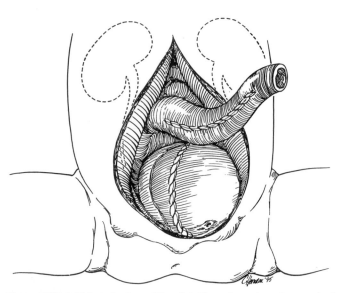

Figure 110–4. Tubularization of the distal bowel employs the terminal ileum and the foreshortened colon to maintain bowel continuity as an end fecal colostomy. The hemibladders are closed posteriorly (as illustrated) and, if possible, closed anteriorly to create a urinary reservoir. (Modified from Warner BW, Ziegler MM. Exstrophy of the cloaca. In Ashcraft KW, Holder TM, eds. Pediatric Surgery, 2nd ed. Philadelphia, WB Saunders, 1993, p 398.)

have a looping course lateral and caudal before entering the bladder). Most of the ureters will reflux, presumably because of the abnormalities of the posterior bladder wall and trigone.

The important components of primary bladder closure include (1) aggressive dissection and mobilization of the bladder to permit relocation deep in the pelvis, (2) extensive dissection of the bladder neck area to permit proper closure of the bladder neck and repositioning behind the symphysis, (3) meticulous bladder closure, (4) symphyseal approximation, (5) abdominal wall closure, and (6) patient immobilization and postoperative care (Fig. 110–6).

The next phase of urinary reconstruction involves procedures to provide for urinary continence and genital reconstruction. These cases can be among the most challenging because of the anatomy, potentially altered innervation, and limitations of available gastrointestinal segments.[5–7] The stomach has become our preferred segment for bladder augmentation or as a gastric continent urinary reservoir. In a review of 14 cloacal exstrophy patients, stomach was used in nine during subsequent reconstruction. Gastrocystoplasty was performed four times, and a gastric continent urinary reservoir with an orthotopic urethra exiting the perineum five times.[8]

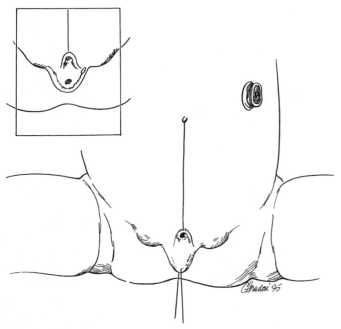

Figure 110–6. Closure of the pubic bones at the midline with heavy polydioxanone suture, followed by closure of the abdominal wall, completes the repair. A perineal stoma for urinary drainage is employed. The suture is placed through the phallus of a 46,XY patient. Further reconstruction will require an extensive epispadias repair and bladder neck reconstruction. The inset depicts a 46,XX patient with a perineal urethral opening and small vaginal inlet. (Modified from Warner BW, Ziegler MM. Exstrophy of the cloaca. In Ashcraft KW, Holder TM, eds. Pediatric Surgery, 2nd ed. Philadelphia, WB Saunders, 1993, p 400.)

Bladder neck or urethral procedures were performed in all 12 reconstructed cases, including reconstruction of a tunneled ureteral urethra (four cases), gastric tube intussuscepted into gastric continent reservoir (one case), Young-Dees-Leadbetter bladder neck reconstruction (three cases), artificial urinary sphincter (two cases), and tapered ileal urethra tunneled into reservoir (two cases). Better than 90 percent continence was achieved. Vaginal reconstruction was performed at the time of bladder reconstruction in several patients by various techniques. Native bladder tissue was used in two patients, previous ileal loop in two, reconfigured distal ureter in one, and an old colon Hartmann pouch in one. The potential for penile reconstruction should not be ruled out a priori. More recently, with complete disassembly and reassembly of the penile components, functional genital reconstruction in boys has been possible. Several cases illustrate the variations and reconstruction used.

CASE REPORTS

Case 1

A 46,XY cloacal exstrophy patient raised as a girl was referred at age 8 years, after having had an attempted pull-through of the hindgut, followed by takedown and ileostomy because of intractable diarrhea. She also had an ileocystoplasty with tapered ileum as a catheterizable stoma created 2 years before presentation. The hindgut was pulled through as a vagina. She had recurrent urinary tract infections (the ileostomy and catheterizable channel were adjacent to one another) and a small-capacity bladder. This patient required greater bladder capacity and separation of the ileostomy and catheterizable channel. To accomplish this, a tubularized neourethra was created from a patch of stomach, an artificial urinary sphincter was placed around the neourethra, and the bladder was augmented with stomach. A subsequent distal urethroplasty and anterior vaginal wall advancement were performed because of urethral stenosis. She now voids by Valsalva maneuver and performs intermittent catheterization every 4 hours. She is dry between catheterizations.

Comments. The extensive use of small bowel for reconstruction in this patient greatly limited further reconstruction potential. In general, we prefer to use as little small bowel as possible for reconstruction in these patients. In our experience, an artificial sphincter should not be used on large or small bowel but can be applied to tubularized bladder and tubularized gastric flap.

Case 2

A 15-year-old girl with cloacal exstrophy was born with a solitary left kidney and underwent delayed closure at 8 months of age. A pull-through procedure of the colon failed, requiring an end colostomy with the distal colon as a Hartmann pouch. The patient was referred for total urinary incontinence. She had a poorly compliant, small-capacity bladder with no urethral resistance and left vesicoureteral reflux but normal renal function. The patient had mild short bowel syndrome, so intestinal cystoplasty was not entertained. To improve compliance and capacity, gastrocystoplasty was performed. A segment of stomach based on the right gastroepiploic artery was used. An artificial urinary sphincter was placed at the bladder neck for continence. The left ureter was submucosally tunneled into the gastric bladder to prevent reflux. Because of the short bowel syndrome, a proximal segment of colon from the Hartmann pouch was isolated and anastomosed to the distal ileum, creating a short colostomy. The remaining colon was used for a vagina. At 9 months postoperatively the patient had normal upper tracts and was free of reflux. She was dry day and night and voided spontaneously with minimal residual urine volumes at intervals of 4 to 6 hours.

Comments. All hindgut should first be placed in the gastrointestinal tract. The most common life-threatening condition of the cloacal exstrophy patient relates to insufficient gastrointestinal resorption. In this patient, placing even a short segment of hindgut at the terminal end of the small bowel corrected a significant problem with chronic fluid loss.

Case 3

A 46,XY cloacal exstrophy patient underwent primary closure as a newborn. He had an adequate phallus for genitourinary reconstruction as a male child. The scrotum was joined in the midline, and an epispadiac penis was present without evidence of diphallus. There was no significant omphalocele. He underwent separation of exstrophy bowel from bladder halves, tubularization of the rudimentary hindgut, and creation of an end-fecal colostomy. The posterior bladder was then closed after paraexstrophy flaps were created, and the urethra was divided distal to the verumontanum. This allowed the proximal urethra to fall back to a dependent position in the pelvis and permit symphyseal closure. Paraexstrophy flaps were anastomosed to the prostatic urethra. Tubularization of the bladder neck region was accomplished, followed by closure of the anterior wall of the bladder.

The patient developed a stricture of the bladder neck that required transurethral incision at 1 year of age. At 2 1/2 years he underwent bladder neck tubularization and epispadias repair with complete division of corporeal bodies and Z-plasties of the dorsal tunica albuginea of the corporeal bodies. Six months after the repair the patient was voiding periodically, not dribbling continuously. He had begun to potty train.

Comment. This patient represents the "good end" of the cloacal exstrophy spectrum, which permitted primary closure and male assignment. Because we were able to bring the bladder neck deep in the pelvis behind the symphysis, there was a good potential for primary urinary continence (he had no spinal malformation).

Summary

The most important operation for the cloacal exstrophy patient is primary closure (staged or not). If this is done well, subsequent procedures are facilitated. Further reconstructive efforts for continence often involve augmentation of the bladder and a continence procedure, depending on innervation and anatomy. The Mitrofanoff principle has proved to be a reliable continence mechanism, and the orthotopic ureteral urethra can be used in this patient group. The disadvantage is the need for intermittent catheterization. In the cloacal exstrophy group, the least effective continence mechanism is the Young-Dees-Leadbetter bladder neck reconstruction. The stomach is ideal for patients requiring cystoplasty or creation of a continent urinary reservoir. All efforts should be made to produce an orthotopic urethra, thus avoiding the "double stoma" once universal to all cloacal exstrophy patients.[9, 10]

Creativity is generally required in the management of these patients, but is particularly important in constructing an adequate vagina in those 46,XY patients converted to the female sex. We recommend using all available tissue other than bowel. A Hartmann pouch, a native bladder, or an isolated segment of ureter for vaginoplasty has been successfully used. Long-term follow-up will be required to permit comment on the ultimate success. The presence of adequate phallic structure may allow the XY cloacal exstrophy patient to function normally in the male role.

Editorial Comment
Craig A. Peters

Cloacal exstrophy is one of the most devastating congenital anomalies compatible with long-term survival. Management requires a thorough understanding of its embryological anatomy and effective reconstructive strategies. Of principal importance is the relationship of the bowel and bladder plates. The former is also descriptively termed the lateral vesicointestinal fissure, and this may be seen when the prolapsed ileum and appendices are reduced into the abdomen. Failure to recognize these relationships may lead to excessive damage during efforts to separate the enteric and vesical components. The embryological descriptions within this chapter should be studied carefully.

The issue of sex reversal in males with cloacal exstrophy is a controversial and difficult one for which little objective information is available. The emphasis by Drs. Mitchell and Carr on individualization of each child is critical. The decision in terms of sex of rearing is a life-long one that must be made quickly and definitively.

Finally, it cannot be overemphasized that preservation and functionalization of as much of the intestinal tract as possible early in life is critical. Not only will this affect the nutritional development of the child, but it will also have a significant impact on later genitourinary reconstructive options. Nothing should be wasted.

REFERENCES

1. Rickham PP. Vesico-intestinal fissure. Arch Dis Child 35:97, 1960.
2. Lund DP, Hendren WH. Cloacal exstrophy: Experience with 20 cases. J Pediatr Surg 28:1360, 1993.
3. Gray SW, Skandalakis JE. Embryology for Surgeons. Philadelphia, WB Saunders, 1972, p 519.
4. Warner BW, Ziegler MM. Exstrophy of the cloaca. In Ashcraft KW, Holder TM, eds. Pediatric Surgery, 2nd ed. Philadelphia, WB Saunders, 1993, p 393.
5. Diamond DA, Jeffs RD. Cloacal exstrophy: A 22-year experience. J Urol 133:779, 1985.
6. Hurwitz RS, Manzoni GAM, Ransley PG, Stephans FD. Cloacal exstrophy: A report of 34 cases. J Urol 138:1060, 1987.
7. Stolar CJH, Randolph JG, Flanigan LP. Cloacal exstrophy: Individualized management through a staged surgical approach. J Pediatr Surg 25:505, 1990.
8. Mitchell ME, Brito CG, Rink RC. Cloacal exstrophy reconstruction for urinary continence. J Urol 144:554, 1990.
9. Gearhart JP, Jeffs RD. Techniques to create urinary continence in the cloacal exstrophy patient. J Urol 146:616, 1991.
10. Husmann DA, McLorie GA, Churchill BM. Phallic reconstruction in cloacal exstrophy. J Urol 142:563, 1989.

Chapter 111

Augmentation Cystoplasty

Richard C. Rink and Mark C. Adams

On the list of major advances in urology over the past several years, the use of gastrointestinal segments for lower urinary tract reconstruction must be near the top. The use of these segments to keep the lower urinary tract intact is now commonplace, and the indications frequently extend to many areas once thought to be absolute contradictions, such as in patients with neurogenic dysfunction or pretransplant patients. Experience with bladder augmentation started a trail that has now led to total lower urinary tract reconstruction in the form of reservoirs and neobladders.

The goals of bladder augmentation are to provide a large-capacity, compliant, and noncontractile urinary storage vesicle. Years of experience have shown the benefits this can provide in protecting the upper urinary tract from high intravesical pressures and in providing continence (the two main indications). Many technical refinements over the years have helped to provide an even more compliant, less contractile bladder. It is now realized that all gastrointestinal segments can achieve these desired results. It is also accepted that each segment has its own inherent advantages and disadvantages. Unfortunately, bowel is not a perfect physiological replacement for native bladder, and some negative effects of bladder augmentation are potentially serious. To avoid these complications and negative side effects, multiple other tissues and synthetic substances have been tried as a bladder substitute, but thus far only the gastrointestinal tract has met with long-term success for bladder augmentation. This chapter focuses on the use of gastrointestinal segments for augmentation cystoplasty, and includes a brief discussion of ureteral cystoplasty.

PREOPERATIVE MANAGEMENT

Evaluation of the total patient is imperative before bladder augmentation. Although it is obviously im-

portant to focus on the anatomy of the lower urinary tract, failure to recognize the patient's physical limitations, social environment, and overall urinary tract dynamics can yield disastrous results. For example, the wheelchair-bound patient may be unable to perform clean intermittent catheterization (CIC) through the native urethra and thus unable to empty the augmented bladder. The patient with poor upper extremity function may be unable to grasp a catheter at all. Another example is that of a standard length of bowel segment used for augmentation that may not provide enough capacity for the child with a severe concentrating defect who generates very high urine volumes.

Appropriately performed urodynamic and radiographical evaluations are essential preoperatively. If bladder augmentation is being performed to achieve continence, not only must the bladder dynamics be well understood, but also the bladder neck/sphincter dynamics. Even with the provision of a large-capacity, compliant reservoir, incontinence may persist if there is inadequate urethral resistance. A voiding cystourethrogram (VCUG) and a functional upper tract study (intravenous pyelogram or radionuclide scan) should be obtained preoperatively. Vesicoureteral reflux or urinary obstruction discovered preoperatively should be corrected at the time of the intestinocystoplasty.

Serum chemistry readings, including creatinine and electrolyte levels, should be evaluated preoperatively, and their implications for the choice of the various gastrointestinal segments understood. The use of ileum or colon will worsen any preexisting acidosis and may result in significant hyperchloremic metabolic acidosis. The reverse is the case when stomach is used, with a potential for hypochloremic metabolic alkalosis. These both appear to be more significant in patients with renal insufficiency. If there is concern regarding a concentrating defect, 24-hour urine volumes should be documented. The patient should not have to empty more often than every 4 hours. In any patient undergoing bladder augmentation, catheterization must be easily achieved or an alternative catheterizable channel must be provided. Some patients may be able to void spontaneously after surgery, but it is much more advisable for all parties involved in the care of the patient to assume that CIC will always be necessary.

All patients undergo mechanical bowel preparation and receive standard antibiotics on the day before surgery. Any urinary tract infection must be treated and sterile urine documented preoperatively.

Selection of a bowel segment is governed partly by the patient's circumstances and partly by the surgeon's choice. A number of patient factors may lead the surgeon to choose a particular portion of the gastrointestinal tract for a particular patient. For example, in a patient who has undergone previous irradiation of the pelvis, it may be best to choose a segment outside the field of radiation, such as transverse colon or stomach. In patients with a potential for development of the short gut syndrome (e.g., those with cloacal exstrophy), the use of stomach would prevent further loss of bowel. In the patient with a neurogenic bladder, the ileocecal valve should not be used, in order to avoid diarrhea. Submucosal tunnels for reimplantation to provide an antireflux or continence mechanism are most easily created in colon or stomach. In patients with significant renal insufficiency, the use of stomach may prevent further acidosis. When achievement of the most compliant, capacious bladder is the only goal, as is the case for most patients, ileum appears to be the best choice.[5]

Lastly, bladder augmentation is a significant operative procedure with lifelong implications, and is frequently part of an even larger total lower urinary tract reconstructive effort. The patient and family must understand the benefits, as well as all the potential risks, and be committed to achieving success in arriving at the desired outcome.

OPERATIVE TECHNIQUE

After administration of general anesthesia, the patient is placed in the dorsal lithotomy position. Cystoscopy is performed to evaluate any potential previously undetected anatomical abnormalities that might affect the surgery or postoperative care. If procedures other than bladder augmentation are to be performed, e.g., ureteral reimplantation or bladder neck reconstruction, the bladder is left full to provide easy exposure of the bladder through the lower abdominal incision. If intestinocystoplasty is the lone procedure, the bladder is emptied to allow easy entrance into the peritoneal cavity. The patient is placed back in the supine position with all pressure points carefully padded, and antibiotic solution is applied to the entire abdomen and genitalia.

Usually a midline incision from pubis to just above the umbilicus is carried out for intestinocystoplasty. This is extended to the xiphoid for gastrocystoplasty. In patients who have had no previous abdominal surgery, a lower abdominal transverse incision can be used, but this is not generally recommended. The peritoneum is not opened until completion of any bladder neck surgery or ureteral reimplantation into the native bladder, to minimize third-space fluid loss. The patient should be well hydrated throughout the procedure.

URETERAL BLADDER AUGMENTATION

Ureteral bladder augmentation has several advantages over intestinocystoplasty. The patient's own urothelium with muscular backing is used, which avoids mucus production, electrolyte changes, and presumably the potential for malignant degeneration.[1] Ureterocystoplasty allows bladder capacity and bladder compliance to be improved to a degree similar to that with intestinocystoplasty.[1, 2] Unfortunately, it is generally applicable only in the patient with a nonfunctioning kidney associated with massive hydroureteronephrosis. Therefore, in spite of the advantages, the potential patient population will remain small.

In general, a midline incision should be used to provide the best exposure and allow for gastric or intestinocystoplasty should the ureter prove unsatisfactory. Ureterocystoplasty has, however, been successfully performed with two separate extraperitoneal incisions, but we would not recommend this. After a midline incision is made, the colon overlying the affected kidney is mobilized to allow complete exposure of the entire kidney and megaureter. Extreme care is taken when mobilizing the kidney to preserve all the blood supply to the ureter and renal pelvis (Fig. 111–1). The gonadal vessels should be preserved with the ureter. After ligation of the renal vasculature, the renal pelvis is preserved with the ureter and the kidney removed. The ureter is then held with stay sutures and mobilized in a "no-touch" fashion to the level of the bladder. If the ureter remains healthy and is large enough to provide adequate capacity, the bladder is opened in a clamshell fashion, extending into the affected ureteral orifice (Fig. 111–2) . The ureter is not detached from the orifice. The ureter is then detubularized throughout its entirety opposite the ureteral blood supply. The detubularized ureter and pelvis are then reconfigured, usually in a U shape, with running, locking 3-0 polyglycolic suture (Fig. 111–3). This ureteral flap is then anastomosed to the bladder in the same fashion as in the following description of intestinocystoplasty. A large-bore suprapubic tube is placed

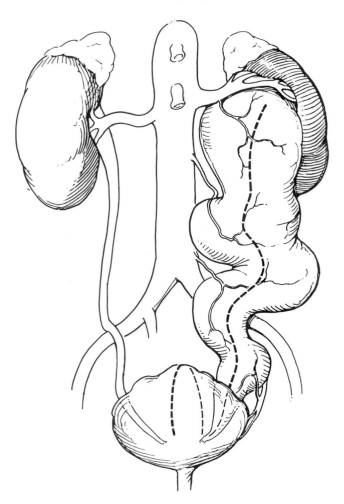

Figure 111–1. Proposed incision for detubularization of the megaureter and hydronephrotic renal pelvis, and for bivalving of the native bladder for ureteral cystoplasty.

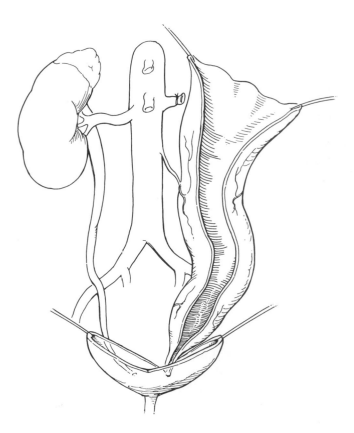

Figure 111–2. Ureteral cystoplasty. The nonfunctioning kidney is removed and the ureteral blood supply preserved. The ureter is detubularized and the bladder opened in the sagittal plane to the ureteral orifice posteriorly.

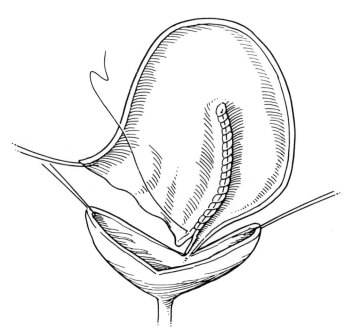

Figure 111-3. The megaureter, which remains attached to the bladder, is reconfigured in a U shape.

through the native bladder wall and secured (Fig. 111–4). Urethral and ureteral catheterization is dependent on the associated procedures.

GASTRIC OR INTESTINAL CYSTOPLASTY

Native Bladder Management

There is controversy regarding how the native bladder should be managed. Many have recommended a supratrigonal excision of the "diseased" bladder. Others have felt that the native bladder can be preserved as long as the bladder is widely opened (Fig. 111–5). This prevents a narrow-mouthed anastomosis, which might result in the augmentation segment acting as a diverticulum with resultant stasis and poor drainage. Both techniques have been successful. We prefer a large sagittal incision of the native bladder without detrusor excision in children. Anastomosis to the bivalved bladder is technically easier than to the trigone alone, and the native bladder adds to overall capacity.

Intestinal Segment Management

At this time, it is clear that the intestinal segment should never be left in its tubular form for anastomosis. Hinman[3] and Koff[4] have demonstrated the advantages of detubularization and reconfiguration of the bowel segment. Detubularization is accomplished with cutting current; reconfiguration is performed with absorbable suture. The resultant reservoir should be as spherical as possible. This will maximize the volume of urine that can be stored, improve overall compliance, blunt bowel contractions, and require a shorter segment of bowel to achieve the same capacity. The bowel segment used must be large enough to provide adequate capacity, and unless this is otherwise contraindicated one should err on the side of making the bladder large. Augmentation cystoplasty with varying segments will be described with ileocystoplasty as the model. The handling of the native bladder, technique of anastomosis, and placement of tubes for bladder and perivesical drainage are the same for each gastrointestinal segment.

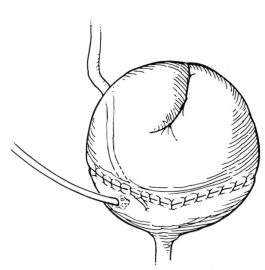

Figure 111-4. Ureteral cystoplasty completed. The suprapubic tube exists through the native bladder.

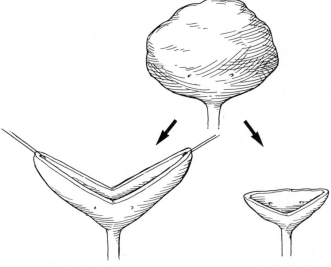

Figure 111-5. Two ways of handling the native bladder: (1) a sagittal incision to bivalve the bladder and (2) supratrigonal cystectomy.

ILEOCYSTOPLASTY

After the abdominal incision is made, a self-retaining ring retractor is placed. The terminal ileum is identified and first inspected by transilluminating its mesentery to identify the vasculature. A segment of ileum at least 10 to 15 cm proximal to the ileocecal valve and measuring 20 to 40 cm in length (depending on patient size and bladder capacity desired) is selected. Vessel loops passed through the mesentery are used as markers at either end of the selected bowel segment. After it is ensured that the segment will easily reach the bladder, the mesentery at each end is cleared from the bowel for a short distance, and a window is created by dividing vessels between small clamps and ligating these vessels with silk suture. Parallel bowel clamps are angled 45 degrees away from the mesentery at either end of the proposed segment. The bowel is divided and the clamps remain on the segment for augmentation. A standard two-layer ileoileostomy is performed, or a stapled bowel anastomosis can be done (Fig. 111–6).

The ileal segment for augmentation is next irrigated clear with 0.25 percent neomycin solution. This segment is incised on its antimesenteric border along the entire length with the cutting current. The opened ileal segment can then be reconfigured in several forms (Fig. 111–7). The most common reconfiguration uses a single fold of the ileum in half, creating a U-shaped flap (Fig. 111–8). Longer segments may be folded a third time into an S shape, or the U-shaped segment may be folded on itself to create a "cup" (Fig. 111–8). The ileal margins may be anastomosed

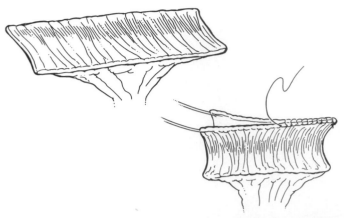

Figure 111–7. The detubularized ileal segment is folded in half and the medial edges are anastomosed to form a U-shaped flap.

by a one- or two-layer technique. The bladder is now opened in the sagittal plane with electrocautery from near the bladder neck anteriorly to a posterior position approximately 2 cm proximal to the trigone. The lateral edges of the bladder are held open by placing stay sutures at the apex and then securing them over the ring retractor. The ileal flap is anastomosed to the bladder by a running, interlocking 3-0 chromic inner layer and an outer layer of running 3-0 polyglycolic suture. This is most easily performed by starting in the midline posteriorly, running up the bladder wall in either direction to the stay sutures (Fig. 111–9).

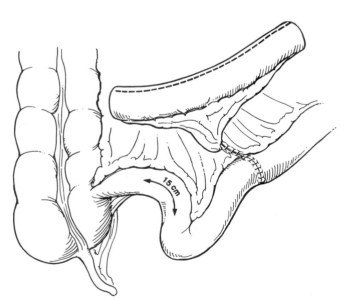

Figure 111–6. Beginning 15 cm from the ileocecal valve, an ileal segment 20 to 40 cm in length is removed from the gastrointestinal tract and a two-layer ileoileostomy is performed. The proposed incision for detubularization of the ileal segment along the antimesenteric border is shown.

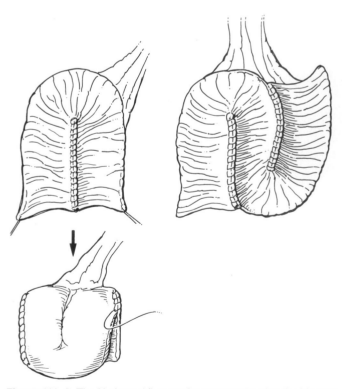

Figure 111–8. The U-shaped flap can be anastomosed to the bladder or further folded into a cup shape. Longer ileal segments may be folded three times to form an S-shaped flap.

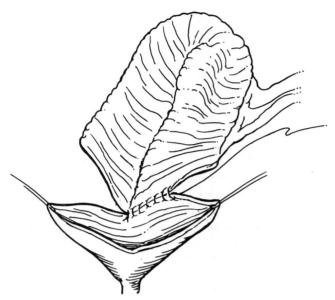

Figure 111–9. A U-shaped ileal flap is anastomosed to the bivalved bladder, beginning in the midline posteriorly.

Next, the outer running layer is created, starting in the midline posteriorly. A suprapubic tube is placed in the native bladder and secured. A urethral catheter may be left indwelling, its size and type dependent on whether urethral or bladder neck surgery was carried out. The ileum is then folded over the bladder anteriorly, and the remainder of the anastomosis is completed by again starting in the midline and working toward the stay sutures on either side. The bladder is filled with saline through the suprapubic tube to make certain the anastomosis is watertight; any leaks are oversewn. The mesenteric window at the bowel anastomosis is closed and the entire wound irrigated. A drain is placed near the bladder and brought out of the pelvis through a separate skin incision. The suprapubic tube is also brought through a separate stab incision. The bladder surrounding the tube is secured to the underside of the abdominal wall, and the abdominal incision is closed in layers.

Sigmoidcystoplasty

The initial exposure for sigmoidcystoplasty is the same as for ileocystoplasty. The sigmoid colon is identified and the small bowel packed superiorly. The sigmoid colon is then mobilized by incising the posterior peritoneum along the white line of Toldt. A 15- to 20-cm segment is necessary and is selected after transilluminating the mesentery and identifying the vascular arcade. One must be certain that the segment will reach the bladder and that the bowel can be easily reanastomosed. The ends of the proposed colonic segment for augmentation are marked with vessel loops as in ileocystoplasty, and the sur-

rounding area of the abdomen is packed to prevent contamination. The mesentery is divided, two bowel clamps are placed perpendicular to the bowel at each end of the isolated segment, and the bowel is divided. A standard two-layer bowel closure is performed using an outer layer of interrupted 4-0 silk and a running interlocking polyglycolic suture layer, starting in the midline and working laterally in either direction (Fig. 111–10). The clamps on the isolated segment are removed and the bowel is irrigated clear with 0.25 percent neomycin solution. The segment is detubularized between the teniae as previously described. This opened segment may be handled in several ways. Mitchell has popularized closing the two ends of the sigmoid segment in two layers, after which the opened antimesenteric boarders can be anastomosed to the sagitally bivalved bladder in either the transverse or sagittal plane (Fig. 111–11).[6] This anastomosis is done in a two-layer manner as described above for ileocystoplasty. Gonzalez has had excellent results reconfiguring the sigmoid segment more in a fashion similar to the previously described ileal segment (Fig. 111–12).[7] The anastomosis to the bladder following this reconfiguration is in two layers as described above for ileocystoplasty, and the sigmoid mesenteric window is closed. Drains and a suprapubic tube are used as previously noted. Omentum is draped over the anastomosis, both the augmented bladder and the abdomen are irrigated, and the abdomen is closed in layers.

Ileocecal Cystoplasty

Simple cecocystoplasty is now rarely performed and therefore will not be discussed. It has been largely replaced by ileocecocystoplasty. The abdomen is opened as previously described. The cecum and

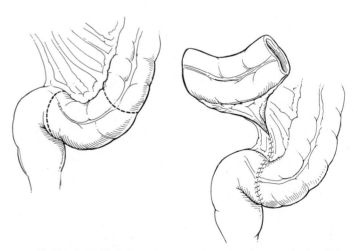

Figure 111–10. The proposed segment for sigmoid augmentation (15 to 20 cm) is identified and removed from the gastrointestinal tract, and a colocolostomy is performed.

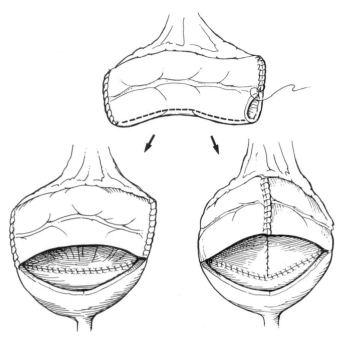

Figure 111–11. The ends of the sigmoid segment may be closed and the antimesenteric border opened. This segment can now be anastomosed to the bivalved bladder in either the sagittal or transverse plane.

right colon are identified and the remainder of the bowel is packed superomedially. The cecum and ascending colon are then mobilized by incising the peritoneum along the white line of Toldt up to and around the hepatic flexure. The mesentery of the cecum and ascending colon is transilluminated, the vasculature is visualized, and a vessel loop is passed through the mesentery distal to the ileocolic artery. This should allow isolation of a 10- to 15-cm segment

of colon. Approximately 15 to 30 cm of ileum is necessary, depending on the technique used (Fig. 111–13). Before isolation of the segment, one must be certain the segment has been mobilized enough to easily reach the bladder. After an appendectomy, unless the appendix is to be used, the mesentery at either end of the proposed segment is divided as previously described. A two-layer ileocolostomy is performed. The bowel clamps on the ileum are angled 45 degrees to allow the ileal opening to equal the size of the ascending colon for end-to-end anastomosis. Likewise, a stapled anastomosis may be performed.

The isolated segment is irrigated clear with 0.25 percent neomycin solution and then opened on its antimesenteric border through its entirety across the ileocecal valve. In the standard ileocecal augmentation, the segment of ileum taken was the same length as that of the cecum. The opened edges of the ileum are folded onto the open cecum as a patch and the two are anastomosed in a one- or two-layer fashion, leaving a large enough opening to fit easily on the bivalved bladder (Fig. 111–14). Alternatively, a Mainz ileocecocystoplasty can be performed by selecting an ileal segment twice the length of the cecal segment (Fig. 111–15). The medial edge of the opened colonic segment is anastomosed to the first portion of the opened ileal segment. The remaining ileum is

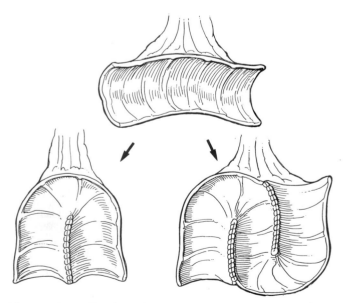

Figure 111–12. The detubularized sigmoid segment may be folded into a U or S shape for anastomosis to the native bladder.

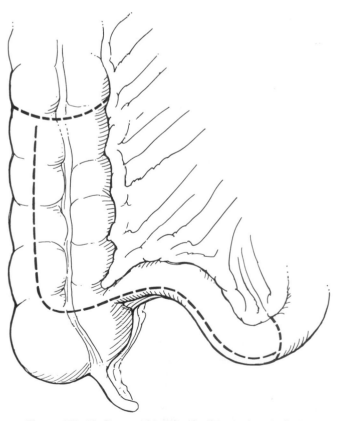

Figure 111–13. Proposed incision for ileocecal cystoplasty.

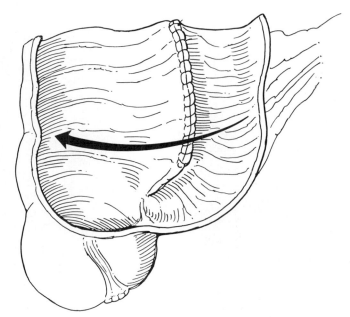

Figure 111–14. The ileum and cecum are detubularized and the two are anastomosed for a composite ileocecal flap.

folded, and the first and second portions of ileum are anastomosed. The mesenteric window at the colostomy is closed. Suprapubic tube placement is through the native bladder wall, and a urethral catheter is placed as previously noted (Fig. 111–16). Perivesical drains exit through separate stab incisions. The bladder and abdomen are irrigated with saline and the abdomen is closed in layers. In a patient with foreshortened ureters, an advantage of ileocecal cystoplasty is that a tail of ileum can be used to bridge the gap between ureters and bladder. In children, ileocecocystoplasty is rarely used because it sacrifices the ileocecal valve. This is particularly true in patients with neurogenic dysfunction, in whom loss of the ileocecal valve may cause diarrhea.

GASTROCYSTOPLASTY

Patient preparation for gastrocystoplasty is the same as for augmentation with other segments. Laparotomy extending to the xiphoid process is necessary for good exposure of the stomach. The stomach is gently grasped to allow inspection. Particular consideration is given to the gastroepiploic vessels, one of which will be used as a vascular pedicle. Once it is determined that the stomach may be used, the greater omentum is mobilized off the transverse colon in an avascular plane. For augmentation with gastric corpus or body, either the right or left gastroepiploic artery may be used as a vascular pedicle. The gastroepiploic anatomy is variable in humans. In most cases the right gastroepiploic artery is predominant and is used as the vascular pedicle.

A wedge-shaped segment, including both the anterior and posterior wall of the stomach, is used for augmentation. This segment does not extend all the way across the stomach to the lesser curvature in order to avoid injury to branches of the vagus nerve, which control gastric emptying. The segment used is 9 to 10 cm in length along the greater curvature. The segment to be isolated must be distal enough on the

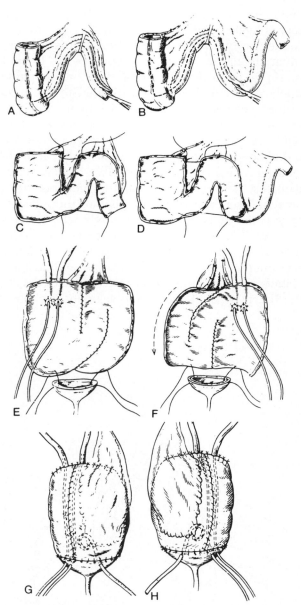

Figure 111–15. Mainz ileocecal augmentation. *A,* The proposed ileocecal segment for augmentation is identified. *B,* The segment is opened on its antimesenteric border. *C* and *D,* The opened ileocecal edyes are anastomosed. *E* and *F,* The segment may be rotated 180 degrees for ease of ureteral implantation if necessary. *G* and *H,* The ileocecal segment is anastomosed to the opened bladder. An ileal segment twice the length of the cecal segment is detubularized and the edges are anastomosed. The ureters can be reimplanted into the cecum if necessary before anastomosis to the bivalved bladder. (From Thuroff JW, et al. In King LR, Stone AR, Webster GD, eds. Bladder Reconstruction and Continent Urinary Diversion. Chicago, Year Book, 1987, pp 257–258.)

gastroepiploic pedicle to reach the pelvis without tension. A silk suture placed along the gastroepiploic pedicle can be held at the origin of that vessel and swung down to the pelvis to make sure that the segment will reach the bladder after isolation. In most cases the right gastroepiploic artery is used as the pedicle, and short branches of the vessel to the pylorus and antrum are divided proximal to the intended segment. These vessels should be ligated near the stomach and away from the gastroepiploic artery to avoid injury to that vessel. The right gastroepiploic artery is ligated and divided distally at the end of the intended segment. A window through the mesentery is then created at that level (Fig. 111–17). If the left gastroepiploic artery is to be used as a pedicle, branches from the vessel are divided to the fundus and high corpus. The pedicle will swing down from its origin at the spleen rather than from the pylorus.

The segment to be isolated is then marked, and parallel bowel clamps are placed on either side of the proposed incision. It is not possible to place clamps adequately across the apex of the incision into the stomach. There are large branches of the left gastric artery at the apex, and these vessels will bleed dramatically if not controlled. It is possible to suture ligate those vessels prospectively before incision of the segment. They should be suture ligated just above the incision where they run in the serosa of the stomach (Fig. 111–18). The isolated segment is rhomboid

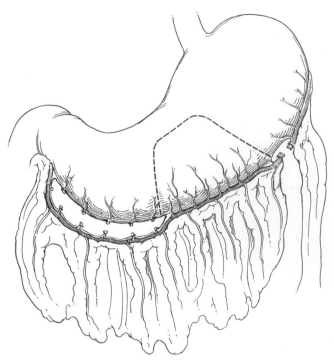

Figure 111–17. A rhomboid-shaped stomach wedge is identified. The right gastroepiploic artery is used as the vascular pedicle and is ligated distal to the wedge.

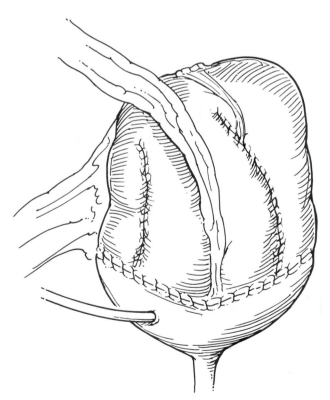

Figure 111–16. Completed ileocecal augmentation. The suprapubic tube is brought out through the native bladder.

shaped when opened and fits nicely on the bivalved bladder. Both the edges of the isolated segment and the native stomach must be carefully inspected to achieve adequate hemostasis. The native stomach is closed in two layers, including an outer seromuscular layer of permanent suture. The isolated segment is then mobilized to the pelvis (Fig. 111–19).

The gastroepiploic vascular pedicle must not be free-floating in the abdomen. There are two ways to place the pedicle in or along the retroperitoneum. With one technique, a window is made in the transverse colon mesentery on the appropriate side of the middle colic vessel. Another window is made through the mesentery of the terminal ileum. The isolated gastric segment and pedicle are then passed through these two windows, and the omentum running along the vessel is approximated to the posterior peritoneum between the two windows with interrupted sutures. Alternatively, the entire cecum and right colon around the hepatic flexure may be mobilized and the gastric segment and pedicle may be truly placed in the retroperitoneum. The right colon can then be loosely reapproximated along the white line. Occasionally, when the segment is brought into the pelvis, the portion of the segment proximal on the gastroepiploic pedicle may not reach the bladder without tension. Further mobilization can be obtained by mobilizing the gastroepiploic artery closer to its origin. It may also be necessary to divide the first few branches of the gastroepiploic artery to that

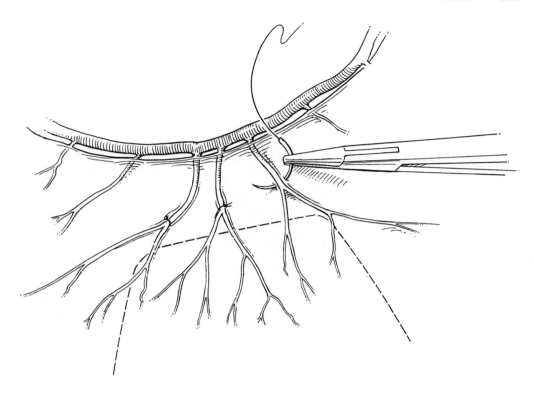

Figure 111–18. Prospective ligation of the branches of the gastric artery near the apex of the gastric wedge.

portion of the isolated gastric segment. The division of these vessels may provide the mobilization necessary and will not devascularize the isolated segment owing to the rich submucosal plexus. Rarely, it has been necessary to close some of the stomach segment to itself to a point that reaches the bladder without tension.

The gastric segment is approximated to the bivalved native bladder in two layers to provide a wide anastomosis (Fig. 111–20). Drainage tubes and drains are used as described. A nasogastric tube is used for bowel decompression only until bowel function returns; no gastrostomy tube is necessary. Postoperative care is not different from that for other patients after augmentation with other segments, except that patients after gastrocystoplasty are maintained on a histamine-2 (H_2) blocker for 6 weeks to decrease acid production and promote healing. Many patients in the immediate postoperative period after gastrocystoplasty have remarkably colored brown urine. This discoloration is probably secondary to blood exposed to acid in the healing bladder and does not represent any problem.

POSTOPERATIVE MANAGEMENT

Care in the postoperative period is similar regardless of the gastrointestinal segment used. Parenteral antibiotics are maintained until the patient is drinking and eating. The fluid and electrolyte status is closely monitored, as large fluid shifts are common in these lengthy procedures. A nasogastric tube remains indwelling until bowel function returns. Copious mucus production is the norm in the early postoperative period, necessitating routine bladder irrigation three times a day and as needed if urinary drainage slows. The patient and family are taught bladder irrigation, which continues twice daily after discharge. Perivesical drains are left in place until a cystogram 1 week postoperatively has demonstrated no extravasation. Any urethral catheter is then removed, and the patient is discharged with the suprapubic tube in place for another 2 weeks. Three weeks postoperatively, CIC is begun every 2 to 3 hours during the day and once at night. This catheterization time interval is increased slowly to every 4 hours during the day and 8 hours at night and continues indefinitely, as do daily bladder irrigations. CIC is discontinued only if the patient repeatedly demonstrates the ability to void to completion. Anticholinergic medications may be necessary in the early postoperative period while the augmentation segment stretches. H_2 blockers, as noted above, are used in the early postoperative period after gastrocystoplasty.

Follow-up evaluation of the upper urinary tract by renal ultrasound is obtained 6 weeks, 6 months, and 1 year postoperatively. A cystogram is repeated at the 6-month visit. Serum electrolyte, blood urea nitrogen, and creatinine values are also obtained at each of these visits. Urine culture and sensitivity is obtained at 3-month intervals during the first year. In the stable patient, yearly evaluation is then carried out by renal ultrasound, KUB (kidney, ureter, and bladder), urine

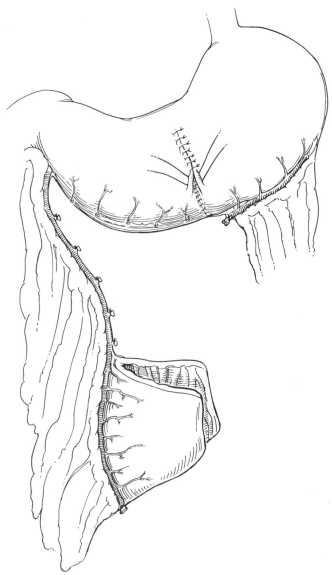

Figure 111–19. The stomach wedge based on the right gastroepiploic artery is brought down to the bladder. The stomach is closed in two layers.

culture and sensitivity, and serum chemistry studies. Urodynamic evaluation is made only when the clinical situation warrants it, such as when there is continued incontinence.

COMPLICATIONS OF GASTROINTESTINAL CYSTOPLASTY

Mucus Production

Mucus production is greatest after colocystoplasty and least after gastrocystoplasty. Ileal mucus production is intermediate. Mucus may become a significant problem in children, in whom small-bore catheters are easily occluded. Mucus production tends to in-

crease with urinary infection. It has also been blamed as constituting a nidus for stone formation. Fortunately, the production is minimal with stomach and decreases over time with ileum. This is not true for colon, however.

We insist on bladder irrigation with normal saline until the mucus clears, three times daily during postoperative hospitalization. This is decreased to twice a day for the next 3 weeks and then continues daily forever, regardless of the gastrointestinal segment used. Hypertonic saline and acetylcysteine sodium (Mucomyst) have been used to disrupt mucous plugs but are not recommended for daily use.

Urinary Tract Infections

Virtually every patient on CIC alone will at some time have bacteriuria. The addition of an intestinal segment increases the frequency with which this occurs. Symptomatic lower urinary tract infections were noted in 22.7 percent of our ileocystoplasty patients, 17.3 percent of our sigmoidcystoplasty patients, and only 8 percent of those with gastrocystoplasty.[5]

As a general rule, we do not recommend treatment of asymptomatic bacteriuria unless the isolated bacteria are capable of splitting urea. Reliable patients are given antibiotics to self-treat for a 2-day course at the first sign or symptom of urinary infection (e.g., dysuria, foul-smelling urine). Alternatively, bladder irrigation with an antibiotic solution may be successful in clearing bacteriuria. Only rarely are patients placed on continual antibiotic therapy. If recurrent symptomatic infections occur, one must be certain the patient is emptying to completion at frequent intervals and that no foreign body or stone is present.

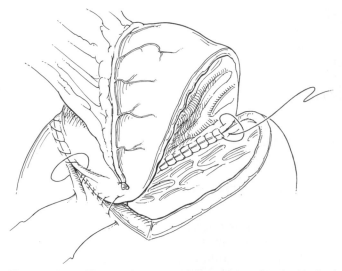

Figure 111–20. The gastric segment is anastomosed to the bivalved bladder.

Bladder Calculi

With further experience and longer follow-up of patients undergoing augmentation cystoplasty, the reported incidence of bladder calculi increases. Palmer et al reported a 52 percent stone incidence.[8] The overwhelming majority of stones are struvite and are found in the augmented bladder. In patients catheterizing through an abdominal wall stoma, the incidence is greater than in those catheterizing through the native urethra.[9] Factors such as urea-splitting bacteria, hypercalciuria, residual urine, mucus, and foreign bodies such as staples have all been implicated as being etiological. Although the exact reason for this high incidence remains unknown, every effort should be made to eliminate these factors in the hope that stone formation may be prevented. Bladder calculi have not been found after gastrocystoplasty.

Electrolyte Imbalance

In virtually all patients after intestinocystoplasty the serum chloride increases from the preoperative level, but this rarely results in significant metabolic acidosis. Patients with preexisting renal insufficiency are much more likely to have these electrolyte problems. Ileum and colon actively transport urinary chloride. The effect on the patient of this chloride transport depends on the length of the bowel segment used, the length of time urine is in contact with bowel, and the renal function status. Any patient becoming acidotic should be given bicarbonate therapy.

Gastric segments result in a net chloride loss with the potential for metabolic alkalosis. Profound hypochloremic metabolic alkalosis has occurred during a viral illness. Nausea and vomiting results in further chloride loss and the patient may be unable to replace the fluid and electrolytes. Those undergoing gastrocystoplasty must be made aware of this potential problem.

Perforation

Perforation of the augmented bladder has been noted in nearly all large series and has occurred with every gastrointestinal segment. Sadly, this has proved lethal in some patients. Any patient with an augmented bladder who has abdominal pain, nausea, vomiting, distention, and fever must be considered to have a bladder rupture until it is proved otherwise. The diagnosis has at times been elusive, but cystography, computed tomography, and ultrasonography have all been helpful.

The cause of perforation is apparently multifactorial. Rupture occurs most often in patients with impaired abdominal sensation who overdistend the bladder. High urethral resistance is generally present, and many patients experience high-pressure intermittent contractions. These factors are thought to result in areas of ischemia susceptible to perforation. In general, immediate exploration and drainage are warranted.

Other Potential Complications

In any patient having a large portion of the terminal ileum removed from the gastrointestinal tract, there is a potential for vitamin B_{12} deficiency and megaloblastic anemia. This is rare in patients undergoing an augmentation procedure; if it does occur, it may not be apparent for 4 to 5 years postoperatively. It should be prevented by leaving an adequate segment of distal ileum.

Tumor formation has been reported rarely after augmentation. The concern regarding neoplasia is present because of the well-known risk of adenocarcinoma after ureterosigmoidostomy and in view of experimental data in animals.[10] As more children undergo augmentation, a population having a very long life span has resulted. One must establish a surveillance program for this group. Furthermore, the need to discuss this risk preoperatively is mandatory.

One third of patients develop the hematuria-dysuria syndrome after gastrocystoplasty.[11] Although generally responsive to oral H_2 blockers, this is sometimes difficult to treat and painful and disruptive for the patient. It has been noted to occur more commonly in those with renal insufficiency.[11] Again, the patient and family must be made aware of this potential problem preoperatively.

Summary

Although all gastrointestinal segments can be used to achieve a large-capacity, compliant reservoir, the clinical situation may warrant use of a particular segment. The surgeon must be comfortable with all the above techniques and fully aware of the advantages and disadvantages of each segment. Meticulous attention to detail in the preoperative evaluation and in the surgical technique will provide the best result. However, ultimate success is also largely dependent on the patient's and family's motivation. This aspect must never be forgotten. Augmentation cystoplasty carries lifelong implications and all parties involved must understand that close follow-up is mandatory forever.

Editorial Comment

Craig A. Peters

Enterocystoplasty is a key component in much of modern pediatric urological reconstruction. The various useful intestinal segments should be familiar to all reconstructive surgeons. Gastrocystoplasty has recently been widely used with good success but some element of complication. While it is very appropriate in the pretransplant patient, caution should be exercised in these patients, who may become anuric. It is in this situation that severe hematuria-dysuria and perforation have been encountered.

Our experience with perforation of augmentation cystoplasty, particularly in the myelodysplastic patient, has given us a very high degree of suspicion. The occurrence of shoulder pain in some of these patients, when associated with urinary infection, fever, sepsis, or hematuria, should be a prominent warning sign of perforation of the augmented bladder. Diaphragmatic irritation by infected intraperitoneal urine is the likely cause of this sensitive clinical sign.

The incidence of stone formation in reconstructed bladders has been reported recently and may be fairly high. We have successfully used percutaneous techniques to remove bladder stones, particularly in patients with a reconstructed bladder neck, an artificial sphincter, or a continent catheterizable stoma.

REFERENCES

1. Landau EH, Jayanthi VR, Khoury AE, et al. Bladder augmentation: Ureterocystoplasty versus ileocystoplasty. J Urol 152:716, 1994.
2. Mitchell ME, Rink RC, Adams MA. Augmentation cystoplasty implantation of artificial urinary sphincter in men and women and reconstruction of the dysfunctional urinary tract. In Walsh PC, Retik AB, Stamey TA, Vaughn ED, eds. Campbell's Urology, 6th ed. Philadelphia, WB Saunders, 1992, p 2630.
3. Hinman F Jr. Selection of intestinal segments for bladder substitution: Physical and physiological characteristics. J Urol 139:519, 1988.
4. Koff SA. Guidelines to determine size and shape of intestinal segments used for reconstruction. J Urol 140:1150, 1988.
5. Rink RC, Hollensbe D, Adams MA. Complications of bladder augmentation in children and comparison of gastrointestinal segments. AUA Update Series 14:122, 1995.
6. Mitchell ME. Use of bowel in undiversion. Urol Clin North Am 13:349, 1986.
7. Hinman F Jr. Colocystoplasty and sigmoidocystoplasty. In Atlas of Pediatric Urologic Surgery. Philadelphia, WB Saunders, 1994, p 444.
8. Palmer LS, Franco I, Kogan SJ, et al. Urolithiasis in children following augmentation cystoplasty. J Urol 150:726, 1993.
9. Blythe B, Ewalt DH, Duckett JW, Snyder HM. Lithogenic properties of enterocystoplasty. J Urol 148:575, 1992.
10. Little JE, Klee LW, Hoover DM, Rink RC. Long-term histopathologic changes observed in rats subjected to augmentation cystoplasty. J Urol 152:720, 1994.
11. Nguyen DH, Bain MA, Salmonson KL, et al. The syndrome of dysuria and hematuria in pediatric urinary reconstruction with stomach. J Urol 150:707, 1993.

Chapter 112

Continent Urinary Diversion in Children

Michael A. Keating

HISTORICAL PERSPECTIVES: CURRENT INDICATIONS

The expectations held for the lower urinary tract are extraordinary ones. The bladder must hold gradually increasing volumes of urine while maintaining low intravesical pressure; its sphincters are required to provide enough resistance to achieve continence; and both must work in concert to enable emptying to completion. Not surprisingly, a number of different pathological conditions can affect this system's unique intrinsic properties, the delicate balance of its complex interactions, or both. Common causes in children include spina bifida, bladder exstrophy, and posterior urethral valves. The progressive upper tract deterioration or relentless urinary incontinence that can result poses a significant threat to the patient's health and well-being.

Diverting urine from inhospitable bladders with noncontinent diversions can provide patients with an effective panacea. However, despite the transient efficacy, long-term follow-up has shown the prognosis for many children with these types of diversions to be suboptimal (see Chap. 104). In addition to the progressive upper urinary tract deterioration that commonly occurs, urologists must deal with patients having stomas and urinary appliances that not only alter body image but can easily scar a fragile psyche.

Historically, these two important considerations were first addressed with ureterosigmoidostomy. This, the oldest of the continent urinary diversions, provided a seemingly ideal solution to bladder exstrophy or cystectomy. In theory, the threat to the kidneys could be eliminated by creating long subtenial tunnels for the ureters and mucosa-to-mucosa anastomoses that prevented reflux. In addition, the psychosocial implications of incontinence or a stoma were obviated by the retention of urine in the rectum.

Despite its seeming simplicity, however, ureterosigmoidostomy can potentially cause as many problems as it solves. Renal deterioration continues, although the improved rates cited in contemporary series probably reflect better methods for creating effective ureterocolonic anastomoses. Another drawback is the hyperchloremic acidosis that results in most patients and can become a serious metabolic complication if renal function is marginal. Finally, the most ominous sequela of the diversion is the appearance of colonic neoplasias at or near the site of the ureteral anastomoses. An incidence estimated at between 6 and 13 percent is not insignificant, although surveillance programs could probably improve the detection and treatment of premalignant lesions. Despite an average 20-year interval between creation of the diversion and the appearance of tumors, placing patients at a 100- to 500-fold risk for developing cancer probably outweighs the benefits of the diversion in most cases. It is also important to remember that ureterosigmoidostomies cannot be used in children with neurogenic bladders who commonly have deficient anal sphincters and who constitute the largest group of potential candidates for continent urinary reconstruction. Despite these drawbacks, some clinicians continue to use ureterosigmoidostomy in select cases (see Chap. 53).

As an alternative, Bricker's ileal conduit became the urinary diversion of choice after its introduction in 1950. Simply constructed and effective, the diversion has been particularly useful in patients with limited life expectancies and remains widely used in adults after cystectomy. In contrast, its performance in children has been less encouraging. One study showed renal deterioration in nearly one half of the children who had an ileal conduit for at least a decade, which is typical of its performance in patients with extended longevity.[1] Nonrefluxing colon conduits, which, theoretically, should do a better job of protecting the upper tracts, have not performed much better. Nevertheless, enteric loops continued to be constructed in a large number of children for nearly 30 years, since a viable alternative was unavailable.

The evolution of continent urinary diversion represents one of the most significant advancements in the field during the past two decades, yet its concept was spawned around the turn of the century when a number of surgeons offered ingenious reconfigurations of the urinary and intestinal tracts. These included variations of rectal bladders, where the isolated rectum serves as a urinary reservoir and the sigmoid colon is pulled through the anal sphincter in an adjacent position (the Gersuny and Heitz-Boyer configurations), and ileocecal reservoirs that used the appendix as an efferent limb (Verhoogen in 1908 and Makkas in 1910).[2] Not surprisingly, these types of complex reconstructions, done in an era before effective antibiotics, microsurgery, and modern anesthesia, typically failed. Retrospectively, it also becomes apparent that most did not fulfill the criteria required of successful continent reservoirs (see below) and as a consequence never became widely used.

Continent reconstruction of the urinary tract did not become an option in the management of children until the 1970s, despite the fact that augmentation cystoplasty had been successfully used for more than 20 years in adults with interstitial cystitis, tuberculosis, and even cancer. In contrast, the most common causes of neuropathic bladders in the pediatric population, neurogenic dysfunction and bladder outlet obstruction, were considered absolute contraindications to enterocystoplasty. Incomplete emptying, already a component of the bladder dysfunction shown by many of these patients, was often amplified after intestinal augmentation and would ultimately defeat the purpose of the reconstruction. It was only with the introduction of clean intermittent catheterization (CIC) that the concepts of cystoplasty, undiversion, and continent enteric reservoirs became a reality for children.[3, 4] Since their reappearance, the configurations of the latter seem limited only by one's surgical creativity and the patient's "available resources."

More than 30 variations of continent diversion are described in the literature. Some have been more effective than others, but each has contributed in some way to the evolution of the field. Like most problems in urology, there is no single reconstruction that is universally applicable to every child. Flexibility is key. Any surgeon who plans to treat these children must be able to apply and even combine a number of different techniques to address patient variability and anatomical nuances. An understanding of the basic principles applicable to any continent urinary reconstruction is the focus of the discussion that follows. Where applicable, specific techniques serve to illustrate those principles.

OPTIONS IN MANAGEMENT

Unless the bladder must be or has been removed, there are two options for surgically achieving continence with a neuropathic bladder: reconstruction with an enteric augmentation or replacement with a continent diversion. The former is far more common in children. Preserving the bladder as a template for enterocystoplasty brings certain advantages. Less bowel is needed to create an adequately sized reservoir, and ureteral reimplantation may be unnecessary if reflux is not present. In many cases, however, the urinary sphincter is deficient and also requires attention. Any one of a number of procedures can be used to provide additional outlet resistance, each with its own particular advantages and drawbacks (Fig. 112–1). These increase the complexity of the reconstruction but, again, preserve apparent normalcy for the patient, since catheterization is done by way of the native urethra.

When catheterization cannot be done through the urethra because of discomfort, body habitus, or a lack of dexterity, another route for emptying must be provided and a continent catheterizable vesicostomy created. Whenever possible, the native urethra should be preserved, especially if it already provides adequate outlet resistance. If salvaged, the urethra can serve as a secondary venue for emptying and as a vent for the elevated intravesical pressures that can occur in children who commonly "forget" to catheterize. For these reasons, the benefits of reconstructing the bladder outlet in concert with enterocystoplasty usually outweigh its risks. However, in some children, especially after a number of unsuccessful surgical procedures on the bladder neck, this becomes difficult, if not impossible. When this is the case, bladder neck closure is preferable if the bladder template is salvageable. Otherwise, total bladder replacement with a continent diversion should be chosen.

Although the technical details of augmentation cystoplasty and bladder neck repair exceed the scope of this discussion, the objectives and principles of successful continent urinary reconstruction remain unchanged regardless of whether the lower urinary tract is being reconstructed or replaced with a continent diversion.

SURGICAL OBJECTIVES

To be effective, continent urinary reconstructions must mimic the characteristics of the native bladder as closely as possible. These include adequate capac-

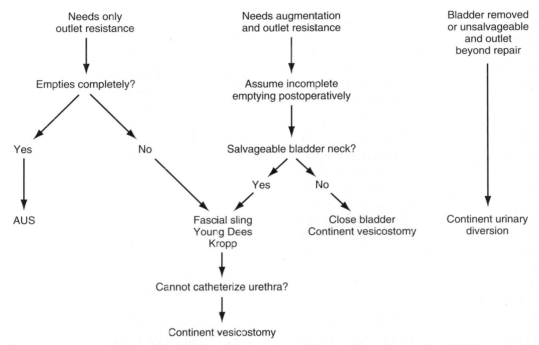

Figure 112–1. Algorithm for continent urinary reconstruction. Management options are dictated by quality of bladder and urinary sphincter and ability to catheterize. AUS, Artificial urinary sphincter.

ity, low pressures, protection of the upper urinary tract, continence, and complete emptying.

ADEQUATE CAPACITY. The size of an enteric reservoir will influence its urodynamic characteristics, the metabolic sequelae, and the frequency of catheterization needed to protect the upper urinary tract. Capacious reservoirs require less frequent emptying and have more volume to buffer the high pressures that occur when filled near capacity or that are sometimes seen from the uninhibited contractions of bowel used in their construction. Yet these advantages must be weighed against the increased absorption of solute and greater potential for bacterial overgrowth that inevitably occur if the frequency of CIC is lessened. An ideal outcome could be obtained with a large reservoir that is frequently emptied to lessen urinary contact time. A rough measure of the bladder capacity expected of a child can be obtained from the calculation: Age + 2 = Capacity (in ounces). Continent reservoirs should be constructed with this volume considered as a minimum (Fig. 112–2). The daily urinary output should also be taken into consideration when deciding on the frequency of catheterization. Asking a patient, especially an adolescent or teenager, to empty more than five or six times a day is probably unrealistic. Some children with nephrogenic diabetes insipidus make such excessive amounts of urine that the requirements of catheterization can be met only by a capacious reservoir.

LOW PRESSURES. The pressures within a continent enteric diversion are dictated by its volume,

configuration, and compliance. Like the native bladder, these reservoirs should exhibit minimal rises in pressure upon filling until capacity is approached. Whether one segment of bowel is significantly more compliant than another remains unclear. Minor differences are probably unimportant if size and shape considerations are fulfilled by an adequate length of reconfigured, detubularized bowel.

PROTECTION OF THE UPPER URINARY TRACT. Continent reconstructions in children should not reflux. Some clinicians have lessened their concerns about reflux with continent diversions, especially in adults in whom large, low-pressure reservoirs can be created. It would seem, however, that they are prone to repeat the errors of the past. The natural history of refluxing systems has been ominously shown by ileal

Volumes of Spheres Created from Cylinders

Length	Radius		
	1.0 cm	1.5 cm	2.5 cm
10	47	86	185
20	132	243	524
30	243	447	963
40	447	688	1,481

Figure 112–2. Capacities expected from different lengths and radii of cylinders. Large bowel yields significantly more volume than small bowel as a consequence of geometrical relationships.

loops, where free drainage should result in little, if any, back pressure. In continent diversions or augmented bladders that are emptied on a periodical basis with catheterization and in which intermittent bacteriuria seems to be the rule rather than the exception, it seems prudent to eliminate reflux in children who have a reasonable life expectancy.

CONTINENCE. The continence of urinary diversions depends on an interplay of pressures. Specifically, those along the catheterizable (efferent) limb should always exceed those within the reservoir itself, irrespective of volume. There are a number of different mechanisms that can be created to effectively maintain this relationship. Like the diversion itself, the selection of a continence mechanism is dictated ultimately by anatomical considerations, ease in construction, long-term performance, and the surgeon's experience and bias.

COMPLETE EMPTYING. The objective of the surgical reconstruction, replacement, or even medical management of neuropathic bladders is urinary retention. Because there is no pharmacological manipulation that facilitates emptying in these cases, consistent intermittent catheterization must be ensured.

SURGICAL PRINCIPLES

Reservoirs: Composition and Configuration

No matter what type of reservoir is being created (Fig. 112–3), the bowel used in its construction should be detubularized and reconfigured to achieve as near a spherical shape as possible. After its antimesenteric border is opened, the bowel can be folded upon itself or patched with adjacent bowel or another similarly opened segment. Reconfiguration serves to maximize the volume yielded from any tubular segment. Cylindrical volume is proportional to the square of the radius but spherical volume is proportional to its radius cubed. Reconfiguration also helps disrupt the peristaltic activity of bowel and dampen the amplitude of phasic pressure waves generated by its contractile nature.

A number of clinical studies have examined the urodynamic characteristics of enterocystoplasties and continent diversions constructed of various types of bowel. If some concession is made for differences in configuration and size, two conclusions can be drawn. The first is that tubular-shaped enteric reservoirs, regardless of source, generate high-pressure contractions. The second is that detubularized ileum appears to be the most compliant and least contractile bladder substitute followed by cecum and sigmoid or stomach. This has not evoked a blanket recommenda-

tion to uniformly construct continent diversions from ileum, however, and other segments should be considered for the following reasons:

ILEOCECAL SEGMENT. Ileocecal segment is easily mobilized and conducive to spherical reconfiguration by simple folding. In addition, the ileocecal valve can be employed as either a continence or antireflux mechanism. One major disadvantage is the diarrhea that occurs in 5 percent of children with spinal dysraphisms, whose fecal continence relies on controlled constipation and the presence of the ileocecal valve.

SIGMOID COLON. Sigmoid colon is usually redundant and easily mobilized in most children who are candidates for these operations. The segment is unavailable in cloacal exstrophy. Its thickened walls and tenia are ideal for implantation of the ureters and creation of flap-valve continence mechanisms using appendix or tapered bowel. Drawbacks include strong unit contractions and mucus secretion, which seems to be higher than that from other segments of bowel. The sigmoid may also be more prone to perforate.

ILEUM. Ileum purportedly has the most favorable urodynamic characteristics but provides only half the diameter of large bowel. Twice as much length is required to create a reservoir of similar size because of this discrepancy. Its absence of tenia also poses problems with the creation of flap valves for ureters and continence. As a consequence, most ileal reservoirs have been combined with ileal nipple valves in complex reconstructions that utilize a significant amount of bowel. This increases the potential for intestinal malabsorption, metabolic deficiencies (vitamin B_{12}) and the disruption of bile salt and lipid metabolism, which results in diarrhea.

STOMACH. Stomach has one major advantage because it provides chloride secretion as opposed to the ammonium and chloride reabsorption seen with other bowel exposed to urine. This benefit comes at the expense of metabolic action that functions autonomously of the body's urinary controls. Serious metabolic alterations can result (see below). The compliance of stomach appears to be comparable with that of other segments, yet it must often be combined with another segment to meet the volume requirements of continent diversion. The concept of a metabolically "balanced" reservoir is attractive yet unproved. Composite reservoirs appear to temper the metabolic acidosis that can occur if stomach is not used, but the detriment of obligate gastric secretion continues.[5] Stomach is currently reserved for patients with short gut syndrome, cloacal exstrophy, and previous pelvic radiation. Mild or moderate renal insufficiency is another common indication for employing stomach, but the procedure must be used with caution in end-

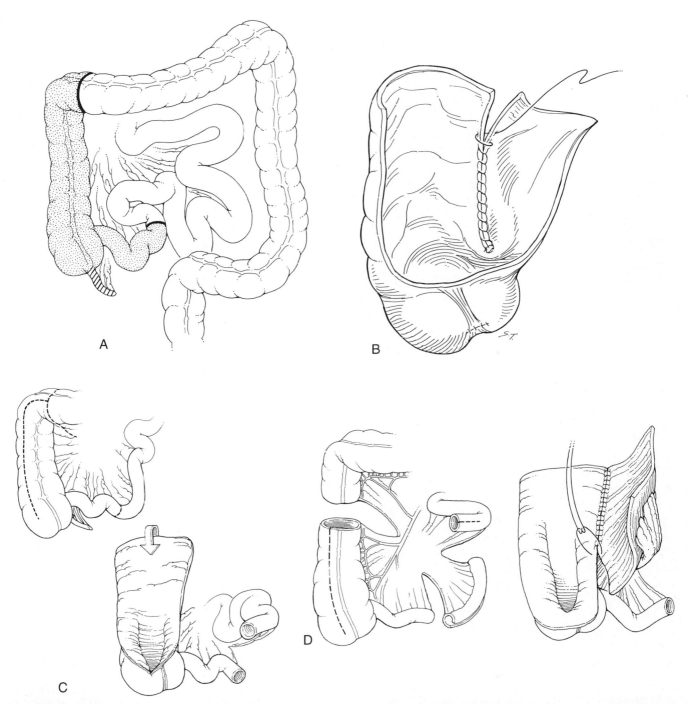

Figure 112–3. Examples of reservoirs. *A,* Ileocecal variants often incorporate the entire ascending colon to achieve adequate capacity. *B,* The entire segment opened along the antimesenteric border. A pouch is created by reapproximating the ileum and cecum. *C,* Indiana pouch. The ileum is intended for an efferent limb. The cecum is detubularized by opening the antimesenteric border and folding the segment upon itself. *D,* Mainz variant. The ileum preserved as an efferent limb. The adjacent ileal segment is mobilized, detubularized, and patched upon the cecal segment.

Illustration continued on following page

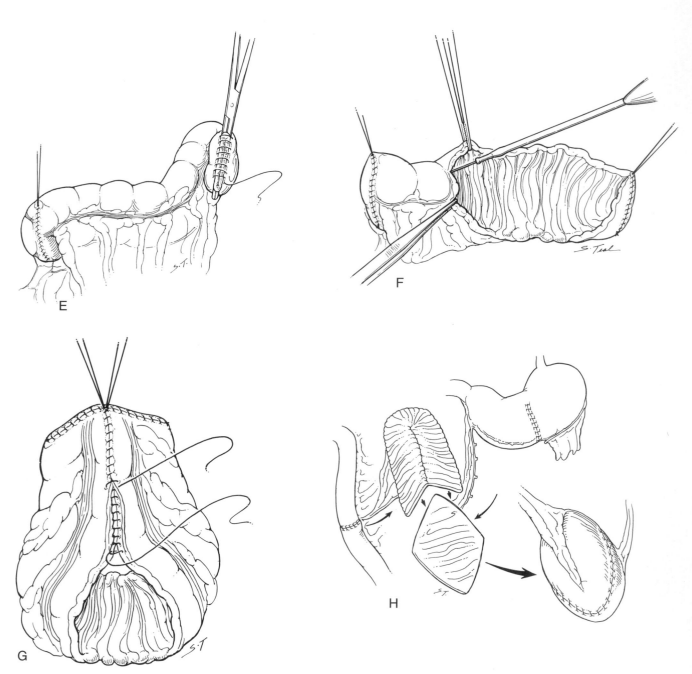

Figure 112–3 *Continued E,* A transverse colon pouch offers an ideal alternative in the setting of previous radiation. The colon is mobilized and the ends are closed. *F,* Segment opened longitudinally. *G,* Transverse closure achieves detubularization. *H,* Composite reservoir. The stomach segment is taken from the greater curvature. The ileal segment is detubularized and reconfigured by approximating one border. Placed together, both yield large capacity and may provide metabolic benefit.

stage renal disease. If the transition to transplantation includes periods of anuria, ulceration from the reservoir can result. Intermittent irrigations with bicarbonate or phosphate buffered saline should be prophylactically used during these episodes.

JEJUNUM. Jejunum should be avoided because of the dramatic fluid and electrolyte shifts that occur across its particularly absorptive surface.

Continence Mechanisms

Four basic mechanisms can be used to achieve the continence required of these diversions. In each case, the pressures along the efferent limb are greater than those within the reservoir. Assuming that the compliance of the reservoir is adequate and that it is being emptied on a regular basis, any of the four should be effective. Nevertheless, when results with the same technique vary widely among institutions, they are often a reflection of its intricacy and the height of the learning curve that must be broached in its application. In order of increasing complexity these include the following:

HYDRAULIC RESISTANCE. The most popular means of providing continence for diversions is by plicating the distal ileum left in continuity with the adjacent cecum (Indiana pouch, see Chap. 59). Small-caliber bowel alone will not provide continence, but in situ tapered ileum generates high resistance and is easy to construct. Components of active contractions and passive resistance from the ileocecal valve, tonic and phasic contractions directed toward the reservoir by the ileum, and its reduced diameter probably all contribute to the barrier against leakage. One advantage of plicated ileum is that leakage will occur when reservoir pressures are exceeded, providing a measure of security.

FLAP VALVES. The efficacy of flap valves in the urinary tract has been repeatedly borne out by ureteroneocystostomy. Their application with continent reconstructions was popularized by Mitrofanoff in 1980, who utilized the appendix and ureter as catheterizable stomas and whose name remains linked with continent diversions that employ flap-valve efferent limbs.[6] To be effective, these consist of a supple, small-diameter tube that is implanted within the wall of a reservoir or the native bladder. In addition, adequate muscular backing is needed to provide the occlusive action that prevents leakage as the reservoir fills. A variety of different structures can be used as a catheterizable conduit, including appendix, tapered ileum, and stomach (see below); fallopian tube; and pedicled skin flaps. When properly constructed, flap valves rarely leak, even at excessive capacities. If compliance with catheterization is suboptimal, this unforgiving nature can increase the risks of upper urinary tract damage or diversion perforation.

NIPPLE VALVES. Nipple valves can be created from intussuscepted ileum and have been widely employed with the Kock and Mainz pouches (see Chaps. 57 and 62). The nipple valve configuration has undergone significant revision since its original description. A pure nipple valve projects into the reservoir and achieves continence by coaptation. Intrinsic contractions also appear to contribute to continence. Protruding nipples, however, are susceptible to lateral forces that occur with reservoir filling. These cause gradual effacement and eventual breakdown with loss of continence. To counteract this problem, the contemporary nipple is now fixed against the wall of the reservoir to create what has become, in essence, a flap valve.

HYDRAULIC VALVES. Both the Benchekroun[7] (see below) and Koff[8] techniques rely on the principle of hydraulic resistance. Ileum is reconfigured to surround the catheterizable limb, either in an invaginating "inkwell" configuration or as a separate "servomechanism" wrap. In both instances, these channels communicate with the reservoir and increase outlet resistance as the reservoir fills. Unfortunately, breakdown of the reconfiguration and difficulty with catheterization have posed problems for the Benchekroun technique, although long-term efficacy may be borne out with continued modification. The complexity of the servomechanism makes it less desirable than other alternatives.

Eliminating Reflux

Ureteral reflux should be eliminated from the diversion to preserve renal function (Fig. 112–4). In most cases this is done by creating a flap-valve mechanism. A healthy, pliable ureter that is implanted along a reservoir bed having adequate length (five times the ureteral diameter) and sufficient muscular backing should not reflux. Subtenial and submucosal tunnels are effective in colon and stomach and are easily constructed. Ileal implantation is more challenging. Submucosal tunnels can be created with some difficulty. LeDuc's open mucosal trough provides another option.[9] In theory, ureters are gradually covered with intestinal mucosa, although complication rates of 20 to 30 percent have been reported. Finally, early results with an extramural tunnel are encouraging. Here the seromuscular layer of two portions of ileum are approximated with nonabsorbable suture behind the ureter to provide backing. The ileal edges are then approximated above the ureter to create a flap-valve mechanism.[10]

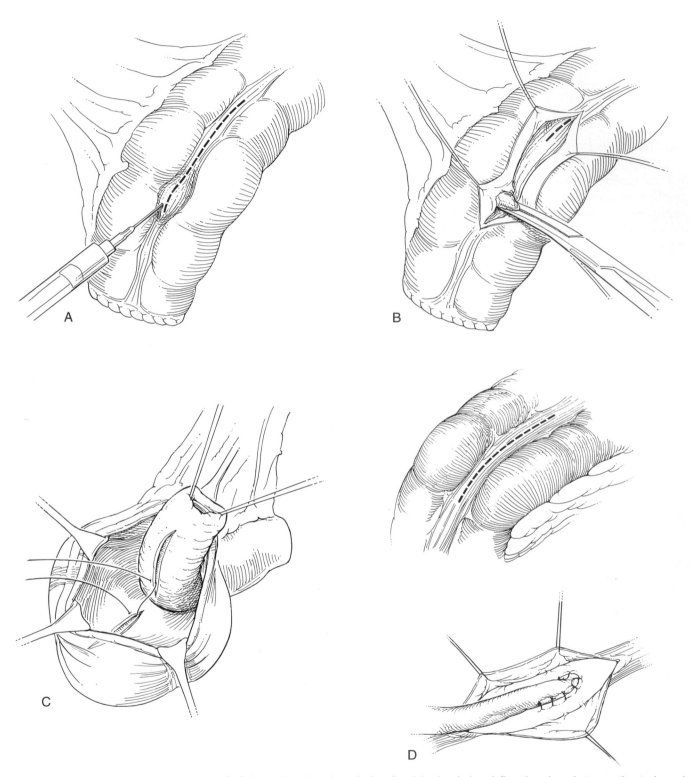

Figure 112–4. Antireflux mechanisms. *A* to *C,* Subtenial implantation. *A,* A saline injection helps define the plane between the tenia and underlying mucosa. *B,* The tenia is elevated using a combination of blunt and sharp dissection. *C,* Anastomosis completed with interrupted sutures. *D* and *E,* Ileal segment as the recipient of megaureters. *D,* The distal ileum is intussuscepted into the cecum. Mucosal counterincisions are made in both segments.

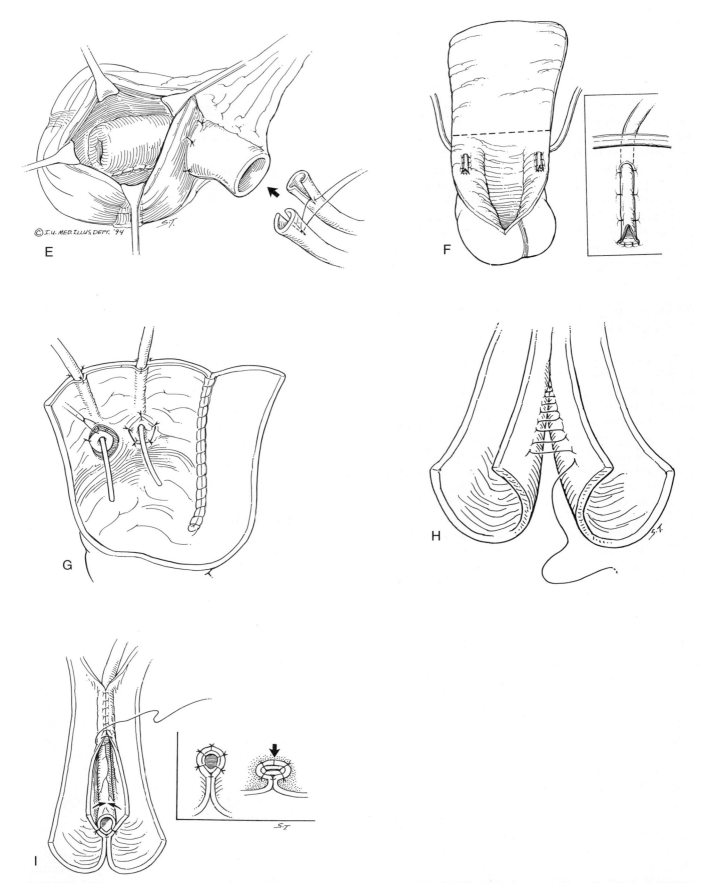

Figure 112–4 *Continued E,* Reapproximation using running sutures on each side of the wounds creates an antirefluxing flap-valve. A Wallace anastomosis of the ureters completes the repair. *F,* LeDuc method. A trough is created by incising the mucosa for 3 or 4 cm. The ureter is anastomosed into position with interrupted sutures of spatulated meatus and along length of ureter. Coverage is ultimately provided from growth of adjacent bowel mucosa. *G,* Intraluminal implantation is created in the cecum by sharply dissecting submucosal tunnels in a technique similar to ureteroneocystostomy. *H* and *I,* Extramural serosal tunnel technique. *H,* Backing for the ureter is created by approximating a seromuscular layer of two portions of bowel. *I,* Ureter positioned along the approximation. Edges of bowel are used as coverage for an effective flap-valve *(arrow).*

The functional characteristics of the ureters must be considered before implantation. Ureters that are congenitally dilated or scarred from chronic infection present a particular challenge. These sometimes fail to drain effectively because of impaired peristalsis or may not coapt with reservoir filling because of intrinsic fibrosis. Although tapering is sometimes done, the better choice is probably to connect the ureters to an ileal nipple valve placed in continuity with a large, low-pressure reservoir. Transureteroureterotomy provides another excellent option in the setting of unilateral ureteral damage. Implantation of a healthy ureter by any one of the above techniques can be used to protect a damaged partner and facilitate its drainage.

PATIENT SELECTION: PREOPERATIVE EVALUATON

The success of continence reconstruction depends as much on a thorough preoperative evaluation as on the correct placement of suture. Any procedure is doomed to fail when applied in unsuitable candidates. The patient and family must be well aware of the life-long care required of these reconstructions. Since intermittent catheterization is usually left up to the patient, some of the worst complications have occurred in cases in which the commitment to catheterization was lax. As a consequence, reconstructions for incontinence, for example, are often deferred for years until a child shows the proper motivation, especially if the child's support systems are marginal and the family dynamics suboptimal. When medical conditions such as increasing hydronephrosis warrant more immediate treatment, a noncontinent diversion should be created until these other considerations improve. A trial of catheterization is particularly helpful. This allows an assessment of the child's and the family's manual dexterity with a catheter, their willingness to comply, and their ability to access and negotiate the native urethra if its preservation is being considered.

Other than patient compliance, an accurate and complete assessment of the anatomy that might be used in the reconstruction is required. Continent diversions have the potential to be lengthy operations, and unanticipated surprises requiring additional procedures can add to one's fatigue and frustration. Ultrasonography and voiding cystourethrography are obtained together with a functional study such as renal scintigraphy. Megaureters require special consideration with continent diversions. Unless reflux is present on the voiding study, excretory urography is preferred in cases in which the degree of ureteral dilatation needs to be defined. Fluoroscopy can also be used to assess the peristalsis of dilated ureters that are potentially fibrotic and poorly draining. Additional

radiography include a gastrointestinal series in children whose histories suggest some limitation of the available bowel (e.g., cloacal exstrophy, radiation exposure, inflammatory bowel disease, previous surgery) and a loopogram when the transformation from a noncontinent to a continent diversion is being considered.

Other studies include an assessment of renal function with a 24-hour creatine clearance study, serum electrolyte analysis, and a urinalysis and culture. Continent reservoirs, which have increased absorptive surface and prolonged urine contact time, probably require better renal function than noncontinent diversions. Patients with creatinine clearances of less than 40 ml/min are more likely to experience metabolic derangements once bowel is interposed in the urinary tract. Serum creatinine alone may not be a valid measure of renal function, especially in children with spina bifida who have decreased muscle mass. When an element of renal failure is present, reconstructions should be deferred or, at the very least, constructed with stomach, the acid-secreting characteristics of which are beneficial. Finally, urodynamic studies should be obtained if preservation or reconstruction of the native bladder and sphincter is being considered.

PREOPERATIVE PREPARATION

Planning the Stoma

The child's habitus and abdomen are examined in different positions, including sitting if wheelchair bound, to plan for placement of the stoma. The recesses of the umbilicus provide the best cosmetic result. It also offers the shortest and most direct route across the abdominal wall, which is an important consideration in the extremely obese child, since the distance to be traversed by an efferent limb can be extreme. Other good options include a skin crease or the depths of an old drain site on the side of the dominant hand. Placement at the beltline should be avoided because irritation can cause the stoma to weep. Despite their small size, some patients eventually wear a Band-Aid or small sponge as coverage.

Bowel Preparation, Prophylaxis, and Other Considerations

A preoperative urine culture is checked and any infection treated. A thorough bowel preparation helps minimize the incidence of wound infections and abcesses. Polyethylene glycol electrolyte solutions are well tolerated by children and are hemodynamically safe and mechanically reliable. Intravenous hydration is begun the night before surgery to avoid problems with dehydration. At completion of the lavage, a bisacodyl suppository is given to evacuate residual fluid from the colon. Enteral neomycin and erythromycin base are also given to further decrease bacterial flora. Finally, a broad-spectrum parenteral antibiotic having anaerobic coverage (cefoxitin for example) is also recommended.

TECHNIQUES

Reservoirs: Indiana, Kock, Mainz, Other

There are a variety of ways to reconfigure bowel to create urinary reservoirs (see Chaps. 57, 58, 59, and 63) (Figs. 112–3 and 112–5). These include the Kock,[11] Mainz,[12] and Indiana[13] techniques. In each instance, large series of adults, who constitute the majority of candidates for continent diversion, are interspersed with occasional children and adolescents. Results are generally excellent. Smaller series composed solely of children have also been carried out with similar results.[14, 15] The details of these different operations are thoroughly covered elsewhere and exceed the scope of this discussion. The only technical adjustments made in children pertain to the lengths of bowel used to create the different pouches and efferent limbs. Alterations depend on age and size (see above). Regardless of the technique chosen, the bowel that is incorporated should be detubularized and closed in a watertight fashion. Single-layer running, locking polyglycolic acid sutures (2-0 or 3-0) are effective. A large Malecot drainage tube (18 or 20 Fr.) should be anchored in place to keep the system decompressed. It is also used to test the integrity of suture lines, the effectiveness of the continence mechanism, and the ease of catheterization by filling the reservoir with saline.

Appendicovesicostomy

Indications

The appendix makes an ideal continent catheterizable stoma.[16] Positioned at the distal extent of the cecum, it has a predictable blood supply emanating from the distal ileocolic artery along the mesoappendix. It can also be mobilized without disrupting the adjacent viscera, although it sometimes becomes necessary to free up the terminal ileum and ascending colon. This allows positioning anywhere in the abdomen or pelvis. The average appendix measures 4.5 cm in neonates and 9 to 10 cm in adults, which is more than enough length to bridge most body walls yet still provide for an effective valvular mechanism.

In addition, the lumen of most appendices accommodates at least a 10 Fr. catheter in all but the youngest patients. This facilitates urinary drainage and the lavage of mucus that is inevitably secreted when other bowel is included in the reconstruction. The supple appendix coapts effectively with filling of a reservoir, yet is durable enough to tolerate the trauma of repeated catheterization. Finally, the organ's uniform diameter minimizes the problems of catheter coiling or false passes that accompany other types of continence mechanisms.

The combination of an appendix and enteric pouch is well suited to children who require bladder replacement. The appendix also provides a useful adjunct to reconstructions of the native bladder in those who are unable or reluctant to catheterize the urethra. The organ can be positioned beneath a tenia, gastric wall, or seromuscular trough (see below). It can also be left in situ and wrapped with adjacent cecum. Mobilization before implantation, however, provides greater flexibility when positioning the stoma and helps eliminate angulations along the route of catheterization. These become important considerations if an umbilical stoma is desired or if the appendix is to be positioned at the introitus to create an orthotopic neourethra.

Operative Technique

MOBILIZING THE APPENDIX. Exposure is provided through a midline incision carried to the left of the umbilicus (Fig. 112–6). If an umbilical stoma is planned, care is taken to preserve a wide cuff of fascia (2.0 cm) around it. This helps avoid later compromise of the appendix during closure.

The appendix is delicately handled and any maneuvers required of its mobilization are directed at the preservation of vascularity. To begin, an initial incision is made in the antimesenteric aspect of the cecum near the base of the appendix. This is extended sharply toward the mesoappendix until the appendix is detached with a cuff or cecum. With the appendix under gentle traction, its mesentery can be fanned out, major blood vessels defined, and any extraneous tethers with the cecum divided. The retrocecal appendix presents a special problem as a consequence of its posterior orientation. For these variants, it is sometimes helpful to create a window in the ileocecal mesentery and carry the appendix through to an anterior position. This avoids kinking or traction of the adjacent bowel, which is freed to lie posterior to the continent stoma. A Doppler ultrasound is a helpful adjunct to identifying vessels and confirming viability.

Once mobilized, the distal tip of the appendix is excised and its lumen cleansed with antibiotic solu-

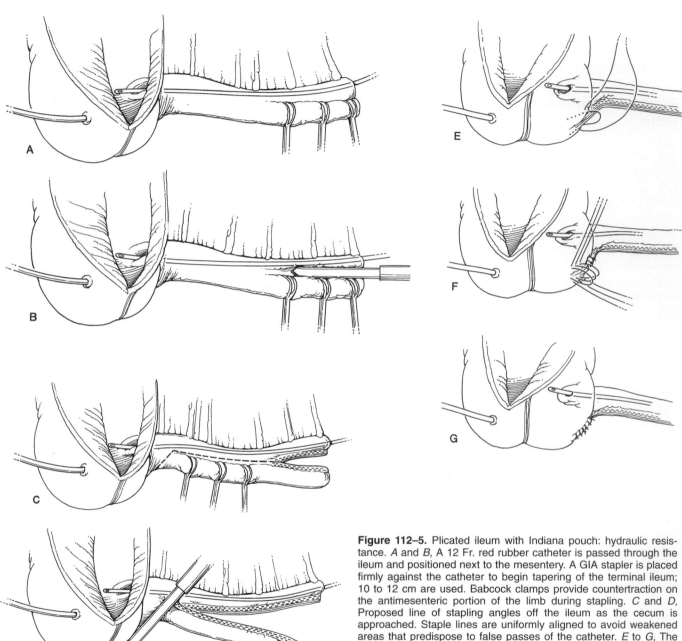

Figure 112–5. Plicated ileum with Indiana pouch: hydraulic resistance. *A* and *B*, A 12 Fr. red rubber catheter is passed through the ileum and positioned next to the mesentery. A GIA stapler is placed firmly against the catheter to begin tapering of the terminal ileum; 10 to 12 cm are used. Babcock clamps provide countertraction on the antimesenteric portion of the limb during stapling. *C* and *D*, Proposed line of stapling angles off the ileum as the cecum is approached. Staple lines are uniformly aligned to avoid weakened areas that predispose to false passes of the catheter. *E* to *G*, The funnel-shaped ileocecal junction is plicated with 3-0 Prolene Lembert sutures. Six or seven sutures are placed along a line indicated by the dotted lines. This maneuver also reinforces the ileocecal valve.

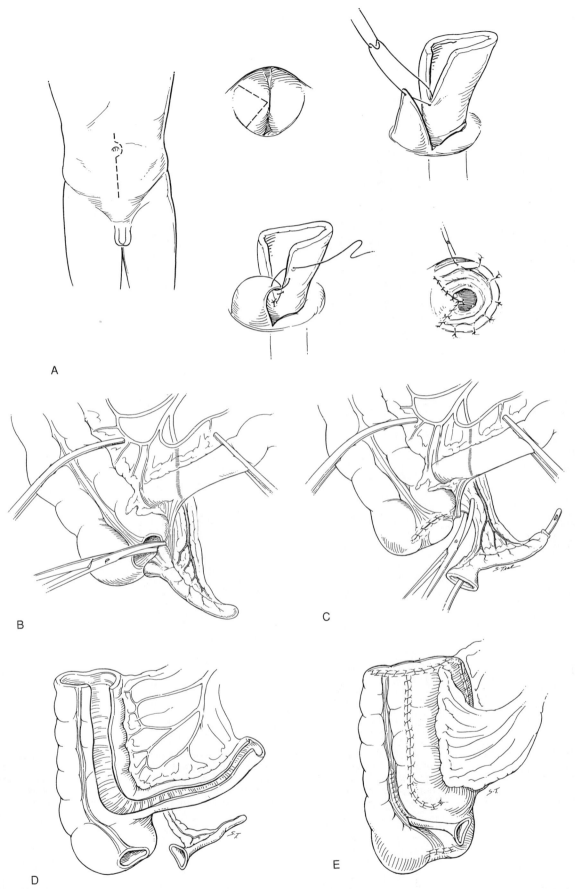

Figure 112–6. Appendicovesicostomy. *A,* Umbilical stoma. The skin incision preserves a wide cuff of skin and fascia to protect the appendicovesicostomy at closure. Maturation can be done before appendiceal implantation. A lateral skin flap is approximated to the appendiceal counterincision to help recess the stoma. *B,* Mobilization of the appendix is begun by approaching the cecum away from the mesoappendix. *C,* Tethers of mesoappendix to the cecum are incised and vascularity is preserved. *D to F,* Continent reservoir. *D,* The reservoir is created from an ileocecal segment. The antimesenteric border is opened and an ileal inlay flap used to detubularize the pouch. *E,* After appendiceal mobilization, subtenial implantation completes the diversion.

Illustration continued on following page

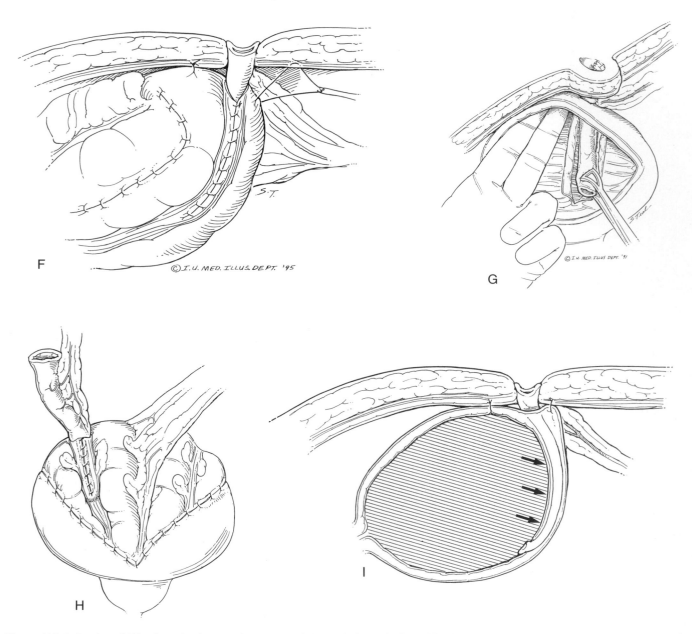

Figure 112–6 *Continued F,* Implantation in a continent reservoir beneath the tenia. Immobilization using an abdominal wall hitch helps eliminate angulations and false passes with catheterization. Pexing sutures are tied at the completion of reconstruction. *G,* Intraluminal implantation in the native bladder is performed before augmentation cystoplasty. Fingers mimic a hitch of the bladder to the abdominal wall as the appendix is drawn within. Placement in a trough created beneath the mucosa completes the repair. *H,* Subtenial implantation in enterocystoplasty by a technique identical to that for a continent reservoir. *I,* A flap-valve mechanism enables compression of the appendix against muscular backing.

tion to remove fecal debris. A 10 or 12 Fr. red rubber catheter is passed to ensure patency. If chronic inflammation has occurred and luminal stenosis is present, the tail of the appendix can be excised back to healthy tissue. In case of marginal length, the cuff of cecum taken in continuity with the appendix can be tubularized as its extension. Otherwise, the entire organ should be discarded and an alternative tube chosen.

COMPLETING THE STOMA. The appendiceal stoma can be completed either before or after its placement in the bladder or reservoir. The former is technically easier because the structures are "up in the air." In addition, a better cosmetic result is given by gently drawing the appendix into the abdominal cavity after it is matured to the skin before implantation, thus recessing the stoma. A laterally based (to preserve vascularity) 1 × 1 cm V-shaped skin flap is made in the umbilicus or lower abdominal wall. A generous hiatus is made in the fascia beneath the flap that allows easy passage of the index finger or a 28 Fr. sound. Peristomal hernias are uncommon because the reservoir is ultimately fixed to the anterior abdominal wall. The appendix is brought through the hiatus after one end is grabbed with a Babcock clamp. It is critical not to twist the mesoappendix. Tension and kinking must also be avoided. Orientation seems unimportant, although antiperistaltic implantation might provide additional continence. Interestingly, appendiceal peristalsis is propagated from the cecum to the tip.

A laterally oriented antimesenteric incision is made in the appendix that mirrors the cutaneous V flap. Skin and stoma are then approximated with interrupted 5-0 polyglycolic acid sutures. The interdigitation of the V flap helps prevent stenosis at the skin level.

IMPLANTATION AND FIXATION. To determine the best site for implantation, the fingers are used to recreate a hitch of the bladder or reservoir to the abdominal wall hiatus. When stomach or native bladder is the recipient, an intraluminal implantation is recommended. A generous ostomy is made in the reservoir that mirrors the hiatus of the abdominal wall. A large red rubber catheter left through the ostomy and laterally positioned retractors provide traction as a bed for the appendix is created from within by elevating the mucosa with cautery or sharp dissection. After the appendix is brought into the reservoir, it is spatulated and circumferentially anastomosed to the distal extent of the bed with fine (4-0) chromic sutures. The repair is completed by approximating the mucosal flaps as coverage with a running chromic suture.

Extraluminal implantation is used if the appendix is intended for an augmentation or enteric reservoir.

Tacking sutures are placed along a colonic tenia to define the proposed tunnel. A 5:1 length-to-width ratio is sufficient. Saline is injected beneath the tenia to help define its plane with the underlying mucosa. After the tenia is incised longitudinally, the plane is developed with tenotomy scissors and a gauze dissector. A small enterotomy is made at the distal extent of the tunnel and the appendix is trimmed to an appropriate length and spatulated. The anastomosis of appendix (full-thickness) and mucosa is completed with 4-0 interrupted chromic sutures. A running 4-0 polypropylene suture is used to reapproximate the tenia and aids in identification if re-exploration is ever necessary. Incising the lip of the tenia beneath the appendix and proximal to its entrance to the reservoir helps avoid angulations along the route of catheterization.

Three or four 2-0 polypropylene sutures are used to pex the seromuscular layer of the reservoir or bladder to the abdominal wall. Fixation ensures a direct route for catheterization and minimizes the false passes that occur when a segment of appendix remains unsupported between the reservoir and the abdominal wall. The fixation sutures are placed in three quadrants around the hiatus. None is positioned where compromise of the mesoappendix and its vasculature might occur. These are left untied until after the appendix is gently drawn into the bladder or is positioned along its subtenial bed or enteric trough before implantation.

COMPLETING THE REPAIR. The appendix must be easily catheterizable at completion of the procedure and should be checked with the reservoir both empty and full. An 8 Fr. feeding tube is left through the appendix to allow for the drainage of secretions.

Tapered Ileal and Gastric Tubes

Indications

Surgeons should think twice before removing structures from children that might become useful in later urinary reconstructions. Typical examples include vaginal remnants, ureters associated with nonfunctioning kidneys, and the appendix. Incidental appendectomies should be avoided in any child who might become a candidate for continent reconstruction. Because this philosophical change has been only recently adopted, patients are still encountered whose appendix has been removed or whose organ is scarred or short and unsuitable for inclusion in a continent diversion. Fortunately, other bowel can be reconfigured to mimic the straight and supple appendix. The same technique maximizes the use of bowel when undiverting an ileal conduit. As opposed to merely discarding the loop, one option is to incorporate it as a portion of the new reservoir. Another is to taper the conduit and employ it as a catheterizable efferent limb, preserving ileum or the ileocecal valve that might otherwise be used to create a continence mechanism.[17] Like appendix, tapered enteric tubes can be combined with a number of different reservoirs. For example, a gastric tube combined with a transverse colonic reservoir is an ideal choice when previous irradiation eliminates more common reservoirs from consideration.[18] Regardless of the type of tube, the technique of implantation is similar to that of the appendix.

Operative Technique

ILEUM. For all but the most obese child, 8 to 10 cm of ileum is adequate. When the appendix is unsuitable or missing, a segment of small bowel is isolated and an ileoileostomy completed using standard techniques. In the case of an ileal loop undiversion, the conduit is identified after laparotomy and its mesentery isolated. Once the stoma is initially freed with a circumferential skin incision, it helps to keep a finger in the distal conduit as subcutaneous and fascial tethers are identified and taken down with the cautery. After the conduit is mobilized, its stomal segment is discarded and the remainder examined for kinks or segmental stenosis. If a significant portion of the loop is affected, it should be discarded and a new section of ileum chosen.

Stay sutures are placed on each end of the ileal segment and a stiff 12 Fr. red rubber catheter placed in its lumen along the mesenteric margin. A GIA 90 stapler is used to taper the segment snugly around the catheter and excise excess bowel (Fig. 112–7). Staple lines are kept in series as close together as possible to avoid weakened areas that might predispose to outpouchings and later false passes. Babcock clamps placed along the antimesenteric border of the bowel are instrumental in keeping the segment taut during stapling and minimizing redundancy. Excess length is trimmed after the segment is completed. In some children, mesentery thick with fat or lymph nodes poses an obstacle to implantation. When this is the case, the end intended for implantation can be debulked and mobilized by cutting the mesentery parallel to the segment but below its intimate vascular arcade. A Doppler flow probe is useful during these manuevers.

STOMACH. Gastric tubes are simultaneously harvested and tubularized from the greater curvature of the stomach. Segments as long as 10 to 12 cm can be mobilized with the right gastroepiploic artery. After the blood supply is identified and the segment marked, its mesentery is defined by carefully ligating branches from the gastroepiploic as it supplies the stomach. Those to the segment itself are preserved, while the left gastroepiploic is ligated beyond the segment to complete its isolation. Fine silk sutures are used to avoid spasm or injury to the main vessel. After the stomach is aspirated with a nasogastric tube and the adjacent bowel covered with towels, a small gastrostomy is made on each side of the segment just above the greater curvature. A stiff 12 Fr. red rubber catheter placed through the gastrostomies and positioned along the greater curve provides countertraction as the stapler is used to tubularize the segment snugly around it. The omentum is then divided to gain additional mobilization of the pedicle, with careful attention paid to its blood supply.

COMPLETING THE REPAIR. The technique for creation of the stoma with enteric tubes is identical to that with the appendix. Like the appendix, tapered bowel can be implanted beneath tenia, along a seromuscular trough, or into the native bladder. Each end of the bowel is spatulated before its maturation to avoid stenosis. Fixation of the recipient reservoir is completed with nonabsorbable sutures, while similar precautions are taken with the alignment of the mesentery, avoidance of tension, and repetitive testing of the new stoma.

Seromuscular Trough

Indications

An effective flap valve provides firm backing for its catheterizable conduit. This guarantees compression as the reservoir fills. In some patients the backing that has been routinely used, colonic teniae or bladder detrusor, is deficient or unavailable. Common examples include existing colonic augmentations, where tenial integrity is often distorted or lost, and ileal reservoirs, where teniae are absent. As an alternative, the seromuscular layers of the recipient reservoir can be simply reconfigured to provide the support required of a continent stoma. The backing created is substantial, effective, and less prone to the lateral forces that are implicated in the breakdown of nipple valve continent stomas or simple plications of these layers.[19]

The trough can be used with any of the catheterizable conduits or different segments of recipient bowel, and offers additional flexibility with continent urinary reconstruction. Possible applications include the revision of existing diversions including the Indiana, Benchekroun, and Kock pouches and undiversion of ileal and colon conduits. The method is also ideally suited to patients whose continent diversion must be constructed with ileum or who need an alternative means of emptying an existing enterocystoplasty.

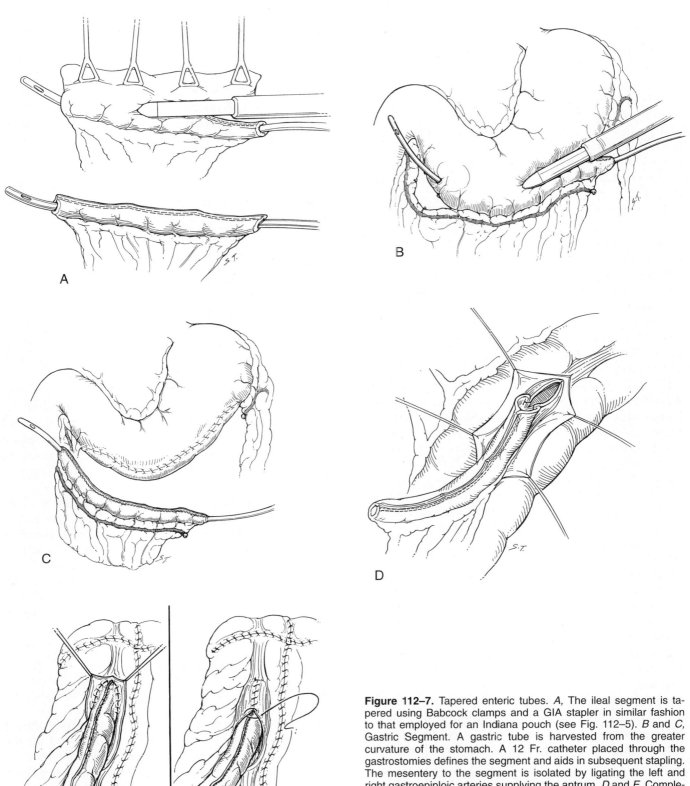

Figure 112–7. Tapered enteric tubes. *A,* The ileal segment is tapered using Babcock clamps and a GIA stapler in similar fashion to that employed for an Indiana pouch (see Fig. 112–5). *B* and *C,* Gastric Segment. A gastric tube is harvested from the greater curvature of the stomach. A 12 Fr. catheter placed through the gastrostomies defines the segment and aids in subsequent stapling. The mesentery to the segment is isolated by ligating the left and right gastroepiploic arteries supplying the antrum. *D* and *E,* Completion of repair. Subtenial implantation is completed after elevating the tenia, creating a small enterotomy, and spatulating the gastric or ileal tube. The reservoir mucosa and a full-thickness tube are joined with fine sutures before reapproximating the tenia above the anastomosis.

Operative Technique

The stoma of the catheterizable conduit (appendix or tapered bowel) can be completed either before or after its implantation into the seromuscular trough. The technique used is identical to that of the appendicovesicostomy. Better recession is achieved by completing the stoma initially and then gently drawing the conduit into the abdominal cavity. This sequence is also helpful in obese patients, in whom the length of the conduit and its mesentery is sometimes questionable.

The site for the trough is initially determined by placing the fingers within the lumen of the augmentation or reservoir to hitch a portion of the bowel to the abdominal wall (Fig. 112–8). Polypropylene sutures (2-0 or 3-0) are then used to secure the recipient bowel on both sides of the conduit's entrance to the abdomen. Tacking sutures help fan out the bowel and define the limits of the trough. Two parallel incisions (5 or 6 cm apart) are planned that are longitudinal to the ultimate position of the conduit. Forceps or additional sutures aid in sizing and can be used to mimic the wraplike effect of the trough. Incisions placed too close together can compromise the underlying conduit and should be avoided. These incisions must also extend beyond the site proposed for the anastomosis to the reservoir to allow for complete coverage of the catheterizable conduit. The length required for effective implantation may not be as great as generally believed, but the 5-to-1 rule held for ureteroneocystostomy is probably a suitable minimum. Both incisions are made through the seromuscular layers alone, with the underlying mucosal layer and reservoir integrity kept intact. After the appendix or enteric tube is spatulated, a small enterotomy is made in the reservoir and an end-to-end anastomosis of the two completed with interrupted polyglycolic acid sutures (5-0) that approximate the full thickness of the conduit and a cuff of mucosa. The lateral edges of two incisions of the trough are reapproximated over the conduit with fine, interrupted polypropylene sutures.

The stoma is checked for ease of catheterization after completion of the implantation and closure of the reservoir. An 8 Fr. feeding tube is left across the repair until catheterization is begun a few weeks later.

Benchekroun Hydrostatic Valve

Indications

The hydraulic ileal valve described by Benchekroun offers another innovative method for creating a continence mechanism. It seems, at times, that understanding its mechanism of action is more difficult than actual construction.

First described in 1977, long-term follow-up has shown good results in a series of 136 patients. Continence was achieved in most, although limb revisions were required of nearly 20 percent.[7] Fistula, stomal stenosis, and devagination of the valve are common complications. The last is most concerning. Because the outer sleeve of the limb is unsupported, the pressures within can cause its gradual dilation as well as compression of the catheterizable channel. The incontinence that results may become more common with extended follow-up.

Operative Technique

An 8- to 10-cm section of ileum is isolated to create the Benchekroun valve. With continent diversions, the ileocecal segment can be detubularized and the valve constructed from adjacent ileum. The antiperistaltic end of the segment is grasped with Allis clamps and intussuscepted through the lumen in a peristaltic fashion (Fig. 112–9). Once the ends are aligned, they are fixed with full-thickness, horizontal mattress absorbable sutures placed at each quadrant. A semicircular running suture completes the fixation. This creates two mucosa-lined channels that allow urine to move between the ileal sleeves, compressing the serosa-lined catheterizable limb as the reservoir fills.

The valve is anastomosed to the reservoir or bladder by incorporating only the outer layer (peristaltic end) of the valve, again using full-thickness absorbable sutures. Stomal maturation is done in a fashion similar to that for a ileal loop. This includes a standard cruciate fascial incision and anchoring sutures. Care is taken at the skin level to incorporate only serosa of the valve with absorbable sutures in order to avoid fistula formation.

POSTOPERATIVE CARE AND FOLLOW-UP

Most children are hospitalized for approximately 1 week. They are encouraged to be out of bed on the first postoperative day, and patients who are not wheelchair-bound are ambulated. Aggressive pulmonary toilet is also encouraged. Nasogastric decompression is continued until any postoperative ileus has resolved, and oral intake is gradually increased once bowel function has returned. Prophylactic antibiotics (a cephalosporin) are continued until all drains are removed.

Stentograms are obtained 5 days after surgery if the ureters have been implanted. These drains are removed if no problems are demonstrated by the

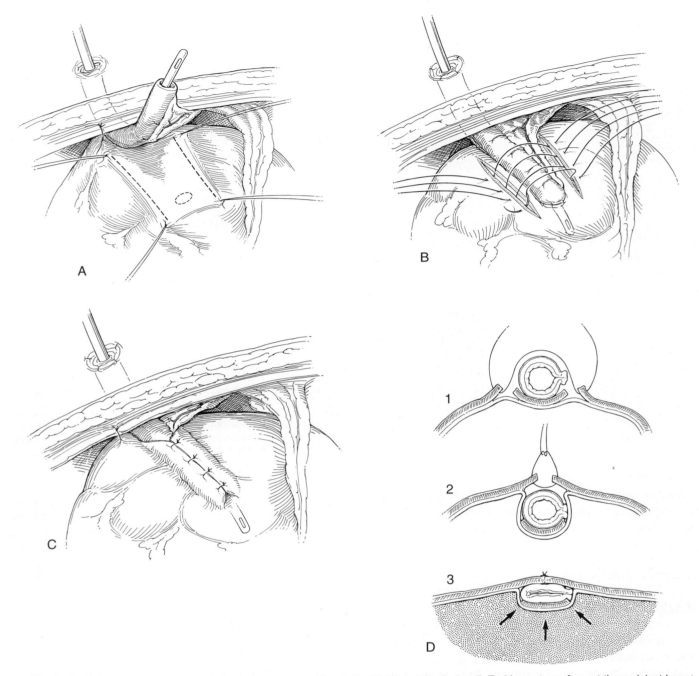

Figure 112–8. Seromuscular trough. *A,* A reservoir or augmentation is fixed to the abdominal wall. Tacking sutures fan out the recipient bowel to define parallel incisions of trough. *B,* Interrupted sutures are placed through the lateral edges of the incisions. *C,* Reapproximation of seromuscular layers covers the catheterizable conduit with backing. *D,* Cross-section of seromuscular trough. 1, Incisions separate the seromuscular layer. The mucosal integrity of the reservoir is kept intact. 2, Reapproximation of seromuscular layers covers the conduit, essentially transferring it to the reservoir lumen. 3, Reservoir filling compresses the conduit against the seromuscular backing.

studies. The Malecot catheter that drains the reservoir and stent of the efferent limb remains for 3 weeks. Before discharge, families are taught to lavage the diversion twice a day with 50 ml normal saline to avoid the accumulation of mucus and clots and ensure catheter patency. Upon the child's return, the stomal stent is removed and a pouchogram obtained. If no leaks are shown, the catheter is clamped and intermittent catheterization begun. It is removed a few days later if all is going well.

Subsequent follow-up consists of periodic radiographs, serum chemistry analyses, and urine cultures. A renal scan is obtained a few weeks after surgery to assess renal function and rule out obstruction. Return visits at 3, 6, and 12 months are also planned. Ultrasound scans provide noninvasive surveillance of the upper urinary tract and are a useful means of assessing diversion emptying. When residuals are significant, patients are instructed to aspirate their catheters at the end of gravity drainage whenever

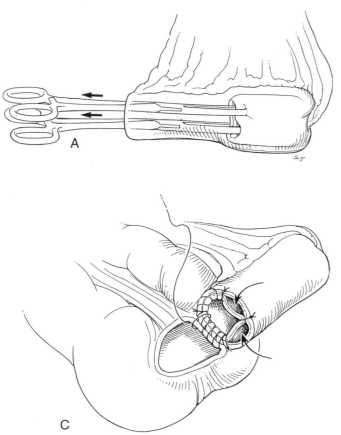

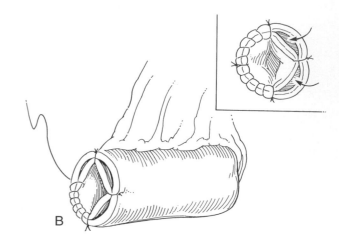

Figure 112–9. Benchekroun hydrostatic valve. *A,* An antiperistaltic end of a 10-cm ileal segment is intussuscepted upon itself using Allis clamps. *B,* The ends of the segment are reapproximated with four quadrant horizontal mattress sutures and a semicircular running suture. The channel of the efferent limb is left lined by serosa. Two mucosa-lined channels are left open to allow urinary inflow, which occludes the catheterizable lumen *(inset). C,* Anastomosis to the cecal reservoir. Reapproximating only an outer layer of segment above the inflow channels preserves the continence mechanism.

possible. Nightly lavage with normal saline is also recommended when collections of mucus are seen on the studies.

COMPLICATIONS

Early

Continent urinary diversions are prone to the same early perioperative complications of any major intra-abdominal operation, including intestinal obstruction, enteric fistula, and wound infection and dehiscence. Unique complications include leaks of the reservoir. This is an uncommon occurrence if the diversion is adequately decompressed. When extravasation is noted on a postoperative ureteral stentogram or pouchogram, drainage is continued for an additional week or two. Repeat studies should document healing of the area in question, unless an unusual, catastrophic event has occurred such as a ureteral slough or a diversion infarction. Conservative therapy can be continued if urinary leakage and infection can be controlled, but exploration is indicated if serious events are suspected, especially in an extremely ill patient. Transureteroureterostomy provides an effective response to unilateral ureteral problems, and the

suture lines of a disrupted reservoir can be freshened up and sewn together. When a diversion infarction has occurred, it is probably wise to temporize and simply divert the urine with a transverse colon or ileal conduit rather than attempt its complete revision.

Late: Reservoirs

Bacteriuria/Urinary Infection

Many children with continent diversions develop intermittent or chronic bacteriuria. This does not seem to be a problem for most patients, and daily oral antibiotics are unnecessary. Host mechanisms such as secretory immunoglobulins (IgA) may play a role in preventing bacterial adherence. An occasional child will develop low-grade fever, abdominal pain, or stomal incontinence during these episodes. These can be treated with a few days of broad-spectrum antibiotic (sulfamethoxazole-trimethoprim). For children who are especially prone to infection, intermittent lavage with antibiotic solution (gentamicin, 480 mg/L of normal saline) is an effective prophylactic having virtually no side effects. More serious symptoms, of course, demand further evaluation. Some infections of the reservoir are so severe that a septic picture results in so-called pouchitis. Diffuse abdominal pain, guarding, vomiting, and fever should raise the suspicion of perforation, yet none is appreciated on subsequent studies. These types of episodes should resolve with aggressive parenteral antibiotics and decompression of the reservoir.

Urinary Calculi

Calculi may ultimately become the most common complication of continent urinary reconstructions. Mucus production and chronic bacteriuria that accompany enteric reservoirs and augmentations provide a fertile milieu for stones, which are typically triple phosphates. Hypocitraturia (a stone inhibitor), impaired renal function, and metabolic acidosis that requires calcium mobilization as a buffer are other risk factors. Incomplete emptying probably also contributes to stone formation and is possibly amplified by superiorly positioned continent stomas that do not provide dependent drainage. Periodical aspiration of residual urine and daily lavage of mucus help minimize these occurrences. When stones do form, a percutaneous or open approach is sometimes necessary if the caliber of the efferent limb is too small to permit endoscopic manipulations through its lumen. In fact, it is probably preferable to deliver larger stones through a simple incision rather than attempt their fragmentation and piecemeal removal, since recurrence rates are higher with the latter.

Carcinogenesis

The predisposition of continent diversions to malignancy is unclear, although the data from augmentation cystoplasties suggest an increased risk to the intestinal mucosa. Contributing factors possibly include chronic infection, mechanical irritation from catheterization, and ischemia. Intestinal mucosa chronically exposed to urine undergoes progressive villous atrophy. Mucin production and composition is also sometimes altered. Whether these changes represent an adaptive benefit or an increased risk for malignant potential will not become apparent for years. In the meantime, periodical surveillance (every 2 to 3 years) with flexible cystoscopy seems reasonable. Urinary cytological studies and flow cytometry may also play a role in the future.

Diversion Perforation

Fortunately, the potentially lethal complication of diversion perforation has not been common with continent diversions, although perforations have been a fairly frequent occurrence with augmentation cystoplasty.[20] The predisposition of different segments has varied among institutions. Stomach appears to be least prone but also has had shorter follow-up. The etiology of perforations is unclear but probably multifactorial. In addition to villous atrophy, the severe depletion of lymphoid elements that is implicated in ileal loop strictures may, in concert with chronic infection, lead to transmural scarring. Hypoperfusion, especially in the face of overdistention, is another real possibility. Urinary retention from mucous plugs, catheter trauma, and high-pressure enteric hyperreflexia may also play a role, while poor compliance with emptying is often suspected.

A high index of suspicion is necessary on the part of the treating physician. The clinical presentation may vary, since many children have neurological deficits that can mask their abdominal findings. Abdominal distention, diaphragmatic or abdominal pain, fever, and decreased urinary output are common signs that warrant further investigation. Low-pressure cystography with drainage films is probably the most accurate study. Computed tomographic scans should be obtained if the perforation has transiently sealed but a collection or abscess is still suspected. Surgical exploration and repair remains the preferred method of management.

Metabolic Alterations

The metabolic acidosis that results from placing ileum or colon in contact with urine is a well-recognized phenomenon that results from the loss of potassium and bicarbonate in exchange for ammonium and chloride. These changes are amplified by marginal renal function but can also continue to deplete buffer stores in the presence of normal serum chemistry values. Oral potassium bicarbonate replacement is given for deficiencies and is prophylactically recommended by some surgeons with concerns about bone changes and overall growth in children. Solute contact time can be lessened by encouraging frequent catheterization.

The stomach can present special metabolic problems. Primary gastric dysfunction has not resulted from removing either the fundus or antrum for urinary reconstruction. To its detriment, stomach in the urinary tract functions autonomously of the body's intrinsic buffer controls and will continue its obligate excretion of acid despite vomiting, diarrhea, or other metabolic changes that cause salt loss. Serious hyponatremic hypochloremic alkalosis can result. This is usually easily correctable with intravenous saline replacement. These episodes can also be arrested in their early stages by the intake of fluids with carbonic acid (soda, pH of 1) that inhibits gastrin secretion from the stomach. Patient awareness is important.

Other Complications

Recurrent rhythmic contractions have posed a problem for some patients and have occurred with every bowel segment, presenting at variable times after surgery. Why these reappear is unclear. Alterations in innervation, incomplete detubularization, and abnormal endocrine response (stomach) have all been implicated. Most do not become clinically significant in the face of generous reservoir capacities. When they are severe, it becomes necessary to augment the existing reservoir. This does not eliminate any abnormal activity but merely serves to dampen its effects by providing more volume.

Late: Continent Stomas

The few complications that do occur with catheterizable limbs are usually minor and easily correctable. The most common arise at the skin level. Stomal prolapse with ectropian formation can be avoided by recessing the appendix or bowel using the flap technique described above. The same maneuver is instrumental in minimizing the incidence of stomal stenosis. Prolapse can be simply revised by excising the redundant tissue flush with the skin and advancing a V-shaped skin flap into a vertical incision made in the end of the conduit. This same technique is used to correct stenosis after opening the stoma by incising its circumferential cicatrix. Difficulty with catheterization was a frequent occurrence in early series of appendicovesicostomy. Angulation or false passes along the appendix can be avoided by the reservoir fixation techniques described above. When the occasional false pass, kink, or stricture does occur, it can sometimes be managed with endoscopic incision, fulguration, or dilation; if not, open revision and replacement become necessary. The same is usually true of efferent limbs that fail to provide continence.

The long-term implications of exposure to urine and trauma from repeated catheterizations for the appendix or other bowel used as an efferent limb is undefined. It is notable that the lumina of ileal segments used to create nipple valves, which are sequestered from urine, do not exhibit the villous atrophy that occurs elsewhere in reservoirs. With the exception of its muscular walls, the appendix is composed largely of lymphatic tissue organized into discrete nodules. Concerns that similar atrophic changes will occur, at least at its interface with the reservoir, are understandable but not borne out by early experience. Fibrous obliteration of the appendiceal lumen, presumably from inflammation, is a fairly common pathological finding after appendectomy. In contrast, the rare occlusions reported in urinary appendices appear to be acutely caused by vascular accidents. It seems reasonable to assume that the organ's propensity to infection (i.e., acute appendicitis) is signifi-

cantly reduced by its conversion from a closed system to an open-ended one.

The malignant potential of continent stomas is even less clear. Primary tumors of the appendix are rare, carcinoid being the most common malignancy (generally cited at less than 0.2 percent). While no malignancy has been described in a continent stoma, benign fibrous polyps have been reported. Additional follow-up is necessary to determine whether the organ exhibits a tendency for malignant transformation similar to that of other bowel used elsewhere in the urinary tract.

Summary

Continent diversions represent a significant advancement in the care of children with difficult urinary problems. Careful selection, attention to surgical detail, and flexible utilization of the anatomical variability that often occurs in these special patients provide the keys to success. When such a reconstruction is properly applied, the benefits will always outweigh the risks.

Editorial Comment
Craig A. Peters

Continent diversion in children has evolved rapidly since the mid-1980s and at present is a routine procedure with predictably excellent results. It requires a broad experience and great flexibility in surgical application, as shown in this chapter. The specific procedures must be tailored to an individual child's anatomy and special requirements. Integrating the various methods for achieving the goals of continent diversion requires careful consideration of the many alternatives to create an effective reservoir and continence mechanism, and to preserve upper urinary tract function. Great attention to technical detail is needed. Most important, however, is patient selection, education, and counseling. The ultimate success of a technically perfect operation will be completely dependent on these elements.

REFERENCES

1. Schwartz GR, Jeffs RD. Ileal conduit urinary diversion in children: Computer analysis of followup from 2 to 16 years. J Urol 114:285, 1975.
2. Studer UE, Casanove GA, Zingg EJ. Historical aspects of continent urinary diversion. In Paulson DF, ed. Problems in Urology, Vol. 5, No. 2. Philadelphia, JB Lippincott, 1991, p 197.
3. Lapides J, Diokno AC, Silber LJ, et al. Clean, intermittent self-catheterization in the treatment of urinary tract disease. J Urol 107:458, 1972.
4. Hendren WH. Reconstruction of previously diverted urinary tracts in children. J Pediatr Surg 8:135, 1973.
5. Lockhart JL, Davies R, Persky L, et al. Acid-base changes following urinary tract reconstruction for continent diversion and orthotopic bladder replacement. J Urol 152:338, 1994.
6. Mitrofanoff P. Cystotomie continente trans-appendiculaire dans le traitement des vessies neurologiques. Chir Pediatr 21:297, 1980.

7. Benchekroun A, Essakalli N, Faik M, et al. Continent urostomy with hydraulic ileal valve in 136 patients: 13 years of experience. J Urol 142:46, 1989.

8. Koff SA, Cirulli C, Wise HA. Clinical and urodynamic features of a new intestinal urinary sphincter for continent urinary diversion. J Urol 142:293, 1989.

9. LeDuc A, Camey M, Teillac P: An original antireflux ureteroileal implantation technique: Long-term followup. J Urol 137:1156, 1987.

10. Abol-enein H, Ghoneim MA. A novel uretero-ileal reimplantation technique: The serous lined extramural tunnel. A preliminary report. J Urol 151:1193, 1994.

11. Skinner DG, Lieskovsky G, Boyd SD. Continent urinary diversion. J Urol 141:1323, 1989.

12. Thuroff JW, Alken P, Riedmiller H, et al. 100 cases of Mainz pouch: Continuing experience and evaluation. J Urol 140:283, 1988.

13. Rowland RG, Mitchell ME, Bihrle R, et al. The Indiana continent urinary reservoir. J Urol 137:1136, 1987.

14. Rink RC, Bihrle R. Continent urinary diversion in children and the Indiana pouch. In Kramer SA, ed. Problems in Urology—Recent Advance in Pediatric Urology, Vol 4. Philadelphia, JB Lippincott, 1990, p 663.

15. Hanna MK, Bloiso G. Continent diversion in children: Modification of Kock pouch. J Urol 137:1206, 1987.

16. Keating MA, Rink RC, Adams MC. Appendicovesicostomy: A useful adjunct to continent reconstruction of the bladder. J Urol 149:1091, 1993.

17. Adams MC, Bihrle R, Foster RS, Brito CG. Conversion of ileal conduit to continent catheterizable stoma. J Urol 147:126, 1992.

18. Birhle R, Klee LW, Adams MC, Foster RS. Early clinical experience with the transverse colon-gastric tube continent urinary reservoir. J Urol 146:751, 1991.

19. Keating MA, Kropp BP, Adams MC, et al. Seromuscular trough modification in construction of continent urinary stoma. J Urol 150:734, 1993.

20. Bauer SB, Hendren WH, Kozakewich H, et al. Perforation of the augmented bladder. J Urol 148:699, 1992.

Chapter 113

Urinary Undiversion: Surgical Considerations and Strategies

Richard N. Schlussel and Craig A. Peters

Despite many impressive innovations in reconstructive urological procedures, none of the end results can rival the native bladder for efficient storage and emptying of urine. The normal urinary bladder is a high-volume, low-pressure distensible reservoir that empties to completion and does so only upon volitional command. It can store urine because of outlet resistance from the urinary sphincters, which work synergistically with the detrusor. The transitional epithelium that lines this reservoir is ideally suited for storage of urine. Finally, urinary expulsion is via the urethra in its normal perineal position. Recognizing these advantages inherent to the bladder, urologists have expended great effort to refunctionalize the lower urinary tract by rerouting the urinary stream from prior diversion back to the native bladder and urethra. This chapter reviews the relevant aspects of urinary diversion and the rationale and approach for urinary refunctionalization or undiversion.

URINARY DIVERSION

Background

Urinary diversion may be defined as the redirection of the urinary stream at any point proximal to the urethra. This has been accomplished in a variety of ways for a number of conditions. One of the earliest diversions was bilateral ureterosigmoidostomy.[1-3] This was usually performed for patients who either were lacking a bladder (exstrophy, cystectomy) or had a bladder that did not provide satisfactory continence. The main advantage of this procedure was the continence achieved by the rectal sphincter. However, as with most novel procedures, the passage of time uncovered unexpected complications, including

metabolic acidosis, urosepsis, and malignant transformation at the ureterocolonic junction.[4-6] These problems dampened the enthusiasm of many surgeons for this procedure.

Bricker[7] introduced a new approach to diversion with his description of the ileal conduit. This procedure was performed for the same indications as ureterosigmoidostomies but had fewer of the abovementioned problems. However, this procedure was not a panacea either, as these patients experienced the disadvantages of loop stenosis, metabolic complications, stones, pyelonephritis, and the need for a prominent external urine collection appliance.[6, 8-13] The same can be said for colon conduits.[14-16]

Cutaneous ureterostomies and pyelostomies were performed most commonly for distal ureteral obstruction (i.e., megaureters, ureterovesical junction obstruction from posterior urethral valves) and even for severe reflux.[17, 18] While ureterostomies were quite easy to manage in a diapered infant, they became unacceptable to the older child who wished to be continent.

Cutaneous vesicostomies have been constructed for a variety of urological conditions, including posterior urethral valves and severe vesicoureteral reflux.[19-21] A vesicostomy is easy to fashion in even the smallest of infants and requires no special care in the diapered infant. Complications such as bladder prolapse and stomal stenosis should be relatively uncommon. While providing effective bladder drainage, a vesicostomy renders the child incontinent and ultimately needs to be closed after correction of the underlying urological problem.

Assorted tubes have been used to deal with the problem of obstruction or incontinence. Many patients had these nephrostomies and suprapubic tubes on a long-term basis. Their care required frequent replacement with eventual problems of stone formation, tube obstruction, dislodgment, infection, and squamous metaplasia of the bladder. In addition, these patients needed an external appliance to collect urine.

The understanding of the complex problems of urinary undiversion has been enhanced by Hendren's contributions.[22-25] In a prominent series of urinary tract refunctionalizations by Hendren,[26] the types of diversions are listed in 182 cases. These included ileal loop (66 patients, or 36 percent), loop ureterostomy (39, 21 percent), vesicostomy (38, 21 percent), end ureterostomy (17, 9 percent), colon conduit (14, 8 percent), nephrostomy (7, 4 percent), and ureterosigmoidostomy (1, 0.5 percent). As mentioned above, such diversions were performed for obstructive processes (posterior urethral valves, urethral stricture, megaureters); severe reflux; incontinence (usually because of myelodysplasia but also from other neurological disorders); absent bladders; and small, scarred, or fibrotic bladders.

Of great significance in the evolution of urinary reconstruction was the demonstration that clean intermittent catheterization could be performed effectively and safely.[27, 28] This became a well-established plinth upon which many operations were built. With catheterization, patients could empty their reservoir in a rapid, easy manner on a regular basis. The fact that this was done on a clean, rather than sterile, basis did not seem to have any significant adverse effect. Catheterization allowed for maintaining other bladder functions (e.g., storage of urine) even if the ability to void was absent.

Assessment

An undertaking as significant and complex as urinary undiversion requires a complete assessment of the anatomy, function, and commitment of the individual patient (Table 113–1).

History

A thorough history is essential to determine the nature of the initial condition, and to what degree it affected normal urinary tract physiology. Previous chemotherapy, pelvic radiation, or pelvic surgery can each contribute to deranged lower urinary tract physiology. Of paramount importance is the assessment of the patient's and family's commitment to a procedure that is lengthy and at times associated with complications and (most important) of their commitment to long-term follow-up.[26, 29, 30] The patient must demonstrate not only the ability to perform catheterization but also the motivation. An irresponsible patient or a

TABLE 113–1. Evaluation for Urinary Undiversion

History and physical examination
Psychological assessment
  Commitment
  Understanding
  Support systems
Imaging
  Kidneys—IVP
  Ureters—IVP
  Diversion—loop-o-gram
  Bladder—VCUG
  Urethra—VCUG or RUG
Renal function
  Serum creatinine
  Acid-base status (CO_2)
  Concentrating ability
Urodynamics
  CMG
  Outlet resistance (UPP or leak point)
Gastrointestinal function
  Previous bowel surgery?
  Radiation?
  Continence?

IVP, intravenous pyelogram; VCUG, voiding cystourethrogram; RUG, retrograde urethrogram; CMG, cystometrogram; UPP, urethral pressure profilometry.

family not compliant with medical advice would be done a disservice by performing an undiversion.

All efforts should be made to obtain previous operative reports to gain insight into the patient's current anatomy. Further anatomical information can be obtained from contrast studies, which should include an intravenous pyelogram to evaluate the upper tracts. This study will show the surgeon some of the most critical information, i.e., the presence, location, and length of the ureters. A cystogram is used to determine bladder capacity and shape and the presence or absence of reflux. "Loop-o-grams" of conduit diversions assess the length of the conduit segment, the presence of stone formation, and reflux.

Imaging

Renal ultrasonography provides data on renal parenchymal thickness and echotexture as well as hydroureteronephrosis when present. Sonography can also identify an ectopic kidney. Cystoscopy should be performed to inspect the bladder, bladder neck, and trigone. Attention should be paid to the ability of the bladder neck and external sphincter to close. Of equal importance is the notation of the length, course, and caliber of the urethra, particularly if penile-urethral reconstruction has occurred. Such information is critical when contemplating postoperative clean intermittent catheterization. At the time of cystoscopy, retrograde pyelograms should be done when relevant to document the length of ureteral stumps available for reconstruction, as well as to assess any possible ureterovesical junction obstruction. An "undivertogram" done at cystoscopy with a simultaneous loop-o-gram can in one image show the anatomical relationships of the functional ureters with the ureteral stumps (Fig. 113–1).

Renal Function

The patient's renal functional status directly influences the surgical options available, especially when the use of different intestinal segments for reconstruction is considered. Functional considerations include glomerular filtration rate, acid-base status, and concentrating ability. Many patients will have suffered renal insufficiency as a result of their underlying urological disorder. In such patients a standard intestinal cystoplasty may result in reabsorption of sodium, chloride, and acidic ions and place further demands on an already stressed system.

Patients with renal insufficiency may be best served by a gastrocystoplasty when bladder augmentation is indicated.[31] Urinary tract refunctionalization

may be performed in preparation for renal transplantation. In some patients it may even slow the progression of chronic renal failure.

Urodynamics

All patients need preoperative formal urodynamic evaluation. If the goal of undiversion is to restore the patient as closely as possible to normal physiology, an accurate picture of current bladder function or dysfunction is crucial.[32–34] A full urodynamic evaluation should assess postvoid residual volume, sensation of fullness, uninhibited contractions, capacity, and compliance, as well as voiding pressures. Urethral pressure profilometry in tandem with electromyography can assess urethral functional length, maximal urethral resistance, the nature of pudendal nerve function, and whether the sphincter is acting in a synergistic fashion. Patients with severe reflux can give a false impression of adequate capacity and compliance, as urine is also stored in their dilated ureters. Ultimately the aim of urodynamics is to determine the degree to which the bladder can function in its storage and emptying capacity. In regard to the former, not only are capacity and compliance pivotal but it is equally crucial to determine whether the bladder neck–sphincter complex can provide adequate resistance, and therefore continence at optimal bladder filling pressures.

Gastrointestinal Function

Gastrointestinal function warrants consideration as well. Intestinal segments may have been used in previous operations or may have been compromised by radiation therapy, precluding their current use. In myelodysplastic patients the removal of colonic segments may result in chronic diarrhea or bicarbonate loss. Removal of the terminal ileum from gastrointestinal continuity can affect vitamin B_{12} absorption. The presence of the appendix affords the surgical option of an appendicostomy (Mitrofanoff procedure).[35]

Surgical Considerations

No two patients who present for undiversion are identical. Therefore, each patient should be approached analytically; once the seeming confusion is distilled to several distinct physiological problems, a rational plan can be formulated.[36–38] A basic plan and possible alternatives should be discussed with patient and family. Undiversion operations do not

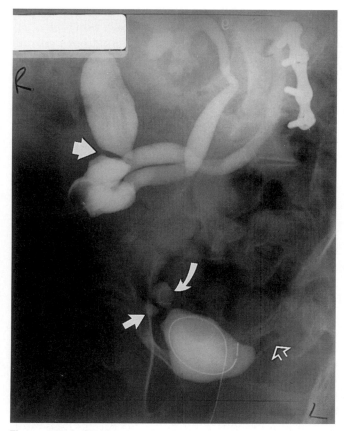

Figure 113–1. Simultaneous loop-o-gram and cystogram in a child with ileal conduit diversion. Ureteral and loop anatomy is clearly demonstrated, including a loop stricture (large arrow), as well as the relative position and length of ureters relative to the bladder. Reflux into the distal dilated ureteral stump (small arrow) and bladder diverticulum (curved arrow) is shown. A small distal left ureteral stump is also demonstrated (open arrow).

proceed identically, yet several general concepts are relevant to all cases.

Preoperatively, all patients should receive a thorough bowel preparation. This affords the surgeon use of the entire bowel with a decreased risk of infection. Preoperative intravenous antibiotics and hydration further diminish infectious complications and maintain the patient in a euvolemic state.

Undiversions can be among the most lengthy procedures in urology and one should plan accordingly. Intraoperative fluid losses far exceed a standard intraperitoneal procedure and all efforts should be made to monitor the patient's volume status regularly. Helpful parameters are central venous pressure, urinary output, and acid-base status. A midline incision from xiphoid to pubis will give the maximal exposure required. Large, oval self-retaining retractors (Denis Browne, Buchwalter) will also help obtain and maintain exposure.

Ureter

Ureteral length should be treated preciously and ureteral tissue should never be sacrificed lightly. If possible, an end-to-end ureteroureterostomy should be created between the proximal ureter and the ureteral stumps. Renal mobilization can allow the proximal ureter to reach more inferiorly and may afford the surgeon the critical extra distance necessary to perform a tension-free anastomosis. In many instances, only one ureter (if any) will be of sufficient length to reach the bladder; therefore, a transureteroureterostomy (TUU)[39] or an ileal interposition[40] may be necessary. As in all TUUs, the donor ureter should be mobilized to preserve the periureteral vasculature and the recipient ureters should be minimally mobilized. The anastomosis should be nonangulated, spatulated, stented, and free of tension. Ileal interpositions require isolation of a segment of ileum on its blood supply; the ileum should be of sufficient length to reach the bladder in a tension-free fashion. Tapering of the ileum is done on its antimesenteric border, with care taken not to remove more than one third of the circumference. The ileum should be maintained in its isoperistaltic orientation. This interposition can also be used to replace both ureters if the need arises by connecting the ileum to both renal pelves.

A psoas hitch can be used to help with short gaps in ureteral distance. This is most effective if the major portion of the ipsilateral bladder wall and a good amount of the contralateral bladder wall are mobilized to allow the bladder to move freely to the psoas. The psoas muscle is cleaned off and its tendon exposed. Sutures are used to fix the bladder to the tendon, just lateral to the iliac vessels, with care not to suture the genitofemoral nerve. A Boari flap can also be used to gain further length (Fig. 113–2A). However, this should be decided at an early stage, as a Boari flap requires an oblique bladder opening to create the flap. Finally, as a last resort, when ureteral length is inadequate and an ileal interposition cannot be performed, an autotransplant can be done. Interposition of a gastric tube for gaps in the ureter has been explored in an animal model. Experience with this approach in humans is limited and it has anecdotally been associated with significant hematuria.

In cases of significant ureteral dilation, the ureter should be tapered on its lateral aspect, as is done in a megaureter repair, to preserve its blood supply. All ureteral reimplants should be done in a tunneled manner to prevent reflux.

Bladder

Bladder augmentation should be considered for any patient whose capacity is insufficient or who demonstrates hypertonicity (filling pressures greater than 40 cm H_2O) on urodynamic testing.[41–43] Lack of consideration of these factors can lead to incontinence and possible reflux. Ileum, ileocecum, sigmoid, and stomach have been used for this purpose. When the bladder is absent, neobladders can be fashioned entirely of detubularized intestine and a continent, catheterizable stoma brought to the abdominal wall or perineum (Fig. 113–2B). In patients with renal insufficiency, gastric augmentation is preferred for its net secretion of hydrogen ions and chloride.[31] All the other segments must be detubularized and reconfigured to prevent high-pressure peristalsis, which will lead to incontinence or upper urinary tract dilation. Our preference is to perform the intestinal-vesical closure in two layers of running Vicryl (polyglactin 910) suture. Both a suprapubic and a urethral catheter should be used to ensure adequate drainage of urine, which will be mixed with clots and mucus. A previous intestinal conduit (if present) may be used as an augmenting patch cystoplasty; this can be coupled with another intestinal segment if needed.

Urethra and Bladder Neck

Frequently, patients need their urethral resistance enhanced (if not created altogether). Pudendal nerve damage from spinal dysraphism or previous surgery may make the urinary sphincter inactive. Previous surgery or radiation may have caused direct damage to the sphincter. To improve on inadequate resistance, several options are available (Fig. 113–2C).

The Young-Dees-Leadbetter bladder neck reconstruction is a urethral lengthening procedure combined with a wrap of detrusor muscle around this tube.[44] Continence results from the increased urethral resistance of the lengthened urethra. Almost uni-

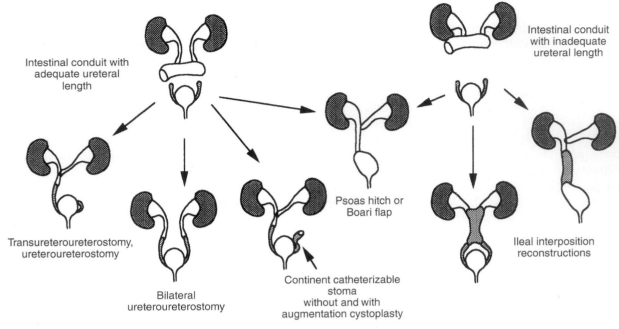

Intestinal conduit with adequate ureteral length

Intestinal conduit with inadequate ureteral length

Transureteroureterostomy, ureteroureterostomy

Bilateral ureteroureterostomy

Continent catheterizable stoma without and with augmentation cystoplasty

Psoas hitch or Boari flap

Ileal interposition reconstructions

A   URETERAL RECONSTRUCTION

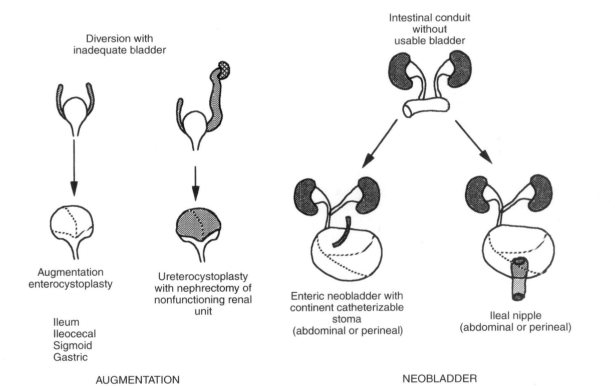

Diversion with inadequate bladder

Intestinal conduit without usable bladder

Augmentation enterocystoplasty

Ileum
Ileocecal
Sigmoid
Gastric

Ureterocystoplasty with nephrectomy of nonfunctioning renal unit

Enteric neobladder with continent catheterizable stoma (abdominal or perineal)

Ileal nipple (abdominal or perineal)

AUGMENTATION   NEOBLADDER

B   BLADDER RECONSTRUCTION

Figure 113–2 *See legend on opposite page*

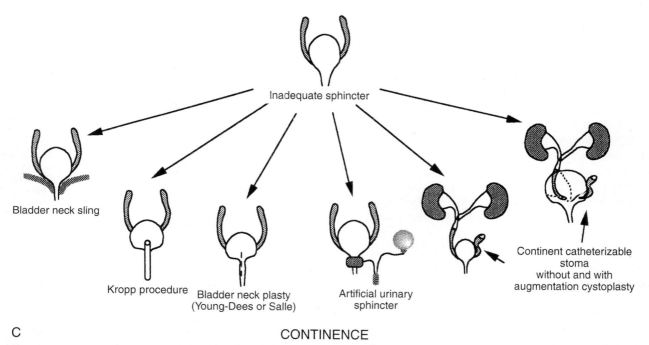

C   CONTINENCE

Figure 113–2. Diagrammatic representation of various reconstructive options available in urinary undiversion to accomplish ureteral reconstruction, perform bladder reconstruction, and achieve continence. *A,* Possible options for ureteral reconstruction to reestablish the connection of the ureters with the urinary reservoir. *B,* The basic bladder reconstructive options are shown in general; each is described in detail elsewhere. *C,* Various techniques to increase continence. In all cases the possibility of intermittent catheterization must be considered and prepared for.

formly the ureters need to be mobilized and reimplanted away from the lengthened urethra positioned on the bladder floor. Because of the detrusor muscle wrap from the base of the bladder, a portion of bladder volume is lost, and this must often be compensated by a bladder augmentation. This procedure has encountered varying rates of continence. It is less effective in the myelodysplastic neurogenic bladder.

Another continence procedure, the Salle,[45] uses an anterior bladder wall flap sutured to a strip of rectangular mucosa on the floor of the bladder. The lengthened urethra is then covered with bladder mucosa lateral to the urethra to create a flap-valve mechanism.

The Kropp procedure involves creating a tube from the anterior bladder wall and tunneling it submucosally in the bladder base.[46] Although continence is achieved, catheterization can be difficult and there is no "pop-off" mechanism.

Fascial slings can support the urethra and add resistance. The end result is usually a need for intermittent catheterization. The fascia can be harvested from either the anterior rectus abdominis fascia or the fascia lata of the thigh. A great deal of care is invested in locating the proper plane behind the bladder neck where the fascia will lie; failure to do so can result in urethral perforation and possible fistula formation.

The Mitrofanoff procedure uses the appendix as a catheterizable conduit that is tunneled under the bladder mucosa to create a flap-valve mechanism of continence.[35] Continence rates have been quite satisfactory. The stoma can be brought to the abdominal wall (which is particularly beneficial to wheelchair-bound patients) or to the perineum. If the appendix is unavailable or unsuitable for use, other organs such as ureter, tapered ileum, gastric, or fallopian tubes can be similarly employed. As with all catheterizable conduits, the path for the catheter should be as straight and as narrow as possible to prevent the catheters kinking or wandering. Creation of a V flap of skin in these stomas will prevent stenoses and further recess the stoma for a better cosmetic result. An umbilical stomal location may be almost invisible.

Artificial urinary sphincters are another tool in the surgeon's armamentarium.[47–49] The bulb for sphincter inflation and deflation can be placed in the scrotum or labia majora. As with the fascial sling procedures, the most important maneuver is getting around the bladder neck without injuring the urethra. This can be difficult in patients with distorted anatomy from myelodysplasia and in reoperative cases. A large metal sound in the vagina may assist in delineating the anatomy.

Reflux

Vesicoureteral reflux needs to be corrected surgically at the time of the undiversion. Ureteral reimplantation can be by either the cross-trigonal or the

Politano-Leadbetter method. Tunnels of 3 to 5 cm are the goal. At times, only one ureter can be reimplanted in a long submucosal fashion; a TUU combined with a psoas hitch is helpful in these situations. Such repairs should be stented and the stents brought through separate stab incisions in the bladder. Some defunctionalized ureteral stumps may have reflux on a preoperative cystogram. This does not necessarily mean they will continue to reflux once urinary flow is resumed after undiversion, as part of the normal physiological prevention of reflux is dependent on the antegrade flow of urine from the kidney; nonetheless, our usual practice is to perform antireflux surgery.

Summary

Urinary continence and preservation of renal function are the goals of urinary undiversion. Each case must be thoroughly analyzed and regarded individually. Careful consideration of normal physiology and how it is altered in these complicated patients will yield the proper plan. Adherence to proper surgical technique plus familiarity with all possible technical options is necessary to ensure optimal results.

REFERENCES

1. Cordonnier JJ. Ureterosigmoid anastomosis. J Urol 63:276, 1950.
2. Nesbit RM. Ureterosigmoid anastomosis by direct elliptical connection: A preliminary report. J Urol 61:728, 1949.
3. Smith T. An account of an unsuccessful attempt to treat extroversion of the bladder by a new operation. St Barth Hosp Rep 15:29, 1879.
4. Altwein JE, Jonas V, Hohenfeller R. Long-term follow-up of children with colon conduit urinary diversion and ureterosigmoidostomy. J Urol 118:832, 1977.
5. Gittes RF. Ureterosigmoidostomy: Pros and cons. Dial Pediatr Urol 5:6, 1982.
6. Koch MO, McDougal WS. The pathophysiology of hyperchloremic metabolic acidosis after urinary diversion through intestinal segments. Surgery 98:561, 1985.
7. Bricker EM. Bladder substitution after pelvic evisceration. Surg Clin North Am 30:1511, 1950.
8. Hendren WH, Radopoulos D. Complications of ileal loop and colon conduit urinary diversion. Urol Clin North Am 10:451, 1983.
9. Mitchell ME, Yoder IC, Pfister RC, et al. Ileal loop stenosis: A late complication of urinary diversion. J Urol 118:957, 1977.
10. Pitts WR Jr, Muecke EC. A 20-year experience with ileal conduits: The fate of the kidneys. J Urol 122:154, 1979.
11. Schwarz GR, Jeffs RD. Ileal conduit urinary diversion in children: Computer analysis of follow-up from 2–16 years. J Urol 114:285, 1975.
12. Shapiro SF, Lebowitz R, Colodny AH. Fate of 90 children with ileal conduit urinary diversion a decade later: Analysis of complications, pyelography, renal function and bacteriology. J Urol 114:289, 1975.
13. Smith ED. Follow-up studies on 150 ileal conduits in children. J Pediatr Surg 7:1, 1972.
14. Elder DD, Moisey CV, Rees RWM. A long-term follow-up of the colonic conduit operation in children. Br J Urol 51:462, 1979.
15. Hendren WH. Non-refluxing colon conduit for temporary or permanent urinary diversion in children. J Pediatr Surg 10:381, 1975.
16. Kelalis P. Urinary diversion in children by sigmoid conduits: Its advantages and limitations. J Urol 129:552, 1983.
17. Perlmutter AD, Tank ES. Loop cutaneous ureterostomy in infancy. J Urol 99:559, 1968.
18. Retik AB, Perlmutter AD. Temporary urinary division in infants and young children. In Walsh PC, Gittes RF, Perlmutter AD, Stamey TA, eds. Campbell's Urology, 5th ed. Philadelphia, WB Saunders, 1986, pp 2116–2136.
19. Allen TD. Vesicostomy for temporary diversion of urine in small children. J Urol 123:929, 1980.
20. Duckett JW Jr. Cutaneous vesicostomy in children: The Blocksom technique. Urol Clin North Am 1:485, 1974.
21. Mandell J, Bauer SB, Colodny AH, et al. Cutaneous vesicostomy in infancy. J Urol 126:92, 1981.
22. Hendren WH. Reconstruction of previously diverted urinary tracts in children. J Pediatr Surg 8:135, 1973.
23. Hendren WH. Urinary diversion and undiversion in children. Surg Clin North Am 56:425, 1976.
24. Hendren WH. Urinary tract refunctionalization after prior diversion in children. Ann Surg 180:494, 1976.
25. Hendren WH. Complications of ureterostomy. J Urol 120:269, 1978.
26. Hendren WH. Urinary undiversion: Refunctionalization of the previously diverted urinary tract. In Walsh PC, Retik AB, Stamey TA, Vaughan ED Jr, eds. Campbell's Urology, 6th ed. Philadelphia, WB Saunders, 1992, pp 2721–2749.
27. Lapides J, Diokno AC, Gould FR, et al. Clean intermittent self-catheterization in the treatment of urinary tract disease. J Urol 107:458, 1972.
28. Lapides J, Diokno AC, Gould FR, Low BS. Further observations on self-catheterization. J Urol 116:169, 1976.
29. Elder JS, Snyder HM, Hubert WC, Duckett JW. Perforation of the augmented bladder in patients undergoing clean intermittent catheterization. J Urol 140:1159, 1981.
30. Rushton HG, Woodward JR, Parrott TS, et al. Delayed bladder rupture after augmentation enterocystoplasty. J Urol 140:344, 1988.
31. Adams MC, Mitchel ME, Rink R. Gastrocystoplasty: An alternative solution to the problem of urological reconstruction in the severely compromised patient. J Urol 140:1152, 1988.
32. Bauer SB, Colodny AH, Hallet M, et al. Urinary undiversion in myelodysplasia: Criteria for selection and predictive value of urodynamics. J Urol 124:187, 1980.
33. Kogan SJ, Kim K, Levitt SB. Preoperative evaluation of bladder function prior to renal transplantation or urinary tract reconstruction in children: Description of a method. J Pediatr Surg 11:1007, 1976.
34. Kogan SJ, Kim K, Levitt SB. Bladder evaluation in pediatric patients before undiversion in previously diverted urinary tracts. J Urol 118:443, 1977.
35. Mitrofanoff P. Cystostomie continente trans-appendiculaire dans le traitement des vessies neurologiques. Chir Pediatr 21:297, 1980.
36. Gonzalez R, Sidi A, Zhang G. Urinary undiversion: Indications, technique and results in 50 cases. J Urol 136:13, 1986.
37. Mitchell ME. Urinary tract diversion and undiversion in the pediatric age group. Surg Clin North Am 61:1147, 1981.
38. Mitchell ME, Rink RC. Urinary diversion and undiversion. Urol Clin North Am 12:111, 1985.
39. Hendren WH, Hensle TW. Transureteroureterostomy: Experience with 75 cases. J Urol 123:826, 1980.
40. Goodwin WE, Winter CC, Turner RD. Replacement of the ureter by small intestine: Clinical application and results of ileal ureter. J Urol 81:406, 1959.
41. Kass EJ, Koff SA. Bladder augmentation in the pediatric neuropathic bladder. J Urol 129:552, 1983.
42. Mitchell ME. Use of bowel in undiversion. Urol Clin North Am 13:349, 1986.
43. Sidi AA, Aliabadi H, Gonzalez R. Enterocystoplasty in the management and reconstruction of the pediatric neurogenic bladder. J Pediatr Surg 22:153, 1987.
44. Leadbetter GW. Surgical correction of total urinary incontinence. J Urol 91:261, 1964.

45. Salle JL, de Fraga JC, Amarante A, et al. Urethral lengthening with anterior bladder wall flap for urinary incontinence: A new approach. J Urol 152 (pt 2):803, 1994.

46. Kropp KA, Angwafo FF. Urethral lengthening and reimplantation for neurogenic incontinence in children. J Urol 135:533, 1986.

47. Mitchell ME, Rink RC. Experience with the artificial urinary sphincter in children and young adults. J Pediatr Surg 18:700, 1983.

48. Rink RC, Mitchell ME. Surgical correction of urinary incontinence. J Pediatr Surg 19:637, 1984.

49. Scott FB, Bradley WE, Trumm GW. Treatment of urinary incontinence by an implantable prosthestic urinary sphincter. J Urol 112:75, 1974.

Part III

GENITALIA/URETHRA

Chapter 114

Circumcision

Steven G. Docimo

Neonatal circumcision is generally performed by obstetricians, pediatricians, or family physicians. The procedure is often done with no anesthesia but is preferably performed after a local penile block.[1] Most commonly, the circumcision is performed using a clamp, bell, or shield, all designed to protect the glans during removal of the prepuce. These procedures are generally safe, but significant complications do occur.[2, 3] The purpose of this chapter is to discuss formal surgical circumcision, usually performed after the first 3 months of life.

The indications for circumcision in the male child are somewhat controversial. Phimosis is often cited as a reason, but a nonretractable foreskin may be a normal condition in a child younger than 4 or 5 years of age (Fig. 114–1).[3] Despite this, in some young boys the prepuce is tight enough to produce ballooning during voiding. These children often present with a discharge from the preputial opening, infection, or both, and these boys will benefit from circumcision. In addition, it has been convincingly demonstrated that an intact prepuce predisposes to a higher incidence of urinary tract infection in boys under 1 year of age.[4] Circumcision is reasonable in boys who have had infection or who have congenital anomalies of the urinary tract, including vesicoureteral reflux, that predispose to infection. Formal circumcision is often performed for cosmetic reasons. Examples include the child whose medical condition precluded elective neonatal circumcision or the child who has an unacceptable cosmetic result from neonatal circumcision.

Little preoperative preparation is necessary for elective circumcision. Taking down preputial adhesions in an awake child preoperatively to allow cleaning under the foreskin seems unnecessary and is clearly painful. No preoperative laboratory studies are necessary in an otherwise healthy child.

SURGICAL TECHNIQUE

The procedure is usually performed in the outpatient setting with the child under general anesthesia and in the supine position. An antiseptic preparation is made of the phallus and lower abdomen, and sterile drapes are employed. If the opening of the prepuce is too narrow to allow visualization of the glans, it can be spread with a fine hemostat, taking care not to enter the urethra. Using proximal traction on the prepuce, adhesions between the foreskin and glans are taken down bluntly with a probe or fine hemostat. Smegma is removed by washing the area under the prepuce with povidone-iodine (Betadine). A dorsal slit of the phimotic ring is seldom required in a young child but may be necessary in an adolescent or adult. If it is performed, the incision should be extended only as far as is necessary for retraction of the prepuce (Fig. 114–2). The remainder of the procedure should be carried out as otherwise described.

A traction suture in the glans is unnecessary for a routine circumcision but may be helpful in more complicated reoperative cases. A skin marker is used to identify the level of the outer preputial incision, as the skin can become distorted during manipulation (Fig. 114–3A). It is important to push down on the prepubic fat pad at the base of the penis to avoid removal of too much shaft skin. In a young boy, it often looks as if too much skin is being left behind when the fat pad is in its natural position. The outer preputial incision can be made in a straight line, or with an inverted V in the ventral side. The inverted V allows a more cosmetic closure with less need for frenuloplasty. The incision is made with the scalpel and carried down almost to Buck's fascia while the first assistant exerts traction on both sides of the incision.

The foreskin is now retracted. The frenulum will

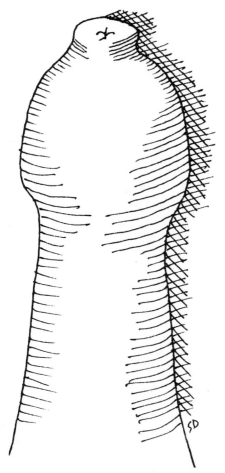

Figure 114–1. The foreskin of a young child may be phimotic and protrude beyond the end of the glans. This does not necessarily represent an abnormal condition in an infant or younger toddler.

most likely tether the urethral meatus at this point (Fig. 114–3*B*). If the frenulum is extremely short and seems to be a superficial web to the meatus, it can be divided superficially with scissors. More commonly, the frenulum can be left undivided and will assume a normal appearance after the inner preputial incision is made. A skin marker is not necessary for the inner preputial incision, as the landmarks are easily followed. The inner preputial incision should be made 4 to 5 mm away from the coronal sulcus to leave a cosmetically pleasing collar between the corona and the shaft skin. This incision should be carried straight across the frenulum, or even low across it. This area will tend to spring up after the incision is made and assume an inverted-V configuration. By carrying the incision low over the frenulum, the need for frenuloplasty will generally be avoided.

After both incisions have been made, a "sleeve" of preputial tissue is created. Two hemostats are placed dorsally on each incision for traction. On the dorsal side, a scissors or hemostat is used to create a plane superficial to Buck's fascia from one incision to the other (Fig. 114–3*C*). The prepuce is incised along this

plane, and the subcutaneous attachments between Buck's fascia and the prepuce are divided with scissors, allowing the prepuce to be removed (Fig. 114–3*D*).

The penile shaft skin is retracted and the electrocautery is used for hemostasis. It is preferable to lift bleeding points with a fine pair of forceps and then coagulate rather than touch the penis directly. The neurovascular bundles run just beneath Buck's fascia and might be injured during cauterization. Bleeding in the skin edge should be handled judiciously; it generally stops after skin closure, and electrocautery can result in focal necrosis along the suture line. Skin closure is carried out with interrupted absorbable suture: plain or chromic catgut in 5-0 or 6-0 is adequate; there should be no need for a longer-lasting suture. Stitches are placed in the area of the frenulum and the dorsum and on both sides, and then held as quadrant traction sutures while intervening sutures are placed. This ensures a symmetrical closure of the penis (Fig. 114–3*E*).

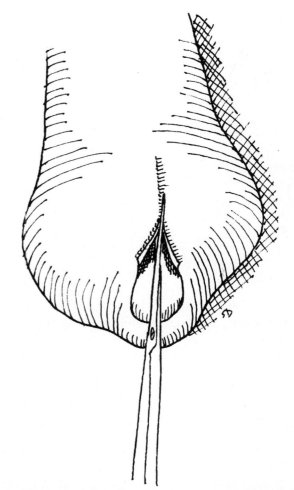

Figure 114–2. When a dorsal slit is necessary, it is made by crushing the midline dorsal prepuce with a straight hemostat. Care is used to avoid placing the clamp into the urethral meatus. The incision is made along the crushed area, minimizing bleeding.

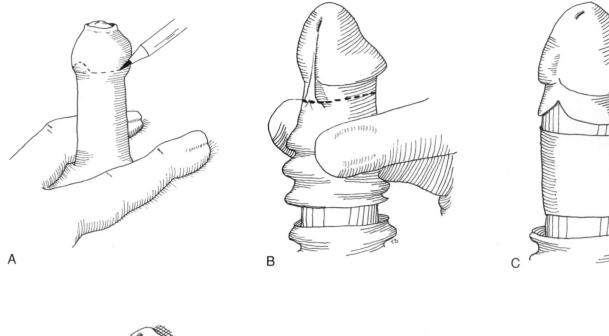

A

B

C

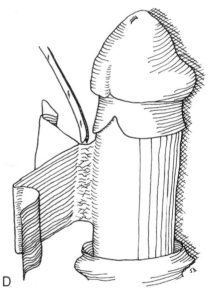

D

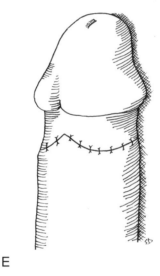

E

Figure 114–3. *A*, An outer preputial incision line is marked while the prepubic fat pad is depressed; this avoids the removal of too much shaft skin. Leaving extra skin in the form of an inverted V ventrally allows reconstruction without frenuloplasty in most cases. *B*, The inner preputial incision is made, leaving an adequate collar for reapproximation. The incision is carried straight or low across the frenulum, which releases the meatus and results in a V-shaped defect. *C*, A plane superficial to Buck's fascia is developed using the scissors on the dorsum of the penis. The skin will then be divided along this line. *D*, Staying close to the skin to be removed, the operator sharply dissects the subcutaneous attachments to the penile shaft, allowing the prepuce to be removed. *E*, Appearance of the penis at the end of the procedure. Note the carefully preserved inner preputial collar.

The dressing for circumcision is not critical. Many practitioners use no dressing at all, with good results. A petrolatum gauze can be used over the incision but should not be wrapped circumferentially. It should be removed on the first postoperative day to prevent sticking. An occlusive plastic dressing does not need to be manipulated by the parents and will fall off on its own in 1 to 2 weeks. The parents should be instructed to remove the dressing if it slips to the base of the penis and forms a tourniquet. If there is persistent oozing from the skin edge, any of the abovementioned dressings can be combined with gentle pressure from a nonadhesive elastic bandage, which should be removed 2 to 12 hours later.

COMPLICATIONS

Complications from a properly performed formal circumcision should be infrequent.[2] Persistent bleeding or subcutaneous hematoma is usually avoided with meticulous attention to hemostasis. Infection is a rare problem, usually amenable to warm soaks and oral antibiotic administration. Severe infection, possibly leading to gangrene, occurs rarely after circumcision[2, 5]; therefore, all infections should be monitored closely. Urethral injury, leading to iatrogenic hypospadias, is more common after clamp circumcisions than after formal circumcisions.[3] To avoid urethral injury, one should dissect close to the prepuce being removed, and take time to be cognizant of the location of the urethra and the plane of dissection at all times. Perhaps the most avoidable complication of formal circumcision is an unacceptable cosmetic result. The desired appearance is obtained by ensuring adequate residual shaft skin and inner preputial skin. Other techniques for performing circumcision, including the guillotine and dorsal slit methods, are less exact than the sleeve technique described. The inexperienced surgeon using these methods is more likely to remove inappropriate amounts of skin or fail to achieve the desired cosmetic appearance.

Editorial Comment
Craig A. Peters

Postoperative patient comfort can be improved with a penile block placed dorsally and ventrally at the start of the procedure, using bupivacaine.

Caution should be exercised in boys with a prominent pubic fat pad, as they are more prone to develop postcircumcision concealment of the penis. This is very distressing to some parents and may progress to a phimotic condition if the shaft skin is not retracted over the head of the penis. Parents should be warned of this possibility and instructed to regularly push the fat pad back with cleaning in the postoperative period.

REFERENCES

1. Fontaine P, Toffler WL. Dorsal penile nerve block for newborn circumcision. Am Fam Physician 43:1327, 1991.
2. Kaplan GW. Complications of circumcision. Urol Clin North Am 10:543, 1983.
3. Clair DL, Caldamone AA. Pediatric office procedures. Urol Clin North Am 15:715, 1988.
4. Wiswell TE. Circumcision—an update. Curr Probl Pediatr 22:424, 1992.
5. Woodside JR. Necrotizing fasciitis after circumcision. Am J Dis Child 134:301, 1980.

Chapter 115

Distal Hypospadias

David H. Ewalt

Hypospadias is a congenital anomaly in which the urethral meatus is located on the ventral aspect of the penis. The incidence of hypospadias from several sources is approximately 1 in 300. Given the bimodal embryological derivation of the male urethra, it is not surprising that it represents a spectrum of disease for which no single method of repair is applicable.[1] Over the years, more than 200 techniques have been described, attesting to the ingenuity of the surgeons dealing with this condition as well as the lack of uniformly optimal cosmetic and functional results. The classification scheme for hypospadias is based on the location of the meatus after correction of associated chordee. Distal hypospadias (at or beyond the distal one third of the penis) constitutes approximately 50 percent of all cases of hypospadias.[2] The contemporary surgical approach to this degree of hypospadias is the subject of this chapter.

PREOPERATIVE EVALUATION

In addition to a standard maternal and postnatal history, specific information regarding a familial history of hypospadias is obtained. Physical examination begins with an assessment of the level and quality of the meatal skin. Although the position of the meatus may be similar in various instances, completely different repairs may be indicated based on anatomical nuances unique to each case. Associated anomalies such as chordee, penile torsion, and penoscrotal transposition are noted. The finding of an undescended testis should always alert the examiner to the possibility of an intersex disorder and warrants a karyotype determination. Although this is extremely uncommon with a distal hypospadias, it has been described and should be ruled out.[3] Upper tract radiological evaluation is not indicated in distal hypospadias unless one or more organ system anomalies are present.[4] Although a prostatic utricle is occa-

sionally associated with a distal hypospadias, voiding studies are rarely indicated before repair.

With refinements in surgical technique and improvements in optical magnification and pediatric anesthesia, correction of hypospadias can be performed at progressively younger ages. The anesthetic risk to infants after 6 months of age is no greater than that for older children when performed by experienced pediatric anesthesiologists. Younger infants are more easily managed (fewer bladder spasms, less discomfort) by parents and have amnesia for the operation. With optical magnification of 2 to 3 power, most repairs can be performed in patients at 6 to 12 months of age on an outpatient basis. If the child has a postoperative complication that requires reoperation, this can be done 6 months after the original repair and will still be performed before 18 months of age when sexual identity begins in the male.

OPERATIVE MANAGEMENT

There are several elements of surgical repair common to all hypospadias procedures. These include meatoplasty, whereby the meatus is positioned on the tip of the glans to permit a straight urinary stream. Glansplasty involves creating a normal conical glans with a normal ventral bridge below the urethral meatus. Orthoplasty ensures that the penis is straight and all chordee is corrected. Urethroplasty involves construction of a hairless urethra of uniform caliber and appropriate size for the patient. Finally, skin coverage should attempt to provide the appearance of a "normal" circumcised penis. All elements of the repair should be met to obtain an optimal cosmetic and functional result.

Many of the basic principles of plastic surgery are utilized during any hypospadias repair. These include liberal use of traction sutures and skin hooks to avoid trauma to the delicate tissues of the infant penis. Hemostasis is obtained by meticulous bipolar electrocautery and fine suture ligatures. Administration of 1 percent lidocaine (Xylocaine) with 1:100,000 epinephrine (maximal lidocaine dose 5 mg/kg) helps provide intraoperative hemostasis and can be used to infiltrate the incision as well as the glans. An elastic tourniquet is usually unnecessary in the techniques described.

The correction of chordee is mandatory for any hypospadias repair. The skin of the shaft of the penis is degloved just superficial to Buck's fascia to the level of the scrotal fat pad. This will relieve most cases of mild chordee secondary to skin tethering. This is confirmed by an artificial erection (placement of a tourniquet at the base of the penis with injection of normal saline [injectable] through a 25-gauge butterfly needle into the side of the corpora cavernosa) demonstrating a straight penis. Persistent chordee requires further ventral dissection to remove any remaining tethering bands. When mild chordee persists, dorsal plication sutures or Nesbit wedge tucks can be used to straighten the area of greatest curvature; 4-0 or 5-0 Prolene or Tevdek suture is used and the knot is buried. When moderate to severe chordee remains, the repairs described in this chapter are unlikely to be suitable.

A variety of different techniques can be used to prevent postoperative urethrocutaneous fistula formation. The avoidance of overlapping suture lines and interposition of healthy tissue between the neourethra and the skin are invaluable aids in preventing fistulas. Additional coverings for the neourethra include portions of the preputial pedicle or areas of deepithelialized shaft skin.[5, 6] A multilayered closure of the urethroplasty can also decrease the rate of fistula formation.[7]

The final elements of all hypospadias repairs include skin coverage. In most repairs, adequate shaft skin remains for coverage of the penis so that a ventral median raphe can be developed to the level of the corona. After the urethroplasty, the dorsal prepuce is split in the midline to the level of the coronal sulcus. This allows for lateral and dorsal shaft skin to be transferred to the ventrum to cover the ventral defect that remains after release of chordee. When there is severe ventral skin deficiency, it may be necessary to split the dorsal prepuce and cover the ventral defect in the Byers manner, which is not as cosmetically appealing as the midline ventral closure. Sutures of 6-0 or 7-0 chromic are used to reapproximate the skin because of the quick reabsorption rate and decreased likelihood of suture sinuses. A horizontal mattress closure gives a more cosmetically appealing result than simple sutures. Another alternative includes a subcuticular closure with 7-0 Vicryl or polydioxanone suture (PDS), but this may be difficult, depending on the thickness of the subcutaneous tissue of the penile skin.

Optimal outcome in hypospadias repair often depends not only on the expertise of the surgeon but also on choosing the appropriate repair for the patient's anatomy. The complications seen after reconstruction are as often related to errors in design and planning as to technique. Versatility and adaptability with a variety of techniques and "tricks of the trade" are key to obtaining consistently successful results. The procedures described in this chapter for distal hypospadias repair include the Magpi procedure, glans approximation procedure (GAP), and Mathieu or flip-flap procedure.

Glanular and Coronal Hypospadias

The meatal advancement and glanuloplasty (Magpi) described by Duckett and Snyder is ideally suited for distal (glanular and coronal) hypospadias without chordee.[8] The success of the procedure depends on proper patient selection. The dorsal urethral plate and ventral urethral meatus must be mobile to allow the urethra to be advanced to the tip of the penis with ventral coverage by glans tissue. The mobility of the ventral urethral meatus can be assessed with fine 0.5-mm tissue forceps. If this tissue will advance to the tip of the penis, the patient is probably a good candidate for the Magpi procedure. Initially, a circumferential skin incision is made 2 to 3 mm proximal to the coronal sulcus, and the shaft skin is degloved just superficial to Buck's fascia (Fig. 115–1A and B). After an artificial erection confirms the absence of chordee, a longitudinal incision is made in the bridge tissue between the dorsal meatus and the tip of the penis (Fig. 115–1B). Occasionally a wedge of tissue must be excised if the bridge tissue is large. The longitudinal incision is then closed transversely with interrupted sutures such as 7-0 Vicryl (Fig. 115–1C). This maneuver not only widens the often stenotic urethral meatus but also advances the dorsal urethral plate to a more normal position. Three traction sutures are then placed on the ventral aspect of the penis, with two in the lateral glanular position and one in the ventral meatal position. The meatal suture is pulled distally, while the two glanular sutures are pulled proximally to give the glans a conical shape (Fig. 115–1D). The redundant medial glanular tissue is then excised. The glans is then reapproximated over the urethral channel in two layers, with a deep layer through the medial aspect of the glanular fascia and a superficial epithelial layer (Fig. 115–1E). Appropriate glans reapproximation ventral to the urethra is paramount to avoid meatal regression. The glanular channel should allow a bougie to 10 to 12 Fr. without any difficulty in a 6- to 12-month-old child. Excess penile skin is then excised as previously described and reapproximated to give

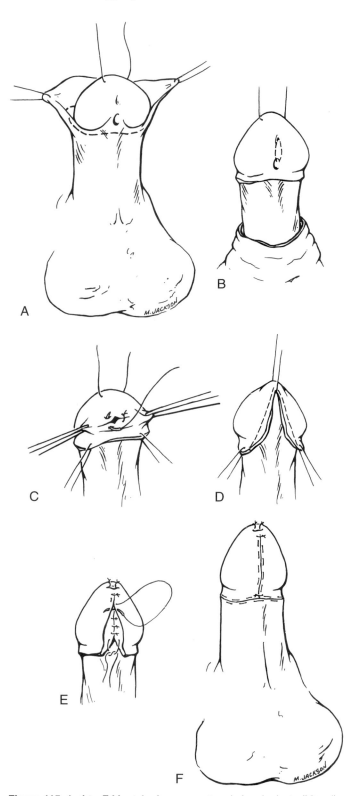

Figure 115–1. A to F, Meatal advancement and glanuloplasty (Magpi) procedure.

a circumcised appearance (Fig. 115–1F). A urethral drainage catheter is generally not necessary with the Magpi procedure.

If the glans is particularly wide and the dorsal urethral groove is deep, the glans approximation pro-

cedure described by Zaontz is appropriate.[9] The circumferential skin incision used is similar to that of the Magpi procedure. After the penis is degloved and the absence of chordee confirmed, two longitudinal incisions are made on the ventral aspect of the glans so that the width between the two incisions is approximately 10 to 12 mm, allowing for a 10 to 12 Fr. urethral channel (Fig. 115–2A and B). The lateral skin margins of the urethral plate are then reapproximated followed by a second-layer closure of glanular tissue (Fig. 115–2C). A standard preputial island flap is then developed from the dorsal penile skin and de-epithelialized. A buttonhole is then made in the dorsal subcutaneous tissue, and the flap is transferred to the ventral aspect of the penis (Fig. 115–2C). It is sutured into place over the repair to prevent overlapping suture lines between the urethra and overlying skin (Fig. 115–2D). The penile skin is then closed in a fashion similar to that of the Magpi procedure (Fig. 115–2E and F). A urinary diversion catheter is left in place for approximately 7 to 10 days.

Distal Shaft Hypospadias

When the meatus is located proximal to the coronal sulcus, the Mathieu or flip-flap procedure is indicated.[6, 7, 10] Because the success of the procedure depends on adequate vascularization from the perimeatal tissue, it should be used only for relatively short defects where healthy ventral shaft skin tissue exists. The meatal-based proximal fasciocutaneous flap can be developed directly over the urethra or off to one side of the penis (Fig. 115–3A). Using a ruler or calipers for measurement, the length of the flap equals the distance between the meatus and the tip of the glans. The flap is then marked on the ventral aspect of the penis as shown in Figure 115–3A. The reconstructed urethra should have a caliber of approximately 12 Fr. The skin incision is made in a circumferential fashion, with care taken to preserve as much of the soft tissue to the flap as possible. The skin of the penis is degloved just superficial to Buck's fascia, and an artificial erection is created to confirm the absence of any associated chordee. Two longitudinal incisions are then made on the ventral aspect of the glans, and glanular wings are developed (Fig. 115–3B). Two traction sutures can be placed at the distal aspect of the fasciocutaneous flap, and dissection is then made between the flap and underlying tissue, with care taken to preserve as much of the vascularity to the flap as possible. The flap is then sutured to the dorsal urethral plate with a running 7-0 PDS or Vicryl suture (Fig. 115–3C). Adjunctive measures that can be taken to prevent fistula formation include a two-layer closure as previously described by Kass, or placement of a portion of the

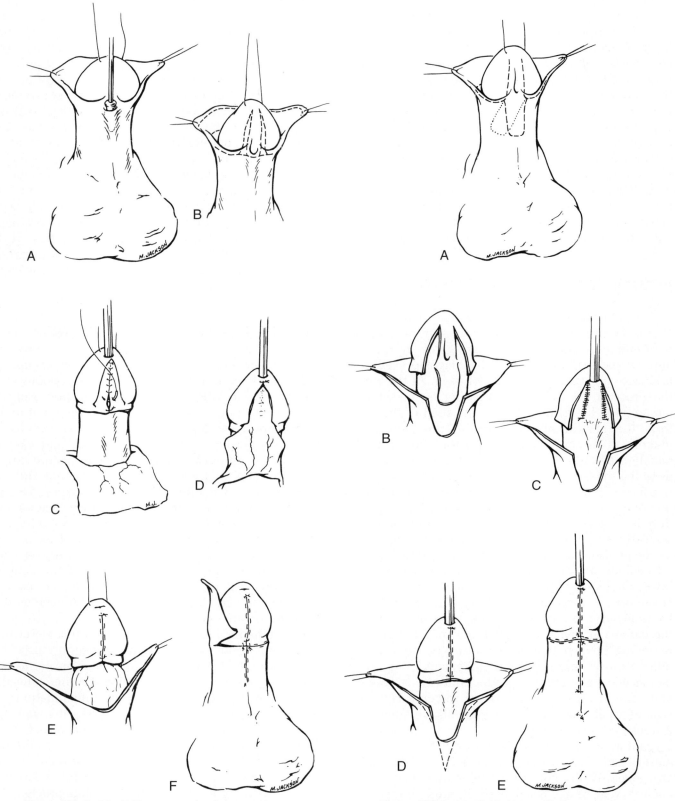

Figure 115–2. *A* to *F*, Glans approximation procedure.

Figure 115–3. *A* to *E*, Mathieu or flip-flap procedure.

dorsal vascular penile pedicle over the repair as described by Retik.[6, 7] The meatus is then reconstructed to have a 12 Fr. caliber with 7-0 chromic suture. The glans is reapproximated in two layers with a deeper layer of glanular tissue and a superficial skin layer closure (Fig. 115–3D). The skin of the penis is reapproximated and closed in a suitable fashion to give the penis a normal circumcised appearance (Fig. 115–3E). In many instances the fasciocutaneous flip-flap removes a significant portion of ventral penile skin so that Byers flaps are often used for ventral skin closure. A urinary diversion catheter is usually left indwelling for approximately 10 days after the repair.[6] We currently place a 6 Fr. urethral catheter into the bladder 2 to 3 cm and suture it to the glans. However, Retik et al have reported excellent results without the use of a diversion catheter.[6]

POSTOPERATIVE MANAGEMENT

The objectives of postoperative management should be minimizing complications, improving patient comfort, and easing the care given by the parents. In patients undergoing the Magpi procedure a drainage catheter is generally not used. At the end of the procedure a Tegaderm dressing is placed in a circumferential fashion around the shaft of the penis from the margin of the glans to the penoscrotal junction. This can be removed in the office approximately 5 to 7 days after the procedure. Patients undergoing the GAP or flip-flap procedure often require a urinary diversion catheter. For those patients who do not, the dressing as described for the Magpi procedure is adequate. Patients who have a urethral drainage catheter can have a compressive dressing placed on the penis to prevent hematoma formation or excessive edema. We currently compress the penis on the lower abdomen with a 4 × 4 gauze pad, which is covered by a Bioclusive dressing. This dressing can be removed 2 to 3 days after the procedure, often by the parents at home. If the parents are reticent about removing this on their own, it can be done in the office. If a urinary diversion catheter is used, it can be placed in a double diaper for continuous drainage and ease of care by the parents. Depending on the type of repair, the catheter is generally removed 1 to 2 weeks postoperatively.

Comfort of the patient is ensured by using acetaminophen (Tylenol) or Tylenol with codeine elixir. We generally do not use codeine in babies under about 1 year of age because of the unpredictable response to narcotic analgesics in this particular age group. In addition, babies under this age do quite well with Tylenol alone. The first several hours of analgesia is often accomplished by a caudal anesthetic, which can be topped off at the end of the procedure by the anesthesiologist. Bladder spasms are often much less severe in the young infant. However, if they are troublesome, oxybutynin (0.2 mg/kg PO twice a day) can be used. We currently do not use belladona and opium suppositories because the manufacturers do not guarantee that the opium is distributed in a uniform fashion throughout the length of the suppository. Since infants require only a portion of the suppository, for medicolegal reasons we do not use this on an outpatient basis when the child is not monitored. Antibiotic prophylaxis for wound infection is generally used at the discretion of the operating surgeon. There are no double-blind randomized studies in initial hypospadias repair that demonstrate the superiority of antibiotic prophylaxis to no antibiotics. In infants with a urethral drainage catheter, we generally do not use antibiotics while the catheter is indwelling, but give a 5-day therapeutic course of nitrofurantoin or Bactrim when the catheter is discontinued.

POSTOPERATIVE COMPLICATIONS

The avoidance of complications often begins by choosing the appropriate repair for the patient's anatomical nuances before the initial incision. Consistently successful results are obtained by attention to detail and preserving the vascularity of all skin flaps. However, despite meticulous planning and careful technique, complications are inevitable. More minor complications include hematoma formation and superficial loss of penile skin. Generally, these can be cared for in a conservative fashion. Even when there is marked loss of penile skin, it often re-epithelializes without hypertrophic scarring. Superficial wound infections occasionally occur and can generally be managed with antibiotics directed at skin flora such as in *Staphylococcus* and *Streptococcus* infections and local wound care. Warm sitz baths and topical antibiotics are invaluable in this regard.

Late complications for the procedures described include persistent or recurrent chordee, urethrocutaneous fistulas, urethral strictures, and meatal stenosis. These are generally dealt with at a time after the healing process is complete and all inflammation has diminished. It is generally appropriate to wait approximately 6 months after initial reconstruction to attempt a repair of any of these particular complications. With the Magpi procedure, meatal regression is the most common complication. Careful reapproximation of the glanular wings will help prevent the retrusive meatus. Fistula and meatal stenosis are rare, and the overall secondary surgery rate should approach approximately 1 percent.[8] The most common complication after the GAP or flip-flap procedure is fistula formation. This can be significantly reduced either by a multilayered closure of the urethra or by placement of interposing tissue between adjacent suture lines.[5-7] The overall reoperation rate after the GAP or flip-flap repair should be less than 5 percent.[6, 7, 9]

Summary

Distal hypospadias repair can generally be performed in children in early infancy, between 6 and 12 months of age, with meticulous technique and optimal magnification. Most contemporary reports of the repairs described suggest that the secondary reoperation rate should be less then 5 percent.[6-9] In the current era of managed care and the importance of successful outcomes, low reoperation rates are mandatory.

Editorial Comment

Craig A. Peters

Both this chapter and Chapter 116 by Drs. Koo and Duckett discuss some of the techniques for the management of distal hypospadias, the most common clinical form of the condition. While the fundamental technical aspects are similar, careful note should be taken of the differences, since they will aid individual surgeons in developing their own nuances to these cases. Selection of the type of repair is important and one should never adopt the approach of one kind of repair for all cases. As Dr. Ewalt emphasizes, the specific anatomy of the patient should be the principal determinant of the technique applied.

We have had good success with the Mathieu (flip-flap) procedure, including performing it without diversion stents. Adjunctive use of the subcutaneous flap of tissue from the dorsal aspect of the prepuce has reduced the incidence of fistulas. When a diversion stent is placed, I have usually preferred a simple, short urethral stent rather than a bladder catheter with its risk of bladder spasm. In children past the age of toilet training who have been referred for repair late, a bladder catheter is needed, because a number of these boys will not void postoperatively.

REFERENCES

1. Hinman F Jr. Atlas of Urosurgical Anatomy. Philadelphia, WB Saunders, 1993, pp 418–429.
2. Duckett J. Successful hypospadias repair. Contemp Urol 4:42, 1992.
3. Rajter J, Walsh PC. The incidence of intersexuality in patients with hypospadias and cryptorchidism. J Urol 116:769, 1976.
4. Khuri FJ, Hardy BE, Churchill PM. Urologic anomalies associated with hypospadias. Urol Clin North Am 8:565, 1981.
5. Belman AB. The de-epithelialized flap and its influence on hypospadias repair. J Urol 152:2332, 1994.
6. Retik AB, Mandell J, Bauer SB, et al. Meatal based hypospadias repair with the use of a dorsal subcutaneous flap to prevent urethrocutaneous fistula. J Urol 152:1229, 1994.
7. Kass EJ, Boling D. Single stage hypospadias reconstruction without fistula. J Urol 144:520, 1990.
8. Duckett JW, Snyder HM. Meatal advancement and glanuloplasty hypospadias repair after 1000 cases: Avoidance of meatal stenosis and regression. J Urol 147:665, 1992.
9. Zaontz MR. The GAP (glans approximation procedure) for glanular/coronal hypospadias. J Urol 141:359, 1989.
10. Mathieu P. Traitment en un temps de l'hypospadias balanique et juxtabalanique. J Chir (Paris) 39:481, 1932.

Chapter 116

Penile Hypospadias

Harry P. Koo and John W. Duckett, Jr.

Hypospadias is a congenital anomaly of the penis resulting in incomplete development of the anterior urethra. It occurs in one in every 300 live male births. The cause is still unknown; it is probably multifactorial (polygenic), given the familial incidence. Fathers of affected boys have an 8 percent incidence of hypospadias; male siblings, 14 percent.

The normal anatomy of the penis consists of paired corpora cavernosa covered by a thick fibrous tunica albuginea with a midline septum. The urethra traverses the penis within the corpus spongiosum. There are three separate portions of the male urethra. The portion above the wolffian duct opening forms the urethra down to and including the verumontanum, utricle, and urogenital sinus. The second anlage forms the segment extending from the verumontanum to the base of the glans. The glans segment is formed separately. The spermatic fascia or dartos fascia is the loose layer of connective tissue immediately beneath the skin. Superficial lymphatics and the dorsal veins of the penis are located in this fascia. Beneath the dartos fascia is Buck's fascia, which surrounds the corpora cavernosa and splits to contain the corpora spongiosum separately. The dorsal neurovascular bundle lies deep to Buck's fascia in the groove between the corpora cavernosa.

Hypospadias results in various degrees of urethral and corpus spongiosum deficiency. The skin on the ventral surface is often thin. The prepuce is deficient ventrally and forms a dorsal hood over the glans. The fibrous tissue found with chordee replaces Buck's fascia and the dartos fascia. Chordee is an entity that still remains poorly understood. The mesenchyme that would normally form the corpus spongiosum and fascial layers distal to the hypospadiac meatus in the normal urethra may persist as fibrous tissue. However, it is clear that the mere presence of this tissue is not responsible for all cases of penile curvature. Often, a growth differential between normally formed dorsal tissue of the corporeal bodies and the deficient ventral tissue and urethra may result in curvature.

PREOPERATIVE EVALUATION

A thorough history is obtained and physical examination performed in each patient. The technical details or complications of any previous genital surgery, including circumcision, have significant implications in planning surgical options at the time of repair. Physical examination assesses the level and quality of the hypospadiac meatus and urethra and identifies elements of the anomaly that will require simultaneous repair, including chordee, meatal stenosis, and penile torsion. The severity of hypospadias cannot always be defined by the original site of the meatus, which may be close to the tip of the glans yet have significant chordee. The location of the meatus after correction of curvature provides the most practical classification of hypospadias. The glanular and coronal types constitute anterior hypospadias, which accounts for 65 percent of all cases; the midshaft type accounts for 15 percent; and penoscrotal, scrotal, and perineal types make up the 20 percent that are classified as posterior.

An overall incidence of cryptorchidism with hypospadias has been cited at 9 percent, the frequency increasing with the severity of the hypospadias. The possibility of intersex should be investigated for severe hypospadias when associated with cryptorchidism. Mixed gonadal dysgenesis is the most common finding in this setting. Enlargement of the prostatic utricle is present in 10 to 15 percent of posterior hypospadias. Most of these are rarely of clinical significance. However, their presence can often result in unexpected difficulty with urethral catheterization at the time of repair.

TIMING OF SURGERY

Refinements in microsurgical technique and improvements in anesthesia have allowed surgeons to perform hypospadias repairs in patients at progressively younger ages. The optimal psychological window for hypospadias repair is between 6 and 18 months, when the emotional effects of surgery are at a minimum. The younger child is easily managed in diapers and probably has amnesia from the operation through subsequent development.

GENERAL PRINCIPLES OF SUCCESSFUL REPAIR

The objectives of hypospadias correction include (1) complete straightening of the penis by orthoplasty (release of chordee), (2) positioning of the neomeatus to the tip of the glans, (3) creation of a symmetrical glans and shaft, and (4) normalization of voiding and erections. In short, the aim of the surgeon is to recreate a "normal" penis while minimizing complications.

Clearly the most important elements for a successful hypospadias outcome are delicate tissue handling, familiarity with mobilizing skin flaps, and compulsive attention to the details of plastic surgical principles. Castroviejo needle holders, fine iris scissors, and optical magnification are invaluable. Tissue handling and trauma to delicate tissues are minimized with traction sutures. Subcutaneous injection of epinephrine (1:100,000) has been very useful for hemostasis without causing tissue ischemia, and is injected along proposed lines of incision and into the glans. Selective low-current electrocautery is used by grasping individual vessels with fine hemostats.

Preparation for each particular repair is made by marking the skin, followed by incision with a sharp, fine blade. The shaft skin is sharply taken down from the penile shaft to its base. The deeper, relatively avascular tissue planes can be opened by spreading the tips of scissors, limiting cutting to only the remaining tissues. Release of the shaft skin will straighten many mild degrees of penile curvature. Adequate orthoplasty is confirmed by placing an elastic tourniquet at the base of the penis and injecting normal saline through a 25-gauge needle through the glans into one corporeal body. When curvature persists, additional fibrous tissue is sharply excised from the corporeal bodies, sometimes extending the dissection into the glans itself. If curvature still persists, dorsal tunica albuginea plication (TAP) with permanent suture material will usually suffice.

Polyglactin sutures (7-0) are normally used for construction of the neourethra. A watertight anastomosis is constructed, inverting the edges toward the lumen when possible, although eversion of suture lines may not pose the threat of fistula formation once widely believed. Skin closure is performed with attention to detail similar to that for neourethral reconstruction. Reapproximation is done without undue tension,

minimizing ischemia. Chromic catgut sutures (7-0) are used for the skin and meatus, as they are resorbed faster than the synthetic fibers. A running mattress suture everts the skin edges and provides an excellent cosmetic result. In most repairs, adequate ventral shaft skin remains to allow realignment of the midline raphe to the corona. When the ventral skin is deficient, the prepuce is split dorsally and transferred ventrally in the Byers method.

MEATAL ADVANCEMENT AND GLANULOPLASTY (MAGPI)

Since its introduction in 1981, the Magpi procedure[1] has withstood the test of time and become the most common hypospadias technique used to date. Approximately 50 percent of the anterior variants, or one third of all hypospadias cases, are suited for the Magpi repair.

There are specific indications for the procedure. Correct case selection is critical to surgical outcome. Cases ideal for the Magpi procedure are usually those in which the meatus is positioned at the coronal margin or subcoronally. Commonly, there is a lip of tissue distal to the meatus, which ventrally deflects the urinary stream to some degree and is the largest functional impairment of these anterior hypospadias anomalies. The glanular groove varies in depth and may require deepening as part of the initial Heineke-Mikulicz maneuver, which advances and flattens the dorsal urethral wall. The importance of the Magpi technique lies in eliminating the bridge, advancing the meatus into the glanular groove, and bringing the glans tissue around the ventrum after elevating the ventral meatal edge.

A holding suture of 5-0 polypropylene is placed in the glans for traction, and a 1:100,000 concentration of epinephrine in 1 percent lidocaine is injected into the subcoronal area and granular groove for hemostasis. A circumferential incision is made subcoronal and proximal to the urethral meatus (Fig. 116–1A). The penile shaft skin is mobilized as a sleeve back to the penoscrotal junction, with freeing of the tethering fibers present in the subdartos fascia, particularly on the ventrum (Fig. 116–1B). An artificial erection is used to check for residual chordee.

The correction of any initial meatal stenosis and the advancement of the dorsal urethral wall are accomplished by a Heineke-Mikulicz vertical incision and horizontal closure (Fig. 116–1C and D) with interrupted 7-0 polyglactin suture. Sometimes, wedge removal of a segment of glanular tissue distal to the meatus is required. A satisfactory glanuloplasty is critical to support the advanced ventral wall of the urethral meatus. This procedure is accomplished by shaping the typically flattened glans into a more nor-

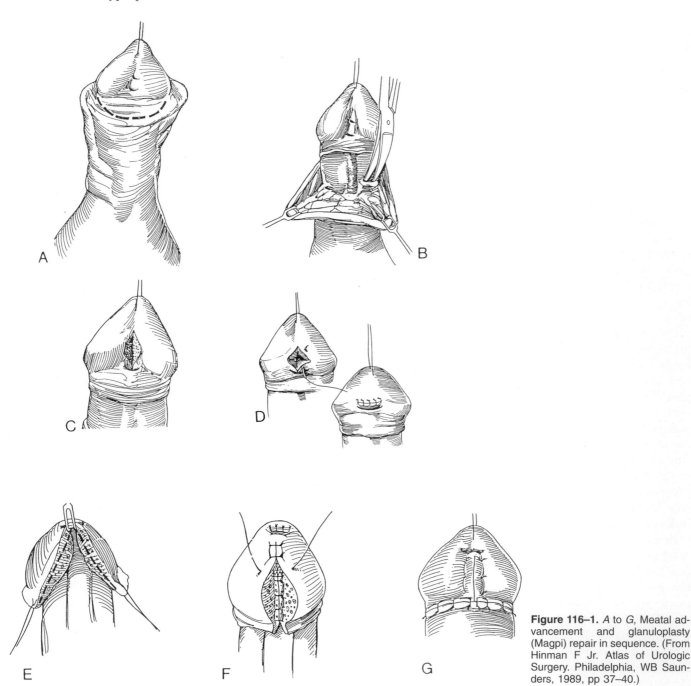

Figure 116–1. *A* to *G*, Meatal advancement and glanuloplasty (Magpi) repair in sequence. (From Hinman F Jr. Atlas of Urologic Surgery. Philadelphia, WB Saunders, 1989, pp 37–40.)

mal conical shape. Reconfiguration is achieved by rotating the lateral aspects of the wings of the glans around to the midline proximal to the advanced ventral wall of the urethral meatus. Skin adjacent to the glanular edges must often be excised to expose glans tissue for reapproximation of the glans wings in the midline ventrally (Fig. 116–1*E* and *F*]. The glanular tissue is brought solidly together with interrupted 7-0 polyglactin sutures, and the superficial epithelial edges are run with 7-0 chromic sutures (Fig. 116–1*G*). A bougie à boule is used to calibrate the meatus and ensure that the glanuloplasty has not compromised the lumen of the distal glanular urethra.

Generally, a sleeve reapproximation of the penile skin is sufficient to complete coverage. Occasionally, a rotation of excessive dorsal preputial skin to the ventrum is used to correct a ventral skin deficiency. Torsion can usually be corrected as part of the initial drop-back of the shaft skin, taking the dissection completely back to the dorsal suspensory ligament and the ventral penoscrotal junction.

PYRAMID PROCEDURE

An unusual although increasingly recognized variant in hypospadias repair is the megameatus intact prepuce (MIP) variant in which the prepuce is intact and the meatus is wide and fish-mouthed (Fig. 116–2*A*). The unusual configuration of the widened distal urethra and meatus poses a special technical challenge. Application of more conventional repairs, including Magpi, to the MIP variant have given less than optimal results. An operation has evolved as a result of our experience with balanitic epispadias, mirroring MIP, which provides a simple technical solution for the problem and an excellent cosmetic result. The procedure is termed the "pyramid," from the description of the exposure and dissection of the "blunderbuss" meatus and wide distal urethra.[2] The patient can remain uncircumcised if desired, although the condition is often not recognized until after circumcision.

Four traction sutures define the megameatus and the base of the pyramid (Fig. 116–2*B*). After infiltration of epinephrine to reduce bleeding, a tennis-racquet incision is made near the glanular groove and around the meatus. The dissection is carried proximally below the coronal level, mobilizing the urethra (to the apex of the pyramid) (Fig. 116–2*C*). Laterally, the edges of the glanular groove are deepened to develop the glans wings from the urethral plate. The distal urethral plate is left wide (12 to 15 mm) and intact dorsally. The excess ventral urethral tissue is removed and the edges are approximated with a continuous 7-0 polyglactin suture to provide a normal caliber to the urethra (Fig. 116–2*D* and *E*). The glans wings are reapproximated in two layers with 7-0 polyglactin sutures (Fig. 116–2*F*). Skin is closed with 7-0 chromic catgut suture. The urethral caliber is tested with a 10 or 12 Fr. bougie à boule. The quality of the stream is observed by

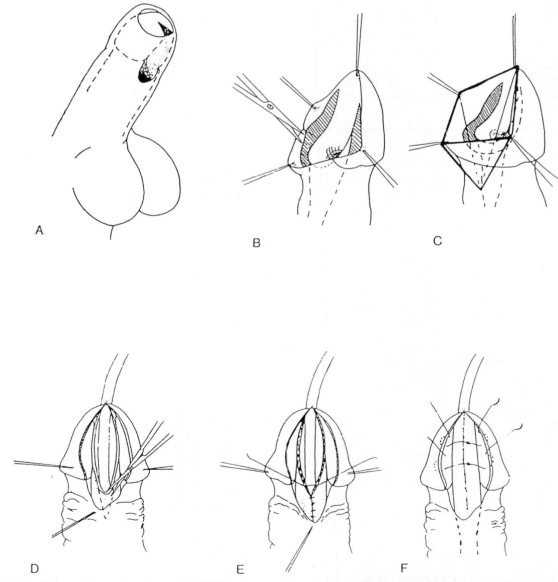

Figure 116–2. *A* to *F*, Pyramid procedure for repair of the megameatus intact prepuce (MIP) variant of hypospadias. (From Duckett JW, Keating MA. Technical challenge of the megameatus intact prepuce hypospadias (MIP) variant: The pyramid procedure. J Urol 141:1407, 1989.)

applying pressure over the bladder. Circumcision may be performed if desired.

ONLAY ISLAND FLAP

Since the mid-1980s, the onlay island flap technique has shown wide versatility and provided excellent results for repair of distal, middle, and even proximal hypospadias. A major increase in the use of this technique stems from a radical change in the concept of the cause of penile curvature.[3] The urethral plate is usually healthy and is not the cause of penile curvature, as proposed many years ago by Mettauer. Rarely is the urethral plate divided. After release of the skin and dartos fascia, a mild residual bend has been found caused by corporeal disproportion (not an abnormal urethral plate), which can be corrected by TAP. Dorsal plications of the tunica albuginea on each side of the penis at the 2 o'clock and 10 o'clock positions are taken at the point of maximal bend. Buck's fascia with the neurovascular bundles is elevated on each side. Parallel incisions (4 to 6 mm) are made into the tunica albuginea about 8 mm apart and are approximated with their lateral edges, using two permanent 5-0 nonabsorbable sutures and burying the knots (Fig. 116–3).

In analyzing the hypospadiac glans penis, the glans configuration may be a reliable indicator for technique selection. Patients with a conical glans penis tend to have a fibrous urethral plate that is best managed with division of the urethral plate, a transverse preputial island tube, and tunneling glanuloplasty. In

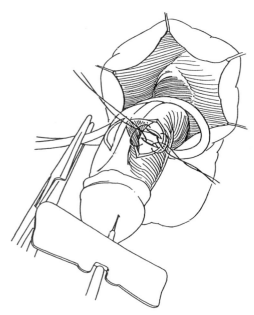

Figure 116–3. Dorsal tunica albuginea plication (TAP) procedure. An artificial erection test is performed by injecting normal saline through a 25-gauge needle that has been placed through the glans into one corporeal body. (From Hinman F Jr. Atlas of Pediatric Urologic Surgery. Philadelphia, WB Saunders, 1994, p 569.)

contrast, patients with a flat glans penis tend to have a normal urethral plate that is amenable to an onlay island flap and a glans wing wrap glanuloplasty.

The onlay island flap is based on the predictable axial blood supply of the dorsal dartos fascia. The preserved urethral plate is healthy and well vascularized with spongiosum beneath it. The onlay island flap provides a more reliable blood supply for the neourethra than do the parameatal skin flaps, which must depend only on the intrinsic blood supply of the hypospadiac meatus.

With the urethral plate outlined about 4 to 6 mm in width with parallel incisions, a strip is made all the way to the tip of the glanular groove, and glanular wings are developed (Fig. 116–4A). The proximal urethra is cut back to good spongiosum and the excess skin edge is excised to make the urethral plate (Fig. 116–4B). Once this is accomplished, a ventral preputial island flap is developed without making any attempt to measure the appropriate size. This is mobilized to the ventrum and placed alongside the urethral plate. A running 7-0 polyglactin suture is used to close one side of the onlay (Fig. 116–4C).

A marking pen is then used to outline the amount of onlay flap. With a 4- to 6-mm strip, the onlay needs to be no more than 6 to 8 mm wide for a 12 Fr. caliber neourethra. Otherwise, a diverticulum may form. The excess epithelium is then excised, leaving the small onlay patch. The pedicle is kept intact, supplying this strip of epithelium. The onlay is rotated over the urethral plate, and interrupted sutures are placed around the horseshoe of the proximal urethra. A running suture is then placed on the lateral side, completing the repair out to the tip of the glans. Bougie à boules are used to calibrate the urethra and make sure it is not too wide to prevent a diverticulum. The urethra is distended with saline to check for leaks.

The lateral glans wings are brought around the ventrum of the urethral onlay and any excess mucosa is excised as an interrupted meatoplasty is performed. The glanular wings are brought over the onlay with deep polyglactin sutures and superficial running 7-0 chromic catgut sutures. This completes the glanuloplasty and the meatoplasty.

The pedicle is splayed over the anastomosis and tacked to the tunica albuginea so that it is flattened out. Excess tissue is excised from the flap to avoid any bulkiness. Skin cover with 7-0 chromic catgut sutures is achieved in the usual manner by dividing the dorsal preputial skin and stretching the skin around to the ventrum for a midline closure up to the glans (Fig. 116–4D).

TRANSVERSE PREPUTIAL ISLAND FLAP TUBULARIZED

If significant fibrous chordee persists, the urethral plate must be divided and the urethra mobilized to

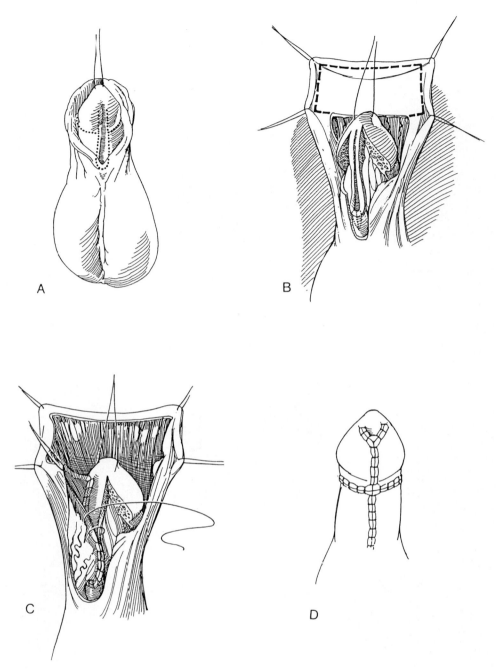

Figure 116–4. *A* to *D*, An onlay island flap is used for cases with minimal or no chordee. The urethral plate is left intact. (From Hinman F Jr. Atlas of Pediatric Urologic Surgery. Philadelphia, WB Saunders, 1994, pp 588–589.)

remove deeper tethering layers from the corpora. In this setting, a tubularized neourethra is needed to bridge the gap to the tip of the penis. This technique has been developed as a modification of the Hodgson III and Asopa procedures. The blood supply to the inner preputial transverse island flap is abundant, with vascularization oriented in a longitudinal fashion. This tissue is dissected from the penile skin and outer preputial skin, leaving the major vasculature attached to the island flap (Fig. 116–5*A*).

As the transverse preputial island flap is developed, a broad skin rectangle is mobilized (Fig. 116–5*B* and *C*). This is then trimmed to fit a template of 12 Fr. caliber so that the neourethra does not bulge

and form diverticula or have redundancy. A length as long as 5 to 6 cm can readily be obtained in young children. The inner portion of the tube is closed with running 7-0 polyglactin suture and the ends are approximated with interrupted sutures so that they may be excised to fit the proper length (Fig. 116–5*D*).

An oblique anastomosis is made, fixing the native urethra to the tunica albuginea. All the skin edges of the native urethra are excised so that good spongiosum is available. Once the neourethra is in place, bougienage with a bougie à boule to 10 or 12 Fr. is done routinely to make sure there are no bumps, kinks, or lips. The glans channel is made by sharp dissection against the corporeal bodies out to the tip

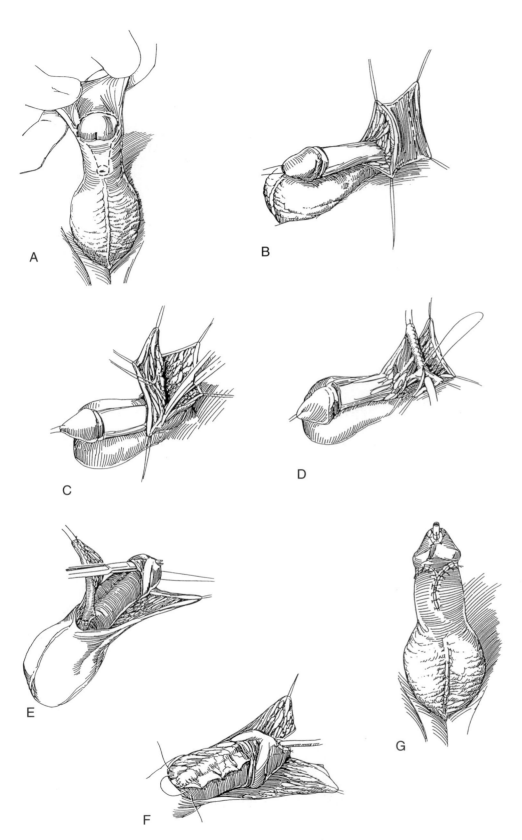

A

B

C

D

E

F

G

Figure 116–5. *A* to *G*, Transverse preputial island flap procedure in sequence. If release of the urethral plate is required to correct the chordee, the missing portion may be replaced with a tube of preputial skin placed as an island flap. (From Hinman F Jr. Atlas of Urologic Surgery. Philadelphia, WB Saunders, 1989, pp 50–52.)

of the glanular groove (Fig. 116–5*E*). A button of glans epithelium is removed and dissection is carried down into the glanular tissue with removal of enough to permit a broad channel through the glans. The most common error is to make the glans channel too narrow, constricting the pedicle of the neourethra as it traverses the glans and causing ischemia and meatal stenosis. Great care must be taken in making a generous glans channel. Interrupted sutures of fine chromic are placed circumferentially to approximate the glans to the end of the neourethra with precision. The pedicle is splayed over the anastomosis and tacked to the tunica albuginea so that it is flattened out (Fig. 116–5*F*).

The skin cover for the transverse preputial flap is made by splitting the dorsal outer prepuce and rotating the lateral wings around to the ventrum so that a midline closure is made with horizontal 7-0 chromic catgut mattress sutures up to the glans. Excess skin is then excised, leading to good, viable penile and preputial skin for cover (Fig. 116–5*G*).

DRAINS, DRESSINGS, AND FOLLOW-UP

Attention to detail in postoperative care should rival that of the surgery itself. Virtually every hypospadias repair can be performed on an outpatient basis without an increase in morbidity. The ability to successfully manage each case is contingent on adequate preoperative parental education and simplified forms of diversion and dressing that minimize side effects such as bladder spasms and the acute complications of edema and hematoma.

Premature voiding is not desirable and may predispose the repair to fistula formation. With the exception of the Magpi repair, which is managed without a diversion, a 6 Fr. Silastic tube is placed through the neourethra and into the bladder. The fine catheter, which is sutured to the glans with 5-0 polypropylene on a taper-point needle, allows continuous drainage of urine into a diaper and appears to minimize bladder spasms. The catheter should be left in place for 7 to 14 days, depending on the extensiveness of the repair and an assessment of healing.

The ideal hypospadias dressing provides three functions: (1) immobilization of the penis and its drainage tube, (2) protection of suture lines, and (3) containment of edema while maximizing hemostasis. For Magpi repairs, a bio-occlusive (Tegaderm) dressing is left in place for 48 hours and then removed at home by the parents. For all other hypospadias repairs that require urethral stents, a sandwich dressing is applied on top of the penis, extending onto the abdominal wall. A Telfa pad on the ventral repair, a 4 × 4 folded four times for pressure on the abdomen, and a bio-occlusive dressing (Tegaderm) compressing the penis against the abdomen form the "sandwich." This dressing is removed in 48 hours by the parents, after residual oozing is controlled. The penis is cared for with polymixin B/bacitracin (Polysporin) ointment placed on the wound without a dressing when the diaper is changed.

A supplemental local block with bupivacaine (Marcaine) at the beginning of the procedure is most helpful. Patients are given oral analgesics (acetaminophen with codeine). For patients with urethral stents, oxybutynin (Ditropan) is given for bladder spasm, and a suppression dose of trimethoprim is given to prevent cystitis when a bladder tube is left to drain in the diaper. Follow-up visits are at 2- and 6-week intervals, and thereafter only as needed. The goal is that the child should grow up without knowing that he had anything "wrong" with his penis.

COMPLICATIONS

Attention to the details that will avoid complications is paramount. To avoid wound infection, povidone-iodine (Betadine) solution is used in preparation. In postpubertal boys, cleansing should begin several days before surgery. Infections seem to be more of a problem in this age group. Prophylactic antibiotics have little value in avoiding wound infection. Poor wound healing is primarily caused by ischemic flaps.

For carefully selected cases, the Magpi procedure has shown excellent success with only 1.2 percent of patients requiring secondary procedures.[1] Potential problems of meatal stenosis and regression can be completely avoided by attention to the details of the Magpi technique. Stenosis is prevented by emphasizing a meatoplasty that extends the dorsal vertical incision into the meatus to widely open its caliber, and an incision sufficiently deep to correct a poorly developed glanular groove. To avoid meatal regression, the glans wings must be brought together ventrally and fixed snugly to ensure solid glans-to-glans healing.

Urethrocutaneous fistulas are likely to remain an inherent risk of hypospadias repairs for many years afterward. Fistulas occurred in 6 percent of patients with onlay island flaps and in 10 to 15 percent with tubularized transverse preputial island flaps. The better fistula rate in the onlay island repair is likely due to better healing of the onlay flap to the spongiosa-supported urethral plate. No attempt should be made to close the fistula for 6 months. To avoid fistulization, it is important to test the repair by injecting saline to identify the gaps in the sutures.

Too wide an epithelial onlay or transverse preputial tube may form a diverticulum, even without meatal stenosis. If meatal stenosis occurs, further dilation may occur. Reduction of such a diverticulum in a longitudinal fashion is necessary.

A stricture at the proximal anastomosis may occur after urethroplasty. This may be due to angulation of the anastomosis and may be avoided by lateral fixation of the anastomosis to the tunica albuginea. Strictures may be repaired by excision and reanastomosis. Optical cold knife urethrotomy is not usually effective. A buccal mucosal graft is the best material for replacement of the complicated hypospadias urethroplasty gone wrong.[4]

Editorial Comment
Fray F. Marshall

Although it is frequently possible to reconstruct even a penoscrotal hypospadias in a single-stage procedure, a two-stage procedure may be useful in the more severe forms of hypospadias. If the chordee is severe, it may be useful and reasonable to initiate a first-stage repair and verify that the penis is straight; the foreskin can often be placed in a more favorable anatomical location for subsequent reconstruction as part of the first-stage repair also.

Editorial Comment
Craig A. Peters

Outpatient management of significant hypospadias repairs is realistic and usually acceptable to most families. This is a marked improvement over the long hospital stays and patient restraint of past years. The successful hypospadias repair depends on meticulous adherence to technical details and the ability to adapt a variety of surgical methods to the particular patient. Different methods may be adapted to various situations and the surgeon should be sufficiently familiar with a variety methods to be able to deal with any situation.

Dorsal plication for chordee in the patient with a short phallus may reduce maximal length. We would favor a corporeal graft when adequate straightening cannot be achieved with thorough ventral dissection of the corpora. Dermis or tunica vaginalis are both useful and may be positioned adjacent to a urethral graft.

REFERENCES

1. Duckett JW, Snyder HM. Meatal advancement and glanuloplasty hypospadias repair after 1,000 cases: Avoidance of meatal stenosis and regression. J Urol 147:665, 1992.
2. Duckett JW, Keating MA. Technical challenge of the megameatus intact prepuce hypospadias variant: The pyramid procedure. J Urol 141:1407, 1989.
3. Baskin LS, Duckett JW, Ueoka K, et al. Changing concepts of hypospadias curvature lead to more onlay island flap procedures. J Urol 151:191, 1994.
4. Duckett JW, Coplen DE, Ewalt DH, Baskin LS. Buccal mucosal urethral replacement. J Urol 153:1660, 1995.

Chapter 117

Proximal Hypospadias

Alan B. Retik

Proximal hypospadias can be treated with a one-stage operative procedure similar to what has been described by Duckett.[1] In some instances, however, the urethral defect may be quite long (greater than 6 cm) after the chordee is corrected, the penis may be very small, and/or there may be persistent significant chordee after the standard measures of correction are employed. In these situations, additional techniques may be necessary for surgery to be successful.

PREOPERATIVE EVALUATION AND MANAGEMENT

Surgery for hypospadias is most often performed between the ages of 4 and 12 months. It is preferable in most babies with hypospadias to perform surgery in the earlier period; however, those with severe proximal hypospadias often have small organs and are more often operated on between the ages of 9 and 12 months. Infants with very small organs are often treated preoperatively with testosterone applied locally or administered parenterally. In infants with severe hypospadias and undescended testes, karyotyping should be obtained. Voiding cystourethrography is advisable in infants with scrotal or perineal hypospadias to determine the frequent presence and extent of a prostatic utricle.

OPERATIVE TECHNIQUES

Duplay Tube Extension

If the urethral meatus is very proximal after correction of chordee, a portion of the scrotum, which is not hair bearing, can be tubularized and anastomosed to either a transverse preputial transverse island flap or a free graft (Fig. 117–1). The Duplay extension tube is 15 mm wide and is tubularized with a running 6-0 or 7-0 Vicryl subcuticular stitch. It is important for the resultant meatus to be wide. This is then anastomosed to the vascularized or free graft with two running locked 6-0 or 7-0 Vicryl stitches.

It is important for these suture lines to be covered with a layer of subcutaneous tissue or a tunica vaginalis graft, which will be described later.

Two-Stage Hypospadias Repair

Despite all the emphasis on single-stage hypospadias repairs, a planned two-stage repair is sometimes advisable.[2, 3] There is a subset of patients with severe proximal hypospadias, chordee, and a small phallus who may benefit best from staging of the repair. In the first stage (Fig. 117–2A and B), a circumferential incision is made proximal to the coronal sulcus and extended ventrally to the urethral meatus. The penile shaft is degloved and chordee is excised. When it is ascertained that the penis is straight (Fig. 117–2C) (the Gittes test),[4] the glans is prepared. The glans is either divided deeply in the midline extending somewhat dorsally, or, alternatively, if the mucosal groove is deep, it is preserved and incisions are made just lateral to the groove on each side (Fig. 117–2D). These incisions must be made deeply. The dorsal foreskin is unfolded carefully and divided in the midline (Fig. 117–2E). The most distal portion of the foreskin is rotated into the glanular cleft and sutured to the mucosa of the glans with interrupted sutures of 6-0 chromic catgut. Closure is midline, and the midline sutures catch a small portion of Buck's fascia. This eliminates dead space and helps create a groove in preparation for the second stage (Fig. 117–2F). The bladder is drained with a No. 8 Foley catheter. The penis is dressed with a modified pressure dressing, which ideally should stay on for 5 to 7 days.

A significant number of children with severe hypospadias have persistent chordee even after extensive removal of the involved tissue by conventional techniques. This can sometimes be corrected by dorsal

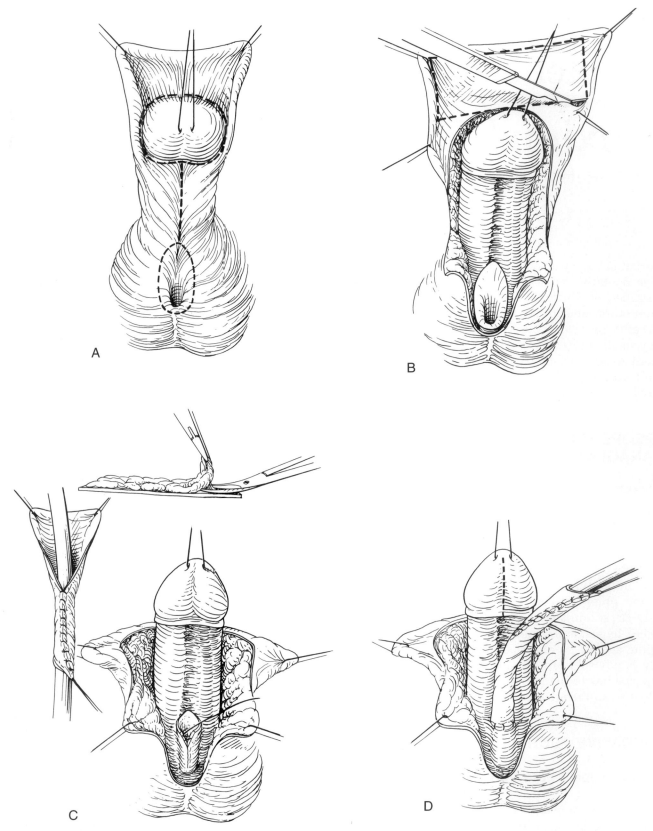

Figure 117–1. Duplay tube extension combined with a free skin graft. *A*, Outline of skin incision. *B*, The chordee is excised, the Duplay tube incised, and a free preputial graft outlined. *C*, The Duplay extension tube is 15 mm wide and tubularized with a running 6-0 or 7-0 Vicryl subcuticular stitch. The free graft is defatted and tubularized. *D*, A wide anastomosis is performed between the Duplay tube extension and the tubed graft.

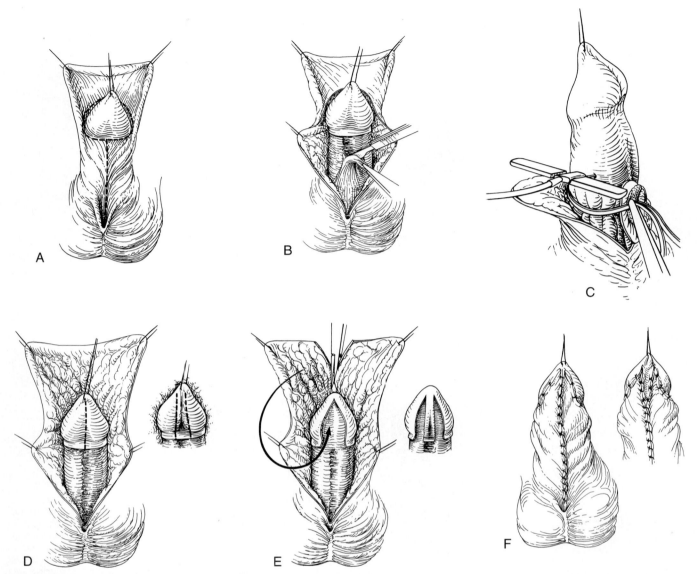

Figure 117–2. First-stage hypospadias repair. *A,* Outline of skin incisions. *B,* The chordee is excised and the penile shaft degloved. *C,* With a rubber band tourniquet at the base of the penis, saline is injected through a fine butterfly needle into the corpora to ascertain that the penis is straight. *D,* The glans is either divided deeply in the midline, extending somewhat dorsally, or, if the mucosal groove is deep, it is preserved and incisions are made just lateral to the groove on each side. *E,* The dorsal foreskin is partially unfolded and divided in the midline. *F,* The most distal portion of the foreskin is rotated into the glanular cleft and sutured to the mucosa of the glans with interrupted sutures of 6-0 chromic catgut. Closure is midline.

plication of the corpora.[5] However, the phallus in most of these babies is very small and would be shortened further by dorsal plication. Therefore, in this group of infants, ventral incision of the corpora and insertion of a dermal graft is usually performed (Fig. 117–3).[6] The graft is obtained from a hairless area in the groin, de-epithelialized and defatted, and sewn in place with two running locked 6-0 Vicryl sutures.

The second stage of the repair is carried out 6 to 12 months later, when complete healing has occurred. A 15-mm diameter strip is measured extending to the tip of the glans (Fig. 117–4A). The strip is tubularized with a running subcuticular stitch of 6-0 or 7-0 Vicryl (Fig. 117–4B). The lateral skin edges are mobilized and the remaining tissues closed over the repair in at least two layers. The subcutaneous and subcuticular tissues are reapproximated with running pull-out stitches of 4-0 nylon tied to themselves (Fig. 117–4C). The bladder is drained with either a small-gauge trocar cystotomy tube or a No. 7 Jackson-Pratt Silastic catheter sutured in at the glans level with two 5-0 Prolene sutures and left draining into a diaper. The child is seen 7 to 10 days after surgery for dressing and catheter removal. At this time one end of each nylon stitch is cut, and the remaining suture material gradually works its way out within a few days.

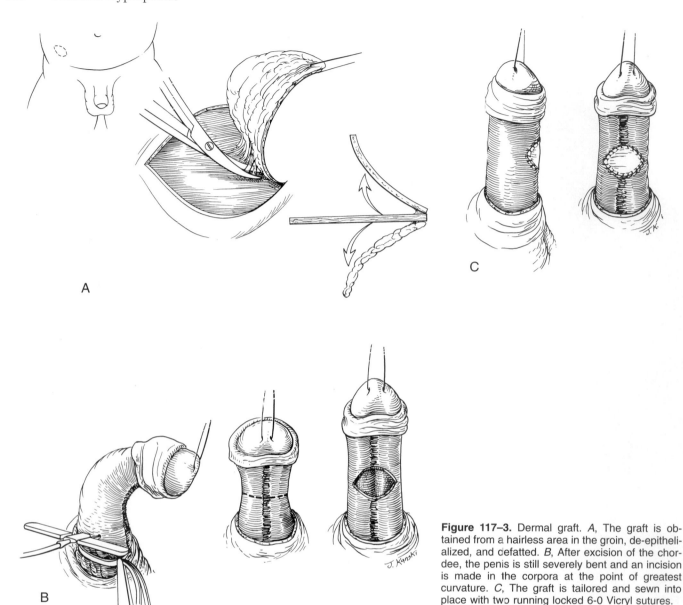

Figure 117–3. Dermal graft. *A*, The graft is obtained from a hairless area in the groin, de-epithelialized, and defatted. *B*, After excision of the chordee, the penis is still severely bent and an incision is made in the corpora at the point of greatest curvature. *C*, The graft is tailored and sewn into place with two running locked 6-0 Vicryl sutures.

Bladder Mucosal Graft

Bladder mucosa tube graft urethroplasty is primarily employed in reoperative surgery for hypospadias when a long defect is present with an inadequate donor skin site.[7, 8] This technique has also been used for some infants with scrotal or perineal hypospadias as a single-stage repair. The bladder mucosa should not be exposed at the meatus because of the very significant incidence of prolapse. Therefore the distal portion of the repair (5 to 10 mm) should be either a free graft of local skin or buccal mucosa sutured to the bladder mucosa, incorporated into the tube, and sutured to the glanular mucosa at the meatus.

As in the previous procedures, incisions are outlined and the penis is straightened by excising chordee. The distance between the new position of the urethral meatus and the tip of the penis is measured so that an appropriate-sized rectangle of bladder mucosa is obtained. The bladder is distended with saline solution and the skin opened with a transverse lower abdominal incision. A linear incision is made in the anterior wall of the bladder extending to the mucosa. The bladder musculature is dissected off the mucosa sharply. An appropriate rectangle of mucosa (Fig. 117–5A) is measured, making it about 10 percent wider and about the same length as measured to be able to accommodate a distal graft of skin or buccal mucosa. Stay sutures of fine silk are placed at the corners and the graft is excised. A 5- to 10-mm graft of local skin or buccal mucosa (see below) of similar width as the bladder mucosal graft is then taken and anastomosed to the bladder mucosal graft with a running 6-0 or 7-0 Vicryl stitch. The entire combined graft then is tubularized (Fig. 117–5B) with a running locked stitch of 6-0 or 7-0 Vicryl and anastomosed to

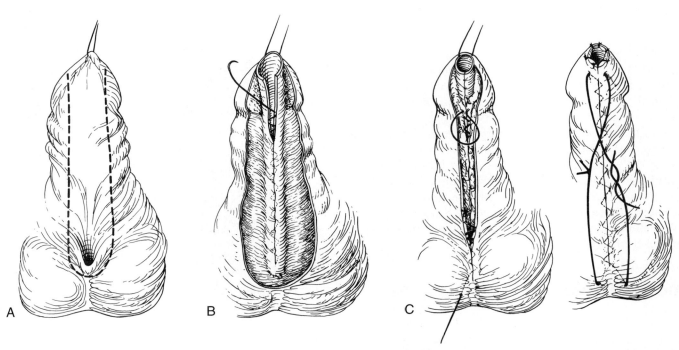

Figure 117–4. Second-stage hypospadias repair. *A,* A strip 15 mm in diameter is measured extending to the tip of the glans. *B,* The strip is tubularized with a running subcuticular stitch of 6-0 or 7-0 Vicryl. *C,* Subcutaneous and subcuticular tissues are reapproximated with running pull-out stitches of 4-0 nylon tied to themselves.

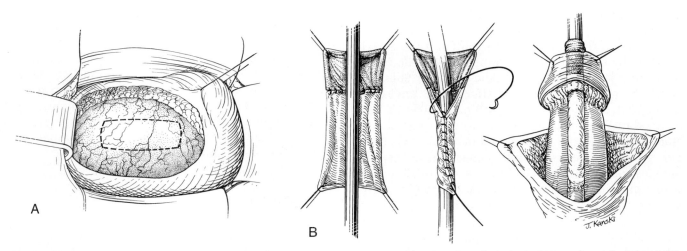

Figure 117–5. Bladder and composite grafts. *A,* The bladder is distended with saline, an incision is made in the anterior wall of the bladder extending to the mucosa, and the bladder musculature is dissected off the mucosa sharply. An appropriate rectangle of mucosa is measured, making it about 10 percent wider and about the same length as measured to be able to accommodate a distal graft of skin or buccal mucosa. *B,* A 5- to 10-mm graft of local skin or buccal mucosa is taken and anastomosed to the bladder mucosal graft with a running 6-0 or 7-0 Vicryl stitch. Then, the entire combined graft is tubularized with a running locked stitch of 6-0 or 7-0 Vicryl and anastomosed to the proximal urethra with two running locked 6-0 or 7-0 Vicryl sutures. The tubularized graft suture line should lie against the corpora. The distal portion of the graft (skin or buccal mucosa) is anastomosed to the glanular meatus with interrupted 6-0 Vicryl.

the proximal urethra with two running locked 6-0 or 7-0 Vicryl sutures, with the tubularized graft suture line lying posteriorly against the corpora. The distal portion of the graft (skin or buccal mucosa) is anastomosed to the glanular meatus with interrupted 6-0 Vicryl after the glans has been prepared by creating a large-caliber tunnel (with excision of some of the glans) or by incising the glans deeply. The tube should fit loosely in the glans whatever technique is used. If the glans is incised, it should be reapproximated over the tube loosely in two layers (subcutaneous and mucosal) with fine Vicryl sutures. The graft is covered with mobilized subcutaneous tissue obtained from the dorsum and swung around ventrally or by local tissue or by a tunica vaginalis flap. The bladder is drained with a Malecot catheter and the newly created urethra is stented with a fine Silastic catheter. The stent is removed 8 to 10 days postoperatively and a trial of voiding begun.

Buccal Mucosal Graft

Buccal mucosa can be used for the entire graft or as the distal portion of a combined graft with bladder mucosa, which is anastomosed to the glans. Grafts are obtained from the cheek or lips.[9, 10] Long composite grafts may be obtained from cheek and lips.

General anesthesia is given by nasal tracheal intubation. With a self-retaining retractor in the mouth, a graft is outlined appropriately on the cheek or lip (Fig. 117–6). The graft is made slightly longer and wider than necessary. Epinephrine (1:200,000) is injected below the mucosa, stay sutures of 5-0 silk are placed on the corners of the graft, and the graft is removed by sharp dissection superficial to the buccinator muscle. Care must be taken to avoid Stensen's duct. The graft is placed in half-strength povidone-iodine (Betadine), placed on cardboard, defatted, and then tubularized in similar fashion as the bladder mucosal graft with a running 6-0 or 7-0 Vicryl stitch. The remaining aspects of the anastomosis are the same as mentioned above. The mucosa of the cheek is reapproximated with running 5-0 chromic catgut. It is not necessary to reapproximate the mucosa of the lip. Mucosa generates very rapidly and there is minimal patient discomfort in the donor area after this procedure. The bladder is drained with a No. 7 Silastic catheter. The remaining aspects of subcutaneous skin coverage are similar to those described earlier.

COMPLICATIONS

The most common complications are similar to those seen in other types of hypospadias repair such

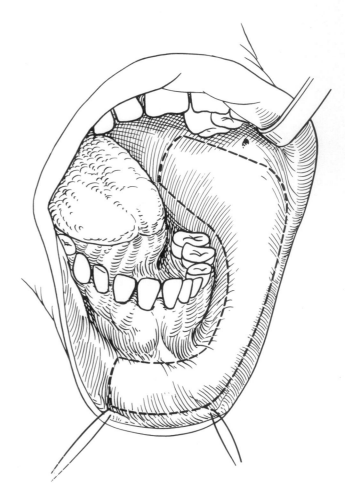

Figure 117–6. Composite buccal mucosal graft from cheek and lip.

as fistula and stricture. It is important not to tubularize hair-bearing skin in order to avoid a hairy urethra with the subsequent sequelae of infection and stones. Occasionally, a urethral diverticulum may occur in a tubularized graft. The complication of prolapse of bladder mucosa can be avoided by not using bladder mucosa at the skin level. Complications can be minimized by careful technique and adequate subcutaneous tissue and skin coverage.

TUNICA VAGINALIS GRAFT

The incidence of fistula can be minimized, as stated above, by adequate coverage over the graft. We have routinely employed a graft of tunica vaginalis (Fig. 117–7) to cover the neourethra in patients with severe hypospadias.[11] The testis is invaginated into the operative field and separated from its scrotal attachments, and the tunica vaginalis is incised. It is then widely mobilized on its own vascular pedicle and sutured over the neourethra with 6-0 Vicryl, covering the entire repair. The testicle is then placed back in the scrotum. This coverage has significantly

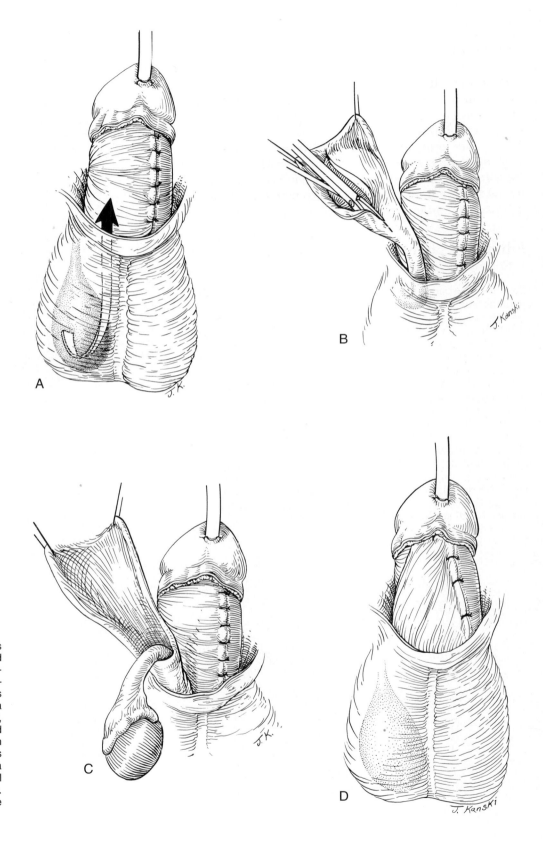

Figure 117–7. Tunica vaginalis graft. *A*, The testis is invaginated into the operative field after completion of a transverse island pedicle flap. The illustration shows coverage of the neourethra by a portion of the pedicle. *B* and *C*, The tunica vaginalis is incised and widely mobilized on its own vascular pedicle. *D*, The graft is then sutured over the neourethra with 6-0 Vicryl as an additional layer covering the entire repair. The testicle is replaced in the scrotum.

reduced the incidence of urethral fistulae after the types of repairs described above.

Summary

Patients with severe proximal hypospadias may be treated in a number of ways. With extensive defects, after chordee correction (greater than 6 cm), one may use a vascularized tube flap anastomosed to a Duplay tube, a free graft of buccal mucosa, or a combined graft of bladder and buccal mucosa or bladder and skin. In children who have very severe hypospadias with a small phallus, it is sometimes better to perform a two-stage repair.

Editorial Comment
Craig A. Peters

Severe hypospadias remains a substantial challenge to all pediatric urologists, and initial surgical intervention will greatly influence the ultimate success of the reconstruction. While it may be attractive to attempt a single-stage repair in all cases, this may not be in the patient's best interests, as indicated by Dr. Retik. A first-stage procedure early in life may ultimately provide the best functional and cosmetic results. We have performed some first-stage operations on children as young as 2 months of age and have seen superb healing.

Penile straightening is essential in boys with severe hypospadias, and we would disagree that most can be made straight with dorsal plications, as suggested in Chapter 116 by Dr. Duckett. Ventral corporeal patching is an effective method of straightening without any loss of penile length. Dr. Retik describes the use of dermal patches; tunica vaginalis has also been a useful material and has further use in supporting a urethral graft. When incising the corpora for straightening, it is important to cut deeply into the corporeal bodies to obtain sufficient ventral length.

While buccal mucosa has received favorable critical analysis recently and it is less morbid to harvest than bladder mucosa, the long-term results remain undefined. Some surgeons are less enthusiastic about its efficacy, particularly in a tubed graft, and have used it only in onlay-type procedures (see Chapter 116). The maintenance of a urethral strip may be practical in less severe hypospadias; it may not be possible in penoscrotal forms. The importance of mechanically and biologically supporting any tube graft with fixed and vascularized tissue in these challenging reconstructions cannot be overemphasized.

REFERENCES

1. Duckett JW. Transverse preputial island flap. Technique for repair of severe hypospadias. Urol Clin North Am 7:423, 1980.
2. Retik AB, Bauer SB, Mandell J, et al. Management of severe hypospadias with a 2-stage repair. J Urol 152:749, 1994.
3. Retik AB, Casale A. Hypospadias. In Libertino JA, ed. Pediatric and Adult Reconstructive Urology. Baltimore, Williams & Wilkins, 1987, p 500.
4. Gittes RF, McLaughlin AP. Injection techniques to induce penile erection. Urology 4:473, 1974.
5. Baskin LS, Duckett JW, Ueoka K, et al. Changing concepts of hypospadias curvature lead to more onlay island flap procedures. J Urol 151:191, 1994.
6. Hendren WH, Keating MA. Use of dermal graft and free urethral graft in penile reconstruction. J Urol 140:1265, 1988.
7. Hendren WH, Reda EF. Bladder mucosa graft for construction of male urethra. Pediatr Surg 21:189, 1986.
8. Ransley PG, Duffy PG, Oesch IL, Hoover D. Autologous bladder mucosa graft for urethral substitution. Br J Urol 59:331, 1987.
9. Burger RA, Muller SC, El-Damanhoury H, et al. The buccal mucosal graft for urethral reconstruction: A preliminary report. J Urol 147:662, 1992.
10. Dessanti A, Rigamonti W, Merulla V, et al. Autologous buccal mucosa graft for hypospadias repair: An initial report. J Urol 147:1081, 1992.
11. Snow BW. Use of tunica vaginalis to prevent fistulas in hypospadias surgery. J Urol 136:861, 1986.

Chapter 118

Reconstruction of Male Epispadias

David A. Diamond

PREOPERATIVE EVALUATION

The repair of male epispadias can be facilitated by preoperative administration of testosterone enanthate (TE). This serves to enlarge the phallus and improve the vascularity and suppleness of penile tissue. The standard approach is to use three separate doses of 50 mg TE intramuscularly 3 months, 2 months, and 1 month before the date of surgery. Because most boys undergoing epispadias repair have classical bladder exstrophy, it is important that their upper tracts be evaluated preoperatively. A well-performed ultrasound scan is usually sufficient. Urinary tract infection should be ruled out before surgery. In certain situations, when the penis seems exceedingly short or a previous epispadias repair has dehisced, iliac osteotomy may be a valuable adjunctive procedure. In this instance, a preoperative orthopedic consultation is valuable.

Postoperative pain control in the epispadias patient has been greatly facilitated by continuous epidural anesthesia, which can also reduce the intraoperative requirement for inhalational anesthetic. This should be given consideration and anesthesia consultation sought, particularly in cases of older patients requiring epispadias repair.

CYSTOSCOPY AND POSITIONING

Cystoscopy is usually performed before epispadias repair, particularly in exstrophy patients. This allows the bladder anatomy to be assessed and problematic lesions such as stones to be ruled out. A cystoscopic aspirate is sent for culture and sensitivity. The patient is then placed in a supine position and prepared and draped to expose the entire lower abdomen from the umbilicus to the genitalia.

OPERATIVE TECHNIQUE

The modified Cantwell approach to epispadias repair incorporates certain elements that Cantwell first described in 1895. These include complete mobilization of the urethral plate from the corporeal bodies and ventral transposition of the reconstructed urethral tube with dorsal rotation of the corpora.

Glans Reconstruction

Glans reconstruction in the modified Cantwell technique of epispadias repair begins with an advancement of the distal urethral plate from its dorsal location on the glans to a more distal location where the urethral meatus should ultimately reside (Fig. 118–1A). The glanuloplasty is begun by first placing two holding sutures on each lateral aspect of the glans. With upward traction on the phallus, epinephrine (1:100,000) is injected judiciously into the tip of the glans as well as along the margins of the urethral plate dorsally and between the corporeal bodies ventrally in the area of the prostate, to facilitate a more bloodless dissection. With lateral traction on each holding suture, a vertical incision approximately 1.5 cm in length is made through the midline of the glans (Fig. 118–1B). This divides the dorsal lip of glans epithelium at the terminal portion of the urethral plate. The incision should be deepened to divide the tough, white, fibrous bands that are encountered subcutaneously (Fig. 118–2A). This dissection results in the creation of a small fossa navicularis. The incised surface, when closed transversely, will ultimately constitute the urethral meatus and thus must be 12 to 14 mm in width. A Heineke-Mikulicz procedure is completed with interrupted 6-0 Vicryl sutures used to close the longitudinal incision transversely

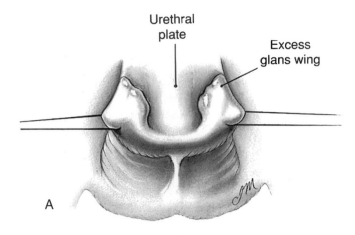

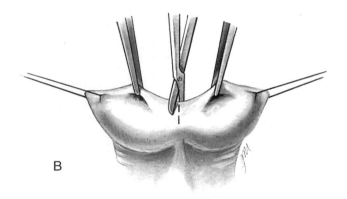

Figure 118–1. *A,* Epispadiac penis with dorsally located urethral plate and excess glans wing tissue splayed laterally. *B,* Vertical incision through the dorsal lip of the glans at the terminal portion of the urethral plate. (From Diamond DA, Ransley PG. Improved glanuloplasty and epispadias repair: technical aspects. J Urol 152:1243, 1994.)

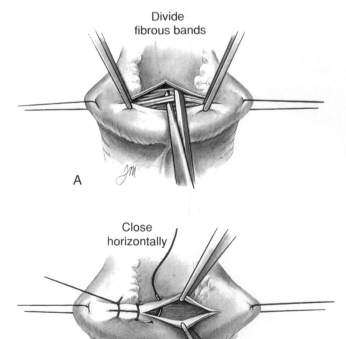

Figure 118–2. *A,* Deepening of the vertical glans incision through tough fibrous bands. *B,* Completion of Heineke-Mikulicz procedure with transverse closure of the glans incision. (From Diamond DA, Ransley PG. Improved glanuloplasty and epispadias repair: technical aspects. J Urol 152:1243, 1994.)

(Fig. 118–2*B*). This results ultimately in a meatus in a more normal, ventral location on the glans. It is most important to leave an adequate bridge of glans tissue ventrally and not to extend the glanular incision too far, or a hypospadiac urethral orifice may result.

Urethral Mobilization

A lower midline abdominal incision is made 3 to 4 cm from the bladder neck up onto the abdominal wall. This creates space for the subsequent penile dissection, allows removal of mons fat where necessary, and enables one to perform a Z-plasty to create flaps for subsequent skin coverage at the base of the phallus. The incision is carried from the midline into the tissue hollow distal to the bladder neck, and is continued laterally along the margins of the urethral plate to the corona of the glans on each lateral aspect (Fig. 118–3). This dorsal incision is linked distally to a ventral transverse incision 1 cm proximal to the corona. This enables the surgeon to thoroughly deglove the penile skin and expose the entire length of the corporeal bodies bilaterally. In so doing, one is able to visualize the neurovascular bundles that run

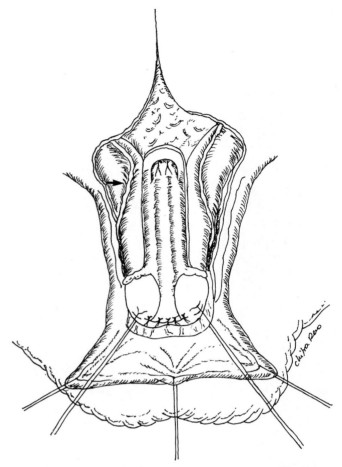

Figure 118–4. Degloved phallus with exposure of corporeal bodies, urethral plate, and neurovascular bundles (*arrow*). (After Snyder HM. The Ransley second stage urethroplasty for exstrophy. In Frank JD, Johnston JH, eds. Operative Paediatric Urology. New York, Churchill Livingstone, 1990, p 173.)

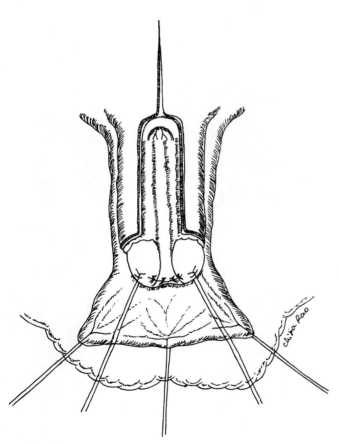

Figure 118–3. Lower midline and penile incision extending around the bladder neck along the urethral plate to the corona bilaterally. (After drawings by Perovic S.)

laterally along the distal aspect of the penis (Fig. 118–4). The corpora are then mobilized proximally from adjacent soft tissue to the level of the pubic bones bilaterally. The midline bridge of tissue from between the corporeal bodies and the dartos layer of the scrotum on the ventral aspect is preserved to maintain this blood supply to the urethral plate (Fig. 118–5). The urethral plate is then separated from the corpora cavernosa on both sides along its entire length. In so doing, the urethra is freed up entirely from the corporeal bodies but retains its attachments to the prostatic urethra proximally and the glans distally.

Dissection is begun on the ventral aspect of the corporeal bodies to avoid the less well defined plane between the urethral plate and the corpora dorsally. To prevent blood from obscuring the surgical field, it is best to begin the dissection proximally and work distally along the corporeal bodies. The dissection is carried around the corner of the corporeal bodies toward the urethra, remaining close to Buck's fascia. Inadvertent entry into the urethral plate can occur

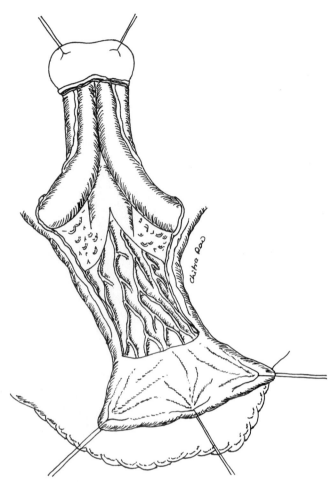

Figure 118–5. Ventral view of the degloved phallus with preservation of the midline tissue bridge to the urethral plate. (After Perovic S.)

during this dissection, and thus patience is particularly rewarding during this part of the procedure. Once the plane of separation between corpora and urethral plate has been clearly established and defined by a vessel loop, it should be extended proximally and distally along the length of the corporeal body with both dorsal and ventral dissection. In so doing, the urethra is freed from the corpora from prostate to glans. At this point, one can readily appreciate the substantial and elastic nature of the urethral plate.

Corporeal Mobilization

For the operation to be successful, the corpora must be adequately mobilized. The corporeal bodies are freed inferiorly and laterally so that they have the freedom to rotate medially. This dissection in an exstrophy patient is in virgin territory and is straightforward. The more difficult dissection is that of the corpora from the distal aspect of the pubic ramus. In an exstrophy patient, there tends to be significant

scarring as a result of the original freeing of the prostatic urethra from the pubic symphysis. Thus, judicious sharp dissection is necessary to free the corpora, which need not be freed completely from the pubic ramus, as has been historically described; this will avoid the risk of vascular injury.

Once the corpora have been mobilized fully, attention is directed to the neurovascular bundles. To avoid injury to the neurovascular bundles during the corporeal reconstruction, they are freed up laterally by developing the plane between Buck's fascia and the tunica albuginea with sharp dissection begun well away from the bundles themselves. The dissection is best begun with sharp iris scissors to enter the proper plane, and then blunt-tipped scissors to develop the plane without injuring the nerves. The neurovascular bundles are freed proximally and distally with their investing layer of Buck's fascia along the length of the corpora. With complete freeing of the neurovascular bundles as well as the corporeal bodies away from the urethral plate, the dismantling portion of the procedure has been completed (Fig. 118–6).

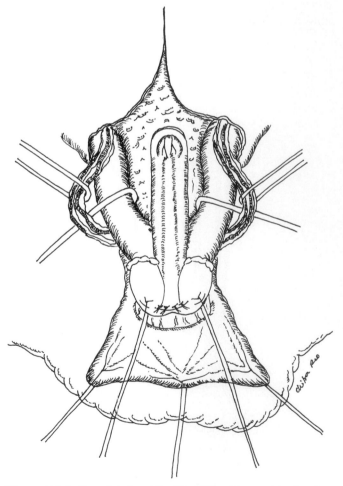

Figure 118–6. Completed mobilization of the corporeal bodies from the urethral plate and the neurovascular bundles off the corpora. (After Perovic S.)

Urethral Reconstruction

The urethral plate is carefully examined and any small rents that may have been produced in the course of the previous dissection are repaired with fine absorbable suture. The urethra is then reconstructed from the prostate to the corona of the glans over a 10 Fr. Silastic tube with multiple side holes placed proximally in the bladder end. Because the tube can slip during the course of the subsequent reconstruction, it is helpful to position it optimally and to mark with a suture the point at which the tube should exit the urethral meatus. The urethral plate is reapproximated with interrupted 6-0 Maxon or polydioxanone (PDS) sutures to preserve its elasticity. Closure of the glanular urethra is deferred until later in the procedure.

Cavernocavernostomy and Correction of Rotational Deformity

Before the corpora are reconstructed, an artificial erection is created. A butterfly needle is used in each corpus because of the absence of cross-circulation between the corporeal bodies. This invariably demonstrates persistent dorsal curvature of the phallus, despite complete freeing of the corporeal bodies from adjacent tethering bands and from the urethral plate. It is important to note the point of maximal corporeal angulation. Correction of the corporeal rotation begins by dropping the urethra into a ventral location relative to the corporeal bodies. This reconstitutes the normal anatomical relationship of urethra to corpora. At the point of maximal corporeal curvature, transverse incisions are made on the dorsolateral aspect of the corpora (Fig. 118–7). At this point the benefit of dissecting the neurovascular bundles away from the corpora is realized, since one can incise the corpora generously (approximately 1.5 cm) and safely. It is interesting to note at this point that the transverse incisions result in diamond-shaped defects as the corpora spring distally approximately 1 to 1.5 cm. The corpora are then rotated dorsomedially over the urethra, and the two diamond-shaped defects, resulting from the transverse incisions in each corporeal body, are approximated in a cavernocavernostomy. A running, double-armed 5-0 Prolene stitch is used with a knot inside the vascular lumen of the corpora (Fig. 118–7, *inset*). This results in a 90-degree rotation of the corpora dorsally and also results in dorsolateral rotation of the neurovascular bundles into a more normal anatomical orientation. One can readily recognize at this point that the penis, rather than having dorsal chordee, now has a more normal, ventral direction.

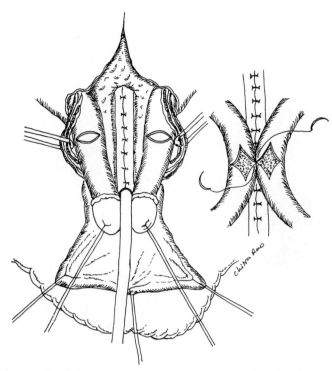

Figure 118–7. Reconstructed urethra over a Silastic tube and transverse incisions in the corpora cavernosa. *Inset*, Cavernocavernostomy with running a double-armed 5-0 Prolene stitch rotates the corpora dorsomedially over the reconstructed urethra. (After Snyder HM. The Ransley second stage urethroplasty for exstrophy. In Frank JD, Johnston JH, eds. Operative Paediatric Urology. New York, Churchill Livingstone, 1990, p 175.)

Glanuloplasty

The glans repair is begun by excising a large triangular area of lateral, irregular glans wing tissue bilaterally. The excision should begin at the ends of the transverse closure and extend proximally to the corona of the glans bilaterally (Fig. 118–8). It is important to be aggressive, because inadequate excision of glans wing tissue may result in a midline dorsal groove. Once the glans wings are excised, two bared areas of glans epithelium result. A deep, urethral layer of glans tissue is then approximated with a running 6-0 Maxon or PDS stitch beginning at the urethral meatus, which has been produced by approximating the ends of the transverse glans closure dorsally (Fig. 118–9A). Before the glans closure is completed, the rotation of the cavernocavernostomy should be reinforced with two or three interrupted Maxon sutures, approximating the corpora distal to the cavernocavernostomy and just proximal to the corona of the glans. The superficial glans skin is then approximated with a subcuticular 6-0 Maxon stitch (Fig. 118–9B). This approach has produced a particularly satisfying cosmetic result with a minimally visible glans scar.

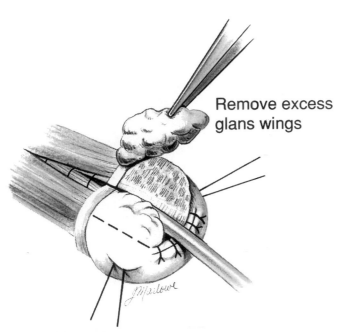

Remove excess glans wings

Figure 118–8. Removal of excess glans wing tissue from transverse closure to the corona bilaterally. (From Diamond DA, Ransley PG. Improved glanuloplasty and epispadias repair: Technical aspects. J Urol 152:1243, 1994.)

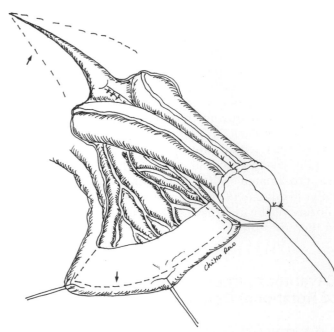

Figure 118–10. Penile skin coverage is achieved by dorsal rotation of a preputial transverse island flap distally and Z-plasty proximally, using a triangular flap created adjacent to the midline incision (*arrows*).

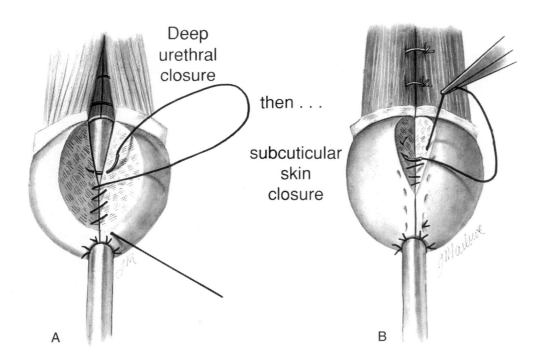

Deep urethral closure

then . . .

subcuticular skin closure

A

B

Figure 118–9. *A,* Closure of the inner glandular urethral layer over an indwelling Silastic stent. *B,* Subcuticular closure of superficial glans epithelium. (From Diamond DA, Ransley PG. Improved glanuloplasty and epispadias repair: Technical aspects. J Urol 152: 1243, 1994.)

Skin Coverage

Reliable dorsal skin coverage is achieved by rotating a transverse island flap of the inner layer of ventral preputial skin dorsally over the distal penile shaft. Proximal penile skin coverage is achieved by rotating the remaining ventral preputial skin to the dorsum bilaterally and performing a Z-plasty of the distal abdominal wall incision (Fig. 118–10). The Z-plasty results in two triangular flaps, which may be approximated at the base of the phallus (Fig. 118–11). This approach provides tissue for proximal penile skin coverage, avoids the hollow that sometimes results at the junction of pubis and penile shaft, and avoids a midline scar extending to the base of the phallus that may be predisposed to contracture.

DRESSING AND POSTOPERATIVE CARE

The penis is encased in a Silastic foam dressing, which is secured to the lower abdominal wall with a six-legged elastic bandage (Elastoplast) wrap. The Silastic stent is allowed to drain into a double diaper postoperatively. The patient is maintained on broad-spectrum oral antibiotics and may be discharged home after 1 or 2 days in the hospital, when pain control with oral analgesics is effective. The child is seen in an outpatient setting at 1-week intervals until the dressing and stent are removed 2 to 3 weeks postoperatively. A thorough bathing of the child facilitates removal of the Silastic foam dressing. If the stent produces bladder spasm, oral oxybutynin (Ditropan) may be of benefit.

POSTOPERATIVE COMPLICATIONS

At 6 months, cystoscopy and examination under anesthesia are performed to rule out stenosis of the urethral tube and urethrocutaneous fistula. The benefits of this approach have included a healthy urethral channel that can be readily catheterized because of maintenance of the continuity of the urethral plate. Urethrocutaneous fistula has been the most common

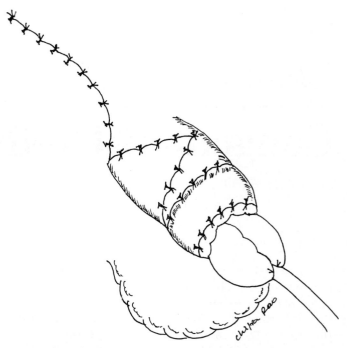

Figure 118–11. Completed repair with skin coverage distally from a transverse preputial island flap and proximally from a Z-plasty.

complication of this repair, occurring in approximately 8 percent of cases. The areas most vulnerable to fistula formation have been the most proximal portion of the urethral reconstruction, as well as the junction of pendulous urethra with the glanular urethra at the level of the corona. Urethral stenosis has been an uncommon complication.

Editorial Comment
Craig A. Peters

An important aspect of the Cantwell-Ransley epispadias technique is the provision of a dependent penis, particularly in patients with bladder exstrophy. This is very often a major cosmetic and functional problem for these boys, especially as they become sexually mature.

REFERENCES

1. Snyder HM. The Ransley second stage urethroplasty for exstrophy. In Frank JD, Johnston JH, eds. Operative Pediatric Urology. New York, Churchill Livingstone, 1990, p 171.
2. Diamond DA, Ransley PG. Improved glanuloplasty and epispadias repair: Technical aspects. J Urol 152:1243–1245, 1994.
3. Gearhart JP, Leonard MP, Burgers JK, Jeffs RD. The Cantwell-Ransley technique for repair of epispadias. J Urol 148:851, 1992.

Chapter 119

Congenital Urethral Duplication

Anthony Atala

Congenital urethral duplication is a well-described but rare entity. The first reference to this condition dates back to Aristotle. The clinical significance of this abnormality is variable. Congenital urethral duplication either can be entirely asymptomatic and diagnosed incidentally, or can have a variety of clinical presentations such as urinary infection, incontinence, and double stream. A complete understanding of this entity is necessary in order to effectively diagnose and treat the patient.

ANATOMICAL CONSIDERATIONS

Since urethral duplication can occur in a wide variety of configurations, many classification systems have been described. A comprehensive, clinically useful classification system is shown in Table 119–1.

Type I urethral duplication describes a blind incomplete duplication or accessory urethra that may or may not have a communication with the functional urethra (Fig. 119–1A). Type I duplications are usually asymptomatic and may be hard to differentiate from a urethral diverticulum or Cowper's duct, depending on their location.

Type II duplications consist of a complete patent

urethral duplication in which both urethras are located within the phallus. Variations in anatomy within this category are numerous. One urethra may arise from the other and course through the penis to either a single meatus (Fig. 119–1B) or two separate meatus (Fig. 119–1C). In some patients, both channels arise separately from the bladder and either unite distally to form a common channel (Fig. 119–1D) or course to their respective meatal openings on the phallus (Fig. 119–1E). The ventral urethral meatus has multiple possible locations within the phallus (Fig. 119–1F), as does the dorsal urethral meatus.

Type III denotes a complete patent urethral duplication wherein the ventral urethra is located outside the phallus. Again, many anatomical variations may exist. More commonly, the ventral urethra may end in the perineum (Fig. 119–1G) or in the anterior wall of the anal canal at the mucocutaneous junction (Fig. 119–1H).

In Type IV, urethral duplication presents as a component of partial or complete caudal duplication syndromes. Usually, the two urethras are located on either side of the midline and course to the penis from separate bladders (Fig. 119–1I).

PREOPERATIVE EVALUATION

The diagnosis is facilitated if the physician has a high index of suspicion for urethral duplication. Presenting complaints may include two meatus, a double stream, recurrent urinary tract infections, or incontinence with no other apparent cause.

The physical examination is helpful only if complete urethral duplication is present and both urethras can be visualized. At times, even this presentation is difficult if the accessory urethra is in an ectopic unsuspected location, such as that seen with type III. A complete history is taken and physical examination performed in all patients. Anesthetic and surgical risks are assessed. The physical exami-

TABLE 119–1. Urethral Duplication: Classification System

Type I
Blind incomplete accessory urethra that may or may not communicate with the functional urethra
Type II
Complete duplication wherein both urethras are located within the phallus
Type III
Complete duplication wherein the ventral urethra is located outside the phallus
Type IV
Urethral duplication is a component of partial or complete caudal duplication syndrome

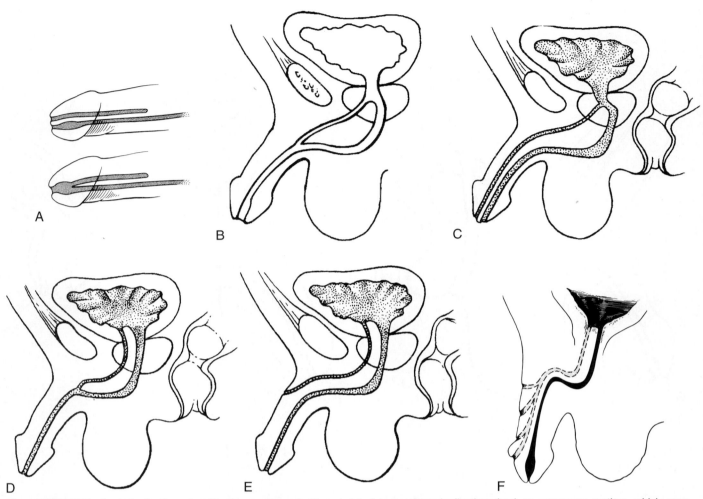

Figure 119–1. Urethral duplication classification system. *A,* Type I, blind incomplete duplication *(top)* or accessory urethra, which may communicate with the functional urethra *(bottom). B* to *F,* Variations in presentation of type II duplications wherein both urethras are located within the phallus.

Illustration continued on following page

nation determines the severity of the duplication and is also aimed at identifying any associated anomalies. The urethras should be inspected and palpated. If a bulge is seen or felt, or if urethral compression produces dribbling, a diverticulum may also be suspected.

A careful radiological evaluation is essential to delineate the exact anatomy of the duplication. A voiding cystourethrogram (VCUG) is the examination of choice and is performed with multiple lateral and oblique views. Retrograde urethrography or antegrade cystography may be necessary if the VCUG fails to delineate the exact anatomy owing to a small-caliber accessory urethra. Renal ultrasound examination should be performed in all patients because of the association of this condition with upper urinary tract anomalies.[1]

Urodynamic studies are indicated if there is urinary incontinence.[2] Particular attention should be directed toward evaluating sphincter function. The continence mechanism is usually located in the more functional ventral urethra.

TREATMENT

Treatment depends on the type of presentation. Asymptomatic patients should be observed. Patients with a double stream, incontinence, or recurrent infections merit excision of the duplicated urethra. The ventral urethra usually contains the sphincter, accessory glands, and verumontanum.[2] The dorsal urethra is usually the least functional and the target for excision.

Although urethral duplication can be classified into distinct types, hundreds of variations in anatomy have been reported. No single technique of urethral duplication repair is suitable for all cases. Therefore, the surgical armamentarium must include a variety of operations to suit the severity of the condition. Surgical management depends on the type of anatomical abnormality present and varies widely from a simple endoscopic procedure to extensive open reconstructive procedures. To describe the surgical approach required for each anatomical variant would be a formidable task beyond the scope of this chapter.

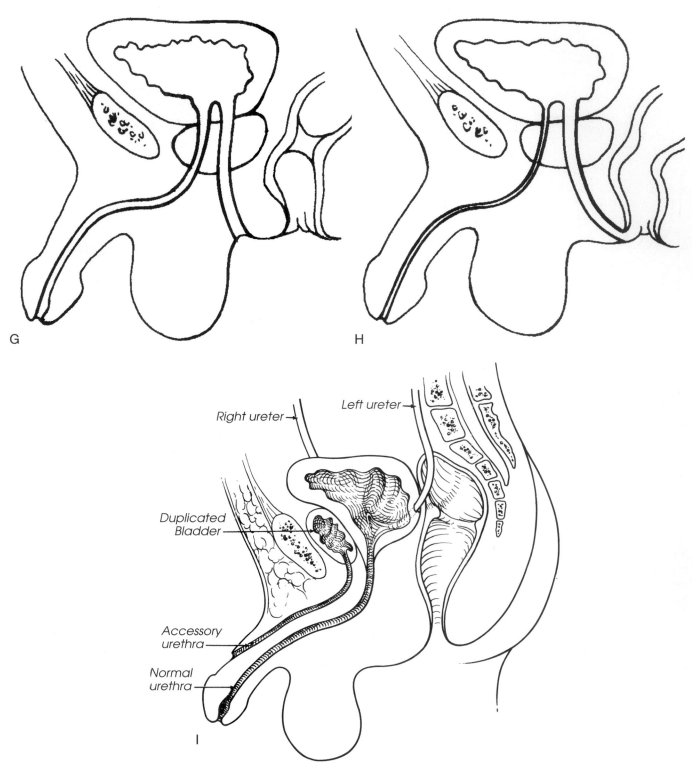

Figure 119–1 *Continued G* and *H*, Type III wherein the ventral urethra is located outside the phallus. *I*, Type IV, a component of partial or complete caudal duplication syndrome; usually the two urethras course to the penis from separate bladders.

However, regardless of the type of anomaly encountered, the patient may always be approached using the same basic decision-making tree. If surgical intervention is indicated, a careful rigid or flexible cystoscopic evaluation is performed immediately before surgery. Both urethras should be stented with indwelling catheters, if possible, to facilitate their identification during surgical dissection. The most functional urethra is preserved (usually the ventral) and the other urethra is either preserved or excised, depending on its location and degree of function. Both urethras may be joined if the anatomy and degree of function of each permits.

Several general principles are important in whatever technique is used. Skin incisions are made using a fine knife blade such as the Weck microsurgical knife. Gentle handling of tissues is mandatory, using tiny skin hooks and fine traction sutures. The tissue should be kept moist at all times. Cautery for hemostasis should be precise, brief, and applied with the pinpoint technique.

Occasionally, the tissue present from both urethras is not enough for the construction of a single functional and anatomically correct urethra. In these patients, a neourethra is constructed by using a flap of penile skin or a full-thickness tube graft from genital or extragenital skin, buccal or bladder mucosa. The use of hair-bearing skin is contraindicated since it may result in a hairy neourethra. The anastomosis should be proximal enough to be in good tissue and not on the thin transparent tissue often seen in the distal urethra because of the lack of corpus spongiosum. The repair is performed with fine absorbable sutures. Urine-tight anastomoses are made and inverted toward the lumen whenever possible. Eversion of suture lines increases periurethral reaction, which contributes both to urinary leakage and to potential fistula or diverticulum formation.[3] The suture lines of tubularized neourethras are placed posteriorly against the shaft of the penis to bury as much of the anastomosis as possible and maximize coverage. Overlying suture lines should be avoided to minimize the possibility of fistula formation. Suture line tension is reduced before closing each layer by generous mobilization and undermining of adjacent tissues.

The new urethra must be wide enough to avoid strictures. It must have a well-vascularized pedicle and/or be covered by well-vascularized layers of subcutaneous tissue and skin for the graft to heal. A dorsal dartos subcutaneous flap may be used to wrap the repair whenever possible.[4] In a similar fashion the tunica vaginalis flap can also be employed to obtain an additional vascularized layer over the repair whenever feasible.[5]

The skin closure is meticulously performed without strangulation to allow for the expected postoperative swelling. Fine absorbable sutures are used. Horizontal mattress stitches are often helpful to evert the skin edges, which minimizes fistula formation.

Type I

Blind-ending urethral duplications are the most common. A lacrimal duct probe can be used to facilitate the diagnosis. Patients with a blind-ending tract wherein both meatus are close together in the glans may be managed, for cosmetic reasons, by excision of the interurethral septum (Fig. 119–2). Lidocaine (1 percent) is injected into the periurethral region; a fine clamp is placed around the septum for approximately 1 minute; the thinned, now avascular, septal tissue is transected; and the edges are approximated with 5–0 chromic sutures. The same procedure can be performed in patients with complete urethral duplication wherein the two meatus are close together at the tip of the glans.

Type II

In some patients the meatus of the dorsal channel may be in an epispadiac position whose location may vary from the glans to the base of the penis. In these cases the ventral channel is the more functional one and its meatus is usually in a normal position. A decision needs to be made whether the dorsal urethra should be either excised or anastomosed to the ventral urethra.

If the dorsal urethra is mostly nonfunctional or rudimentary, excision is preferred and should be made as close to its origin as possible. This may be accomplished by a penile or combined pubic and penile approach.

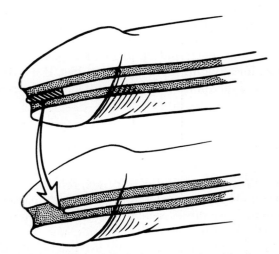

Figure 119–2. Patients with both meatus close together may be managed by excision of the interurethral septum. A fine clamp is placed around the septum and the tissue is transected. The edges are approximated with fine absorbable sutures.

If the dorsal urethra originates proximally, one may start with a retropubic approach, making an infraumbilical abdominal incision. The prevesical space is entered. Fingers over the bladder will help direct the retropubic dissection anteriorly toward the apex of the prostate, staying close to the retropubic peritoneum until the accessory urethra is reached.

If the dorsal urethra is not easily localized in this fashion, an inferior pubectomy may be necessary (Fig. 119–3A). The surface of the pubis is exposed, the periosteum is reflected, and a hand-held osteotome may be used to transect the pubis. Occasionally, a small 1- to 2-cm wedge of bone may be excised. The pubic bones are retracted laterally at the prostatic apex, and the origin of the accessory urethra is visualized (Fig. 119–3B). After the accessory urethra is isolated, it is transected and ligated proximally (Fig. 119–3C). The dorsal urethra is dissected distally until the penile entry site is reached, where it is again excised. The phallic aperture is then closed in several layers. The pubis is closed with two or three figure-of-eight heavy sutures.

If the dorsal urethra is functional, it may be preserved by anastomosing it to the ventral urethra. Depending on the urethral anatomy, a penile or combined pubic and penile approach may be necessary, as described above. Regardless of the approach required, the anastomosis is performed in the same fashion. The ventral urethra is incised dorsally (anteriorly) for 1 cm, and the dorsal urethra is spatulated posteriorly in the midline (Fig. 119–4). Either interrupted or continuous 6–0 absorbable sutures are used for the anastomosis.

Occasionally, in type II duplications, the dorsal urethra and its meatus are in a normal anatomical position and the ventral urethra opens in a hypospadiac location ranging from the glans to the penoscrotal junction. In these instances, one must again remember that the ventral urethra is usually the more functional even though the anatomy does not suggest it. If the dorsal urethra is rudimentary, it should be excised, and additional surgical management is the same as for any child with hypospadias. If the dorsal urethra is functional, the hypospadiac urethra can be anastomosed to the dorsal urethra.

Type III (To Perineum)

Type III urethral duplication, wherein the ventral urethra ends in the perineum, is more complex, but the surgical principles remain the same. If the dorsal urethra is not functional, its excision may be necessary. In these patients the ventral urethra is mobilized and brought to the penoscrotal junction.

A perineal approach is initiated. The patient is placed in an exaggerated dorsal lithotomy position,

the legs well padded to avoid peroneal nerve injury. The ventral urethral meatus is circumscribed in the perineal region with a superior midline extension (Fig. 119–5A). A suture, with or without a silicone catheter, is placed through the outer edge of the ventral urethra to facilitate the dissection. The bulbocavernous muscle is exposed medially (Fig. 119–5B) and the ventral urethra is sharply dissected off the underlying bulbocavernous muscle (Fig. 119–5C). Hugging the bulbocavernous muscle, a passage is made between the inferior margin of the scrotum and the penoscrotal junction (Fig. 119–5D). The ventral urethra is repositioned in the region of the penoscrotal junction (Fig. 119–5E) and secured with interrupted absorbable 6–0 sutures (Fig. 119–5F). The perineal incision is closed in several layers.

With the patient under the same anesthetic, the prepuce is incised in the midline dorsally. The preputial flap is advanced ventrally and distally to the tip of the glans, in a fashion similar to the first stage of a two-stage hypospadias repair.[6] After 6 to 12 months the tissues have usually softened sufficiently to permit the second-stage repair with a Duplay tube.

If the dorsal urethra is functional, it may be possible to anastomose the ventral urethra to it proximally. For these patients a perineal approach is also used. A midline perineal incision is made and extended to the circumference of the ventral urethra (Fig. 119–6A). A suture is placed through the distal end of the ventral urethra to facilitate its dissection (Fig. 119–6B) down to the bulbocavernous muscle. The latter is exposed, divided along its raphe (Fig. 119–6C), and retracted laterally. This exposes the underlying corpus spongiosum and dorsal urethra, which are easily identifiable with an indwelling catheter (Fig. 119–6D). The corpus spongiosum tissue is sharply dissected off the underlying dorsal urethra and a 1-cm longitudinal incision is made in the midline posteriorly, exposing a previously inserted indwelling catheter (Fig. 119–6E). The end of the ventral urethra is trimmed back to normal tissue. The ventral urethra is then spatulated and anastomosed to the dorsal urethra in a tension-free manner with 6–0 absorbable sutures (Fig. 119–6F). Figure 119–6G shows the completed urethral repair. The perineal incision is closed in several layers.

Type III (To Anus)

The most extensive reconstructive surgery is required in patients with a type III defect in which the ventral channel exits onto the anus. Fortunately, this is rare. The patient is again approached using the same basic decision-making tree. The most functional urethra is preserved (usually the ventral) and the

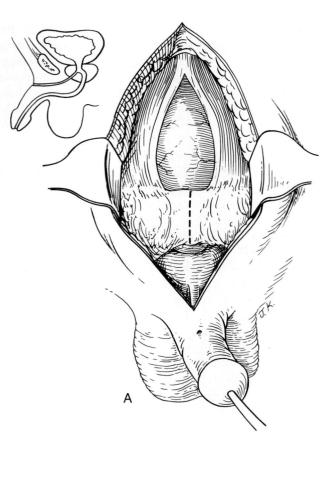

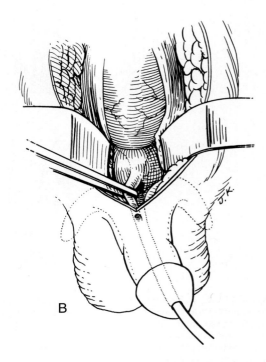

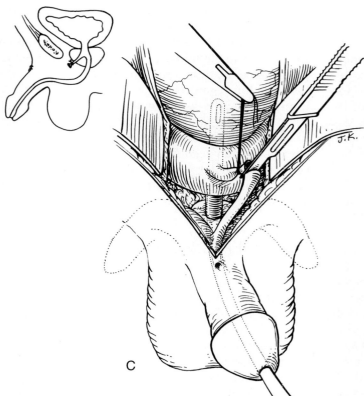

Figure 119–3. Excision of the dorsal urethra in a type II urethral duplication. *A,* An infraumbilical abdominal incision is made to gain retropubic access to the dorsal urethra. If the dorsal urethra is not easily localized, an inferior pubectomy may be necessary. The surface of the pubis is exposed and the periosteum is reflected. An osteotome is useful for transection. *B,* The pubic bones are retracted laterally and the origin of the dorsal urethra is visualized. *C,* The dorsal urethra is transected and ligated both proximally and distally. The phallic aperture is closed in two layers of absorbable suture. The pubis is closed with two or three figure-of-eight heavy sutures.

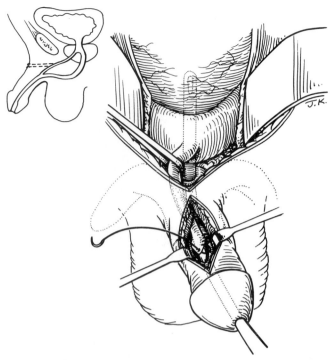

Figure 119–4. A functional dorsal urethra may be preserved by anastomosing it to the ventral urethra with either interrupted or continuous 6–0 absorbable sutures. The ventral urethra is incised anteriorly for 1 cm and the dorsal urethra is spatulated posteriorly. A pubectomy is necessary only if additional dorsal urethral length is needed for a tension-free anastomosis. Otherwise, a direct phallic approach may be sufficient.

other urethra is either preserved or excised, depending on its location and degree of function.

If the dorsal urethra is nonfunctional, it may require excision. The ventral urethra needs to be mobilized to the penoscrotal junction, thus converting the defect to a proximal hypospadias in preparation for a later second-stage repair. This procedure may be accomplished by using a perineal approach as described above or a posterior sagittal (Peña) approach. These patients should have the bowel prepared before surgery. If the posterior sagittal approach is preferred, the child is turned into the prone jackknife position. A circumferential incision is made around the anus with a midline extension superiorly and inferiorly (Fig. 119–7A). The anus and distal part of the rectum are dissected free until the external portion of the ventral urethra is identified (Fig. 119–7B). The distal end of the ventral urethra is transected with a small cuff of bowel. The remaining defect is closed with one continuous mucosal layer of 4–0 chromic and a second serosal layer of interrupted 4–0 silk sutures (Fig. 119–7C). A stay suture is placed through the distal end of the ventral urethra for traction. Sharp and blunt dissection is maintained. A small incision is made in the penoscrotal junction (Fig. 119–7D). Hugging the bulbocavernous muscle, a passage is made between the inferior margin of the

scrotum and the penoscrotal junction, and the ventral urethra is tunneled to its new location in the penoscrotal region (Fig. 119–7E). The urethra is anastomosed in a circumferential fashion using interrupted absorbable 6–0 sutures. The perineal region is closed with two or three layers of absorbable sutures, taking particular care to replace the rectum in its proper position (Fig. 119–7F).

As with other cases described above, if the dorsal urethra is functional, the ventral urethra can be joined to the dorsal urethra, forming a common channel. In these instances a posterior sagittal approach is also preferable (Fig. 119–8A). The ventral urethra is dissected off the distal end of the rectum or anus (Fig. 119–8B). The distal segment of the ventral urethra is transected along with a small cuff of bowel (Fig. 119–8C). The end of the ventral urethra is trimmed back to normal tissue. The bulbocavernous muscle is exposed, divided along its raphe, and retracted laterally until the proximal aspect of the dorsal urethra is visualized. The dorsal urethra is incised dorsally (anteriorly) for 1 cm and the ventral urethra is spatulated posteriorly in the midline (Fig. 119–8D). Either interrupted or continuous absorbable 6–0 sutures are used for the anastomosis. The perineum is closed as described above.

Type IV

Type IV duplications are also varied in terms of their anatomy. Usually, the two urethras are located on either side of the midline and course to the penis from separate bladders. The anomalies are more complex, since bladder emptying also plays a role in the decision regarding how to approach the urethral duplication. The achievement of adequate bladder drainage and of urethral function is equally important in these patients, and the surgical management decisions are made accordingly. The major principles described above for urethral duplication surgery still apply, as long as adequate bladder drainage is either achieved or maintained.

POSTOPERATIVE MANAGEMENT

Attention to detail in postoperative care should rival that during the operation itself. A transparent biomembrane (Tegaderm) is usually selected as a surgical penile dressing and applied to the penile shaft and the glans in a circumferential fashion without tension. If there is excessive bleeding during the procedure, a circumferential gauze dressing is applied over the Tegaderm for compression and removed 12 to 24 hours after surgery, leaving the Tegaderm dressing in place.

Text continued on page 1003

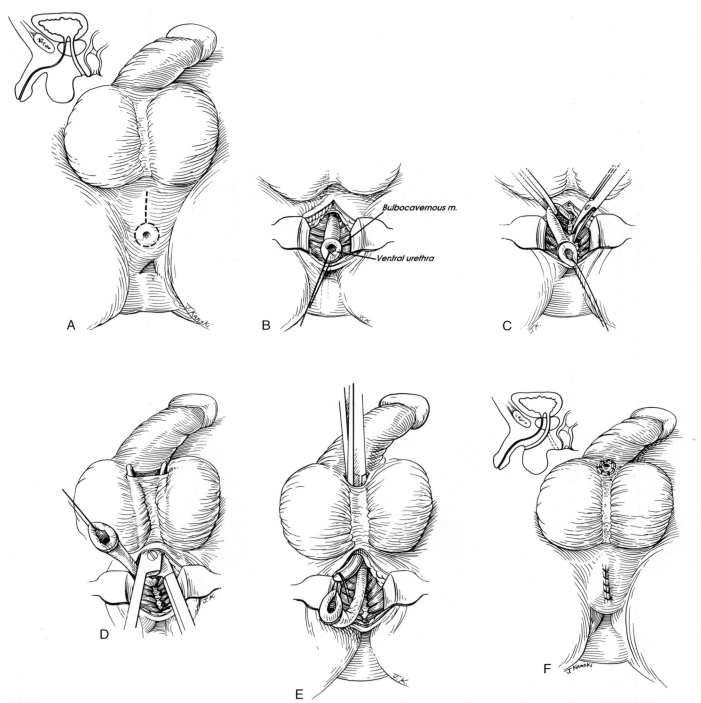

Figure 119–5. Conversion of a perineal ventral urethral defect to a penoscrotal hypospadias in patients with a rudimentary dorsal urethra. *A,* The patient is placed in an exaggerated dorsal lithotomy position. The ventral urethral meatus is circumscribed with a superior midline extension. *B,* A suture is placed through the outer edge of the ventral urethra and proximal dissection is initiated. *C,* The ventral urethra is dissected off the underlying bulbocavernous muscle. *D,* Hugging the bulbocavernous muscle, a passage is made between the inferior portion of the scrotum and the penoscrotal junction. *E,* The urethra is tunneled to the penoscrotal location. *F,* The ventral urethra is secured to its new location in the penoscrotal junction in a tension-free manner with interrupted absorbable sutures. The perineal incision is closed in several layers. The penis is prepared for a subsequent second-stage repair.

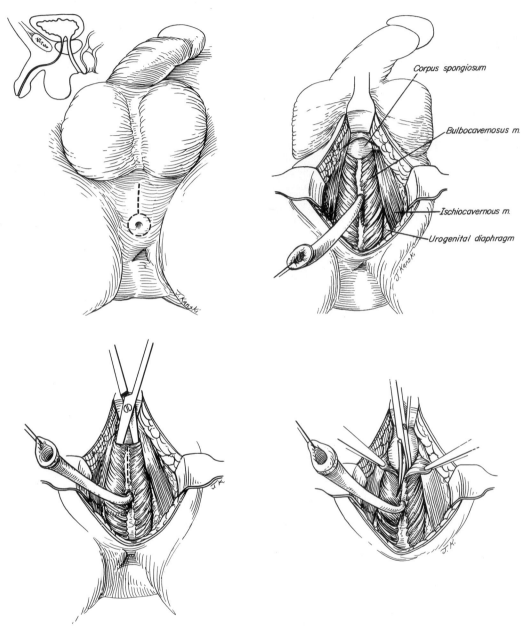

Figure 119–6. Anastomosis of the perineal ventral urethra to a functional dorsal urethra. *A,* A perineal approach is initiated. *B,* With a suture through the ventral urethral meatus and gentle traction, the ventral urethra is dissected to the level of the bulbocavernous muscle. *C,* An indwelling catheter is placed in the dorsal urethra to facilitate its identification perineally. The bulbocavernous muscle is divided along its raphe, exposing the underlying corpus spongiosum and dorsal urethra. *D,* The bulbocavernous muscle is dissected off the underlying corpus spongiosum and dorsal urethra.

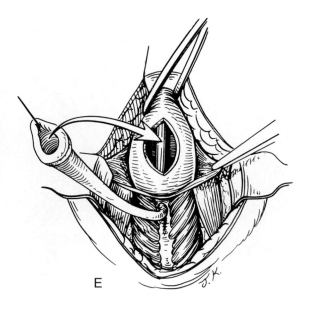

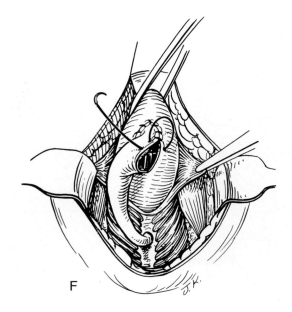

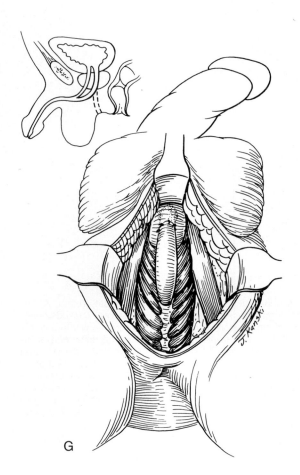

Figure 119–6 *Continued E,* The corpus spongiosum tissue is dissected free, exposing the dorsal urethra. A 1-cm longitudinal incision is made in the midline posteriorly, exposing the indwelling catheter. *F,* The end of the ventral urethra is trimmed back to normal tissue and spatulated. A tension-free anastomosis is initiated with the dorsal urethra. *G,* Before the closure is completed, the indwelling urethral catheter is placed through the ventral urethra to "stent" the anastomoses. The perineum is closed in several layers.

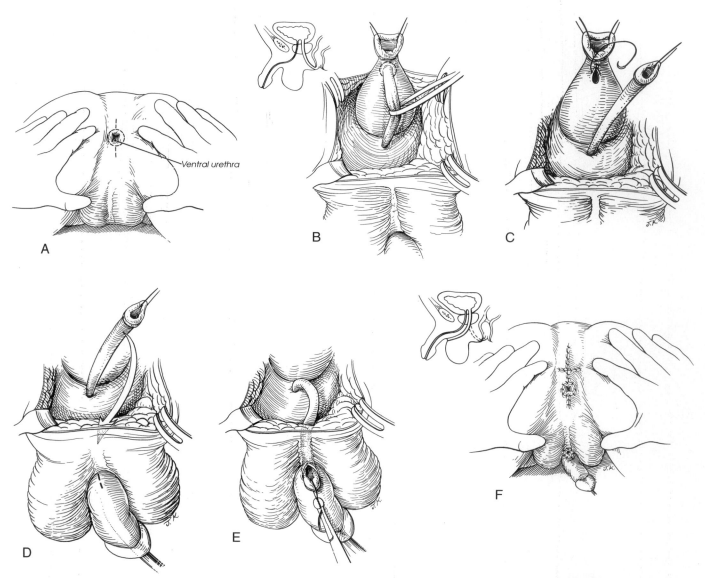

Figure 119–7. Conversion of a ventral urethroanal defect to a penoscrotal hypospadias in patients with a rudimentary dorsal urethra. *A,* The child is placed in a prone jackknife position in preparation for a posterior sagittal (Peña) approach. A povidone-iodine (Betadine) soaked sponge is packed into the distal portion of the rectum to avoid fecal contamination. A circumscribing incision is made around the anus with a superior and inferior midline extension. *B,* The anus and distal rectum are dissected free until the ventral urethra is identified. The distal end of the urethra is transected with a small cuff of bowel. *C,* The bowel defect is closed with a mucosal layer of absorbable chromic and a serosal layer of silk sutures. A traction suture is placed through the distal end of the ventral urethra and gentle dissection is performed until adequate urethral length is obtained. *D,* A passage is made between the inferior margin of the scrotum and the penoscrotal junction. *E,* The ventral urethra is tunneled to its new location in the penoscrotal junction. The distal end of the urethra is trimmed back to normal tissue. The ventral urethra is secured with interrupted absorbable 6–0 sutures. *F,* The rectum is replaced in its proper position. The perineum is closed with several layers of absorbable sutures. The anocutaneous margin is approximated in a circumferential fashion with interrupted 5–0 chromic sutures. The penis is prepared for a subsequent second-stage repair.

If a suprapubic or perineal incision is made, a gauze covered with Tegaderm is applied. If extensive dissection has been performed, drainage with a small Penrose drain for 2 or 3 days should be considered.

Premature voiding may not be desirable and may lead to complications. The choice for urinary diversion varies with the technique used. No drainage is required for simple septal resections. Children who undergo any type of urethroplasty usually require urinary diversion, performed with a 7 Fr. soft Jackson-Pratt urethral "splent." This acts as an effective conduit for the urine during voiding and also decreases the accumulation of secretions given off by the traumatized urethra, which may be predisposed to infection.[7] An additional advantage of this form of diversion is the elimination of external collection devices and lessening of the bladder spasms often seen with Foley catheters. The tube is well tolerated and the child no longer requires restraints and complete bed rest.

In more extensive repairs in which long-term diversion is necessary, a round 7 Fr. soft silicone drain can be positioned in the bladder, and the urine can drain freely into protective diapers or a urinary reservoir. Ten to 14 days of urinary diversion is usually maintained. Radiographical visualization of the repair may be achieved with a "pull-out" urethrogram through the urethral catheter as it is being removed.

If a major reconstructive procedure is undertaken, a suprapubic catheter may also be inserted for temporary urinary diversion. Ten to 14 days after surgery, the suprapubic catheter is clamped. The urethral stent is removed and the patient is allowed to void per urethram. Radiographical visualization of the repair can be achieved with a VCUG through the suprapubic catheter before its removal.

COMPLICATIONS

Even in the hands of the most experienced surgeons, urethral duplication repair is associated with a number of complications, including urethrocutaneous fistula, stricture, chordee, and diverticula. A careful preoperative evaluation, precise surgical technique, and appropriate postoperative care are required to achieve the desired objectives of surgery.

Perioperative bleeding can be minimized during dissection by intermittent use of an elastic penile tourniquet for periods of up to 30 minutes. After release, cauterization ensures hemostasis. The glanular, periurethral, and subcutaneous injection of epinephrine (1:200,000) has also been useful in maintaining hemostasis without causing tissue ischemia. The anesthesiologist should be informed when epinephrine is used because halothane, a common inhalational anesthetic, sensitizes the heart to catecholamines, and ventricular arrhythmia may result.

Penile chordee may be present in some patients with urethral duplication. Failure to create a straight phallus is one of the avoidable complications of surgery. Penile straightening and removal of full chordee must be confirmed before beginning the urethral repair by use of the artificial erection test.[8] After an elastic band is securely placed at the base of the penis or after use of perineal compression, injection of normal saline with a 25-gauge butterfly needle placed in one corporeal body will fill the entire organ and identify any restraining fibrous bands that remain. Multiple tests may be necessary to ensure complete excision. If the penis remains bent despite resection of all chordee, an alternative approach may be needed, such as insertion of a dermal or tunica vaginalis graft into the shaft, or dorsal plication.

Fistulas may develop after surgical repair and may be small, large, and multiple. Although their exact cause cannot be defined, two avoidable factors usually underscore the problem: infection and tissue ischemia. Patients empirically receive broad-spectrum antibiotics perioperatively and for 10 days postoperatively. Tissue ischemia can be minimized by excision of any devitalized tissue at the time of initial surgery.

A fistula may be suspected before the voiding trial when an area of inflammation or wound breakdown is noticed along a urethral course. Often, fistulas are observed shortly after the initiation of spontaneous voiding. Patients who still have a urinary diversion catheter present when the fistula is first noticed may have the urinary drainage period extended for several days in an attempt to encourage closure of the fistula (although the chance of a fistula closing spontaneously is small). If urinary diversion is not present, placement of a catheter to bypass the fistula is not recommended. Additional damage may be caused by placing a catheter in a nonanesthetized patient. If the fistula is small and there is no evidence of a distal obstruction or inflammation, it may close spontaneously in a few instances.

Fistulas are often associated with distal strictures. The distal phallic urethra should be examined for early stenosis, edema, or plugging with secretions. Liberal use of antibiotic ointment postoperatively helps eliminate any secretions. No attempt at surgical repair should be undertaken until all edema and induration have subsided and the surrounding tissues are soft and pliable. This usually occurs about 6 months postoperatively, although it is not uncommon for surgery to be deferred for as long as 1 year. The method of correction depends on the location, size, and number of fistulas present.

Silver nitrate cautery of small fistulas is usually not successful in my experience. It is useful to inject

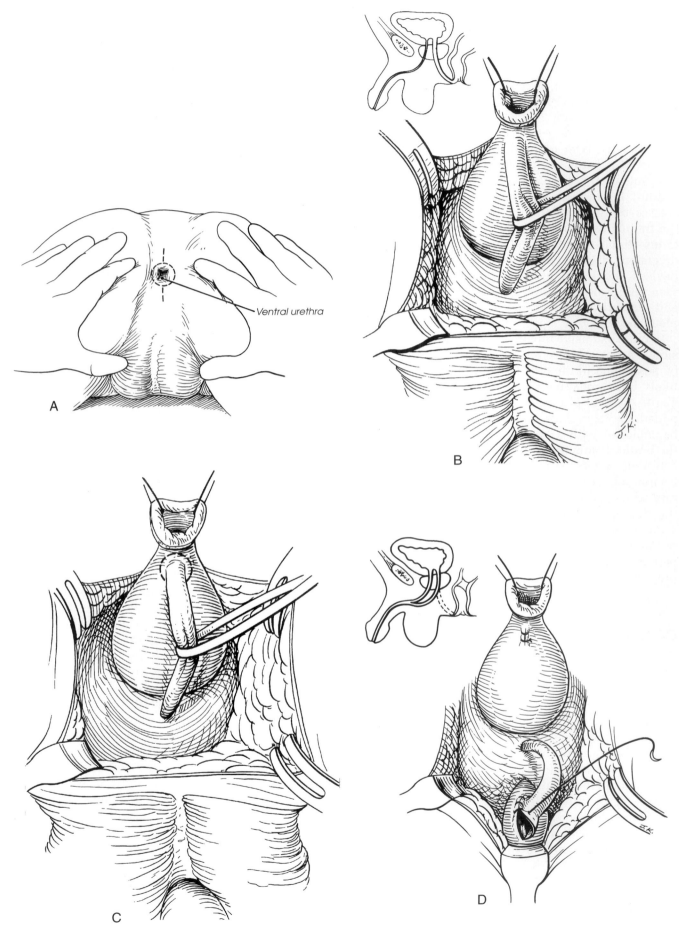

Ventral urethra

A

B

C

D

Figure 119–8 *See legend on opposite page*

Chapter 120

Ambiguous Genitalia

John P. Gearhart

INDICATIONS

An infant with ambiguous genitalia poses a great dilemma for parents and physician, even if the child has a normal 46,XX or 46,XY karyotype. Gender assignment is often difficult and requires a full understanding of all factors involved, including chromosomal sex, hormonal sex, exogenous hormonal influence, anatomy of the internal and external genital structures, ultimate gonadal function, potential fertility, predilection of the gonads for malignancy, and parental attitudes. However, in all cases the sex of rearing should be determined as rapidly as possible after birth so that early perineal reconstruction can be performed, preferably within the first 3 to 6 months of life.

PREOPERATIVE MANAGEMENT

Evaluation of a newborn with ambiguous genitalia should include a careful family history, physical examination, and karyotyping. Contrast studies of the urogenital system, biochemical evaluation, endoscopy, laparoscopy, and gonadal biopsy may be indicated. History taking should include inquiries concerning maternal ingestion of possible androgenic substances during pregnancy. A history of an unexpected death of a sibling in the first week or two of life can pinpoint the likelihood of the adrenogenital syndrome with salt wasting. Some of these syndromes can be sex-linked recessive traits. Therefore, it may help to learn whether sterility, amenorrhea, or a hernia containing a gonad is part of the family history.

On physical examination, one should look for the following: (1) bifid scrotum, (2) rugated labia, (3) hypospadias, (4) chordee, (5) gonads above or below the inguinal ring, (6) a palpable epididymis on the gonad, and (7) a midline uterus detectable during the rectal examination. The presence of vaginal epithelial cells in the smear of the urethral discharge, obtained by milking the vagina during the rectal examination, is taken into consideration.

The possibility of other major associated anomalies should be considered. Karyotyping can help differentiate mixed gonadal dysgenesis (relatively common) from true hermaphroditism (very rare). If the buccal smear results are positive with masculinized external genitalia, biochemical studies, including urinary ketosteroids, pregnanetriol, serum 17-hydroxyprogesterone, and electrolyte analyses, should be performed to ascertain the presence of an enzymatic defect. Ultrasonography, retrograde urethrography, and endoscopy can determine where the vagina is attached to the urogenital sinus. Laparotomy and gonadal biopsy may be necessary for definite diagnosis of mixed gonadal dysgenesis, male pseudohermaphroditism, or true hermaphroditism.

It is important to define the types of male pseudohermaphroditism so that the males who do not respond to testosterone production or replacement at puberty are reared as females. Because the phallus may appear reasonably adequate at birth but not respond at puberty, it is essential to rear infants who have severe deficiency in male genital development as females. Androgen receptors can be measured in cultured fibroblasts from genital skin. If receptor levels are low or absent, complete androgen insensitivity must be considered. Type 1 familial incomplete pseudohermaphroditism also occurs and is characterized by different degrees of hypospadias, hypogonadism, and gynecomastia. In 5-alpha-reductase deficiency, testosterone cannot be converted to dihydrotestosterone. The patient is characterized by severe hypospadias, bifid scrotum, blind-ending vagina, failure of breast development, and incomplete masculinization at puberty.

The choice of sex of rearing should be based on the infant's anatomy and not on the chromosomal karyotype. Information gained from preoperative studies helps the surgeon plan a surgical repair and decide whether it should be done from a perineal, combined perineal, or abdominal exposure, or even from a posterior sagittal approach. It is not difficult to create a vagina if one is absent, but it is difficult to create a satisfactory penis if the phallus is diminutive or rudimentary. Only those patients with a stretched penile length of at least 2.5 cm that will respond to testosterone should be considered for male sex of rearing. Otherwise, female gender assignment should be considered.

SURGICAL OPTIONS

Intersex patients who require feminine reconstruction of the perineum can be divided into two groups: (1) females with extreme masculinization of the external genitalia, i.e., the adrenogenital syndrome; and (2) others with incomplete masculinization of the sexual structure (male pseudohermaphrodites, those with mixed gonadal dysgenesis, and those with some forms of true hermaphroditism).[1] Surgical repair of these infants who are to be reared as females includes phallic reduction, creation of labia majora and minora, and construction of a neovagina. Originally the enlarged clitoris or diminutive phallus was managed by clitorectomy, and the entire structure was excised.[2] Since that time, some conservative procedures have been implemented, including excision of the

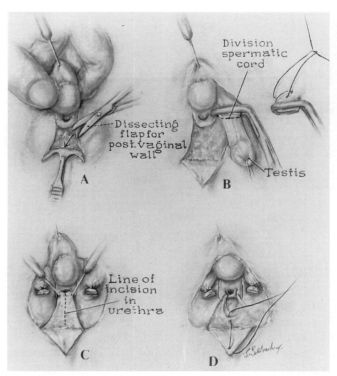

Figure 120–2. *A,* Dissection of a perineal flap. *B,* Removal of an inappropriate gonad via the lateral border of the perineal incision. *C,* Incision into the urethral floor. *D,* The apex of the perineal flap is secured to the floor of the bulbar urethra.

corporeal bodies without removal of the glans, and symmetrical wedge resection of the tunica albuginea to shorten the corpora.[3, 4] Subsequently, methods to resect the entire corporeal body while preserving innervation to the glans have been developed.[5, 6] A modified approach to phallic reduction has been developed by Kogan et al and popularized by other groups.[7, 8] A recent neurometric study by Gearhart et al has shown preservation of clitoral innervation by means of the above technique.[9]

OPERATIVE TECHNIQUE

The surgical repair is similar whether the diagnosis be female pseudohermaphroditism secondary to the adrenogenital syndrome, male pseudohermaphroditism, mixed gonadal dysgenesis, or true hermaphroditism. First and most important, endoscopic examination of the lower genitourinary tract is performed to supplement the preoperative genital radiographs. If a vagina is present that enters the urethra or urogenital sinus distal to the external urinary sphincter, a flap vaginoplasty is performed provided that endoscopic examination reveals this to be feasible. If there is any doubt about the feasibility of early vaginoplasty, it can easily be delayed. If construction of a neovagina is to be deferred, as in some patients whose vaginal entry is proximal to the external sphincter or who

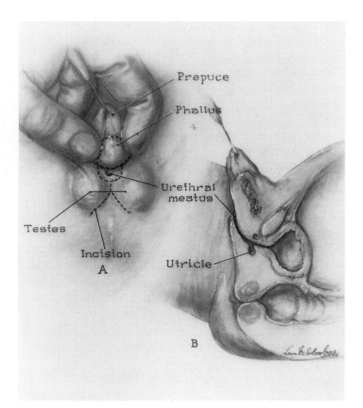

Figure 120–1. *A,* Circumcision incision around the phallus and *B,* the resultant perineal flap.

have no vagina, phallic reduction and recession are the initial procedures of perineal reconstruction.

Surgical repair is begun by making a circumferential incision at the phallus at the coronal level, sparing the ventral mucosal groove (Fig. 120–1). The perineal flap is outlined and dissected carefully from the underlying tissues to ensure an adequate blood supply (Fig. 120–2A). Any inappropriate gonads present can be removed easily through this incision at this time (Fig. 120–2B). Because no vagina exists in some male pseudohermaphrodites, the urethra, which may be of variable length, is opened ventrally from the meatus to the posterior bulbar area (Fig. 120–2C). The perineal flap is then brought into the bulbus urethra to provide a feminine appearance (Fig. 120–2D). Next, the dorsal skin of the prepuce is dissected from the penile shaft, starting at the glans and continuing to the base of the phallus (Fig. 120–3A and B). The skin is divided in the midline in preparation for construction of the labia minora (Fig. 120–3C). After the suspensory ligament is taken down, a 2-0 polyglycolic acid suture ligature is placed in each corporeal

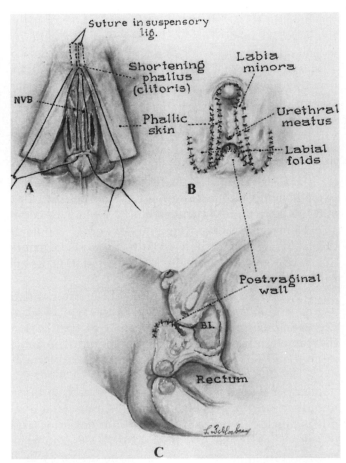

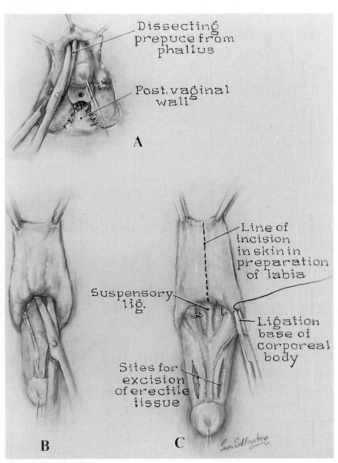

Figure 120–3. *A,* The dorsal skin of the prepuce is freed from the shaft of the phallus. *B,* Dissection of the dorsal skin is extended cephalad to the base of the phallus. *C,* Ligation of each corporeal body at the base of the phallus and lateral incision into the tunica albuginea.

Figure 120–4. *A,* The dorsal skin split in the midline is to be used as labia minora. Phallic recession sutures from the base of the glans to the anterior pubis place the glans in a hidden recessed position. *B,* Completed perineal reconstruction with glans and body of the phallus recessed beneath the mons pubis. *C,* Lateral view of completed perineal construction.

body near the base of the penis, to occlude the central corporeal artery and reduce blood flow into the erectile tissue (Fig. 120–3C). This maneuver minimizes the amount of bleeding during subsequent manipulation of the corporeal tissues. Care is taken to avoid the neurovascular bundles.

Reduction of the phallus to a normal-appearing clitoris is accomplished by making an incision into each corporeal body as lateral as possible to avoid injury to the neurovascular bundles (Fig. 120–3C). Enough erectile tissue is removed to create a clitoris of appropriate size via these two incisions. In this manner, the phallic structure can be markedly reduced without excising the tunica albuginea or manipulating the neurovascular bundles supplying the glans. Sutures are placed starting at the anterior aspect of the pubic symphysis and running through the apex of the dissected dorsal skin flap to the base of the glans (Fig. 120–4A). When they are tightened the clitoris recesses to a concealed position near the mons pubis (see Fig. 120–4B). In this manner, a midline scar over the mons is avoided. After excision of the erectile tissue, if the clitoris still appears to be too large, it can easily be reduced before recession by excision of a dorsal wedge of tissue from the glans.

The two flaps that have been created previously by dividing the phallic skin are draped around the sides of the clitoris to create the labia minora (Fig. 120–4*B* and *C*). The medial border of these flaps is sutured to the trimmed glans and to the edges of the ventral phallic urethral strip. The lateral aspect of the same dorsal skin flap is sutured to the labioscrotal folds (Fig. 120–4*B* and *C*). The labioscrotal flap is then extended into the angle formed by the perineal flap and the labia minora (labioscrotal Y-V plasty) to construct the labia majora (Fig. 120–4*B* and *C*). Some of the labioscrotal skin may have to be excised before the Y-V plasty is completed to prevent this tissue from having a rugated appearance.

When there is a low confluence of the urethra and vagina in the urogenital sinus, as in the typical adrenogenital syndrome, the vagina can be exteriorized at the same time as the phallic reduction. The labia minora and labia majora can be created without endangering the external urinary sphincter. A flap vaginoplasty is performed with incisions similar to those described previously (Fig. 120–5). The urogenital sinus is opened in the midline until the posterior wall of the vagina is reached (Fig. 120–5). Care must be taken at this juncture not to injure the rectum, which lies immediately posterior to the vagina. The posterior flap of the vagina is opened to the midline, and the perineal flap is advanced to exteriorize the vagina. The labioscrotal folds are sutured to the lateral borders of the urogenital sinus and vagina, using the dorsal phallic skin, which has been divided previously in the midline (see Fig. 120–4*A* and *B*). Some authors recommend routine dilation of this newly constructed vaginal orifice, but in my experience this has not usually been necessary.

If the vaginal entry into the urogenital sinus is proximal to the external urinary sphincter and if adequate drainage of the müllerian system is evident, the vaginoplasty is deferred to avoid injury to the sphincter and subsequent stress incontinence. In these cases, several options exist that allow the vagina to be exteriorized when the surgeon feels that the surgery is indicated.[11–14] However, if the müllerian tract on either side is obstructed or serves as a diverticulum for urine, a reconstructive procedure may need to be performed in early life. Clean intermittent vaginal catheterization may be necessary in some patients until a definitive operation can be performed. For an individual in whom the vagina is absent, creation of the neovagina is deferred until late adolescence or young adulthood. At this time the person is mature and regular dilation of the vagina can be accomplished. This delay also allows time for the

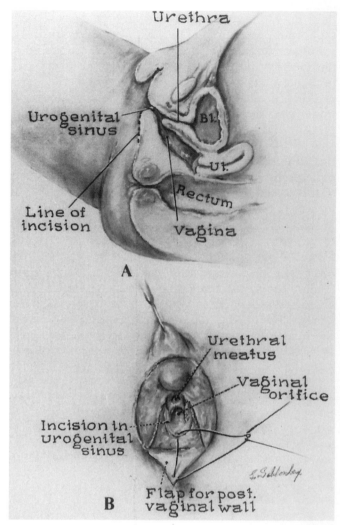

Figure 120–5. *A*, Lateral view shows the extent of the perineal flap incision. *B*, Incision of the urogenital sinus and perineal flap is secured to the floor of the urogenital sinus to create a posterior vaginal wall.

pelvis and perineal tissues to develop fully before reconstruction is performed.

POSTOPERATIVE MANAGEMENT AND COMPLICATIONS

The cosmetic and functional outcomes from this technique have been excellent, and recent clinical evidence shows that clitoral sensation is preserved thereby.[9] No episodes of glans sloughing, flap necrosis, urinary tract infections, or wound infections have been reported. It should also be noted that no patient in my series has stress incontinence as a result of this reconstruction. Of all patients in whom a flap vaginoplasty was performed at the time of the original perineal reconstruction, none has required regular dilation to maintain an adequately sized vaginal orifice.

Most patients have had few immediate postoperative complications. A Y-shaped perineal pressure dressing is made from an adhesive elastic dressing and left in place for 48 hours. A Foley catheter is placed at the time of surgery and left in the bladder until the dressing is removed and the wound is examined. After 5 days the child is given sitz baths twice daily, and a blow dryer is used to dry the perineal wound after bathing. If all is well, the Foley catheter is removed and the suture lines are cleaned daily with hydrogen peroxide solution by the parent.

SUMMARY

This approach to surgical reconstruction of the perineum can be used in all patients with ambiguous genitalia, regardless of the diagnosis, who are to be reared as females. The only aspect of reconstruction that varies among patients is the timing of the vaginoplasty.[10] However, in all cases the phallic reduction, creation of the labia minora, and majora, and gonadectomy if indicated are performed when the child is approximately 3 to 6 months old. Early genitoplasty ensures that the appearance of the external genitalia is consistent with the female sex of rearing and relieves the parents' anxiety about the child in regard to the concerns of relatives and friends.[15]

In this procedure, phallic reduction with phallic recession is demonstrated. The erectile tissue is removed using two lateral corporeal incisions without manipulation of the neurovascular bundles. The newly constructed, appropriately sized clitoris is placed beneath the mons pubis without an overlying scar. In addition, the phallic foreskin is employed to create the labia minora. A labioscrotal Y-V plasty reduces the enlarged labioscrotal folds to produce normal-appearing labia majora. A posterior perineal flap provides access to the vagina when present and to the urethra when the vagina is absent. This unified approach is applicable to a variety of patients with different types of intersexual abnormalities.

Editorial Comment

Craig A. Peters

The management of the newborn with ambiguous genitalia can be one of the most challenging, yet rewarding of all pediatric urological cases. We have recently seen children with prenatal sex identification that proved to be erroneous owing to an intersex condition. This can add an extra degree of confusion and anxiety to an already complex situation.

Early feminizing genitoplasty can be very helpful to parents who may have difficulty dealing with a masculinized child who is to be raised as a girl. There is probably no reason not to undertake these cases as early as the first few months of life if appropriate. Similarly, early vaginoplasty may be appropriate to limit the amount of major reconstructive genital surgery in the teenage years.

REFERENCES

1. Donahoe PK, Hendren WH III. Perineal reconstruction in ambiguous genitalia in infants raised as females. Ann Surg 200:363, 1984.
2. Gross RE, Randolph J, Kriggler JF Jr. Clitorectomy for sexual abnormalities: Indications and technique. Surgery 59:300, 1966.
3. Spence HM, Allen TD. Genital reconstruction in the female with adrenogenital syndrome. Br J Urol 45:126, 1973.
4. Glassburg KI, Laungani G. Reduction clitoroplasty. J Urol 17:604, 1981.
5. Barrett TM, Gonzalez ET Jr. Reconstruction of the female external genitalia. Urol Clin North Am 7:455, 1980.
6. Snyder HMc III, Retik AB, Bauer SB, Coloday AH. Feminizing genitoplasty: A synthesis. J Urol 129:1024, 1983.
7. Kogan SJ, Smey P, Levitt SB. Subtunical total reduction clitoroplasty: A safe modification of existing techniques. J Urol 130:746, 1983.
8. Oesterling JE, Gearhart JP, Jeffs RD. A unified approach to early reconstructive surgery of the child with ambiguous genitalia. J Urol 130:1079, 1987.
9. Gearhart JP, Burnett A, Owen G. Preservation of clitoral innervation during reduction clitoroplasty: A neurometric study. J Urol 153:487, 1995.
10. Bailez MM, Gearhart JP, Migeon C, Rock J. Vaginal reconstruction after initial construction of the external genitalia in girls with salt-wasting adrenal hyperplasia. J Urol 148:680, 1992.
11. Hendren WH. Reconstructive problems of the vagina and the female urethra. Clin Plast Surg 7:207, 1980.
12. Hendren WH, Donahoe PK. Correction of congenital anomalies of the vagina and the perineum. J Pediatr Surg 15:751, 1980.
13. Pena P, Devries P. Posterior sagittal anorectoplasty: Important technical considerations and new applications. J Pediatr Surg 17:796, 1982.
14. Passeri-Giazel G. A new 1-stage procedure for clitorovaginoplasty in severely masculinized female pseudohermaphrodites. J Urol 142:565, 1989.
15. Snyder HMc III. Clitoroplasty, part II. Dial Pediatr Urol 8:2, 1985.

Chapter 121

Colovaginoplasty for Vaginal Reconstruction in Children and Adults

Terry W. Hensle and Eric K. Seaman

Vaginal aplasia is a rare congenital anomaly, occurring in only about 1 in every 5000 to 10,000 births.[1] The major causes of vaginal agenesis include varying degrees of müllerian failure, including Mayer-Rokitansky syndrome (XX), intersex states (XY),[2] and patients who have undergone pelvic exenteration for tumor (e.g., rhabdomyosarcoma). Although vaginal agenesis is a rare disorder, its description dates back to antiquity. Hippocrates described obstruction of the vaginal canal in *On the Nature of Woman*. Celsus, a first-century Roman medical writer, described the conditions of imperforate hymen and vaginal atrium as well as the technique of surgical correction wherein the vaginal space was opened and packed with a wool tampon dipped in vinegar.[3]

The first modern approach to replacement vaginoplasty is attributed to Abbe who, in 1898, introduced the technique of inlay split-thickness skin grafting.[4] McIndoe and Banister[5] later modified and expanded this technique. Experience with the skin grafting technique has revealed a few relative disadvantages, the most common being the use of vaginal dilators, which are required for several months. There is also a significant rate of neovaginal stenosis, inadequate vaginal length, and poor lubrication. In 1904, Baldwin first proposed the use of bowel for vaginal replacement.[6] Since Abbe and Baldwin published their techniques, several different approaches have been utilized in an attempt to construct a functional substitute, including a nonoperative method, or Frank technique[7]; an amnion graft[8]; and bowel vaginoplasty.[9–11]

The goals of any procedure are to provide a vagina that has an appropriate length and that requires minimal, if any, dilation. Ideally, the tissue should not scar, stenose, or contract, and the neovagina should not require additional lubrication. In addition, to provide a satisfactory cosmetic result, the external genitalia should be intact. In appropriate surgical candidates, we believe colovaginoplasty offers the best surgical means to achieve these goals.

INITIAL PATIENT EVALUATION

The initial evaluation consists of obtaining a complete medical history and physical examination, followed by appropriate imaging.

History

Young women with complete müllerian failure (Mayer-Rokitansky syndrome) develop normal secondary sex characteristics at the appropriate time, but present in the early to midteenage years with failure to initiate menstruation; patients with partial müllerian syndrome (vaginal atresia) may present in infancy with hydrometrocolpos.[12] Approximately 8 percent of girls with müllerian abnormalities have a functional uterus associated with vaginal agenesis and present early in adolescence (age 11 to 12 years) with abdominal pain and distention resulting from hematometria.[13]

Patients with male pseudohermaphroditism who are not discovered in infancy during evaluation for ambiguous genitalia usually present in late adolescence with primary amenorrhea. All patients with female-appearing external genitalia and a short or absent vagina should undergo a chromosomal evaluation to rule out androgen insensitivity syndrome.[12]

Physical Examination

Initial attention should be directed to body habitus, breast development, external genitalia, and rectal examination. A eunuchoid habitus, truncated breast development, an enlarged clitoris, and ambiguous genitalia suggest male pseudohermaphroditism. In Mayer-Rokitansky syndrome the mons pubis, clitoris, pubic hair, labia majora, labia minora, and perineum are normal. The vaginal introitus, however, is usually covered by a thick membrane where the vagina failed to canalize.

Rectal examination is especially important in this group. Mayer-Rokitansky patients have a sling of tissue at the level of the peritoneal reflection; presumably, this represents the atretic müllerian ducts that failed to fuse and canalize. Male pseudohermaphrodites may have remnants or immature structures from the wolffian ducts that may impede dissection of the potential vaginal space when the vaginoplasty is performed. These must be identified on evaluation before surgery.[13]

Imaging

Ultrasound, computed tomography scanning, or magnetic resonance imaging can be used to visualize the gonads and pelvic anatomy, as well as the urinary tract. Urinary tract anomalies occur in roughly 30 percent of women with vaginal agenesis. Most commonly, patients have unilateral renal agenesis. It is important to identify the existence of a pelvic kidney before operation in order to prevent injury.[14] Skeletal abnormalities are recognized in 12 percent of women with Mayer-Rokitansky syndrome, and two thirds of these are abnormalities of the spine, with the rest involving the limbs and ribs.[14] Vaginal agenesis is sometimes associated with Klippel-Feil syndrome (congenital fusion of the cervical spine, short neck, low posterior hairline, and painless limitation of cervical movement). Unless demonstrable skeletal deformities are seen on physical examination, however, a skeletal survey is unnecessary.

Counseling

The management of intersex patients with respect to subsequent gender assignment is complex and requires careful counseling of the parents by the primary care physician, pediatric endocrinologist, pediatric urologist, and psychiatrist. From the outset, the family should understand that their child's anomaly is not unique and that their physicians can clarify and treat the problem. The parents will need help and support in coping with the delay in announcement of the infant's sex, as this delay affects the most basic communication they can make to friends and family about their new baby. In patients with Mayer-Rokitansky syndrome, counseling is further complicated by the late age at which the diagnosis is usually made. Issues that need to be discussed include future fertility, capacity for future sexual intercourse, and external genital appearance, as well as surgical and medical options.

COLOVAGINOPLASTY

In 1904, Baldwin described using a "U-shaped" sigmoid segment anastomosed to the perineum at one operation with subsequent division of the septum performed 6 weeks later.[6] Since that time, several different colovaginoplasty techniques have been described.

Operative Technique

The patient is given a mechanical bowel preparation consisting of 1 gallon of GoLYTELY (polyethylene glycol–electrolyte solution) by mouth the night before surgery. Broad-spectrum antibiotic prophylaxis is begun before the incision is made.

At the time of surgery, the patient is placed in the lithotomy position with legs extended in Allen stirrups so that the abdomen and perineum can be prepared in one field (Fig. 121–1). A Foley catheter is placed in the bladder, and the abdomen and pelvis can be approached through either a Pfannenstiel or midline abdominal incision.

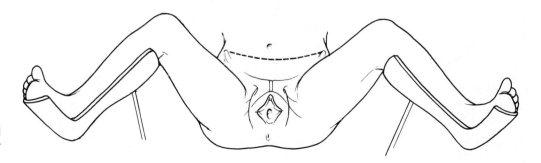

Figure 121–1. Patient positioned in Allen stirrups for a Pfannenstiel incision.

In most patients presenting with Mayer-Rokitansky syndrome, exploration may reveal bifid remnants of uterine horns along with portions of fallopian tubes, both of which should be removed. In addition, there is a normal distal portion of the vagina that enables extension of that tissue into the pelvic cul-de-sac, where it can be used for anastomosis to the bowel segment. In Mayer-Rokitansky syndrome, the ovaries are often normal in size and position and should remain in place. In patients with androgen insensitivity (testicular feminization), the gonads should be removed.

It is our preference to use a sleeve of distal sigmoid colon for vaginal replacement. When use of this segment is contraindicated, as when there has been previous surgery or pelvic irradiation, the cecum is an acceptable alternative. The small bowel is also acceptable; however, when utilizing small bowel, a double-lumen U-shaped portion should be used with the common septum divided in order to have an adequate lumen in the neovagina. In most cases, an 8- to 10-cm sleeve of distal sigmoid based on the left colic or superior hemorrhoidal vessels is sufficient for adequate vaginal length (Fig. 121–2). Segments of greater length can be associated with excessive mucus production.

The sigmoid segment is taken between noncrushing Allen-Kocher clamps, or, alternatively, by using

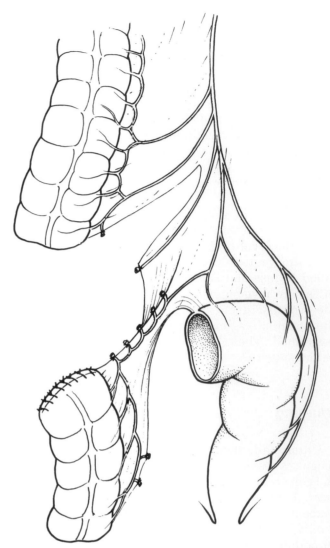

Figure 121–3. Isolated bowel segment rotated into the pelvis, medial to the sigmoid colocolostomy.

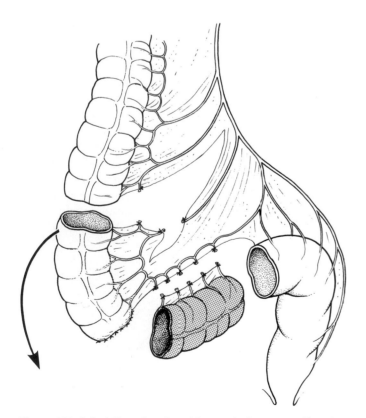

Figure 121–2. Isolation of an 8- to 10-cm colonic segment based on the left colic or superior hemorrhoidal vessels.

the GIA stapler. A hand-sewn or stapled colocolostomy is used to re-establish bowel continuity. Once isolated, the sigmoid segment can be brought down in an isoperistaltic fashion to the perineum or rotated 180 degrees on its mesentery, depending on the length of the vessels (Fig. 121–3). The direction of peristalsis does not affect operative success. The proximal end of the loop is closed with two layers of absorbable suture material, and the distal end of the segment is then brought to the perineum for anastomosis.

Utilizing the technique originally described by Radhakrishan, a Hegar dilator can be used to push the rudimentary anterior vagina into the pelvic cul-de-sac, where it can be grasped with Allis clamps and opened widely for a capacious anastomosis to the bowel segment (Fig. 121–4).[9] The open sigmoid loop is pulled down to this opening with stay sutures. In patients with an inadequate distal third of the

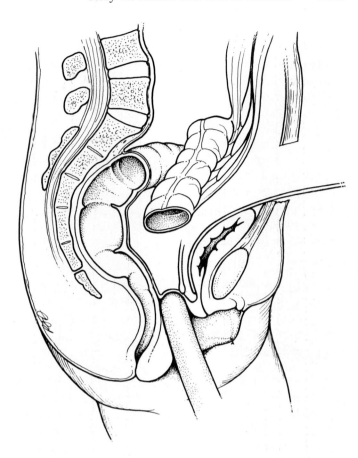

Figure 121–4. Pushing the anterior vagina up to meet the isolated bowel segment.

vagina or in those who have undergone previous exenteration or gender reassignment, the bowel segment can be anastomosed directly to the perineum (Fig. 121–5). When a direct perineal anastomosis is required, it is of utmost importance to create a space

large enough distally for the bowel to fit comfortably (Fig. 121–6).

In patients who have undergone previous pelvic surgery or irradiation, or in whom the distal sigmoid is inadequate, cecum can be used. The cecal segment

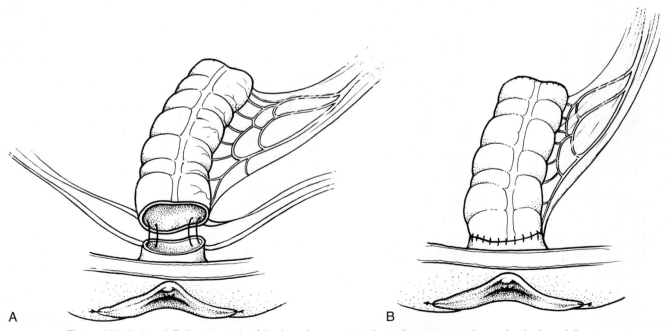

A   B

Figure 121–5. A and B, Anastomosis of the bowel segment to the rudimentary anterior vagina in the cul-de-sac.

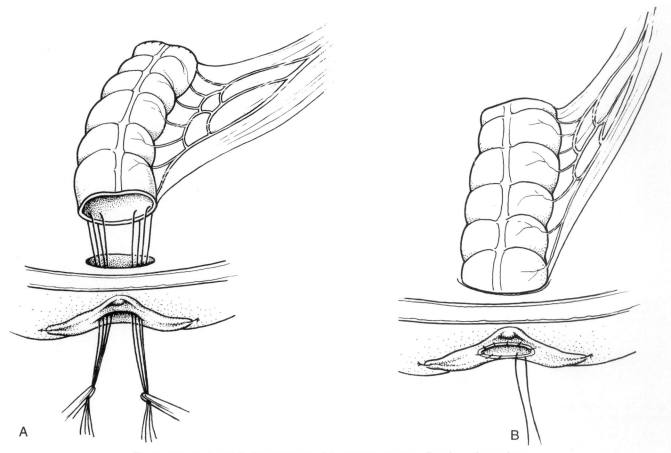

Figure 121–6. *A* and *B,* Anastomosis of the bowel segment directly to the perineum.

is isolated on the ileocolic vessels and rotated 180 degrees into the perineum for anastomosis.

After anastomosis of either the sigmoid or ileocolic segment, the position of the bowel is evaluated to ensure a capacious, well-vascularized, and tension-free anastomosis. With sigmoid and cecal segments, great care is taken to provide adequate two-point posterior fixation of the bowel segment to the retroperitoneum (Figs. 121–7 and 121–8). This two-point

fixation with nonabsorbable suture prevents "wandering" of the neovagina as well as prolapse of the segment. A pelvic Jackson-Pratt drain is placed before closure.

Postoperatively, the neovagina is stented with a device using the barrel of a 10- or 20-ml syringe wrapped with antibiotic-soaked gauze and left in place for 5 days. The size of the stent used varies with patient age. Patients are examined under anesthesia at 3 weeks and 3 months postoperatively. If there is any suggestion of introital stenosis at the first visit, manual dilation with the patient under anesthesia is performed at 3 weeks. No home dilation is usually necessary.

RESULTS

Hensle and Dean,[9] in 1992, reported 17 patients undergoing bowel vaginoplasty, 15 of whom had colovaginoplasty with either sigmoid colon or cecum. Two cases were complicated by prolapse of the bowel segment. One of these patients required reoperation and fixation; the other required only fulguration and excision of the small amount of prolapsed tissue.

Fourteen patients responded to a questionnaire re-

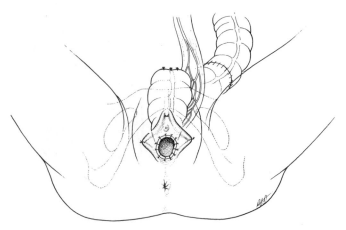

Figure 121–7. Final position of the bowel neovagina with posterior fixation, anteroposterior view.

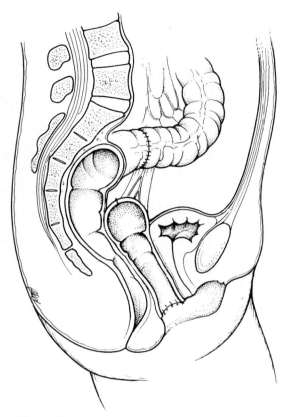

Figure 121–8. Final position of the bowel neovagina with posterior fixation, lateral view.

lating to sexual activity. In that group, ten patients were sexually active and only one described any dyspareunia. No patient had vaginal stenosis or required periodic dilation. There were also two patients in the series who had stenosis of the bowel segment; in these, small bowel had been used as the isolated bowel segment for vaginoplasty. The authors conclude that the mesentery of the ileum may have been too short to provide an adequate tension-free anastomosis in the perineum, and that, in their hands, reconstruction with cecum or sigmoid colon provides the best results.

Wesley and Coran[11] reported six sigmoid vaginoplasties, four in adolescents and two in infants. They described no operative complications, and in follow-up three of the patients were currently sexually active, none requiring lubrication. In addition, Turner-Warwick and Kirby[15] reported 13 patients who underwent "colocecal" vaginoplasty. Three patients required minor revisions to adjust the introitus, and one patient had a protrusion of the neovagina that required a simple circumferential resection of the redundant intestine. Seven of the 13 patients in their series were sexually active.

Summary

Patients with vaginal agenesis are confronted with two important medical and social difficulties. One is

the inability to bear children; however, patients with normal ovaries may have oocytes harvested for pregnancy in a surrogate mother. The other is inability to engage in sexual intercourse. By means of replacement vaginoplasty techniques, patients can be offered the construction of a functional neovagina.

Because of dissatisfaction and complications with skin graft vaginoplasty, we prefer the use of a bowel segment (sigmoid colon or cecum) for the creation of a neovagina. The advantages of a bowel segment are minimal likelihood of graft failure or later contraction, maintenance of patency and sufficient length without a mold and with minimal dilation, spontaneous mucus production from bowel mucosa matching that of the normal vagina and facilitating sexual intercourse, and finally, avoidance of the dyspareunia sometimes seen with skin grafts achieved by the ability of the intestinal segment to withstand local trauma.

We believe the sigmoid colon is the best choice for colovaginoplasty because of size, location, and ease of preserving the blood supply. Above all, to optimize results of reconstruction, one must take into consideration not only the patient's anatomy, but also her intelligence, support system, and motivation.

Editorial Comment
Craig A. Peters

The functional outcomes of sigmoid vaginoplasty have been so good as to outweigh the relatively minor complication of mucous secretion, and this is our preferred modality for vaginal reconstructions. After transecting the sigmoid colon distally, it may be useful to ensure that the planned segment can reach the perineum before performing the proximal colonic transection. Further colonic mobilization can then be performed to guarantee a well-vascularized, tension-free sigmoid segment. The perineal dissection can be facilitated by splitting the fibers of the urogenital diaphragm in the midline, as with anorectal pullthrough procedures. There is probably no reason not to perform the vaginoplasty in children around the age of 4 or 5 years if appropriate. Any revisions may be after puberty but would be only minor operations, in contrast to a major genital reconstruction in a teenage girl.

REFERENCES

1. Rock JA, Azziz R. Genital anomalies in childhood. Clin Obstet Gynecol 30:682, 1987.
2. Evans PN, Poland NL, Boving RL. Vaginal malformations. Am J Obstet Gynecol 141:910, 1981.
3. Goldwyn RM. History of attempts to form a vagina. Plast Reconstr Surg 57:319, 1977.
4. Abbe R. New method for creating a vagina in a case of congenital absence of the vagina. Med Rec 54:836, 1898.
5. McIndoe AH, Banister JB. An operation for the cure of congenital absence of the vagina. J Obstet Gynaecol Br. Common 45:490, 1938.
6. Baldwin JF. The formation of an artificial vagina by intestinal transplantation. Ann Surg 40:398, 1904.

7. Frank RT. The formation of an artificial vagina without operation. Am J Obstet Gynecol 35:1053, 1938.

8. Ashworth MF, Morton KE, Dewhurst J, et al. Vaginoplasty using amnion. Obstet Gynecol 67:443, 1986.

9. Hensle TW, Dean GE. Vaginal replacement in children. J Urol 148:677, 1992.

10. Pratt JH. Sigmoidovaginostomy: A new method of obtaining satisfactory vaginal depth. Am J Obstet Gynecol 81:535, 1961.

11. Wesley JR, Coran AG. Intestinal vaginoplasty for congenital absence of the vagina. J Pediatr Surg 27:885, 1992.

12. Stephens FD. The Mayer-Rokitansky syndrome. J Urol 135:106, 1986.

13. Wiser WL, Bates GW. Management of agenesis of the vagina. Surg Gynecol Obstet 159:108, 1984.

14. Griffin JE, Edwards C, Madden JD, et al. Congenital absence of the vagina: The Mayer-Rokitansky-Küster-Hauser syndrome. Ann Intern Med 85:244, 1976.

15. Turner-Warwick R, Kirby RS: The construction and reconstruction of the vagina with the colocecum. Surg Gynecol Obstet 170:132, 1990.

Chapter 122

Orchiopexy and Herniorrhaphy; Diagnostic Laparoscopy for the Impalpable Testis

Jack S. Elder

INDICATIONS

Cryptorchidism is a common disorder, affecting 3 to 6 percent of male newborns and 0.8 to 1.6 percent of 1-year-old male infants.[1, 2] Important long-term sequelae of cryptorchidism include infertility and testicular tumor. By light microscopy, the undescended testis shows a diminished number of germ cells, diminished seminiferous tubular size, and peritubular hyalinization and fibrosis by 18 months of age.[3] Abnormalities are evident by electron microscopy at 1 year of age.[4] Therefore, orchiopexy is generally recommended when the child is 12 to 18 months old.

The patient should be examined in a warm room by an examiner with warm hands to minimize the risk of testicular retraction. One hand should be placed at the level of the anterosuperior iliac spine, which is superolateral to the internal inguinal ring. This hand should then be swept firmly down the inguinal canal while the other hand is positioned at the scrotum. In most cases the testis may be palpated with the lower hand or by ballottement. If the testis seems impalpable, it may be helpful to lubricate the patient's groin and the examiner's hand with soap to reduce friction. The child should also be in the sitting or squatting position during the examination. Commonly, a testis that is impalpable when the child is supine may be palpated when he is in a sitting or squatting position, because the upright position seems to inhibit the cremasteric reflex, and the increased abdominal pressure allows the testis to drop down from a position high in the inguinal canal inferiorly to the external inguinal ring.

If the clinician is uncertain whether the testis is retractile, human chorionic gonadotropin (hCG), 3000 IU, may be administered by intramuscular injection weekly for 4 weeks. One week after the final injection, the patient is re-examined. If the testis has "descended" into the scrotal sac, it is probably retractile. However, the child should be re-examined 6 months after completion of hormonal therapy to reassess the exact location of the testis. If it has returned to an apparent undescended position, an orchiopexy should be performed.

PREOPERATIVE PREPARATION

In general, orchiopexy may be performed safely as an outpatient procedure if the child has an American Society of Anesthesiologists' Physical Status of 1 or 2.[5] Contraindications to outpatient orchiopexy include prune-belly syndrome; congenital heart disease; and preexisting conditions that affect respiratory function, such as asthma and bronchopulmonary dysplasia. The child is allowed to ingest solid food until 8 hours before surgery, formula until 6 hours before surgery, and clear liquids until 3 hours before the scheduled operation.[6] Administration of a caudal block by the anesthesia staff or infiltration of the incision with bupivacaine or lidocaine allows the child to awaken with minimal discomfort.

SURGICAL OPTIONS

The usual therapy for an undescended testis is orchiopexy through an inguinal incision. If the testis is impalpable, the surgeon should be prepared to perform a peritoneotomy; therefore, a slightly higher skin incision will be necessary. Laparoscopy is a helpful adjunctive procedure at the time of planned inguinal-abdominal exploration for an impalpable testis.[7] If the testis is intra-abdominal, the testis may be mobilized and brought down to the scrotum using the conventional techniques of orchiopexy. Other options include the Fowler-Stephens orchiopexy (either one-stage or two-stage), conventional two-stage orchiopexy, testicular autotransplantation, and orchiectomy.[8] If the testis is atrophic, is abnormal in appearance, or cannot be brought down to the scrotum satisfactorily, or if the patient is postpubertal, orchiectomy is recommended.

OPERATIVE TECHNIQUE

Standard Orchiopexy

The testicular artery normally assumes a triangular course from its origin at the aorta through the internal ring down to the base of the scrotum. The testicular artery to an undescended testis is usually short and an associated hernial sac is adherent to the spermatic

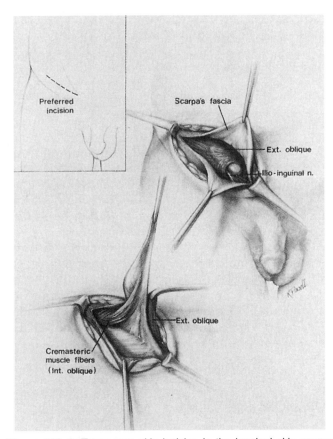

Figure 122–1. Transverse skin incision in the inguinal skin crease. Scarpa's fascia is opened. The external oblique fascia is opened, avoiding the ilioinguinal nerve, and the testis is identified. (From Marshall GG, Elder JS. Cryptorchidism and Related Anomalies. New York, Praeger, 1982.)

cord. Mobilizing the spermatic cord with division and high ligation of the hernial sac usually allows the testis to reach the scrotum. In general, the vas deferens has sufficient length to reach the scrotum easily.

An incision is made in the inguinal skin crease, with the medial aspect of the incision approximately 2 fingerbreadths above the pubic tubercle (Fig. 122–1). The incision should be long enough to provide sufficient exposure of the cord structures; a difficult dissection is often attributable to inadequate exposure. The subcutaneous fat is separated to expose Scarpa's fascia, which in children is well developed and may be confused with the external oblique fascia. Scarpa's fascia is picked up with two forceps and incised with scissors. Small retractors and blunt dissection allow visualization of the external oblique fascia. This fascial layer is opened through the external ring and up to the internal inguinal ring, and the ilioinguinal nerve is protected by retracting it medially over the fascia. With compression of the abdomen, the testis will most commonly be evident near the external ring, enveloped by the processus vaginalis. The longitudinal cremasteric fibers are then separated bluntly to free the testis and spermatic cord. If the testis is ectopic in the superficial inguinal pouch, it may need to be mobilized before opening the external oblique fascia.

The processus vaginalis is incised sharply to expose the testis, with great care not to cut the testis or epididymis. Next, a traction stitch is placed through the gubernaculum, the distal aspect of the processus, or through the testis itself. Studies of the microvasculature of the testis indicate that placement of a stitch through the middle of the testis is unlikely to cause significant damage.[9] The distal gubernacular attachments are then transected. Next, it is important to examine the epididymis for abnormalities and to identify the vas deferens, because either of these structures may loop down several centimeters toward the scrotum. Between 35 and 50 percent of children with an undescended testis have an associated epididymal abnormality.[10, 11] Next, the entire spermatic cord, surrounded by external spermatic fibers, can be mobilized up to the internal inguinal ring.

In almost all cases a patent processus vaginalis is present with a canalicular testis, whereas the processus is often obliterated with an ectopic testis. Assuming a patent processus is present, it is usually quite thin and extremely adherent to the vas (Fig. 122–2). It is easier to free the sac off the spermatic cord near the internal ring rather than near the testis where the sac is open. Some have found that injecting a small amount of saline under the sac facilitates dissection. After the sac has been separated from the vas and spermatic cord, it is suture ligated twice at the internal ring with 3–0 polyglycolic acid suture.

Inferomedial traction is placed on the testis, and

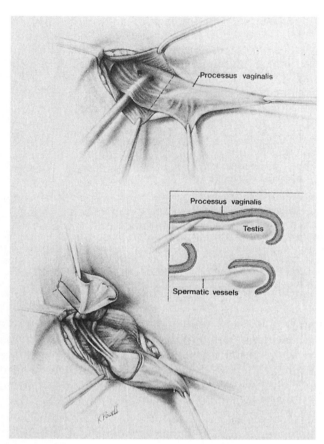

Figure 122–2. The processus vaginalis (hernia sac) is dissected from the remainder of the spermatic cord and a high ligation is performed, allowing mobilization of the testis. (From Marshall GG, Elder JS. Cryptorchidism and Related Anomalies. New York, Praeger, 1982.)

the cremasteric and spermatic fibers attached to the spermatic cord are divided. This maneuver is accomplished by using a fine pair of Adson forceps to identify these lateral fibers. One must be careful not to pick up either the testicular vessels or the vas deferens. Transection of the fibers lateral to the cord allows optimal mobilization of the testis. The dissection is carried into the retroperitoneum beyond the point where the testicular artery and vas diverge. In most cases, this dissection allows the testis to reach the scrotum without tension. Occasionally, further mobilization in the retroperitoneum is necessary, separating the peritoneum from the testicular artery and dividing the fibers lateral to the artery in the retroperitoneum.

If the testis still does not reach the scrotum easily, the floor of the inguinal canal (transversalis fascia) may be divided (Fig. 122–3). This requires division of the inferior epigastric artery and vein, which are in the floor of the inguinal canal. Alternatively, the testis may be brought posterior to these vascular structures. The purpose of this maneuver (Prentiss) is to allow the testicular artery to assume a more direct course to the scrotum.[12, 13]

The testis is then placed in a pouch in the scrotal wall between the skin and dartos.[14] A transverse inci-

sion is made through the dermal layer of skin in the inferior aspect of the scrotum, and the pouch is developed by blunt dissection, first with a small curved mosquito clamp and subsequently with a larger mosquito clamp. It is important that the pouch not be developed laterally beyond the edge of the scrotum, or the testis may migrate out of the scrotal area postoperatively. The mosquito clamp is passed retrograde through the scrotal incision up to the inguinal incision, and the traction suture on the testis is grasped. The testis is brought down through the scrotal incision. When the testis is brought down, it is important to be certain that the spermatic cord is not twisted. The neck of the dartos pouch is closed with a 4–0 polyglycolic acid stitch to prevent retraction of the testis. Usually this stitch is also passed through the tunica vaginalis layer of the spermatic cord to help fix the testis in place. If tension is noted on the testis, it may be helpful to place a traction stitch with 3–0 polyglycolic acid or silk suture through a small external pledget, which is used for temporary fixation. This stitch should penetrate only

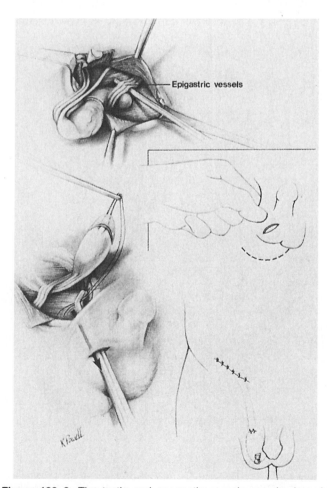

Figure 122–3. The testis and spermatic vessels may be brought behind the inferior epigastric artery and vein, or the vessels may be ligated. A dartos scrotal pouch is created into which the testis is placed. The external bolster is optional. (From Marshall GG, Elder JS. Cryptorchidism and Related Anomalies. New York, Praeger, 1982.)

the gubernaculum or the capsule of the testis, and the pledget should be removed 1 week postoperatively.

The scrotal skin is closed with a running 5–0 chromic stitch. Attention is then directed to the inguinal incision. If the floor of the inguinal canal was taken down during the orchiopexy, it is reconstructed with interrupted 2–0 polyglycolic acid sutures between the transversus abdominis arch superiorly and Poupart's ligament inferiorly. Usually three or four sutures are needed. Next, the external oblique fascia is closed with a running 3–0 polyglycolic suture. Scarpa's fascia is closed with interrupted 4–0 chromic sutures, and the skin is closed with interrupted 5–0 polyglycolic acid subcuticular stitches.

The Intra-Abdominal Testis

If the testis is not identified in the inguinal canal, the incision must be extended to allow intraperitoneal exposure. The retroperitoneum should not be explored further, as the testis, if present, is usually found in the peritoneal cavity just inside the internal

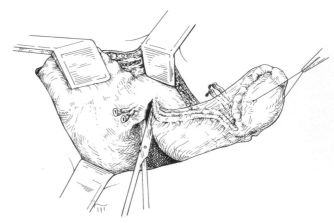

Figure 122–5. The testis is mobilized by incising the peritoneal reflection lateral and superior to the testis. (From Elder JS. Laparoscopy and Fowler-Stephens orchiopexy in the management of the impalpable testis. Urol Clin North Am 16:399, 1989.)

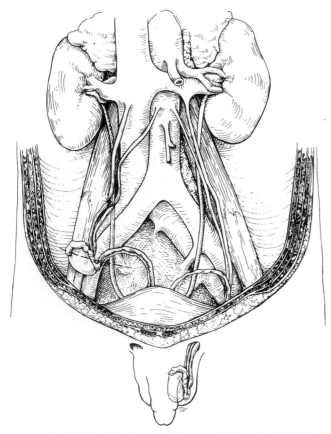

Figure 122–4. Fowler-Stephens orchiopexy (right testis). Dashed line indicates incision. The testicular vessels are doubly ligated in situ 1 to 2 cm above the testis, allowing collateral arterial flow to develop through the deferential artery. (From Elder JS. Laparoscopy and Fowler-Stephens orchiopexy in the management of the impalpable testis. Urol Clin North Am 16:399, 1989.)

ring. When it is identified, several surgical options are available. One possibility is a two-stage orchiopexy, in which the testis is mobilized and brought into the inguinal canal as far as possible. The testis and spermatic cord are wrapped with a silicone sheath to prevent adhesions to the testis and spermatic cord. The second stage is performed 6 to 12 months later. Another option is testicular autotransplantation. This procedure is difficult technically in a child younger than 2 years of age. If the child is postpubertal or if the testis is abnormal, orchiectomy is recommended. Another option is the Fowler-Stephens procedure, in which the testicular artery is divided in the hope that the testis will retain sufficient vascularity based on collateral flow through the deferential artery.[15]

After the peritoneal cavity is opened, the small bowel is retracted superiorly and the testis identified. If a long vascular mesentery to the testis is seen, the testis may be brought down with a standard orchiopexy, although the Prentiss maneuver will probably be necessary.[12] If the testis seems fixed in position and a Fowler-Stephens procedure is planned, the testicular artery and vein should be identified coursing to the testis from a cephalad position, and the vas should be identified entering the testis medially. The testicular vessels are ligated 2 cm above the testis, incorporating all vessels between the posterior abdominal wall and the testis, leaving maximum local collateral circulation to the testis and epididymis (Fig. 122–4). The testicular artery and vein are transected distal to the ligature, allowing back-bleeding to occur. This bleeding is helpful for assessing testicular perfusion during the remainder of the procedure. Traction is placed on the testis and an incision is made in the lateral peritoneal reflection (Fig. 122–5). The peritoneum medial to the testis should not be incised, as it contains other important collateral testicular vessels. As the testis and vas are mobilized

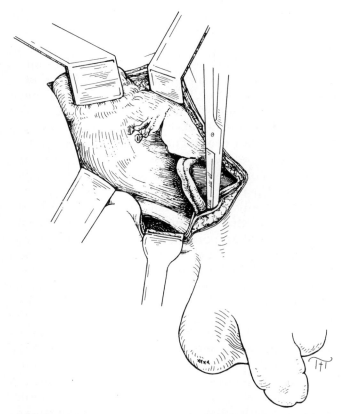

Figure 122–6. The testis has been mobilized and brought through the lower abdominal wall at the junction between the lateral border of the rectus muscle and the superior pubic ramus, and is placed in a dartos pouch. When a long looping vas deferens is found coursing down the inguinal canal, the testis is brought down through the inguinal canal rather than medial to it. (From Elder JS. Laparoscopy and Fowler-Stephens orchiopexy in the management of the impalpable testis. Urol Clin North Am 16:399, 1989.)

together, care should be taken not to injure the ureter, which lies deep to these structures. The testis, vas, and peritoneal attachments are mobilized and brought medial to the inguinal canal (Figs. 122–6 and 122–7). The testis is brought through a small incision through the posterior wall of the inguinal canal just above the pubic tubercle and is placed in a dartos pouch in the ipsilateral hemiscrotum. If a long-looping vas courses down the inguinal canal, the testis should be placed in the scrotum along this route rather than brought medial to the inguinal canal.

A technique that has been popularized since 1984 is the *staged* Fowler-Stephens procedure.[16] The concept is that preliminary ligation of the gonadal vessels allows collateral circulation through the deferential artery to develop with minimal risk of arterial spasm. During the initial stage, the testicular artery and vein are ligated but the testis is not mobilized. In the second stage, performed 6 to 12 months later, the testicular vessels are transected and a Fowler-Stephens orchiopexy is performed. Usually the deferential artery is seen to have enlarged considerably, approximating the size of the testicular artery.

If inguinal exploration fails to identify the testis or spermatic cord structures a peritoneotomy must be performed to try to find the testis. In 4 percent of boys with cryptorchidism, the testis is absent. This usually occurs secondary to testicular torsion in utero rather than as a result of testicular agenesis. To make the diagnosis of an absent testis, both the vas deferens and testicular vessels should be identified. It is insufficient to identify only the vas, because the epididymis and vas may be completely separated from the testis. Occasionally, a patient has an intra-abdominal testis with a vas deferens that loops down the inguinal canal. Therefore, if an inguinal dissection reveals a vas deferens that appears to end in a nubbin of tissue at the external ring or scrotum, the peritoneum should be opened to be absolutely certain that a testis is not associated with a long-looping vas. In the past, in a boy with an absent testis, consideration was given to inserting a testicular prosthesis, regardless of his age.[17] Currently, however, these prostheses are gel-filled, and implantation of these prostheses is not advised until their safety has been proved.

Diagnostic Laparoscopy for the Impalpable Testis

Approximately 20 percent of undescended testes are impalpable, and 20 to 65 percent of impalpable

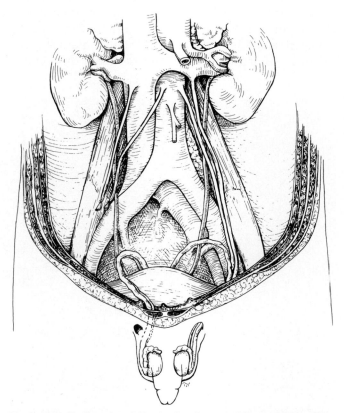

Figure 122–7. Completed Fowler-Stephens orchiopexy. (From Elder JS. Laparoscopy and Fowler-Stephens orchiopexy in the management of the impalpable testis. Urol Clin North Am 16:399, 1989.)

testes are absent.[18, 19] Several clinical approaches to a boy with an impalpable testis are possible.[18, 19] Numerous radiological techniques have been developed to localize the impalpable testis preoperatively. Ultrasound is used commonly but is extremely unreliable in identifying the testis if it is intra-abdominal. In contrast, computed tomography (CT) scanning and magnetic resonance imaging (MRI) can localize an impalpable testis. No imaging study can be relied on to *prove* that the testis is absent simply because it fails to visualize the testis. Consequently, routine imaging studies in boys with an impalpable testis are discouraged.[20]

Laparoscopy has been used as an intraoperative method of aiding localization of the impalpable testis. The procedure takes 10 to 15 minutes and may avoid the need for peritoneotomy. Laparoscopy may be performed in children of any age, even those under 6 months old. It is also useful in the older child or teenager who has previously undergone an inadequate inguinal exploration, in which no testicular tissue was identified or in which only a vas deferens and no testicular vessels were present without inspecting the peritoneal cavity. Relative contraindications include prune-belly syndrome, any bleeding disorder, previous abdominal surgery, obesity, and umbilical hernia.[7]

The equipment necessary for laparoscopy includes the Veress needle; a pediatric trocar sleeve or cannula, 5 mm in diameter; a Hasson cannula; a lens sheath; and an automatic CO_2 insufflator (Fig. 122–8).

Laparoscopy is performed in the ambulatory surgical unit. After the child is anesthetized, the bladder is drained with a small pediatric feeding tube. The patient is re-examined carefully to make absolutely certain that the testis is impalpable. He is placed in the supine position, and a semicircular incision is made in the inferior margin of the umbilicus with a No. 11 scalpel blade. The incision is carried down to and just slightly through the rectus fascia. The infraumbilical abdominal wall is grasped to increase the distance between the umbilicus and sacral promontory, and the Veress needle is held by its spring chamber or collar to allow free movement of the inner needle as it penetrates the fascial and peritoneal layers (Fig. 122–9). The insufflation port should be directed toward the abdomen, because this is directly opposite the sharp point of the needle. The needle is held at a right angle to the abdominal wall and pushed forcefully through the fascia; resistance is felt at the fascial and peritoneal layers. Next, a saline aspiration test is performed by injecting 5 ml of saline through the needle and gently withdrawing on the plunger (Fig. 122–10). If the needle is in the correct position, no saline will be aspirated, whereas if the needle is extraperitoneal, fluid is aspirated. To eliminate the risk of bowel injury, some clinicians always use the Hasson cannula to gain access to the peritoneal cavity rather than the Veress needle and trocar.

The insufflation tubing is attached to the needle. The insufflator is set on the low or manual position and insufflation with CO_2 is begun. The abdomen is filled until it is moderately tense, when the intraperitoneal pressure is approximately 15 mm Hg. Most children require 1.0 to 1.5 L, and it takes approximately 30 to 60 seconds for the peritoneal cavity to fill.

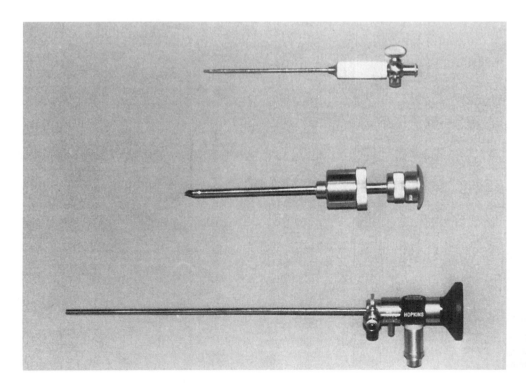

Figure 122–8. Equipment for laparoscopy. *Top,* Veress needle. *Middle,* 5-mm cannula with trocar. *Bottom,* Pediatric cystoscope lens with adapter (sheath) for laparoscopy. (From Elder JS. Laparoscopy and Fowler-Stephens orchiopexy in the management of the impalpable testis. Urol Clin North Am 16:399, 1989.)

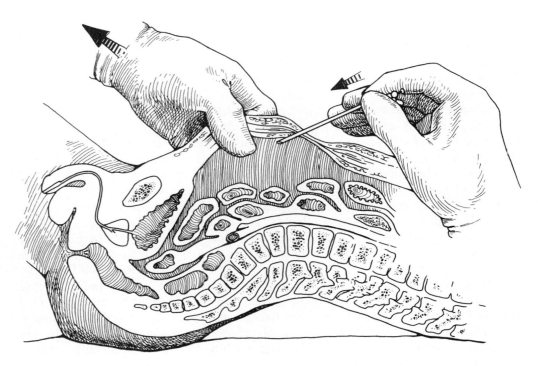

Figure 122–9. Insertion of Veress needle. As the needle passes through the fascial layers, the blunt inner round-ended needle (not shown) retracts into the sharp outer sleeve. Note that the insufflation port is directed toward the abdomen. (From Elder JS. Laparoscopy and Fowler-Stephens orchiopexy in the management of the impalpable testis. Urol Clin North Am 16:399, 1989.)

The Veress needle is then removed. The abdominal wall is again grasped and the trocar is inserted at an angle similar to that of the Veress needle, approximately 45 degrees toward the hollow of the sacrum (Fig. 122–11). The ulnar border of the dominant hand should be placed on the abdominal wall to encircle the cannula in order to act as a stop if a sudden thrust forces the cannula through the abdominal wall. Rotating the trocar as it is passed allows it to traverse the fascia more smoothly. Usually one feels a single distinct pop when the trocar is inserted. As the trocar

and cannula are advanced, gas can be heard escaping as the trocar tip enters the peritoneal cavity. The trocar is then removed and the lens inserted into the sheath. The insufflator is set on the low/automatic or maintain position and the laparoscope is attached to a high-intensity light source.

The peritoneal cavity may be inspected with a 0- or 30-degree lens. An antifog agent should be applied to the lens and eyepiece before inspection. In a boy with a unilateral impalpable testis, the normal side is examined first. The vas deferens is identified as a

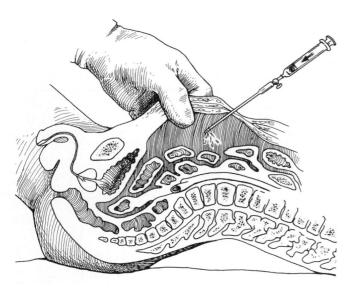

Figure 122–10. In the saline aspiration test, 5 ml of saline is injected, which one should not be able to aspirate if the needle is in the appropriate position. (From Elder JS. Laparoscopy and Fowler-Stephens orchiopexy in the management of the impalpable testis. Urol Clin North Am 16:399, 1989.)

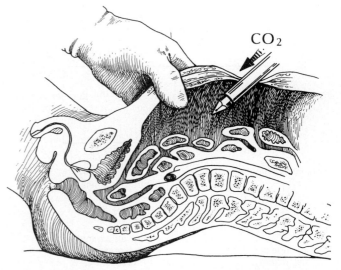

Figure 122–11. After the peritoneal cavity has been filled with carbon dioxide, the trocar cannula is inserted. (From Elder JS. Laparoscopy and Fowler-Stephens orchiopexy in the management of the impalpable testis. Urol Clin North Am 16:399, 1989.)

small white cord that rises out of the pelvis and joins the gonadal vessels at a 60- to 90-degree angle just proximal to the internal ring.

After the normal side is identified, the affected side should be examined. Again, one should look for the testicular vessels and vas. An indirect inguinal hernia is usually obvious and generally indicates that an undescended testis is present.[19, 21] If the vessels enter the internal ring and an inguinal hernia is present, the groin should be manipulated with the nondominant hand to try to milk the testis back into the peritoneal cavity, because many nonpalpable testes may pop in and out of the internal ring. The laparoscopic findings allow one to guide further management according to the status of the processus vaginalis (Fig. 122–12).

If laparoscopy discloses a patent processus vaginalis with the vas and vessels entering the internal ring, a viable testis is likely to be distal to the internal ring. Standard inguinal exploration and orchiopexy should be performed, although extensive mobilization of the internal spermatic vessels and the Prentiss maneuver may be necessary. If the patient is postpubertal, orchiectomy and herniorrhaphy should be considered.

If the vas deferens enters the inguinal canal with a patent processus vaginalis but the internal spermatic vessels are not identified, there is probably an intra-abdominal testis with a long-looping vas that will need to be mobilized during orchiopexy. If there is a patent processus vaginalis and neither vas nor vessels enter the internal ring, an intra-abdominal testis is likely to be present and can usually be identified endoscopically. At times it is necessary to insert a second trocar into the ipsilateral lower quadrant through which grasping forceps may be inserted to facilitate identification of the nonpalpable testis. In this situation a variety of options are available, as described previously. In recent years, there has been interest in the complete laparoscopic orchiopexy.[22] If the testis is abnormal, laparoscopic orchiectomy may be performed.[23] If one chooses to perform an intra-peritoneal exploration, CO_2 should be left within the abdominal cavity, as this facilitates opening the peritoneum. However, if abdominal exploration is not anticipated, all the CO_2 should be expressed from the peritoneal cavity before removing the sheath, because CO_2 is a peritoneal irritant.

If laparoscopy discloses that the vas and vessels enter the inguinal canal through the internal ring with no associated hernia, the testis is probably absent. Remnant testicular nubbins should be removed through a small low inguinal incision. Although one might be inclined to avoid inguinal exploration simply to remove the nubbin, removal of the remnant seems advisable in view of a 1992 report that 13 percent of such nubbins contain viable tubular structures that conceivably could become malignant in the future.[24] Furthermore, at times a normal testis may be in an ectopic position, such as in the perineum or through the femoral ring. In boys in whom a nubbin is removed, contralateral scrotal orchiopexy should be considered to protect the solitary functioning testis from future torsion. If the vas and vessels terminate blindly in the abdominal cavity, one may assume that the testis underwent in utero torsion prior to testicular descent, and no further exploration is necessary. Finally, if neither testis nor vas and vessels are seen, depending on the surgeon's experience with laparoscopy, abdominal exploration may not be necessary if the peritoneum is visualized to the level of the kidney.

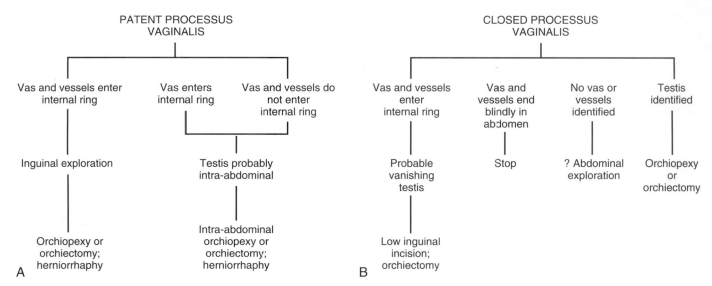

Figure 122–12. Management algorithm based on laparoscopic findings. (From Elder JS. Laparoscopy for impalpable testes. Significance of the patent processus vaginalis. J Urol 152:778, 1994.)

POSTOPERATIVE MANAGEMENT AND COMPLICATIONS

After an orchiopexy, the child is usually discharged from the ambulatory surgery unit with adequate analgesia and instructions to remain at bed rest for 1 to 2 days. Ecchymosis of the scrotum or groin, or both, and transient scrotal swelling are common. The child is re-examined 2 to 3 weeks after orchiopexy and again after 4 months.

The most common complication of orchiopexy is probably testicular retraction.[25] In one series of 336 orchiopexies, ten (3.4 percent) had a testis that was high-riding in the scrotum, although only three (1 percent) required reoperation.[26] This complication generally results from inadequate mobilization of the testis during orchiopexy or from failure to perform the Prentiss maneuver, although it also occurs with testes that were originally intra-abdominal or high in the inguinal canal. In children who have a testis that is not in the scrotum after orchiopexy, a second orchiopexy is recommended. In most cases, division of the floor of the inguinal canal is necessary for successful secondary orchiopexy. In one series, all of the testes deemed viable during secondary orchiopexy were brought down successfully.[27]

Other potential complications of orchiopexy include testicular atrophy, transection of the vas deferens, inguinal (indirect or direct) hernia, hematoma, and wound infection. Testicular atrophy usually results from transection of the testicular artery. If transection of the vas is discovered during an orchiopexy, immediate microsurgical vasovasostomy should probably be performed.

Men with a history of cryptorchidism have an increased incidence of infertility. Men who have undergone orchiopexy for a unilateral undescended testis have a 65 to 80 percent paternity rate; the rate is only 50 to 60 percent in men treated for bilateral cryptorchidism.[25, 28] Since microscopic pathological changes are present in the cryptorchid testis by 1 to 2 years, it is hoped that performing the orchiopexy when the child is 12 to 18 months old will improve the chances of fertility. The other long-term potential sequela of cryptorchidism is testicular cancer, and it is not thought that orchiopexy diminishes the potential for malignancy. However, having the testis in a scrotal position allows early detection of a testicular mass, and it is important to counsel families of boys with an undescended testis that malignant degeneration may occur.

Summary

In the child with an undescended testis, abnormal histological changes are present by the time he is 12 to 18 months old. Early orchiopexy is recommended with the intention of allowing normal testicular development. In a boy with an impalpable testis, laparoscopy may aid in its localization. In 97 percent of cases, orchiopexy is successful.

Editorial Comment
Craig A. Peters

Laparoscopy provides anatomical information on the presence and location of cryptorchid testes. This can facilitate surgical decision making and should not be viewed as simply a means to avoid "surgery." We have been using laparoscopy for diagnostic purposes for 10 years and have been performing operative orchiopexy for 2 years with good results. We have also identified several intra-abdominal testes after reportedly negative inguinal explorations. The complication rate of laparoscopy in pediatric urological applications should be low, but significant complications have been reported. On the basis of a survey representing over 5000 cases, the experience of the operator, as well as the technique used, influenced the incidence of complications. The open cannula technique was associated with fewer complications, even in experienced hands.

REFERENCES

1. Scorer G, Farrington GH. Congenital Deformities of the Testis and Epididymis. New York, Appleton-Century-Crofts, 1971.
2. John Radcliffe Study Group. Clinical diagnosis of cryptorchidism. Arch Dis Child 63:587, 1988.
3. Huff DS, Hadziselimovic F, Duckett JW, et al. Germ cell counts in semi-thin sections of biopsies of 115 unilaterally cryptorchid testes: The experience from the Children's Hospital of Philadelphia. Eur J Pediatr 146(Suppl 2):S25, 1987.
4. Mininberg DT, Rodger JC, Bedford JM. Ultrastructural evidence of the onset of testicular pathological conditions in the cryptorchid human testis within the first year of life. J Urol 128:782, 1982.
5. Siegel AL, Snyder HM, Duckett JW. Outpatient pediatric urological surgery: Techniques for a successful and cost-effective practice. J Urol 136:879, 1986.
6. Schreiner MS. Preoperative and postoperative fasting in children. Pediatr Clin North Am 41:111, 1994.
7. Elder JS. Laparoscopy and Fowler-Stephens orchiopexy in the management of the impalpable testis. Urol Clin North Am 16:399, 1989.
8. Elder JS. The undescended testis: Hormonal and surgical management. Surg Clin North Am 68:983, 1988.
9. Lee LM, Johnson HW, McLoughlin MG. Microdissection and radiographic studies of the arterial vasculature of the human testes. J Pediatr Surg 19:297, 1984.
10. Marshall FF, Shermeta DW. Epididymal abnormalities associated with undescended testis. J Urol 121:341, 1979.
11. Elder JS. Epididymal anomalies associated with hydrocele/hernia: Implications regarding testicular descent. J Urol 148:624, 1992.
12. Prentiss RJ, Weickgenant CJ, Moses JJ, et al. Undescended testis: Surgical anatomy of spermatic vessels, spermatic surgical triangles, and lateral spermatic ligament. J Urol 83:686, 1960.
13. Gross RE, Replogle RL. Treatment of the undescended testes. Opinions gained from 1967 operations. Postgrad Med 34:266, 1963.
14. Benson CD, Lotfi MW. The pouch technique in the surgical correction of cryptorchidism in infants and children. Surgery 62:967, 1967.
15. Fowler R, Stephens FD. The role of testicular vascular anatomy

in the salvage of the high undescended testes. Aust N Z J Surg 29:92, 1959.

16. Elder JS. Two-stage Fowler-Stephens orchiopexy in the management of intra-abdominal testes. J Urol 148:1239, 1992.

17. Elder JS, Keating MA, Duckett JW. Infant testicular prostheses. J Urol 141:1413, 1989.

18. Diamond DA, Caldamone AA, Elder JS. Prevalence of the vanishing testis in boys with a unilateral impalpable testis: Is the side of presentation significant? J Urol 152:502, 1994.

19. Elder JS. Laparoscopy for impalpable testes: Significance of the patent processus vaginalis. J Urol 152:776, 1994.

20. Hrebinko RL, Bellinger MF. The limited role of imaging techniques in managing children with undescended testes. J Urol 150:458, 1993.

21. Weiss RM, Seashore JH. Laparoscopy in the management of the nonpalpable testis. J Urol 138:382, 1987.

22. Bogaert GA, Kogan BA, Mevorack RA. Therapeutic laparoscopy for intra-abdominal testes. Urology 42:182, 1993.

23. Thomas MD, Mercer LC, Saltzstein EC. Laparoscopic orchiectomy for unilateral intra-abdominal testis. J Urol 148:1251, 1992.

24. Plotzker ED, Rushton HG, Belman AB, Skoog SJ. Laparoscopy for nonpalpable testes in childhood: Is inguinal exploration also necessary when vas and vessels exit the inguinal ring? J Urol 148:635, 1992.

25. Elder JS, Marshall FF. Complications of orchidopexy. In Marshall FF, ed. Urologic Complications, 2nd ed. St. Louis, Mosby-Year Book, 1990, p 545.

26. Moul JW, Belman AB. A review of surgical treatment of undescended testes with emphasis on anatomical position. J Urol 140:125, 1988.

27. Maizels M, Gomez F, Firlit CF. Surgical correction of the failed orchiopexy. J Urol 130:955, 1983.

28. Marshall FF, Elder JS. Cryptorchidism and Related Anomalies. New York, Praeger, 1982.

Chapter 123

Surgical Management of Testicular Torsion

Craig A. Peters

Acute torsion of the testicle represents a surgical emergency in any age group, requiring a high index of suspicion to achieve early diagnosis and a satisfactory result with surgical management. Clinical decisions should be based on history and clinical examination as well as a recognition of the consequences of untreated torsion, rather than an excessive reliance on adjunctive diagnostic testing. Neonatally detected testicular torsion poses no less a threat to the well-being of the child and warrants prompt attention and treatment.

ANATOMY AND ETIOLOGY

The normal testis is attached to the scrotal wall by the gubernaculum and the mesorchium with its peritoneal investment. The latter is a broad band oriented vertically along the side of the testis with the epididymis, holding the testis in a near vertical orientation (Fig. 123–1A). The gubernaculum or scrotal ligament attaches the inferior aspect of the testis to the base of the scrotum. When the gubernacular attachments are deficient and the reflection of the tu-

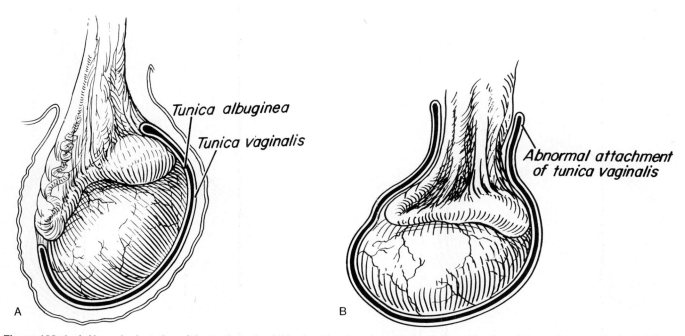

Figure 123–1. *A*, Normal orientation of the testis and epididymis with a broad mesorchium. The reflection of the tunica vaginalis (parietal) onto the tunica albuginea (serosal) spreads over a wide area of the epididymis and testis. *B*, The "bell-clapper" deformity is created by the abnormal location of the reflection of the parietal surface (tunica vaginalis) onto the serosal surface around the entire spermatic cord, leaving the testis and epididymis unattached within the pocket of the parietal tunica vaginalis. This is depicted with a transverse orientation that may also be seen.

nica vaginalis onto the testis and epididymis is high on the spermatic cord (the bell-clapper deformity), the testis has a greater tendency to rotate about a vertical axis (Fig. 123–1B). The testis may also be oriented more horizontally (transverse lie), increasing the torquing force of the testis itself about its vertical axis.

The contribution of these factors is evidenced by the two peaks of occurrence of torsion.[1, 2] In the perinatal period the gubernacular attachments are poorly developed and may permit twisting of the entire spermatic cord and its investing visceral tunica vaginalis (peritoneum) (Fig. 123–2A). Thus, in the neonate, torsion is usually extravaginal. In the pubertal boy, rapid testicular growth increases the risk of twisting about a narrowly attached mesorchium (Fig. 123–2B), creating an intravaginal torsion. The distinction between these two entities is somewhat academic and has been called into question.[3]

Ischemic damage to the testis occurs from venous occlusion with subsequent arterial obstruction or outright arterial occlusion.[1] The number of turns of the spermatic cord may determine the mechanism of injury. The rapidity of irreversible damage may therefore be determined by this factor. It should be emphasized that dogmatic adherence to a time period of testicular salvage is not justified in that the different mechanisms of injury progress with different time courses.

CLINICAL APPEARANCE

The clinical evidence of torsion is usually sudden, excruciating pain, although more gradual progression or less severe pain may be reported.[2, 4] There may be a predisposing factor such as vigorous activity, yet its absence does not in any way rule out torsion. Patients have often reported being awakened from sleep with the pain. Pain may radiate into the groin and abdomen, and nausea may be present.[1] The clinical picture of a patient with acute torsion in the early stages is usually distinctive. The young or poorly communicative child, however, may simply evidence abdominal pain. Unfortunately, many patients do not present promptly for medical attention, and the clinical picture may be less distinct.

Initially, the scrotum appears normal, without erythema or swelling. The testis, however, is tender, hard, and smooth. With time, the local tissues become inflamed and boggy, erythematous and indurated. Late torsions may present with skin fixation over a hard mass that may mimic a tumor. Differentiation of testicular torsion from that of torsion of a testicular or epididymal appendage may be a challenge in the prepubertal child. Gradual onset of moderately severe pain, focal tenderness at the superior aspect of the testis, a testis that is not hard, scrotal erythema, and a boggy epididymis are more indicative of torsion of an appendix than of torsion of

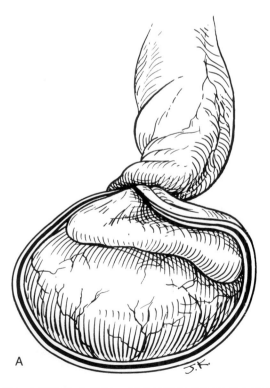
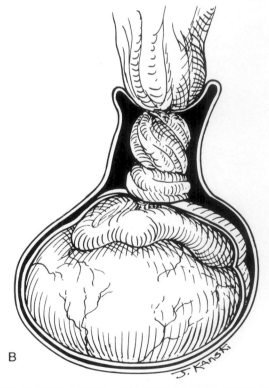

Figure 123–2. *A*, Extravaginal torsion, typical of a neonatal testicular torsion. The tunica vaginalis is involved with the twist of the spermatic cord. *B*, Intravaginal torsion, usually seen after the neonatal period, involves the spermatic cord below the reflection of the tunica vaginalis onto the spermatic cord.

the testis. The classic blue dot sign of an infarcted appendix may occasionally be seen. Torsion of an appendix usually induces a reactive epididymitis, which should not be confused with bacterial epididymitis. Treatment is nonoperative if the diagnosis is clear, with adjunctive anti-inflammatory agents rather than antibiotics.

The neonate with a firm and enlarged testicle, often without evidence of distress, may have suffered a torsion. This has probably occurred in utero or at birth and represents an infarcted testicle. A reactive hydrocele is common. There may be little in the clinical examination to distinguish this from a hydrocele, tumor, or even an inguinal hernia, and adjunctive measures are useful. Scrotal ultrasound imaging is the most efficient and accurate method of evaluation. When a previously normal testis has been well documented in a neonate presenting with a swollen scrotum and hard testis, acute, reversible torsion must be considered and exploration undertaken. The incidence of bilateral torsion is not high but its consequences are disastrous, and our practice has evolved to consider testicular torsion in the neonate as an emergency.[5]

NATURAL HISTORY

Untreated testicular torsion may appear as a prolonged episode of epididymitis, for which it has often been mistaken, unresponsive to antibiotics. This may be significantly debilitating to the patient, persisting for weeks. Theoretical questions have been raised, with some supportive data, about the long-term consequences of a retained infarcted testis upon fertility of the contralateral testis.[6-8] This concept has not been proved in humans. Rarely, an infarcted testis will suppurate.

EVALUATION OF THE ACUTE SCROTUM

The presentation of a child with scrotal pain should immediately bring to mind the diagnosis of testicular torsion. Clinical evaluation usually quickly confirms the diagnosis of torsion when present but is not as specific or reliable in ruling out a torsion of the testicle. While this review is ongoing, preparations should be made for scrotal exploration. Historical review with the patient or parent should focus on the time and rapidity of onset of symptoms, previous similar symptoms, a history of torsion in the father, and any previous surgery of the genitalia.

Physical examination should document the character and location of *both* testes. The typical testis in torsion is exquisitely tender in its entirety, firm to

hard, and drawn up somewhat into the groin; it frequently has some surrounding fluid, and with delay the scrotum may become edematous and erythematous. The cremasteric reflex has been reported to be absent in torsion. Its presence has been said to rule out torsion,[2, 9] although cases of torsion with the cremasteric reflex present have been reported. Any of these findings serve to further convince the clinician of the correctness of the suspicion of torsion, yet their absence must not dissuade one from the diagnosis. Overinterpretation of the significance of clinical findings only serves to increase the risk of missing the diagnosis of torsion. The avoidance of minor surgery in a few patients is hardly worth the risk of losing the testis of a young boy.

Adjunctive diagnostic measures may help further confirm the diagnosis of torsion but should not delay the definitive diagnostic test of scrotal exploration. When the index of suspicion for torsion is so low as to warrant observation, these tests are very useful in documenting the validity of this course. Doppler flow studies of the testicular artery may be performed in the emergency room and have been reported to be reliable,[10] yet reactive scrotal hyperemia in delayed cases may mimic testicular flow. Nuclear scintigraphy with technetium 99m tracer may be used to document blood flow to the testis,[11, 12] yet false-negative results may also be caused by reactive hyperemia, particularly in the smaller child in whom resolution decreases.

If clinical suspicion is low and a definitive diagnosis is being sought, the nuclear scan is used, but most patients undergo ultrasonographic imaging with duplex pulsed-flow Doppler assessment of testicular blood flow.[13-17] This newer modality holds significant promise for rapid and specific diagnosis of scrotal abnormalities in children. In addition to providing information on intratesticular blood flow, the echotexture of the testis may be assessed, as well as that of peritesticular tissues. In the unlikely situation of a testicular tumor presenting acutely (as with hemorrhage), ultrasonographic imaging will permit a preoperative diagnosis. Ultrasonographic imaging may also distinguish between torsion and the testicular manifestations of Henoch-Schönlein purpura, which may present with an acutely painful scrotum.[17] Testicular torsion produces changes in echotexture after 24 to 48 hours, with slow evolution of heterogeneous echotexture associated with necrosis.

Early in the course of testicular torsion, however, there are no consistent differences in the echotexture of the testis. Intratesticular blood flow, however, is not detectable. Its absence, when a strong signal has been obtained on the contralateral testis, should be considered a strong indication of testicular torsion. The presence of intratesticular blood flow is a good indication that there is no torsion of the testis. This may be reinforced by temporary extinction of the signal by cord compression over the pubic tubercle. The well-recognized operator dependence of ultrasound imaging is particularly relevant in this use. As with any imaging study, the clinical context must be considered. Formal trials of the utility of testicular ultrasound imaging in the evaluation of the acute scrotum are needed before this method is widely applied and relied on.[18, 19]

Magnetic resonance imaging may demonstrate infarction[20] but has not yet been brought into the realm of emergent diagnostics.

The differential diagnosis of acute scrotal pain includes torsion of the testicle or appendices, testicular rupture, testicular tumor (particularly with acute bleeding), and incarcerated hernia. Each of these entities is properly and definitively treated with surgical exploration. Any suspicion of tumor warrants preoperative ultrasonography, tumor markers, and a high inguinal approach for exploration. The presence of a hernia is usually evident on careful examination. Other entities to be considered include epididymitis, orchitis, acute infarction, Henoch-Schönlein purpura, insect bites, and idiopathic or allergic scrotal edema. These are usually evident on careful history and examination, but the most certain diagnostic measure is surgical exploration, with more specific testing guided by the surgical findings.

EXPLORATION

If the diagnosis of testicular torsion has been considered and cannot be quickly and completely ruled out, immediate exploration is indicated. Confirmatory testing should not delay exploration. The fact that the clinical history has been prolonged should not lessen the urgency for exploration, as partial torsion and venous obstruction may have a slower course toward irreversible testicular damage. There is seldom an indication for manual detorsion or spermatic cord block; these maneuvers may only cloud the clinical picture. Manual detorsion should be used only after a commitment has been made to explore the child and only if there is a truly unavoidable delay in taking him to the operating room. The patient and family must be informed of the possibility of testicular loss and can be offered the option of a testicular prosthesis, although we have recently discouraged such placement.

General endotracheal anesthesia is preferred, particularly in the younger child. Preanesthetic gastric aspiration has been advocated by some.[21] Antibiotics are usually administered preoperatively only in consideration of the possibility of orchiectomy and placement of a testicular prosthesis. A full bilateral scrotal and inguinal surgical preparation should be performed.

A vertical midline incision is used to explore both hemiscrota. After incision to the level of the dartos muscles, the affected testis is moved under the incision and further dissection continued until the tunicae are incised along the vertical line. The character of the fluid should be noted. The testis with torsion is usually dark blue or black, but spontaneous detorsion with anesthesia is not uncommon. The tunic is fully opened, detorsion is performed, and the testis is inspected. The surface is typically smooth, and an exudate or adhesions to the tunica suggest a prolonged ischemic injury or an inflammatory process.

An obviously viable testis will "pink up" promptly, but many do so slowly over 10 to 15 minutes. If there is no sign of recovery, a small nick is made in the tunica albuginea to expose seminiferous tubules. There should be some fresh bleeding and the tubules should appear dusky to pink; if they are black and friable, there is little likelihood of the testis regaining viability. Time is allowed for the testis, wrapped in a warm moist sponge, to recover, while the contralateral testis is being fixed to the scrotal wall. Intraoperative Doppler flow study may help assess perfusion; fluorescein injection may be tried.[22]

A nonviable testis should be removed to avoid continued symptoms and possible superinfection, and to minimize the theoretical concern of contralateral testicular damage from an in situ infarcted testis. If viability is uncertain, the testis may be left in place to permit the chance of any endocrine function recovery, despite loss of spermatogenic function. The neonatal testicle in torsion is usually infarcted and should be removed.[5, 23] A normal contralateral testis should always be confirmed before orchiectomy. The appendices of the testis and epididymis are removed with cautery or suture.

A testicular prosthesis may be placed at the time of orchiectomy, with antibiotics added to the treatment regimen in the perioperative period. Acute placement of a prosthesis at this time does carry a risk of extrusion of the prosthesis from the scrotum owing to the more friable condition of the tissues. Delayed placement through a low inguinal incision is preferable. Although there are no reports of complications from silicone testicular prostheses, we have discouraged their placement. Many families have chosen not to have them placed.

The viable testis is still at risk for torsion, and fixation with nonabsorbable sutures is required.[24] Numerous methods have been described.[4, 25, 26] The method shown in Figure 123–3 provides three-point fixation into the septum of the scrotum. A finger in the contralateral hemiscrotum exposes the septum very well, permits deep sutures to be placed without concern for dimpling of the skin, and makes position-

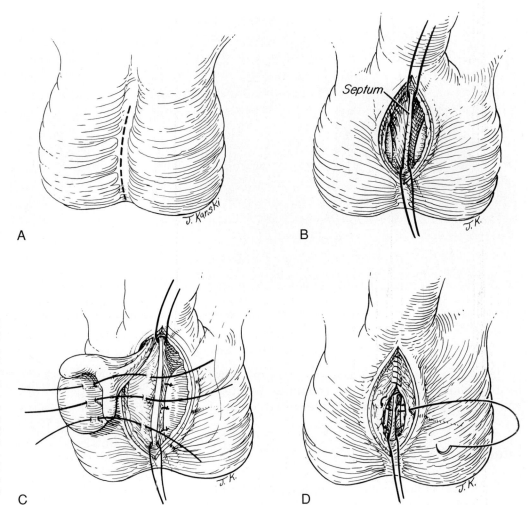

Figure 123–3. *A*, Midline scrotal incision for scrotal exploration of presumed testicular torsion. *B*, Exposure of the scrotal septum to facilitate placement of testicular fixation stitches. *C*, The three septopexy stitches are of nonabsorbable suture material and oriented vertically. They should pass through the tunica albuginea of the testis. The left testis fixed into position and the three fixation sutures between the right testis and scrotal septum are shown. *D*, The scrotum is being closed in two layers after testicular fixation.

ing of the sutures easier (Fig. 123–3*A*). A nonabsorbable suture of the appropriate size should be used (4-0 for infants, 3-0 for children and young adults). Three sutures are placed for each testis before being tied down. The tunica does not need to be closed. The scrotum is closed in two layers, closing both hemiscrota simultaneously, and is not drained (Fig. 123–3*B*). An everting skin closure improves wound healing.

Cotton fluff dressing and a scrotal support minimize discomfort. The patient is discharged later that day or the following morning. Minimal postoperative analgesia is needed.

COMPLICATIONS

Nonviable Testis

Testicular loss has been reported to occur in 25 to 55 percent of cases of torsion.[2, 27–30] The primary reasons are delay in presentation and delay in diagnosis and treatment. With a proper index of suspicion and prompt exploration when indicated, testicular loss should be minimized. In the postpubertal patient, epididymo-orchitis is more frequent, yet torsion still occurs, probably more so than has been classically described. Torsion of the testis has been reported in adults.

Contralateral Torsion

This complication has been seen either when contralateral fixation has not been performed or when inadequate fixation was used.[24] Absorbable sutures have been associated with torsion of testes that have undergone orchiopexy. Routine contralateral fixation with several permanent sutures should prevent this. Contralateral torsion has also been seen in the newborn patient who has had testicular torsion and in whom fixation of the contralateral testis has been delayed. Although not a regular occurrence, metachronous contralateral torsion of the testis has been described.[5, 23] The consequences are disastrous: the patient becomes a eunuch, dependent on exogenous androgen. Although there is rarely a chance of salvaging the testis with initial torsion, protecting the now

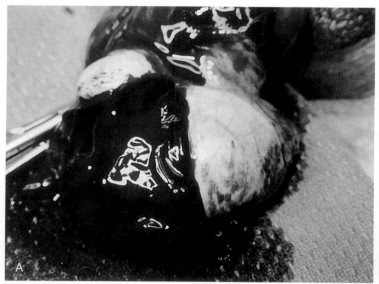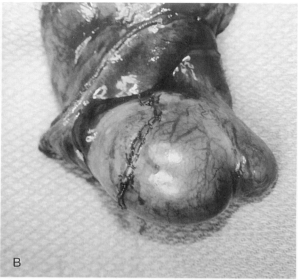

Figure 123–4. *A,* Appearance of the ruptured testicle in an 18-year-old patient who sustained a kick to the genitals. The hemorrhagic seminiferous tubules are seen outside the ruptured tunica albuginea. *B,* The same testicle after debridement of devitalized tubules. The tunica albuginea has been primarily repaired.

solitary contralateral testis is a priority. Contralateral fixation should be carried out promptly, within several days or weeks of detecting the initial torsion.

Infertility

Theoretical concerns have been raised that contralateral testicular damage occurs with torsion. The mechanism is hypothesized to be an immunological response to the disrupted blood-testis barrier. Published reports may reflect species idiosyncrasies, but the possibility of a comparable effect in humans cannot be discounted at this time.[6–8]

TESTICULAR RUPTURE

Although not common, testicular rupture often presents with a clinical appearance similar to that of testicular torsion. Ultrasonography often demonstrates a hematocele and may show the disrupted tunica albuginea. The presence of the hematocele is strongly suggestive of rupture, and exploration is advisable.[31, 32] Exploration should be prompt, within 12 to 18 hours. Debridement of nonviable seminiferous tubules with repair of the tunical tear has generally yielded a satisfactory result (Fig. 123–4).

REFERENCES

1. Skoglund R, McRoberts J, Radge H. Torsion of the spermatic cord: A review of the literature and an analysis of 70 new cases. J Urol 104:604, 1970.
2. Melekos MD, Asbach HW, Markou SA. Etiology of acute scrotum in 100 boys with regard to age distribution. J Urol 139:1023, 1988.
3. Friedman RM, Flashner SC, Akwari OE, King LR. An experimental model of neonatal testicular torsion: Evidence against an exclusively extravaginal etiology. J Urol 150:246, 1993.
4. Retik AB, Colodny AH, Bauer SB. Pediatric urology. In Paulson DF, ed. Genitourinary Surgery, Vol. II, New York, Churchill Livingstone, 1984, p 863.
5. LaQuaglia MP, Bauer SB, Eraklis A, et al: Bilateral neonatal torsion. J Urol 138 (pt 2):1051, 1987.
6. Nagler HM, White RD. The effect of testicular torsion on the contralateral testis. J Urol 128:1343, 1982.
7. Janetschek G, Heilbronner R, Schachtner W, et al: Unilateral testicular disease: Effect on the contralateral testis (morphometric study). J Urol 138:878, 1987.
8. Fisch H, Laor E, Reid RE, et al: Gonadal dysfunction after testicular torsion: Luteinizing hormone and follicle-stimulating hormone response to gonadotropin releasing hormone. J Urol 139:961, 1988.
9. Rabinowitz R. The importance of the cremasteric reflex in acute scrotal swelling in children. J Urol 132:89, 1984.
10. Levy B. The diagnosis of torsion of the testicle using the Doppler ultrasonic stethoscope. J Urol 113:63, 1975.
11. Valvo JR, Caldamone AA, O'Mara R, Rabinowitz R. Nuclear imaging in the pediatric acute scrotum. Am J Dis Child 136:831, 1982.
12. Brehmer B, Grunig F, von Berger L. Radionuclide scrotal imaging: A useful diagnostic tool in patients with acute scrotal swelling? Scand J Urol Nephrol Suppl 104:119, 1987.
13. Meza MP, Amundson GM, Aquilina JW, Reitelman C. Color flow imaging in children with clinically suspected testicular torsion. Pediatr Radiol 22:370, 1992.
14. Cohen HL, Shapiro MA, Haller JO, Glassberg K. Torsion of the testicular appendage. Sonographic diagnosis. J Ultrasound Med 11:81, 1992.
15. Kass EJ, Stone KT, Cacciarelli AA, Mitchell B. Do all children with an acute scrotum require exploration? J Urol 150:667, 1993.
16. Wilbert DM, Schaerfe CW, Stern WD, et al: Evaluation of the acute scrotum by color-coded Doppler ultrasonography. J Urol 149:1475, 1993.
17. Laor T, Atala A, Teele RL. Scrotal ultrasonography in Henoch-Schönlein purpura. Pediatr Radiol 22:505, 1992.
18. Chinn DH, Miller EI. Generalized testicular hyperechogenicity in acute testicular torsion. J Ultrasound Med 4:495, 1985.
19. Mueller DL, Amundson GM, Rubin SZ, Wesenberg RL. Acute

scrotal abnormalities in children: Diagnosis by combined sonography and scintigraphy. AJR Am J Roentgenol 150:643, 1988.

20. Landa HM, Gylys-Morin V, Mattery RF, et al: Detection of testicular torsion by magnetic resonance imaging in a rat model. J Urol 140 (pt 2):1178, 1988.

21. Schurizek B, Bøggild-Madsen B, Juhl B. Do patients with torsion of the testis have an increased risk of pulmonary aspiration during general anaesthesia? Br J Anaesth 56:312, 1984.

22. Schneider HC, Kendall AR, Karafin L. Fluorescence of the testicle: An indication of viability of spermatic cord after torsion. Urology 5:133, 1975.

23. Burge DM. Neonatal testicular torsion and infarction: Aetiology and management. Br J Urol 59:70, 1987.

24. Kossow AS. Torsion following orchiopexy. N Y State J Med 80:1136, 1980.

25. Harrison RH III. Testicular torsion. In Glenn JF, ed. Urologic Surgery. Philadelphia, JB Lippincott, 1983, p 1067.

26. Hamdy FC, MacKinnon AE. Technique of testicular fixation for torsion of the testis. Br J Surg 74:1174, 1987.

27. Krorup T. The testes after torsion. Br J Urol 50:43, 1978.

28. Thomas WE, Williamson RC. Diagnosis and outcome of testicular torsion. Br J Surg 70:213, 1983.

29. Bennett S, Nicholson MS, Little TM. Torsion of the testis: Why is the prognosis so poor? Br Med J 294:824, 1987.

30. Sethia KK, Bickerstaff KI, Murie JA. Changing pattern of scrotal exploration for testicular torsion. Urology 31:408, 1988.

31. Cass AS. Testicular trauma. J Urol 129:299, 1983.

32. Vaccaro JA, Davis R, Belville WD, Kiesling V. Traumatic hematocele: Association with rupture of the testicle. J Urol 136:1217, 1986.

Chapter 124

Posterior Urethral Valves

H. Norman Noe

Posterior urethral valves constitute the most common significant obstruction to the bladder outlet in children. Although a few isolated cases in girls have been reported, this occurs almost exclusively in boys. For the purposes of this discussion, I am assuming that valves occur exclusively in male children, realizing that the same destructive techniques for the valve can be applied in either case.

Normal urethral anatomy in a male child includes the inferior crest (crista urethralis) arising from the distal end of the verumontanum and terminating in two finlike structures that insert laterally into the wall of the urethra (plicae colliculi). These structures are normally readily identifiable at endoscopy in a child, do not meet in the anterior midline, and are not obstructive. Embryologically, the plicae colliculi are believed to represent the path of regression of the wolffian ducts as they move to terminate at the verumontanum as ejaculatory ducts. Incomplete re-

gression of these ducts can leave substantial folds of tissue, which could act as posterior urethral valves (Fig. 124–1). Thus, valves can appear to be an exaggeration of normally present anatomy, the distinguishing characteristic being the fusion of the valve cusps anteriorly, leaving a posterior and proximal opening that is significantly restricted in size.

Young's original classification described three types of valves (Fig. 124–2).[1] Type I valves extend from the inferior verumontanum distally and superiorly, forming an oblique obstruction to the posterior urethra. Type II valves were thought to be folds extending from the verumontanum back proximally to the bladder neck, but are now believed to be nonexistent. The type III valve is a more distal diaphragmatic type of obstruction, similar to a congenital urethral membrane. In this chapter, type I urethral valves are the ones discussed for treatment since they constitute the majority of cases encountered clinically.

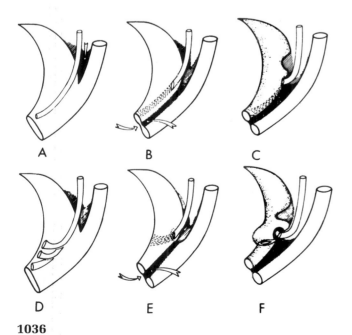

Figure 124–1. Development of type I valves. *A* to *C*, Normal urethral crest development. The orifice or the wolffian duct migrates from its anterolateral position in the cloaca to the site of Müller tubercle on the posterior wall. Dots denote the pathway of migration, which remains as the normal inferior crest and plicae culliculi. *D* to *F*, Abnormal anterior positions of wolffian duct orifices and consequent abnormal migration of the terminal ends of the ducts. This results in circumferential, obliquely oriented ridges that persist as valvular obstruction. (From King LR. Posterior urethra. In Kelalis PP, King LR, Belman AB, eds. Clinical Pediatric Urology, 2nd ed. Philadelphia, WB Saunders, 1985, p 530.)

INDICATIONS FOR TREATMENT

The diagnosis of posterior urethral valves is one that can be made definitely only by radiography. The findings on voiding cystourethrography (VCUG) regarding valvular obstruction are characteristic (Fig. 124–3).

Previously, approximately half of the cases of posterior urethral valves were diagnosed in the neonatal period. They were found as a result of a palpable flank or abdominal mass representing a distended bladder, or in the course of an investigation for sepsis and urinary tract infections. Occasionally, a weak urinary stream was noted or a full-term infant with respiratory distress was evaluated and found to have posterior urethral valves. Commonly, cases are now being discovered by prenatal ultrasonography, which identifies hydronephrosis in the fetus and allows the diagnosis to be made before clinical deterioration can occur or urinary tract infection arises. Of particular importance in those cases discovered prenatally is the presence or absence of oligohydramnios. Children with diminished amniotic fluid representing poor uri-

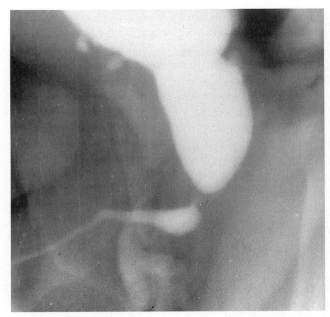

Figure 124–3. Radiographical appearance of posterior urethral valvular obstruction: a typical dilated posterior urethra with widened bladder neck and bladder diverticula.

nary output usually have a high degree of renal dysplasia and a much poorer prognosis. Accompanying pulmonary hypoplasia can occur in these cases also.

Older boys are usually diagnosed during the course of a work-up for obstructive voiding symptoms, weak urinary stream, wetting disorders, failure to thrive, urinary tract infection, or (infrequently) detection of a flank mass on physical examination.

Thus, the indication for surgical removal of a urethral valve is verification of its presence. The course of action is dictated by patients' clinical status as well as their age and size. While in most cases there is clearly upper tract alteration with hydronephrosis or reflux, or both, it is still the primary objective to first remove the urethral obstruction.

PREOPERATIVE MANAGEMENT

In newborns or infants presenting with posterior urethral valves, it is necessary to establish bladder drainage, correct any metabolic disturbances present, and treat any infection before undertaking a definitive treatment course for removal of urethral obstruction. Bladder drainage can be established with either urethral feeding catheters, suprapubic punch catheters, or, in the older child, the appropriate size of urethral Foley catheter. In addition to bladder drainage, attention must be paid to the metabolic status of the child. Many children present with failure to thrive, acidosis, electrolyte abnormalities, and dehydration. Electrolyte problems can be diagnosed by appropriate serum measurements, and dehydration diagnosed

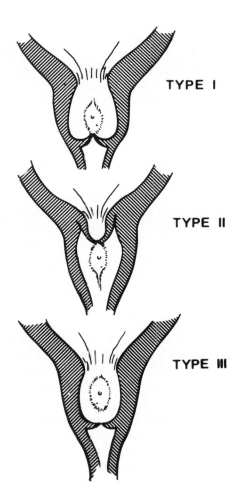

TYPE I

TYPE II

TYPE III

Figure 124–2. Young's classification of valvular type. (From King LR. Posterior urethra. In Kelalis PP, King LR, Belman AB, eds. Clinical Pediatric Urology, 2nd ed. Philadelphia, WB Saunders, 1985, p 531.)

clinically. Appropriate fluid and electrolyte administration can be completed once bladder drainage has been established, to prepare the child for surgery. An occasional child develops considerable diuresis with loss of fluids and electrolytes after the establishment of bladder drainage. In such cases, careful management and replacement of fluids and electrolytes and close monitoring of body weight and serum electrolytes and osmolality are necessary. Specific treatment with antibiotics for any urinary tract infection or sepsis is also mandatory.

In the otherwise healthy or older child in whom posterior valves have been diagnosed and normal renal function is still present, no preliminary drainage is necessary. One can then move at once to remove the urethral obstruction.

Thus, the goal of preoperative management is to have a child who is optimally prepared for surgery with control of any metabolic disturbances and infection before anesthesia and surgery are undertaken.

SURGICAL OPTIONS

Ideally, the primary surgical approach should be directed toward relief of the urethral obstruction. In some infants who are deemed either too ill or too small, some form of temporary diversion is believed to be best. Cutaneous vesicostomy by the Blocksom technique has been used to provide tubeless, readily reversible drainage in such a sick infant to allow for growth and development until such time as primary valve ablation can be undertaken.[2] Another potential advantage of cutaneous vesicostomy is the situation in which an infant's urethra is so small that endoscopic treatment would have an increased chance of resulting in urethral stricture, and thus vesicostomy would allow time to pass and the infant to grow before valve ablation is undertaken.[3] In a few infants, drainage at the bladder level is insufficient either to improve renal function or to clear infection from large, dilated upper tracts. In these instances, supravesical diversion by cutaneous ureterostomy or pyelostomy can be performed.

Several options are available for dealing with urethral valves, although some of these are now of historical interest only.

Open Removal

Open removal can be accomplished by splitting the symphysis pubis and then opening the anterior commissure of the prostate and destroying the valves under vision. This higher-risk approach no longer has a place in modern pediatric urology because of the improvement in endoscopic instruments.

Destruction by Sounds or Catheter

Passage of sounds antegrade from the bladder through the bladder neck and out through the urethra could lead to mechanical disruption of the valves but is a blind technique that seems to have little use today. Likewise, it was noted early in the treatment of valves that some children, after being catheterized for a long period, ultimately had their valves necrose and disappear to the point at which they could not be demonstrated on follow-up studies. This was thought to be due to direct pressure necrosis from a large-bore indwelling catheter. The need to leave the catheter for a long period, with its attendant complications of either infection or stricture, seem to rule against this form of treatment.

Perineal Urethrostomy With Visual Ablation of the Valves

This technique employs the use of a perineal urethrotomy into which is inserted a plastic aural speculum.[4] By this means, the valves can be directly viewed and engaged with a metal hook and either disrupted mechanically or destroyed with electrocoagulation. This has been advocated in underdeveloped countries where the more sophisticated endoscopic equipment is not available. The usefulness of this technique has been documented, but its place would seem to be only in those situations in which endoscopic equipment is not readily available.

Radiographically Controlled Valve Destruction

A modified crochet hook has been used to destroy valves by passing it up the urethra and then withdrawing it, snagging and disrupting the valve directly. The original technique described by Williams and associates was successful, but complications were encountered in that the hook would engage tissues other than the valves.[4a] A modification of this technique has been described with a redesigned hook so that the tip is now much less likely to snare any urethral tissue other than the obstructing valve leaflet (Fig. 124–4).[5] Additionally, the terminal portion of the hook is bare metal, so that diathermy can be used and can aid in the destruction of the valve. More recently, another technique has been described involving a modified venous valvulotome under fluoroscopic guidance.[6] A variation of this principle is to use a Fogarty balloon catheter, which is inflated superior to the obstructing valves and then withdrawn sharply to rupture the anterior obstructing membrane and thus clear the urethral obstruction.[7]

These techniques may have their greatest use for those who prefer to avoid a preliminary vesicostomy in a very-low-birthweight infant yet would still like to proceed with ablation of the urethral valve. Although claimed to be not as traumatic as direct endoscopic resection of the valve, these closed techniques have potential for urethral damage, and postoperative urinary extravasation has been demonstrated. Long-term results must be evaluated to see how they compare with endoscopic treatment.

Endoscopic Valve Ablation

Destruction of posterior urethral valves by endoscopic means is the standard treatment today. Access to the posterior urethra is either through the existing meatus, if the anterior urethra is large enough to permit it, or by perineal urethrotomy, if the anterior urethra is judged too small (Fig. 124–5). Care must be taken to avoid either dilating or traumatizing the delicate anterior urethra of the male child to prevent strictures from forming in that area. Improved instrumentation and optics today allow use of either a 6.9 or 8 Fr. fulgurating cystoscope or a 9.5 to 10.5 Fr. pediatric resectoscope to destroy the valves. Although the indications for perineal urethrotomy have

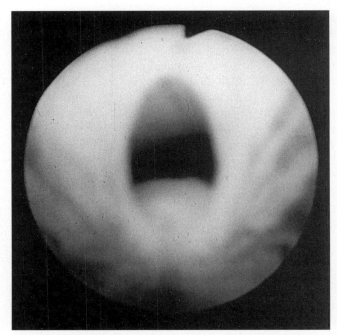

Figure 124–5. Endoscopic appearance of the posterior urethral valve. Note the valvular leaflets clearly joining at the 12 o'clock position.

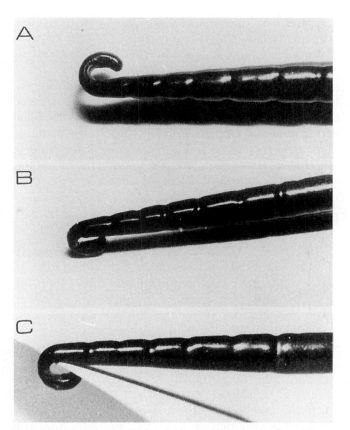

Figure 124–4. Modified crochet hook for use in destroying posterior urethral valves. (From Whitaker RH, Sherwood T. An improved hook for destroying posterior urethral valves. J Urol 135:531, 1986.)

become fewer with the advent of smaller instruments, it is still my preference to gain access to the posterior urethra by this means rather than risk trauma to the anterior urethra by passing a scope that is too snug in its fit. If the miniature cystoscopes are to be used, a small Bugbee electrode can be employed to directly fulgurate and destroy the valve cusps. An alternative is to use a woven 3 Fr. ureteral catheter through which is protruded a hooked wire stylet connected to operating current for the same purpose. The fulgurating cystoscope has its greatest application when either resectoscopes are not available or the urethra is deemed too small to accommodate the larger resectoscope.

I prefer to use one of the miniature resectoscopes and a right-angled electrode to disrupt the annular nature of the posterior urethral valve and thus remove the obstruction. Some surgeons prefer to begin incision of the valvular ring at the 12 o'clock position; others prefer to begin at the 5 and 7 o'clock positions where the valve cusps arise at the level of the verumontanum (Fig. 124–6). Since the valves insert most distally and nearest the sphincter at the 12 o'clock position, it has been argued that this is the area in which damage is most likely to occur. If the valve can be clearly seen and only valve tissue is to be incised, there appears to be no danger in destroying the valve at this position. The advantage of the 5 and 7 o'clock positions is that they allow, in most cases, the clearest delineation of valve tissue, with the resectoscope loop usually clearly seen through the valvular tissue, and a controlled incision can be made in this area. The starting point for valve destruction should depend on the surgeon's experience, preference, and ability to clearly delineate valvular extent and normal landmarks. When disrupting the valve, a cutting mode is used to try to minimize the spread of current and thus damage to surrounding tissues. Once the valves are disrupted, light fulguration of any bleeding points can be undertaken to ensure hemostasis. If large valve cusp remnants are evident within the lumen of the urethra, light fulguration can be used to destroy these, taking care not to allow thermal injury into the deeper levels of the urethral tissue. In most cases, a catheter is left in place for 24 to 72 hours. If the adequacy of valve resection is in question, an expression cystogram can be obtained on the operating table before terminating the procedure.

Alternative techniques to transurethral valve obstruction have arisen as the field of percutaneous endourology has matured. Originally the technique was employed to insert a resectoscope through an existing vesicostomy through the bladder neck and into the posterior urethra, where the valves can be viewed from above and destroyed from that position.[8] This technique has subsequently been modified in that it is performed through a percutaneous cystotomy trocar sheath and a vesicostomy is not required (Fig. 124–7).[9] Incision of the valve can then proceed in a distal to proximal direction and theoretically avoid sphincteric injury. The patient's pelvis and sacrum may have to be repositioned to allow adequate visualization of the posterior urethra, and a period of time and experience may be required to become comfortable with this endoscopic approach. However, it does offer an advantage in the low-birthweight

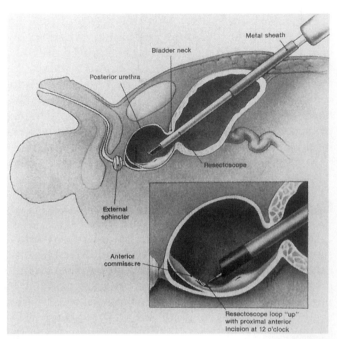

Figure 124–7. Diagram of percutaneous antegrade valve obstruction. (From Zaontz MR, Firlit CF. Percutaneous antegrade ablation of posterior urethral valves in premature or underweight term neonates: an alternative to primary vesicostomy. J Urol 134:139, 1985. © by Williams & Wilkins.)

or premature child in that vesicostomy can be avoided.

A variation of this technique has been to use the laser to destroy the valvular tissue.[10] Laser destruction offers a theoretical advantage of reduced scarring and reaction at the ablation site with a better-defined and better-controlled level of tissue damage. Visualization can be difficult, however, and the increased cost of such a mode of treatment may be a disadvantage compared with established forms of treatment. More experience with this technique is required to see if laser disruption offers a significant advantage over what is currently being employed.

POSTOPERATIVE COMPLICATIONS

With improved instrumentation and operative techniques, complications have become minimal. Intraoperative bleeding can be controlled by direct light fulguration, and postoperative catheter drainage can allow for continued tamponade of any bleeding points in the urethra. Infection accompanying urinary stasis and posterior urethral valves is always a possibility, and prophylaxis seems to be advisable in this at-risk group of patients. An unusual and infrequently encountered complication is oliguria and renal failure secondary to transient obstruction at the ureterovesical junction after valve fulguration and bladder manipulation.[11] This can be managed by temporary ureteral catheterization, percutaneous neph-

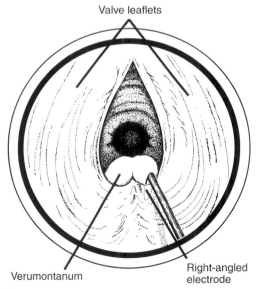

Figure 124–6. Diagram showing engagement of valve cusps at the 5 o'clock position using the miniature resectoscope. The right-angled electrode is used to cut the leaflet at this point and at the 7 o'clock position.

rostomy drainage, or, in some cases, simply removing the Foley catheter from the bladder and reducing bladder spasm, which contributes to the ureterovesical junction obstruction.

Most commonly, the complications after valve ablation have been either stricture or urinary incontinence. Although in some series the stricture rates have been reported to be quite high, my experience has not borne this out. Strictures occurring in the anterior urethra may result from trying to use too large an instrument, whereas those in the membranous urethra may be due to overzealous resection or thermal injury to the surrounding urethral tissues at the time of resection. As with any complication, prevention is the best treatment. Use of a right-angled electrode to provide simple disruption of the valve with a low cutting current seems to be superior to an attempt at complete loop resection of the valves. The latter appears to lead to the greatest amount of thermal injury and thus predisposes to scarring and fibrosis. Urethral strictures usually occur several weeks after valve fulguration and may be discovered either on the follow-up VCUG or upon resumption of an obstructive voiding pattern in the child. It seems wise to avoid valve fulguration in any child with vesicostomy or supravesical diversion until planned reconstruction, so as to prevent scarring of the so-called dry urethra. If strictures do occur, they can usually be managed endoscopically.[12]

Incontinence is another frequently mentioned complication after valve fulguration and is presumably due to sphincteric injury. It is my opinion that this occurs rarely, if at all, in experienced hands, the incontinence being primarily related to abnormal bladder and sphincteric function as demonstrated in urodynamic studies of such children.[13] Surgical manipulation of the bladder neck in children with posterior urethral valves should be avoided if at all possible, to minimize the risk of internal sphincteric damage and incontinence. It thus seems unlikely that incontinence would result from simple controlled ablation of the posterior urethral valves.

As mentioned previously, in the child in whom valve ablation or simple catheter drainage of the bladder does not improve renal function, or in whom infection intervenes, higher diversion will be necessary, usually by ureterostomy or pyelostomy.

POSTOPERATIVE MANAGEMENT

In the immediate postoperative period, renal function is closely monitored, and once the catheter is removed it is confirmed whether the child will be able to void adequately. Maintenance of sterile urine can be ensured by prophylaxis. A follow-up VCUG is usually obtained about 6 weeks after valve ablation.

Once it is determined that obstruction has been removed, long-term management centers on upper tract considerations (i.e., reflux or obstruction), bladder dysfunction, and long-term renal function prognosis.[14–16]

Some children who exhibit vesicoureteral reflux at the time of the valve discovery cease refluxing once the valves have been successfully removed. In those in whom high-grade reflux persists, particularly with difficult-to-control infections, tailoring and reimplantations of the ureters and urinary reconstruction seem appropriate. In children with persistent bilateral high-grade reflux, the prognosis appears to be somewhat worse, and in some cases may be related to the degree of renal dysplasia. Dilation, without reflux, of the upper urinary system usually remains in most of these children for years, but in most cases it is usually not representative of high-grade obstruction. In the child in whom ureterovesical obstruction can be demonstrated by either diuretic renography or pressure perfusion studies, urinary reconstruction may be indicated.

Problems with urinary incontinence may be related to a poorly compliant, overactive, or somewhat spastic bladder and may require specific pharmacological therapy. In some patients with the so-called valves bladder syndrome, the entire bladder is a high-pressure, poorly compliant system acting as an obstruction to the upper urinary tracts. In such cases, an augmentation cystoplasty may be required to relieve high pressures within the urinary system, reduce hydronephrosis, and help establish continence.

Additionally, a long-term prognosis in regard to renal function must be made based on the degree of renal function impairment at discovery, how quickly renal function improves, the presence or absence of reflux, the control of infections, and urodynamic considerations of the entire lower urinary system.

Thus, the management of the child with posterior urethral valves extends well beyond simple ablation of the valve. As newer techniques and instrumentation have allowed us to treat these children with greater degrees of success and lower rates of complication, there are still factors that must be considered over the long term. In many cases, simple destruction of the posterior urethral valves may be the easiest task the surgeon has to perform.

Editorial Comment
Craig A. Peters

Even with improvements in miniature endoscopic instruments, transurethral resection of valves (TURV) is not a trivial procedure. Visualization of the valve leaflets may be enhanced by filling the bladder with irrigant and establishing antegrade flow by pressure on the abdomen, with the drainage port on the cystoscope open. The leaflets may be seen to fill like sails, and more precise cutting is possible.

During valve ablation, visualization may deteriorate because of blood and edema. It is always preferable to exercise caution in valve ablation even if it means needing to repeat the TURV rather than cause sphincteric injury or stricture from a poorly controlled endoscopic procedure. When antegrade valve ablation is being performed, it can be useful to have a blunt-tipped catheter in the urethra positioned with its tip at the level of the valves. It shows the leaflets well and offers a backstop for fulguration.

REFERENCES

1. Young HH, Frontz WA, Baldwin JC. Congenital obstruction of the posterior urethra. J Urol 3:289, 1919.
2. Noe HN, Jerkins GR. Cutaneous vesicostomy experience in infants and children. J Urol 134:301, 1985.
3. Meyers DA, Walker RD III. Prevention of urethral strictures in the management of posterior urethral valves. J Urol 126:655, 1981.
4. Johnston JH. Posterior urethral valves: An operative technique using an electric auriscope. J Pediatr Surg 1:583, 1966.
4a. Williams DI, Whitaker RH, Barratt TM, Keeton JE. Urethral valves. Br J Urol 45:200, 1973.
5. Whitaker RH, Sherwood T. An improved hook for destroying posterior urethral valves. J Urol 135:531, 1986.
6. Cromie WJ, Cain MP, Bellinger MF, et al: Urethral valve incision using a modified venous valvulotome. J Urol 151:1053, 1994.
7. Diamond DA, Ransley PG. Fogarty balloon catheter ablation of neonatal posterior urethral valves. J Urol 137:1209, 1987.
8. Zaontz MR, Gibbons MD. An antegrade technique for ablation of posterior urethral valves. J Urol 132:982, 1984.
9. Zaontz MR, Firlit CF. Percutaneous antegrade ablation of posterior urethral valves in premature or underweight term neonates: An alternative to primary vesicostomy. J Urol 134:139, 1985.
10. Ehrlich RM, Shanberg A, Fine RN. Neodymium:YAG laser ablation of posterior urethral valves. J Urol 138:959, 1987.
11. Noe HN, Jerkins GR. Oliguria and renal failure following decompression of the bladder in children with posterior urethral valves. J Urol 129:595, 1983.
12. Noe HN. Long term follow up of endoscopic management of urethral strictures in children. J Urol 137:951, 1987.
13. Bauer SB, Dieppa RA, Labib KK, Retik AB. The bladder in boys with posterior urethral valves: A urodynamic assessment. J Urol 121:769, 1979.
14. Warshaw BL, Hymes LC, Turlock TS, Woodard JR. Prognostic features in infants with obstructive uropathy due to posterior urethral valves. J Urol 133:240, 1985.
15. Tejani A, Butt K, Glassberg K, et al: Predictors of eventual end stage renal disease in children with posterior urethral valves. J Urol 136:857, 1986.
16. Parkhouse HF, Barratt TM, Dillon MJ, et al: Long term outcome of boys with posterior urethral valves. Br J Urol 62:59, 1988.

Part IV

MISCELLANEOUS

Chapter 125

Surgical Management of Pediatric Neoplasms

Stephen A. Kramer

WILMS TUMOR

Wilms tumor is the most common malignant neoplasm in the urinary tract of children. It develops in approximately 1 in 100,000 children, and more than 500 new cases occur annually in the United States.[1] The peak incidence of sporadic unilateral Wilms tumor is at age 3.5 years, whereas hereditary and bilateral tumors occur at a mean age of 2.5 years.[2] There is no apparent sex predominance, but black children are more prone to develop Wilms tumor than white children.[3, 4]

A specific constitutional chromosome abnormality has been identified in children with aniridia and Wilms tumor and is present in 30 to 50 percent of all Wilms tumors.[5, 6] This abnormality—a deletion of band 13 on the short arm of chromosome 11 (11p13)—is known as the "Wilms tumor 1 (WT1) gene."[7, 8] This 11p13 chromosomal deletion may represent a mutation that results in loss of a tumor-suppressor function. Deletion of 11p13 has been identified in specimens of nephroblastomatosis, in patients with bilateral Wilms tumor, and in virtually all examples of Wilms tumor associated with Denys-Drash syndrome.[9] A second Wilms tumor gene (WT2) was initially identified in patients with Beckwith-Wiedemann syndrome and has been mapped to chromosome 11p15.[10] More recent investigations suggest the existence of a third Wilms tumor gene at the 16q locus in up to 20 percent of patients with Wilms tumor.[11, 12]

Although most patients with Wilms tumor have no associated congenital abnormalities, significant associations with congenital urinary tract defects (4.5 percent), hemihypertrophy (3 percent), and sporadic an-iridia (1.1 to 2.2 percent) have been well documented.[2, 13] Wilms tumor occurs eight times more frequently in patients with horseshoe kidneys than in the general population.[14] Ten percent of patients with Beckwith-Wiedemann syndrome are diagnosed to have Wilms tumor, and those who develop hemihypertrophy are particularly at risk of tumor formation.[15] Gonadal dysgenesis and male pseudohermaphroditism are also associated with Wilms tumor.[16, 17]

Most patients with Wilms tumor are thriving young children who present with an asymptomatic upper abdominal mass that bulges into the flank. The mass is smooth and firm and often extends across the midline of the abdomen. Vague abdominal pain is a common presenting complaint, occurring in about 30 percent of children with this tumor. The pain is often the result of capsular distention as a consequence of acute hemorrhage into the neoplasm. Patients may have nonspecific symptoms such as anorexia, malaise, or fever. Weight loss and vomiting from displacement or invasion of the intestinal tract occur infrequently and usually reflect advanced disease. Infrequently, the diagnosis of Wilms tumor may be established during the investigation of hematuria after minor renal trauma. Gross hematuria occurs rarely, but microscopic hematuria has been detected in 50 percent of patients at the time of diagnosis. Hypertension is present in up to 60 percent of children with this tumor and is due to either encroachment on the blood supply producing ischemia or renin secretion by the tumor itself.[18]

Preoperative Evaluation and Staging

The main differential diagnosis lies in distinguishing Wilms tumor from neuroblastoma, but other considerations include clear cell sarcoma; rhabdoid tumor; congenital mesoblastic nephroma; cystic, partially differentiated nephroblastoma; lymphoma; angiomyolipoma; solitary multilocular cyst; and renal cell carcinoma.[19] The initial laboratory evaluation of any child with a retroperitoneal mass includes a complete blood cell count, urinalysis and culture, serum electrolytes, and renal and liver function tests. Urinary catecholamines should be measured to rule out neuroblastoma. An abnormal level of serum creatinine suggests the possibility of bilateral Wilms tumor, solitary kidney, or significant congenital or acquired renal disease.

Abdominal ultrasonography has supplanted excretory urography as the primary imaging technique for Wilms tumor. This noninvasive technique is the best method for detecting extension of the tumor into the renal vein or vena cava.[20] Routine evaluation of the inferior vena cava (IVC) is important because half of the patients with extension of the tumor into the IVC are asymptomatic at presentation.[21, 22] Inferior venacavography is indicated in patients in whom ultrasonography suggests involvement of the vena cava or does not show a normal vena cava. Superior venacavography and right atrial catheterization are reserved for cases in which the IVC is completely occluded.

Abdominal computed tomography (CT) is the best imaging modality for determining the location and extent of the primary tumor. Furthermore, CT is excellent for evaluating function of the contralateral kidney and for determining whether the contralateral kidney has any nephrogenic rests or frank tumor. The most important limitation of CT is its inability to assess reliably the status of the lymph nodes.[23]

Chest radiography with frontal and lateral views is essential because the thorax is the most common site of metastatic disease. In a series of 2500 patients from the National Wilms' Tumor Study group III, only 31 (1 percent) had negative findings on chest radiography and positive findings on CT.[23] The National Wilms' Tumor Study reported no difference in prognosis between these 31 patients and those with positive findings on CT when given appropriate treatment.[24] Therefore, routine CT scanning of the chest does not appear to be cost effective; furthermore, positive CT findings are not associated with any survival advantage.

Operative Techniques

Proper preoperative preparation of the patient is essential to avoid intraoperative complications. All intravenous access routes should be established through the neck and upper extremities to permit adequate fluid replacement in case of extensive blood loss or caval resection. Careful preoperative staging,

meticulous attention to surgical detail, and judicious use of adjuvant chemotherapy and radiation therapy to avoid morbidity and mortality are mandatory.[19] Specific intraoperative complications resulting from inadvertent damage to normal portions of the arterial tree or adjacent organs have been described elsewhere.[25, 26]

The study design for treatment of patients in National Wilms' Tumor Study group IV is shown in Table 125–1. Surgical extirpation is the cornerstone of therapy for all children with Wilms tumor.[19, 27] The child is placed in the supine position and then rotated slightly so that the involved side is up. It is important to make a generous transverse transperitoneal incision to afford maximal exposure and to prevent intraoperative spillage of tumor (Fig. 125–1). This incision allows for en bloc resection of the tumor and involved kidney with the least risk of rupture of the tumor during its removal from the abdominal cavity. A thoracoabdominal incision may be used with very large tumors that involve the upper pole and for excision of ipsilateral pulmonary metastatic lesions. The flank approach should never be used in children with Wilms tumor because (1) adequate

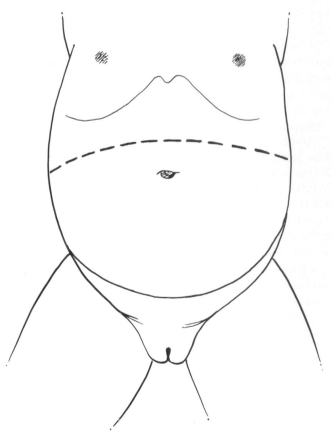

Figure 125–1. A transverse upper abdominal incision is used to gain access to the peritoneal cavity and contralateral kidney. (From Kramer SA. Surgical management of pediatric neoplasms. In Marshall F, ed. Operative Urology. Philadelphia, WB Saunders, 1991, pp 547–554. By permission of Mayo Foundation.)

TABLE 125–1. National Wilms' Tumor Study IV Protocol

Disease	Initial Therapy	Radiotherapy	Chemotherapy Regimen
Stage I Favorable histology Anaplastic	Surgery	None	EE—actinomycin D + vincristine (24 wk) EE-4—pulsed, intensive actinomycin D + vincristine (15 wk)*
Stage II—favorable histology	Surgery	None	K—actinomycin D + vincristine (22 and 65 wk) K-4—pulsed, intensive actinomycin D + vincristine (24 and 60 wk)*
Stage III—favorable histology	Surgery	1080 cGy	DD—actinomycin D, vincristine, and doxorubicin (26 and 65 wk) DD-4—pulsed, intensive actinomycin D, vincristine, and doxorubicin (24 and 52 wk)*
High risk (clear cell sarcoma, all stages) and stage IV—favorable histology	Surgery	Yes†	DD—actinomycin D, vincristine, and doxorubicin (26 and 65 wk) DD-4—pulsed, intensive actinomycin D, vincristine, and doxorubicin (24 and 52 wk)*

*Refer to latest National Wilms' Tumor Study protocol for dosage and length of treatment.
†Clear cell sarcoma patients receive 1080 cGy and stage IV–favorable histology cancer patients are given 1080 cGy if the primary tumor would qualify as stage III were there no metastases.
From Mesrobian H-GJ. Wilms tumor: Past, present, future. J Urol 140:231, 1988. By permission of Williams & Wilkins.

staging cannot be performed; (2) the abdomen, contralateral kidney, and lymph nodes cannot be assessed accurately; and (3) the likelihood of tumor spillage is increased.[28]

After the peritoneal cavity has been entered, the extent of the tumor is assessed, the liver is inspected, and the periaortic area and vena cava are palpated to determine whether primary excision is advisable. The incidence of bilateral synchronous Wilms tumors is 4.2 percent; therefore, the status of the opposite kidney must be assessed before dissection of the tumor is begun.

The use of newer imaging techniques may obviate contralateral renal exploration. Advances in noninvasive imaging techniques, including ultrasonography, CT, and magnetic resonance imaging (MRI), have led to an accurate definition of intrarenal lesions. Koo et al[29] reviewed the cases of 48 consecutive children who underwent radiological and operative staging of Wilms tumor. Imaging modalities used preoperatively included CT, ultrasonography, and MRI. In five patients the diagnosis of bilateral Wilms tumor was made preoperatively and confirmed at operation. Radiological imaging of the 43 other patients showed unilateral Wilms tumor only, without any contralateral abnormality. Operative exploration of the contralateral kidney in these 43 patients showed no evidence of Wilms tumor. Thus, in this study, radiological investigation was accurate in demonstrating the laterality of the disease.

The National Wilms' Tumor Study protocol continues to recommend bilateral renal exploration, with palpation and formal inspection of the contralateral kidney. Gerota's fascia should be opened, and the contralateral kidney should be mobilized from its perirenal fat and fascia to allow thorough inspection and palpation of both the anterior and posterior surfaces. Suspicious-looking lesions require careful biopsy. The presence of bilateral Wilms tumor alters significantly the surgical approach (see below).

The colon is mobilized and reflected medially, with care taken to preserve the colonic blood supply (Fig. 125–2). The renal vein, often splayed over the tumor, must be handled with extreme caution. Large tumors may compress and distort the vena cava, and the apparent "ipsilateral renal vein" may actually be the contralateral renal vein! It is important to ligate the renal vein and artery separately and early to avoid tumor manipulation and possible dissemination (Fig. 125–3). Ideally, the renal artery should be ligated first to decrease venous pressure within the tumor, because increased pressure may predispose to dissemination or rupture.

Wilms tumor extends into the renal vein in 11 percent of patients,[20] into the IVC in 6 percent,[30] and into the right atrium in 1 percent. The four types of tumor thrombus within the vena cava are (1) free-floating tumor thrombus, (2) tumor thrombus adherent to the wall of the inferior vena cava, (3) infiltration of the wall of the IVC by tumor thrombus, and (4) extension of tumor thrombus into the right atrium.[19] In patients with free-floating tumor thrombus, vascular control is established, a cavotomy is performed, and the tumor is extracted. This should be performed with the patient in the Trendelenburg position to avoid air embolus.

Tumor thrombus adherent to the wall of the IVC can be extracted with a Fogarty or Foley balloon catheter. The catheter is placed into the vena cava, and the intracaval thrombus is extracted through the venotomy site.

In patients with retrohepatic extension of tumor

into the IVC, it is necessary to release the liver by division of the triangular, coronary, and falciform ligaments. This technique involves systematic clamping of the superior mesenteric artery, porta hepatis, distal IVC, contralateral renal vein, and proximal IVC before suprahepatic clamping of the IVC (Pringle maneuver). This technique is important in decreasing hemorrhage and sequestration of blood in the liver.

Infiltration of the wall of the IVC by tumor thrombus often requires resection of the vena cava. If the pressure in the occluded contralateral renal vein is increased after nephrectomy and caval resection, it is necessary to reanastomose the renal vein to another vein to establish adequate drainage. In right-sided Wilms tumor, collateralization to the left renal vein is often inadequate, and resection of the cava should be combined with revascularization of the left renal vein to the splenic vein or to the IVC by an interposition vein graft or Dacron graft. In left-sided Wilms tumor, the right renal vein can be anastomosed to the portal vein or to the superior portion of the divided IVC with a vein graft or prosthetic interposition graft.

In patients with endocardiac extension of the tumor, a median sternotomy and midline abdominal incision or a combined median sternotomy and thoracoabdominal approach provides excellent exposure

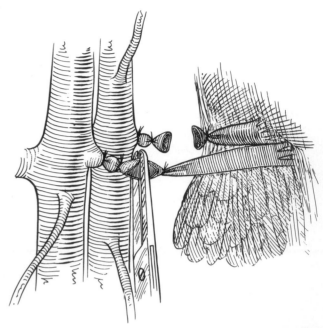

Figure 125–3. After the posterior peritoneum is excised and the renal vasculature exposed, the ipsilateral renal artery is double ligated with nonabsorbable sutures and divided before ligation of the renal vein. (From Kramer SA. Surgical management of pediatric neoplasms. In Marshall F, ed. Operative Urology. Philadelphia, WB Saunders, 1991, pp 547–554. By permission of Mayo Foundation.)

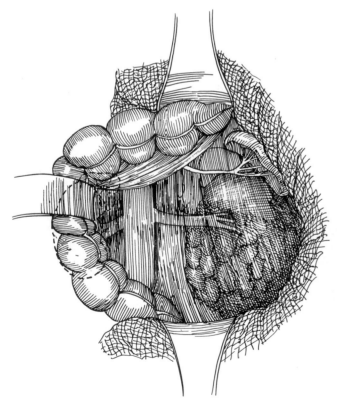

Figure 125–2. The colon is mobilized and reflected medially. The renal vein is often spread out over the tumor and must be handled with extreme caution. (From Kramer SA. Surgical management of pediatric neoplasms. In Marshall F, ed. Operative Urology. Philadelphia, WB Saunders, 1991, pp 547–554. By permission of Mayo Foundation.)

of the right atrium and intrapericardial portion of the vena cava. Extracorporeal circulation is required in these situations, and it is necessary that a combined operation be performed with a cardiac surgeon. Tumor that has extended into the atrium can be removed directly by the thoracic team, and thrombus in the IVC can be removed with a Fogarty or Foley balloon catheter passed up through a venotomy in the abdominal vena cava. A detailed description of cardiopulmonary bypass, hypothermia with temporary cardiac arrest, and total exsanguination is given in Chapter 4.

Complete surgical extirpation implies removal of the perirenal fascia, adrenal gland (with upper pole tumors), and tumor without opening Gerota's fascia. Although excision of all the tumor should be attempted, heroic efforts to remove all of it surgically are not necessary because small amounts of tumor have not been associated with more frequent abdominal recurrence or decreased survival rate.[28]

Regional lymphadenectomy should be performed for accurate staging and selection of appropriate postoperative therapy. The presence or absence of lymph node metastasis is a major factor in determining relapse-free survival. However, aggressive lymph node resection does not alter the outcome in patients with Wilms tumor; therefore, lymph node dissection should be confined to the perihilar and periaortic regions only (Fig. 125–4).

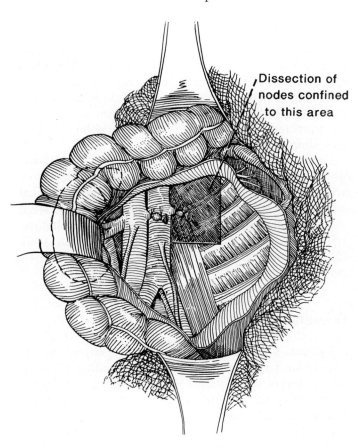

Dissection of
nodes confined
to this area

Figure 125–4. The tumor is removed with Gerota's fascia intact. A regional lymphadenectomy is accomplished by excision of the hilar and periaortic nodes. (From Kramer SA. Surgical management of pediatric neoplasms. In Marshall F, ed. Operative Urology. Philadelphia, WB Saunders, 1991, pp 547–554. By permission of Mayo Foundation.)

Alternative Therapeutic Techniques

The alternative therapies in the surgical management of Wilms tumor are controversial. In patients with massive Wilms tumor suspected on preoperative evaluation, the National Wilms' Tumor Study recommends formal exploration for accurate staging to avoid overtreatment or undertreatment due to either inaccurate assessment of nodal status or nonrecognition of unfavorable histological type in the tumor biopsy specimens (sampling error). Primary cytoreductive chemotherapy can then be instituted to decrease the size of the tumor and to allow for partial nephrectomy in selected patients. Confirmation of malignancy and identification of the cell type allow appropriate preoperative chemotherapeutic management without risk of mistaken diagnosis, and eliminate the possibility of benign disease.

Although preoperative therapy is used routinely in many European medical centers, it is not the preferred method in most North American medical centers, where its use is restricted to tumors too large to be removed without considerable surgical risk and to bilateral tumors. Preoperative chemotherapy may decrease the size of such tumors and make excision less hazardous, but it also produces a thick capsule around the tumor, thus decreasing the possibility of intraoperative spillage. It does allow enucleation in selected patients. This is the approach taken by the International Society of Pediatric Oncology and their successive clinical trials. However, these trials have been based on clinical diagnosis without pretreatment biopsy findings and thus have been associated with a pretreatment diagnostic error of about 2 percent.[31] This error can be avoided if percutaneous fine needle aspiration biopsy is performed before chemotherapy is initiated.

McLorie et al[32] have used CT scanning for staging and percutaneous needle biopsy for confirming the diagnosis, followed by pretreatment with systemic chemotherapy in patients with either unilateral or bilateral Wilms tumor. The subjective opinion of the authors was that the tumors were more confined, less vascular, and less friable after initial chemotherapy. There were no instances of needle track seeding or tumor rupture. A sampling error was present in 6 percent of their patients. (Initial biopsy results showed favorable histological patterns, and the surgical specimens showed anaplasia.)

In a review of a large series of patients with Wilms tumor seen at the Children's Hospital in Boston, Green and Jaffe[33] showed that patients younger than 24 months of age with stage I tumors had an excellent prognosis but did not show any improvement in disease-free survival after local radiation or systemic chemotherapy. In a prospective study of eight patients, Larsen et al[34] confirmed that patients under 24 months of age at presentation with small (less than

550 gm of total kidney and tumor weight), favorable stage I lesions had an excellent survival rate with surgical treatment alone (100 percent overall survival and 88 percent disease-free survival). In this selected subgroup of patients, perhaps adjuvant chemotherapy could be withheld, with the presumption that if surgical treatment alone failed, salvage could be by effective chemotherapy.

Hanna and Samowitz[35] suggested that partial nephrectomy should be considered in selected patients with small polar tumors and favorable histological patterns. They reported four patients who underwent partial nephrectomy and postoperative chemotherapy with actinomycin D and vincristine; all four were alive without evidence of disease from 1 to 11 years postoperatively.

Bilateral Wilms Tumors

Patients with bilateral synchronous Wilms tumors should undergo transperitoneal exploration with bilateral biopsy and lymph node sampling.[19, 36] In patients with *favorable histological patterns*, excisional biopsy can be performed if two thirds or more of the renal parenchyma can be preserved. Chemotherapy is administered postoperatively and is continued as long as an objective response is detected with ultrasonography, CT, or (if necessary) subtraction angiography. A second-look procedure is performed within a period not to exceed 6 months. Early intervention (e.g., at 6 weeks) may be appropriate if there is an excellent response to chemotherapy or, conversely, if there is tumor growth. If there is no objective response or only minimal response (less than 50 percent reduction in tumor size) at the end of 3 months, second-look exploration is accomplished. At this procedure, partial nephrectomy or excisional biopsy can be performed if all the tumor can be removed. If resection of all the tumor is not possible, only biopsy specimens are taken and nephrectomy is deferred. Chemotherapy is continued and radiation therapy is given to one or both kidneys.

At an interval not to exceed 6 months, a third-look procedure is undertaken. The therapeutic options include bilateral excisional biopsy, nephrectomy and contralateral partial nephrectomy or excisional biopsy, bilateral partial nephrectomy, bench surgery, and (as a last resort) bilateral nephrectomy. Interestingly, residual tumor has been left behind in about 60 percent of patients with bilateral Wilms tumor despite repeated surgical resections.[37, 38] However, the 2-year survival rate of 76 percent for this subgroup of patients is encouraging. When one or both tumors demonstrate unfavorable histological patterns, treatment is more aggressive and includes triple-agent chemotherapy and radiation therapy (1500 cGy) to one or both flanks. Second-look procedures may involve nephrectomy or bilateral nephrectomy if nonoperative measures fail to remove all tumors.

In a review of 185 patients with bilateral Wilms tumor registered with National Wilms' Tumor Study groups II, III, and IV, the overall survival was 83, 73, and 70 percent at 2, 5, and 10 years, respectively.[37] The important prognostic variables were unfavorable histological pattern, age at diagnosis, and the most advanced stage of the individual tumors. No significant difference in survival was noted between patients undergoing initial surgical resection of the tumor and those undergoing initial tumor biopsy followed by chemotherapy and subsequent surgical resection. Survival did not appear to be compromised with kidney-sparing operations. The excellent survival may be the result of several factors, including the earlier age at which bilateral lesions occur, the high incidence of favorable histological patterns, the excellent response to chemotherapeutic agents, and the different biological behavior of bilateral tumors.

Results

Clinical trials in the United States by the National Wilms' Tumor Study group and in Europe by the International Society of Pediatric Oncology have produced cure rates of more than 80 percent in patients with Wilms tumor. This coordinated multidisciplinary effort to study surgical extirpation, chemotherapy, and selected methods of radiation therapy has produced excellent survival rates in children with localized disease and favorable histological type and has served as a model for cooperative clinical studies of other malignant tumors. The objectives of National Wilms' Tumor Study group III were to decrease chemotherapy exposure of Wilms tumor patients at low risk and to develop more aggressive chemotherapy protocols for patients at high risk. The presence of nodal disease and the histological pattern have been the two most important primary determinants of survival. Analysis of tumor nuclear DNA pattern by flow cytometry has been used to identify patients at high risk for treatment failure.[39–41] The results in more than 2500 patients from National Wilms' Tumor Study group III are shown in Table 125–2. Children with stage I disease and favorable histological pattern treated with actinomycin D and vincristine for 10 weeks after nephrectomy had a 4-year relapse-free survival of 97 percent. Those with stage II disease had a 4-year relapse-free survival of 92 percent. This includes a subgroup of 77 patients with gross involvement of the IVC (stage II), in whom there was no effect on prognosis. Furthermore, 16 patients had extension of thrombus into the right atrium but had a 3-year survival of 100 percent![30] Patients with stage III disease had a 4-year disease-free survival between

TABLE 125–2. Survival in National Wilms' Tumor Study III

	4-Year Survival Rate (%)
Favorable histology	
Stage I	97
Stage II	92
Stage III	84
Unfavorable histology	
Stage I	87*
Stages II–IV	55*

*ADR, AMD, VCR, RT ± cyclophosphamide.
ADR, doxorubicin (Adriamycin); AMD, dactinomycin; RT, radiation therapy; VCR, vincristine.
From McMahon DR, Kramer SA. Pediatric urological oncology. In Whitfield H, Kirby R, Hendry WF, Duckett J, eds. Textbook of Genito-Urinary Surgery, 2nd ed. London, Blackwell (in press), as adapted from D'Angio GJ, Breslow N, Beckwith JB, et al. Treatment of Wilms' Tumor Study. Cancer 64:394, 1989. By permission of Blackwell Scientific Publications and JB Lippincott.

71 and 88 percent, depending on the chemotherapy regimen. Finally, more than 80 percent of patients with stage IV disease were long-term survivors.

GENITOURINARY RHABDOMYOSARCOMA

Rhabdomyosarcoma is the most common soft tissue sarcoma of childhood, accounting for 10 to 15 percent of all solid tumors in children; 15 to 20 percent of these tumors arise from the genitourinary tract.[42] The estimated annual incidence of rhabdomyosarcoma of the urogenital tract is 0.5 to 0.7 per 1 million children younger than age 15 years.[19] Boys are affected more often than girls in a ratio of 3:1.

Rhabdomyosarcomas arise from undifferentiated mesenchyme that differentiates into myxomatous tissue, fibrous tissue, or striated muscle.[43] The term *sarcoma botryoides* refers to a polypoid form of embryonal rhabdomyosarcoma that grossly appears as a cluster of grapes projecting into the vagina or bladder. Histological subtypes include both favorable and unfavorable patterns.[42] Unfavorable variants include anaplastic, monomorphous round cell, and alveolar rhabdomyosarcomas.[44] All other gross or cellular features are categorized as favorable.[45] An embryonal histological pattern, the most common favorable variant, occurs in 80 percent of patients with genitourinary rhabdomyosarcoma.[42]

Rhabdomyosarcoma of the bladder usually originates in the submucosa and superficial layers at the trigone. Extension of the tumor into the urethra, prostate, vulva, and vagina occurs before lymphatic or hematogenous metastatic lesions develop.[46] Bladder tumors often present in a botryoid form and may reach massive size before producing symptoms. The most common method of presentation is bladder outlet obstructive symptoms and, often, acute urinary retention. Gross hematuria occurs infrequently and results from disruption of the overlying bladder mucosa. The excretory urogram reveals ureteropyelocaliectasis in more than 50 percent of the patients, and the cystogram shows the characteristic polypoid lesions and filling defects within the bladder.[19] Cystoscopy permits evaluation of the bladder, bladder neck, and urethra, and multiple biopsy specimens are taken from suspicious-looking areas during endoscopy. If cystoscopy is not possible because of an obstructed and tortuous urethra, transperineal or transrectal biopsy is acceptable.

Prostatic rhabdomyosarcoma tends to be solid rather than botryoid. Contiguous spread into the bladder often makes it difficult to distinguish histologically whether this tumor originates primarily in the prostate or in the bladder. The tumor infiltrates the neck of the bladder and the posterior portion of the urethra and causes bladder outlet obstruction. Infiltration of the rectum by tumor may produce constipation as a presenting symptom. Excretory urography demonstrates elevation of the bladder base, and voiding cystourethrography shows distortion of the prostatic urethra. The diagnosis is established by transurethral biopsy (if possible) or perineal biopsy.

Primary vaginal rhabdomyosarcoma is the most common tumor of the female genital tract in children.[47] The tumor usually occurs on the anterior vaginal wall adjacent to the cervix, but it may arise from the distal portion of the vagina or from the labia. The tumor often extends through the vesicovaginal septum into the bladder and urethra. Patients present with a prolapsing vaginal mass or bleeding. The diagnosis of vaginal and uterine rhabdomyosarcomas is established by cystoscopy, vaginoscopy, and biopsy.

Staging

Clinical staging is based on the local extent of tumor, the presence or absence of metastatic disease, and the microscopically verified completeness of surgical removal (Table 125–3). CT and ultrasonography are used routinely to determine the size and anatomical extent of disease. More recently, MRI has been extremely helpful in accurately staging the extent of a pelvic tumor.[48]

Therapy

Combined therapy, including extirpative surgery, local irradiation, and 2-year multiagent chemotherapy, has produced survival rates greater than 90 percent in patients with localized disease.[42, 49, 50] Chemotherapy is important to treat the primary tumor and also to control clinically evident metastasis or micrometastasis. Vincristine (V), actinomycin D (A), and cyclophosphamide (C) have traditionally been the

TABLE 125–3. Staging of Rhabdomyosarcoma

Group	Features
1	Localized disease, completely excised
A	Confined to organ of origin
B	Outside organ of origin; regional nodes not involved
2	Grossly excised tumor with microscopic residual disease
A	No evidence of gross residual tumor or regional node involvement
B	Completely excised tumor, no microscopic residual, regional nodes are positive or adjacent organ is involved
C	Regional nodes are positive with evidence of microscopic residual disease
3	Incomplete resection or biopsy with gross residual disease
4	Distant metastases at presentation

From McMahon DR, Kramer SA. Pediatric urological oncology. In Whitfield H, Kirby R, Hendry WF, Duckett J, eds. Textbook of Genito-Urinary Surgery, 2nd ed. London, Blackwell (in press) as adapted from Leuschner I, Newton WA Jr, Schmidt D, et al. Spindle cell variants of embryonal rhabdomyosarcoma in the paratesticular region: A report of the Intergroup Rhabdomyosarcoma Study. Am J Surg Pathol 17:221, 1993. By permission of Blackwell Scientific Publications and Raven Press.

most effective chemotherapeutic agents, and combination chemotherapy (VAC) has been superior to single-agent treatment.[49] The treatment design for Intergroup Rhabdomyosarcoma Study (IRS) IV is shown in Table 125–4. The diagnosis is confirmed by biopsy, and pulsed multiagent chemotherapy with VAC is repeated twice, at 4-week intervals.[40] Clinical evaluation is undertaken at the end of 8 weeks, and if there is complete or partial response (tumor shrinkage of at least 50 percent), pulsed VAC is continued for an additional 8 weeks. At 16 weeks, exploratory laparotomy is performed and residual tumor is excised. In patients with no residual disease, pulsed VAC is continued for 2 years.

Radiation therapy is added postoperatively if there is evidence of microscopic or gross residual disease. If there is evidence of progressive disease or there is no response to treatment at 8 weeks, radiation therapy is begun. At 16 weeks, exploration is performed. In patients with no microscopic residual disease, pulsed VAC is alternated with vincristine, doxorubicin, and cyclophosphamide for 2 years. Patients with microscopic or gross residual disease undergo pulsed VAC alternating with pulsed vincristine, doxorubicin, cyclophosphamide, and radiation therapy.

In females with pelvic rhabdomyosarcoma, anterior exenteration is reserved for complicated recurrent disease. When hysterectomy is required for tumors of the proximal vagina, the ovaries should be preserved and repositioned to minimize the effects of radiation therapy. Fortunately, dilation and curettage is adequate initially for the 60 percent of uterine tumors that are polypoid.[47]

Alternatively, we have used vincristine, doxorubicin, and cyclophosphamide, alternating this treatment with etoposide and ifosfamide for patients with bladder and prostatic rhabdomyosarcoma. Doxorubicin was not given during radiation therapy. This neoadjuvant chemotherapy regimen has been very effective and appears to facilitate local control in selected patients (Arndt C., unpublished data). In a subset of patients with prostatic rhabdomyosarcoma, we have been successful in performing either transurethral resection of tumor or radical prostatectomy without cystectomy. In our small series, local control has been achieved in all patients, and tumor deaths were associated with distant pulmonary metastases rather than with local recurrence.

Results

The overall patient survival and bladder salvage rates have improved significantly from IRS I to IRS III (Table 125–5). Current survival data from IRS III for patients with group 1, 2, or 3 disease at diagnosis indicate that the survival rate is about 90 percent. Sixty percent of the patients were alive with a functional bladder 3 years after diagnosis.[50] The best prognostic indicators of survival are (1) clinical stage, (2) histological findings, and (3) site of the primary tumor. Other factors associated with favorable outcome have included age less than 5 years, nonprostate primary tumor, botryoid tumors, and female sex.[49] Flow cytometry has been effective for stratifying favorable versus unfavorable tumors.[51] In an IRS review of 34 patients with clinical group 3 tumors, the 5-year progression-free survival rate was 91 percent for hyper-

TABLE 125–4. Intergroup Rhabdomyosarcoma Study IV Treatment Design

Stage	Chemotherapy	Radiation
I*	Vincristine, actinomycin D, cyclophosphamide *or* Vincristine, actinomycin D, ifosfamide	None
II	Vincristine, actinomycin D, cyclophosphamide *or* Vincristine, actinomycin D, ifosfamide *or* Vincristine, ifosfamide, etoposide	None
III	Vincristine, actinomycin D, cyclophosphamide *or* Vincristine, actinomycin D, ifosfamide *or* Vincristine, ifosfamide, etoposide	Conventional
IV	Vincristine, melaphan *or* Ifosfamide, etoposide *or* Ifosfamide, doxorubicin } Vincristine, actinomycin D, cyclophosphamide	Conventional

*Excludes group 1 paratesticular patients who received vincristine and actinomycin D.

From Mandell LR. Ongoing progress in the treatment of childhood rhabdomyosarcoma. Oncology 7:71, 1993. By permission of PRR, Inc.

TABLE 125–5. Survival Rates for Intergroup Rhabdomyosarcoma Studies (IRS) I, II, and III*

	Survival (%)		
	IRS I	IRS II	IRS III
Overall survival	81	70	90
NED × 3 years	70	52	—
Bladder salvage rate	22	22	60

*Excludes patients with clinical grade IV disease.
NED, no evidence of disease.

diploid tumors compared with 17 percent for diploid tumors.[52]

Paratesticular Rhabdomyosarcoma

Paratesticular rhabdomyosarcoma accounts for about 75 percent of all rhabdomyosarcomas. It is the most frequent spermatic cord tumor of childhood; 17 percent of malignant intrascrotal tumors are paratesticular rhabdomyosarcomas.[53, 54] This neoplasm presents as a unilateral, painless, firm, and nontender mass in the scrotum, lying superior to the testis.

Staging

Clinical staging is based on the local extent of the tumor, the presence or absence of metastatic disease, and the microscopically verified completeness of surgical removal (see Table 125–3). Appropriate metastatic evaluation includes CT scans of the abdomen and chest, a bone scan or skeletal survey, and a bone marrow aspirate or biopsy (or both).[46]

Therapy

Radical inguinal orchiectomy with early vascular occlusion at the level of the internal inguinal ring is still the first line of treatment. Transscrotal procedures should be avoided to prevent the likelihood of tumor spillage and contamination of local tissues. Staging should be done carefully with thin-cut CT scans of the abdomen and pelvis. In the protocol for IRS IV, node dissection is not recommended in patients with localized, completely excised paratesticular rhabdomyosarcoma (clinical stage I) without clinical or radiographical evidence of lymph node involvement at diagnosis. Retrospective reviews show that the risk of lymph node involvement or nodal relapse is minimal in this group of patients.

In the IRS series, only three of 57 patients (5 percent) undergoing retroperitoneal lymph node dissection have had pathologically positive nodes (un-

suspected clinically and radiographically). In a retrospective series of 20 patients from Germany and 11 patients from Italy undergoing retroperitoneal lymph node dissection, no positive nodes were found in children with clinical stage I disease. Therefore, initial retroperitoneal lymph node dissection sampling was helpful in only three of 88 patients (3 percent; IRS III, Germany, and Italy) in determining the need for additional therapy.[55] All children received maintenance chemotherapy, and the 5-year survival rate for this combined group of patients was 92 percent.

Results

Ninety-five patients with paratesticular rhabdomyosarcomas were entered into IRS I and II. The overall survival was 89 percent at 3 years and 80 percent at 5 years. The 3-year relapse-free survival for stages I, II, and III tumors was 93, 90, and 67 percent, respectively.[45] Distant metastases at presentation and bulky retroperitoneal disease are most frequently associated with a fatal outcome.[53] Spindle cell variants are associated with fewer metastases (16.3 percent) than the classical embryonal variant (35.7 percent). The 5-year survival in patients with the spindle cell histological pattern was 95 percent compared with 80 percent in those with embryonal patterns.[56]

Editorial Comment
Craig A. Peters

The efficacy of multimodal therapy for Wilms tumor remains a superb model of what may be achieved with a carefully integrated treatment plan for a once lethal malignancy. Continued refinements in the selection of therapy permit more precisely tailored treatment with minimal morbidity without sacrificing efficacy. Although partial nephrectomy for bilateral Wilms tumors is an accepted treatment strategy, it has yet to become a part of the regimen for unilateral disease. In all likelihood, it will eventually become an accepted means of treatment with early diagnosis, improved chemotherapy, and a better understanding of the biology of this neoplasm.

The reconstructive options for pediatric genitourinary rhabdomyosarcomas continue to evolve and should be considered in the treatment planning for children with these tumors. While bladder-sparing treatment is an admirable goal, the functional consequences of the intensive radiotherapy that is often required to achieve this result may be counterproductive. A scarred, radiated bladder may have little real functional potential; similar considerations should be given to the effects of intensive radiation on the rectum. Continent urinary diversions have permitted many of these patients to achieve excellent functional urinary results with durable cures.

REFERENCES

1. Young JL Jr, Miller RW. Incidence of malignant tumors in U.S. children. J Pediatr 86:254, 1975.

2. Breslow NE, Beckwith JB. Epidemiological features of Wilms' tumor: Results of the National Wilms' Tumor Study. J Natl Cancer Inst 68:429, 1982.

3. Breslow NE, Langholz B. Childhood cancer incidence: Geographical and temporal variations. Int J Cancer 32:703, 1983.

4. Matsunaga E. Genetics of Wilms' tumor. Hum Genet 57:231, 1981.

5. Brown KW, Wilmore HP, Watson JE, et al. Low frequency of mutations in the WT1 coding region in Wilms' tumor. Genes Chromosom Cancer 8:74, 1993.

6. Wang-Wuu S, Soukup S, Bove K, et al. Chromosome analysis of 31 Wilms' tumors. Cancer Res 50:2786, 1990.

7. Riccardi VM, Sujansky E, Smith AC, et al. Chromosomal imbalance in the aniridia-Wilms' tumor association: 11p interstitial deletion. Pediatrics 61:604, 1978.

8. Francke U, Holmes LB, Atkins L, et al. Aniridia-Wilms' tumor association: Evidence for specific deletion of 11p13. Cytogenet Cell Genet 24:185, 1979.

9. Coppes MJ, Huff V, Pelletier J. Denys-Drash syndrome: Relating a clinical disorder to genetic alterations in the tumor suppressor gene WT1. J Pediatr 123:673, 1993.

10. Koo HP, Hensle TW. Molecular biology of Wilms' tumor. Urol Clin North Am 20:323, 1993.

11. Partin AW, Gearhart JP, Leonard MP, et al. The use of nuclear morphometry to predict prognosis in pediatric urologic malignancies: A review. Med Pediatr Oncol 21:222, 1993.

12. Newsham I, Cavenee W. Tumors and developmental anomalies associated with Wilms tumor. Med Pediatr Oncol 21:199, 1993.

13. Miller RW, Fraumeni JF Jr, Manning MD. Association of Wilms's tumor with aniridia, hemihypertrophy and other congenital malformations. N Engl J Med 270:922, 1964.

14. Mesrobian HG, Kelalis PP, Hrabovsky E, et al. Wilms' tumor in horseshoe kidneys: A report from the National Wilms' Tumor Study. J Urol 133:1002, 1985.

15. Clericuzio CL. Clinical phenotypes and Wilms tumor. Med Pediatr Oncol 21:182, 1993.

16. Beheshti M, Mancer JF, Hardy BE, et al. External genital abnormalities associated with Wilms tumor. Urology 24:130, 1984.

17. Rajfer J. Association between Wilms tumor and gonadal dysgenesis. J Urol 125:388, 1981.

18. Ganguly A, Gribble J, Tune B, et al. Renin-secreting Wilms' tumor with severe hypertension: Report of a case and brief review of renin-secreting tumors. Ann Intern Med 79:835, 1973.

19. Kramer SA, Kelalis PP. Pediatric urologic oncology. In Gillenwater JY, Grayhack JT, Howards SS, et al, eds. Adult and Pediatric Urology, 2nd ed, vol 2. St Louis, Mosby-Year Book, 1991, p 2245.

20. Ritchey ML, Othersen HB Jr, de Lorimier AA, et al. Renal vein involvement with nephroblastoma: A report of the National Wilms' Tumor Study–III. Eur Urol 17:139, 1990.

21. Clayman RV, Sheldon CA, Gonzales R. Wilms' tumor: An approach to vena caval intrusion. Prog Pediatr Surg 15:285, 1982.

22. Nadas AS, Ellison RC. Cardiac tumors in infancy. Am J Cardiol 21:363, 1968.

23. D'Angio GJ, Rosenberg H, Sharples K, et al. Position paper; imaging methods for primary renal tumors of childhood: Costs versus benefits. Med Pediatr Oncol 21:205, 1993.

24. Green DM, Fernbach DJ, Norkool P, et al. The treatment of Wilms' tumor patients with pulmonary metastases detected only with computed tomography: A report from the National Wilms' Tumor Study. J Clin Oncol 9:1776, 1991.

25. Kramer SA. Complications of Wilms' tumor and neuroblastoma. In Marshall FF, ed. Urologic Complications: Medical and Surgical, Adult and Pediatric, 2nd ed. St Louis, Mosby-Year Book, 1990, p 421.

26. Ritchey ML, Kelalis PP, Breslow N, et al. Surgical complications after nephrectomy for Wilms' tumor. Surg Gynecol Obstet 175:507, 1992.

27. Woodard JR. Wilms' tumor. In Glenn JF, ed. Urologic Surgery, 4th ed. Philadelphia, JB Lippincott, 1991, p 79.

28. Leape LL, Breslow NE, Bishop HC. The surgical treatment of Wilms' tumor: Results of the National Wilms' Tumor Study. Ann Surg 187:351, 1978.

29. Koo AS, Koyle MA, Hurwitz RS, et al. The necessity of contralateral surgical exploration in Wilms tumor with modern noninvasive imaging technique: A reassessment. J Urol 144:416, 1990.

30. Ritchey ML, Kelalis PP, Breslow N, et al. Intracaval and atrial involvement with nephroblastoma: Review of National Wilms' Tumor Study–III. J Urol 140:1113, 1988.

31. Tournade MF, Com-Nougué C, Voûte PA, et al. Results of the Sixth International Society of Pediatric Oncology Wilms' Tumor Trial and Study: A risk-adapted therapeutic approach in Wilms' tumor. J Clin Oncol 11:1014, 1993.

32. McLorie GA, McKenna PH, Greenberg M, et al. Reduction in tumor burden allowing partial nephrectomy following preoperative chemotherapy in biopsy proved Wilms tumor. J Urol 146:509, 1991.

33. Green DM, Jaffe N. The role of chemotherapy in the treatment of Wilms' tumor. Cancer 44:52, 1979.

34. Larsen E, Perez-Atayde A, Green DM, et al. Surgery only for the treatment of patients with stage I (Cassady) Wilms' tumor. Cancer 66:264, 1990.

35. Hanna MK, Samowitz HR. Rationale for partial nephrectomy in selected cases of Wilms' tumor. Dial Pediatr Urol 14:3, 1991.

36. Blute ML, Kelalis PP, Offord KP, et al. Bilateral Wilms tumor. J Urol 138:968, 1987.

37. Montgomery BT, Kelalis PP, Blute ML, et al. Extended followup of bilateral Wilms tumor: Results of the National Wilms' Tumor Study. J Urol 146:514, 1991.

38. Shaul DB, Srikanth MM, Ortega JA, et al. Treatment of bilateral Wilms' tumor: Comparison of initial biopsy and chemotherapy to initial surgical resection in the preservation of renal mass and function. J Pediatr Surg 27:1009, 1992.

39. Rainwater LM, Hosaka Y, Farrow GM, et al. Wilms tumors: Relationship of nuclear deoxyribonucleic acid ploidy to patient survival. J Urol 133:974, 1987.

40. O'Meara A, Gururangan S, Ball R, et al. Ploidy changes between diagnosis and relapse in childhood renal tumours. Urol Res 21:345, 1993.

41. Gearhart JP, Partin AW, Leventhal B, et al. The use of nuclear morphometry to predict response to therapy in Wilms' tumor. Cancer 69:804, 1992.

42. Shapiro E, Strother D. Pediatric genitourinary rhabdomyosarcoma. J Urol 148:1761, 1992.

43. Mostofi FK, Morse WH. Polypoid rhabdomyosarcoma (sarcoma botryoides) of the bladder in children. J Urol 67:681, 1952.

44. Kodet R, Newton WA Jr, Hamoudi AB, et al. Childhood rhabdomyosarcoma with anaplastic (pleomorphic) features: A report of the Intergroup Rhabdomyosarcoma Study. Am J Surg Pathol 17:443, 1993.

45. Crist WM, Garnsey L, Beltangady MS, et al. Prognosis in children with rhabdomyosarcoma: A report of the Intergroup Rhabdomyosarcoma Studies I and II. J Clin Oncol 8:443, 1990.

46. LaQuaglia M: Genitourinary rhabdomyosarcoma in children. Urol Clin North Am 18:575, 1991.

47. Hays DM, Shimada H, Raney RB Jr, et al. Clinical staging and treatment results in rhabdomyosarcoma of the female genital tract among children and adolescents. Cancer 61:1893, 1988.

48. Fletcher BD, Kaste SC. Magnetic resonance imaging for diagnosis and follow-up of genitourinary, pelvic, and perineal rhabdomyosarcoma. Urol Radiol 14:263, 1992.

49. Raney RB Jr, Gehan EA, Hays DM, et al. Primary chemotherapy with or without radiation therapy and/or surgery for children with localized sarcoma of the bladder, prostate, vagina, uterus, and cervix: A comparison of the results in Intergroup Rhabdomyosarcoma Studies I and II. Cancer 66:2072, 1990.

50. Maurer HM, Gehan EA, Beltangady M, et al. The Intergroup Rhabdomyosarcoma Study–II. Cancer 71:1904, 1993.

51. Boyle ET Jr, Reiman HM, Kramer SA, et al. Embryonal rhabdomyosarcoma of bladder and prostate: Nuclear DNA patterns studied by flow cytometry. J Urol 140:1119, 1988.

52. Pappo AS, Etcubanas E, Santana VM, et al. A phase II trial of ifosfamide in previously untreated children and adolescents with unresectable rhabdomyosarcoma. Cancer 71:2119, 1993.

53. LaQuaglia MP, Ghavimi F, Heller G, et al. Mortality in pediatric

paratesticular rhabdomyosarcoma: A multivariate analysis. J Urol 142:473, 1989.

54. Blyth B, Mandell J, Bauer SB, et al. Paratesticular rhabdomyosarcoma: Results of therapy in 18 cases. J Urol 144:1450, 1990.

55. Rodary C, Gehan EA, Flamant F, et al. Prognostic factors in 951 nonmetastatic rhabdomyosarcoma in children: A report from the International Rhabdomyosarcoma Workshop. Med Pediatr Oncol 19:89, 1991.

56. Leuschner I, Newton WA Jr, Schmidt D, et al. Spindle cell variants of embryonal rhabdomyosarcoma in the paratesticular region: A report of the Intergroup Rhabdomyosarcoma Study. Am J Surg Pathol 17:221, 1993.

Chapter 126

Surgical Considerations in Pediatric Renal Transplantation

Craig W. Lillehei and Craig A. Peters

Renal transplantation has emerged as the optimal treatment for children with end-stage renal disease (ESRD).[1] Although peritoneal dialysis or hemodialysis can be performed, even in small infants, neither modality maintains a constantly normal physiological state. Growth and development are clearly impaired in children on chronic dialysis compared with those who have functional allografts.[1, 2] Currently, nearly 26 percent of pediatric transplants are performed preemptively before the initiation of dialysis.[3] The goal of most pediatric ESRD programs is timely transplantation.

PRETRANSPLANT UROLOGICAL EVALUATION

Structural anomalies are the most common causes of ESRD in children (Table 126–1). Urological evaluation must therefore be undertaken in all transplant candidates.[4–6] The extent of the evaluation is guided by the likelihood of significant urological pathology. Historical clues such as voiding dysfunction and urinary tract infections must be sought. One cannot assume that the given diagnoses are either correct or complete. For example, a child's renal dysplasia may in fact be secondary to severe posterior urethral valves. A complete history of all previous urological procedures is essential.

Voiding cystography is performed routinely. Ultrasound examination of the kidneys is often the most helpful test, as functional imaging of the upper urinary tract is seldom possible. If there is any suspicion of bladder dysfunction, urodynamic evaluation should be undertaken. Assessment of compliance, capacity, and postvoid residual is essential. Children with myelodysplasia or other neuropathic bladder conditions, previous posterior urethral valves, or bladder reconstructions should be studied. It is criti-

cal that significant bladder dysfunction be identified to permit appropriate pretransplant management. In children with minimal urinary output, bladder cycling may be required to determine true bladder capacity and function. Endoscopic evaluation is not routine but should certainly be made whenever relevant diagnostic uncertainties warrant.

Native Nephrectomy

The decision to remove native kidneys before transplantation remains controversial. One clearly sacri-

TABLE 126–1. Causes of End-Stage Renal Disease in Children*

Diagnosis	%
Aplastic/hypoplastic/dysplastic condition	17.0
Obstructive uropathy	16.8
Focal segmental glomerulosclerosis (FSGS)	11.5
Reflux nephropathy	5.7
Systemic immunological diseases	4.7
Chronic glomerulonephritis (GN)	4.3
Prune-belly syndrome	3.1
Congenital nephrotic syndrome	3.1
Hemolytic-uremic syndrome	2.8
Polycystic kidney disease	2.8
Cystinosis	2.7
Medullary cystic disease/juvenile nephronophthisis	2.6
Familial nephritis	2.2
Pyelonephritis/interstitial nephritis	2.2
Membranoproliferative GN type I	2.1
Renal infarct	2.1
Unknown	3.7
Other (less than 2% each)	
Idiopathic crescentic GN	1.7
Membranoproliferative GN type II	1.0
Oxalosis	0.8
Wilms tumor	0.5
Drash syndrome	0.5
Membranous nephropathy	0.5

*A total of 3176 renal transplant patients from 83 participating centers.
Data from the North American Pediatric Renal Transplantation Cooperative Study. Personal communication, Amir Tejani, 1995.

fices residual hormonal or fluid output. The former may be supplemented with exogenous vitamin D or erythropoietin. However, the loss of urinary output may complicate subsequent fluid management on dialysis. Potential indications for nephrectomy include residual infection, severe vesicoureteral reflux, poorly controlled hypertension, large polycystic kidneys, and excessive proteinuria. Native nephrectomy in infants may reduce the risk of subsequent graft thrombosis.[7]

Bilateral flank incisions have been our routine, but dorsal lumbar incisions, laparoscopic nephrectomy, and transabdominal removal at the time of transplantation are definite options.

Urinary Reconstructive Options

The bladder is the best reservoir for placement of the transplant ureter. Bladder reconstruction may be necessary in some patients to ensure adequate capacity, low pressure, and continence, and this has been well demonstrated in the pediatric transplant population.[8–10] Patients who have been previously diverted but have a satisfactory bladder may be undiverted, ideally well before transplantation to avoid the risks of immunosuppression.[11]

A satisfactory outlet should be ensured (Fig. 126–1).

Clean intermittent catheterization is invaluable. If bladder dysfunction dictates, clean intermittent catheterization may be required to ensure a low residual volume. The ability to reliably catheterize should be assured before transplant.

If necessary, a continent catheterizable stoma can be constructed using appendix, tapered ileum, or native ureter into an appropriate reservoir. Options for continent urinary diversion are addressed elsewhere (see Chap. 113) and are well documented in the renal transplant population.

Children at risk for bladder dysfunction include those with previous posterior urethral valves, myelodysplasia, or multiple failed ureteral reimplants. If bladder noncompliance or small capacity persists despite mechanical (e.g., bladder cycling) and/or pharmacological interventions, bladder augmentation may be required. Augmentation cystoplasty itself may be beneficial to native renal function and may delay the need for dialysis. If transplantation is anticipated, augmentation is best performed at least 6 weeks before the transplant.

A variety of options are available for augmentation including detubularized bowel (ileum, ileocecum, sigmoid), stomach, or ureter (see Chap. 111). Most centers favor detubularized bowel. One must be aware that sacrifice of the ileocecal valve may exacerbate diarrhea.

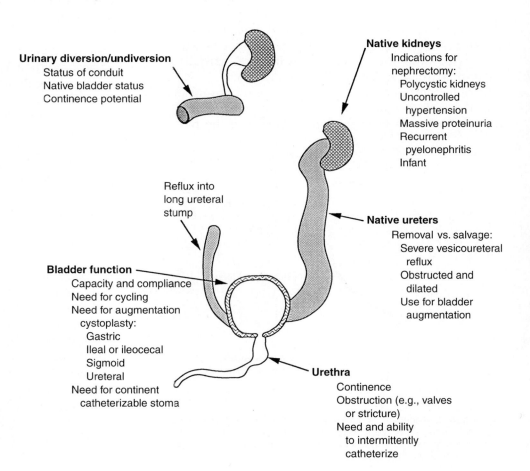

Figure 126–1. Aspects of the native urinary tract requiring pretransplant surgical evaluation and intervention.

Urinary diversion/undiversion
Status of conduit
Native bladder status
Continence potential

Native kidneys
Indications for nephrectomy:
Polycystic kidneys
Uncontrolled hypertension
Massive proteinuria
Recurrent pyelonephritis
Infant

Reflux into long ureteral stump

Native ureters
Removal vs. salvage:
Severe vesicoureteral reflux
Obstructed and dilated
Use for bladder augmentation

Bladder function
Capacity and compliance
Need for cycling
Need for augmentation cystoplasty:
Gastric
Ileal or ileocecal
Sigmoid
Ureteral
Need for continent catheterizable stoma

Urethra
Continence
Obstruction (e.g., valves or stricture)
Need and ability to intermittently catheterize

If the position of the anticipated renal allograft is known, the pedicle of the augmented segment can be positioned on the opposite side. In any case, careful description of the anatomy should be documented. Ideally, the surgeon responsible for the augmentation should be present for the transplant.

Gastrocystoplasty has been used successfully in renal transplantation. Its advantages include absence of mucus production, avoidance of hyperchloremic or hypochloremic acidosis, and possibly fewer infections secondary to the acidic environment. Unfortunately, a very troublesome hematuria-dysuria syndrome may develop with risk of perforation, particularly if there is minimal urinary output to buffer the acid production.[12]

An alternative to enterocystoplasty when a dilated ureter is present is ureterocystoplasty.[13] Such consideration must be made before nephrectomy in order to preserve the ureteral vasculature.

TRANSPLANT

Preparation

Large-volume vascular access is essential to maintain adequate perfusion pressure to the allograft. A central venous line is useful to ensure reliable venous access. Intra-arterial monitoring is advisable if cross-clamping of the aorta is anticipated. A Silastic Foley catheter is inserted at the onset, the bladder is irrigated with antibiotic solution, and it is left partially filled to facilitate subsequent cystotomy.

In older children, as in adults, a retroperitoneal curvilinear lower quadrant incision is made (Fig. 126–2). It extends from the lateral border of the rec-

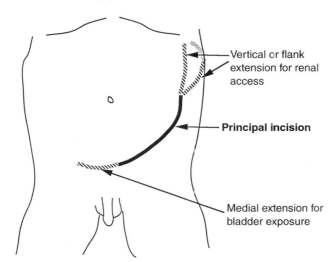

Figure 126–2. Placement of incision for pediatric renal transplant. The proximal aspect of the incision may be extended into the flank or vertically for native nephrectomy. The incision may be extended across the midline inferiorly to improve access to the bladder.

[Figure labels:] Vertical or flank extension for renal access; **Principal incision**; Medial extension for bladder exposure

tus, 1 to 2 cm above the pubis, laterally above the anterosuperior iliac spine. We favor medial extension across the rectus to facilitate bladder exposure. The incision may also be extended laterally, either cephalad to the costal margin or into the flank to allow an ipsilateral native nephrectomy or improved exposure of the allograft bed. The abdominal muscles are divided with electrocautery, and the retroperitoneum is entered. In males the spermatic cord is mobilized and retracted; in females the round ligament is ligated and divided. The lymphatics overlying the iliac vessels are divided between ligatures. The common, external, and internal iliac arteries are mobilized. The common iliac vein usually does not require circumferential mobilization, although restrictive small branches may need division.

Vascular Anastomoses

In most children, anastomoses of the allograft vessels to the larger iliac vessels are preferred, but anastomoses to the external or internal iliac arteries may be indicated. In infants and young children (<10 to 15 kg) a midline transperitoneal approach is used that allows end-to-side anastomoses to the infrarenal abdominal aorta and inferior vena cava (Fig. 126–3A and B).

Multiple renal vessels in cadaveric donors are usually managed with a Carrel patch of donor aorta. However, in living donors, the more common donor source in children, this is not possible. Multiple arteries are best reconstructed in the cold to allow a single anastomosis and thereby minimize warm ischemic time. However, separate implantation is certainly an option. Our preference is an end-to-side anastomosis, although end-to-end anastomosis to the internal iliac artery may be used, especially when additional arterial length is desired (Fig. 126–4). Multiple veins may be implanted jointly or separately, again end to side. Small venous branches can be sacrificed.[14]

While the vascular anastomoses are being performed, the kidney is kept cold with iced saline. A child is more susceptible to cooling than an adult; core temperature should be monitored. Given that an adult allograft may represent a significant fraction of a child's intravascular volume, adequate preload should be established before reperfusion of the allograft. Central venous pressure (CVP) is a reliable gauge of volume status in otherwise healthy children. CVP greater than 15 cm H_2O is recommended to avoid significant hypotension with unclamping and perfusion of this additional vascular bed.

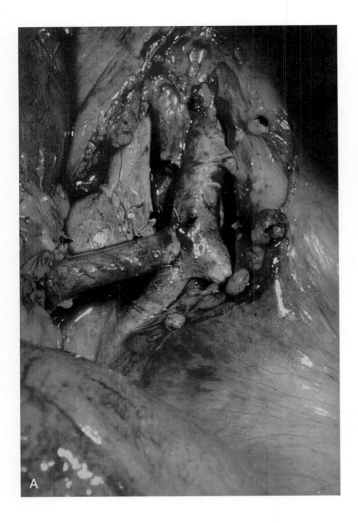

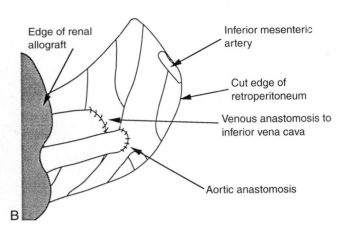

Figure 126–3. In addition to the standard anastomoses to the iliac vessels, placement of the arterial segment onto the aorta may be necessary. *A,* Operative photograph showing an adult renal graft being placed into a child. The aortic anastomosis of the renal artery is evident at the arrow in *B.* The anastomosis is performed low on the aorta to avoid injury to the inferior mesenteric artery, which should be spared when possible. *B,* Position of the opened retroperitoneum and the vena cava. (*A,* From Lillehei CW. Renal transplantation. In Ashcraft KW, Holder TM, eds. Pediatric Surgery, 2nd ed. Philadelphia, WB Saunders, 1993, p 769.)

Ureteral Anastomosis/Bladder Management

After the vascular anastomosis, the bladder is dissected free and prepared for the ureteral implantation. Our preference is an intravesical (Politano-Leadbetter) ureteroneocystostomy. Although the effectiveness of extravesical techniques has been well proven in transplantation,[15] the need to ensure a successful reimplantation without reflux or obstruction has compelled us to continue this intravesical technique. It is particularly effective in the abnormal bladder. The procedure can be performed in a transtrigonal or the more traditional vertical orientation.

The bladder is left partially full with a Silastic Foley catheter in place. Careful exposure of the bladder and opening is performed through a vertical cystotomy. The bladder base is exposed for ureteral reimplantation. If the native ureter(s) remain, their lumen(s) are identified. Large or bulky ureteral stumps may require removal but otherwise may not be harmful. The position for the neohiatus is carefully chosen: it should permit a sufficiently long tunnel without relative obstruction at high bladder volumes. If the ureter is short or if a very long tunnel is

desired because of the condition of the bladder, the psoas hitch is a useful adjunct to fix the position of the ureterovesical anastomosis. As in repeat ureteral reimplantation, a combined intra- and extravesical dissection is employed. The neohiatus is opened with passage of a soft catheter for subsequent countertraction. The intravesical ureteral tunnel is dissected. In trabeculated or fibrotic bladders, it has been our practice to open the tunnel completely to permit adequate mobilization of the bladder epithelium. This also facilitates meticulous hemostasis. In children who have been anticoagulated, such hemostasis may be critical. We have seen acute ureteral obstruction due to a submucosal tunnel hematoma. The ureter should be examined for any periadventitial bleeding and any such vessels controlled with suture ligation rather than cautery, to avoid ureteral ischemia. Minimal periureteral fat is removed unless it is very bulky. The ureter is positioned through the neohiatus. If extra length is present, it is trimmed. Anastomosis is similar to that for a standard ureteral reimplantation. The bladder epithelium is closed over the ureter and should be under no tension. The bladder is closed in three layers with absorbable suture, usually polydiaxanone (PDS) or polyglycolic acid sutures. The con-

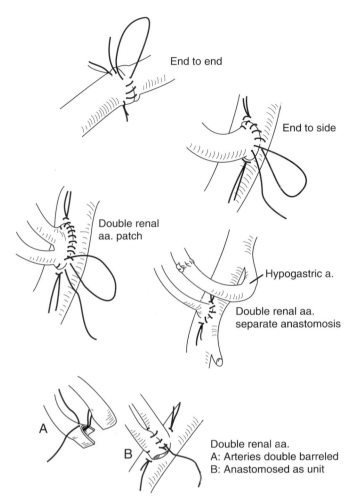

Figure 126–4. Diagram of possible arterial anastomoses used in pediatric transplantation. (From Lee HM. Surgical techniques of renal transplantation. In Morris PJ, ed. Kidney Transplantation: Principles and Practice, 3rd ed. Philadelphia, WB Saunders, 1988, p 220.)

figuration of the ureter relative to the bladder should be examined with the bladder full and empty, and any bladder wall leaks closed. Ureteral stents are not routinely used. The Silastic Foley catheter should be of an appropriate size for satisfactory drainage. Closed suction drainage is used.

POST TRANSPLANT

Management of immunosuppression is beyond the scope of this chapter. Careful fluid monitoring is essential. Diuresis by the allograft may produce substantial fluid and electrolyte loss, which should be quantitatively replaced to avoid significant imbalances within the recipient.

Bladder irrigation may be necessary to prevent clot retention and ensure adequate bladder drainage. Antispasmodics (oxybutynin) may reduce bladder spasms. Catheter drainage is usually maintained for 5 to 7 days. If the child was on intermittent catheter-

ization before surgery, it must be reinstituted initially at a greater frequency, since the bladder will not regain its full capacity for several weeks.

COMPLICATIONS

VASCULAR OCCLUSION. Potential complications must be anticipated to allow prompt recognition and management.[16] Vascular thrombosis, either arterial or venous, is a significant cause of graft loss in children (Table 126–2). Meticulous intraoperative vascular technique is mandatory. Radionuclide renal imaging and duplex Doppler ultrasound are useful to assess postoperative renal perfusion, particularly if multiple vessels were encountered. Evidence of thrombosis requires immediate intervention, although the prospects for salvage are poor.

FLUID COLLECTIONS. Pelvic or perirenal fluid collections are identified by routine postoperative ultrasound examinations. The fluid may represent serum, lymph, urine, or pus. Ultrasound- or computed tomography–guided aspiration may be required for diagnosis or treatment. Drainage alone may be sufficient. However, persistent lymphoceles have been successfully managed with chemical sclerosis.[17]

URINE LEAKS. Recognition of urinary extravasation is best accomplished by comparing the fluid creatinine concentration with that of urine and serum. The mode of urinary reconstruction should focus attention on the potential sites of difficulty. Careful imaging and occasional endoscopy are necessary to identify the source and guide management. If the leak is small, reinstitution of bladder drainage may be sufficient, but large or persistent leakage usually necessitates operative intervention.

TABLE 126–2. Causes of Renal Graft Failure in Children*[3]

Cause	Total Graft Failures	
	n	%
Primary nonfunction	21	3
Vascular thrombosis	87	13
Miscellaneous technical failure	14	2
Hyperacute rejection (<24 hr)	8	1
Accelerated acute rejection (2–7 days)	24	3
Acute rejection	145	21
Chronic rejection	174	25
Recurrence of original disease	50	7
Death	67	10
Other	96	14

*From a total of 686 total graft failures.
Modified from Avner ED, Chavers B, Sullivan EK, Tejani A. Renal transplantation and chronic dialysis in children and adolescents: The 1993 annual report of the North American Pediatric Renal Transplant Cooperative Study. Pediatr Nephrol 9:61, 1995.

URETERAL OBSTRUCTION. In the early postoperative period, ureteral obstruction may be manifested as graft dysfunction or simply hydronephrosis. Prompt evaluation is needed to minimize the possible functional effects, but one should not be too quick to instrument a fresh ureteral anastomosis. A certain amount of edema is to be expected. Temporary ureteral stenting may be useful in the early postoperative period. However, late onset of obstruction secondary to ureteral stenosis usually requires open surgical intervention to achieve a lasting remedy.

As with any ureteral stricture, the method of repair depends on the location. Distal stenoses necessitate a repeat ureterovesical anastomosis, often with a psoas hitch (see Chap. 106). More proximal stenoses may require a ureteroureterostomy with stenting or pyeloureterostomy if the native ureter is satisfactory. Stenting may be helpful.

VESICOURETERAL REFLUX. The incidence and significance of reflux after transplantation are controversial. However, recurrent episodes of pyelonephritis, particularly with altered renal function, are an indication for surgery if reflux is present. The presence of reflux should prompt consideration of bladder dysfunction, which, if present, must also be treated. Repeat ureteral reimplantation in the transplant patient is similar to that in other children. Care must be taken to minimize dissection of the ureter and to provide an intravesical tunnel of adequate length. A psoas hitch is useful, as noted above. The transplant ureter may be stiff and fibrotic, and such a segment should be removed if possible.

BLADDER DYSFUNCTION. Bladder dysfunction in the post-transplant child may be manifested by graft dysfunction associated with bladder hypertonicity, hydronephrosis, incontinence, or infections. Significant bladder dysfunction can lead to graft loss. Anticipation and management of this possibility is one of the chief responsibilities of the urologist on the transplantation team. The principles of evaluation and treatment are well described elsewhere. Therapeutic options include behavioral modification, pharmacological therapy, augmentation cystoplasty, and intermittent catheterization with any of the others. All of these may be applied in the pediatric transplant patient with excellent results.

Summary

Renal transplantation in children can be achieved with excellent patient and graft survival.[3, 18–20] *Equivalent outcomes are possible even in infants.*[21, 22] *Nonetheless, attention to the relevant and unique pediatric management issues described above is mandatory.*

REFERENCES

1. Harmon WE, Jabs K. Special issues in pediatric renal transplantation. Semin Nephrol 12:353, 1992.
2. Davis ID, Chang P, Nevins TE. Successful renal transplantation accelerates development in young uremic children. Pediatrics 86:594, 1990.
3. Avner ED, Chavers B, Sullivan EK, Tejani A. Renal transplantation and chronic dialysis in children and adolescents: The 1993 annual report of the North American Pediatric Renal Transplant Cooperative Study. Pediatr Nephrol 9:61, 1995.
4. Waltzer WC. The preoperative evaluation of the urinary tract for adults and children undergoing solid-organ transplantation. Semin Urol 12:84, 1994.
5. Reinberg Y, Bumgardner GL, Aliabadi H. Urological aspects of renal transplantation. J Urol 143:1087, 1990.
6. Marshall FF, Smolev JK, Spees EK, et al. The urological evaluation and management of patients with congenital lower urinary tract anomalies prior to renal transplantation. J Urol 127:1078, 1982.
7. Harmon WE, Stablien D, Alexander S, et al. Graft thrombosis as a cause of graft failure in pediatric renal transplant recipients. Transplantation 51:406, 1991.
8. Sheldon CA, Gonzalez R, Burns MW, et al. Renal transplantation into dysfunctional bladder: Role of adjunctive bladder reconstruction. J Urol 152:972, 1994.
9. Thomalla JV, Mitchell ME, Leapman SB, Filo RS. Renal transplantation into the reconstructed bladder. J Urol 141:265, 1989.
10. Koyle MA, Pfister RR, Woo H, et al. Management of the lower urinary tract in pediatric transplantation. Semin Urol 12:74, 1994.
11. Gonzalez R, LaPointe S, Sheldon CA. Undiversion in children with renal failure. J Pediatr Surg 19:632, 1984.
12. Reinberg Y, Manivel JC, Froemming C, Gonzalez R. Perforation of the gastric segment of an augmented bladder secondary to peptic ulcer disease. J Urol 148:369, 1992.
13. Churchill BM, Aliabadi H, Landau EH, et al. Ureteral bladder augmentation. Part 2. J Urol 150:716, 1993.
14. Benedetti E, Troppmann C, Gillingham K, et al. Short- and long-term outcomes of kidney transplants with multiple renal arteries. Ann Surg 221:406, 1995.
15. Gibbons WS, Barry JM, Hefty TR. Complications following unstented parallel incision extravesical ureteroneocystostomy in 1,000 kidney transplants. J Urol 148:38, 1992.
16. Zaontz MR, Hatch DA, Firlit CF. Urological complications in pediatric renal transplantation: Management and prevention. J Urol 140:1123, 1988.
17. Gilliland JD, Spies JB, Brown SB, et al. Lymphoceles: Percutaneous treatment with povidone-iodine sclerosis. Radiology 171:227, 1989.
18. Broyer M, Chantler C, Donckerwolke R, et al. The paediatric registry of the European Dialysis and Transplant Association: 20 years' experience. Pediatr Nephrol 7:758, 1993.
19. Shapiro R, Tzakis A, Scantlebury V, et al. Improving results of pediatric renal transplantation. J Am Coll Surg 179:424, 1994.
20. Churchill BM, Sheldon CA, McLorie GA, Arbus GS. Factors influencing patient and graft survival in 300 cadaveric pediatric renal transplants. J Urol 140:1129, 1988.
21. Najarian JS, Frey DJ, Matas AJ, et al. Renal transplantation in infants. Ann Surg 212:353, 1990.
22. Briscoe DM, Kim MS, Lillehei C, et al. Outcome of renal transplantation in children less than two years of age. Kidney Int 42:657, 1992.

Chapter 127

Surgical Management of Fetal Uropathies

Craig A. Peters

BACKGROUND

Current indications for the surgical management of fetal uropathies remain incompletely defined. With the advent of routine prenatal detection of congenital uropathies, therapeutic fetal intervention has remained controversial. The principal point of question remains the inability to accurately predict the outcome of a specific fetus in order to justify an intervention. The risks of fetal intervention, as well as the outcomes, remain poorly defined. Initial enthusiasm for fetal interventions for congenital uropathies occurred in the early 1980s and the results were summarized in 1986.[1] It was apparent from this registry that fetal interventional therapy was being applied in an inconsistent manner, without well-documented indications and with incomplete assessment of the clinical outcomes. Few institutions engaged in a careful, protocol-guided program. The work at the University of California, San Francisco (UCSF) Fetal Treatment Center was a carefully documented program of fetal interventions for obstructive uropathies, coupled with an experimental research program.[2] The results suggested that in some cases fetal decompression of an obstructive condition was beneficial in terms of preventing the anticipated life-threatening pulmonary hypoplasia. This has been confirmed in anecdotal fashion at other centers.

Nonetheless, even with the careful documentation practiced at UCSF, controversy regarding the appropriateness of fetal interventions remains.[3, 4] The reported application has been minimal in recent years. The issues remain the same: the natural history and the ability to predict outcomes remain incompletely known. Consequently, it is difficult, if not impossible, to predict which children will benefit from fetal intervention, and which will not require intervention until after birth. The long-term effects of interventions in the fetal period are essentially unknown. The broader application of fetal shunting of obstructions to less severe obstructions is being considered in some centers but is incompletely defined.[5] At present, fetal intervention for obstructive uropathies remains an experimental management approach. With continued investigation into the pathophysiology of congenital obstructive uropathies and improved interventional techniques, it is likely that some element of fetal therapeutic intervention will be a part of perinatal urology in the future.

INDICATIONS

Therapeutic fetal intervention for an obstructive uropathy is indicated when the newborn is likely to die from respiratory compromise due to pulmonary hypoplasia secondary to renal obstruction (Table 127–1). It is also essential that there be a reasonable likelihood that the fetus will benefit from such an intervention, i.e. there must be evidence of salvageability of both pulmonary and renal development and function.[6, 7] The setting for this is usually posterior urethral valves, diagnosed before 20 to 22 weeks of gestation. The ultrasonographic appearance is characterized by bilateral hydroureteronephrosis; renal parenchyma without ultrasound evidence of dysplasia; a dilated, thick-walled bladder; and oligohydramnios (Fig. 127–1). The assessment of salvageability is based on aspirated urine electrolytes from freshly produced urine (Fig. 127–2). The absence of new urine production after bladder aspiration is indicative of a poor prognosis despite any therapy. Urine chemistry values that indicate a reasonable degree of fetal renal function may indicate that renal development is salvageable and therefore that pulmonary development may be salvaged. Normal fetal urine is hypo-

TABLE 127–1. Indications for In Utero Intervention for Obstructive Hydronephrosis

Bilateral hydroureteronephrosis	Pattern consistent with posterior urethral valves: male fetus, thick-walled bladder
Risk of pulmonary hypoplasia	Oligohydramnios before 26–28 weeks' gestation
Sufficiently early to benefit	Before 24–26 weeks' gestation
Absence of renal dysplasia	Sonographic appearance of healthy parenchyma; no cystic changes; minimal to no increased echogenicity
Salvageable renal function	"Good prognosis" biochemical evaluation: Na$^+$ <100 mEq/L, Cl$^-$ <90 mEq/L, Osm <210 mOsm/L
No major associated anomalies	By fetal survey and karyotype
Uncomplicated pregnancy	Nontwin
Informed consent	Including risk of partial treatment (i.e. renal failure, respiratory insufficiency)

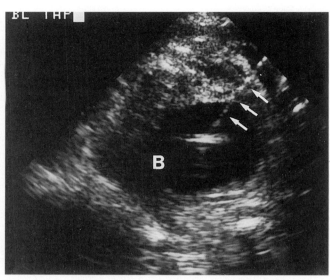

Figure 127–2. Ultrasonographic image of a percutaneous fetal bladder tap as would be performed to obtain urinary biochemistry values. A similar percutaneous tap would be performed to place a vesicoamniotic shunt. (From Mandell J, Peters CA. Antenatal diagnosis and treatment of genitourinary abnormalities. Curr Probl Urol 2:82, 1992.)

tonic and the sodium should be below 100 mEq/L during the mid–second trimester; the normal level is gestation dependent and this must be factored into the evaluation. Urine osmolarity should be less than 210 mOsm/L and chloride less than 90 mEq/L.[8–10] Some evidence has been presented to include the use of beta$_2$-microglobulin, and this may be indexed against urine sodium as a more precise indicator of ultimate renal outcomes.[5, 11] There are numerous reports demonstrating the potential inaccuracies of these measurements as absolute indicators of the fetal prognosis, yet they remain the only real indicators available.[12]

Equally important as the indications are the contra-

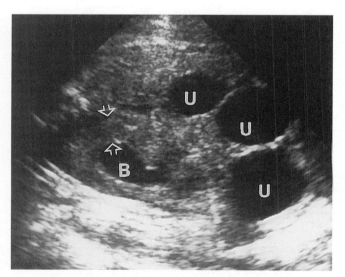

Figure 127–1. Ultrasonographic appearance of severe posterior urethral valves. The bladder (B) is not markedly distended but has a very thick wall (between arrows). The ureters (U) are markedly dilated and seen in multiple cross-sections owing to tortuosity. They might be mistaken for a dilated bladder.

indications to fetal intervention. The condition of the renal parenchyma must be assessed, since cystic or severely echogenic kidneys may signify renal dysplasia that is unlikely to be altered by in utero decompression. The fetus must undergo a total body survey to look for other major life-threatening defects, and karyotyping is necessary to rule out major chromosomal defects. The presence of a healthy twin is a contraindication. A complete explanation of the potential risks and uncertain benefits of the procedure must be provided to the parents and consent obtained.

It is also important to recognize the limitations of fetal interventions. A fetus with an ultrasound appearance consistent with severe bladder obstruction from valves with oligohydramnios late in the second trimester (after 25 weeks) is unlikely to benefit from in utero shunting, as the potential for adequate pulmonary development may be very low. When oligohydramnios is detected after 30 weeks and associated with an apparent obstructive uropathy, it is unlikely that shunting would affect in a positive way either renal or pulmonary development.[13] New-onset oligohydramnios after 30 weeks is unlikely to be associated with significant pulmonary hypoplasia. Whether shunting or early delivery of a fetus with obstruction is preferable remains unclear.

It is critical to recognize the difference between the ultrasonographic appearance of posterior urethral valves and the megacystis-megaureter syndrome of massive bilateral reflux in a male fetus.[14] These fetuses have a massively dilated bladder and hydroureteronephrosis with a thin-walled bladder and are not obstructed. They do not usually have oligohydramnios and are not at risk for pulmonary insufficiency. Unilateral obstructive processes with a normal contralateral kidney and no oligohydramnios should not be considered for fetal intervention (Fig. 127–3).

Indications for fetal therapy of bladder obstructive processes without oligohydramnios, yet with a risk of significant renal impairment, are developing slowly, yet hold the theoretical potential to prevent or delay the onset of end-stage renal failure in small children. The precise prognosis needed to select those cases needing intervention from those in which it is an unnecessary risk remains incompletely developed.[5]

TECHNIQUES

The earliest fetal interventions for obstructive uropathy were performed using direct surgical creation of a cutaneous vesicostomy to decompress the bladder into the amniotic cavity. With careful fetal-maternal monitoring and anesthesia, several of these procedures were successfully carried out through an open hysterotomy. The technique of vesicostomy was similar to that used in newborns. With meticulous control of preterm labor, these fetuses were carried well into the third trimester.[15]

Vesicoamniotic shunting using small double-J stent tubes has subsequently been applied more frequently. Initially, these procedures were fraught with technical problems. A trocar is passed under ultrasound control into the fetal bladder (see Fig. 127–2). Often this was hindered by fetal positioning or movement. The bladder is often massively enlarged and projects into the abdomen, and some of the shunts passed through the peritoneum. The shunts were passed over the trocar, often pushed away the fetal tissues, and could not be accurately positioned. The retention coils on the outside of the fetus projected outward and were frequently dislodged, occasionally by the fetus. The small caliber of the shunts permitted frequent clogging with debris, and the longevity of the

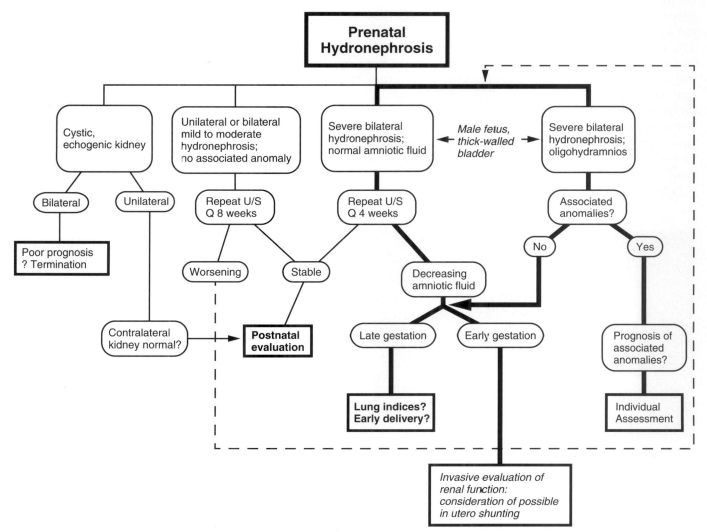

Figure 127–3. Algorithm showing an approach to prenatal evaluation and intervention for hydronephrosis. Bold lines indicate pathways leading to possible fetal interventions.

shunts was limited. Consequently, success rates with the original shunts were less than perfect and multiple passages or shunts were needed to produce sustained decompression. A modification of the original concept has been an improvement with a larger shunt placed through a larger cannula and retained by a coil lying flat against the fetal abdomen. With proper placement, these shunts have provided more consistent decompression. They have had problems owing to the large size of the tube and insertion cannula, with several reports of bowel herniation through the insertion sites noted at delivery.[16]

At present the technique is performed using maternal sedation and local anesthesia for the maternal abdominal puncture site. Under ultrasound guidance,

a 15 Fr. cannula with internal trocar is passed into the fetal bladder (see Fig. 127–2). Often it is necessary to produce an artificial echo window by filling the amniotic space with a small amount of warm amniotic fluid. This has the adverse consequence of allowing the fetus to move about more, however. If the fetus is particularly mobile, a fetal injection of intramuscular pancuronium may be used. The large caliber of the cannula and trocar makes placement somewhat challenging, but it is usually possible to enter the bladder. When the bladder has been entered, the internal trocar (stylet) is removed and the shunt is placed through the cannula using a blunt pusher device (Fig. 127–4). An internal coil keeps the shunt in the bladder, and an external coil is posi-

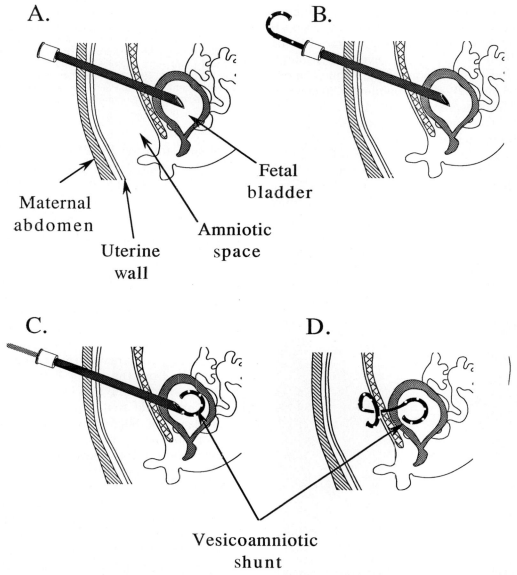

Figure 127–4. Placement of a vesicoamniotic shunt for bladder outlet obstruction. *A*, The introducing cannula with stylette is passed into the fetal bladder under ultrasonographic guidance. The amniotic space has been created with saline infusion to provide a sonographic window. *B*, The stylet is removed and replaced by the shunt passed within the introducing cannula. *C*, The shunt is pushed into the bladder where a pigtail curl maintains its position. *D*, As the introducing cannula is removed, the amniotic coil of the shunt is positioned outside the fetal abdomen, creating the vesicoamniotic communication.

tioned just outside the fetal abdomen to allow urine to drain into the amniotic cavity. The cannula is removed, and the uterine and maternal abdominal puncture sites seal spontaneously. The fetus is observed for distress and the mother for evidence of preterm labor. Prophylactic antibiotics are given for the procedure.

The efficacy of the procedure is assessed ultrasonographically by the amount of amniotic fluid present and the state of filling of the bladder. An empty bladder and the presence of amniotic fluid indicate a successful decompression. As with vesicostomy in the newborn, upper tract decompression is anticipated but not assured, and should be assessed. Perinephric urinomas have been aspirated on occasion.[17] This condition should be maintained until there is evidence of fetal lung maturation or term. There is no particular benefit to early delivery unless there is a change in status. Delivery needs to be by cesarean section, and we have adopted the practice of being present for all deliveries in the event of a shunt complication and to initiate adequate urinary drainage (Figs. 127–5 and 127–6). Subsequent management is similar to that of a premature child (as they most often are) with severe posterior urethral valves.

New techniques are being explored for shunt placement, including fetoscopically controlled insertions.[18] Such techniques may also permit more specific therapeutic interventions to be carried out in the fetus, such as creation of a cutaneous vesicostomy without foreign material.

Adjunctive techniques available to the maternal fetal medicine physician include various diagnostic techniques such as chorionic villus sampling for very early chromosomal diagnosis, percutaneous umbili-

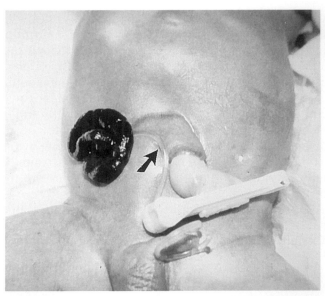

Figure 127–6. A newborn in whom effective shunt placement for bladder outlet obstruction was complicated by perinatal small bowel herniation through the puncture site of the vesicoamniotic shunt. The herniated bowel was urgently reduced in the operating room and found to be viable. The shunt was then removed and a vesicostomy created. (From Mandell J, Peters CA. Antenatal diagnosis and treatment of genitourinary abnormalities. Curr Probl Urol 2:89, 1992.)

cal blood sampling (PUBS), and needle aspiration and decompression of various fluid-filled spaces. These may include perinephric urinomas as well as bladders, kidneys, and ureters.

RESULTS

Reported results of fetal interventions are generally anecdotal and with only short-term follow-up. The assessment of risk to the mother and fetus is not well defined. This is particularly important in consideration of an inaccurate diagnosis and the added risk of performing an unnecessary intervention in a fetus. The reports from the UCSF Fetal Treatment Center are the most complete and extensive, yet are limited in their urological analysis and follow-up. In a number of cases, the diagnosis leading to the intervention was not known.

The report of the Registry of Fetal Intervention published in 1986[1] presented a somewhat negative view of the efficacy of in utero therapy for uropathies. Subsequently a de facto moratorium occurred, and relatively little activity has been reported and is likely to be occurring only occasionally. The principal elements of the 1986 report included 73 fetuses undergoing intervention, with an overall survival rate past the neonatal period of 45 percent. In newborns with a confirmed diagnosis of valves, however, survival was 76.5 percent. In the 33 fetuses in whom a specific cause of obstruction was not identified, sur-

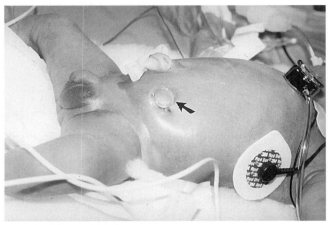

Figure 127–5. Immediately postnatal photo of a baby in whom a vesicoamniotic shunt had been placed at 22 weeks' gestation. The infant was delivered at 33 weeks because of increasing oligohydramnios. The shunt was seen to be dripping urine in the delivery suite and was confirmed to be in adequate position at the time of exploration and vesicostomy creation. (From Mandell J, Peters CA. Antenatal diagnosis and treatment of genitourinary abnormalities. Curr Probl Urol 2:89, 1992.)

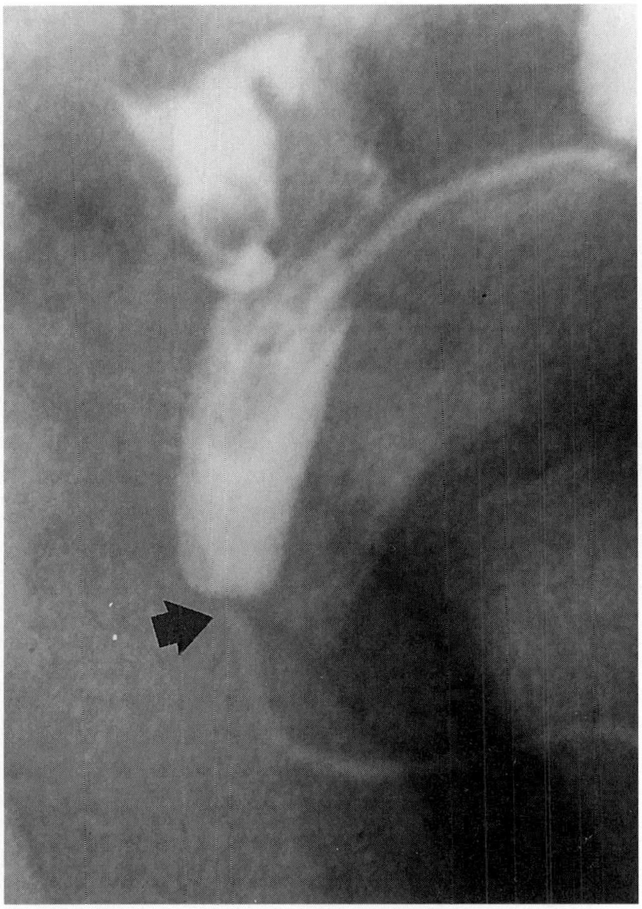

Figure 127–7. Radiographical demonstration of the presence of posterior urethral valves *(arrow)* in the newborn shown in Figure 127–5. Careful documentation of the urological pathology is critical in any fetal intervention.

vival was only 30 percent. The procedural mortality was 4.5 percent. Multiple shunt placements were necessary in 92 percent, ranging from two to seven shunts. Of 21 reporting centers, 14 performed only one procedure, which raises concern about the experience of practitioners of this technique. These data did not include any open vesicostomies in utero. The results from the UCSF group have been reported in a number of places.[8, 19–21] The results of open surgical intervention with five cases of vesicostomy show a survival of three patients, with one having normal renal function at 1 year of age. There were two girls and three boys. The diagnoses included prune-belly syndrome in one, and in the other four the urological diagnosis is unspecified, except for congenital hydronephrosis (Fig. 127–7). There were no maternal complications.[22] A larger series of vesicoamniotic shunting procedures for apparent bladder outlet obstruction with 40 patients is reported, comparing those with good-prognosis urine indices and those with poor prognosis. Those with good prognosis who were shunted had a survival rate of 100 percent, excluding one fetus who was aborted. All eight of these children were reported to have normal renal function; six had been found to have oligohydramnios. No intervention was performed in seven patients with good prognosis, and two died in the newborn period; both had oligohydramnios. Two of the five survivors have chronic renal failure. Of the cases with a poor prognosis, no intervention was performed in 14, 11 were terminated, and 3 died in the neonatal period. Ten with poor prognosis underwent intervention and seven were followed to term; three survived and two have renal failure, while four died. This was not a controlled, randomized study, and it is clear that the comparison groups were not strictly equivalent and that elective termination eliminates the possibility of observing the natural history.

It is clear, however, that some children who would otherwise have died of pulmonary insufficiency have been salvaged as a result of in utero urinary decompression. These observations are compelling in two ways. First, they indicate the need for more detailed multidisciplinary evaluation and follow-up of these patients. More important, they show that fetal intervention for obstructive uropathies can be lifesaving and very likely may be able to spare renal development. With improved prognostic accuracy[5] and decreased risk to the mother and fetus, development of this treatment may benefit children otherwise likely to die in the newborn period or suffer chronic renal insufficiency.

REFERENCES

1. Manning F, Harrison M, Rodeck C. Catheter shunts for fetal hydronephrosis and hydrocephalus. N Engl J Med 315:336, 1986.
2. Adzick NS, Harrison MR, Flake AW. Experimental studies on prenatal treatment of congenital anomalies. Br J Hosp Med 34:154, 1985.
3. Elder JS, Duckett JWJ, Snyder HM. Intervention for fetal obstructive uropathy: Has it been effective? Lancet 2:1007, 1987.
4. Sholder AJ, Maizels M, Depp R, et al. Caution in antenatal intervention. J Urol 139:1026, 1988.
5. Muller F, Dommergues M, Mandelbrot L, et al. Fetal urinary biochemistry predicts postnatal renal function in children with bilateral obstructive uropathies. Obstet Gynecol 82:813, 1993.
6. Nakayama DK, Glick PL, Harrison MR, et al. Experimental pulmonary hypoplasia due to oligohydramnios and its reversal by relieving thoracic compression. J Pediatr Surg 18:347, 1983.
7. Nakayama DK, Harrison MR, de Lorimier AA. Prognosis of posterior urethral valves presenting at birth. J Pediatr Surg 21:43, 1986.
8. Harrison MR, Golbus MS, Filly RA, et al. Fetal hydronephrosis: Selection and surgical repair. J Pediatr Surg 22:556, 1987.
9. Nicolini U, Tannirandorn Y, Vaughan J, et al. Further predictors of renal dysplasia in fetal obstructive uropathy: Bladder pressure and biochemistry of "fresh" urine. Prenat Diagn 11:159, 1991.
10. Nicolini U, Fisk NM, Rodeck CH, Beacham J. Fetal urine biochemistry: An index of renal maturation and dysfunction. Br J Obstet Gynaecol, 99:46, 1992.
11. Mandelbrot L, Dumez Y, Muller F, Dommergues M. Prenatal prediction of renal function in fetal obstructive uropathies. J Perinat Med 1:283, 1991.

12. Elder JS, OGrady JP, Ashmead G, et al. Evaluation of fetal renal function: Unreliability of fetal urinary electrolytes. J Urol 144(part 2):574, 1990.
13. Mandell J, Benaceraff BB, Peters CA, Estroff J. Late onset oligohydramnios. J Urol 148:515, 1992.
14. Mandell J, Lebowitz RL, Peters CA, et al. Prenatal diagnosis of the megacystis-megaureter association. J Urol 148:1487, 1992.
15. Crombleholme TM, Harrison MR, Langer JC. Early experience with open fetal surgery for congenital hydronephrosis. J Pediatr Surg 23:1114, 1988.
16. Robichaux AI, Mandell J, Greene M, et al. Fetal abdominal wall defect: A new complication of vesicoamniotic shunting. Fetal Diagn Ther 6:11, 1991.
17. Mandell J, Greene MF, Peters CA, Benacerraf BR. Aspiration of bilateral perinephric urinomas and vesicoamniotic shunt placement in fetal bladder outlet obstruction. J Ultrasound Med 11:679, 1992.
18. Estes JM, MacGillivray TE, Hedrick MH, et al. Fetoscopic surgery for the treatment of congenital anomalies. J Pediatr Surg 27:950, 1992.
19. Crombleholme TM, Harrison MR, Longaker MT, Langer JC. Prenatal diagnosis and management of bilateral hydronephrosis. Pediatr Nephrol 2:334, 1988.
20. Glick PL, Harrison MR, Golbus MS, et al. Management of the fetus with congenital hydronephrosis II: Prognostic criteria and selection for treatment. J Pediatr Surg 20:376, 1985.
21. Golbus MS, Harrison MR, Filly RA. Prenatal diagnosis and treatment of fetal hydronephrosis. Semin Perinatol 7:102, 1983.
22. Longaker MT, Golbus MS, Filly RA, et al. Maternal outcome after open fetal surgery. JAMA 265:737, 1991.

Index

Note: Page numbers in *italics* refer to illustrations; page numbers followed by t refer to tables.

ISBN 0-7216-5510-6